STEVENS'S CLINICAL IMMUNOLOGY

A Laboratory Perspective

SIXTH EDITION

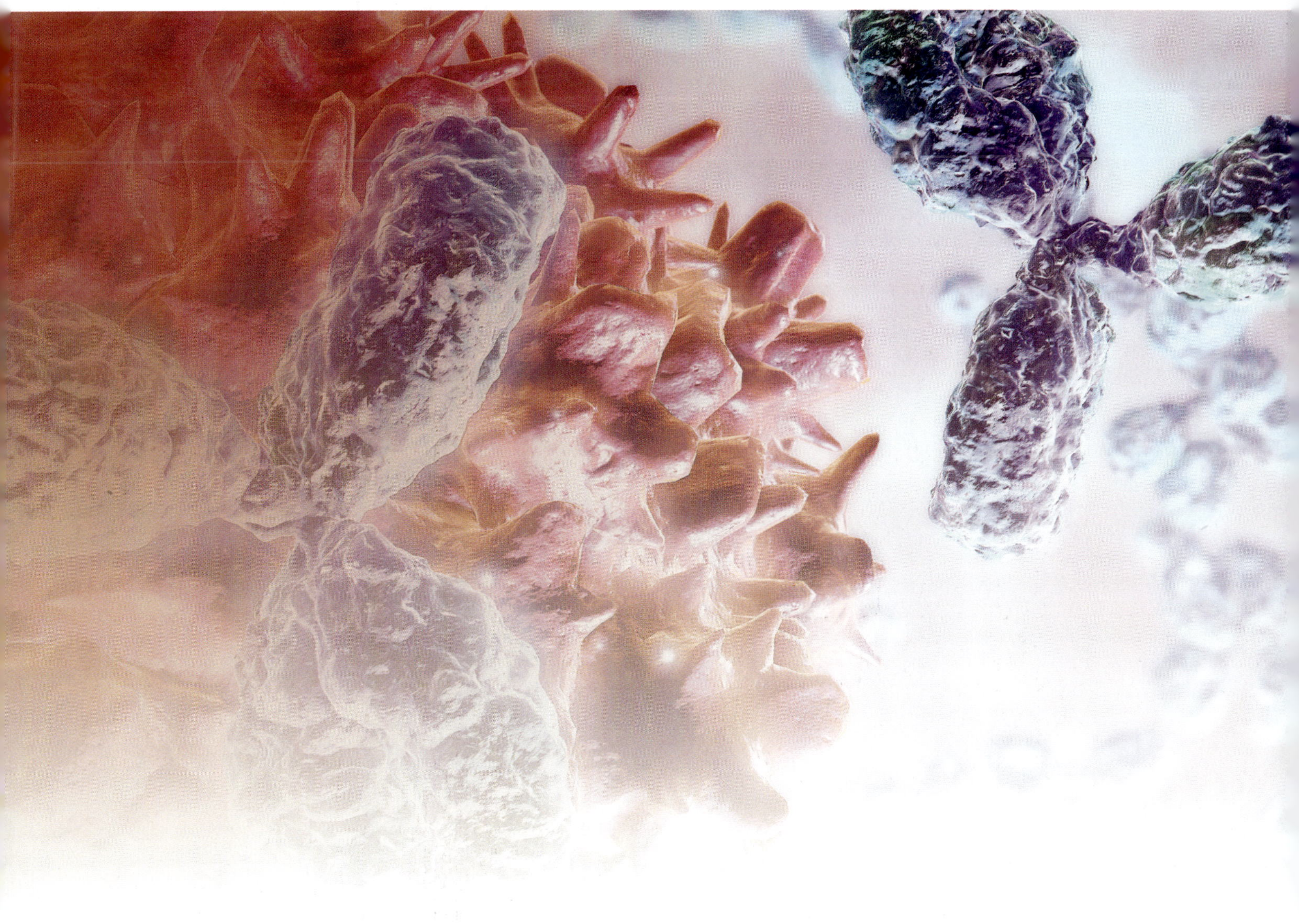

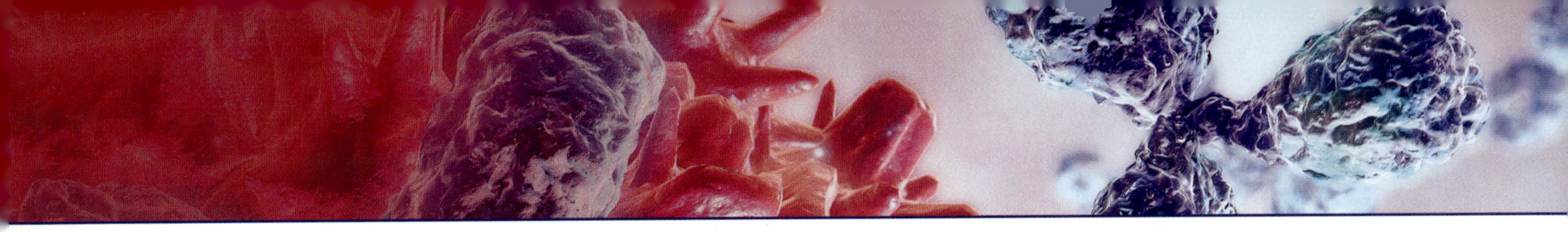

STEVENS'S CLINICAL IMMUNOLOGY

A Laboratory Perspective

SIXTH EDITION

Linda E. Miller, PhD, I, MB^{CM}(ASCP)SI
Professor Emeritus
Dept. of Clinical Laboratory Science
College of Health Professions
SUNY Upstate Medical University
Syracuse, New York

F.A. DAVIS
Philadelphia

F.A. Davis Company
1915 Arch Street
Philadelphia, PA 19103
www.fadavis.com

Printed in the United States of America.

10 9 8 7 6 5 4 3 2 1

Publisher, Health Professions: Christa Fratantoro
Director of Content Development: George W. Lang
Senior Developmental Editor: Jill Rembetski
Content Project Manager: Elizabeth Stepchin
Senior Manager of Design and Illustration: Carolyn O'Brien

Library of Congress Cataloging-in-Publication Data is available upon request.

To Christine Dorresteyn Stevens, for creating the original edition of this series through her expertise, innovation, and hard work, and for providing me with the opportunity to participate in subsequent editions; and to my students, who inspired me to share my passion for immunology over the years.

— L.E.M.

Preface

The sixth edition of *Stevens's Clinical Immunology: A Laboratory Perspective* is built on the foundation laid by the first five editions of this textbook. The book is designed to meet the needs of students enrolled in 4-year medical laboratory science and 2-year medical laboratory technology programs but may also serve as a valuable source of information about basic and clinical immunology for other students and health professionals.

As in the previous editions, the sixth edition combines fundamental immunology concepts with information about laboratory testing and its applications to the diagnosis and management of immune disorders. Over the years, immunology testing in the clinical laboratory has evolved from primarily manual serological methods to include advanced techniques such as automated immunoassays, flow cytometry, molecular diagnostics, and functional cellular assays. Therefore, while serology testing remains a focus in the sixth edition, we have dropped the words, "and Serology" from the title of the book to reflect the broader range of laboratory tests that are now performed in clinical immunology.

The sixth edition continues to be readable and user friendly and includes features designed to enhance student learning. Because educational research has shown that students learn better when they are actively engaged in the material, the chapters now include two new features—Knowledge Check (KC; recall) questions and Critical Thinking questions—as well as more review questions. The answers to the KC and chapter Review Questions are located at the end of each chapter to provide immediate feedback, while the answers to the Critical Thinking questions and the chapter Case Studies appear in an Answer Key at the end of the book.

The chapters also include new figures and additional study guides, which summarize major concepts and may serve as study tools to reinforce concepts. Based on instructor feedback, we have simplified sentence structure, provided definitions of difficult medical terms, and condensed information where possible to facilitate student comprehension of immunology concepts. Additionally, we expanded and grouped the bulleted Key Concepts at the end of each chapter under their corresponding section titles for easier reference to the more detailed text. Finally, we attempted to increase inclusivity by removing gender- and race-associated information from the case studies and text, as appropriate.

The organization of the chapters within the table of contents is based on our experience of many years of teaching clinical immunology to undergraduate students. The book is divided into four major sections: I. Nature of the Immune System; II. Basic Immunologic Procedures; III. Immune Disorders; and IV. Laboratory Diagnosis of Infectious Disease. The sections build on one another, and the chapters relate previous material to new material. For this reason, we have reordered some of the chapters in Section I by placing Antibody Structure and Function (now Chapter 3) before the chapters on Antigens and the MHC, and Adaptive Immunity.

All chapters in this edition have been thoroughly researched and updated to reflect the growing knowledge of immunology concepts and advances in laboratory techniques and their applications. In Section I, major revisions to Chapters 2, 5, and 6 provide more in-depth discussions on basic immune mechanisms. Updates to Sections II, III, and IV include new information about laboratory testing and treatments for immunologic diseases, for example,

- Chapter 12 presents a new section on nucleic acid isolation and expanded information on CRISPR-Cas9 and next-generation sequencing.
- Chapter 15 includes new anti-nuclear antibody (ANA) images.
- Chapters 18 and 19 include updates on classification systems for immunoproliferative diseases and immunodeficiency diseases.
- Chapter 20 contains a new section on tuberculosis and corresponding laboratory testing. The section on ***Helicobacter pylori*** has been removed, as antibody tests for this organism are no longer performed in the clinical laboratory.
- Chapter 21 presents a new section on relapsing fever.
- Chapter 23 includes information on influenza viruses A and B, RSV, and SARS-CoV-2.
- Chapter 24 has been renamed "Laboratory Diagnosis of Human Retroviruses" and includes a new introduction to retroviruses and the section on human T-cell lymphotropic viruses (which was previously in Chapter 23).
- Chapter 25 includes information on mRNA and viral vector vaccines.

FADavis.com provides many online resources to support the sixth edition of this text to assist instructors with course development. These resources serve as valuable tools for developing course materials that can be used in in-person teaching, online instruction, and hybrid learning environments. They include an Instructor's Guide with suggested learning activities, updated PowerPoint slides, additional case studies, new laboratory exercises, and an expanded bank of test questions that can be used for review or test preparation.

Because the field of clinical immunology continues to grow so rapidly, the challenge in writing this book has been to ensure adequate coverage but to keep it at an introductory level. Every chapter has been revised to include current practices as of the time of writing. We hope that this book will kindle an interest in students and serve as a valuable reference for laboratory professionals in this exciting and dynamic field.

Contributors

Lela Buckingham, PhD, MB(ASCP), DLM(ASCP)
Director, Medical Oncology (retired)
Rush Medical Laboratories
Rush University Medical Center
Chicago, Illinois

Marjorie Schaub Di Lorenzo, MLS(ASCP)SH
Program Coordinator (retired)
Phlebotomy Technician Program
Nebraska Methodist College
Omaha, Nebraska

Bradley Dixon, MD, FASN
Renal Section Head, Department of Pediatrics
School of Medicine
University of Colorado
Denver, Colorado

Ashley Frazer-Able, PhD, D(ABMLI)
Director, Exsera BioLabs
Associate Professor
School of Medicine
University of Colorado
Denver, Colorado

Aaron Glass, PhD, MB^CM(ASCP)
Assistant Professor
Chair, Department of Clinical Laboratory Science
SUNY Upstate Medical University
Syracuse, New York

Audrey Grimaldi, DHSc, MS, MLS(ASCP)
Vice Chair and Clinical Assistant Professor
Department of Clinical Laboratory Sciences
Stony Brook University: The State University of New York
Stony Brook, New York

Rachael Hagerman, MA, MLS(ASCP)^CM MB^CM
Clinical Assistant Professor
Department of Clinical Laboratory Science
SUNY Upstate Medical University
Syracuse, New York

Marnie Imhoff, MA, MBA, MLS(ASCP)^CM
Associate Program Director
Assistant Professor
Medical Laboratory Science
Department of Clinical, Diagnostic and Therapeutic Sciences
University of Nebraska Medical Center
Omaha, Nebraska

Paul R. Johnson, PhD, MBA, MT(ASCP), DABCC
Associate Professor
Department of Clinical Laboratory Science
Upstate Medical University
State University of New York
Syracuse, New York

Deborah Josko, PhD, MLT(ASCP)M,SM
Associate Professor and Director
Medical Laboratory Science Program
Clinical Laboratory and Medical Imaging Sciences
Rutgers University–School of Health Professions
Newark, New Jersey

Magenta Love, MS, MLS(ASCP) SCYM
Clinical Assistant Professor
Department of Clinical Laboratory Science
SUNY Upstate Medical University
Syracuse, New York

John L. Schmitz, PhD, D(ABMLI), F(ACHI)
Professor
Department of Pathology and Laboratory Medicine
University of North Carolina at Chapel Hill
Chapel Hill, North Carolina

James L. Vossler, MS, MLS^CM(ASCP)SM^CM
Assistant Professor
Department of Clinical Laboratory Science
SUNY Upstate Medical University
Syracuse, New York

Stephen M. Wiesner, PhD, MT(ASCP), FACSc
Associate Professor
Medical Laboratory Science Program
Center for Allied Health Programs
University of Minnesota
Minneapolis, Minnesota

Reviewers

Lauren Brooks, PhD, MLS(ASCP)^{CM}

Assistant Professor
Chemistry and Biochemistry Department
Nazareth University
Rochester, New York

Jennifer Bushnell, MEd, MT(ASCP)

Program Director
Medical Laboratory Science
McNeese State University
Lake Charles, Louisiana

Tiffani Bussie, MLS(ASCP)^{CM}

Adjunct Faculty
Medical Laboratory Technology
University of St Francis
Crown Point, Indiana

Sonny Carapella, MLS(ASCP)

Adjunct Faculty
Medical Laboratory Technology
Community College of Allegheny County
Jefferson Hills, Pennsylvania

Leslie A. Cooper, MS, MLS(ASCP)^{CM}, AHI(AMT)

Medical Laboratory Technology Program Director
Health and Sciences, Medical Laboratory Technology Program
Wiregrass Georgia Technical College
Valdosta, Georgia

Rosemary Duda, MS, MLS(ASCP)^{CM}

Medical Laboratory Science Program Director
Medical Laboratory Science Program
Franciscan Health
Dyer, Indiana

Nancy Eckert, MS, BS, MT(ASCP), PBT

Program Director and Professor
Medical Laboratory Technology
River Valley Community College
Claremont, New Hampshire

Michelle Fahs, MHPTT, MLS(ASCP)

Program Director
School of Clinical Laboratory Science
Mercy Hospital
St. Louis, Missouri

Karen Gatewood, MEd, MLS (ASCP)^{CM} PBT(ASCP)^{CM}

Associate Professor, Area Coordinator for Medical Laboratory Technology and Phlebotomy
Health Science Department
Bucks County Community College
Bristol, Pennsylvania

Jennifer Guriel, MS, MLS(ASCP)^{CM}

Program Director
Medical Laboratory Technology
Ivy Tech Community College
South Bend, Indiana

Uyen T. Ha, MLS(ASCP)

Medical Laboratory Science Specialist
Medical Laboratory Science
The Methodist Hospital
Houston, Texas

Rachel R. Hulse, EdD, MS, MLS(ASCP)^{CM}

Program Director and Associate Professor
Medical Laboratory Science Department
Idaho State University
Pocatello, Idaho

Marnie Imhoff, MA, MBA, MLS(ASCP)^{CM}

Associate Program Director, Assistant Professor
Medical Laboratory Science Program
University of Nebraska Medical Center
Omaha, Nebraska

Steven M. Johnson, MS, MT(ASCP)

Program Director
School of Medical Laboratory Science
AHN Saint Vincent Hospital
Erie, Pennsylvania

Amy R. Kapanka, MS, MLS(ASCP)SC

Medical Laboratory Technology Program Director
Health Science Department
Hawkeye Community College
Waterloo, Iowa

Jennifer Knight, MHS, MLS(ASCP)^{CM}

Program Director
Medical Laboratory Science
Mississippi Baptist Medical Center
Jackson, Mississippi

Michael Lacy, MLS(ASCP)

Assistant Professor
Medical Laboratory Science
Virginia Commonwealth University
Richmond, Virginia

Mylene L. Lampano, RMT, MSMT, PhS

Faculty
Medical Technology
University of Perpetual Help System
Binan, Philippines

Christine Laviolette, MT(ASCP)

Professor
Medical Laboratory Technology
Middlesex Community College
Lowell, Massachusetts

Lacey Murphy, MS, MLS(ASCP)CM

Assistant Professor
Pathology Department
Spencer Fox Eccles School of Medicine
University of Utah
Salt Lake City, Utah

Lynn Poth, MS, MLS(ASCP)

Medical Laboratory Science Program Director
Medical Laboratory Science Program
Hennepin Healthcare–HCMC
Minneapolis, Minnesota

Juan U. Rojo, PhD, MLS(ASCP)CMMBCM

Assistant Professor
Clinical Laboratory Sciences Department
University of Texas Medical Branch
Galveston, Texas

Teri J. Ross, MS, MLS(ASCP)SBB

Faculty
Clinical Laboratory Science
Loma Linda University
Loma Linda, California

Jean Rudell, MLS(ASCP)CM, SBB

Faculty
Clinical Laboratory Technology
Sinclair Community College
Dayton, Ohio

John K. Scariano, PhD, MT(ASCP)

Lecturer III
Pathology Department
University of New Mexico
Albuquerque, New Mexico

Lynne Shetron-Rama, PhD, MLS(ASCP)

Professor
School of Health Sciences
Eastern Michigan University
Ypsilanti, Michigan

Donna Spannaus-Martin, PhD, MLS

Professor
Medical Laboratory Sciences
University of Minnesota
Minneapolis, Minnesota

Acknowledgments

I am very grateful for the assistance I received from many individuals during the preparation of the sixth edition of this book. I would like to express a special appreciation to our chapter contributors for sharing their valuable expertise: Lela Buckingham, Marjorie Di Lorenzo, Bradley Dixon, Ashley Frazer-Able, Aaron Glass, Audrey Grimaldi, Rachael Hagerman, Marnie Imhoff, Paul Johnson, Deborah Josko, Magenta Love, John Schmitz, James Vossler, and Stephen Wiesner. I would also like to thank our reviewers for their helpful suggestions for improving the chapters.

I would like to acknowledge everyone at F.A. Davis for their hard work in making this book a reality. A special thank-you goes to Christa Fratantoro, Publisher for Health Professions, for her passion and innovative ideas for the sixth edition, and for gathering valuable feedback from MLS and MLT faculty to help the book achieve its educational goals. I especially appreciate the opportunity to work with Jill Rembetski, Senior Developmental Editor, whose creative ideas for improving the chapters were invaluable, and Content Project Manager, Elizabeth Stepchin, for her role in the review process and for keeping this project on track. I extend thanks to Senior Manager of Design and Illustration Carolyn O'Brien and her team for designing the front cover and working on the figures for this edition. I would like to extend much appreciation to the following faculty for their extensive reviews and innovative ideas in revising the online resources that accompany this book: Lacey Murphy - Instructor's Guide and Branching Case Studies; Audrey Grimaldi - Test Bank Questions; and Marnie Imhoff - Laboratory Exercises. A special thanks goes to Christine Becker, Project Manager with Apex CoVantage, for her efficient coordination of the production of this book. Thanks to George Lang, Director of Content Development, and everyone else behind the scenes at F.A. Davis who helped this book come to life.

Immunology students—past, present, and future—are the reason for writing this book. I hope that this text will inspire interest in the field of immunology and help to make a very complex subject easier to understand.

Finally, a big thank-you goes to my family, whose love, support, and patience made it possible for me to engage in this labor of love.

Contents

SECTION II

SECTION III

I

Nature of the Immune System

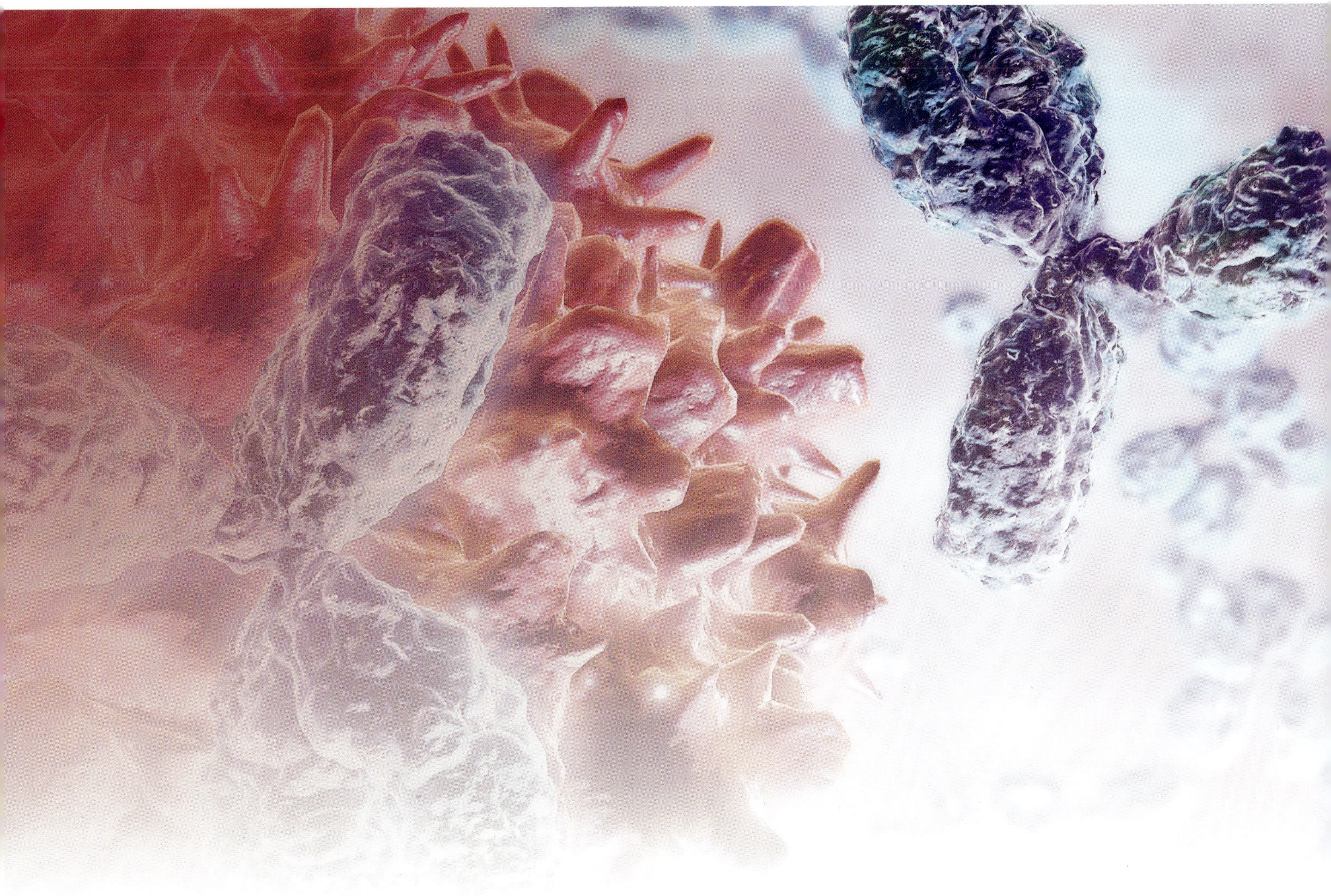

1 Introduction to Immunity and the Immune System

Christine Dorresteyn Stevens, EdD, MT (ASCP), and
Linda E. Miller, PhD, I, MB^{CM}(ASCP)SI

LEARNING OUTCOMES

After finishing this chapter, you should be able to:

1.1 Define *immunology, immunity, antigen, attenuation*.

1.2 Discuss early scientific discoveries that contributed to the understanding of immunology.

1.3 Contrast innate immunity and adaptive immunity.

1.4 Describe how leukocytes are formed during the process of hematopoiesis.

1.5 List the types of white blood cells capable of phagocytosis.

1.6 Discuss the roles of neutrophils, eosinophils, basophils, mast cells, macrophages, and dendritic cells in the immune system.

1.7 Identify the two primary lymphoid organs and discuss the main functions of each.

1.8 List four secondary lymphoid organs and discuss their overall importance to immunity.

1.9 Describe the function and architecture of the lymph nodes and spleen, including the locations of the B and T lymphocytes.

1.10 Define "cluster of differentiation" (CD) and recognize major CD markers on T cells, B cells, and natural killer (NK) cells.

1.11 Differentiate the functions of T cells, B cells, and NK cells in the immune response.

CHAPTER OUTLINE

You can go to **fadavis.com** keyword stevens for the laboratory exercises that accompany this text.

Although humans have been trying for centuries to unravel the secrets of preventing disease, the field of immunology is a relatively new science. **Immunology** can be defined as the study of a host's reactions to foreign substances that are introduced into the body. The foreign substances that induce an immune response are called **antigens.** Antigens are all around us in nature. They vary from substances that trigger allergies, like pollen, to serious pathogens that can cause life-threatening illnesses, such as group A *Streptococcus* or the coronavirus, SARS-CoV-2. The study of immunology has given us the ability to prevent diseases such as smallpox, polio, diphtheria, and measles through the development of vaccines.

Immunology is also important to many other areas of medicine. Understanding how the immune system works has made successful organ transplantation possible and has given us new tools to treat diseases such as cancer and autoimmune diseases. Automated immunologic techniques have made testing in many areas of the clinical laboratory more precise, leading to more accurate patient diagnoses and improved health care.

We begin this chapter by providing a brief look at the history of immunology. An introduction to the cells and organs of the immune system follows to help you develop an understanding of how immune responses work. In later chapters, we apply this knowledge to principles of laboratory testing for specific diseases.

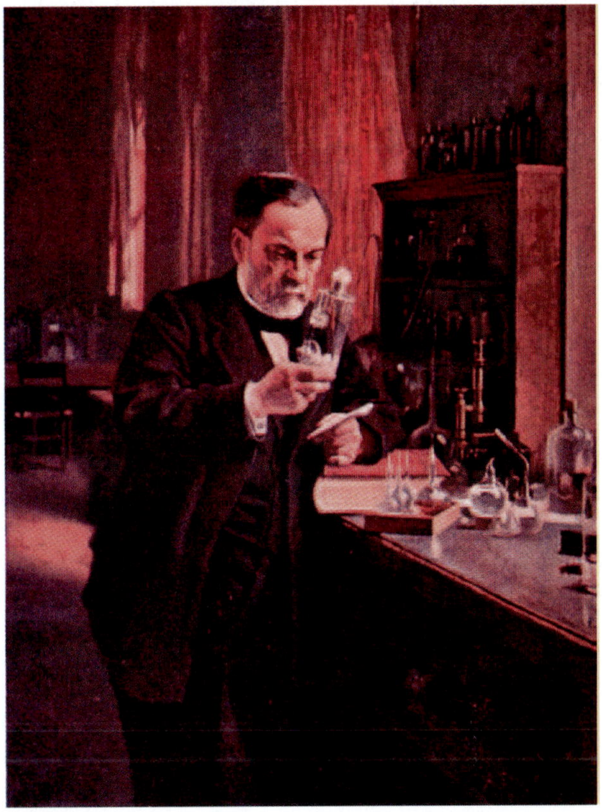

FIGURE 1–1 Louis Pasteur. (*Courtesy of the National Library of Medicine.*)

Immunity and Immunization

Immunology as a science has its roots in the study of **immunity:** the condition of being resistant to infection. The first recorded attempts to deliberately induce immunity date back to the 15th century when people living in China and Turkey inhaled powder made from smallpox scabs to produce protection against this dreaded disease. The hypothesis was that if a healthy person was exposed as a child or a young adult, the effects of the disease would be minimized. However, rather than providing protection, exposure to the material had a fatality rate of 30%. Further refinements did not occur until the late 1700s when Edward Jenner, an English country doctor, was able to successfully prevent infection with smallpox by injecting a less harmful substance—cowpox—from a milder disease affecting cows and humans who handle infected animals. Details about this first vaccine can be found in Chapter 25.

The next major development in disease prevention did not occur until almost a hundred years later when Louis Pasteur, often called the "Father of Immunology," observed that older bacterial cultures accidentally left out on a laboratory bench for the summer would not cause disease when injected into chickens **(Fig. 1–1).** Subsequent injections of more virulent organisms had no effect on the birds that had been previously exposed to the older cultures. In contrast, chickens that were not exposed to the older cultures died after being injected with fresh cultures. In this manner, the first attenuated vaccine was discovered; this event can be considered the birth of immunology. *Attenuation* means "to weaken," making a pathogen less virulent; it takes place through heat, aging, or chemical treatment. Attenuation remains the basis for several vaccines that are used today. Pasteur applied this same principle of attenuation to prevent rabies in exposed individuals. He was the first scientist to introduce the concept that vaccination could be applied to any microbial disease.

Innate Versus Adaptive Immunity

In the late 1800s, scientists began to identify the actual mechanisms that produce immunity in a host. Looking under a microscope, Élie Metchnikoff, a Russian scientist, observed that foreign objects introduced into transparent starfish larvae became surrounded by motile amoeboid-like cells that attempted to destroy the penetrating objects. This process was later termed *phagocytosis,* after the Greek terms to describe the means by which cells "eat" other cells. Metchnikoff hypothesized that immunity to disease was based on the action of these scavenger cells and was a natural, or innate, host defense. He was eventually awarded a Nobel Prize for his pioneering work.

Other researchers argued that noncellular elements in the blood were responsible for protection from microorganisms. Emil von Behring demonstrated that diphtheria and tetanus toxins, which are produced by specific microorganisms as they grow, could be neutralized by the noncellular portion of the blood, or serum, of animals previously exposed to the microorganisms. In 1901, von Behring was awarded the first Nobel Prize in Physiology or Medicine for his work with serum therapy. The theory of **humoral immunity** was thus born and sparked a long-lasting dispute over the relative importance of cellular immunity versus humoral immunity.

In 1903, English physician Almroth Wright showed that the immune response involved both cellular and humoral elements. He observed that certain humoral, or circulating, factors called *opsonins* acted to coat bacteria so they became more susceptible to ingestion by phagocytic cells. These serum factors include specific proteins known as **antibodies,** which are serum proteins produced by certain lymphocytes when exposed to a foreign substance, and which react specifically with that foreign substance (see Chapter 3). Other humoral factors include *complement* and *acute phase reactants,* which increase nonspecifically in any infection.

These discoveries showed that there were two major branches of immunity, *innate immunity* and *adaptive immunity.* **Innate,** or **natural immunity,** is the individual's ability to resist infection by means of normally present physical, chemical, and biological barriers such as the skin, and certain blood proteins (e.g., *cytokines, complement, acute phase reactants*). Innate defenses have limited specificity and are similar for all pathogens or foreign substances to which one is exposed. No prior exposure is required, and the response is immediate. Therefore, innate immunity is considered to be the body's first line of defense against an attack by a foreign invader. Innate responses involve cells such as macrophages, which are capable of recognizing a limited number of structures on pathogens, and neutrophils, which can engulf microbes and destroy them, a process called **phagocytosis.** A limitation of innate responses is that **immunologic memory,** or the ability of the immune system to respond more effectively after reexposure to the same foreign substance, is not induced. The components and underlying mechanisms of innate immunity are discussed in detail in Chapter 2.

In contrast, **adaptive immunity,** also referred to as *acquired immunity*, is a type of resistance characterized by precise specificity for each individual pathogen or nonmicrobial foreign substance because of specialized receptors on lymphocytes that recognize antigens. Because these receptors are diverse, the immune system can respond to a vast number of antigens. The immune responses involved are delayed as the lymphocytes "adapt" to the presence of an antigen and become activated to eliminate it. **Cytokines,** small proteins that act as chemical messengers, are released by cells of the innate immune response and play a major role in activating the lymphocytes. Although the responses of adaptive immunity are delayed, they are more effective because the lymphocytes generated have the ability to remember a prior exposure to the same antigen. As a result, an increased response to the antigen is mounted, and the resulting immunity is long lasting. This characteristic, immunologic memory, serves as the basis for vaccination, as we will discuss in Chapter 25. See Chapter 5 for a more detailed discussion of the components and underlying mechanisms of adaptive immunity.

Both the innate and adaptive branches of the immune system can differentiate between foreign antigens and those that are part of one's own body (i.e., "self") to prevent the immune response from injuring the host. They operate in combination and depend on one another for maximal effectiveness. Reviewing the Study Guide at the end of this chapter will help you compare and contrast key features of innate and adaptive immunity. In the next section, we discuss the cells of the immune system and their important roles in the innate and adaptive immune responses.

Knowledge Check 1-1

Innate immune defenses are characterized by:
a. Specificity for antigen
b. Generation of a memory response
c. Natural barriers and rapid responses to infection
d. Diversity of lymphocyte receptors

Cells of the Immune System

Leukocytes

White blood cells (WBCs), or **leukocytes,** play a key role in both innate immunity and adaptive immunity. Leukocytes can be found in the peripheral (circulating) blood, lymph, and tissues, where they defend against invasion by bacteria, viruses, fungi, and other foreign substances. The five principal types of leukocytes in peripheral blood are neutrophils, eosinophils, basophils, monocytes, and lymphocytes. Mast cells, macrophages, and dendritic cells are WBCs that are located in the tissues.

All blood cells arise from an undifferentiated type of cell called a *hematopoietic stem cell* (HSC) in the bone marrow. The bone marrow produces approximately one and one-half billion WBCs daily. During a process known as **hematopoiesis,** the HSC differentiate into two distinct types of precursor cells: *common myeloid precursors* (CMPs) and *common lymphoid precursors* (CLPs) **(Fig. 1–2)**. The CMPs differentiate further into mature red blood cells (RBCs), platelets, and WBCs of the **myeloid** lineage: neutrophils, eosinophils, basophils, monocytes, and most dendritic cells. Myeloid cells participate in phagocytosis and are key to innate immunity, but they are also important in processing antigens for the adaptive immune response. CLPs give rise to cells of the **lymphoid** lineage, T and B lymphocytes, which play essential roles in the adaptive immunity, natural killer (NK) cells, and innate lymphoid cells. Mature lymphocytes are found in the tissues as well as in the peripheral blood.

Myeloid Cells and Mast Cells

Granulocytes

The **granulocytes** are so named because they contain numerous distinct granules in their cytoplasm. This group of cells is composed of neutrophils, eosinophils, basophils, and mast cells. These cells play an important role in innate immunity and in regulation of the adaptive immune response. Their granules contain specific proteins that function in various aspects of these immune responses, including destruction of pathogens, inflammation, attraction of WBCs, and modulation of adaptive immune responses. In the next sections, we take a closer look at each cell type in this group.

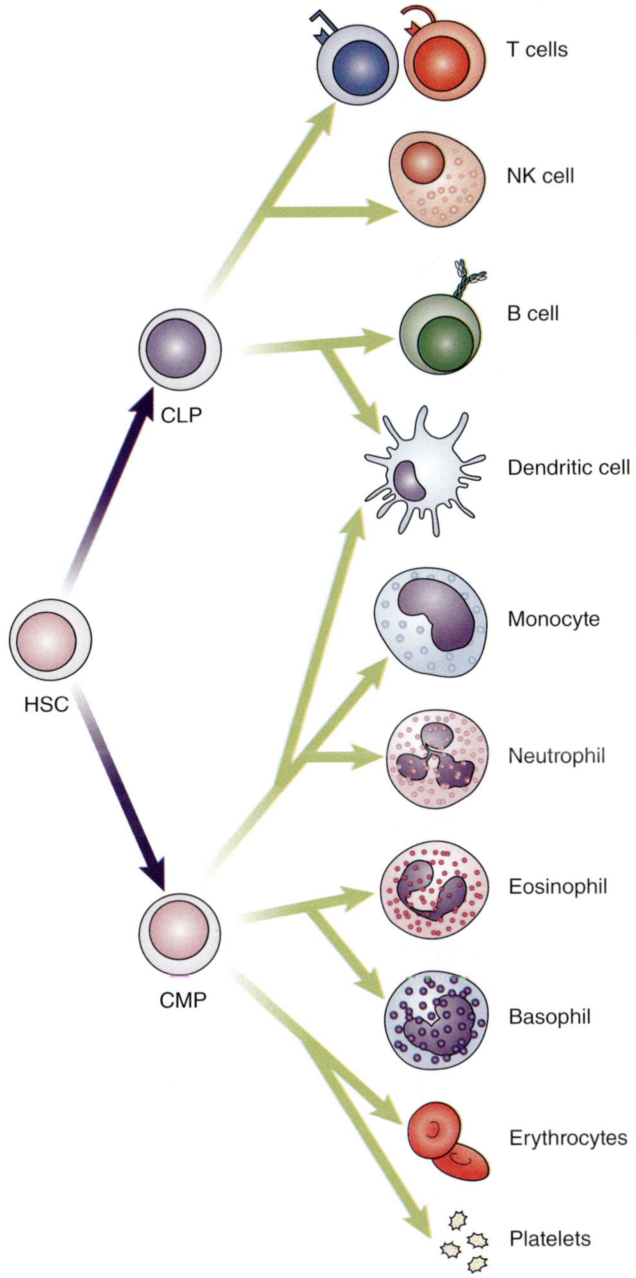

FIGURE 1–2 Simplified scheme of hematopoiesis. In the bone marrow, HSCs give rise to two different lines—a CLP and a CMP. CLPs give rise to T cells, B cells, NK cells, and some dendritic cells. The CMP differentiates into another type of dendritic cell, monocytes/macrophages, neutrophils, eosinophils, basophils, erythrocytes, and platelets.

Neutrophils

The **neutrophil** represents the most abundant type of leukocyte in the blood, about 50% to 70% of the total peripheral WBCs in adults. Neutrophils are the key cell type involved in acute inflammatory responses, where they function in phagocytosis and destruction of foreign particles.

Mature neutrophils are also known as *polymorphonuclear* (PMN) leukocytes because of their nuclear morphology. They are approximately 10 to 15 μm in diameter with a nucleus that has between two and five lobes, which are connected by thin, threadlike filaments **(Fig. 1–3).** Hence, they are also called *segmented neutrophils*, or "segs." Their cytoplasm contains a large number of neutral (violet-pink)-staining granules when stained with Wright stain. The granules contain enzymes and other proteins that have various roles in neutrophil function. While these proteins play an essential role in the destruction of engulfed microbes, they can also be released outside of the cell and cause damage to surrounding tissues in some cases (see Chapter 14).

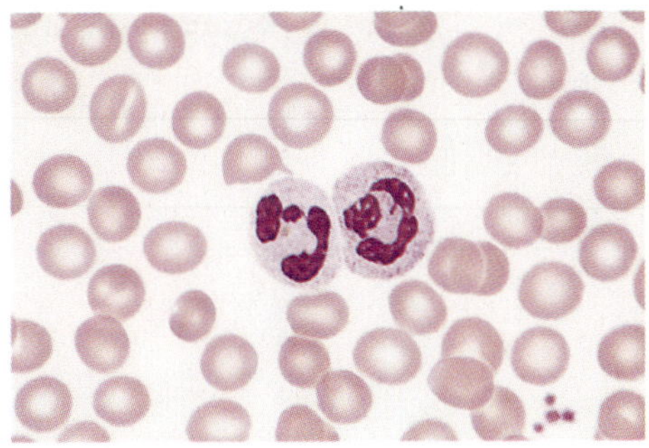

FIGURE 1–3 Neutrophils. Note the neutral granules and variations in morphology of the nucleus.

The most abundant type of granules are the neutrophil-*specific granules*, also known as *secondary granules*, which contain enzymes that break down bacterial cell walls (e.g., lysozyme); proteins that bind iron to prevent its utilization by bacteria (i.e., lactoferrin); and components essential for the oxidative burst (a process that occurs during phagocytosis and results in the formation of reactive oxygen molecules that are toxic to bacteria; see Chapter 2). Another type of granule is the *azurophilic* or *primary* granule, which contains antimicrobial proteins (e.g., myeloperoxidase, lysozyme, elastase, proteinase-3, cathepsin G, defensins). The other types of granules present are the *tertiary granules*, which contain enzymes that degrade extracellular matrix proteins (e.g., gelatinase, collagenase) to facilitate neutrophil migration into the tissues, and *secretory granules* or *vesicles*, which contain proteins needed for neutrophil adhesion to the vessel walls and movement into the tissues (e.g., selectins).

Normally, half of the total neutrophil population in peripheral blood is found in a marginating pool adhering to blood vessel walls, whereas the rest of the neutrophils circulate freely for about 6 to 8 hours. There is a continuous interchange, however, between the marginating and the circulating pools. Margination allows neutrophils to move from the circulating blood, through the vessel walls, to the tissues. They are attracted to a specific area by chemotactic factors that cause cells to migrate in a particular direction. Once in the tissues, neutrophils have a life span of up to several days. Normally, the influx of neutrophils from the bone marrow equals the output from the blood to the tissues to maintain a steady state. However, in the case of acute infection, the number of neutrophils in the circulating blood increases almost immediately. These cells are then driven rapidly to the site of an infection.

Eosinophils

Eosinophils are approximately 10 to 15 μm in diameter and normally make up between 1% and 4% of the circulating WBCs in a nonallergic person. Their number increases in an allergic reaction or in response to certain parasitic infections. The nucleus is usually bilobed or ellipsoidal and is often eccentrically located **(Fig. 1–4).** Eosinophils take up the acid eosin dye, and

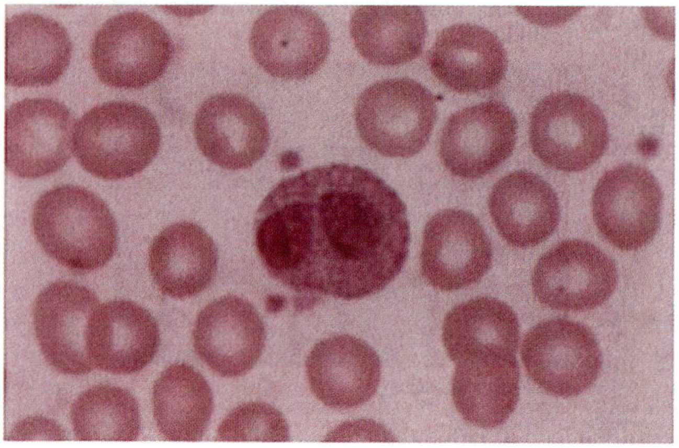

FIGURE 1–4 Eosinophil. Note the red granules.

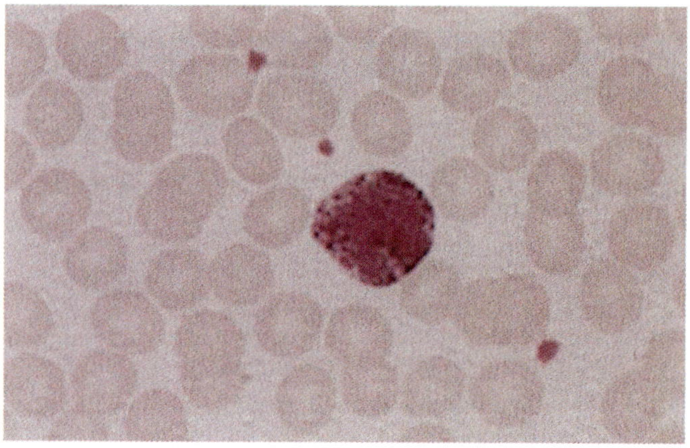

FIGURE 1–5 Basophil. Note the bluish-purple granules.

the cytoplasm is filled with large orange to reddish-orange granules after treatment with Wright stain. The granules are spherical and evenly distributed throughout the cell, and they contain a large number of previously synthesized proteins, including eosinophil-derived neurotoxin, peroxidase, histamine, proteases, growth factors, cationic proteins, and cytokines, which act as chemical messengers between cells of the immune system.

Eosinophils are capable of phagocytosis but are much less efficient than neutrophils because they are present in smaller numbers and lack digestive enzymes. Eosinophils release mediators that contribute to allergic reactions (see Chapter 14). They can also use cationic proteins released during degranulation to damage cell membranes and kill larger parasites, such as helminth worms, that cannot be phagocytized (see Chapter 22). In addition, eosinophils produce cytokines that play important roles in modulating immune responses and maintaining tissue integrity.

Basophils

Basophils are the least numerous of the WBCs in peripheral blood, representing less than 1% of all circulating WBCs. The smallest of the granulocytes, basophils are slightly larger than RBCs (between 10 and 15 µm in diameter) and with Wright stain, show coarse, deep-bluish-purple granules that often obscure the bilobed nucleus **(Fig. 1–5)**. Constituents of these granules include histamine, cytokines, growth factors, and a small amount of heparin, all of which have an important function in inducing and maintaining allergic reactions. Histamine contracts smooth muscle, and heparin is an anticoagulant. Basophils also regulate some T-helper (TH) cell responses and stimulate B cells to produce the antibody, immunoglobulin E (IgE). They have a life span of only a few hours in the bloodstream, after which they are removed and destroyed by macrophages in the spleen.

Mast Cells

Mast cells resemble basophils, but they come from a different lineage. They originate in the bone marrow, are released into the blood, and mature in the tissues. Mast cells are distributed in various tissues throughout the body, notably the skin, connective tissue, and mucosal epithelial tissue of the respiratory, genitourinary, and digestive tracts. Mast cells are larger than basophils, with a diameter of up to 20 µm, and have a small ovoid nucleus with many granules **(Fig. 1–6)**. Unlike basophils, they have a long life span of between 9 and 18 months. The enzyme content of the granules in mast cells helps to distinguish them from basophils because they contain serine proteases, heparin, and neutrophil chemotactic factor, in addition to histamine. Histamine and other proteins released by mast cells promote inflammation by increasing vascular permeability and blood flow to the affected area. The chemical mediators produced by mast cells also play important roles in regulating innate and adaptive immune responses as well as vascular homeostasis. Mast cells possess a diverse set of receptors, including receptors for IgE antibody. They are versatile cells that can detect a variety of pathogens and initiate innate defenses against them. They are best known for their principal role in allergic reactions (see Chapter 14).

Monocytes and Macrophages

Monocytes are the largest cells in the peripheral blood, with a diameter that can vary from 12 to 20 µm (the average is 18 µm). In the clinical laboratory, they can be identified by their surface expression of a myeloid cell antigen called *CD14*. Another distinguishing feature of monocytes is an irregularly folded or horseshoe-shaped nucleus that occupies almost one-half of the entire cell volume **(Fig. 1–7)**. The abundant

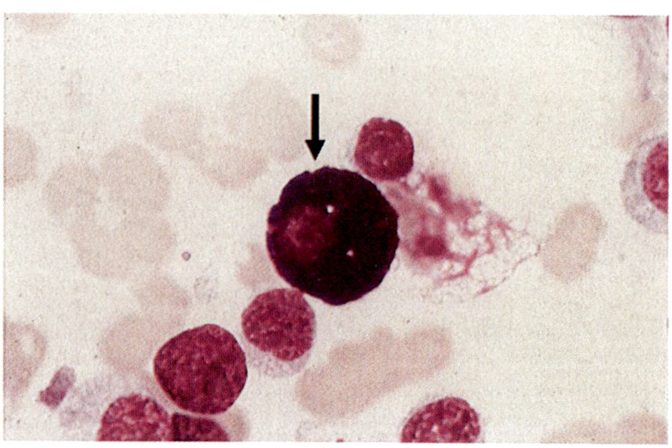

FIGURE 1–6 Mast cell.

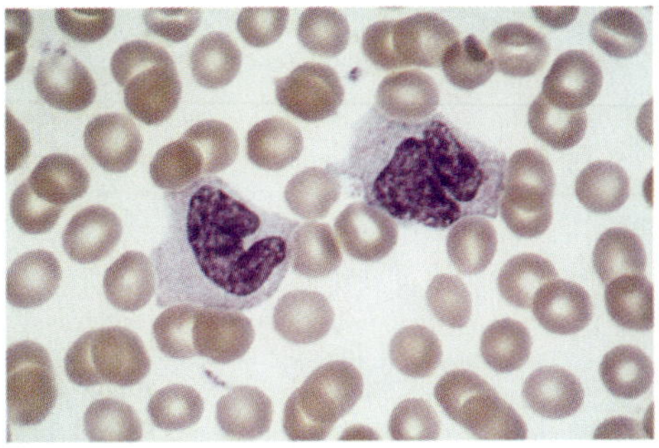

FIGURE 1–7 Two monocytes.

cytoplasm stains a dull grayish blue and has a ground-glass appearance because of the presence of fine, dustlike granules which contain various antimicrobial enzymes. Digestive vacuoles may also be observed in the cytoplasm. Monocytes make up between 2% and 10% of total circulating WBCs; however, they do not remain in circulation for long. They stay in peripheral blood for up to 30 hours; then, they migrate to the tissues and become known as **macrophages.** The transition from monocyte to macrophage in the tissues is characterized by progressive cellular enlargement to between 25 and 80 μm. Unlike monocytes, macrophages contain no peroxidase. Tissue distribution appears to be a random phenomenon.

Macrophages have specific names according to their particular tissue location. Macrophages in the lungs are called *alveolar macrophages;* in the liver, *Kupffer cells;* in the brain, *microglial cells;* in the bone, *osteoclasts;* and in connective tissue, *histiocytes.* Macrophages may not be as efficient as neutrophils in phagocytosis because their motility is slow compared with neutrophils. Some macrophages progress through the tissues by means of amoeboid action, whereas others are immobile. However, their life span appears to be in the range of months rather than days.

Macrophages play an important role in initiating and regulating both innate and adaptive immune responses. Their innate immune functions include phagocytosis, microbial killing, anti-tumor activity, intracellular parasite eradication, and secretion of cytokines. Killing activity is enhanced when macrophages become "activated" by contact with microorganisms or cytokines that are released by lymphocytes during the immune response. Macrophages play a major role in the adaptive immune response by presenting phagocytosed antigens to T lymphocytes (see Chapters 4 and 5).

Dendritic Cells

Dendritic cells are so named because they are covered with long, membranous extensions that resemble nerve cell dendrites. Progenitors in the bone marrow give rise to dendritic cell precursors that travel to lymphoid as well as nonlymphoid tissues. Like macrophages, dendritic cells are classified according to their tissue location. After capturing an antigen in the tissue by phagocytosis or endocytosis, they travel to the nearest lymph node and present the antigen to T lymphocytes to initiate the adaptive immune response in a similar way to macrophages. Dendritic cells, however, are considered the most effective antigen-presenting cells in the body, and the most potent phagocytic cell.

Knowledge Check 1-2

Phagocytosis is the primary function of which cell?
a. Lymphocyte
b. Neutrophil
c. Basophil
d. Mast cell

Knowledge Check 1-3

Which of the following cells are the most effective at antigen presentation to T cells?
a. Neutrophils
b. Macrophages
c. B cells
d. Dendritic cells

Lymphoid Cells

Lymphocytes, innate lymphoid cells, and special population of dendritic cells comprise the lymphoid cell population. The **lymphocyte** is the key cell type involved in the adaptive immune response and will be the main focus of this section. Lymphocytes represent between 20% and 40% of the circulating WBCs. The typical small lymphocyte is similar in size to RBCs (7 to 10 μm in diameter) and has a large, rounded nucleus that may be somewhat indented. The nuclear chromatin is dense and tends to stain a deep blue **(Fig. 1–8).** Cytoplasm is sparse, containing few organelles and no specific granules, and consists of a narrow ring surrounding the nucleus. The cytoplasm stains a light to dark blue with Wright stain. Lymphocytes are unique because they arise from an HSC and then are further differentiated in the primary lymphoid organs, namely, the bone marrow and the thymus.

Lymphocytes can be divided into three major populations—T cells, B cells, and NK cells—based on their functions and the proteins on their cell surfaces. In the peripheral blood of adults, about 10% to 20% of lymphocytes are B cells, 60% to 80% are T cells, and 10% to 20% are NK cells. T and B lymphocytes are difficult to distinguish visually. In the laboratory, antigens on cell surfaces can be used to

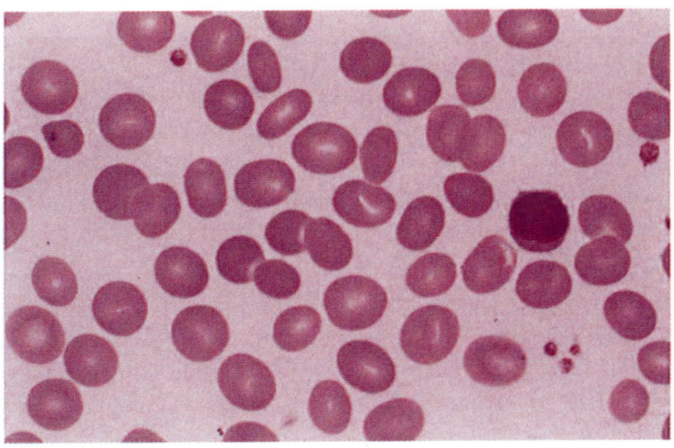

FIGURE 1–8 Typical lymphocyte in peripheral blood.

Table 1-1 Surface Markers on Lymphocytes

CELL TYPE	MAJOR SURFACE MARKERS
B cells	CD19, CD20, CD21, CD22, surface immunoglobulin
All T cells	CD2, CD3
Helper T cells	CD2, CD3, CD4
Cytotoxic T cells	CD2, CD3, CD8
T regulatory cells	CD2, CD3, CD4
NK cells	CD16, CD56
All leukocytes	CD45

identify each lymphocyte subpopulation. To standardize the nomenclature for these antigens, scientists held the Human Leukocyte Differentiation Antigens Workshops to relate their research findings. Panels of antibodies from different laboratories were used for analysis, and antibodies reacting similarly with standard cell lines were said to define **clusters of differentiation (CD).** As each antigen, or CD, was found, it was assigned a number. **Table 1–1** lists the major lymphocyte populations and some of the surface markers commonly used to identify them. A more detailed discussion of these markers is presented in Chapter 13.

B Cells and Plasma Cells

B cells are derived from a lymphoid precursor in the bone marrow that differentiates to become a T cell, B cell, or NK cell depending on exposure to different cytokines. B cells remain in the environment provided by bone marrow stromal cells. B-cell precursors go through a developmental process that prepares them for their role in antibody production and, at the same time, restricts the types of antigens to which any one cell can respond. They are able to generate highly specific cell surface receptors through genetic recombination of their immunoglobulin genes (see Chapter 3 for details). The end result is a **B lymphocyte** that is genetically programmed to produce a unique antibody molecule. B cells can be recognized by the presence of membrane-bound antibodies of two types, namely, immunoglobulin M (IgM) and immunoglobulin D (IgD). Other surface proteins that appear on the B cell include CD19, CD20, CD21, CD22, and class II major histocompatibility complex (MHC) molecules (see Chapter 5).

Plasma cells represent the most fully differentiated B lymphocyte, and their main function is antibody production. They are not normally found in the blood; rather, they are located in germinal centers in the peripheral lymphoid organs, or they reside in the bone marrow. Plasma cells are spherical or ellipsoidal cells between 10 and 20 µm in size that are characterized by the presence of abundant cytoplasmic immunoglobulin and little to no surface immunoglobulin **(Fig. 1–9).** The nucleus is eccentric or oval with heavily clumped chromatin that stains darkly. An abundant endoplasmic reticulum and a clear, well-defined Golgi zone are present in the cytoplasm. CD38 is a marker that is routinely used in the clinical

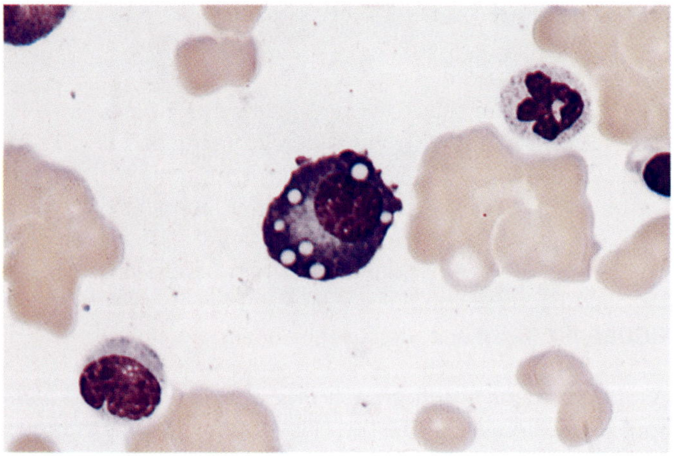

FIGURE 1–9 A typical plasma cell.

laboratory to identify plasma cells. Plasma cells can be long-lived in lymphoid organs and continually produce antibodies. Antibodies are the major component of humoral immunity, and their functions are described in detail in Chapter 3.

T Cells

T lymphocytes are so named because they differentiate in the thymus. Lymphocyte precursors from the bone marrow enter the thymus through the bloodstream. As they mature, the T cells express unique surface markers that allow them to recognize foreign antigens bound to cell membrane proteins called *MHC molecules.* T cells have multiple roles in the immune system. They produce cytokines that stimulate B cells to make antibodies; they kill tumor cells and virus-infected cells; and they regulate innate and adaptive immune responses. The processes in which T cells have a primary role are collectively known as **cell-mediated immunity.**

Three main subtypes of T cells can be distinguished according to their unique functions: **helper T (TH) cells, cytotoxic T (TC) cells,** and **regulatory T (Treg) cells.** TH cells help B cells to make antibody and other T cells to carry out cell-mediated immune responses, TC cells kill virally infected cells and tumor cells, and Treg cells help to control the actions of B cells and other T cells. A small population of T cells called NKT shares some of the properties of NK cells and recognizes lipid and glycolipid antigens.

All T cells possess the CD3 marker on their cell surface, and the T-cell subtypes can be identified by the presence of either CD4 or CD8 as well. T cells bearing the CD4 protein are mainly either TH or Treg cells, whereas the $CD8^+$ population consists of TC cells. The normal ratio of $CD4^+$ to $CD8^+$ cells is about 2:1 in peripheral blood.

Natural Killer Cells and Innate Lymphoid Cells

NK cells and innate lymphoid cells are related types of cells that have important roles in innate immunity and tissue remodeling. These cells share three main properties: (1) they have a lymphoid morphology, (2) they do not possess antigen-specific receptors, and (3) they do not have myeloid and dendritic cell markers. Both cell types originate from a common innate lymphocyte precursor (CILP) that is derived from the CLP.

NK cells are so named because they serve as an early defense against altered host cells. NK cells mature in the bone marrow and are generally larger than T cells and B cells, at approximately 15 µm in diameter. They contain kidney-shaped nuclei with condensed chromatin and prominent nucleoli. Described as large granular lymphocytes, NK cells are found mainly in the liver, spleen, and peripheral blood.

There are no surface markers that are unique to NK cells, but they express a specific combination of antigens that can be used for identification. Two such antigens are CD16 and CD56. CD16 is a receptor for the antigen-nonspecific part of antibody molecules (see Chapter 3). Because of the presence of CD16, NK cells are able to make contact with and then lyse abnormal cells coated with antibodies (see Chapter 2). NK cells continuously scan for protein irregularities on host cells, and they represent the first line of defense against virally infected cells and tumor cells. NK cells destroy these target cells in a manner similar to the Tc cell, except that they are not antigen-specific. Granules found in NK cells contain serine proteases called *granzymes*, and release of these enzymes causes target cell death.

Innate lymphoid cells (ILCs) are functionally similar to TH cells. They have been classified into three groups, based on the cytokines they produce. Although the functions of these cells are not completely understood, they appear to respond to cytokines released during the early stages of an infection or tissue injury by secreting additional cytokines that play a role in adaptive immune responses.

Although NK cells and ILCs are considered part of the innate immune system because they are not antigen specific and respond quickly to a variety of stimuli, they are thought to play important roles as transitional cells that bridge the innate and the adaptive immune responses against pathogens.

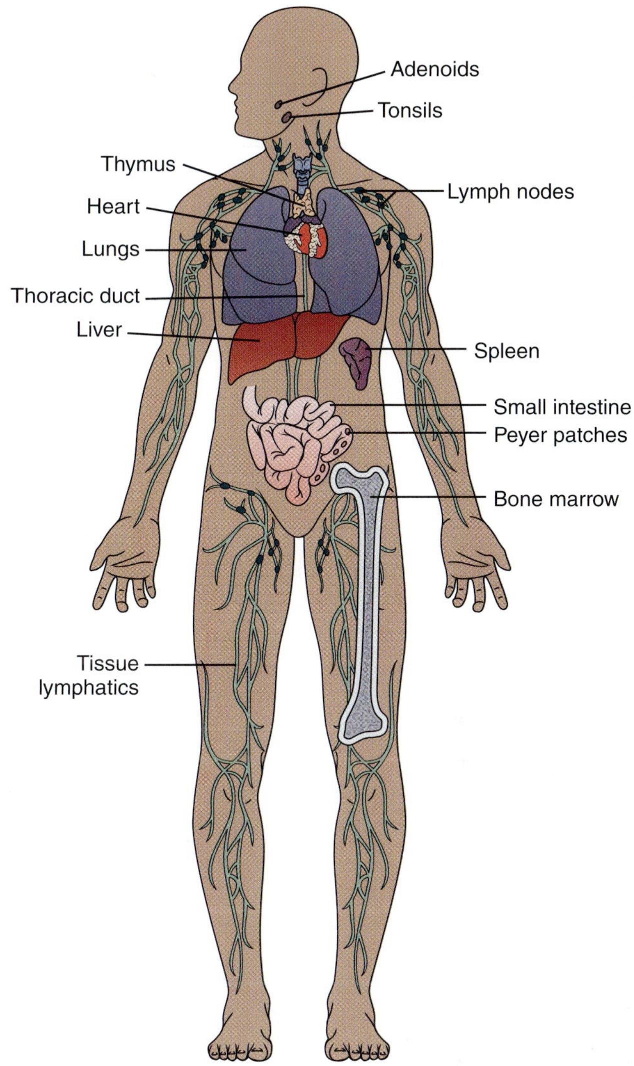

FIGURE 1–10 Organs and tissues of the immune system. The primary lymphoid organs are the bone marrow and the thymus. Secondary lymphoid organs are distributed throughout the body and include the spleen, lymph nodes, and mucosal-associated lymphoid tissue. The spleen filters antigens in the blood, whereas the lymph nodes filter fluid from the tissues.

Knowledge Check 1-4

Antibody production is the primary function of which cell?

a. B lymphocyte
b. T lymphocyte
c. NK cell
d. Monocyte

Critical Thinking 1-1

Suppose a patient acquired an infection with a virus that destroys $CD4^+$ lymphocytes. What parts of the immune response would be affected by the infection?

Organs and Tissues of the Immune System

Just as the cells of the immune system have diverse functions, so too do key organs that are involved in the development of the immune response **(Fig. 1-10)**. The bone marrow and thymus are considered the **primary lymphoid organs** where maturation of B lymphocytes and T lymphocytes takes place, respectively. Lymphocytes go through complex maturation pathways in the bone marrow and thymus, during which they acquire specific surface antigens and their characteristic functions. We discuss these processes briefly in the section that follows and in more detail in Chapter 5. Formation of lymphocytes in the primary lymphoid organs is antigen independent, meaning that lymphocytes are constantly being produced without the presence of specific antigens. This characteristic allows the immune system to be prepared before an encounter with a foreign antigen occurs. Mature lymphocytes released from the bone marrow or thymus are called *naïve* before they come into contact with foreign antigens.

The **secondary lymphoid organs** provide a location where contact with foreign antigens can occur. Secondary lymphoid organs and tissues include the spleen, lymph nodes, skin-associated lymphoid tissue (SALT), and various types of mucosal-associated lymphoid tissue (MALT); see Fig. 1-10. In these organs, lymphocytes derived from the bone marrow and thymus are activated by antigen to proliferate and differentiate into *effector cells,* which carry out specific functions of the immune response. Some of the lymphocytes in the secondary lymphoid organs develop into long-lived *memory cells,* which are capable of responding faster and more efficiently if re-exposed to the same antigen at a later time.

Primary Lymphoid Organs

Bone Marrow

Bone marrow is considered one of the largest tissues in the body, and it fills the core of all long flat bones. It is the main source of HSCs, which develop into erythrocytes, granulocytes, monocytes, platelets, and lymphocytes. Each of these lineages has specific precursors that originate from the pluripotent stem cells.

Some lymphocyte precursors remain in the marrow to mature and become B cells or NK cells. B cells received their name because they were originally found to mature in birds in an organ called the *bursa of Fabricius,* which is similar to the human appendix. After searching for such an organ in humans, it was discovered that B-cell maturation takes place within the bone marrow itself. Thus, the naming of these cells was appropriate. Other lymphocyte precursors go to the thymus and develop into T cells, so named because of where they mature. Lymphocyte differentiation takes place very early in fetal development and is essential to acquisition of immunocompetence by the time the infant is born.

Thymus

T cells develop their identifying characteristics in the **thymus,** a small, flat, bilobed organ found in the thorax, or chest cavity, right below the thyroid gland and overlying the heart. In humans, the thymus reaches a weight of 30 to 40 g by puberty and then gradually shrinks in size. Although the thymus diminishes in size as humans age, it is still capable of producing T lymphocytes, although at a reduced rate.

Each lobe of the thymus is divided into smaller lobules filled with epithelial cells that play a central role in the differentiation process. T-cell maturation occurs during a 3-week period as cells filter through the outer portion of the thymus, called the *cortex*, to its inner portion, the *medulla.* Different proteins and antigen-specific receptors are expressed on the T-cell membrane as these cells mature, creating a repertoire of T cells to protect the body from foreign invaders. The medulla then releases mature T lymphocytes.

Secondary Lymphoid Organs

Once lymphocytes mature in the primary lymphoid organs, they are released and travel through blood vessels to the secondary lymphoid organs such as the spleen and lymph nodes. In these organs, the main contact with foreign antigens takes place, and the immune response is initiated. Lymphocytes that do not encounter their specific antigen remain in a resting, or nondividing, state. Encounter with an antigen induces specific lymphocytes to be transformed into an activated state and divide to produce a large number of effector cells. The effector cells then migrate to sites in the body where they are needed to perform their specialized functions: B cells develop into plasma cells that produce specific antibodies to provide humoral immunity, whereas T cells regulate the humoral immune response and are effectors of cell-mediated immunity. Some of the lymphocytes develop into long-lived memory cells, as mentioned earlier.

Because each individual possesses only a small number of lymphocytes that have specific receptors for any given antigen, many lymphocytes continuously circulate throughout tissues in the body to increase the likelihood of coming into contact with their corresponding antigen. Lymphocyte circulation occurs through blood vessels and the lymphatic system (Fig. 1–10). In the circulatory system, arteries carry blood away from the heart, and veins transport blood back to the heart. The vessels are lined with endothelial cells to which the WBC can bind via different cell surface adhesion molecules. Specific cytokines and other factors will then guide the WBC to travel through small gaps between the endothelial cells to the tissue site where a foreign antigen is located.

The lymphatic system consists of the lymph nodes (see section that follows) and a network of vessels that contain a protein-rich fluid known as *lymph.* Lymph is a filtrate of the blood that arises from the passage of water and low molecular weight solutes out of blood vessel walls and into the interstitial spaces between cells. The interstitial fluid is collected in thin-walled *lymphatic vessels,* pumped through a series of progressively larger vessels, enters and travels through the lymph nodes, and is eventually returned to the blood. Lymphatic vessels also transport lymphocytes and carry microbial antigens from the site of an infection to the secondary lymphoid organs, where an immune response is initiated. Lymphocytes travel through the secondary organs and flow through a series of progressively larger vessels that culminate in the *thoracic duct,* the largest lymphatic vessel in the body. The thoracic duct collects most of the body's lymph fluid and returns it to the blood via the left subclavian vein, thus maintaining steady fluid levels in the tissues and circulatory system.

Lymphocytes are segregated within the secondary lymphoid organs according to their functions. These organs contain distinct but neighboring regions of B cells and T cells, allowing them to interact with each other in an organized manner that results in a productive immune response. The lymph nodes and spleen have the most highly organized structures and are discussed in more detail in the sections that follow. Most of the lymphoid tissues in the skin and mucous membranes are more loosely organized.

Lymph Nodes

Lymph nodes are small bean-shaped organs that filter lymph fluid from adjacent tissues. There are 500 to 600 lymph nodes located throughout the human body, and they are especially numerous in the armpits *(axillary nodes),* groin *(inguinal nodes),* and neck *(cervical nodes)* (Fig. 1–10).

The lymph nodes are connected to both lymphatic vessels and blood vessels, allowing lymphocytes and foreign antigens from the tissues to enter the organ and interact. Lymphocytes and any foreign antigens in the lymph fluid enter the lymph nodes through *afferent lymphatic vessels.* Numerous lymphocytes also enter the nodes from the bloodstream through specialized venules called *high endothelial venules.* Lymph fluid flows slowly through spaces called *sinuses,* which are lined with macrophages, creating an ideal location where phagocytosis can take place.

Structurally, lymph nodes are surrounded by a fibrous capsule, and the tissue under the capsule is organized into three regions: an outer *cortex,* a *paracortex,* and an inner *medulla* **(Fig. 1–11).** The outermost layer, the **cortex,** contains macrophages and aggregations of B cells in **primary follicles.** These are mature, resting B cells that have not yet been exposed to antigens. Specialized cells called *follicular dendritic cells* are also located here. These cells have a large number of antibody receptors that help capture antigens to present to T cells and B cells.

Following exposure to an antigen, B lymphocytes with specific receptors are stimulated to divide, forming a colony of B cells that can respond to the antigen, and the primary follicles are transformed into **secondary follicles.** The interior of a secondary follicle is known as a **germinal center** because it is here that transformation of the B cells takes place. When exposed to an antigen, the activated B cells develop into plasma cells (see Fig. 1–9), which secrete antibodies, and **memory cells,** which can quickly respond to a foreign substance previously encountered by the immune system.

T lymphocytes are mainly located in the **paracortex,** the region between the follicles and the medulla. T lymphocytes are in close proximity to dendritic cells, which can take up antigens, process them, and present them to T cells that possess antigen-specific receptors. The innermost layer of the lymph nodes is the **medulla.** It is less densely populated than the cortex but contains some T cells, B cells, macrophages, and numerous plasma cells.

Particulate antigens are removed from the fluid as it travels across the lymph node from cortex to medulla. Fluid and lymphocytes exit the node by way of the *efferent lymphatic vessels.* These vessels meet to form a larger duct that eventually connects with the thoracic duct and the venous system. Therefore, lymphocytes are able to recirculate continuously between lymph nodes and the peripheral blood.

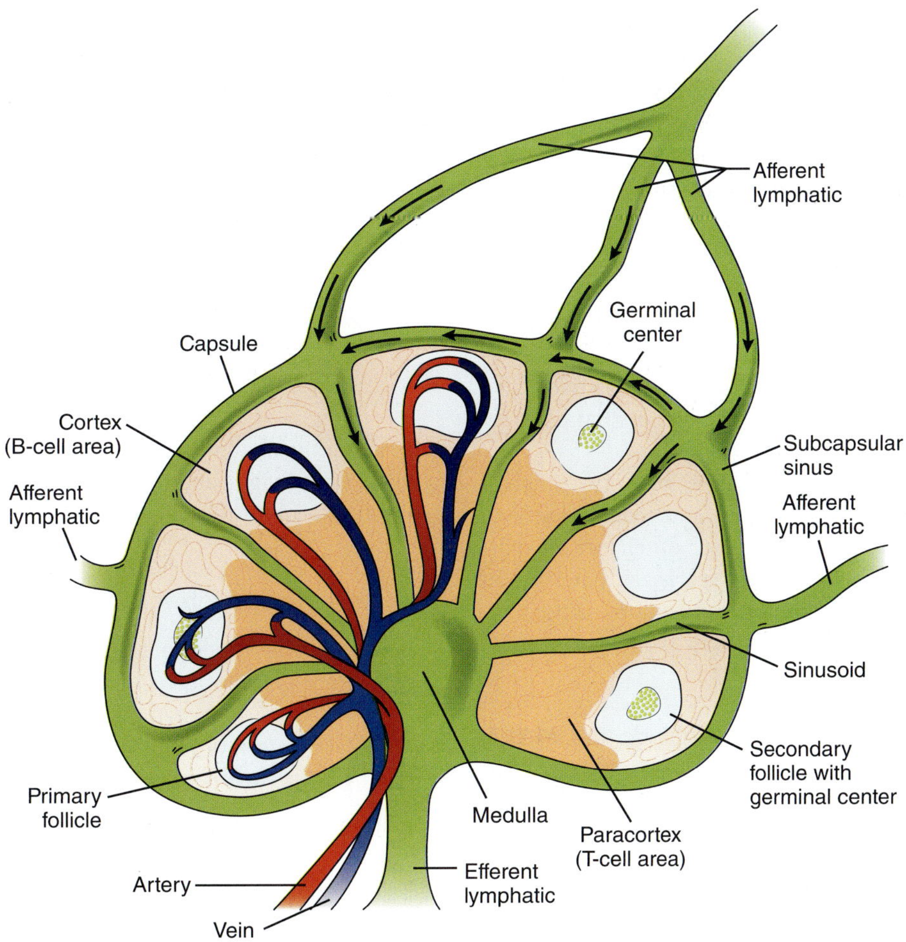

FIGURE 1–11 Structure of a lymph node. A lymph node is surrounded by a fibrous outer capsule. Right underneath is the subcapsular sinus, where lymph fluid drains from afferent lymphatic vessels. The outer cortex contains collections of B cells in primary follicles. When stimulated by antigens, secondary follicles are formed. T cells are found in the paracortical area. Fluid drains slowly through sinusoids to the medullary region and out the efferent lymphatic vessel to the thoracic duct.

If contact with an antigen takes place, lymphocyte traffic stops. Lymphocytes that are able to respond to a particular antigen proliferate in the node. Accumulation of lymphocytes and other cells causes the lymph nodes to become enlarged, a condition known as *lymphadenopathy*. As lymphocyte traffic resumes, recirculation of expanded numbers of lymphocytes occurs.

Spleen

The **spleen**, the largest secondary lymphoid organ, has a length of approximately 12 cm and weighs 150 g in the adult. It is located in the upper-left quadrant of the abdomen just below the diaphragm and is surrounded by a thin capsule of connective tissue. The organ acts as a large discriminating filter, removing old and damaged cells and foreign antigens from the blood.

Splenic tissue can be divided into two main types: red pulp and white pulp. The red pulp makes up more than one-half of the total volume of the spleen. It contains numerous small vessels called sinusoids that are filled with blood, and it is rich in macrophages. The major function of the red pulp is to destroy old RBCs, platelets, and some pathogens. Blood flows from the arterioles into the red pulp and then exits by way of the splenic vein.

The white pulp comprises approximately 20% of the total weight of the spleen and contains the lymphoid tissue, which is arranged around arterioles to form a **periarteriolar lymphoid sheath (PALS) (Fig. 1–12).** The PALS contains mainly T cells. Attached to the sheath are primary follicles containing B cells that are not yet stimulated by antigens. As in the lymph nodes, exposure to specific antigen induces the primary follicles to develop germinal centers and become transformed into secondary follicles. Surrounding the PALS is a region called the marginal zone, which separates the red pulp from the white pulp. The marginal zone contains macrophages and dendritic cells that trap antigens, and a specialized type of B lymphocyte. Lymphocytes enter and leave this area through the many capillary branches that connect to the arterioles.

The spleen receives a blood volume of approximately 350 mL/minute, allowing lymphocytes and macrophages to constantly survey for infectious agents or other foreign matter. Surgical removal of the spleen, or *splenectomy*, results in increased susceptibility to bloodborne infections caused by encapsulated bacteria.

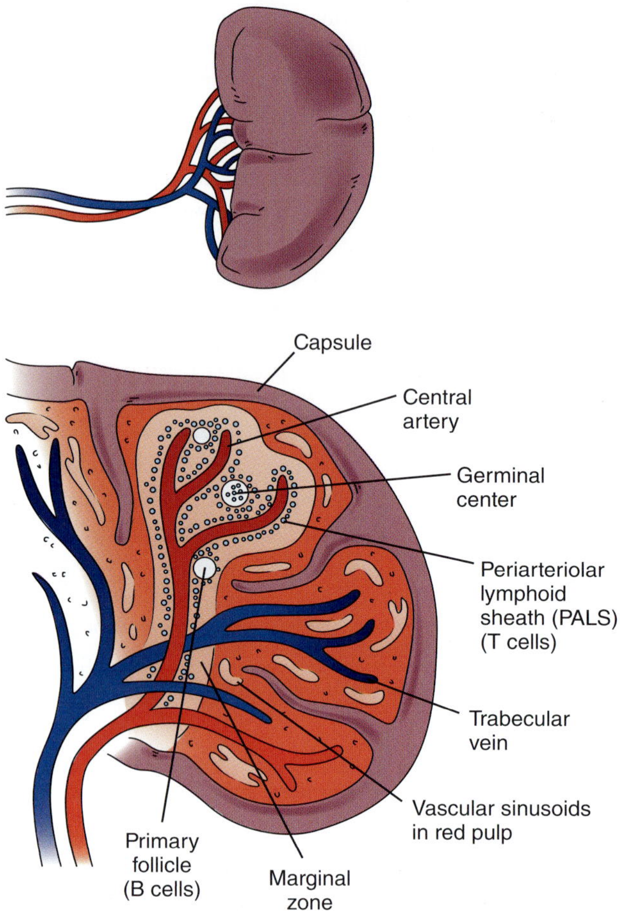

FIGURE 1–12 Cross section of the spleen showing organization of the lymphoid tissue. T cells are located in the PALS surrounding the central arteries. Follicles containing B cells are positioned close to the PALS. When stimulated by antigens, the B cells form germinal centers. All the lymphoid tissue in the spleen is referred to as the *white pulp*.

Secondary Lymphoid Tissues

Additional areas of lymphoid tissue include the **MALT.** MALT is found in the gastrointestinal, respiratory, and urogenital tracts. Some examples of MALT are the tonsils; appendix; and *Peyer patches*, a specialized type of organized MALT located at the lower part of the small intestine. These mucosal surfaces are some of the main ports of entry for foreign antigens, and thus, numerous macrophages and lymphocytes are located here.

The skin is considered the largest organ of the body, and the epidermis layer contains several intraepidermal lymphocytes. Most of these are T cells, which are uniquely positioned to combat any antigens that enter the body through the skin. Monocytes, macrophages, and dendritic cells are also found here. The collective term for these tissues is the **SALT.**

Knowledge Check 1-5

What is the function of the primary lymphoid organs?

a. Receipt of antigens from lymph fluid
b. Removal of foreign antigens from the blood
c. Generation of mature B and T lymphocytes
d. Contact with antigens at mucosal surfaces

Critical Thinking 1-2

Suppose a boy was born with an immunodeficiency in which lymph node follicles and germinal centers are underdeveloped or absent. What part of the immune system would be affected?

KEY CONCEPTS

Immunity and Immunization

- Immunology has its roots in the study of immunity—the condition of being resistant to disease.
- Edward Jenner performed the first vaccination against smallpox by using material from cowpox lesions.
- Louis Pasteur is considered the "Father of Immunology" for his use of attenuated vaccines.
- Élie Metchnikoff was the first to observe phagocytosis, the process by which cells engulf other cells.

Innate Versus Adaptive Immunity

- Immunity has two branches: innate and adaptive. Innate immunity is the ability of the body to resist infection through means of preexisting barriers or nonspecific mechanisms that can be activated quickly. Adaptive immunity is characterized by specificity for antigen, memory, and dependence on lymphocytes.
- There are two main types of adaptive immune responses: (1) humoral immunity, which involves production of antibodies by B lymphocytes and plasma cells, and (2) cell-mediated immunity, which is carried out by T lymphocytes to destroy intracellular pathogens.

Cells of the Immune System

- All blood cells arise from multipotent HSCs in the bone marrow during a process called *hematopoiesis.*
- The five principal types of leukocytes in the peripheral blood are neutrophils, eosinophils, basophils, monocytes, and lymphocytes.
- Tissue cells involved in immunity include mast cells, dendritic cells, and macrophages which arise from monocytes.
- Cells that are involved in the innate immune response and are actively phagocytic include neutrophils, monocytes, macrophages, and dendritic cells.
- Lymphocytes are the key cells involved in the adaptive immune response because they have antigen-specific receptors.
- *CD* stands for "clusters of differentiation," which are proteins found on cell surfaces that can be used to identify specific cell types and stages of differentiation.
- B cells are lymphocytes that develop in the bone marrow and are capable of secreting antibody when they mature into plasma cells. They can be identified by the presence of CD19, CD20, CD21, CD22, and surface antibody.
- T cells acquire their antigen specificity in the thymus and consist of two main subtypes: $CD4^+$, which are primarily TH or Treg cells, and $CD8^+$, which are Tc cells. The CD3 and CD2 markers are present on all T-cell subtypes.
- NK cells are lymphocytes that arise from a lymphocyte precursor but do not develop in the thymus. NK cells can kill virally infected or cancerous target cells without previous exposure to them.

Organs and Tissues of the Immune System

- In humans, the bone marrow and the thymus are the primary lymphoid organs where lymphocytes mature. B cells remain in the bone marrow to mature, whereas T cells develop their specific characteristics in the thymus.
- The secondary lymphoid organs are the sites in which lymphocytes come into contact with foreign antigens and become activated in the adaptive immune response. Secondary lymphoid organs and tissues include the lymph nodes, spleen, MALT, and SALT.

Study Guide: Innate Versus Adaptive Immunity

KEY FEATURES	INNATE IMMUNITY	ADAPTIVE IMMUNITY
Alternative names	Natural immunity	Acquired immunity
Specificity	Nonspecific	Specific for a particular antigen
Timing	Immediate or rapid, due to preexisting barriers or quick cell activation	Delayed
Memory	No	Yes, following re-exposure to an antigen
Diversity	Limited	Creates responses to a large variety of antigens
Ability to differentiate between self and non-self	Yes	Yes
Primary cells involved	Neutrophils, eosinophils, basophils, monocytes/macrophages, mast cells, dendritic cells, natural killer cells	B cells, T cells, plasma cells, macrophages, dendritic cells
Major blood proteins involved	Cytokines, complement, acute phase reactants	Antibodies, cytokines, complement

Study Guide: Cells of the Immune System

CELL TYPE	WHERE FOUND	FUNCTION	
Neutrophils	50%–70% of circulating WBCs, also in tissues	First responders to infection, phagocytosis	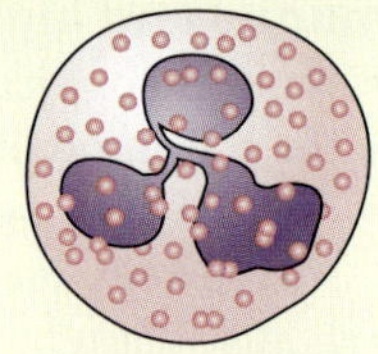
Eosinophils	1%–4% of circulating WBCs	Kill parasites, neutralize basophil and mast cell products, regulate mast cells	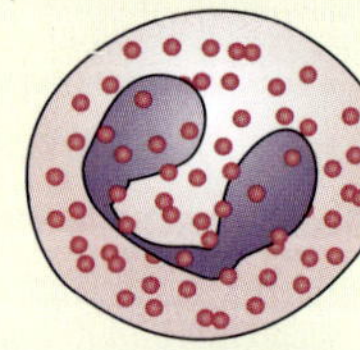
Basophils	Less than 1% of circulating WBCs	Produce inflammatory mediators that induce and maintain allergic reactions	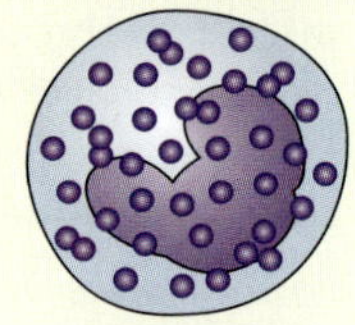
Mast cells	Skin, connective tissue, mucosal epithelium	Produce inflammatory mediators that induce and maintain allergic reactions	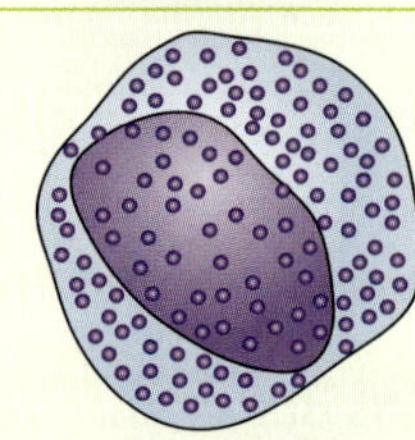
Monocytes	2%–10% of circulating WBCs	Phagocytosis; migrate to tissues to become macrophages	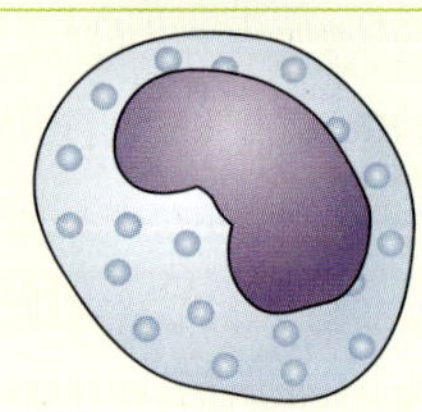
Macrophages	Lungs, liver, brain, bone, connective tissue, other tissues	Phagocytosis; kill intracellular parasites; tumoricidal activity; antigen presentation to T cells	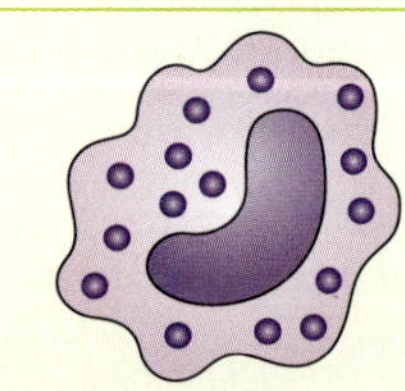
Dendritic cells	Skin, mucous membranes, heart, lungs, liver, kidney, other tissues	Most potent type of phagocytic cell; cell most effective at antigen presentation	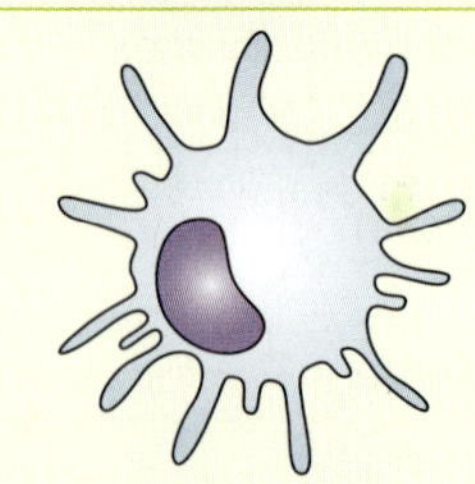
Lymphocytes	20%–40% of circulating WBCs; also found in lymph nodes, spleen, other secondary lymphoid organs	Key cells in adaptive immune responses; major types: T cells, B cells, and NK cells	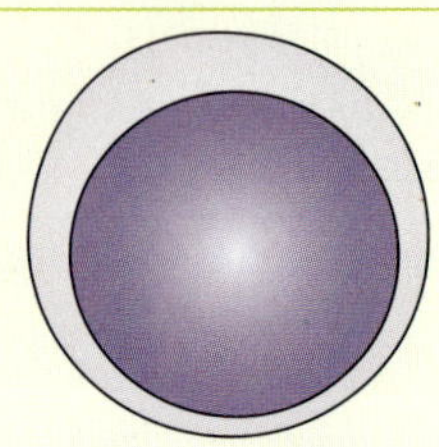

Study Guide: Cells of the Immune System—cont'd

CELL TYPE	WHERE FOUND	FUNCTION
B lymphocytes	Develop in bone marrow and migrate to secondary lymphoid organs; found in peripheral blood and follicles in lymph nodes and spleen	Key role in humoral immune response; possess antibody receptors that bind to specific antigen; mature into plasma cells 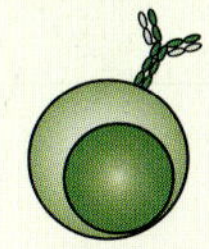
Plasma cells	Bone marrow; germinal centers in secondary lymphoid organs	Secrete antibodies into blood and other body fluids 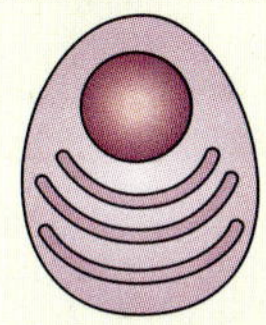
T lymphocytes	Mature in thymus; also found in peripheral blood and secondary lymphoid organs; located in paracortex in lymph nodes and PALS in spleen	Key role in cell-mediated immunity; different subtypes produce cytokines that help or suppress adaptive and innate immune responses 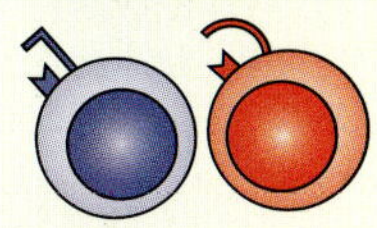
NK cells	Develop in bone marrow; found in peripheral blood, liver, and spleen	Kill target cells such as tumors or virus-infected host cells in an antigen-nonspecific manner 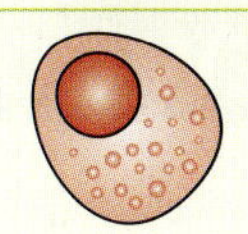

Study Guide: Comparison of T Cells, B Cells, and NK Cells

T CELLS	B CELLS	NK CELLS
Develop in the thymus	Develop in the bone marrow	Develop in the bone marrow
Found in thymus, lymph nodes, spleen, thoracic duct fluid; 60%–80% of circulating lymphocytes in blood	Found in bone marrow, lymph nodes, spleen; 10%–20% of circulating lymphocytes in blood	Found in spleen, liver; 10%–15% of circulating lymphocytes in blood
Adaptive immunity: end products of activation are cytokines	Adaptive immunity: end product of activation is antibody	Bridge innate and adaptive immunity: lysis of virally infected cells and tumor cells
Antigens include CD2, CD3, CD4, and CD8	Antigens include CD19, CD20, CD21, CD22, surface antibody	Antigens include CD16, CD56

Study Guide: Primary and Secondary Lymphoid Organs

LYMPHOID ORGAN CATEGORY	ORGANS INVOLVED	FUNCTION
Primary		Organs in which B- and T-cell maturation takes place
	Bone marrow	Produces HSCs; maturation of B cells and NK cells
	Thymus	Maturation of T cells
Secondary		Sites where contact between T cells, B cells, and antigens occurs
	Spleen	Filters antigens from the blood
	Lymph nodes	Filter antigens in the lymphatic fluid
	MALT SALT	Protects mucosal surfaces Prevents antigens from penetrating the skin

CASE STUDIES

1. After an ear piercing at a jewelry store in a mall, a 13-year-old forgot to clean the area around the earrings with alcohol for the first 2 days, despite instructions to do so. On the third day, the teenager noticed redness, swelling, and pus in the area around one earlobe.

Questions

a. Are the teenager's symptoms most likely caused by innate immunity or adaptive immunity?
b. What types of cells would you expect to see in the affected earlobe tissue?

2. You and your friends are discussing the relative merits of immunizations. Your friends say that they do not want to get a tetanus booster shot because they have a good immune system and their natural defenses will take care of any possible infection. You have just been studying this subject in your immunology class.

Questions

a. What argument could you make to convince them that a tetanus booster is a good idea?
b. What would you tell them about the types of cells involved in the response to a vaccine?

REVIEW QUESTIONS

1. Which scientist is considered to be the Father of Immunology based on his work with attenuated vaccines?
   a. Edward Jenner
   b. Élie Metchnikoff
   c. Louis Pasteur
   d. Almroth Wright

2. Which WBCs differentiate into macrophages in the tissues?
   a. Neutrophils
   b. Eosinophils
   c. Basophils
   d. Monocytes

3. Innate defenses include all of the following *except:*
   a. Phagocytosis of bacteria by neutrophils
   b. Lymphocyte responses to antigen
   c. Production of acute phase reactants
   d. The skin as a barrier to pathogens

4. Where does hematopoiesis take place?
   a. Bone marrow
   b. Spleen
   c. Thymus
   d. Lymph nodes

5. How do NK cells differ from T cells?
   a. NK cells are better at phagocytosis than T cells.
   b. NK cells require the thymus for development, and T cells do not.
   c. NK cells are found in lymph nodes; T cells are not.
   d. NK cells are not antigen specific.

6. A foreign substance that induces an immune response is called a(an):
   a. Antigen
   b. Antibody
   c. Cytokine
   d. Cluster of differentiation

7. The ability of an individual to resist infection using normally present body functions is called:
   a. Innate immunity
   b. Humoral immunity
   c. Adaptive immunity
   d. Cross-immunity

8. A cell characterized by a nucleus with two to five lobes, a diameter of 10 to 15 μm, and a large number of neutral-staining granules is identified as a(n):
   a. Eosinophil
   b. Monocyte
   c. Basophil
   d. Neutrophil

9. Which of the following is a primary lymphoid organ?
   a. Lymph node
   b. Spleen
   c. Thymus
   d. MALT

10. Which of the following would be found in a primary follicle?
    a. Unstimulated B cells
    b. Germinal centers
    c. Plasma cells
    d. Memory cells

11. What is a distinguishing feature of B cells?
    a. Act as helper cells
    b. Are identified by presence of surface antibody
    c. Are able to nonspecifically recognize target cells
    d. Are active in phagocytosis

12. Where do lymphocytes mainly come in contact with antigens?
   a. Secondary lymphoid organs
   b. Bloodstream
   c. Bone marrow
   d. Thymus

13. Which marker is found on the surface of helper T cells?
   a. CD19
   b. CD4
   c. CD8
   d. CD56

14. Which statement best characterizes adaptive immunity?
   a. Relies on normally present body functions
   b. Responds similarly to each exposure
   c. Has specificity for each individual pathogen
   d. Involves only cellular immunity

15. An important function of T cells in the immune response is to:
   a. Produce antibodies
   b. Produce cytokines that regulate both innate and adaptive immunity
   c. Participate actively in phagocytosis
   d. Respond to target cells in an antigen-nonspecific manner

16. Which of the following is the central component of humoral immunity?
   a. T cells
   b. Antibodies
   c. Lymph
   d. Neutrophils

17. Immunity can be defined as:
   a. The study of medicines used to treat diseases
   b. A specific population at risk for a disease
   c. The condition of being resistant to disease
   d. The study of the noncellular portion of the blood

18. A blood cell that has reddish-staining granules and is able to kill large parasites describes:
   a. Basophils
   b. Monocytes
   c. Neutrophils
   d. Eosinophils

19. Which statement best describes a lymph node?
   a. It is a primary lymphoid organ.
   b. It removes old RBCs.
   c. It collects fluid from the tissues.
   d. It is where B cells mature.

20. Antigenic groups identified by different sets of antibodies reacting in a similar manner to particular standard cell lines best describes:
   a. Cytokines
   b. Clusters of differentiation
   c. Neutrophilic granules
   d. Opsonins

21. Which of the following cells are *incorrectly* matched with their function?
   a. Plasma cells—antibody production
   b. Macrophages—phagocytosis
   c. Neutrophils—antigen presentation to T cells
   d. NK cells—destruction of tumor cells

22. Which of the following cells are *correctly* matched with their location in the lymphoid organs?
   a. B lymphocytes—cortex of the thymus
   b. B lymphocytes—paracortex of the lymph nodes
   c. T lymphocytes—follicles in the lymph nodes
   d. T lymphocytes—PALS in the spleen

Chapter 1 Answer Key

Answers to Knowledge Checks

1.1 c 1.2 b 1.3 d 1.4 a 1.5 c

Answers to Review Questions

1. c	2. d	3. b	4. a	5. d	6. a	7. a
8. d	9. c	10. a	11. b	12. a	13. b	14. c
15. b	16. b	17. c	18. d	19. c	20. b	21. c
22. d						

2 Innate Immunity

Linda E. Miller, PhD, I, MB^CM^(ASCP)SI

LEARNING OUTCOMES

After finishing this chapter, you should be able to:

2.1 Define the principal characteristics and components of innate defenses.

2.2 Discuss the major functions of innate immunity.

2.3 Discuss the roles of the skin and other anatomical barriers in defense against pathogens.

2.4 Recognize examples of pattern recognition receptors (PRRs) and describe their relationship with pathogen-associated molecular patterns (PAMPs) or damage-associated molecular patterns (DAMPs).

2.5 Explain how interactions between toll-like receptors (TLRs) and PAMPs activate innate immune responses.

2.6 Describe the steps involved in the inflammatory response and their clinical effects.

2.7 Describe the process of phagocytosis and killing of pathogens, indicate the types of white blood cells capable of this function, and explain the effect of opsonins on the process.

2.8 Discuss positive and negative outcomes of the inflammatory response.

2.9 Describe the mechanisms used by type I interferons and natural killer cells to destroy virus-infected host cells.

2.10 Discuss ways in which innate immune responses can stimulate adaptive immunity.

2.11 Explain the basic principle of the erythrocyte sedimentation rate (ESR).

2.12 Define "acute phase reactant" and explain the general purpose of measuring this type of protein in the laboratory.

2.13 Specify the roles of the following acute phase reactants in innate immunity and determine the clinical significance of abnormal levels of each: C-reactive protein, procalcitonin, serum amyloid A, complement, $alpha_1$-antitrypsin, haptoglobin, ferritin, fibrinogen, ceruloplasmin.

CHAPTER OUTLINE

You can go to **fadavis.com** keyword stevens for the laboratory exercises that accompany this text.

As we discussed in Chapter 1, humans are protected by two systems of immunity—innate and adaptive. **Innate immunity** consists of the defenses that are always present, ready for immediate action when a host is attacked by a pathogen. Thus, innate immunity is the first line of defense against infectious microbes, and these defenses are so efficient that many pathogens are destroyed before they encounter cells of the adaptive immune response.

Characteristics and Functions of Innate Defenses

Unlike adaptive immune responses, innate defenses are not antigen specific, and they do not exhibit immunologic memory. The innate defenses consist of (1) anatomical barriers that keep microorganisms from entering the body, (2) cells with receptors that recognize pathogens, and (3) soluble factors that play important roles in the immune response. Anatomical barriers are the first line of defense, and if microbes are able to penetrate these barriers, then cells of the innate immune system are triggered within minutes to clear the invaders as quickly as possible. Pathogens are recognized by specialized receptors on these cells, activating intracellular signals that result in inflammation or an anti-viral response. During these processes, humoral factors are produced, and phagocytic cells are attracted to the injured tissues, attacking the microbes and orchestrating the healing process. If healing begins and inflammation is resolved quickly, the tissues are less likely to be damaged.

In summary, the innate defenses have several important functions:

- Blocking the entry of microbes into the body
- Providing initial responses such as inflammation, phagocytosis, and anti-viral defenses to attack pathogens that have invaded the body, in order to control or eliminate the infection
- Removing damaged cells from the body and initiating tissue repair
- Alerting the adaptive immune system to respond to an infection

In this chapter, we discuss the components of the innate immune system and their important functions in more detail.

Specialized Barriers to Infection

The skin and the mucosal membranes that line the respiratory, gastrointestinal, and genitourinary tracts are important physical and chemical barriers to infection **(Fig. 2–1).** These surfaces block entry of pathogens that encounter the host by physical contact, inhalation, ingestion, or sexual activity. They are able to function as structural barriers because they are lined with tightly adherent epithelial cells that prevent microbes from invading the body.

For example, the outer layer of the skin, the *epidermis,* contains several sublayers of tightly packed epithelial cells. The outermost sublayer is composed of dead cells that are coated with a protein called *keratin,* making the skin impermeable to most infectious agents. Exposed to the outside environment, these cells are shed periodically and replaced by cells in the deeper sublayers of the epidermis to keep the skin intact. If injury disrupts the skin's integrity, the individual is predisposed to infection. The importance of the skin becomes evident when one considers how vulnerable victims of severe burns are to life-threatening infections. Likewise, a break in the mucous membranes lining the gastrointestinal tract can cause leakage of bacteria into the abdominal cavity, causing a serious inflammatory condition called peritonitis.

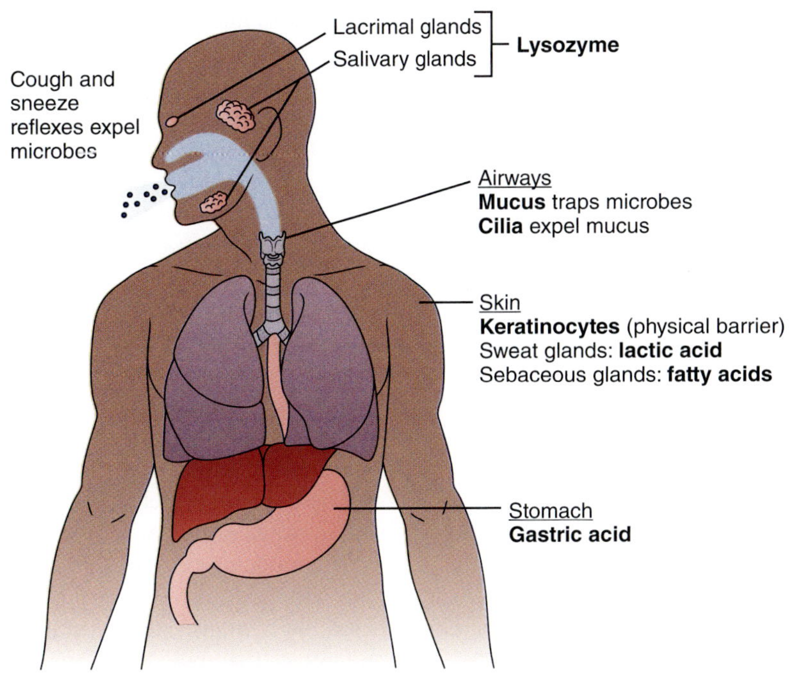

FIGURE 2–1 Specialized barriers of the innate immune system.

The skin and mucosal membranes also function as chemical barriers to infection because the epithelial cells that line these surfaces and some types of leukocytes produce substances that have anti-microbial activity. Two major classes of anti-microbial peptides (AMPs) produced by these cells are the **defensins** and the **cathelicidins.** These families of small peptides have broad-spectrum anti-microbial activity and can kill bacteria and viruses by a variety of mechanisms involving direct toxicity to the microbes or activation of an inflammatory response. Another type of AMP, the *histatins,* are found in saliva and have potent antifungal activity.

Additionally, each organ system in the body has its own unique defense mechanisms. For example, the skin has a thicker layer just underneath the epidermis called the *dermis*, which is composed of connective tissue with blood vessels, hair follicles, sebaceous glands, sweat glands, and white blood cells (WBCs), including macrophages, dendritic cells, Langerhans cells, and mast cells. Not only does the skin serve as a major structural barrier, but the presence of several secretions originating from the dermis discourages the growth of microorganisms on the skin. Lactic acid in sweat, for instance, and fatty acids from sebaceous glands (sebum) maintain the skin at a pH of approximately 5.6. This acidic pH keeps most microorganisms from growing. Sebum is also thought to prevent entry of microbes into the deeper layers of the skin by acting as a seal for the hair follicles.

In the respiratory tract, mucous secretions block the adherence of bacteria to epithelial cells. These secretions contain small proteins called *surfactants* that are produced by the epithelial cells and bind to microorganisms to promote the clearance of pathogens. The motion of the cilia that line the nasopharyngeal passages clears away most of the deposited material by moving it up toward the pharynx, where it is coughed up or swallowed. Sneezing also helps to move pathogens out of the respiratory tract.

The flushing action of urine, plus its slight acidity, helps to remove many potential pathogens from the genitourinary tract. Lactic acid production in the female genital tract keeps the vagina at a pH of about 5, another means of preventing colonization by pathogens. In the digestive tract, the stomach's hydrochloric acid keeps the pH as low as 1. Many microorganisms are ingested with food and drink, and the low pH serves to halt microbial growth. Lysozyme—an enzyme found in many bodily secretions, including tears and saliva—attacks the cell walls of microorganisms, especially gram-positive microorganisms.

In addition, the presence of microbiota, commonly known as "normal flora," in many locations of the human body helps to keep pathogens from establishing themselves in these areas. **Microbiota** consist of a mixture of large, diverse communities of microorganisms that are normally found at specific body sites and do not typically cause disease. These microbes help to inhibit the growth of pathogens in many ways, including competing for growth space and nutrients, producing certain metabolites, and stimulating maturation of the immune system. The significance of microbiota is readily demonstrated by looking at the side effects of anti-microbial therapy. For example, women who take an antibiotic for a urinary tract infection (UTI) frequently develop a yeast infection because of the presence of *Candida albicans.* In this case, anti-microbial therapy depletes not only the pathogenic bacteria that caused the UTI but also the microbiota. Knowledge about interactions between resident microbes of the digestive tract (the gut microbiome) and the innate immune system has inspired research on therapies for a variety of conditions, including inflammatory bowel disease, obesity, *Clostridioides difficile* infection, and arthritis.

Knowledge Check 2-1

Which of the following is not an example of innate immunity?

a. The skin acting as a barrier to pathogenic bacteria
b. Inflammation induced by an infection
c. Production of defensins by leukocytes
d. Specific antibodies neutralizing activity of a virus

Recognition of Microbes and Damaged Cells

If microorganisms penetrate the anatomical barriers in the body, additional mechanisms of the innate immune system are activated to destroy foreign invaders and eliminate damaged tissues. These second lines of defense, discussed in detail in later sections of this chapter, involve phagocytosis and destruction of pathogens that enter the body, induction of the inflammatory response, and production of certain soluble mediators. The first step in these processes is identification of foreign invaders and differentiation of pathogens from self. In the sections that follow, we discuss key receptors involved in the recognition of microbial components by cells of the innate immune system.

Pattern Recognition Receptors

The innate defense system is designed to recognize structures that are commonly found in infectious organisms and distinct from the host. Macrophages and dendritic cells are the most important cells involved in pathogen recognition. They are able to distinguish pathogens from normally present molecules in the body by means of receptors known as **pattern recognition receptors (PRRs),** which are also found on neutrophils, eosinophils, monocytes, mast cells, and epithelial cells. These receptors act as sensors for cellular infection. Once PRRs bind to a pathogen, phagocytic cells become activated and are better able to engulf and eliminate microorganisms. Activated cells then secrete pro-inflammatory cytokines and chemokines, chemical messengers that make capillaries more permeable and recruit additional phagocytic cells to the area of infection. Cytokines and chemokines also stimulate the adaptive immune responses.

PRRs are able to differentiate invading pathogens from healthy host cells by recognizing substances known as **pathogen-associated molecular patterns (PAMPs),** which are found only in microorganisms. Some examples of PAMPs include peptidoglycan in gram-positive bacteria, lipopolysaccharide in gram-negative bacteria, zymosan in yeast, and flagellin in bacteria with flagellae. PRRs can also identify substances such as heat-shock proteins, altered membrane phospholipids, and DNA that are released by stressed, injured, or transformed cells; such substances are called **damage-associated molecular patterns (DAMPs).** There are several different types of PRRs. Some are found on the plasma membranes of host cells, where they recognize extracellular pathogens, while others are on the intracellular membranes of the endoplasmic reticulum, endosomes, and lysosomes, enabling them to identify bacteria and viruses located inside of host cells. In the next sections of this chapter, we discuss different families of PRRs that are involved in the innate defenses.

Toll-Like Receptors

The most thoroughly studied family of PRRs are the **toll-like receptors (TLRs).** TLRs were so named because they resembled the toll protein originally discovered in the fruit fly *Drosophila,* where it plays important roles in embryonic development and innate responses against fungal and bacterial infections. There are 10 different TLRs in humans, and they are found in highest concentration on monocytes, macrophages, and dendritic cells. TLR1, TLR2, TLR4, TLR5, and TLR6 are found on surfaces of these cells, whereas TLR3, TLR7, TLR8, TLR9, and TLR10 are found in the endosomal compartments. Each of these receptors recognizes a different microbial product. **Table 2–1** lists the human TLRs along with major examples of PAMPs and types of microorganisms they recognize.

TLRs are membrane-spanning glycoproteins that share a common structural element called *leucine-rich repeats* (LRRs). The LRRs form a horseshoe-shaped domain that is involved in binding to the PAMP. This region is connected to a membrane-spanning domain, which, in turn, is connected to an interior domain called TIR (toll/interleukin [IL]-1 receptor) **(Fig. 2–2).** The TIR domain provides molecular signals to the inside of the cell, which ultimately lead to the production of proteins that are essential to innate immune responses.

After binding to their corresponding PAMP or DAMP ligand, TLRs are induced to form dimers (two molecules linked together), either with a TLR of the same type (homodimers; e.g., TLR-4 with TLR-4) or with a different TLR (heterodimers; e.g., TLR-2 with TLR-1). Dimerization brings the cytoplasmic tails of the TLRs close together, facilitating the binding of adaptor proteins, which recruit and activate protein kinases. These enzymes activate different transcription factors that lead to the expression of host genes that code for proteins important to innate immune responses.

Thus, once TLRs bind to their corresponding PAMP or DAMP, complex cell signaling pathways are activated. The specific pathways that follow depend on the type of TLR and adaptor protein involved. General concepts of TLR pathways are illustrated in **Figure 2–3.** The ultimate result of these pathways is the production of numerous cytokines, chemokines, and other molecules involved in the inflammatory response or the production of type I interferons (IFNs), which are involved in anti-viral immunity.

Table 2-1 The 10 Human Toll-Like Receptors

RECEPTOR	PAMPS RECOGNIZED	TARGET MICROORGANISMS
TLR Receptors Found on Cell Surfaces		
TLR1	Lipopeptides	Mycobacteria, gram-negative bacteria
TLR2	Peptidoglycan, lipoteichoic acid, lipoproteins, zymosan, mannan	Gram-positive bacteria, mycobacteria, yeast, and other fungi
TLR4	Lipopolysaccharide, fusion proteins, mannan	Gram-negative bacteria, respiratory syncytial virus, fungi
TLR5	Flagellin	Bacteria with flagellae
TLR6	Lipopeptides, lipoteichoic acid, zymosan	Mycobacteria, gram-positive bacteria, yeast, and other fungi
TLR Receptors Found in Endosomal Compartments		
TLR3	Double-stranded RNA	RNA viruses
TLR7	Single-stranded RNA	RNA viruses
TLR8	Single-stranded RNA	RNA viruses
TLR9	Unmethylated microbial DNA	DNA viruses, bacteria
TLR10	Unknown	Unknown

PAMPs = pathogen-associated molecular patterns; TLR = toll-like receptor.

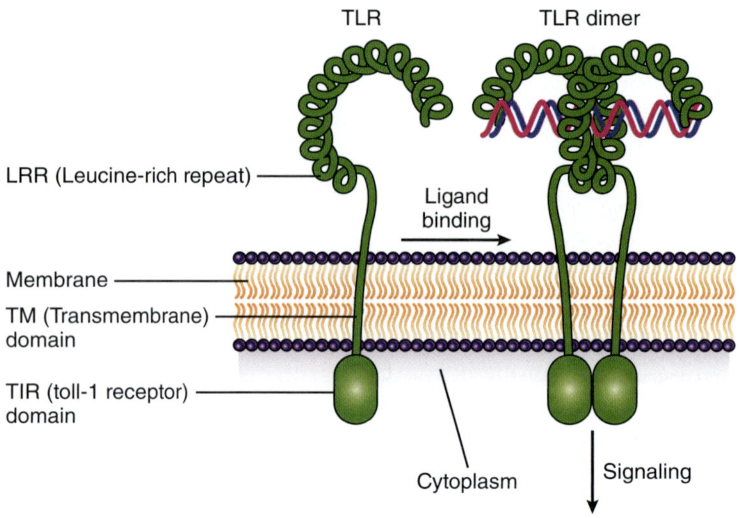

FIGURE 2–2 General structure of a TLR. TLRs possess a leucine-rich PAMP-binding domain, a transmembrane component, and an intracellular TIR domain, which is involved in cell signaling. Binding of TLRs to their corresponding ligand induces them to form dimers.

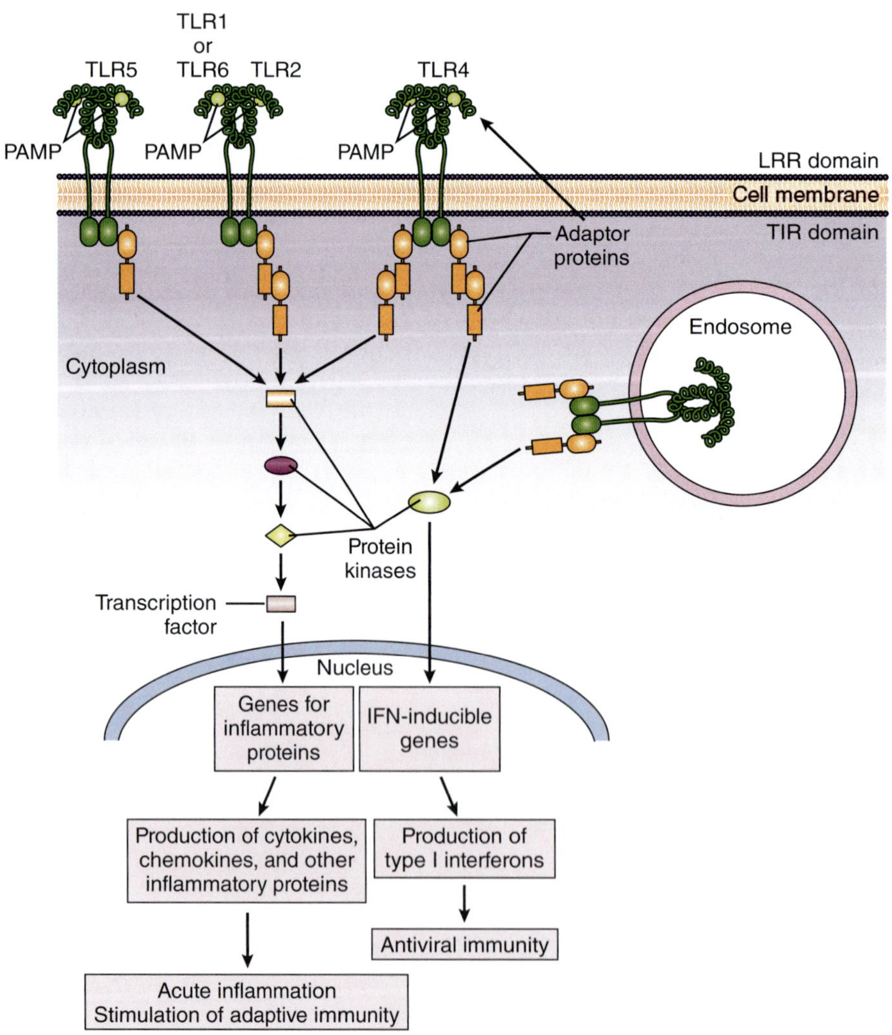

FIGURE 2–3 General concept of TLR cell signaling pathways. Binding of TLRs to their corresponding PAMP or DAMP results in recruitment of adaptor proteins and activation of transcription factors that turn on genes coding for the production of inflammatory proteins and type I interferon gamma.

Other Pattern Recognition Receptors

In addition to TLRs, several other families of receptors activate innate immune responses. Although the cell signaling pathways activated by these other PRRs differ from those of the TLRs, the end result is the same—the production of inflammatory cytokines and type I IFNs. Type I IFNs are cytokines that inhibit viral replication and induce *apoptosis* (a process of cell death that minimizes tissue injury) in infected cells (see Chapter 6).

Two families of cell surface PRRs are the *C-type lectin receptors (CLRs)* and the *scavenger receptors.* CLRs are membrane-bound receptors found mainly on macrophages, dendritic cells, and neutrophils. These receptors bind to carbohydrates such as mannan and beta-glucans found in fungal cell walls (see Chapter 22). Scavenger receptors are a diverse group of cell surface proteins that can bind to a range of PAMPs and DAMPs, including lipoteichoic acid from gram-positive bacteria, lipopolysaccharide from gram-negative bacteria, and beta-glucan from fungal cell walls. Some scavenger receptors, such as CD36 and SR-A, found on macrophages, help to mediate phagocytosis of pathogens.

Three other families of receptors recognize pathogens found in the cytosol: *retinoic acid–inducible gene-I-like receptors (RLRs), nucleotide-binding oligomerization domain (NOD)-like receptors (NLRs),* and *cytosolic DNA sensors (CDSs).* The RLR family recognizes viral RNA in the cytoplasm of infected cells. NLRs provide immune surveillance in the cytoplasm, where they bind ligands from microbial pathogens, such as peptidoglycan, flagellin, viral RNA, and fungal hyphae. CDSs detect double-stranded DNA from viruses and bacteria in the cytosol of infected cells and trigger cell signaling that results in type I IFN production. NLRs and a type of CDS called AIM-2 can also assemble with other proteins to form large complexes called **inflammasomes,** which enzymatically cleave precursors of the pro-inflammatory cytokines, IL-1β and IL-18, to generate their active forms and induce death of host cells infected with intracellular pathogens by a lytic process called *pyroptosis.*

Although PRRs are essential for protection against pathogens, inappropriate PRR responses have been found to contribute to acute and chronic inflammation and systemic autoimmune diseases. For example, mutations in NLRs may result in Crohn disease, a painful inflammatory disease of the bowel. Additionally, in systemic lupus erythematosus, there is a high concentration of antibodies to self–nucleic acids, which activate dendritic cells through TLR9. Therefore, a tight regulatory network of PRR signaling is critical to ensure the elimination of invading pathogens while avoiding harmful immune reactions that can cause pathology.

2-1 Clinical Correlations

Adjuvants

Contact of PRRs with the appropriate ligand not only stimulates innate immunity but can also lead to enhancement of adaptive immune responses. Therefore, some of these ligands are being used in vaccines as *adjuvants.* Adjuvants are substances that are administered together with a vaccine antigen to boost immunity to a potential pathogen (see Chapter 25 for details).

Knowledge Check 2-2

The function of TLRs is to:

a. Recognize pathogenic bacteria and viruses
b. Specifically attack RNA viruses
c. Destroy tumor cells
d. Participate in the formation of inflammasomes

Inflammation

As we discussed in the previous sections, an important consequence of the interaction between PRRs and their corresponding PAMPs or DAMPs is initiation of the inflammatory response. **Inflammation** is a biological process by which vascularized tissue responds to injury or invasion by an infectious agent. The goals of this innate immune response are to destroy invading pathogens, remove damaged cells, and repair injured tissues. Inflammation is a complex, highly orchestrated series of events that involves WBCs, blood vessels, and plasma proteins. Each component of the reaction plays an important role in initiating, amplifying, or sustaining inflammation, and a delicate balance must be maintained for the process to be quickly and efficiently resolved.

The five cardinal signs of inflammation were originally described in the first and second centuries by the physicians Celsus and Galen. They are (1) redness or erythema *(rubor),* (2) swelling or edema *(tumor),* (3) heat *(calor),* (4) pain *(dolor),* and (5) loss of function *(functio lasea).* The first four characteristics occur rapidly after tissue injury and are caused by a coordinated cascade of events, which are summarized in **Figure 2–4** and described in more detail in the paragraphs that follow. Loss of function may result if inflammation persists and causes significant tissue damage.

The inflammatory response can be triggered by pathogenic microbes as well as a variety of nonmicrobial inducers, including substances that trigger allergic reactions, toxic or irritating chemical compounds, ionizing radiation, frostbite, burns, and physical injury. As we discussed in the previous sections, when pathogens breach the anatomical barriers or when other injurious agents cause tissue damage, PAMPs and DAMPs are detected by cells of the innate immune system through binding to sensing receptors, or PRRs. As a result, macrophages, dendritic cells, and mast cells residing in the tissues produce a variety of soluble inflammatory mediators, including cytokines, chemokines, and vasoactive amines, and additional leukocytes are recruited to the site of the injury.

Activated mast cells quickly degranulate and release chemical mediators such as histamine, leukotrienes, and prostaglandins, which cause dilation and increased permeability of the blood vessels. Vasodilation results in increased blood flow to the affected area, producing redness and heat. Increased capillary permeability, caused by contraction of the endothelial cells lining the vessels, creates gaps that allow fluids in the plasma to leak into the tissues, resulting in swelling and pain. These changes to the blood vessels promote increased delivery of WBCs and key plasma proteins to the site of inflammation.

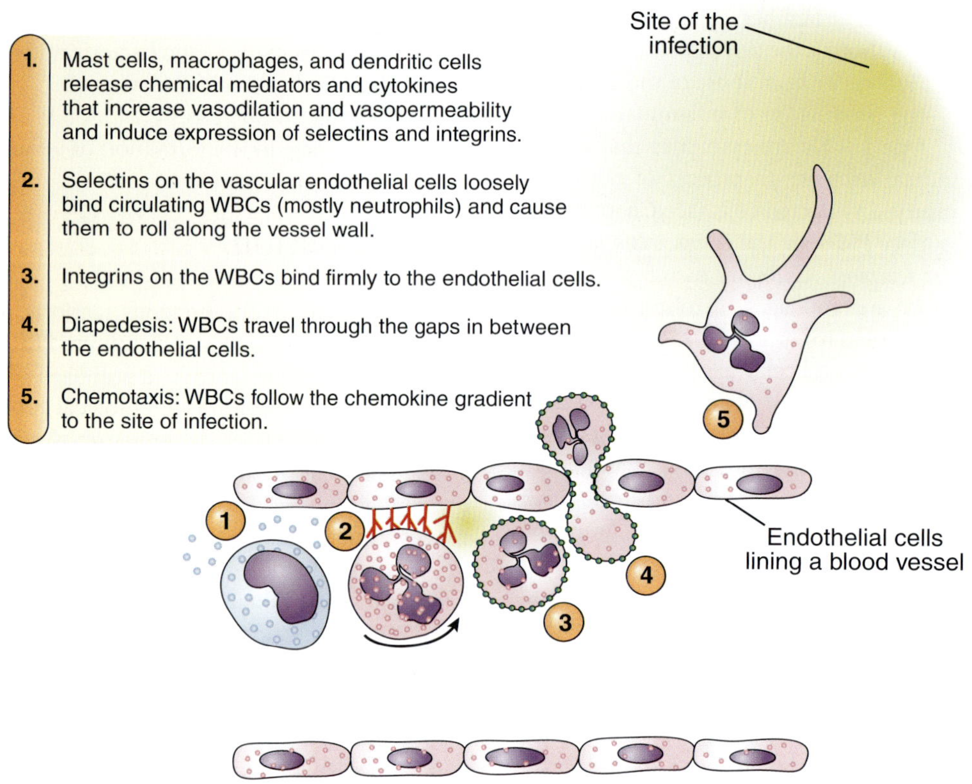

FIGURE 2–4 Major steps of the local inflammatory response.

In addition, tissue-residing mast cells, dendritic cells, and macrophages, and the endothelial cells lining the vessels produce several cytokines that have many effects on the response. Tumor necrosis factor alpha (TNF-α), IL-1, and IL-6 are among the most important pro-inflammatory cytokines. TNF-α and IL-1 induce the expression of adhesion molecules called **selectins** on the surface of the vascular endothelial cells and other adhesion molecules called **integrins** on the surface of WBCs in the blood. Physical contact occurs as the WBCs bind loosely to the selectins, causing the neutrophils to roll along the vascular wall in a random pattern. Integrins then strengthen the binding of the leukocytes by causing them to spread along the vessel wall.

These changes are followed by migration of WBCs through the gaps between the endothelial cells lining the capillaries out to the surrounding tissues in a process called **diapedesis.** The WBCs are then attracted to the site of injury as they follow concentration gradients of certain substances, including chemokines produced by tissue macrophages, the complement protein C5a, and bacterial peptides. This process, called **chemotaxis,** causes the WBCs to migrate out of the vessels and into the tissues.

The first WBCs to migrate to the site of injury are the neutrophils, because they are the most abundant type of WBC and respond rapidly to the chemotactic signals (Fig. 2–4). Neutrophils are mobilized within 30 to 60 minutes after the injury, and their emigration may last 24 to 48 hours. Several hours later, monocytes begin to migrate out of the vessels and into the tissues, where they develop into macrophages. Additional macrophages and dendritic cells from surrounding tissues are also recruited to the injured area. A major function of the neutrophils, macrophages, and dendritic cells is to engulf pathogens and damaged host cells by phagocytosis and destroy the ingested material. In the section that follows, we describe the processes of phagocytosis and pathogen destruction.

The acute inflammatory response acts to eliminate an infection or other injurious agent and typically lasts for a few days. If the immune system fails to remove a pathogen quickly or tissue injury persists, adaptive immunity is triggered, and chronic inflammation can develop. Lymphocytes are recruited to the site of injury and mount a potent immune response against the inciting pathogen. In most cases, the healing process is completed with a return to normal tissue structure. However, if inflammation persists, it can lead to further tissue damage and loss of function. The tissue damage resulting from chronic inflammation is the basis for the pathogenesis of many autoimmune diseases, in which the body mounts an immune response against self-antigens (see Chapter 15).

Phagocytosis and Pathogen Destruction

Phagocytosis can be defined as the process by which certain WBCs engulf and destroy microbes, dead or aging cells, or other large particles (greater than 0.5 μm in diameter). As we discussed in Chapter 1, the cells that are most active in phagocytosis are the neutrophils, macrophages, and immature dendritic cells.

Phagocytosis can be performed by macrophages or dendritic cells that reside in the tissues or by phagocytic cells (mostly neutrophils) that are attracted to the site of inflammation.

The process of phagocytosis is energy dependent and consists of several steps, which are illustrated in **Figure 2–5.** Phagocytosis begins with physical contact between the WBC and the particle or cell to be engulfed. Contact can occur when PRRs on the plasma membrane of the phagocytic cell membrane bind to their corresponding PAMPs or DAMPs. In addition to receptors for pathogens, phagocytic cells have high-affinity receptors for certain immunoglobulins, complement components, and C-reactive protein (CRP), which serve as opsonins (see Chapters 3 and 7). **Opsonins** are serum proteins that attach to a foreign cell or pathogen and make the process of phagocytosis much more efficient by initiating contact and ingestion.

After attachment to a foreign cell or pathogen has occurred, the cell membrane of the phagocytic cell invaginates, and pseudopodia (outflowing of cytoplasm) surround the pathogen. The pseudopodia fuse to completely enclose the pathogen, forming a structure known as a **phagosome.** The phagosome is moved toward the center of the cell. Lysosomal granules quickly migrate to the phagosome, and fusion between granules and the phagosome occurs. At this point, the fused elements are known as a **phagolysosome.** The granules contain AMPs such as the defensins and the cathelicidins, and proteolytic enzymes, including lysozyme, myeloperoxidase, and elastase (see Chapter 1). The anti-microbial activity of these agents is enhanced by the low pH of the phagolysosome. The contents of the granules are released into the phagolysosome, and digestion of the pathogen occurs. Undigested material is excreted from the cells by exocytosis. Heavily opsonized particles are taken up in as little as 20 seconds, and killing is almost immediate.

The elimination of pathogens also occurs by oxygen-dependent mechanisms that generate **reactive oxygen species (ROS)** and **reactive nitrogen species (RNS),** which are highly toxic to phagocytized microbes. ROS are unstable, highly reactive molecules that contain oxygen. They are generated in activated phagocytic cells by an oxygen-dependent process known as the **oxidative burst (Fig. 2–6).** This process occurs within the phagocytic cell as it increases its oxygen consumption, and pseudopodia enclose the engulfed particle in a vacuole. The mechanism generates considerable energy through oxidative metabolism. The hexose monophosphate shunt is used to convert nicotinamide adenine dinucleotide phosphate (NADP) to its reduced form (NADPH) by adding a hydrogen atom. Electrons pass from NADPH to oxygen in the presence of NADPH oxidase, a membrane-bound enzyme complex that is only formed in activated phagocytes, and the radical, superoxide anion (O_2^-) is then made. Superoxide anion is highly toxic to microbes and can be rapidly converted to even more lethal products. By adding hydrogen ions, the enzyme superoxide dismutase (SD) converts O_2^- to hydrogen peroxide (H_2O_2), which can then react with iron to produce hydroxyl radicals (•OH). The anti-microbial effect of H_2O_2 is further enhanced when it combines with chloride ions to form hypochlorite (OCl–) in the presence of the enzyme myeloperoxidase. Hypochlorite is the main component of household bleach used to disinfect surfaces. The ROS generated by these pathways are all powerful oxidizing agents that are highly toxic for microorganisms.

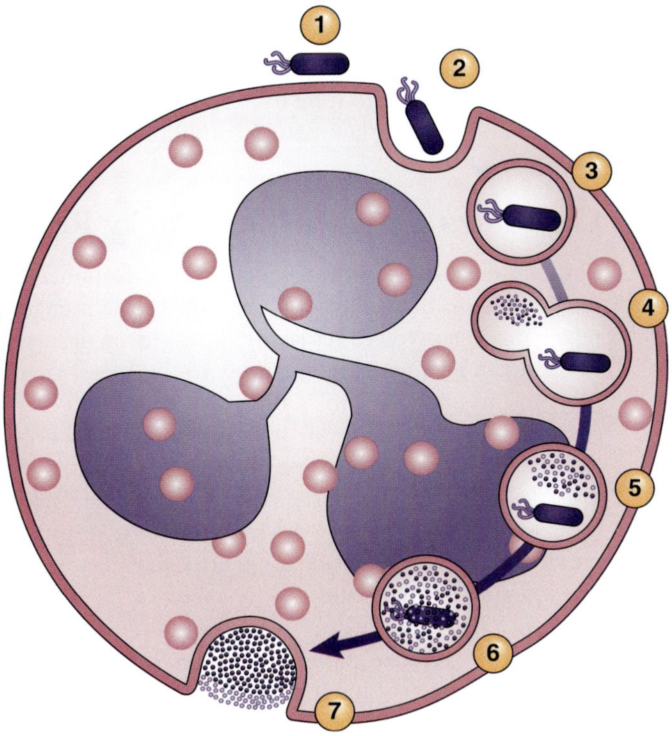

1. Adherence: physical contact between the phagocytic cell and the microorganism occurs, aided by opsonins.
2. Engulfment: outflowing of cytoplasm to surround the microorganism.
3. Formation of phagosome: microorganism is completely surrounded by a part of the cell membrane.
4. Granule contact: lysosomal granules contact and fuse with the phagosome.
5. Formation of the phagolysosome: contents of the lysosome are emptied into this membrane-bound space.
6. Digestion of the microorganism by hydrolytic enzymes.
7. Excretion: contents of phagolysosome are expelled to the outside by exocytosis.

FIGURE 2–5 Steps involved in phagocytosis.

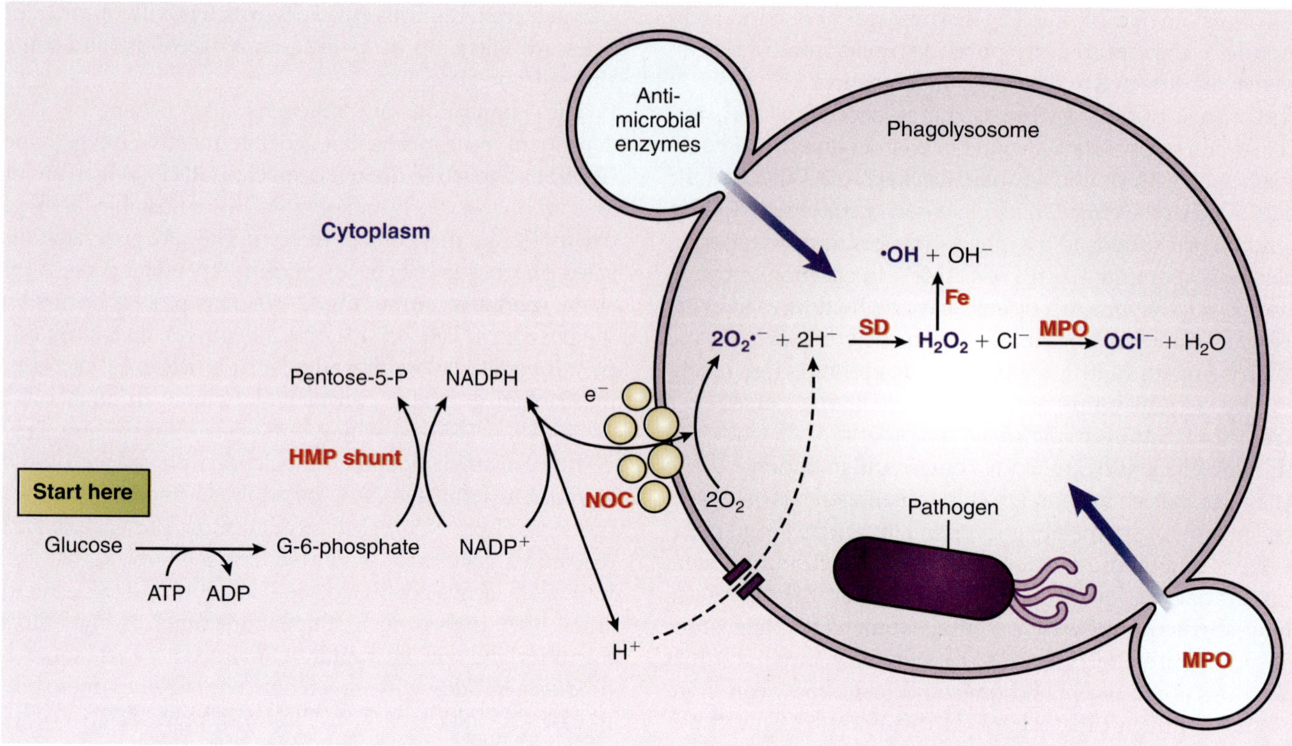

FIGURE 2–6 Creation of ROS in the activated phagocytic cell. HMP = hexose monophosphate; NADP = nicotinamide adenine dinucleotide phosphate; O_2-= superoxide anion; NOC = NADPH oxidase complex; SD = superoxide dismutase; H_2O_2 = hydrogen peroxide; MPO = myeloperoxidase; OCl- = hypochlorite; •OH = hydroxyl radicals (•OH).

2-2 Clinical Correlations

Chronic Granulomatous Disease

The importance of NADPH oxidase in the elimination of microbes is demonstrated by the fact that a lack of it may lead to an increased susceptibility to infection. Patients with chronic granulomatous disease have a genetic mutation that causes a defect in NADPH oxidase, resulting in an inability to kill bacteria during the process of phagocytosis. Patients with this disease experience recurring, severe bacterial infections (see Chapter 19).

RNS are a group of anti-microbial molecules that include nitric oxide (NO) and its derivatives. RNS are produced mainly in macrophages that have been activated as a result of phagocytosis. NO is generated when the enzyme, inducible nitric acid synthase (iNOS) acts on the amino acid, L-arginine to produce L-citrulline. NO can further react with O_2^- to produce additional RNS, which can destroy pathogens through a variety of mechanisms.

Other mechanisms of microbial killing also exist. For example, when inflammasomes are activated, macrophages can undergo pyroptosis (a type of regulated cell death mentioned earlier), which prevents any ingested microbes from replicating intracellularly. Another important mechanism involves extracellular killing of pathogens by neutrophils. Following activation through contact of PRRs with their corresponding microbial ligand, neutrophils can produce structures called **neutrophil extracellular traps (NETs)**. NETs are composed of strands of DNA bound to histone proteins, to which high concentrations of anti-microbial substances from the neutrophil granules are attached. NETs are extruded from the activated neutrophils into the extracellular environment, where they trap and kill bacteria, fungi, and parasitic cells. Neutrophils die in the process, and damage to the surrounding tissues can occur, contributing to the pathology of autoimmune diseases and other inflammatory conditions.

Outcomes of the Inflammatory Response

The tissues affected by the inflammatory response must be repaired once the source of the injury is eliminated. The repair process involves replacing damaged or dead cells and restoring an adequate blood supply to the area. Macrophages play several important roles in this process. They ingest and eliminate cell remnants, debris, and foreign material. They also produce various cytokines that stimulate proliferation of fibroblasts and residual tissue cells, promote angiogenesis (the formation of new blood vessels), and direct formation and remodeling of the extracellular matrix that restores strength and integrity to the tissue.

Ideally, the inflammatory response should act quickly and efficiently to remove pathogens and other harmful agents, because prolonged or intense inflammation can harm the host. Therefore, several mechanisms exist to regulate the response, including the production of cytokines that inhibit activation of macrophages and dendritic cells, and proteins that block cell signals generated by PRRs and inflammatory cytokines. However, if the injurious agent is unable to be eliminated and persists in the body, these regulatory mechanisms can be overcome, resulting in chronic or excessive inflammation. Such responses can lead to a variety of conditions that can be detrimental, or in some cases, even deadly, to the host, including overgrowth of scar tissue and loss of normal tissue function, hypersensitivity, autoimmune diseases, septic shock associated with certain systemic infections, and "cytokine storm," a dangerous condition resulting from overproduction of proinflammatory cytokines (see Chapters 6, 14, and 15).

Knowledge Check 2-3

What is the correct order of steps in inflammation?

a. Attachment of WBCs to vessel walls, migration of neutrophils to injured tissue, release of proteolytic enzymes and ROS, release of vasoactive amines by mast cells, tissue repair
b. Attachment of WBCs to vessel walls, release of vasoactive amines by mast cells, migration of neutrophils to injured tissue, release of proteolytic enzymes and ROS, tissue repair
c. Release of vasoactive amines by mast cells, attachment of WBCs to vessel walls, migration of neutrophils to injured tissue, release of proteolytic enzymes and ROS, tissue repair
d. Release of vasoactive amines by mast cells, migration of neutrophils to injured tissue, release of proteolytic enzymes and ROS, attachment of WBCs to vessel walls, tissue repair

Critical Thinking 2-1

Suppose a child was born with a genetic defect that affected the function of his neutrophilic granules. How do you expect that this would affect the child's innate immune response to bacteria?

Anti-Viral Defenses

As we mentioned previously, another function of the innate immune system is to provide early protection against viral infections. The two major mechanisms by which this occurs are through the actions of type I IFNs and natural killer cells.

Type I Interferons

IFN-α and IFN-β, or the type I IFNs, are produced by many types of virus-infected cells as a result of signaling pathways stimulated by contact of certain TLRs or other PRRs with viral nucleic acids. These cytokines bind to receptors on the infected cells and nearby uninfected cells and induce other signaling pathways that lead to the production of enzymes that interfere with different steps of the virus replication cycle. As a result, synthesis of viral proteins is inhibited, viral RNA is degraded, and assembly of intact viruses is prevented. Type I IFNs also enhance the activity of natural killer cells.

Natural Killer Cells

Another way in which the innate immune system protects against viral infections is through the action of natural killer (NK) cells. These cells localize in tissues where inflammation is occurring and where dendritic cells are found. Although phagocytosis is important in eliminating extracellular infectious agents, NK cells represent the first line of defense against virally infected cells, tumor cells, and cells infected with other intracellular pathogens. NK cells constantly monitor the body for potential target cells and are able to eliminate such target cells quickly, because, unlike lymphocytes, they do not need to differentiate further before becoming functional.

Destruction of abnormal target cells by NK cells requires direct cell-cell contact followed by release of cytotoxic proteins from the NK cell. Target cell destruction occurs outside of the NK cell and does not involve phagocytosis or complement fixation. Unlike T and B lymphocytes, NK cells are not antigen specific. However, NK cells have two types of receptors on their surface that allow them to recognize their targets: inhibitory receptors, which deliver signals that block NK cell activity, and activating receptors, which deliver signals to activate cytotoxic mechanisms that destroy the target cells. The balance between activating and inhibitory signals enables NK cells to distinguish healthy cells in the body from infected or cancerous ones.

The inhibitory signal is based on recognition of class I major histocompatibility complex (MHC) proteins, which are expressed on all healthy nucleated cells (see Chapter 4 for details). If inhibitory receptors on the surface of NK cells bind to class I MHC proteins on another cell in the body, the natural killing process is blocked because that cell is more likely to be normal **(Fig. 2–7A)**. Examples of inhibitory receptors include killer cell immunoglobulin-like receptors (KIRs) and CD94/NKG2A receptors.

Diseased and cancerous cells may lose their ability to produce MHC proteins. In the absence of class I MHC antigens, NK cell activity is allowed to occur; this is sometimes referred to as recognition of "missing self." The lack of inhibition is combined with an activating signal that is switched on through the binding of activating receptors on the NK cells to various proteins produced by cells under stress, namely, those cells that are cancerous or infected with a pathogen. Examples of activating receptors that bind stress proteins are CD16, NKG2D, and other KIRs.

Thus, depending on the signals, the NK cell either proceeds to activate cell destruction or detaches and moves on to search for another target cell. To attack their targets, activated NK cells release cytotoxic proteins called *perforins* and *granzymes* from their cytoplasmic granules into the extracellular space between the NK cell and the target cell **(Fig. 2–7B)**. Perforins are proteins that form channels (pores) in the target cell membrane. Granzymes are packets of enzymes that enter through the channels and induce cell death by activating the process of apoptosis. The elimination of target cells can occur in as little as 30 to 60 minutes. The cytotoxic activity of NK cells

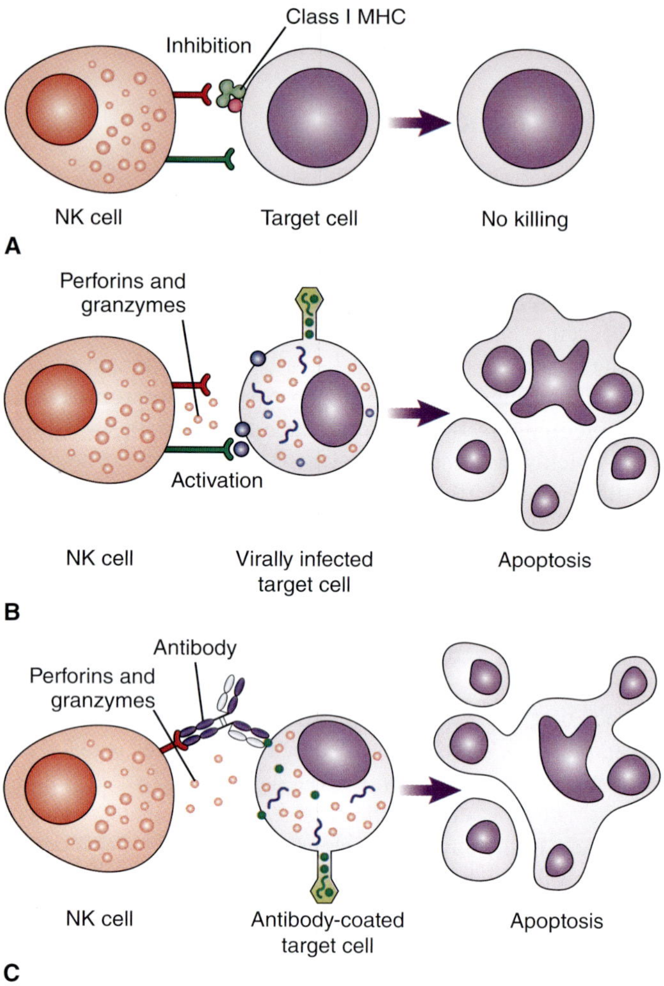

FIGURE 2–7 NK cell recognition and lysis of abnormal target cells. NK cells are constantly surveying cells in the body. **(A)** If class I MHC protein is present and there are no foreign or stress proteins, then an inhibitory signal is sent to the NK cell, no killing occurs, and the normal cell is released. **(B)** If an activating receptor is engaged by a foreign or stress protein and class I MHC is altered or missing ("missing self"), then no inhibitory signal is given, granzymes and perforins are released, and the infected or diseased cell is eliminated by apoptosis. **(C)** Alternatively, infected cells may express foreign proteins on their surface that are recognized by antibody. NK cells express CD16 receptors that bind the immobilized antibody and activate the release of perforins and granzymes. This process is called *antibody-dependent cellular cytotoxicity.*

is enhanced by exposure to cytokines such as IL-12, IFN-α, and IFN-β, which rise rapidly during a viral infection.

The ability of NK cells to recognize target cells is increased when the target cells have previously bound antibody, which has been produced during an adaptive immune response. NK cells recognize and lyse antibody-coated target cells through a process called **antibody-dependent cellular cytotoxicity (ADCC)** (see **Fig. 2–7C** and Chapter 3). Contact of the NK cell with antibody occurs through the surface receptors, CD16 (FcγIII) and CD32 (FcγRIIC), which bind to the Fc portion of human immunoglobulins. After binding, the NK cell is stimulated to release perforins and granzymes from its granules, and destruction of the target cell occurs, as we described previously. ADCC is not unique to NK cells, as monocytes, macrophages, and neutrophils also have such receptors and act in a similar manner.

NK cells are able to respond early during an infection, and their activity peaks in about 3 days, well before antibody production or an initial cytotoxic T-cell response. By quickly engaging infected target cells, NK cells give the immune system time to activate the adaptive responses of specific T and B cells. NK cells are also thought to play a key role in immunosurveillance by continually patrolling the body for cancerous cells and eliminating them before they become clinically apparent (see Chapter 17). We can appreciate the overall importance of NK cells as a defense mechanism by considering the fact that patients who lack these cells have recurring, serious viral infections, and an increased incidence of cancer.

Knowledge Check 2-4

Important innate mechanisms against viral pathogens are:

a. Antibodies and T cells
b. T cells and interferon gamma
c. NK cells and type I interferons
d. ADCC and B cells

Stimulation of Adaptive Immune Responses

While innate defenses provide the first line of protection mounted by the immune system, they are not always successful in preventing infections because microbes may sometimes be able to penetrate the anatomical barriers, and many pathogens have developed mechanisms to escape innate immunity (see Chapters 20, 22, and 23). Activation of potent, antigen-specific adaptive immune responses is therefore often necessary to eliminate an infection. Certain cells and molecules of innate immune responses play important roles in initiating adaptive immunity. In this section, we present some key examples of the many ways in which this can occur.

Phagocytosis is a crucial link between innate and adaptive immunity. Following phagocytosis of microbes, macrophages and dendritic cells begin to mature into antigen-presenting cells (APCs) and migrate to nearby lymph nodes or other peripheral lymphoid organs. There, the APCs process peptides from the pathogens and present them to antigen-specific T cells they encounter (see Chapter 4). This step is needed because T cells are unable to respond to intact pathogens. The activated T lymphocytes then interact with B cells to produce antibodies and with other T cells to mount cell-mediated immune responses (see Chapter 5).

NK cells provide another link between innate immunity and adaptive immune responses. Once activated, NK cells become major producers of cytokines such as interferon gamma (IFN-γ) and TNF-α. IFN-γ enhances antigen presentation to T cells by increasing macrophage activation and expression of MHC class I and class II molecules. TNF-α increases the inflammatory response and stimulates other cells to produce chemokines that help recruit leukocytes to the area. NK cells also release the granulocyte-macrophage colony-stimulating factor, GM-CSF, which promotes the development of granulocytes and macrophages from stem cells in the bone marrow. Innate lymphoid cells (ILCs) residing in the epithelial barrier tissues are also on the alert for signals of tissue injury. ILCs are not antigen specific but have receptors for cytokines released early in the inflammatory response, such as IL-12. Upon exposure to these cytokines, ILCs are thought to respond by rapidly releasing other cytokines, including IFN-γ, IL-4, and GM-CSF. These are the same cytokines that are produced later by activated T cells during the adaptive immune response.

Many of the soluble proteins generated during innate immune responses play important roles in adaptive immunity. For example, cytokines such as IL-1 and IL-25 activate signaling pathways that stimulate naïve T lymphocytes to differentiate into various helper T-cell subsets or regulatory T cells, as we describe in Chapter 6. IL-4 stimulates the proliferation of B cells and their differentiation into antibody-secreting plasma cells. Proteins of the complement system that are generated during innate responses can interact with the antibodies produced to help eliminate pathogens (see Chapters 3 and 7). As we describe in the sections that follow, acute phase reactants have many activities that affect adaptive immune responses and other body systems that work together to eliminate an injurious agent and promote healing.

Laboratory Detection of Inflammation and Acute Phase Reactants

A systemic inflammatory response is often accompanied by many changes in the body, including development of fever and alterations in leukocyte blood counts, hormone production, metabolism, and hepatic activity. Such changes may be associated with infections, trauma, autoimmune diseases, some hematologic malignancies, or other causes of systemic inflammation. While these changes are not disease specific in most cases, many of these parameters can be measured by the laboratory to detect presence of acute inflammation, monitor patient response to treatment, or predict recovery from an illness.

Among the oldest markers of inflammation is the erythrocyte sedimentation rate (ESR). This test is based on the formation of rouleaux (stacks or aggregations of red blood cells [RBCs]) caused by increased production of positively charged plasma proteins during inflammation. These proteins hinder the negatively charged RBCs from repelling each other. The resulting aggregates settle more quickly in a tube than individual RBCs, thus increasing the ESR value. While the ESR remains helpful in the diagnosis of selected conditions, several factors can influence test results, and measurement of actual plasma proteins associated with inflammation is generally more accurate.

The most commonly measured humoral markers of inflammation are the acute phase reactants. **Acute phase reactants** are normal plasma proteins that rapidly increase or decrease in concentration by at least 25% during an inflammatory response. Those that increase are termed *positive acute phase reactants*, whereas those that decrease, such as albumin and transferrin, are known as *negative acute phase reactants*. In this chapter, we discuss positive acute phase reactants. These proteins are produced mainly by hepatocytes (liver parenchymal cells) within 12 to 24 hours in response to an increase in cytokines. Many of the proteins have functions that help the body defend against injurious agents and perform tissue repair, for example, by binding to microorganisms and promoting adherence to phagocytic cells or limiting tissue destruction caused by the release of proteolytic enzymes from neutrophils. Other functions of the acute phase reactants include participation in the coagulation system, iron metabolism, and transport of other proteins, lipids, or elements in the body.

The positive acute phase reactants that are most commonly measured in clinical practice are C-reactive protein (CRP) and procalcitonin (PCT). Other acute phase reactants that may be quantified by the laboratory include serum amyloid A (SAA), complement components, α_1-antitrypsin (AAT), haptoglobin, ferritin, fibrinogen, and ceruloplasmin. **Table 2–2** summarizes characteristics of these acute phase reactants, and they are described in more detail in the sections that follow. A variety of automated methods are routinely used to measure these proteins, including nephelometry, immunoturbidimetry, chemiluminescent immunoassay, and ELISA (see Chapters 10 and 11). These assays detect complexes of an acute phase protein with antibody reagents and are highly sensitive. Results are available within minutes. More recently, laboratories have begun to measure some of the cytokines involved in inflammation, such as IL-1, IL-6, and TNF-α. Laboratory assays for cytokines are discussed in Chapter 6.

C-Reactive Protein

CRP is an acute phase protein that is made in the liver and normally circulates in the blood in low concentrations. It is a member of the family of proteins known as the *pentraxins,* which are each composed of five identical subunits. The subunits of CRP are arranged together to form a ring-shaped structure that has a molecular weight of approximately 120,000 Da. The name CRP was derived after the discovery of Tillet and Francis in 1930 that serum from patients with *Streptococcus pneumoniae* infection formed a precipitate upon reaction with C-polysaccharide from the capsule of the *Streptococcus* bacteria.

CRP is produced during the innate immune response, and binding to its substrate is nonspecific and calcium dependent. The main ligand of CRP is phosphocholine, a common constituent of bacterial membranes. CRP can also bind to small ribonuclear proteins; phospholipids; peptidoglycan; and other constituents of bacteria, fungi, and parasites. After binding to such a substance, CRP can participate in processes important in the early defense against microbes. Notably, CRP is capable of *opsonization,* a process in which the protein promotes phagocytosis by binding to specific receptors on monocytes, macrophages, and neutrophils (see Chapter 3). In addition, CRP-ligand complexes can activate the classical pathway of

Table 2-2 Characteristics of Acute Phase Reactants

PROTEIN	RESPONSE TIME (HOURS)	NORMAL CONCENTRATION	INCREASE	FUNCTION
C-reactive protein	6–8	3–10 mg/L	100–1,000×	Opsonization, complement activation
Procalcitonin	4	<0.05 ng/mL	100–1,000×	Reduces calcium concentration in plasma
Serum amyloid A	24	20–50 mcg/mL	1,000×	Activates monocytes and macrophages; transports cholesterol
Alpha$_1$-antitrypsin	24	100–400 mg/dL	2–5×	Protease inhibitor
Ferritin	*	30–300 ng/mL (males) 10–200 ng/mL (females)		Storage of intracellular iron
Fibrinogen	24	200–400 mg/dL	2–3×	Clot formation
Haptoglobin	24	30–200 mg/dL	2–10×	Binds hemoglobin
Ceruloplasmin	48–72	20–40 mg/dL	1.5×	Binds copper and oxidizes iron
Complement C3	48–72	60–140 mg/dL	2×	Opsonization, lysis

**Elevation is seen in iron overload, liver diseases, and chronic inflammatory conditions.*

complement to destroy bacteria (see Chapter 7). Also, the binding of CRP to phospholipids and small ribonuclear proteins released from damaged cells is thought to help the body eliminate these cells by apoptosis.

CRP is a relatively stable serum protein, with a half-life of about 18 hours. CRP levels increase in response to cytokines such as IL-1, IL-6, and TNF-α produced during the innate immune response. The increase is rapid, within 6 to 8 hours following infection, surgery, or other trauma to the body. Levels increase dramatically, as much as a hundredfold to a thousandfold, reaching a peak value within 48 hours. CRP also declines rapidly with cessation of the stimuli. Elevations in CRP concentrations are associated with active systemic inflammation caused by various conditions, including severe bacterial infections, sepsis, myocardial infarction, rheumatoid arthritis and other autoimmune disorders, cancer progression, extensive burns, and surgery. Smaller elevations in CRP may be seen in viral infections, coronary artery disease, pregnancy, diabetes, and other conditions.

CRP is more sensitive than ESR, and because its levels rise and then decline so rapidly, CRP is the most widely used indicator of acute inflammation. In the laboratory, assays for CRP can be used to quickly identify or monitor a variety of conditions in which there is systemic inflammation. For example, a significant elevation in CRP is an early indicator of complications after surgery, such as an infected incision, thrombosis, or pneumonia. Studies evaluating the use of CRP as a prognostic marker have found that very high levels of CRP correlate with the likelihood of patients with severe acute respiratory syndrome coronavirus 2 (SARS-CoV-2) infection to progress to severe disease. Monitoring CRP levels can be useful clinically to follow a disease process and observe patient response to treatment of inflammatory conditions and/or infection. For example, serial measurements of CRP can be used to observe patients for progression or remission of certain autoimmune diseases and their response to anti-inflammatory therapies. Along with clinical examination and microbiology testing, monitoring CRP levels can also be helpful in determining the effectiveness of antibiotic therapy when treating patients with severe infections. CRP levels can also be used to follow the course of malignancy and organ transplantation because a rise in the level may mean a return of the malignancy or, in the case of transplantation, the beginning of organ rejection.

2-3 Clinical Correlations

CRP and Rheumatoid Arthritis

Rheumatoid arthritis (RA) is an autoimmune disease characterized by inflammation of the joints. CRP is often used to monitor patients with RA because the CRP concentration reflects the intensity of the inflammatory response. CRP levels decrease when therapy is successful in reducing inflammation.

CRP has also received attention as a risk marker for cardiovascular disease, the leading cause of mortality. CRP has been found in atherosclerotic lesions, and it may contribute to the pathogenesis of atherosclerosis (coronary artery disease) in several ways, including complement activation, recruitment and stimulation of monocytes, vascular cell activation, and promotion of thrombosis (clot formation). In accord with the finding that atherosclerosis may be the result of a chronic inflammatory process, an increased level of CRP has been shown to be a significant risk factor for myocardial infarction, ischemic stroke, and peripheral vascular disease in men and women who are at an intermediate risk for cardiovascular disease.

Experts consider a serum CRP concentration of lower than 1 mg/L to be associated with a low risk for cardiovascular disease, 1 to 3 mg/L to be associated with an average risk, and greater than 3 mg/L to be associated with a high risk. While measurement of CRP is not recommended as a general screen for cardiovascular disease, it may be used in conjunction with other laboratory parameters, such as cholesterol and triglyceride levels, to assess risk of cardiovascular disease in certain populations. Knowing the potential risk of developing a heart attack, stroke, or other manifestation of vascular disease may alert doctors to monitor or treat high-risk patients more aggressively and to motivate such patients to change lifestyle factors such as diet, exercise, and smoking.

Reference ranges for CRP have not been standardized, but normal levels in adults usually range from less than 3 mg/L to less than 10 mg/L, depending on the assay used and the laboratory conducting the assay. Most healthy adults have a CRP level less than 3 mg/L. The median CRP value for an individual increases with age, reflecting an increase in subclinical inflammatory conditions. CRP testing as a risk factor for cardiovascular disease requires high-sensitivity CRP assays (hs-CRP) that have the necessary lower level of detection of 0.01 mg/L, which enables measurement of much smaller increases in the protein.

Procalcitonin

Procalcitonin (PCT) is a peptide of 116 amino acids and a molecular weight of 14.5 kDa. It is the precursor of the hormone, calcitonin, which is made exclusively by C-cells in the thyroid gland and functions to lower calcium levels in the blood to maintain homeostasis.

In healthy individuals, the serum concentration of PCT is low (less than 0.05 mg/L) because PCT is rapidly converted into calcitonin. However, during a systemic bacterial infection, cytokines such as TNF-α, IL-1, and IL-6 stimulate PCT synthesis in tissues other than the thyroid gland such as the liver, pancreas, kidneys, lungs, and intestines. Because these tissues lack the enzymes needed to process PCT into calcitonin, PCT levels in the serum can increase a hundredfold to a thousandfold. PCT becomes detectable by 4 hours after infection, peaks at 6 to 12 hours, and declines to 50% by 24 hours after successful treatment and resolution of the infection. The PCT serum concentration can also rise in response to other conditions, including major surgery, severe trauma, severe burns, and prolonged cardiac shock.

Because PCT synthesis is usually suppressed during a viral infection, PCT levels can be used in context with clinical findings to help clinicians differentiate between bacterial and viral infections and guide antibiotic therapy in conditions such as bacterial sepsis, meningitis, and community-acquired pneumonia. PCT test results can help physicians decide to begin antibiotic treatment if the source of the infection is likely to be bacterial. PCT levels can then be monitored to help determine when antibiotic treatment can be safely discontinued. Guided therapy can improve patient outcomes, while reducing side effects and emergence of antibiotic resistance.

In the laboratory, PCT is measured by automated, sensitive immunoassays. Results can be available within 20 to 30 minutes, leading to earlier initiation of antibiotic therapy in appropriate cases and improvement of clinical outcomes.

Serum Amyloid A

Serum amyloid A (SAA) is a family of apolipoproteins synthesized by the liver. Two of the four SAA isoforms, SAA1 and SAA2, are acute phase reactants and are collectively known as A-SAA. A-SAA has a high affinity for high-density lipoprotein (HDL) and transports cholesterol from the plasma to the site of infection, where it is used in tissue repair. A-SAA has also been found to have cytokine-like functions such as chemotaxis and activation of macrophages. It can also promote clearance of pathogens through opsonization and stimulate cells of the immune system to make products that regulate inflammation.

The normal circulating concentration of A-SAA is low (20 to 50 mcg/mL) but can increase more than a thousandfold in response to infection or injury. Levels reach a peak between 24 and 48 hours after an acute infection and decline rapidly as inflammation resolves. A-SAA increases significantly more in bacterial infections than in viral infections. A-SAA can also be increased as a result of other inflammatory conditions, including RA, cardiovascular disease, acute pancreatitis, cancer, and SARS-CoV-2 infection. Chronic inflammation with persistently high levels of A-SAA can lead to amyloidosis, a condition in which the proteins form fibrils that deposit in the tissues, causing impaired function of several organs, including the kidneys, spleen, and liver. A-SAA has also become a well-established inflammatory marker in veterinary medicine.

Complement

Complement refers to a series of serum proteins that participate in immune defenses against pathogens but can also contribute to pathological inflammatory responses. Nine complement proteins are activated by antibodies bound to antigen in a sequence known as the *classical pathway*. Additional complement proteins are involved in the alternative and lectin pathways that are triggered by the presence of microorganisms during the innate immune responses. Several of the complement proteins are upregulated during the acute phase response. The major functions of complement are cell lysis, opsonization, anaphylatoxin activity, and chemotaxis of WBCs. Complement is discussed in detail in Chapter 7.

Alpha$_1$-Antitrypsin

Alpha$_1$-antitrypsin (AAT) is a 52-kDa protein that is primarily synthesized in the liver. It is the major component of the alpha band when serum is electrophoresed. The main function of AAT is to inhibit the activity of the enzyme elastase, which is released by neutrophils during inflammation and degrades elastin, a connective protein in the lungs. Excess neutrophil elastase can also increase the expression of other proteolytic enzymes. Thus, AAT counteracts the effects of neutrophil invasion during an inflammatory response and protects the lungs from proteolytic damage. AAT is also an anti-inflammatory agent that regulates the expression of pro-inflammatory cytokines such as TNF-α, IL-1β, and IL-6. As a result, chemotaxis and activation of neutrophils and monocytes are inhibited, limiting the harmful side effects of inflammation.

AAT is coded for by the *SERPINA1* gene on chromosome 14. More than 100 mutations in this gene have been discovered, and, depending on the type, can result in a lack of production, degradation, or misfolding of the AAT protein. The mutations are inherited in an autosomal codominant fashion, meaning that the genes inherited from each parent are equally expressed; therefore, the severity of AAT deficiency can vary among patients. As a result of this deficiency, elastase is allowed to damage the lung tissue, especially in people who smoke or who have frequent exposure to noxious chemicals. Uninhibited proteases remain in the lower respiratory tract, leading to destruction of parenchymal cells in the lungs and to the development of chronic obstructive pulmonary disease (COPD), with shortness of breath, chronic cough, increased mucous production, and wheezing. The abnormal AAT polymers can also accumulate in the liver, causing dysfunction of that organ and possibly leading to liver cirrhosis and increased risk for hepatocellular carcinoma. Less commonly, people with AAT deficiency can develop a condition called panniculitis, in which painful subcutaneous nodules develop in the skin as a result of neutrophil infiltration.

It has been estimated that as many as 100,000 Americans suffer from AAT deficiency, although many of them are undiagnosed. Laboratory testing for the condition begins with measurement of the AAT level in the serum of symptomatic patients or their relatives using an automated immunoassay. People with AAT deficiency typically have an AAT concentration of less than 1.1 g/L (100 mg/dL). If the AAT level is low, AAT phenotyping can be performed to characterize the forms of circulating AAT present by isoelectric focusing in an agarose gel (see Chapter 11). If the results are inconclusive, genetic sequencing can be done to identify specific *SERPINA1* mutations.

Haptoglobin

Haptoglobin is an α_2-globulin with a molecular weight of 100,000 Da. It binds irreversibly to free hemoglobin released by damaged RBCs. Haptoglobin acts as an antioxidant to provide protection against oxidative damage mediated by free hemoglobin. Once bound, the complex is cleared rapidly by macrophages in the liver. In innate immunity, haptoglobin also protects against tissue damage by inhibiting prostaglandin production and promoting angiogenesis.

Haptoglobin testing is mainly performed to confirm the presence of intravascular hemolysis associated with conditions such as hemolytic anemias. In these conditions, haptoglobin concentrations decrease because the protein is complexed to hemoglobin. However, a 2- to 10-fold increase in haptoglobin can be seen following inflammation, stress, or tissue necrosis. Early in the inflammatory response, haptoglobin levels may drop because of intravascular hemolysis, consequently masking the protein's behavior as an acute phase reactant. Thus, plasma levels must be interpreted in light of other acute phase reactants. Normal plasma concentrations range from 30 to 200 mg/dL.

Ferritin

Ferritin is a 450-kDa protein whose main function is the storage of intracellular iron. It is found in the cytosol of all cells and protects the body from the toxic effects of iron caused by the formation of iron-mediated free radicals. The concentration of ferritin in the serum reflects the total iron stores in the body. Normally, serum ferritin is present in a low concentration and varies significantly with age, race, and gender; levels in adult males are commonly considered to range from 30 to 300 ng/mL, while those in adult females are between 10 to 200 ng/mL. The concentration of ferritin is decreased in iron deficiency anemia, and measurement of the protein is essential in the diagnosis of this condition. In contrast, ferritin levels can increase significantly as a result of disorders in which there is an iron overload, for example, hereditary hematochromatosis and hemolytic anemia. Ferritin levels are also increased in patients with liver diseases and a variety of conditions involving inflammation, including chronic infections, autoimmune disorders, and malignancies. As an acute phase reactant, ferritin is thought to play a protective role against invading pathogens and tumors by restricting the availability of iron to these cells.

Fibrinogen

Fibrinogen is an acute phase protein involved in blood clot formation. The molecule is a dimer with a molecular weight of 340,000 Da. In the final step of the coagulation pathway, a small portion of the protein is cleaved by thrombin to form fibrils that cross-link and form a fibrin clot. The clot functions to stop bleeding caused by injury, promotes wound healing, and stimulates endothelial cell adhesion and proliferation. Formation of a clot also creates a barrier that helps prevent the spread of microorganisms further into the body. The normal plasma concentration of fibrinogen ranges from 200 to 400 mg/dL. Levels of the protein increase two- to threefold during inflammation, making blood more viscous and promoting aggregation of RBCs and platelets. Elevated levels may contribute to an increased risk for developing coronary artery disease. Hereditary defects resulting in decreased fibrinogen levels or function are associated with an increased risk of bleeding. Fibrinogen deficiency can also be acquired as a result of acute or decompensated intravascular coagulation and fibrinolysis (DIC), advanced liver disease, or certain therapies.

Ceruloplasmin

Ceruloplasmin consists of a single polypeptide chain with a molecular weight of 132,000 Da. It is the principal copper-transporting protein in human plasma, binding more than 95% of the copper in plasma by attaching six to eight copper atoms per molecule. Additionally, ceruloplasmin acts as an enzyme, converting toxic ferrous ion (Fe^{2+}) to a nontoxic ferric form (Fe^{3+}). Thus, ceruloplasmin can limit the growth of pathogenic bacteria by reducing the amount of iron available for their metabolism.

The normal plasma concentration of ceruloplasmin for adults is 20 to 40 mg/dL. A decrease or absence of ceruloplasmin is found in Wilson disease, an autosomal recessive genetic disorder characterized by a massive increase of copper in the tissues. Normally, circulating copper is absorbed out of the circulation by the liver and either combined with ceruloplasmin and returned to the plasma or excreted into the bile duct. In Wilson disease, toxic amounts of copper accumulate in the liver and subsequently in other tissues, such as the brain, corneas, kidneys, and bones. Treatment involves long-term chelation therapy to remove the copper or a liver transplant. Decreased levels of ceruloplasmin can also be found in Menkes disease or dietary copper insufficiency.

As an acute phase reactant, plasma levels of ceruloplasmin can increase, typically by about 50%, as a result of inflammation, trauma, or infection. Caution must be used in interpreting test results, as such an elevation in the protein can mask a ceruloplasmin deficiency.

Knowledge Check 2-5

Match each acute phase reactant with its major function:

a. C-reactive protein (CRP)	____	1. Degrades neutrophil elastase
b. Procalcitonin (PCT)	____	2. Storage of intracellular iron
c. Serum amyloid A (SAA)	____	3. Clot formation
d. Haptoglobin	____	4. Lowers blood calcium levels
e. Alpha$_1$-antitrypsin (AAT)	____	5. Binds hemoglobin
f. Fibrinogen	____	6. Opsonization and complement activation
g. Ceruloplasmin	____	7. Transports cholesterol
h. Ferritin	____	8. Principal copper-transporting protein

Critical Thinking 2-2

Suppose a patient underwent surgery for gallbladder removal. Three days later, the patient developed a fever as well as redness, swelling, and pus at the incision site. The CRP level was 1,000 mg/L (normal = 3–10 mg/L). What does this result indicate in light of the patient's clinical presentation? What other key laboratory findings would you expect to see?

KEY CONCEPTS

Characteristics and Functions of Innate Defenses

- Innate immunity encompasses all the body's normally present defense mechanisms for resisting disease. It is characterized by lack of antigen specificity and does not induce immunologic memory.
- Innate defenses include cells capable of phagocytosis and acute phase reactants that enhance the process of phagocytosis. Cells that are most active in phagocytosis include neutrophils, monocytes, macrophages, and dendritic cells.
- Innate immunity is important in blocking the entry of microbes into the body, providing initial responses to pathogens such as inflammation and anti-viral defenses, removing damaged cells and initiating tissue repair, and alerting the adaptive immune system to an infection.

Specialized Barriers to Infection

- Innate defenses consist of structural barriers (the skin and mucous membranes), cells with receptors that recognize pathogens, and a variety of soluble factors.

Recognition of Microbes

- PRRs are molecules on host cells that recognize substances found only on pathogens. These receptors are found on neutrophils, macrophages/monocytes, eosinophils, mast cells, dendritic cells, and epithelial cells.
- PAMPs are molecules found only on pathogens but not on host cells, allowing the host cells to distinguish them from self. They are recognized by PRRs.
- DAMPs are substances released by stressed, injured, or transformed cells that are recognized by PRRs.
- The most well-studied family of PRRs are the TLRs. When TLRs bind to their corresponding PAMPs, complex cell signaling pathways are activated, resulting in the production of numerous cytokines, chemokines, and other molecules involved in inflammation, or in the production of type I IFNs, which are important for anti-viral immunity.

Inflammation

- Inflammation is the body's initial response to injury or invasion by a pathogen. This innate immune response is characterized by an increased blood supply to the affected area, increased capillary permeability, and migration of neutrophils to the injured area (a process called chemotaxis).
- Once they arrive at the inflammatory site, neutrophils, along with dendritic cells and macrophages from surrounding tissues, come into physical contact with the foreign invader via PRRs or other receptors and perform phagocytosis.
- During the process of phagocytosis, cytoplasm from the phagocytic cell flows around the foreign particle to form a phagosome. Fusion of the phagosome with lysosomal granules creates a phagolysosome. Inside this structure, enzymes such as lysozyme and

myeloperoxidase are released, and the foreign particle is digested.

- Activated phagocytic cells can also eliminate pathogens by oxygen-dependent mechanisms that generate ROS and RNS, which are highly toxic to microbes.
- When the inflammatory response acts quickly to eliminate a pathogen, the injured tissue can be repaired. However, persistent inflammation can harm the host by leading to pathological conditions.

Anti-Viral Defenses and Stimulation of Adaptive Immune Responses

- Two mechanisms of innate immunity against viral infections involve type I IFNs and NK cells.
- The type I IFNs, IFN-α and IFN-β, bind to receptors on virally infected host cells and nearby uninfected cells. This results in activation of cell signaling pathways that leads to production of enzymes that block viral replication.
- NK cells target abnormal host cells for destruction, such as malignant cells and cells that are infected with a virus or another intracellular pathogen.
- NK cells recognize abnormal target cells through a lack of class I MHC protein and presence of proteins produced by cells under stress. Once binding to the target cell occurs, NK cells release perforins, which create pores in the target cell membrane, and granzymes, which enter the pores and induce apoptosis.
- NK cells can also bind to and destroy antibody-coated target cells through a process called ADCC.
- The cells activated during innate immunity and the products they release stimulate more potent, antigen-specific, adaptive immune responses.

Laboratory Detection of Inflammation and Acute Phase Reactants

- The clinical laboratory can detect systemic inflammation by testing for alterations in WBC counts, elevations in the ESR, and increased concentrations of acute phase reactants.
- Acute phase reactants are mostly produced by hepatocytes in the liver in response to cytokines. They function in various ways to help the body defend against pathogens and repair injured tissues.
- Positive acute phase reactants are serum proteins that increase rapidly in response to infection or injury. They include CRP, procalcitonin, A-SAA, complement components, AAT, haptoglobin, ferritin, fibrinogen, and ceruloplasmin.
- CRP is the acute phase reactant that is most widely monitored by the laboratory; it increases 100 to 1,000 times in response to infection or trauma, acts as an opsonin, and is able to bind complement.

Study Guide: Mechanisms of Innate Immunity

TYPE OF DEFENSE	EXAMPLES	FUNCTION
Anatomical barriers	Skin and mucous membranes	Block entry of pathogens into the body Produce anti-microbial chemicals such as lysozyme Have special features that reduce growth or remove pathogens (e.g., cilia in respiratory tract, low pH of stomach acid, microbiota that compete with pathogens for nutrients)
Cells that quickly recognize and destroy pathogens	Neutrophils, macrophages, dendritic cells	Recognize PAMPs and DAMPs through binding to PRRs (e.g., TLRs) Phagocytize and destroy extracellular pathogens Activate inflammation and anti-viral defenses
Inflammation	Rapid response to infection, trauma, toxic chemicals, ionizing radiation, frostbite, burns	Steps include: (1) Release of vasoactive amines and cytokines by mast cells, macrophages, and dendritic cells following binding to PAMPs or DAMPs (2) Attachment of WBCs to blood vessel wall endothelial cells (3) Migration of neutrophils and monocytes out of blood vessels into the injured tissue, where they phagocytize and destroy pathogens and damaged host cells through release of proteolytic enzymes, ROS, and RNS (4) Repair of injured tissues
Anti-viral defenses	Type I interferons NK cells	Trigger virus-infected and nearby host cells to produce enzymes that interfere with viral replication Bind to virus-infected host cells and tumor cells and destroy such abnormal targets by extracellular release of perforins and granzymes
Cytokines and chemokines	TNF-α, IL-1, IL-6	Many functions, including enhancing inflammation, recruiting WBCs to injured tissues, activating adaptive immune responses
Acute phase reactants	CRP, procalcitonin, A-SAA, AAT, ferritin, fibrinogen, haptoglobin, ceruloplasmin, complement protein C3	Destroy pathogens through opsonization or complement activation; limit tissue damage from neutrophil enzymes; participate in coagulation, iron metabolism, and transport of various substances

CASE STUDIES

1. A 30-year-old adult underwent a splenectomy because of an injury to the spleen that caused uncontrollable bleeding. One year later, the patient presented to the emergency room with severe pain in the upper abdomen and a fever of 102.2°F (normal = 98.6°F). The patient's abdomen was swollen, and a CT (computed tomography) scan showed fluid accumulation in the large intestine. Laboratory results were as follows: WBC count, $20.50 \times 10^3/\mu L$ (normal = $4–10 \times 10^3/\mu L$); ESR = 40 mm/hr (normal = 0–15 mm/hr); CRP = 108 mg/L (normal = 3–10 mg/L); procalcitonin = 4.5 ng/mL (normal = less than 0.05 ng/mL). Suspecting sepsis, the patient's doctors administered a broad-spectrum antibiotic intravenously. Blood cultures were ordered and came back the next day as positive for *Streptococcus pneumoniae*. Antibiotic treatment was continued for 5 days, and the patient recovered.

Questions

a. What is causing the patient's abdominal edema?
b. What does the increased WBC count indicate, and which type of WBC would be expected to be the most elevated?
c. Why was it beneficial for the laboratory to measure CRP and procalcitonin?

2. A 45-year-old adult went to a physician for an annual checkup. Although the patient was slightly overweight, laboratory results indicated that the total cholesterol and HDL cholesterol were within normal limits. The fibrinogen level was 450 mg/dL, and the CRP level was 35 mg/L. The physical examination was normal. The physician cautioned the patient that the laboratory results might indicate a higher risk for a future heart attack and counseled the patient to be sure to exercise and eat a healthy, low-fat diet. The patient's spouse said that as long as the cholesterol level was normal, the patient did not have to be concerned.

Question

a. Is the patient's spouse correct? Explain your answer.

REVIEW QUESTIONS

1. Phagocytosis can be enhanced by the coating of foreign particles with serum proteins called:
   a. Antigens
   b. Agglutinins
   c. Opsonins
   d. Chemotaxis

2. Which of the following plays an important role as an innate defense mechanism?
   a. Phagocytosis
   b. Antibody
   c. T lymphocytes
   d. Antigen-specific recognition

3. The process of inflammation is characterized by all of the following *except:*
   a. Increased blood supply to the area
   b. Migration of WBCs
   c. Decreased capillary permeability
   d. Increased acute phase reactants

4. Skin, lactic acid secretions, stomach acidity, and the motion of cilia represent which type of immunity?
   a. Innate
   b. Cross
   c. Adaptive
   d. Auto

5. The structure formed by the fusion of engulfed material and enzymatic granules within the phagocytic cell is called a:
   a. Phagosome
   b. Lysosome
   c. Vacuole
   d. Phagolysosome

6. The presence of human microbiota (normal flora) acts as a defense mechanism by which of the following methods?
   a. Maintaining an acid environment
   b. Competing with potential pathogens
   c. Keeping phagocytes in the area
   d. Coating mucosal surfaces

7. Measurement of CRP levels can be used for all of the following *except:*
   a. Monitoring drug therapy with anti-inflammatory agents
   b. Tracking the progress of an organ transplant
   c. Diagnosing a specific bacterial infection
   d. Determining active phases of rheumatoid arthritis

8. Pattern recognition receptors act by:
   a. Recognizing molecules common to both host cells and pathogens
   b. Recognizing molecules that are unique to pathogens

c. Helping to spread infection because they are found on pathogens
d. All recognizing the same pathogens

9. Which of the following are characteristics of acute phase reactants?
   a. Rapid increase following infection
   b. Enhancement of phagocytosis
   c. Nonspecific indicators of inflammation
   d. All of the above

10. Which is the most potent agent formed in the phagolysosome for the elimination of microorganisms?
   a. Proteolytic enzymes
   b. Hydrogen ions
   c. Hypochlorite ions
   d. Superoxide

11. Which acute phase reactant helps to prevent the formation of peroxides and free radicals that may damage tissues?
   a. Haptoglobin
   b. Fibrinogen
   c. Ceruloplasmin
   d. Serum amyloid A

12. Which statement best describes TLRs?
   a. They protect adult flies from infection.
   b. They are found on all host cells.
   c. They only play a role in adaptive immunity.
   d. They enhance phagocytosis.

13. CRP is considered part of the innate immune system because it:
   a. Is a negative acute phase reactant
   b. Is not specific for a particular antigen
   c. Binds complement
   d. Acts as an opsonin

14. How does innate immunity differ from adaptive immunity?
   a. Innate immunity requires prior exposure to a pathogen.
   b. Innate immunity depends on normally present body functions.
   c. Innate immunity develops later than adaptive immunity.
   d. Innate immunity is more specific than adaptive immunity.

15. A 40-year-old individual who is a smoker develops symptoms of premature emphysema. The symptoms may be caused by a deficiency of which of the following acute phase reactants?
   a. Haptoglobin
   b. Alpha$_1$-antitrypsin
   c. Fibrinogen
   d. Ceruloplasmin

16. Which statement best describes NK cells?
   a. Their response against pathogens is specific.
   b. They only react when an abundance of MHC antigens is present.
   c. They react when both inhibitory and activating signals are triggered.
   d. They kill virus-infected cells in an antigen-nonspecific manner.

17. **Which of the following cytokines plays a major role in anti-viral immunity?**
   a. IL-1
   b. IL-6
   c. TNF-α
   d. IFN-α

18. **Which of the following is/are clinical signs indicating inflammation in an injured tissue?**
   a. Swelling
   b. Redness
   c. Pain
   d. All of the above

19. **Which cell type is not involved in phagocytosis?**
   a. NK cell
   b. Macrophage
   c. Neutrophil
   d. Dendritic cell

20. **How does inflammation affect the concentration of positive acute phase reactants in the blood?**
   a. Concentrations will mostly be unaffected.
   b. Concentrations will increase.
   c. Concentrations will decrease.
   d. Concentrations will only change if the inflammation is chronic.

Chapter 2 Answer Key

Answers to Knowledge Checks

2.1 d **2.2** a **2.3** c **2.4** c **2.5** 1-e; 2-h; 3-f; 4-b; 5-d; 6-a; 7-c; 8-g

Answers to Review Questions

1. c	2. a	3. c	4. a	5. d	6. b	7. c
8. b	9. d	10. c	11. a	12. d	13. b	14. b
15. b	16. d	17. d	18. d	19. a	20. b	

3 Antibody Structure and Function

Linda E. Miller, PhD, I, MB^CM(ASCP)SI

LEARNING OUTCOMES

After finishing this chapter, you should be able to:

3.1 Diagram the general structure of an immunoglobulin and recognize its major components.

3.2 Identify the electrophoretic fraction of serum that contains the majority of immunoglobulins.

3.3 Differentiate between isotypes, allotypes, and idiotypes.

3.4 Differentiate between the light chains and heavy chains of an immunoglobulin molecule and indicate the Greek letters that denote each type.

3.5 Describe the fragments that result from treating an immunoglobulin molecule with papain, pepsin, or mercaptoethanol.

3.6. Describe the structures and functions of the five immunoglobulin classes found in humans.

3.7 Discuss how the immunoglobulin G (IgG) subclasses differ in functional capability.

3.8 Describe the functions of the J chain and the secretory component (SC) and indicate in which immunoglobulin classes they are found.

3.9 Discuss how immunoglobulin D (IgD) differs from other immunoglobulin types.

3.10 Identify the types of cells that immunoglobulin E (IgE) binds to in allergic reactions.

3.11 Compare and contrast the primary and secondary antibody responses to antigen.

3.12 Describe the genes that code for the immunoglobulin proteins and explain how they combine to code for a unique antibody molecule.

3.13 Explain how immunoglobulin class switching occurs on a genetic level.

3.14 Explain how the clonal selection hypothesis contributes to antibody specificity.

3.15 Outline the traditional process of mouse monoclonal antibody production.

3.16 Discuss some clinical and research applications of monoclonal antibodies.

CHAPTER OUTLINE

You can go to **fadavis.com** keyword stevens for the laboratory exercises that accompany this text.

In 1890, scientists Emil von Behring and Shibasaburo Kitasato described a substance in the blood that could neutralize the toxin produced by the bacteria that cause diphtheria. The substance responsible for this and similar activities was later termed **antibody.** As we mentioned in Chapter 1, antibodies are the main element of the humoral arm of the adaptive immune response. Located on the surface of B cells, they serve as receptors that specifically recognize foreign antigens to initiate the immune response. When B lymphocytes are stimulated by antigen, they undergo differentiation into plasma cells, which secrete antibodies into the blood and other body fluids. There, antibodies perform biological activities that inactivate antigens like toxins and help to eliminate harmful microorganisms from the body.

Another term for antibody is **immunoglobulin** because these molecules are globular proteins that play a role in immunity. Immunoglobulins are glycoproteins composed of 86% to 98% polypeptide and 2% to 14% carbohydrate. They constitute about 20% of plasma proteins in healthy individuals and can be detected by performing serum protein electrophoresis. In this process, serum is placed on an agarose gel, and an electrical current is applied to separate the proteins. If electrophoresis is carried out at pH 8.6, most serum proteins can be separated based on size and charge. Five distinct bands are obtained in this manner. Immunoglobulins are the slowest-moving proteins and appear mostly in the gamma (γ) band **(Fig. 3–1).** Because the gamma band contains most of the antibody activity, antibodies have also been referred to as *gamma globulins.*

Electrophoresis of immunoglobulins and testing for specific antibodies by other laboratory methods are helpful in the diagnosis of many diseases. Knowledge about the type of immunoglobulin produced by a patient is important in blood banking and in interpretating laboratory tests based on a patient's immune response to a specific antigen. Testing for specific antibodies assists in the diagnosis of a variety of diseases, including infections, allergies, autoimmune diseases, and immunoproliferative diseases. In later chapters, we discuss laboratory tests to detect antibodies for the purpose of diagnosing these diseases in more detail.

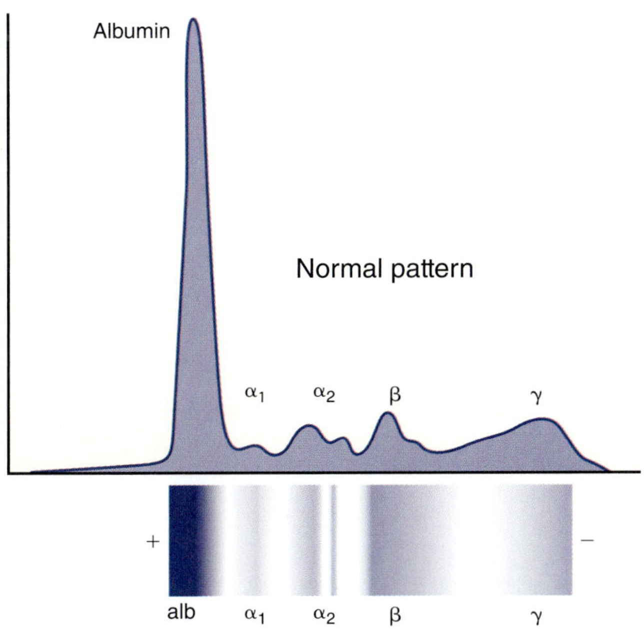

FIGURE 3–1 Serum electrophoresis. Serum is subjected to an electrical charge, and proteins are separated based on size and charge. Antibodies are found in the gamma region because they are the slowest-migrating proteins and have a charge that is close to neutral. Hence, they do not move far from the origin.

Immunoglobulins are divided into five major classes based on a part of the molecule called the heavy chain: IgG, IgM, IgA, IgD, and IgE (with *Ig* being the abbreviation for *immunoglobulin*). The heavy chains within these classes are denoted by the Greek letters γ (gamma), μ (mu), α (alpha), δ (delta), and ε (epsilon), respectively. Some of the Ig classes also contain subclasses, which have slight differences in their heavy chains. Although each class has distinct properties, all immunoglobulin molecules share many common features and a similar basic structure.

In this chapter, we present the nature of this generalized structure and the characteristics of each immunoglobulin type. We examine specific functions for each of the classes in relation to their structural differences and then proceed to explain the cellular and genetic basis by which the specificity and diversity of antibodies arise. In the final section of this chapter, we describe how highly specific antibodies, called *monoclonal antibodies,* can be produced in the laboratory and used in a variety of clinical and research situations.

General Structure of Immunoglobulins

The basic structure of immunoglobulins was first discovered in the 1950s and 1960s because of biochemical analyses performed by two scientists—Gerald Edelman, of the Rockefeller Institute in the United States, and Rodney Porter, at Oxford University in England. These scientists chose to work with IgG, the most abundant of all the antibodies. For their contributions, they shared the Nobel Prize in Physiology and Medicine in 1972. **Table 3-1** summarizes the key findings of these scientists and others.

Two-Dimensional Structure

Because of this research, scientists developed an understanding of the basic structure of the IgG molecule. In its two-dimensional form, IgG can be visualized as a Y-shaped molecule consisting of two larger peptide chains, known as **heavy (H) chains,** bound to two smaller peptide chains, called **light (L) chains (Fig. 3–2).** The molecule is symmetrical, with the two heavy chains being identical to each other and the two light chains identical to each other. The heavy chains of IgG are denoted by the Greek letter for G (gamma or γ); they have a molecular weight of approximately 50,000 and are unique to the IgG molecule. The light chains have a molecular weight of about 22,000 and can be one of two types: **kappa (κ) chains** or **lambda (λ) chains.** The κ and λ chains differ by just a few amino acid substitutions along their length, and there are no functional differences between the two types. Both κ and λ light chains are found in all five classes of immunoglobulins, but only one type is present in a given molecule.

Table 3-1 Scientific Discoveries: Understanding the Structure and Function of Immunoglobulins

SCIENTIST(S) (YEAR OF DISCOVERY)	DISCOVERY
Henry Bence Jones, 1847	Discovered monoclonal light chains in the urine of patients with multiple myeloma, facilitating the characterization of the Ig light chains
Von Behring and Kitasato, 1890	Discovered that a substance in blood could neutralize activity of diphtheria toxin
Arne Tiselius and Elvin Kabat, 1939	Separated serum into protein fractions by electrophoresis and identified the gamma globulin fraction as the main source of immunoglobulins
Gerald Edelman, 1959	Performed analytic ultracentrifugation to separate immunoglobulins based on molecular weight; unfolded the IgG molecule with urea, and disrupted the disulfide bonds with mercaptoethanol
Rodney Porter, 1959	Used the enzyme papain to cleave IgG into the fragments Fab and Fc
Alfred Nisonoff, 1960	Used the enzyme pepsin to cleave IgG to produce the fragment $F(ab')_2$

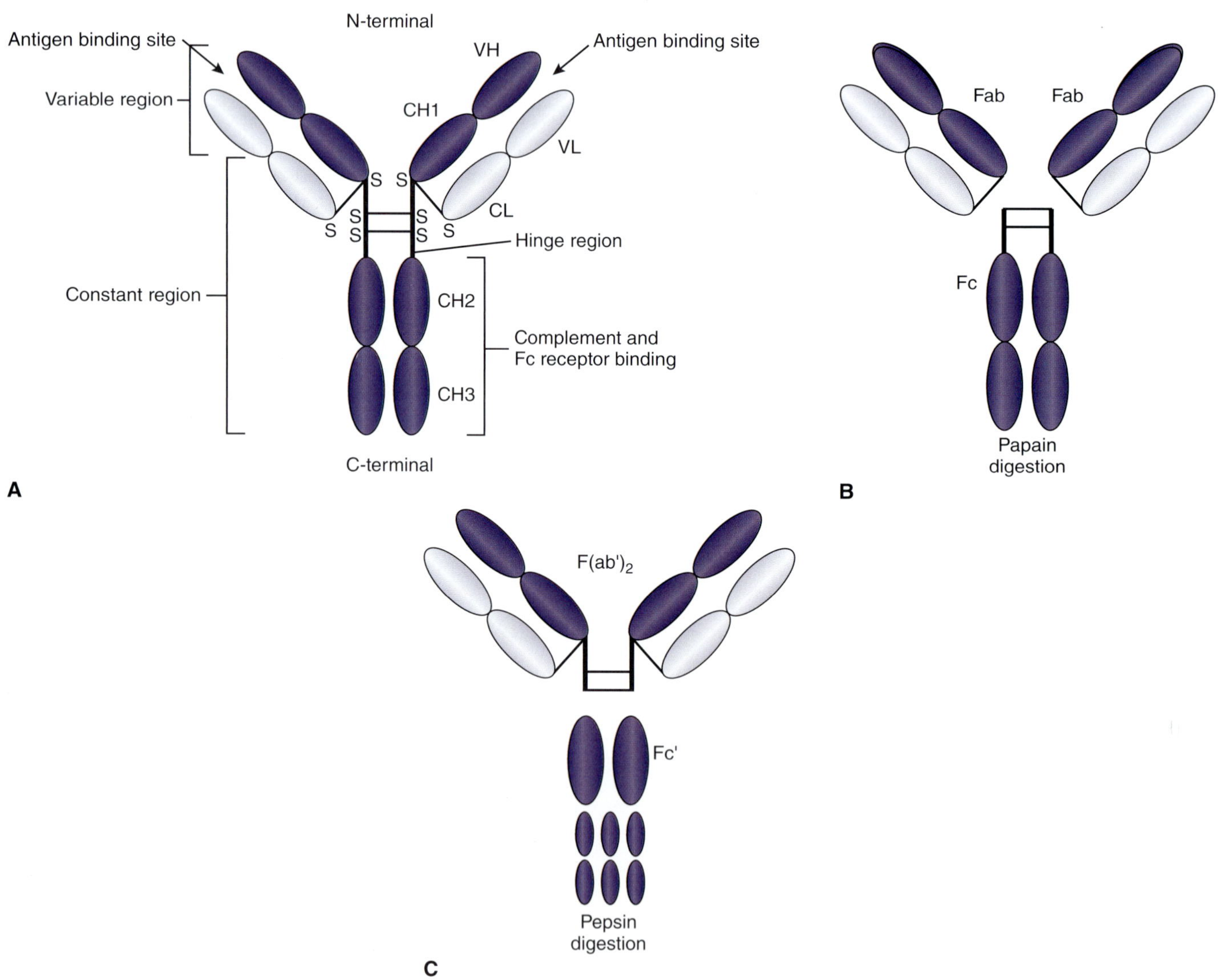

FIGURE 3–2 Basic two-dimensional structure of an immunoglobulin molecule. (A) Immunoglobulin G is a Y-shaped molecule made up of two identical heavy chains (shown in dark blue) and two identical light chains (light blue), held together by disulfide bonds. Intrachain disulfide bonds create looped regions or domains. The amino-terminal end of each chain is a variable region, whereas the carboxy-terminal is at the end of the constant regions. (B) Papain digestion yields two Fab fragments and an Fc portion. (C) Pepsin digestion yields an $F(ab')_2$ fragment with all the antigen binding activity, as well as an Fc′ portion.

The heavy and light chains are held together by disulfide (S–S) bonds and other forces, including hydrogen bonds, hydrophobic forces, and electrostatic attractions. The sulfhydryl bonds can be broken by treatment of the molecule with a reducing agent, such as mercaptoethanol. The exact number of disulfide bonds differs among antibody classes and subclasses. The **tetrapeptide** structure of an antibody, indicated by the formula H_2L_2, serves as the basic structural unit of all the immunoglobulin classes, although the type of heavy chain is unique to each class, and the number of units may vary, depending on the class.

Sequencing of the amino acids in the immunoglobulin molecule revealed that each light chain has a single variable region (V_L) and one constant region (C_L). Each of the heavy chains consists of one variable region (V_H) and three or four constant regions (C_H), depending on the Ig class. The **variable region** is located in the first 110 amino acids of the molecule at the amino terminal. It is unique to each antibody molecule and allows the molecule to bind specifically to a particular antigen. The **constant regions** of the molecule, from amino acid 111 to the carboxyl terminal, are the same in each molecule within an immunoglobulin class or subclass and are responsible for the biological functions that play a role in immune defense against an antigen. The IgG heavy chain has three constant regions, C_H1, C_H2, and C_H3. C_H2 and C_H3 are responsible for binding to complement and Fc receptors on phagocytic cells, respectively. We discuss the importance of these functions in the later section on IgG.

Treatment With Proteolytic Enzymes

Porter and another scientist, Alfred Nisonoff, used the proteolytic enzymes papain and pepsin, respectively, to elucidate the structure of IgG. As shown in Figure 3–2, papain cleaves the IgG molecule below the set of disulfide bonds that holds the two heavy chains together, resulting in the formation of three fragments. Two of these fragments, located at the amino-terminal end of the molecule, are identical and have antigen binding capability; hence, they are known as the **Fab fragments** (fragment antigen binding). Each Fab fragment consists of one light chain and one-half of a heavy chain held together by disulfide bonding. The third fragment, consisting of the carboxy-terminal halves of two heavy chains held together by S–S bonds, was designated as the **Fc fragment** because it spontaneously crystallized at 4°C. The Fc portion of the molecule does not bind antigen and contains the constant regions C_H2 and C_H3, which are responsible for important biological activities, such as binding to complement and phagocytic cells.

In contrast to papain, the enzyme pepsin cleaves IgG at the carboxy-terminal side of the interchain disulfide bonds, yielding a single fragment with a molecular weight of 100,000 Da that contains two antigen binding sites, known as a **$F(ab')_2$ fragment.** An additional fragment called *Fc′* is created in the carboxy-terminal portion of the molecule, which disintegrates into several smaller pieces and has no biological activity. The enzymes papain and pepsin are still used today to obtain immunoglobulin fragments with the desired activities, and the terms *Fab, Fc,* and *$F(ab')_2$* are commonly used to describe various portions of the antibody molecule.

Hinge Region

The segment of heavy chain located between the C_H1 and C_H2 regions is known as the **hinge region.** It is rich in hydrophobic residues and has a high proline content that makes the molecule flexible. The ability to bend lets the two antigen binding sites operate independently and engage in an angular motion relative to each other and to the Fc stem. Thus, two Fab arms can bind simultaneously to parts of the antigen that are separated by varying distances. Such flexibility also assists in effector functions, including initiation of the complement cascade (see Chapter 7) and binding to cells with specific receptors for the Fc portion of the molecule. Gamma, delta, and alpha chains all have a hinge region, but mu and epsilon chains do not. However, the C_H2 domains of these latter two chains are paired in such a way as to confer flexibility to the Fab arms.

Carbohydrate Portion

In addition to the four polypeptide chains, all types of immunoglobulins contain a carbohydrate portion, which is localized between the C_H2 domains of the two heavy chains. The carbohydrate has several important functions, including (1) increasing the solubility of an immunoglobulin, (2) providing protection against degradation of the molecule, and (3) enhancing functional activity of the Fc domains. Glycosylation appears to be critical for recognition by Fc receptors that are found on phagocytic cells.

Isotypes, Allotypes, and Idiotypes

Amino acid sequencing of the immunoglobulin peptide chains revealed the presence of antigenic determinants that can react with other antibodies produced by immunization of heterologous species. These antigenic determinants can be classified into one of three groups: isotypes, allotypes, and idiotypes **(Fig. 3–3).**

Isotypes are unique amino acid sequences that are common to all immunoglobulin molecules of a given class or subclass. They are identical in all individuals of a given species and differ from one species to another. Isotypes are the constant regions of the heavy chains that are unique to each immunoglobulin class and give each type its name. Hence, the isotypes of the classes are known as γ for IgG, μ for IgM, α for IgA, δ for IgD, and ε for IgE. Antibodies to human isotypes can be prepared by immunizing animals with human serum. For example, goat antibodies directed against human IgG can be prepared after immunizing goats with human serum, and these antibodies can be used as reagents in immunoassays (see Chapter 11).

Allotypes are minor variations of amino acid sequences that are present in some individuals of the same species but

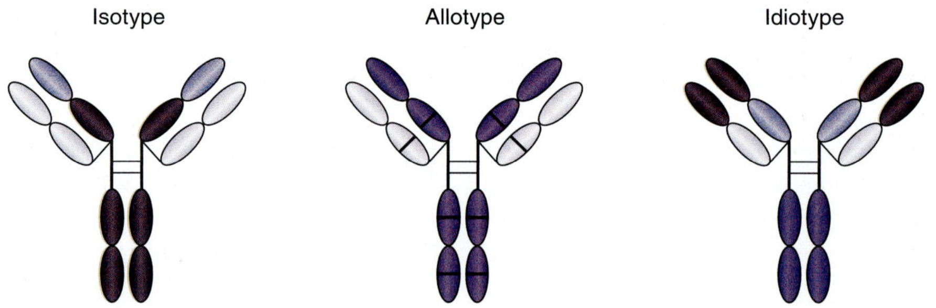

FIGURE 3–3 Antibody variations (shown in black). (A) Isotype—the heavy chain that is unique to each immunoglobulin class. (B) Allotype—genetic variations in the constant regions. (C) Idiotype—variations in variable regions that give individual antibody molecules specificity for antigen.

not others. Allotypes occur in the four IgG subclasses, in one IgA subclass, and in the λ light chain. These genetic markers are found in the constant region and are inherited in a simple Mendelian fashion. Some of the best-known examples of allotypes are variations of the γ chain known as G1m3 and G1m17. Individuals can produce antibodies against allotypes they do not have if they are exposed through pregnancy or transfusion.

Idiotypes are composed of the variable portions of each immunoglobulin chain that are unique to a specific antibody molecule. The amino-terminal ends of both heavy chains and light chains contain these regions, which are essential to the formation of the antigen binding site. Together, they serve as the antigen-recognition unit.

Three-Dimensional Structure of Antibodies

The immunoglobulin structure is similar to other molecules belonging to the *immunoglobulin superfamily,* a group of glycoproteins that share a common ancestral gene. Each type of immunoglobulin chain is made up of several regions called **domains.** Each domain is a globular structure that consists of approximately 110 amino acids. Although the different immunoglobulin classes may have differing numbers of domains, the three-dimensional structure of each is essentially the same.

Thus, the basic four-chain structure of all immunoglobulin molecules does not exist as a straight *Y* shape but is folded into compact globular subunits (i.e., domains) that are stabilized by intrachain disulfide bonds. The polypeptide chain within each of these domains consists of segments called *β strands* that fold back and forth on themselves to form what is called a *β-pleated sheet.* An Ig domain is made up of two layers of β-pleated sheets, each containing three to five antiparallel β strands **(Fig. 3-4).**

Short, protruding, balloon-shaped loops connect adjacent strands of each β-pleated sheet. Some of these loops are very diverse in their amino acid sequence and are known as *hypervariable regions.* These regions contain about 10 amino acids and are also called **complementarity-determining regions (CDRs)** because they form a surface that is complementary to the shape of the bound antigen. The heavy and light chains each contain three CDRs—CDR1, CDR2, and CDR3. The

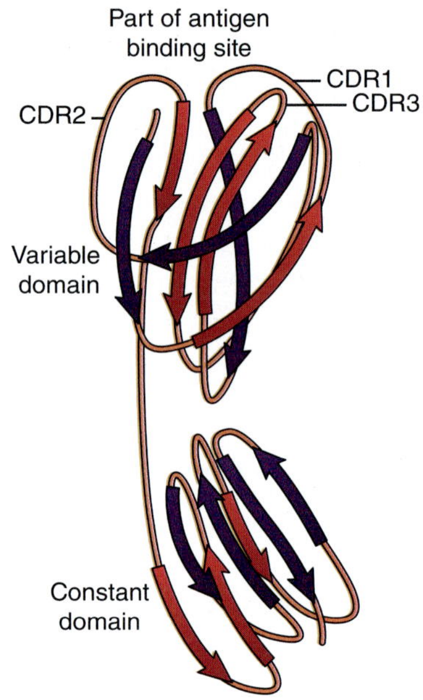

FIGURE 3–4 Three-dimensional structure of a light chain. In this diagram tracing the polypeptide backbone, the antiparallel β strands are shown as wide red or blue ribbons and other regions as narrow strings. The three hypervariable regions (CDR1, CDR2, and CDR3) are flexible loops that project outward from the amino-terminal end of the V_L domain.

antigen binding site, or **paratope,** is determined by the apposition of the six CDRs, three from the heavy chain and three from the light chain. Antigen is captured in the middle of the CDRs in a cylindrical structure called an *immunoglobulin fold.* Remarkably, an immense diversity of antigen binding sites can be created by variations in the small number of amino acids in the CDRs.

Knowledge Check 3-1

The basic structural unit of all immunoglobulin classes consists of which of the following?

a. Two light chains and two heavy chains
b. Four light chains and two heavy chains
c. Four light chains and four heavy chains
d. Two light chains and four heavy chains

Knowledge Check 3-2

Papain digestion of an IgG molecule results in which of the following?

a. Two Fab′ fragments and one Fc′ fragment
b. One $F(ab')_2$ fragment and one Fc′ fragment
c. Two Fab fragments and two Fc fragments
d. Two Fab fragments and one Fc fragment

Antibody Classes

As we mentioned previously, there are five major classes of immunoglobulins—IgG, IgM, IgA, IgD, and IgE—and some of these can be further divided into subclasses. The structural and functional properties of the individual antibody classes are summarized in **Table 3–2** and are discussed in the following sections.

Immunoglobulin G (IgG)

IgG is the predominant immunoglobulin in humans, comprising about 70% to 75% of the total serum immunoglobulins. In adults, the normal serum concentration of IgG ranges from 800 to 1,600 mg/dL. As shown in Table 3–2, IgG has the longest half-life of any immunoglobulin class, approximately 23 days, which may help to account for its predominance in human serum.

IgG is a monomer, consisting of one tetrapeptide unit, with a molecular weight of 150,000 and a sedimentation coefficient of 7S. The *sedimentation coefficient*, or number of Svedberg units, is a measure of the rate by which the molecule sediments in a high-speed ultracentrifuge, and the S-value reflects the molecular weight of the molecule. There are four major IgG subclasses with the following distribution: IgG1, 66%; IgG2, 23%; IgG3, 7%; and IgG4, 4%. The γ heavy chains of these subclasses have slight variations in their constant-region amino acid sequences and differ in the number and position of disulfide bridges, as shown in **Figure 3–5.** Variability in the hinge region affects the ability of the antibody to reach for antigen and its effectiveness in initiating important biological functions. In general, IgG1 and IgG3 are produced in response to protein antigens, whereas IgG2 and IgG4 production is associated with polysaccharide antigens. All subclasses can cross the placenta except IgG2.

IgG has many important functions in the humoral immune response. Its major functions include the following:

1. **Binding to complement.** The C_H2 region of IgG can bind to complement, a series of proteins that interact with antibodies to combat foreign antigens (see Chapter 7). Activation of complement occurs when complement binds to the C_H2 regions of two adjacent IgG molecules (Fig. 7–1). This results in an enhanced inflammatory response and destruction of foreign cells such as bacteria. IgG3 is the most efficient subclass to bind complement because it has the largest hinge region and the largest number of interchain disulfide bonds. IgG1 is the second most efficient subclass to perform this function. In contrast, IgG2 and IgG4 have shorter hinge segments, which tend to make them poor mediators of complement activation.
2. **Opsonization.** IgG is an important mediator of **opsonization,** or the coating of a foreign antigen that

Table 3-2 Properties of Immunoglobulins

IMMUNOGLOBULIN PROPERTY	IgG	IgM	IgA	IgD	IgE
Molecular weight (in daltons)	150,000	900,000	160,000—monomer; 390,000—dimer	180,000	190,000
Sedimentation coefficient	7 S	19 S	7 S	7 S	8 S
Serum half-life (days)	23	6	5	1–3	2–3
Serum concentration (mg/dL)	800–1,600	120–150	70–350	1–3	0.005
Percentage of total immunoglobulin	70–75	10	10–15	≤1	0.02
Heavy chain	γ	μ	α	δ	ε
Heavy chain subclasses	γ1, γ2, γ3, γ4	None	α1, α2	None	None
Heavy chain molecular weight	50,000–60,000	70,000	55,000–60,000	62,000	70,000–75,000
Number of constant domains in heavy chain	3	4	3	3	4
Carbohydrate content (percentage)	2–3	12	7–11	9–14	12
Electrophoretic migration	γ2–α1	γ1–β2	γ2– β1,2	γ1	γ1
Complement fixation	Yes	Yes	No	No	No
Crosses placenta	Yes	No	No	No	No

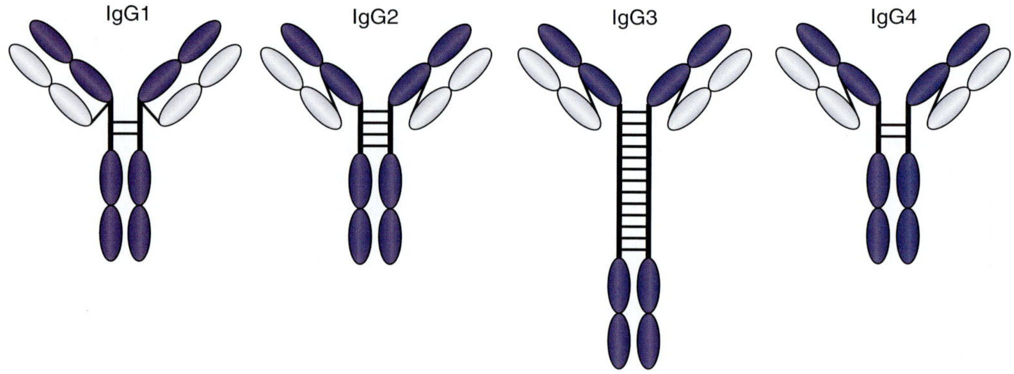

FIGURE 3–5 The four IgG subclasses are IgG1, IgG2, IgG3, and IgG4. These differ in the number and linkages of the disulfide bonds.

leads to enhanced phagocytosis. This process occurs because macrophages, monocytes, and neutrophils have receptors on their surfaces that are specific for the Fc region of IgG. Binding of the C_H3 region of IgG to the Fc receptor enhances contact between the antigen and phagocytic cells and increases the efficiency of phagocytosis **(Fig. 3–6).** IgG1 and IgG3 are particularly good opsonins because they bind most strongly to Fc receptors.

3. **Antibody-dependent cellular cytotoxicity (ADCC).** In this process, IgG binds to Fc receptors on the surface of macrophages, monocytes, neutrophils, and natural killer (NK) cells. Unlike in opsonization, however, the antigen is not engulfed; instead, binding triggers the release of enzymes by the cells, which destroy the antigen extracellularly **(Fig. 3–7).**
4. **Neutralization of bacterial toxins and viruses.** This process involves the inactivation of bacterial toxins and viruses after binding to IgG. IgG is effective at neutralization because it has a high diffusion coefficient that allows it to enter extravascular spaces more readily than the other immunoglobulin types.
5. **Crossing the placenta.** IgG is the only type of antibody that can cross the placenta. This ability is present because the placenta possesses receptors for the Fc region of IgG molecules, which take up the antibodies by receptor-mediated endocytosis and transport them to the fetal blood. This function is mediated mainly by IgG1, IgG3, and IgG4; IgG2 is much less efficient at crossing the placenta. Passive transfer of maternal IgG to the fetus is especially important in providing immunity to the newborn during the first few months of life, when the immune system is immature. The level of maternal IgG declines steadily according to its half-life, so by about 6 months of age, its levels are very low; however, the infant will have started to make its own IgG by that time. IgG concentrations gradually increase until about 6 or 7 years of age, when adult levels are reached.
6. **Agglutination and precipitation.** IgG participates in *agglutination* reactions, or clumping of large particles, and *precipitation,* which involves immune complexes falling out of a solution; see Chapter 10. These reactions occur in some laboratory tests, but it is not known how significant a role they play in the body. IgG is better at precipitation reactions than at agglutination because precipitation involves small soluble particles, which are brought together more easily by the relatively small IgG molecules.

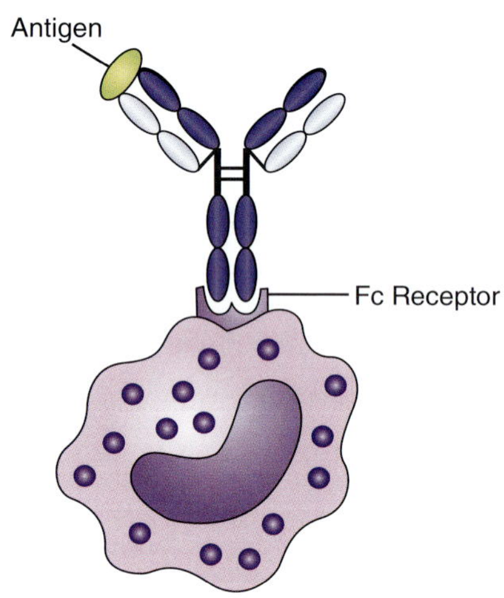

FIGURE 3–6 Opsonization. The Fab portion of IgG binds to the antigen, and the Fc portion binds to receptors on phagocytic cells.

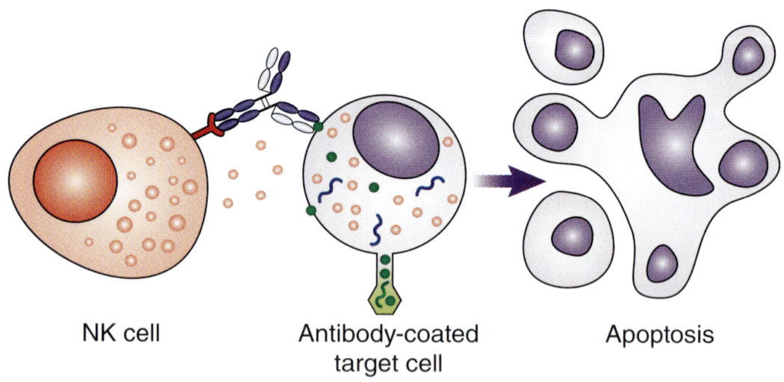

FIGURE 3–7 Antibody-dependent cellular cytotoxicity (ADCC). The Fab portion of IgG antibody binds to an antigen, whereas the Fc portion binds to receptors on macrophages, neutrophils, or NK cells, triggering the release of enzymes that destroy cells expressing the antigen. The figure shows an NK cell destroying an antibody-coated virus-infected host cell by ADCC.

Immunoglobulin M (IgM)

IgM is known as a *macroglobulin* because it is the largest of all the immunoglobulin classes, having a sedimentation rate of 19 S, which represents a molecular weight of approximately 900,000 Da. In the serum, IgM exists as a pentamer of five monomeric units held together by a glycoprotein known as the **J** or **joining chain,** whose cysteine residues form disulfide bonds that link the carboxy-terminal ends of adjacent monomers together to form a starlike shape **(Fig. 3–8).** Each monomer contains μ heavy chains and either κ or λ light chains. The μ heavy chains possess one more constant domain, C_H4, adding to the large size of the molecule. Treatment of the pentamer with mercaptoethanol dissociates the molecule into its monomeric units. The μ heavy chain monomer can also be found on the surface of B cells, and its expression is important to the process of B-cell maturation.

The half-life of IgM is about 6 days, and it accounts for between 5% and 10% of all serum immunoglobulins. In healthy adults, serum concentrations range from 120 to 150 mg/dL. IgM shares some of the same functions as IgG but performs them more effectively because of its multiple binding sites. For example, IgM is the most efficient of all the immunoglobulins at triggering the classical pathway of complement because a single molecule can initiate the reaction when complement binds to two adjacent C_H2 regions (see Chapter 7, Fig. 7–1). This probably represents the most important function of IgM. The larger number of binding sites also makes IgM more efficient at agglutination reactions than IgG. Because IgM is a pentamer, it can bind up to 10 separate antigens or bind to multivalent antigens. The high valency of IgM antibodies helps to overcome the fact that they tend to have a low affinity for antigen.

Because of its large size, IgM is found mainly in the intravascular pool and not in other body fluids or tissues. It can neutralize bacterial toxins and viruses, but it cannot cross the placenta. IgM is known as the *primary response antibody* because it is the first to appear after antigenic stimulation and the first to appear in the maturing infant. It is synthesized only as long as antigen remains present because there are no memory cells for IgM. As we discuss in later chapters, IgM can be used to diagnose an acute infection because its presence indicates a primary exposure to antigen.

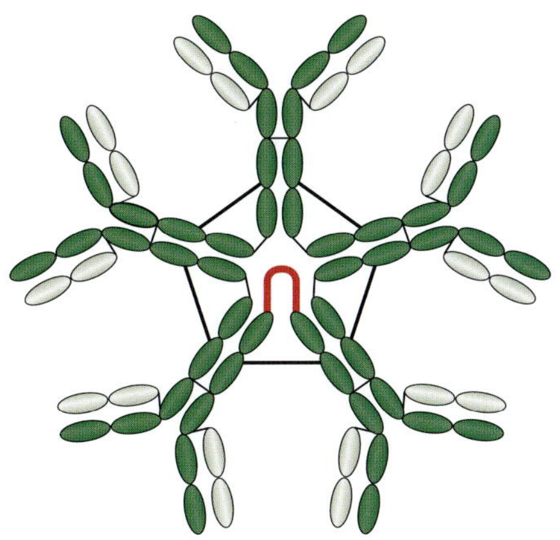

FIGURE 3–8 The pentameric structure of IgM is linked by a J chain (shown in red). Each arm can bend out of the plane to capture antigen.

3-1 Clinical Correlations

IgM Testing for Congenital Infections

The presence of antigen-specific IgM antibodies can be helpful in the diagnosis of congenital infections. This is because, unlike IgG, IgM cannot cross the placenta. Thus, IgM in a newborn's serum reflects the infant's own immune response to an intrauterine infection rather than passive transfer of maternal antibodies. The human fetus can start producing IgM antibodies at about 20 weeks of gestation.

Immunoglobulin A (IgA)

IgA represents 10% to 15% of all immunoglobulins circulating in the blood, with a normal adult serum concentration of 70 to 350 mg/dL. IgA exists in the serum as a monomer with a molecular weight of approximately 160,000 Da and a sedimentation coefficient of 7 S. Upon electrophoresis, IgA migrates between the β and γ regions. The heavy chain of IgA is called α, and it contains one variable and three constant regions. The two subclasses of IgA are designated IgA1 and IgA2. They differ in content by 22 amino acids; 13 of these are located in the hinge region and are deleted in IgA2. The lack of this region appears to make IgA2 more resistant to some bacterial proteases that are able to cleave IgA1. Hence, IgA2 is the predominant form in secretions at mucosal surfaces, whereas IgA1 is mainly found in serum. Serum IgA's major role is as an anti-inflammatory agent. Serum IgA appears to downregulate IgG-mediated phagocytosis, chemotaxis, bactericidal activity, and cytokine release.

IgA2 is found as a dimer along the respiratory, urogenital, and intestinal mucosa; it also appears in breast milk, colostrum, saliva, tears, and sweat. The dimer consists of two monomers held together by a J chain, as seen in IgM. The J chain is essential for the polymerization and secretion of IgA. Secretory IgA is synthesized in plasma cells found mainly in mucosal-associated lymphoid tissue and is released in dimeric form. IgA is synthesized at a much greater rate than that of IgG—about 3 g per day in the average adult—but because it is mainly in secretory form, the serum concentration is much lower.

Another protein, called the **secretory component (SC),** is later attached to the Fc region around the hinge portion of the α chains. This protein is derived from epithelial cells found near the plasma cells. As **Figure 3–9** indicates, an SC precursor is present on the surface of epithelial cells and serves as a specific receptor for IgA. Plasma cells are attracted to subepithelial tissue, where they secrete IgA, which binds to the precursor. Once binding takes place, the IgA and SC precursor are taken inside the cell and released at the opposite surface by a process known as *transcytosis.* The vesicle carrying IgA and the SC receptor fuses with the membrane on the cell's opposite side; a small fragment of SC is then cleaved to

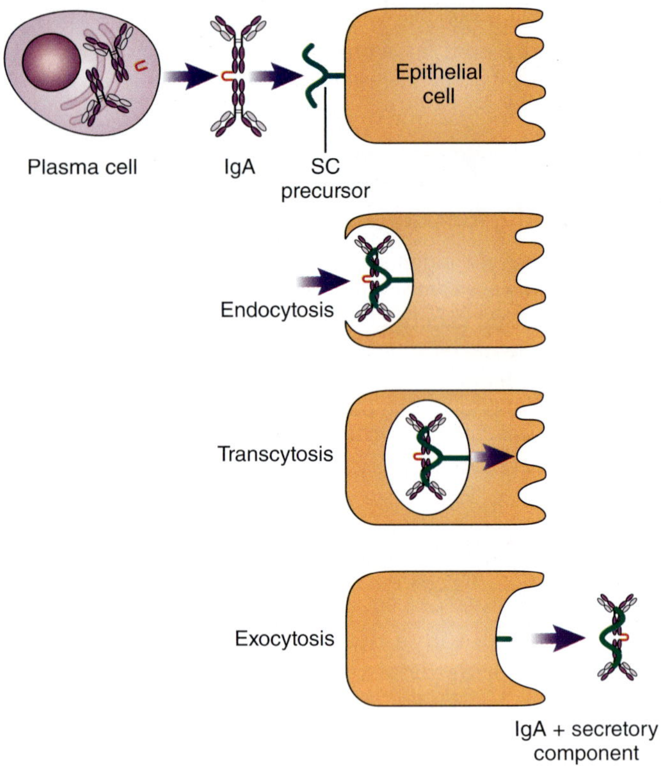

FIGURE 3–9 Formation of secretory IgA. IgA is secreted as a dimer from plasma cells and is captured by specific receptors on epithelial cells. The receptor is actually a secretory component, which binds to IgA and exits the cell along with it.

liberate the IgA dimer with the remaining SC. The SC may thus act to facilitate transport of IgA to mucosal surfaces. It also makes the dimer more resistant to enzymatic digestion by masking sites that would be susceptible to protease cleavage.

The main function of secretory IgA is to patrol mucosal surfaces and act as an early defense by preventing antigens from penetrating farther into the body. IgA plays an important role in neutralizing toxins produced by microorganisms and helps to prevent bacterial and viral adherence to mucosal surfaces. Complexes of IgA and antigen are easily trapped in mucus and then eliminated by the ciliated epithelial cells of the respiratory or intestinal tract. This prevents pathogens from colonizing the mucosal epithelium.

Furthermore, because IgA is found in breast milk, breast-feeding helps to maintain the health of newborns by passively transferring antibodies, thus protecting infants from respiratory and gastrointestinal infections. It appears that IgA is not capable of fixing complement by the classical pathway, although aggregation of immune complexes may trigger the alternative complement pathway (see Chapter 7). Lack of complement activation may help to clear antigen without triggering an inflammatory response, thus minimizing tissue damage.

Immunoglobulin D (IgD)

IgD was not discovered until 1965, when it was found in a patient with multiple myeloma, a cancer of the plasma cells. It is extremely scarce in the serum, representing less than 0.001% of total immunoglobulins. It is synthesized at a low level and has a half-life of only 1 to 3 days. The molecule has a molecular weight of approximately 180,000 Da and migrates as a fast γ protein. The delta (δ) heavy chain has a molecular weight of 62,000 and appears to have an extended hinge region consisting of 58 amino acids.

Because of its unusually long hinge region, IgD is more susceptible to proteolysis than other immunoglobulins. This may be the main reason for its short half-life. The protective functions of circulating IgD have been puzzling because IgD does not have typical antibody functions, such as binding to complement, attaching to neutrophils or macrophages, or crossing the placenta. Studies suggest that secreted IgD may play a role in differentiating between commensal microbes and invasive pathogens in the mucosa. In addition, IgD is thought to interact with basophils, stimulating their release of cytokines that can enhance humoral immunity in the respiratory tract.

Most of the IgD is found on the surface of mature but unstimulated B lymphocytes. It is the second class of immunoglobulin to appear (IgM being the first), and it may play a role in B-cell activation, although its function is not completely understood. The high level of surface expression and its intrinsic flexibility make IgD an ideal early responder to antigen. Unlike B cells bearing only IgM receptors, those with both IgM and IgD receptors can respond to T-cell help and switch to synthesis of IgG, IgA, or IgE. Thus, IgD may play a role in regulating B-cell maturation and differentiation.

Immunoglobulin E (IgE)

IgE is best known for its very low concentration in serum and its ability to activate mast cells and basophils. It is the least abundant immunoglobulin in the serum, accounting for only 0.0005% of total serum immunoglobulins, with a normal adult serum concentration of about 0.005 mg/dL. The molecular weight of IgE is approximately 190,000 Da, making it an 8S molecule, and it has a carbohydrate content of 12%. The epsilon (ε) heavy chain is composed of one variable and four constant domains. A single disulfide bond joins each ε chain to a light chain, and two disulfide bonds link the heavy chains to one another.

IgE is the most heat labile of all immunoglobulins; heating to 56°C for 30 minutes to 3 hours results in conformational changes and loss of ability to bind to target cells. Similar to IgD, IgE does not participate in typical immunoglobulin reactions such as complement fixation, agglutination, or opsonization. Additionally, it is incapable of crossing the placenta. Instead, shortly after synthesis, it attaches to basophils, Langerhans cells, eosinophils, and tissue mast cells through high-affinity receptors for the Fc portion of the ε chain (Fc ε RI), which are found exclusively on the surface of these cells. The molecule binds at the C_H3 domain, leaving the antigen binding sites free to interact with specific antigen **(Fig. 3–10).** Plasma cells that produce IgE are located mostly in the lungs and in the skin.

Mast cells are found mainly in the skin and in the linings of the respiratory and gastrointestinal tracts. One such cell may have several hundred thousand receptors, each capable of binding to an IgE molecule. When two adjacent IgE

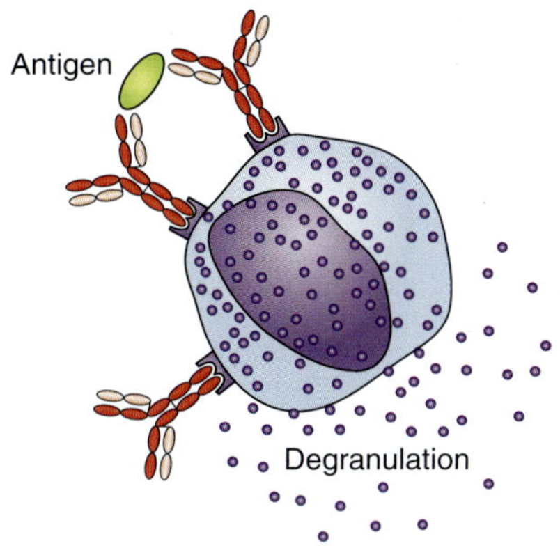

FIGURE 3–10 IgE binds to specific Fc ε receptors on mast cells. When antigen bridges two nearby IgE molecules, the membrane is disturbed, degranulation results, and chemical mediators are released.

molecules on a mast cell bind specific antigen, this initiates a cascade of cellular events that results in degranulation of the mast cells with the release of vasoactive amines such as histamine and heparin. The release of these mediators induces what is known as a *type I* immediate hypersensitivity or allergic reaction (see Chapter 14). Typical reactions include hay fever, asthma, vomiting and diarrhea, hives, and life-threatening anaphylactic shock.

IgE appears to be a nuisance antibody; however, it may serve a protective role by triggering an acute inflammatory reaction that recruits neutrophils and eosinophils to the area to help destroy invading antigens that have penetrated IgA defenses. Eosinophils, in particular, play a major role in destroying large antigens, such as parasitic worms, that cannot be easily phagocytized (see Chapter 22).

Knowledge Check 3-3

Match each antibody class with its major characteristic:

a. IgA ____ 1. Found mainly on surface of B cells

b. IgD ____ 2. Crosses the placenta

c. IgE ____ 3. Most effective in complement activation

d. IgG ____ 4. Predominant Ig in secretions

e. IgM ____ 5. Binds to mast cells in allergic reactions

Critical Thinking 3-1

Suppose a patient had a deficiency in IgA production but normal levels of all other immunoglobulins. How might this condition affect the patient's immune response to pathogens?

Immunologic Memory: Primary and Secondary Antibody Responses

As we discussed in earlier chapters, one of the key features of the adaptive immune response is immunologic memory, or the ability of the immune system to respond more rapidly and effectively to an antigen after repeated exposure. The first time an individual is exposed to an antigen, they mount what is called a **primary antibody response.** This response is characterized by a long time period, or *lag phase*, between encounter with the antigen and production of detectable antibody. During the lag phase, which typically lasts between 4 and 7 days, T and B lymphocytes are being activated to respond to the antigen by the T-dependent mechanism of antibody production (see Chapter 5). This process results in the generation of antibody-secreting plasma cells. Antigen-specific IgM antibody is produced first, followed by specific IgG antibody **(Fig. 3–11).** The amounts of antibody produced are relatively low and decline during the span of a few weeks.

Some of the activated B cells from the primary response will not develop into plasma cells but, rather, expand into clones of long-lived memory cells. Memory cells have undergone genetic changes that allow them to resist apoptosis (a type of cell death); they express high-affinity antigen receptors and switch their production from IgM to another isotype, predominantly IgG. Therefore, if memory B cells are exposed to the same antigen weeks, months, or even years later, they can rapidly differentiate into plasma cells, and larger amounts of antibody are produced. The memory response is also referred to as the **secondary antibody response,** or **anamnestic response.** As you can see in Figure 3–11, this response has a shorter lag phase than the primary response (~1 to 2 days) followed by production of low levels of IgM that rapidly decline. However, higher levels of another immunoglobulin isotype, usually IgG, are produced. IgG levels decline slowly and persist in the body for longer periods, sometimes providing lifelong immunity to the antigen. Antibodies produced in the secondary response also have a higher affinity for antigen (i.e., they can bind more strongly) than antibodies in the primary response. **Table 3–3** summarizes the key differences between the primary and secondary antibody responses. The memory response serves as the basis for the booster injections given in routine vaccination schedules to optimize the recipient's immunity to potentially harmful pathogens (see Chapter 25).

3-2 Clinical Correlations

Serologic Testing

The antibody responses shown in Figure 3–11 are the basis for serology testing for infectious diseases. The antibody classes can be used to differentiate an acute immune response, characterized by IgM only, from the response occurring later in the course of an infection (IgM plus IgG) and a past infection (IgG only). See Chapters 20 through 23.

Knowledge Check 3-4

How does the memory response differ from the primary antibody response?

a. There is a larger delay in antibody production.

b. IgM antibodies persist.

c. A higher titer of IgG antibody is produced.

d. Antibody of lower affinity is produced.

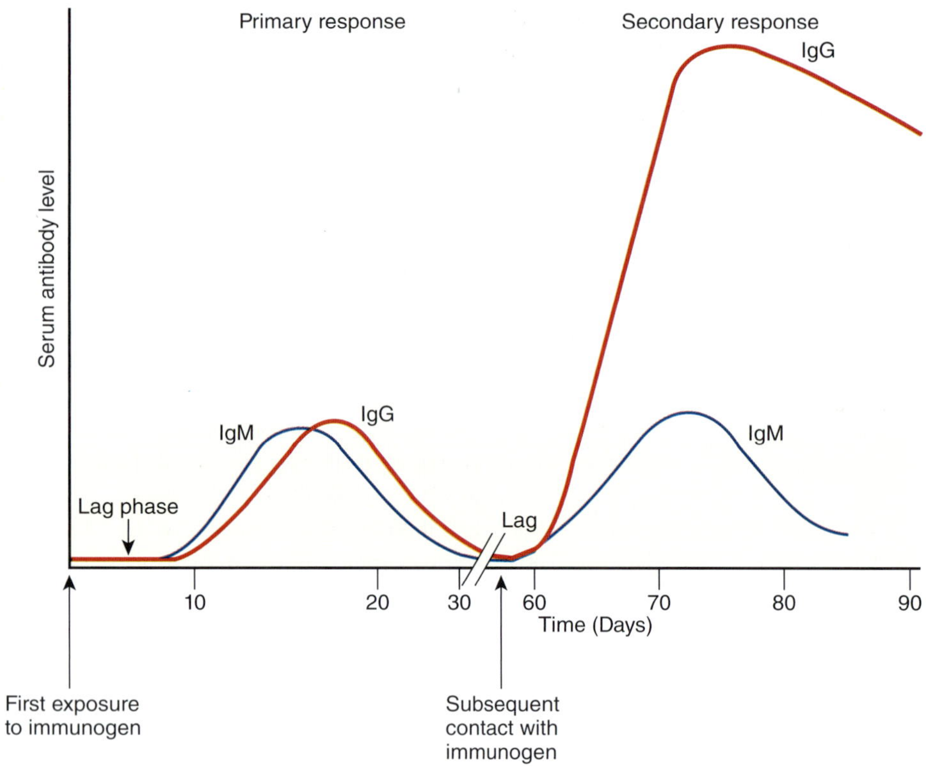

FIGURE 3–11 Primary and secondary antibody responses. Memory lymphocytes are generated during the primary response, and these cells can respond more effectively upon subsequent exposure to the same antigen. As compared with the primary response, the secondary or anamnestic response has a shorter lag phase; a much more rapid increase in antibody titer, mainly IgG; and greater persistence of IgG over time.

Table 3-3 Comparison of Primary and Secondary Antibody Responses

CHARACTERISTIC	PRIMARY RESPONSE	SECONDARY RESPONSE
Time to antibody production	Longer lag phase	Shorter lag phase; faster appearance of antibody
Antibody classes	IgM, followed by IgG	IgM, followed by a greater predominance of IgG
Antibody titer	Relatively low; declines in a few weeks	High IgG titer, which declines slowly and persists for a long time
Antibody affinity for antigen	Low affinity	High affinity

Critical Thinking 3-2

Suppose a symptomatic patient was tested for an infection with a certain virus. Antibody tests indicated the presence of IgM antibody to the organism, along with a low titer of specific IgG. What do these results indicate?

Antibody Specificity and Diversity

Important features of adaptive immunity are its specificity for a particular antigen and its ability to respond to a diverse array of antigens in our environment. It is estimated that humans have the potential to respond to between 10^7 and 10^9 different antigens. Yet, when an individual is exposed to a particular antigen, the immune system produces antibodies that are specific for that antigen and not for unrelated antigens. For example, a person infected with group A *Streptococcus* bacteria will make antibodies to antigens possessed by those bacteria and not to *Staphylococcus* bacteria. How is this possible? In this section, we explore the genetic basis for antigen specificity and diversity and discuss how these characteristics are achieved on a cellular level.

Clonal Selection

As we discussed previously, in addition to their presence in the blood and other body fluids, immunoglobulins are found on the surface membrane of B cells, where they serve as receptors for antigens. Through the years, scientists discovered that the body has numerous clones of lymphocytes, each possessing surface receptors with a unique antigen specificity. When an antigen enters the body, it selectively binds to receptors on the B cells capable of responding to that antigen, causing only those cells to proliferate and mount the antibody responses discussed in Chapter 5. This process, first hypothesized by the scientist Paul Ehrlich in the early 1900s and confirmed independently by Niels Jerne and Macfarlane Burnet in the 1950s, is called the **clonal selection hypothesis.** Today, clonal selection is considered a fundamental concept of the immune response **(Fig. 3–12).**

Furthermore, as we discuss in the next section, individual lymphocytes are genetically preprogrammed to produce an immunoglobulin receptor with a single antigen specificity. This process occurs before contact with antigen, during maturation of the B cells in the bone marrow. In a similar fashion, antigen-specific T-cell receptors are generated during maturation of the T cells in the thymus (see Chapter 5). Because

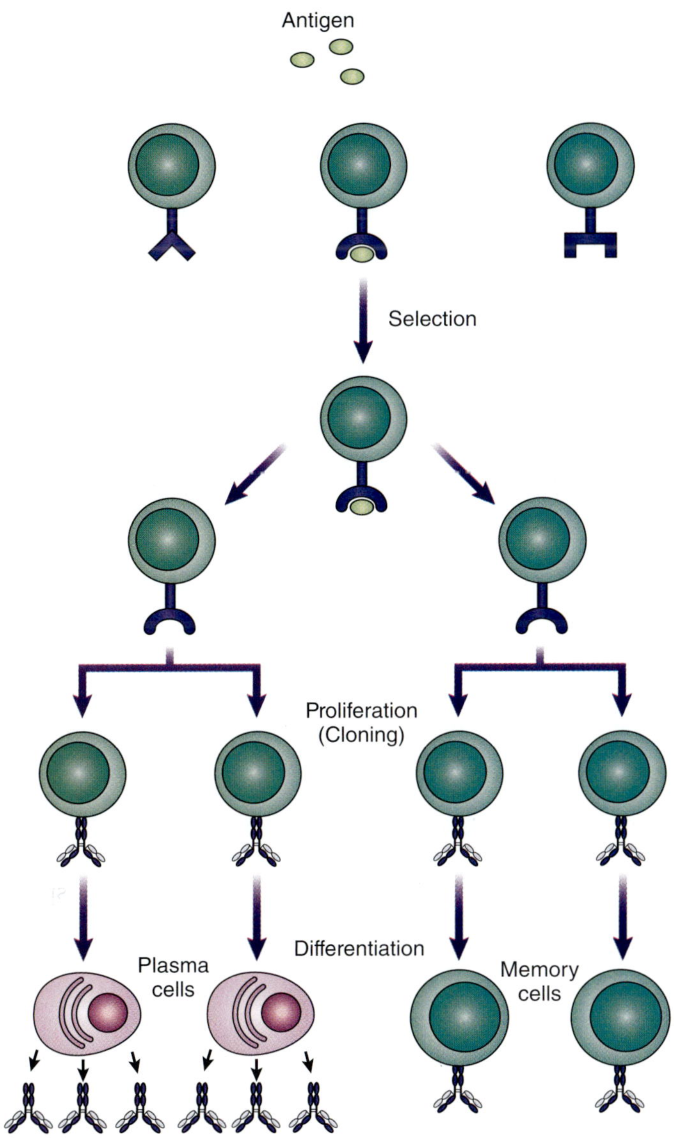

FIGURE 3–12 Clonal selection. Antigen binds only to B lymphocytes expressing receptors specific for the antigen (in this example, the B cell in the middle). Those B cells are stimulated to divide and differentiate into plasma cells that secrete antibody specific for the antigen. Some of the B cells develop into long-lived memory cells.

of this remarkable process, mature lymphocytes that have seeded the lymphoid tissues are prepared to respond to a diverse array of potentially harmful antigens long before the body encounters them.

Immunoglobulin Genes

Before the concept of clonal selection became established, scientists wondered how to reconcile this hypothesis with the genetic basis for antibody diversity. The central dogma of molecular genetics is that one gene codes for one polypeptide. However, if there were separate genes to code for all the antibody molecules to every possible antigen, an overwhelming amount of DNA would be needed, much more than could be packaged into a cell nucleus. In 1965, Dreyer and Bennett suggested that the constant and variable portions of immunoglobulin chains are actually coded for by separate genes. They hypothesized that there was a small number of genes coding for the constant region and a larger number of genes coding for the variable region. This notion implied that although all lymphocytes originate with identical germline DNA, diversity is created by a series of events whereby separate gene segments are selected and joined together as the B cell matures. Susumu Tonegawa's pioneering work provided scientific evidence for this hypothesis, and he was awarded the Nobel Prize in 1987 for his monumental discovery.

Tonegawa's experiments with DNA revealed that chromosomes do not contain intact immunoglobulin genes but, rather, building blocks from which genes can be assembled. Human immunoglobulin genes are found in three unlinked clusters: Heavy chain genes are located on chromosome 14, κ light chain genes are on chromosome 2, and λ light chain genes are on chromosome 22. Within each of these clusters, a selection process occurs. The genes cannot be transcribed and translated into functional antibody molecules until rearrangement, assisted by special recombinase enzymes, takes place. Gene rearrangement involves a cutting-and-splicing process that removes much of the intervening DNA and joins the ends together, resulting in a functional gene that codes for a specific antibody. Once gene rearrangement occurs in a B lymphocyte, it permanently changes its DNA.

Rearrangement of Heavy Chain Genes

The selection process begins with rearrangement of the genes that code for the immunoglobulin heavy chains. All heavy chains are derived from a single region on the long arm of chromosome 14. The genes that code for the variable region of the heavy chain are divided into three groups—V_H, D, and J. There are approximately 45 functional V_H (variable) genes, 23 D (diversity) genes, and six J (joining) genes. All the V, D, and J genes are present in the germline DNA of a bone marrow stem cell. Another set of genes codes for the constant region (C). This set includes one gene for each heavy chain isotype. The genes are located in the following order: Cμ, Cδ, Cγ3, Cγ1, Cα1, Cγ2, Cγ4, Cε, and Cα2, as shown in **Figure 3–13.** Only one of these constant regions is selected at any one time.

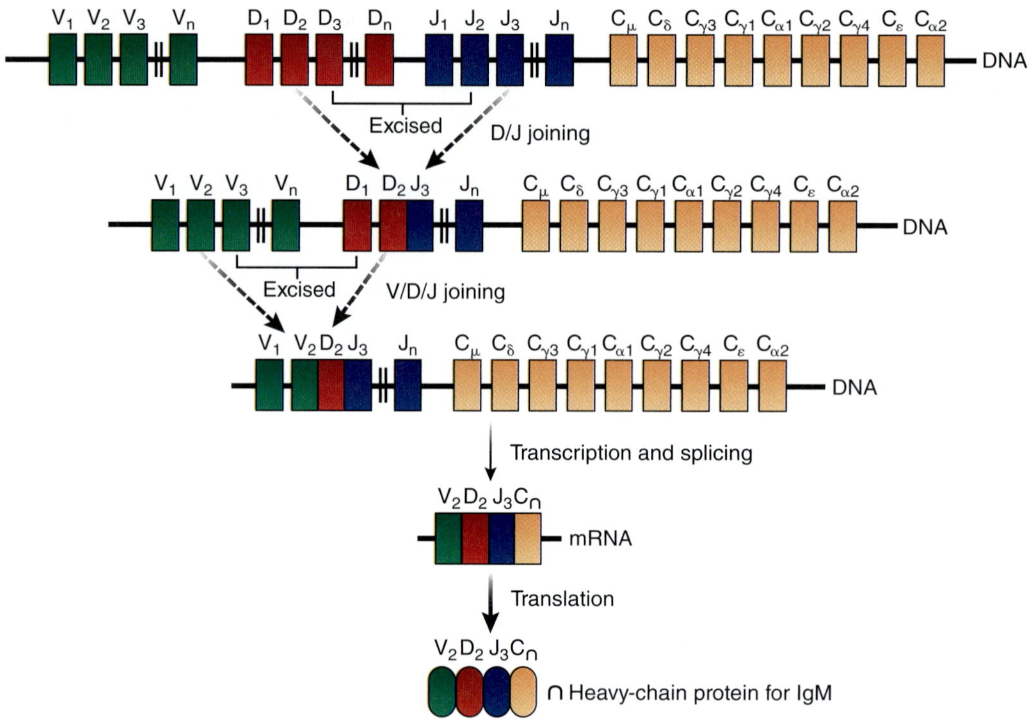

FIGURE 3–13 Genes coding for immunoglobulin heavy chains. Four separate regions on chromosome 14 code for heavy chains. DJ regions are spliced first, and then this segment is joined to a variable region. When RNA synthesis occurs, one constant region is attached to the VDJ combination; μ heavy chains are made first, but the cell retains its capacity to produce immunoglobulin of other classes.

As the B cell matures and the heavy chain is constructed, a random choice is made from each of the sections to include one V_H gene, one D gene, one J gene, and one constant-region gene. Joining of these segments occurs in two steps: First, in pro-B cells, one D gene and one J gene are randomly chosen and are joined by means of a recombinase enzyme after the intervening DNA is deleted (Fig. 3–13). Next, in the pre–B cell stage, a V gene is joined to the DJ complex, resulting in a rearranged VDJ gene. The VDJ gene combination codes for the entire variable region of the heavy chain. Thus, during the process of B-cell maturation, the pieces are spliced together to commit each B lymphocyte to making antibody of a single specificity.

If a successful rearrangement of DNA on one chromosome 14 occurs, then the genes on the second chromosome are not rearranged; this phenomenon is known as **allelic exclusion.** If the first rearrangement does not result in a functional immunoglobulin chain, then rearrangement of the second set of genes on the other chromosome 14 occurs. This mechanism maintains clonal specificity by ensuring that each B cell only expresses a single antigen receptor.

Next, the variable- and constant-region genes are joined. This process occurs at the ribonucleic acid (RNA) level, thus conserving the DNA of the constant regions. During transcription and synthesis of messenger ribonucleic acid (mRNA), a constant region is spliced to the VDJ complex. Because Cμ is the region closest to the J region, μ heavy chains are the first to be synthesized, and they appear in the cytoplasm of the pre-B lymphocytes. In mature B cells, the Cδ region, which lies closest to the Cμ region, is often transcribed along with Cμ. The presence of DNA for both the Cμ and Cδ regions allows for mRNA for IgD and IgM to be transcribed at the same time. Thus, a B cell could express both IgD and IgM with the same variable domain on its surface.

Light Chain Gene Rearrangement

Because light chain rearrangement occurs only after μ chains appear, μ-chain synthesis represents a pivotal step in the process. Light chain genes exhibit a similar rearrangement, except they lack a D region. Recombination of segments on chromosome 2, coding for κ chains, occurs before that on chromosome 22, which codes for λ chains.

The κ locus contains approximately 35 V_κ, 5 J_κ, and one functional C_κ segment. The process of VJ joining is accomplished by cutting out intervening DNA. This results in the V_κ and J_κ segments becoming permanently joined to one another on the rearranged chromosome. Transcription begins at one end of the V_κ segment and proceeds through the J_κ and C_κ segments. J segments that have not been rearranged are removed by RNA splicing, which occurs during translation **(Fig. 3–14).**

A productive rearrangement of the κ genes with subsequent protein production keeps the other chromosome 2 from rearranging and shuts down any recombination of the λ -chain locus on chromosome 22. Only if a nonfunctioning gene product arises from κ rearrangement does λ-chain synthesis occur. The λ locus contains about 30 V_λ, 4 J_λ, and 4 functional C_λ segments. If functional heavy and light chains are not produced in a B lymphocyte by these rearrangements, then that cell dies by apoptosis.

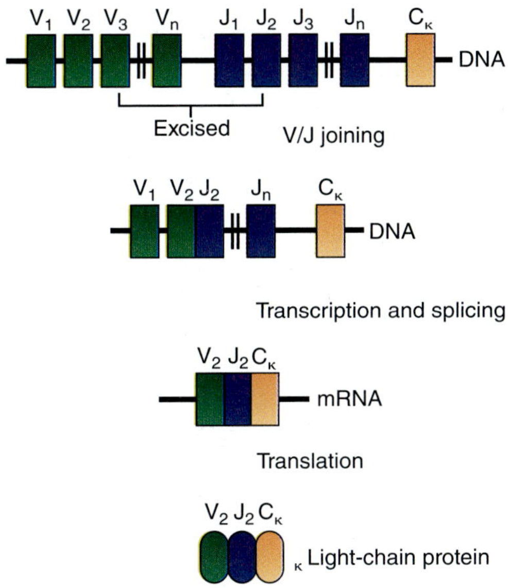

FIGURE 3–14 Assembly and expression of the κ–light chain locus. A DNA rearrangement fuses one V segment to one J segment. The VJ segment is then transcribed along with a unique C_κ region to form mature κ mRNA. Unarranged J segments are removed during RNA splicing.

Two of the light chains are subsequently joined with two μ chains to form an IgM monomer, which first appears on the surface of immature B cells. Once IgM and IgD are present on the surface membrane, the B lymphocyte is fully mature and capable of responding to antigen (see Chapter 5).

Additional Sources of Diversity

Thus, a main source of antibody diversity involves the formation of unique immunoglobulin gene sequences from the large variety of possible combinations of the V, D, and J segments that code for the variable portion of the antibody molecule. However, this process is just one way in which diversity is generated in the creation of B-cell antigen receptors. The recombinase enzymes RAG-1 and RAG-2 are essential for initiating VDJ recombination during B-cell maturation. These enzymes recognize specific recombination signal sequences in the DNA that flanks the immunoglobulin gene segments. However, joining of the V, J, and D segments does not always occur at a fixed position, so each sequence can vary by a small number of nucleotides. This variation, called *junctional diversity,* is a major contributor to diversity in the variable-region genes. Furthermore, nucleotides may be added to or deleted from the junctions.

Another source of variation occurs at the protein level. Once the immunoglobulin chains are synthesized, different heavy chains can combine with different light chains to produce functional antibody molecules.

A final source of variation, called *somatic hypermutation,* can occur after the B cell makes contact with the antigen. During the T cell–dependent antibody response, cytokines are produced that stimulate the B cells to divide so that the response to the antigen is enhanced. Genetic mutations occur at a very high rate in the variable regions of the immunoglobulin genes during this period of rapid B-cell proliferation. Mutations in some of these B cells result in immunoglobulin receptors that can bind the antigen more strongly, and these B cells become the dominant clones as the immune response evolves. This process, called **affinity maturation,** results in a more effective response to the antigen.

Thus, there are several sources of immunoglobulin diversity: (1) the large variety of V, J, D, and C combinations for each type of chain; (2) junctional diversity; (3) different possibilities for light and heavy chain combinations; and (4) somatic hypermutation. All these processes, taken together, result in a tremendous number of antibody configurations, allowing humans to effectively respond to any antigen in the environment.

Immunoglobulin Class Switching

As we discussed earlier, the first immunoglobulin to be synthesized during the immune response is IgM. This occurs because the Cμ gene is the constant-region gene that is closest to the VDJ genes. As the immune response progresses, B cells may become capable of producing antibody of another class, a phenomenon called **class switching.**

Production of other immunoglobulin isotypes occurs because of a process called *switch recombination,* whereby a portion of the constant-region DNA is deleted, and the remaining C_H genes are placed adjacent to the variable-region genes. This allows the same VDJ region to be coupled with a different C region to produce antibody of a different class (i.e., IgA, IgG, or IgE) but with identical specificity for antigen. Contact with T cells and cytokines determines where switching takes place and which C_H gene will be transcribed. For example, the cytokine IL-4 provides the signal for transcription of the Cε gene and deletion of the intervening sequences. The resulting production of IgE antibody might be helpful in defense against parasitic infections. In contrast, a switch to IgA would be more effective in combating a bacterial infection of the gut. Thus, class switching allows B cells to change their production to a different antibody isotype, tailoring the immune response so that it will be most effective in defending against a particular type of pathogen in a specific location in the body.

Knowledge Check 3-5

Diversity in antibody specificity results from:
a. The switching of C genes
b. Recombination of V, D, and J genes
c. Alteration of surface Ig on B cells by antigen
d. Selective expression of a single gene

Monoclonal Antibodies

The normal response to an antigen results in the production of polyclonal antibodies because even a purified antigen has multiple epitopes that stimulate a variety of B cells. Polyclonal antibodies have been produced for use in the laboratory or as therapeutic agents by immunizing animals such as goats or horses with the desired antigen, and after a period of time, collecting and purifying blood from the animals. The resulting antiserum contains a mixture of antibodies, directed against different parts of the immunizing antigen. While polyclonal antibodies have been useful for some applications, they are variable in terms of their ability to bind to the antigen and may react with related but nonidentical antigens as well.

In contrast, **monoclonal antibodies** are derived from a single parent antibody-producing cell that has reproduced many times to form a clone. All the cells in the clone are identical, and the antibody produced by each of these cells is the same as that produced by every other cell in the clone. Monoclonal antibodies are directed against a specific epitope on an antigen. The knowledge that B cells are genetically preprogrammed to synthesize a specific antibody has been used to produce monoclonal antibodies for diagnostic testing and for treating patients with various diseases (see Chapter 25).

Hybridomas

In 1975, Georges Kohler and Cesar Milstein developed a technique to produce antibody arising from a single B cell, and this method has revolutionized laboratory testing and immunotherapy. They were awarded the Nobel Prize in 1984 for their pioneering research.

A normal B cell can only survive for a short time in culture. To develop a cell line that produces antibody but can live for a long period of time, Kohler and Milstein combined an activated B cell with a myeloma cell, a cancerous plasma cell that can be grown indefinitely in the laboratory. The fusion product of these two cell types is called a **hybridoma.** The particular myeloma cell line that was chosen to make the hybridoma was not capable of producing its own antibody. This cell line was also deficient in the enzyme hypoxanthine-guanine phosphoribosyltransferase (HGPRT), making it incapable of synthesizing nucleotides from hypoxanthine and thymidine, substances needed for DNA synthesis. The fact that these myeloma cells could not make their own DNA meant that they would die unless they were fused to a B cell that had the enzymes necessary to synthesize DNA. This deficiency kept the myeloma cells from reproducing on their own.

The technique Kohler and Milstein developed to generate hybridomas is the traditional method of making monoclonal antibodies. The production of hybridomas begins by immunizing a mouse with the desired antigen. After a time, the mouse's spleen cells are harvested because the spleen is a rich source of B lymphocytes. The spleen cells are combined with HGPRT-deficient myeloma cells in the presence of polyethylene glycol (PEG), a surfactant that brings about fusion of the cells to produce a hybridoma. Only a small percentage of the cells actually fuse, and some of these are not hybridomas but, rather, two myeloma cells or two spleen cells combined together **(Fig. 3–15).**

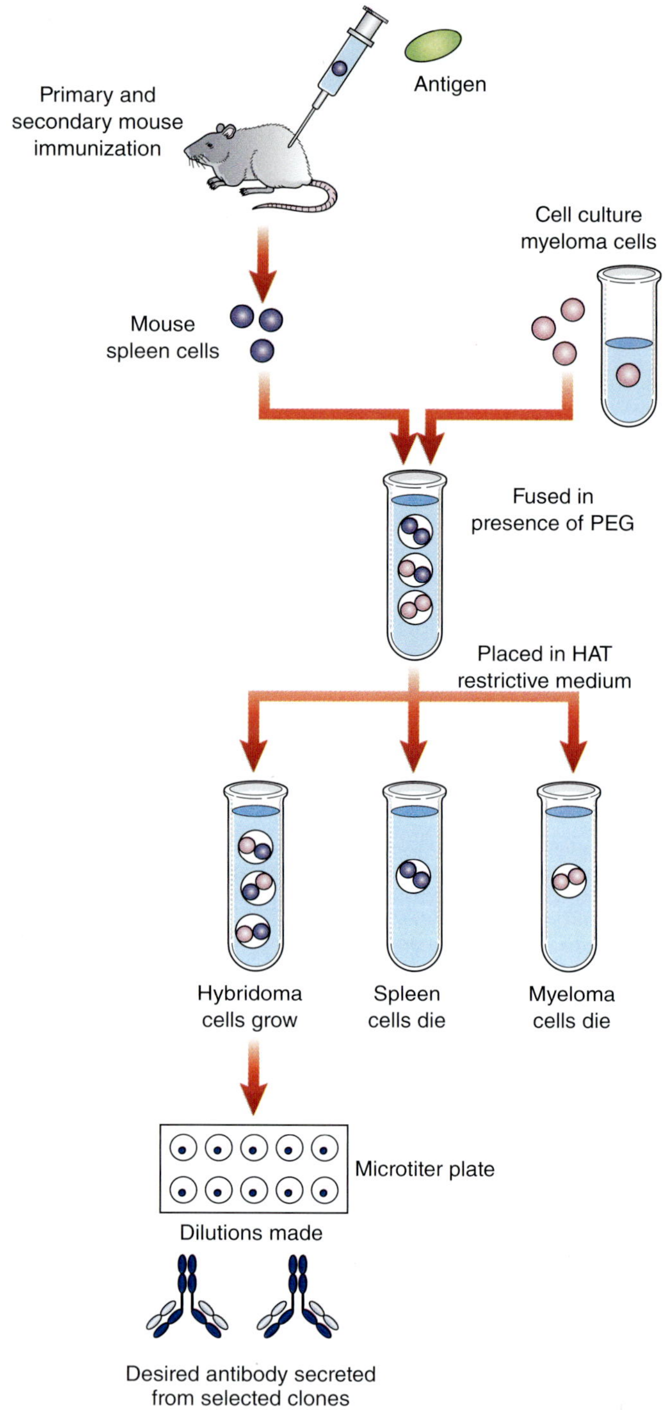

FIGURE 3–15 Formation of a hybridoma in monoclonal antibody production. A mouse is immunized, and spleen cells are removed. These cells are fused with nonsecreting myeloma cells and then plated in a selective culture medium (HAT). Only the hybridoma cells can grow in this medium. Hybridomas producing the desired antibody are isolated, and the monoclonal antibody is obtained from the culture medium.

After fusion, all the cells are placed in culture using a selective medium called *HAT,* which contains hypoxanthine, aminopterin, and thymidine. The culture medium allows the hybridoma cells to grow but does not allow the fused myeloma cells or fused spleen cells to survive. The myeloma cells die because the two pathways of nucleotide synthesis (the de novo pathway and the salvage pathway) are blocked under these conditions. The de novo pathway, which makes DNA from new nucleotides, is blocked by the presence of aminopterin. The salvage pathway, which builds DNA from degradation of old nucleic acids, is blocked because the myeloma cell line is deficient in the required enzymes HGPRT and thymidine kinase. Consequently, the myeloma cells die. Normal B cells cannot be maintained continuously in cell culture, so these die as well. This leaves only the fused hybridoma cells, which can reproduce indefinitely in culture (acquired from the myeloma cell) and can synthesize nucleotides by the HGPRT and thymidine kinase pathway (provided by the B cell).

At this point, the culture contains a mixture of hybridoma cell lines, each producing a unique antibody. To isolate the cells producing antibody to the desired antigen, dilutions are made, and individual hybridomas are placed in microtiter wells, where they replicate in the presence of culture medium to form a clone. The supernatants from each clone are screened for the desired antibody. Those cultures producing the antibody are grown in larger quantities, and the monoclonal antibody is collected from the culture supernatant and purified. The hybridomas can be maintained in cell culture indefinitely and produce an abundant supply of monoclonal antibody that reacts with a single antigen epitope.

Other Methods of Monoclonal Antibody Production

A major limitation of using mouse monoclonal antibodies as therapeutic agents is that they are highly immunogenic for humans, inducing the development of human–anti-mouse antibodies (HAMAs) that can cause severe hypersensitivity reactions (see Chapters 14 and 25). Therefore, several techniques have been developed to reduce such reactions by constructing monoclonal antibodies that have a larger human protein component and less mouse protein. Chimeric and humanized monoclonal antibodies have been generated by using molecular techniques to graft the entire antibody-combining site or CDRs from mouse antibodies onto the rest of a human immunoglobulin. More recently, fully human monoclonal antibodies have been produced by transgenic mice in which the mouse immunoglobulin genes have been replaced by human immunoglobulin genes. The spleen cells from the transgenic mice immunized with a specific antigen can be used to generate hybridoma cell lines, as we described previously. Libraries of genetically engineered bacteriophages (viruses that infect bacteria), yeast, or mammalian cells can also be used to clone the antibody genes of interest, and along with next-generation sequencing (see Chapter 12), select for antibodies that have a high binding affinity for antigen.

Clinical and Research Applications

Monoclonal antibodies have a wide range of applications in clinical laboratory testing, therapeutics, and research. We present some of the major uses of monoclonal antibodies briefly in the following paragraphs.

Use as reagents in laboratory tests for circulating antigens. Before the development of monoclonal antibodies, antibody reagents could only be produced by immunizing animals such as horses or goats with the desired antigen and isolating polyclonal antibodies from the animal serum. The main advantages of monoclonal antibody reagents are that they provide decreased lot-to-lot variation and increased specificity toward a single epitope, rather than multiple epitopes of an antigen. These advantages have led to the widespread use of monoclonal antibodies in a variety of laboratory tests. A familiar example is pregnancy testing, which uses antibody specific for the β chain of human chorionic gonadotropin, thereby eliminating many false-positive reactions. Other examples include tests that detect tumor antigens, identify infectious agents, or measure hormone levels.

Use as reagents in laboratory tests for cell surface markers. Monoclonal antibodies are used routinely in laboratory tests that identify different types of lymphocytes and other white blood cells based on their cell surface antigens, most notably, the CD markers. These tests are essential for the diagnosis of hematologic malignancies and for monitoring the immune status of patients with HIV infection (see Chapters 18 and 24).

3-3 Clinical Correlations

CD4 T-Cell Quantitation

An example of a laboratory test that uses monoclonal antibodies to detect lymphocytes is CD4 T-cell quantitation. CD4 T cells (i.e., T-helper cells) are the main target of HIV, and a decrease in the number of CD4 T cells in the peripheral blood is a hallmark characteristic of HIV infection and its end stage, AIDS. The CD4 T cells are detected by fluorescent-labeled monoclonal antibodies to the T-cell antigen, CD3, and the helper-T-cell marker, CD4. The amount of fluorescence emitted by the cells is recorded by an instrument called a *flow cytometer* (see Chapters 13 and 24).

Monoclonal antibodies as therapeutic agents. Monoclonal antibodies are being used as therapeutic agents to treat a variety of diseases, especially cancer and autoimmune disorders. Some examples include the antibody trastuzumab (Herceptin), directed against the HER-2 protein, which is amplified in some patients with breast cancer; rituximab (Rituxan), which targets the B-cell marker CD20 and is used to treat patients with non-Hodgkin lymphoma and other B-cell malignancies; and adalimumab (Humira), a monoclonal antibody that blocks the action of tumor necrosis factor-α (TNF-α), a cytokine that plays a pathogenic role in rheumatoid arthritis. The use of monoclonal antibodies as therapeutic agents continues to grow. This represents a rapidly developing area in pharmacology that is impacting several fields of medicine by changing treatment options for many diseases (see Chapter 25).

Research applications. Monoclonal antibodies have been an important tool in biological research, and they have played a major role in many scientific discoveries. For example, binding of monoclonal antibodies to cell surface antigens has been used in defining the roles of various proteins in cell function. Monoclonal antibodies have also been used to isolate different cell populations from a mixture of cells so that their properties and functions can be analyzed more accurately.

Knowledge Check 3-6

Monoclonal antibodies differ from other antibodies in that they are:

a. Produced by a single cell
b. Derived from a clone of identical cells
c. Obtained from cultures of B cells
d. Coded for by different genes

KEY CONCEPTS

General Structure and Functions of Immunoglobulins

- Most immunoglobulins migrate to the gamma region upon serum electrophoresis.
- The basic structural unit for all immunoglobulins is a tetrapeptide composed of two light chains and two heavy chains joined together by disulfide bonds.
- The five classes of antibodies are IgM, IgG, IgA, IgD, and IgE. IgG, IgD, and IgE exist as monomers. IgA has a dimeric form in the secretions, whereas IgM is a pentamer. The subunits of IgM and dimeric IgA are held together by a J chain.
- Kappa and lambda light chains are found in all types of immunoglobulins, but the heavy chains differ for each immunoglobulin class.
- The enzyme papain cleaves IgG above the set of disulfide bonds that hold the heavy chains together. This creates two Fab fragments that can bind antigen and an Fc fragment that contains the constant regions of the molecule that are responsible for its biologic functions. The enzyme pepsin cleaves IgG below that set of disulfide bonds, creating a fragment with two antigen binding sites called "F(ab')$_2$."
- Each immunoglobulin molecule has constant and variable regions. The variable region is at the amino-terminal end, within the Fab fragment; this determines the specificity of the molecule for a particular antigen.
- The constant region, located at the carboxy-terminal end of the molecule, contains the Fc fragment and is responsible for binding to complement and to effector cells such as neutrophils, basophils, eosinophils, and mast cells.
- Opsonization refers to the coating of a foreign antigen by antibody to enhance phagocytosis through binding of the Fc portion of the antibody to receptors on neutrophils and macrophages.
- ADCC is a process by which IgG binds to Fc receptors on macrophages, monocytes, neutrophils, and NK cells, triggering the release of enzymes that cause extracellular destruction of antigen.
- The five different types of heavy chains are called "isotypes." Isotypes are unique to each Ig class or subclass within a species.
- Allotypes are minor variations in a particular type of heavy chain. They are genetically determined markers that are shared by some individuals of the same species.
- Idiotypes are the variable portion of the heavy and light chains unique to a particular immunoglobulin molecule; they are essential to the formation of unique antigen binding sites.

Antibody Classes

- IgG is relatively small and easily penetrates tissues. IgG is a monomer that is capable of binding to complement, mediating opsonization, participating in ADCC, and neutralizing bacterial toxins. It is the only immunoglobulin that can cross the placenta.
- IgM is a large pentamer whose subunits are held together by a protein known as the "J chain." IgM is more efficient at complement fixation than IgG because it has more binding sites for complement. IgM is also very efficient in agglutinating antigens. IgM is known as the "primary response antibody" because it is the first Ig to appear in the maturing infant and the first to be produced by the host during an immune response.
- IgA is the main immunoglobulin in the body's secretions. Secretory IgA is a dimer that contains a J chain and a secretory component, which protects it from enzymatic digestion while it patrols mucosal surfaces. IgA is also found in breast milk and thus is involved in the passive transfer of immunity from mother to infant.
- IgD exists mainly as a surface receptor for antigen on B cells, and its level in the serum is low.
- IgE binds to mast cells and basophils to initiate an inflammatory response that plays a role in allergic reactions.

Immunologic Memory: Primary and Secondary Antibody Responses

- The primary antibody response is mounted after the first time an individual is exposed to an antigen. It has a relatively long lag phase (usually 5 to 7 days before antibody can be detected) and results in low levels of IgM and IgG, which decline during a period of a few weeks.
- The secondary response to antigen, also known as the "memory" or "anamnestic response," occurs after a second or subsequent exposure of the host to the same antigen. The secondary response occurs more rapidly than the primary response because

memory lymphocytes are activated. The amount of IgM is similar to that of the primary response, whereas IgG levels are much greater than in the primary response. The IgG levels decline slowly and provide long-term immunity to the antigen. IgG produced in the secondary response also has a higher binding affinity for the antigen.

Antibody Specificity and Diversity

- Clonal selection is a fundamental concept of the immune response. In this process, when antigen is introduced into the body, it binds to unique receptors on selected B cells, stimulating only those B cells to divide and differentiate into plasma cells that produce antibody specific for that antigen.
- Several genes code for the variable and constant regions of a particular immunoglobulin: The V_H, D, and J genes code for the variable portion of the Ig heavy chains, and there is one constant-region gene for each Ig class; a similar set of genes codes for the Ig light chains, except they do not include the D genes. Through a random selection process, the individual gene segments are joined to make antibody of a single specificity. The antibody appears on the surface of B lymphocytes, where it serves as a receptor for antigen.
- Antibody diversity results from several different mechanisms: VDJ gene recombination, junctional diversity, various combinations of heavy and light chains, and somatic hypermutation.
- During the course of the immune response, Ig production switches from IgM to another Ig class because of genetic recombination between the constant-region genes for the different heavy chains.

Monoclonal Antibodies

- In the traditional method, monoclonal antibodies are made by hybridoma cells, which are created by fusing an antibody-producing B cell with a malignant myeloma cell line that contributes the property of immortality. The fused cells are isolated in a selective medium called "HAT." Those hybridomas secreting the desired antibody are selected and grown in larger quantities.
- More recently, molecular methods, transgenic mice, and genetically engineered bacteriophages have been developed to produce monoclonal antibodies. These techniques have made it possible to produce antibodies that are partially or fully human, thus reducing or eliminating the chance of hypersensitivity reactions to mouse proteins in patients who are given these antibodies as therapeutic agents.
- Monoclonal antibodies are used as reagents in laboratory tests and as therapies for the treatment of various diseases.

Study Guide: The Five Classes of Immunoglobulins

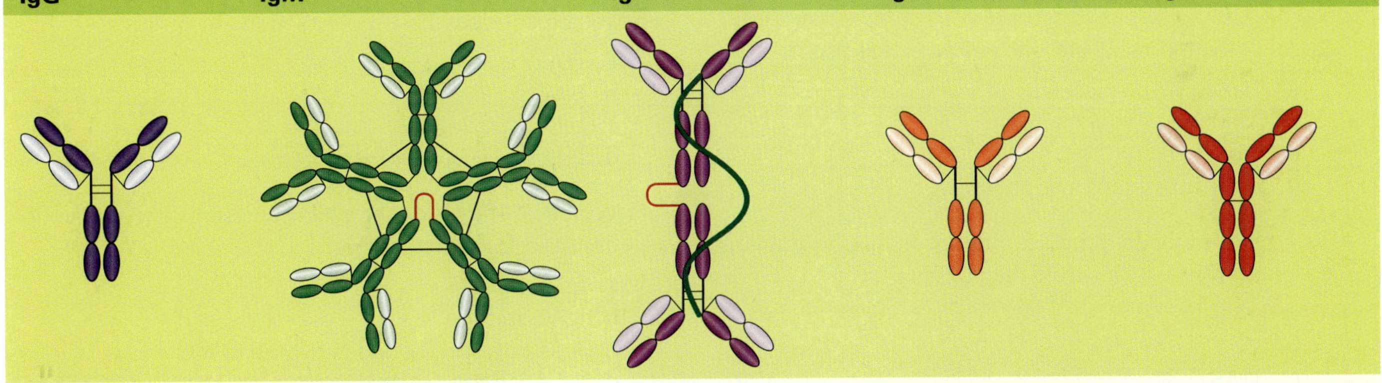

IgG	IgM	IgA	IgD	IgE
Most abundant in serum Binds complement Opsonization—binds to receptors on phagocytic cells Able to cross placenta Increases with second exposure to antigen	Primary response antibody; indicates acute infection First Ig to be produced by fetus; specific IgM in newborn serum indicates congenital infection Pentamer with 10 antigen binding sites Subunits held together by a J chain Binds efficiently to complement Causes efficient agglutination of antigens	Monomer in serum and dimer in secretions Protects mucosal surfaces Present in breast milk J chain holds subunits of the dimer together Dimer has secretory component	Present as an antigen receptor on B-cell membrane Role in B-cell activation Identifies mature B cells	Binds to mast cells and basophils Triggers allergic response Role in immune response to parasites

CASE STUDIES

1. A 15-year-old patient exhibited symptoms of fever, fatigue, nausea, and sore throat. The patient went to a primary care physician, who ordered a rapid strep test and a test for infectious mononucleosis to be performed in the office. The rapid strep test result was negative, but the test result for infectious mononucleosis was faintly positive. The patient mentioned the possibility of having had mononucleosis about 2 years earlier, but it was never officially diagnosed. A serum sample was sent to a reference laboratory to test for antibodies to specific Epstein-Barr viral antigens. The results indicated the presence of IgM only.

Questions

a. Is this a new or reactivated case of mononucleosis? Explain your answer.
b. How do the results relate to the difference between a primary and a secondary response to exposure to the same antigen?

2. A 10-year-old child experienced one cold after another in the springtime. The child had missed several days of school, and the mother, who was greatly concerned, took the child to the pediatrician, worried that the child might be immunocompromised because they could not seem to fight off infections. A blood sample was obtained and sent to a reference laboratory to determine antibody levels, including an IgE level. The patient's IgM, IgG, and IgA levels were all normal for child's age, but the IgE level was greatly increased.

Questions

a. What does the increase in IgE signify?
b. Should there be a concern about the patient being immunocompromised?

REVIEW QUESTIONS

1. Which of the following is characteristic of the variable domains of immunoglobulins?
   a. They represent the complement-binding site.
   b. They are at the amino-terminal ends of the molecules.
   c. They are found only on heavy chains.
   d. They are found only on light chains.
2. All of the following are true of IgM *except* that it:
   a. Can cross the placenta
   b. Can bind complement
   c. Has a J chain
   d. Is a primary response antibody
3. Which antibody provides protection to the growing fetus because it can cross the placenta?
   a. IgA
   b. IgG
   c. IgM
   d. IgE
4. How many antigen binding sites does an IgM molecule in the serum have?
   a. 2
   b. 4
   c. 6
   d. 10
5. A Fab fragment consists of:
   a. Two heavy chains
   b. Two light chains
   c. One light chain and one-half of a heavy chain
   d. One light chain and an entire heavy chain
6. Which antibody best protects mucosal surfaces?
   a. IgA
   b. IgG
   c. IgD
   d. IgM
7. Which of the following pairs represents two different immunoglobulin allotypes?
   a. IgM and IgG
   b. IgA1 and IgA2
   c. Anti-human IgM and anti-human IgG
   d. IgG1m3 and IgG1m17
8. Which of the following components is found in all five classes of immunoglobulins?
   a. J chain
   b. κ and λ light chains
   c. Binding sites for complement
   d. Binding sites for macrophages

9. Which of the following are light chains of antibody molecules?
   a. Kappa
   b. Gamma
   c. Mu
   d. Alpha

10. If the results of serum protein electrophoresis show a significant decrease in the gamma band, which of the following is a likely possibility?
   a. Normal response to active infection
   b. Multiple myeloma
   c. Immunodeficiency of antibody production
   d. Monoclonal gammopathy

11. The subclasses of IgG differ mainly in:
   a. The type of light chain
   b. The arrangement of disulfide bonds
   c. The ability to act as opsonins
   d. Molecular weight

12. Which best describes the role of the secretory component of IgA?
   a. A transport mechanism across epithelial cells
   b. A means of joining two IgA monomers together
   c. An aid to trapping antigen
   d. Enhancement of complement fixation by the classical pathway

13. Amino acid sequences in the variable portion of the antibody molecule that constitute the antigen binding site are called:
   a. Allotypes
   b. Isotypes
   c. Idiotypes
   d. Crosstypes

14. Which best characterizes the secondary antibody response?
   a. Equal amounts of IgM and IgG are produced.
   b. There is an increase in IgM only.
   c. There is a large increase in IgG but not IgM.
   d. The lag phase is the same as in the primary response.

15. Which of the following can be attributed to the clonal selection hypothesis of antibody formation?
   a. Each plasma cell can make antibodies to many antigens.
   b. B cells are preprogrammed for specific antibody synthesis.
   c. Antibodies can alter their shape to conform to an antigen.
   d. Cell receptors break off and become circulating antibody.

16. All of the following are true of IgE *except* that it:
   a. Cannot bind complement
   b. Is heat stable
   c. Attaches to tissue mast cells
   d. Is increased in the serum of allergic persons

17. Which best describes the genes that code for immunoglobulin molecules?
   a. All genes are located on the same chromosome.
   b. Light chain gene rearrangement occurs before heavy chain gene rearrangement.
   c. Four different gene segments are involved in coding for heavy chains.
   d. Lambda gene rearrangement occurs before kappa gene rearrangement.

18. What is the purpose of HAT medium in the production of a monoclonal antibody?
   a. Fusing the two cell types
   b. Restricting the growth of myeloma cells
   c. Restricting the growth of spleen cells
   d. Restricting antibody production to the IgM class

19. How would cleavage of an antibody molecule with the enzyme pepsin affect the function of the antibody?
   a. It would be unable to bind antigen.
   b. It could bind to a greater number of antigens.
   c. It would have increased complement-binding activity.
   d. It could not bind to macrophages.

20. Suppose a patient was tested for an infection with a particular microorganism. Antibody tests indicated the presence of high-affinity IgG antibody to the organism but absence of specific IgM. These results indicate:
   a. Early-stage infection
   b. An active infection
   c. A past infection
   d. An incubation period

Chapter 3 Answer Key

Answers to Knowledge Checks

3.1 a 3.2 d 3.3 1-b; 2-d; 3-e; 4-a; 5-c 3.4 c
3.5 **b** 3.6 b

Answers to Review Questions

1. b	2. a	3. b	4. d	5. c	6. a	7. d
8. b	9. a	10. c	11. b	12. a	13. c	14. c
15. b	16. b	17. c	18. b	19. d	20. c	

Nature of Antigens and the Major Histocompatibility Complex

4

Aaron Glass, PhD, MB^CM(ASCP)

LEARNING OUTCOMES

After finishing this chapter, you should be able to:

4.1 Define and characterize the nature of immunogens.

4.2 Differentiate an immunogen from an antigen.

4.3 Describe four important traits of immunogens that affect their ability to stimulate a host response.

4.4 Discuss biological properties of individuals that influence the nature of the immune response.

4.5 Define *haptens* and describe some of their characteristics.

4.6 Describe the relationship between an epitope and an antigen.

4.7 Discuss the functions of adjuvants.

4.8 Differentiate autoantigens, alloantigens, and heterophile antigens.

4.9 Describe the inheritance of the major histocompatibility complex (MHC) and human leukocyte antigen (HLA) genes and define the term *haplotype* in this context.

4.10 Compare and contrast class I and class II MHC antigens in terms of their association with HLA genes, cellular expression, molecular structure, source of peptide antigens, and interaction with $CD4^+$ vs. $CD8^+$ T lymphocytes.

4.11 Describe the intracellular pathways leading to the presentation of peptide antigens at the cell surface by class I and class II MHC molecules.

4.12 Explain the clinical significance of the class I and class II MHC molecules.

CHAPTER OUTLINE

You can go to **fadavis.com** keyword stevens for the laboratory exercises that accompany this text.

As we discussed in Chapter 2, a hallmark of innate immunity is the ability of the host to respond nonspecifically to infection by recognizing broad classes of molecular patterns found within a pathogen or on its surface. In contrast, adaptive immunity targets highly specific molecules that are usually unique to each pathogen. While a wide range of immune cells and molecules are involved in the innate response, the key cells responsible for the specificity, diversity, and memory associated with adaptive immunity are the T and B lymphocytes.

Two key terms used to define the substances targeted by adaptive immune responses are *antigen* and *immunogen*. An **antigen** is a substance that is specifically recognized by the adaptive immune system, whereas an **immunogen** is a substance capable of causing an adaptive response. The main distinction between an antigen and an immunogen is the latter's ability to successfully stimulate an immune response. To achieve immunogenicity, certain conditions must be met, meaning that some antigens are not immunogenic. Thus, all immunogens are antigens, but not all antigens are necessarily immunogens. Despite this distinction, immunologists often use these terms interchangeably.

One of the most exciting areas of immunologic research focuses on how and why certain antigens act as immunogens. Multiple factors influence our response to antigens: unique biological properties of the individual, the nature of the antigen itself, antigen processing in conjunction with inherited *major histocompatibility complex (MHC)* molecules (discussed later), and antigen presentation to T cells. In this chapter, we focus on all these areas and discuss clinical implications of some recent findings.

Factors Influencing the Immune Response

Many factors are known to influence immunogenicity. These factors can arise from the biology of the host, the way antigen is encountered, and the nature of the antigen itself. Outbred populations such as humans exhibit diverse biological properties, meaning that each person has unique traits, and certain traits strongly influence the nature of the immune response. Factors including age, health status, and genetics are all important in determining whether an immune response is mounted against a particular antigen. Similarly, the antigen dose and route of exposure also influence immunogenicity. Finally, and fundamentally, not all antigens are equivalent in their ability to stimulate an immune response.

In general, older adults are more likely to exhibit *immunosenescence,* or a decreased response to antigenic stimulation with age. Similarly, neonates do not fully respond to immunogens because their immune systems are not completely developed. For people of all ages, overall health strongly influences immunity because those who are malnourished, fatigued, or stressed are less likely to mount a successful immune response.

An individual's genetic composition plays a major role in determining the immune response, or lack thereof, to an antigen. Although many genes influence innate and adaptive immunity, the **major histocompatibility complex (MHC)** genes exert perhaps the most profound overall influence. The MHC is a system of genes that code for cell surface molecules that play an important role in antigen recognition. Further details are found later in this chapter.

To stimulate an adaptive immune response, a certain amount of antigen must be introduced into the body. Small quantities of antigen, as would be found in very minor infections, simply do not meet the threshold of stimulation required for activation of an adaptive immune response. Throughout the human life span, such minor infections occur continuously and are quickly and efficiently cleared by innate immune mechanisms, reserving adaptive immunity for persistent infections that involve relatively greater quantities of antigen. Conversely, very large quantities of antigen can be detrimental to the development of an immune response by encouraging lymphocyte *tolerance,* or a state of ignorance, toward a particular antigen.

There are many ways that we encounter antigens in nature. How and where antigens enter our bodies can impact the amount of antigen required to generate an immune response. Possible routes of exposure include airborne inhalation of aerosol droplets or particles, intravenous (into a vein), intradermal (into the skin), subcutaneous (beneath the skin), intramuscular (into a muscle), and oral (into the mouth). One mechanism explaining the differential response to antigens is that each of these routes ultimately shuttles antigens to different secondary lymphoid tissues, where they encounter distinct populations of immune cells. For example, a deep puncture wound may introduce antigens intravenously, where they are carried by the blood to the spleen, where an immune response will be mounted. On the other hand, superficial cuts and scratches may lead antigens to enter subcutaneously, in which case they are delivered to local lymph nodes. Oral introduction of an antigen can be counterproductive to immunity, as this route of entry is associated with the development of *oral tolerance,* a phenomenon where cells of the adaptive immune system ignore antigens delivered via the gastrointestinal tract. This mechanism is believed to have evolved so that we do not mount immune responses against the foods we eat.

Knowledge Check 4-1

Which of the following antigen exposures would you expect to elicit the strongest immune response?

a. Oral ingestion of a substance
b. Inoculation with an extremely small quantity of a substance
c. Intradermal exposure of a substance by an older adult
d. Intramuscular exposure to a substance by a *healthy* individual

Traits of Antigens and Immunogens

In general, **immunogenicity**—the ability of an antigen to stimulate a host response—depends on the following characteristics:

- Molecular size
- Foreignness
- Chemical composition and complexity
- The ability to be processed and presented within MHC molecules

Usually, an immunogen must have a molecular weight of at least 10,000 Da to be recognized by the immune system, and the most effective immunogens typically have a molecular weight of more than 100,000 Da. Although a few substances with molecular weights less than 1,000 Da are known to induce immune responses, generally the greater the molecular weight, the more potent is a substance's immunogenicity.

Another characteristic shared by strong immunogens is *foreignness,* or unrelatedness to the host. To prevent the immune system from attacking the body's own cells and tissues, lymphocytes are carefully selected during their development to ensure that the pool of mature lymphocytes responds only to antigens *not* recognized as self (see Chapter 15 for details). Typically, the more taxonomically distant an antigen's source is from the host, the greater the likelihood that host lymphocytes will react to it, dramatically increasing the probability that the antigen will be a successful immunogen. For example, plant protein is a better immunogen for an animal than is material from a related animal.

Immunogenicity is also determined by a substance's chemical composition and molecular complexity. Proteins are the most effective immunogens. In contrast, synthetic polymers are composed of a few simple repeating units with no bending or folding within the molecule, and these materials are nonimmunogenic. For this reason, they are used in making artificial heart valves, joint replacements, and other medical devices.

The immunogenicity of a substance is also strongly influenced by the type of molecules it is composed of. Proteins are highly immunogenic when compared with other biomolecules, such as polysaccharides, nucleic acids, and lipids. The mechanisms underlying the strong immunogenicity of proteins are related to (1) differences in how the T and B lymphocytes detect antigens and (2) a requirement for interactions between B cells and T cells for an effective antibody response to occur. We discuss these concepts in Chapter 5.

Proteins are composed of subunits known as *amino acids,* which are covalently linked together in polypeptide chains of varying length. The linear sequence of amino acids comprises the *primary* structure of a protein. Each type of amino acid incorporated into a protein possesses distinct chemical properties, and interactions between the amino acids within a protein's primary structure cause the chain to bend, kink, and loop, forming basic three-dimensional shapes, or *secondary* structures. Two common secondary structures found in proteins are the *α helices,* which have peptide chains that twist to form a spiral, and *β-pleated sheets,* in which chains form undulating zigzags that coalesce into a planar shape. In the third, or *tertiary,* level of protein structure, these basic secondary structures fold on themselves once again, bringing distant regions of the primary amino acid chain together and representing the spatial or three-dimensional orientation of the entire molecule. At the final level of protein structure, known as *quaternary,* two or more polypeptide chains come together, forming a multimeric unit **(Fig. 4–1)**. The interactions between amino acids that dictate the overall three-dimensional shape of a protein are very complex but can ultimately be traced back to the sequence of peptides found in the primary structure.

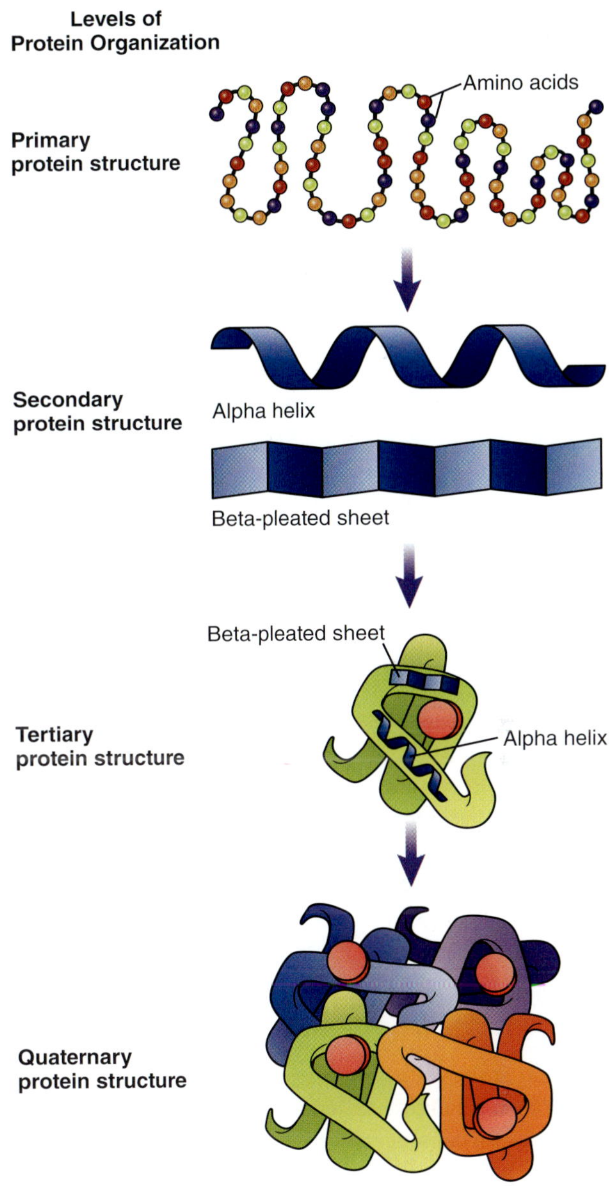

FIGURE 4–1 Levels of protein organization.

The activating receptors of both T and B lymphocytes can recognize proteins, but the levels of protein structure at which this recognition occurs are very different. T cells, as you will learn later in this chapter, detect small fragments of a protein, known as *peptides,* and rely on MHC molecules to cradle these peptides for antigen recognition to occur. Thus, T cells "see" the primary structures, or amino acid sequences, of small pieces of a protein. The receptors on B cells, on the other hand, are activated by binding to a protein's exterior-facing amino acids. In this way, B cells "see" the exposed tertiary or quaternary structures of a protein.

An effective B-cell response to most antigens (one that involves the production of high-affinity antibodies and results in immunologic memory) requires "help" from T cells. In other words, to mount an appropriate B-cell response, T cells must also be activated so that they can provide necessary physical and chemical signals to the B cell.

Polysaccharides are less immunogenic than proteins because of their smaller relative size and because T cells do not recognize carbohydrates. Therefore, exposure to pure polysaccharide does not result in T-cell activation, and B cells that respond to a particular polysaccharide antigen may not receive crucial T-cell help. As immunogens, carbohydrates most often occur in the form of glycolipids or glycoproteins. Many of the blood group antigens are composed of such carbohydrate complexes. For example, the A, B, and H blood group antigens are glycolipids, and the Rh and Lewis antigens are glycoproteins. Other carbohydrates that are important immunogens are the capsular polysaccharides of bacteria such as *Streptococcus pneumoniae*. Pure nucleic acids and lipids are not immunogenic by themselves, although a response can be generated when they are attached to a suitable carrier protein (see *Haptens*). This is the case for autoantibodies to DNA that are formed in systemic lupus erythematosus (SLE). These autoantibodies are stimulated by a DNA-protein complex rather than by DNA itself.

Finally, for a substance to elicit a successful adaptive response, it must undergo antigen processing, which involves enzymatic digestion to create small peptides or pieces that can be complexed to MHC molecules for presentation to responsive T lymphocytes. The particular MHC molecules expressed by an individual also govern responsiveness to specific antigens. Each person inherits genes encoding only a limited repertoire of MHC molecules, as we discuss in the section on the genes coding for MHC molecules.

Knowledge Check 4-2

Which of the following answers best describes how T lymphocytes detect antigens?

a. T cells recognize carbohydrate antigens.
b. Receptors on T cells bind to amino acids on a protein's exterior.
c. T cells detect the tertiary structures of antigens.
d. T-cell receptors recognize antigen peptide fragments bound to MHC molecules.

Epitopes

Although an immunogen must have a molecular weight of at least 10,000 Da, only a small portion of the overall molecule is recognized by each individual lymphocyte. This key portion of the immunogen is known as an *antigenic determinant* or *epitope*. **Epitopes** are the precise molecular shapes or configurations recognized by receptors on B cells or the peptide sequences detected by T-cell receptors. Large molecules may contain many epitopes, and each epitope is capable of triggering the production of a specific antibody or activating a T cell. B cells may recognize two types of epitopes: (1) **linear epitopes** that consist of sequential amino acids on a single polypeptide chain or (2) **conformational epitopes** that result from the folding of one or more polypeptide chains, bringing together amino acids that may be distant from each other so that they are recognized together **(Fig. 4–2).** Stimulation of a B-lymphocyte response requires that epitopes be found on the surface of a molecule, accessible to the B-cell receptor, and that these sites contain more than one copy of the epitope so that *cross-linking* of the B-cell receptors may occur; in other words, the receptors are connected by their attachment to the antigen (see Fig. 4-3B). This can be accomplished by as few as 6 to 15 amino acids. In contrast, T cells detect only linear epitopes that are liberated once a protein has been degraded during antigen processing. This means that many T cells respond to cryptic epitopes found deep within the interiors of large proteins that are not available for B-cell recognition. As mentioned previously, T-cell recognition also requires that these peptide antigens are presented by MHC molecules.

Critical Thinking 4-1

Heat and certain chemical treatments can cause protein denaturation, a permanent change in three-dimensional shape. Would you expect denaturation to have a greater impact on protein antigen recognition by B cells or T cells?

Haptens

Many substances are too small to be recognized by B cells but can stimulate a response if bound to a larger molecule. A **hapten** is a substance that is nonantigenic by itself but becomes antigenic when combined with, or *conjugated* to, a larger carrier molecule such as a protein. The hapten-carrier complexes can initiate the production of antibodies by cross-linking receptors on the surface of the B cell **(Fig. 4–3)**; these antibodies can then react with the hapten even in the absence of the carrier. Small size and the presence of a solitary determinant site also make haptens incapable of participating in antibody-mediated precipitation or agglutination reactions because cross-linking with more than one antibody molecule is not possible.

Examples of haptens found in nature are the *catechol* compounds in the urushiol sap of plants such as poison ivy (*Toxicodendron radicans* and *rydbergii*). Once in contact with the skin, oily catechols diffuse deep into the dermis and bind to skin proteins, instantly becoming recognizable to immune cells. The strong immunogenicity and antigenicity of the catechol-protein conjugate stimulates B and T cells, giving rise to the contact dermatitis associated with poison ivy exposure. Other clinically relevant examples of haptens include certain pharmaceutical drugs that can bind to host proteins to provoke an immune response in the form of a drug allergy.

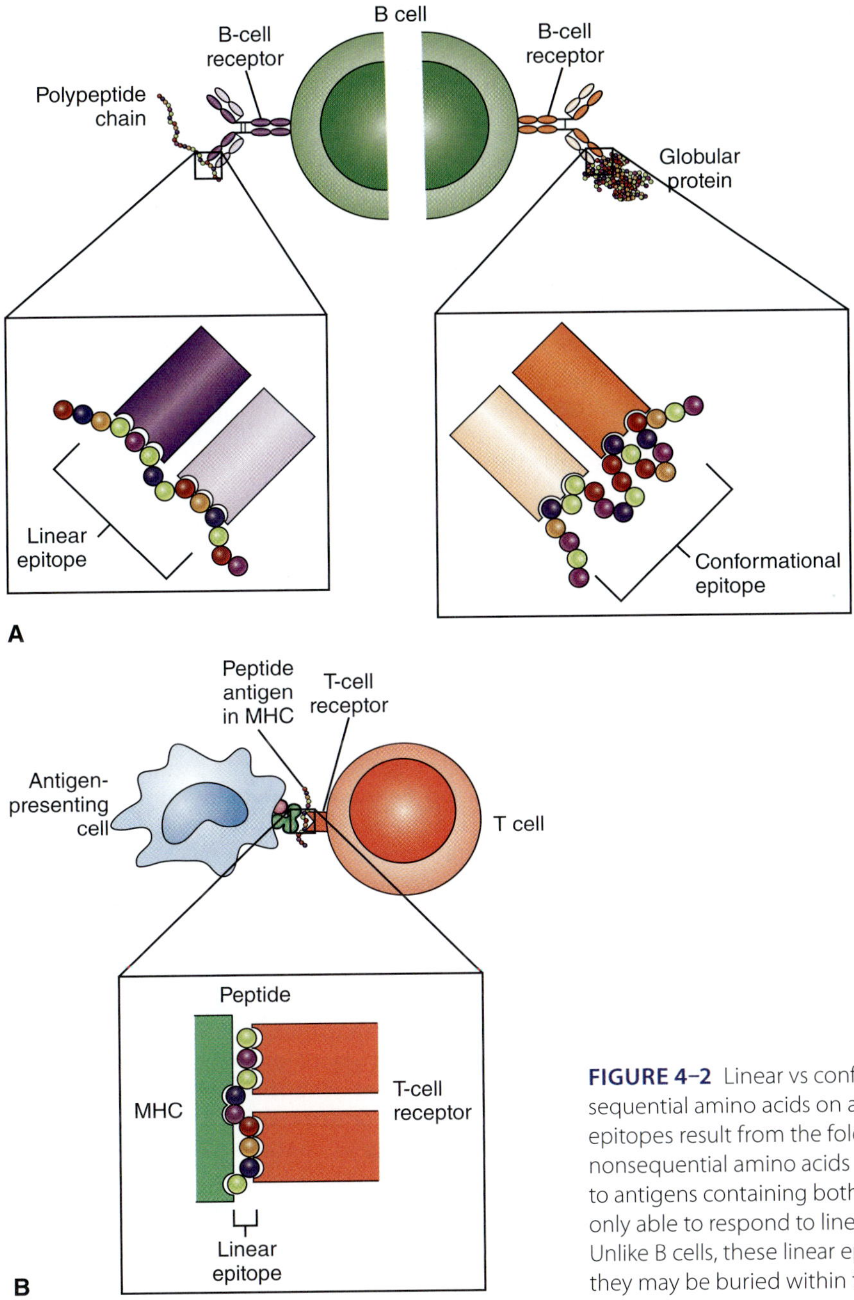

FIGURE 4–2 Linear vs conformational epitopes. (A) Linear epitopes consist of sequential amino acids on a single polypeptide chain, whereas conformational epitopes result from the folding of a polypeptide chain or chains, placing nonsequential amino acids in close proximity. B cells are capable of responding to antigens containing both linear and conformational epitopes. (B) T cells are only able to respond to linear epitopes that are displayed in MHC molecules. Unlike B cells, these linear epitopes need not be found at the surface of a protein; they may be buried within the molecule.

4-1 Clinical Correlations

Haptens: A Double-Edged Sword

Drug hypersensitivities (allergies) can theoretically occur with any pharmaceutical compound capable of binding to human proteins after administration. One common example is the immune reaction that occurs in some people in response to antibiotic compounds containing a β-lactam ring, such as penicillin. Under certain conditions, these compounds can form covalent bonds with plasma proteins such as albumin. Not only does the binding of the comparatively tiny hapten (penicillin, 334 Da) to the more massive carrier protein (albumin, ~66,000 Da) provide a larger epitope for B-cell receptor recognition, but the hapten also remains bound to antigenic peptides throughout antigen processing, providing a powerful signal for T-cell activation.

Clever vaccinologists have taken advantage of the hapten-carrier phenomenon by developing *conjugate vaccines*. The surface antigens of many encapsulated pathogens, such as *Haemophilus influenzae*, are composed of complex polysaccharides, which do not elicit a strong or long-lasting immune response. Conjugate vaccines combine weakly antigenic capsular polysaccharides with a carrier protein, such as tetanus toxoid, to induce strong immunity against the hapten (capsular polysaccharide). Millions of lives have been saved by effective conjugate vaccines targeting the bacteria that cause pneumonia and meningitis (see Chapter 25).

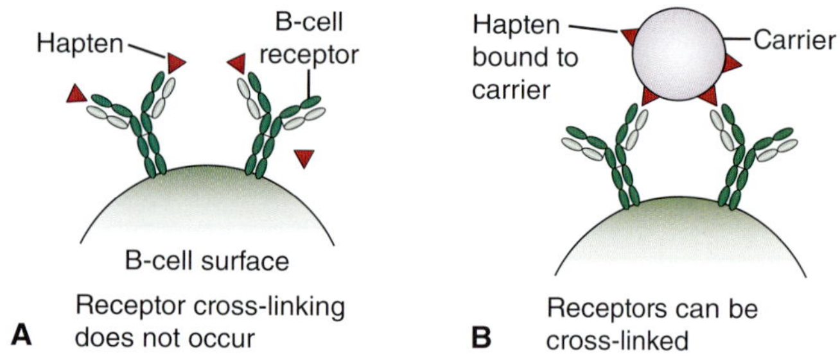

FIGURE 4–3 Characteristics of haptens. (A) Haptens bind B-cell receptors, but the receptors are not cross-linked; therefore, no activation occurs. (B) Hapten-carrier complexes cross-link receptors, leading to B-cell activation and antibody production.

Adjuvants

For the purpose of vaccination, pathogen-derived proteins and glycoproteins often represent ideal antigens. However, proteins are not necessarily highly immunogenic. The generation of a robust immune response against proteins requires stimulation of innate immunity, especially antigen-presenting cells (APCs), such as dendritic cells. Substances delivered simultaneously with an antigen for the purpose of *potentiating*, or enhancing, the immune response are known as **adjuvants.**

Adjuvants are substances that increase the immunogenicity of an antigen by stimulating innate immune receptors, such as toll-like receptors, that detect the presence of infection or danger. Adjuvants are also thought to work by preventing antigens from diffusing away from an inoculation site, allowing innate immune cells to accumulate in the site. In this way, adjuvants deceive the immune system that an infection is under way, even if the vaccine antigens are essentially harmless.

Many vaccines use adjuvants to achieve protective immunity against the target antigen (see Chapter 25). Vaccines that do not require adjuvants are usually composed of whole pathogens or substances derived from pathogens that have been killed or weakened. Some vaccines consist of microbes that have been altered so that they are capable of limited replication within a human host but cannot establish a productive infection. In vaccines composed of such live or killed pathogens, no adjuvant is required, because the pathogen itself supplies the immune danger signals necessary to stimulate an immune response.

Many newer vaccines consist of recombinant antigenic proteins or nucleic acids that encode antigens. These forms of antigen are carefully developed and manufactured in sterile laboratory settings and are not ideal immunogens; they require the inclusion of adjuvants to trigger an immune response. The improvement of existing adjuvants and the design of new adjuvants is a rapidly developing field in immunology.

Critical Thinking 4-2

The synthetic adjuvant AS04 has a chemical structure similar to that of the bacterial structural molecule lipopolysaccharide (endotoxin). Based on your knowledge of innate immune receptors (Chapter 2 and Table 2–1), which toll-like receptor is most likely to be activated by AS04?

Relationship of Antigens to the Host

Antigens can be broadly categorized according to their relationship to the host. **Autoantigens** are those antigens that belong to the host (i.e. self-antigens). These do not evoke an immune response under normal circumstances. However, if an immune response does occur to autoantigens, it may result in an autoimmune disease (see Chapter 15). **Alloantigens** are from other members of the host's species and are capable of eliciting an immune response. Alloantigens are important considerations in transplantation immunology and in blood transfusions. **Heteroantigens** are from other species, such as other animals, plants, or microorganisms.

4-2 Clinical Correlations

Inoculation With Animal Antigens and Serum Sickness

In the late 1800s, immunologists began using animal serum to protect against toxins and venoms. In one famous example, Emil von Behring identified the protective activity of serum against diphtheria toxin. In a series of experiments, von Behring treated laboratory animals with small doses of the toxin. Anti-toxin antibodies generated in vaccinated animals could then be used to rescue other animals, or even humans, from diphtheria infection by binding to and neutralizing the toxin. Throughout the beginning of the 20th century, many different anti-toxins and anti-venoms were prepared, most commonly by using horse serum. As the therapeutic use of animal anti-toxins grew in popularity, adverse events, including rash, fever, joint pain, and even anaphylactic shock, were observed in some individuals after treatment. These reactions, termed *serum sickness*, were later understood to be immune reactions against heteroantigens contained within the anti-toxin inoculum.

Today, clinical use of animal anti-toxins is rare, but anti-venoms against snake and spider bites are still prepared by horse immunization. Manufacturers have taken several precautionary steps to reduce the antigenic strength of these life-saving medications, such as preparing purified anti-venom antibodies treated with enzymes to isolate only the region of the immunoglobulin molecules that neutralizes venom.

Despite the dramatic progress, serum sickness reactions can still be observed in patients receiving some animal-derived drugs. One example is the immunosuppressant drug anti-thymocyte globulin, which consists of antibodies from rabbits or horses that have been immunized with immature human T cells (thymocytes). Although this drug suppresses T-cell activity, some people can experience an immune response targeting the animal immunoglobulins. Additionally, some monoclonal antibody therapies consist of immunoglobulins that are partially mouse derived (see Chapter 25). Serum sickness reactions can be mounted by patients against the mouse-derived portions of these antibodies.

Heterophile antigens are antigens expressed by bacteria or by virally infected cells with structures similar to certain alloantigens or heteroantigens. The human blood group A and B antigens are examples of heterophile antigens that share a high degree of similarity to bacterial polysaccharides. In individuals who express only the A or the B antigen, or individuals who express neither the A nor B antigen (those with blood group O), exposure to common bacteria stimulates the production of antibodies that can target the A or B alloantigens on other individuals' erythrocytes. The presence of these naturally occurring antibodies is an important consideration in selecting the appropriate blood type for transfusion purposes.

The classical heterophile antigens (for which the term was coined) are produced by cells infected with Epstein-Barr virus (EBV), which causes infectious mononucleosis (IM; see Chapter 23). During EBV infection, an immune response is initiated against cell membrane glycoproteins expressed by infected cells. The historical Paul-Bunnell test for EBV IM relied on the fact that similar glycoproteins are found on erythrocytes from nonhuman animals. By observing the agglutination of sheep erythrocytes, a titer of EBV heterophile antibodies could be determined, providing a reasonable confirmation of IM. Current rapid screening tests for IM detect similar antibodies against heterophile antigens found in the sera of EBV-infected patients that cross-react with horse or bovine antigens.

While EBV heterophile antibodies are helpful in the diagnosis of IM, other heterophile antibodies can confound clinical immunoassays. In many assays for specific analytes, animal antibodies are used as reagents. Such antibody reagents may be bound to a surface and used to capture an analyte from a patient sample, or they may be covalently bound to reporter molecules, such as enzymes or fluorescent dyes, and used to detect the presence and quantity of an analyte. In rare cases, patient-produced heterophile antibodies can link together the reagent antibodies used for antigen capture and the reagent antibodies used for detection of the analyte, falsely elevating its apparent level. This concept is discussed in more detail in Chapter 11.

Major Histocompatibility Complex

The capacity to mount a T-cell response to an antigen is largely determined by an individual's MHC genes. The MHC genes encode glycoproteins that determine whether transplanted tissue is *histocompatible,* or accepted by the recipient, or if it is instead rejected as foreign. MHC molecules are found on all nucleated cells in the body, and they are pivotal in the development of both humoral and cell-mediated immunity. Although MHC molecules were initially identified by their antigenicity in the context of organ transplantation, their main immune function is to serve as carriers of peptide antigens for recognition by T cells. Unlike B cells, whose surface receptors recognize antigen directly, T-cell receptors require antigens to be bound to, or *presented* by, MHC molecules for recognition to occur.

In humans, the MHC genes and their glycoprotein products are referred to as **human leukocyte antigens (HLA)**; see Chapter 16. In most cases, immunologists use the terms MHC and HLA interchangeably with the caveat that animal models, such as mice *(Mus musculus),* possess MHC but not HLA (because they are not human).

Genes Coding for MHC Molecules (HLA Antigens)

The HLA genes are found on the short arm of chromosome 6 and are divided into three classes. Class I genes are found at three different locations (loci), termed *A, B,* and *C.* Class II genes are found in the D region, where there are several different loci, including *DR, DQ,* and *DP.* Only one gene codes for each MHC class I molecule. Class II molecules, in contrast, have one gene that codes for the α chain of the molecule and one or more genes that code for the β chain. The class III gene region lies between the class I and class II gene regions on chromosome 6. Class III genes code for the complement proteins, C4a, C4b, C2, and B, and cytokines such as tumor necrosis factor (TNF) **(Fig. 4–4).**

The class I and class II MHC proteins are involved in antigen recognition by T cells. In this role, they influence the varied collection, or *repertoire,* of antigens to which lymphocytes can respond. In contrast, class III molecules are secreted proteins that have important immune functions but are not expressed on cell surfaces.

MHC/HLA genes are highly polymorphic, meaning that many alternate forms, or **alleles,** of each MHC gene are found throughout the human population. In fact, the MHC is considered the most polymorphic system in the human genome. Different HLA alleles encode slightly different versions of each MHC protein. Thousands of different HLA-A alleles, HLA-B alleles, HLA-C alleles, and HLA-D alleles have been identified within the human population. This high degree of genetic variation, or *polymorphism,* is thought to improve survival of a species from infections. Having a diverse HLA repertoire among the human population allows for effective immune responses to essentially unlimited numbers of different pathogens, even if some individuals are unable to respond. Conversely, the antigenic uniqueness of MHC proteins is a major obstacle when matching organ donors to recipients.

Expression of MHC genes is *codominant* in nature, meaning that all an individual's MHC genes can be expressed. Since humans possess two copies of chromosome 6, each with genes encoding three MHC class I proteins (HLA-A, HLA-B, and HLA-C) and genes encoding at least three MHC class II proteins (HLA-DP, HLA-DR, and HLA-DQ), every person has the potential to produce at least 12 different MHCs. Occasionally, an individual will have two identical MHC alleles at a particular location, but such homozygosity is rare.

The proximity of the MHC genes to each other on the chromosome leads to their inheritance as a group, or **haplotype,** that consists of a specific combination of genes for HLA-A, HLA-B, HLA-C, HLA-DR, HLA-DP, and HLA-DQ. Individuals inherit one MHC haplotype from each parent. Because the number of unique haplotypes in the population is enormously large, knowing a person's haplotype can be useful in forensics, molecular genealogy, and paternity determination.

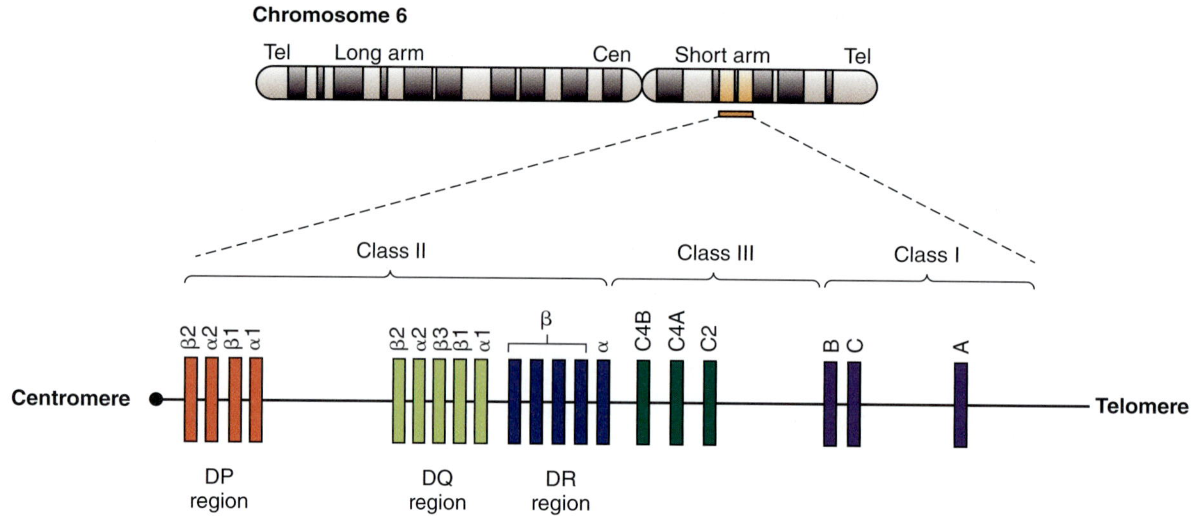

FIGURE 4–4 The major histocompatibility complex. Location of the class I, II, and III genes on chromosome 6. The class I MHC consists of loci A, B, and C, whereas the class II MHC has at least three loci: DR, DQ, and DP.

Knowledge Check 4-3

How many different class I molecules will be expressed on a cell from a person that inherits unique HLA alleles for all MHC genes?

a. 0
b. 3
c. 6
d. 12

Expression of Class I and II MHC Molecules

The class I and II MHC (HLA) genes encode proteins that localize to the cell surface. All the proteins of a particular class share structural similarities and are expressed by similar types of cells. Class I MHC molecules are expressed widely throughout the body. In contrast, class II MHC molecules are found primarily on *antigen-presenting cells (APCs),* which include monocytes, macrophages, dendritic cells, B lymphocytes, and thymic epithelial cells.

Although class I MHC molecules are expressed on all nucleated cells, expression levels can vary between different cell types. Class I expression is highest on lymphocytes and myeloid cells and is low or undetectable on liver hepatocytes, neural cells, muscle cells, and sperm. This may explain why engraftment of HLA-mismatched livers can be quite successful, whereas other solid-organ transplants require a much closer MHC match between donor and recipient. Additionally, HLA-C antigens are expressed at a much lower level than HLA-A and HLA-B antigens, so the latter two are the most important class I MHC antigens to consider for transplantation.

Class II MHC molecules are expressed in high levels on the surface of APCs, especially on dendritic cells, which are considered the most effective APCs. Among the class II antigens, HLA-DR is expressed at the highest level and accounts for about one-half of all the class II molecules found on an APC. Conversely, HLA-DP molecules are found in the lowest abundance.

Structure of Class I MHC Molecules

Each class I antigen is a glycoprotein dimer made up of two noncovalently linked polypeptide chains **(Fig. 4–5).** The class I α chain has a molecular weight of 44,000 Da, while an associated chain, β_2-*microglobulin,* has a molecular weight of 12,000 Da. β2-microglobulin is encoded by a single nonpolymorphic gene on chromosome 15 and is essential for the function of the class I molecule and stabilizes the MHC I-peptide complex. The class I α chain is folded into three domains—α1, α2, and α3—and it is inserted into the cell membrane via a hydrophobic transmembrane segment. The α chain also features a short cytoplasmic tail region that functions in localization to the cell membrane. β_2-Microglobulin does not traverse the cell membrane but is incorporated into the tertiary structure of MHC class I through noncovalent interactions. Functionally, the α1 and α2 domains cooperate to bind antigen, while the α3 domain interacts with CD8 molecules on cytotoxic T cells.

X-ray crystallographic studies indicate that two critically important α helices are present in the secondary structures of the class I α1 and α2 domains. In the overall class I tertiary structure, these α helices align to form the walls of a deep groove. Found at the top of the MHC molecule (facing away from the cell membrane), this furrow functions as a peptide-binding site capable of holding peptide antigens between 8 and 11 amino acids in length.

Structure of Class II MHC Molecules

The major class II molecules—HLA-DP, HLA-DQ, and HLA-DR—each consist of two noncovalently bound polypeptide chains called α and β, which are encoded by separate genes. This type of quaternary protein structure is often referred to as a *heterodimer* because it is made up of two ("dimer") dissimilar polypeptide chains ("hetero").

Both the class II MHC α chain, with a molecular weight of 34,000 Da, and the β chain, with a molecular weight of 29,000 Da, are anchored to the cell membrane **(Fig. 4–6).**

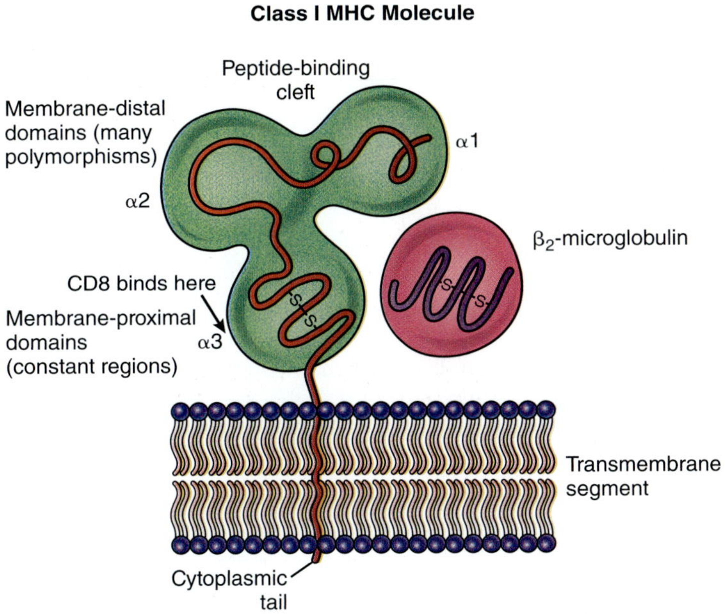

FIGURE 4–5 General structure of a class I MHC molecule. Class I MHC molecules consist of an α chain with three domains and a shorter chain, β_2-microglobulin, common to all class I molecules.

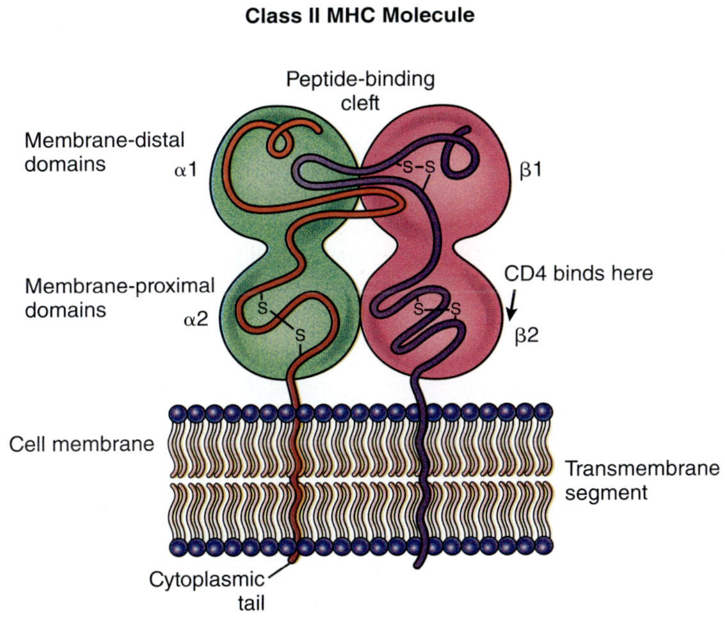

FIGURE 4–6 General structure of a class II MHC molecule. Class II MHC molecules consist of an α chain and a β chain, each of which has two domains.

The α chain and the β chain each contain two domains, numbered 1 and 2. In the quaternary structure of class II MHC molecules, the α1 and β1 domains vary among different class II MHC molecules, and each contributes an α helix in formation of the peptide-binding groove. Both ends of the peptide-binding cleft are open, enabling the capture of longer peptides, in comparison to class I MHC molecules. The α2 domains and the β2 domains are evolutionarily conserved among different class II molecules. Similar to MHC class I, class II α and β chains both contain transmembrane domains and short cytoplasmic tails.

Knowledge Check 4-4

Which of the following proteins or domains would you expect to exhibit the highest degree of polymorphism, or differences between different individuals?

a. Class I α2 domain
b. Class I α3 domain
c. Class II α2 domain
d. β_2-Microglobulin

Roles of Class I and II Molecules in the Immune Response

The primary immune function of class I and II MHC molecules is **antigen presentation,** the process by which peptide fragments derived from degraded proteins are transported to the plasma membrane, allowing recognition by T lymphocytes. As we mentioned previously, T cells can only "see" and respond to peptide antigens that are bound to MHC molecules.

The two classes of MHC have evolved to respond to two distinct types of infections: those that attack cells from the outside (such as most bacteria) and those that attack from the inside (viruses and other intracellular pathogens). Class I MHC molecules present cytoplasmic peptide antigens to $CD8^{+}$ (cytotoxic) T cells and are the watchdogs of viral, tumor, and intracellular parasitic antigens synthesized *within* the cell. In contrast, class II molecules present extracellular antigens to $CD4^{+}$ (helper) T cells, permitting immune responses to bacterial infections or other pathogens commonly found *outside* of cells. To trigger a T-cell response, peptides must be available in adequate supply to bind MHC, able to bind to MHC effectively, and recognized by a T cell's antigen receptor. Some viruses, such as herpes simplex and adenovirus, have managed to escape the immune response by interfering with one or more processes involved in antigen presentation, allowing them to maintain a lifelong presence in the host.

In contrast to the *classical* class I MHC described earlier, HLA-E, HLA-F, and HLA-G are considered *nonclassical* class I MHC molecules. HLA-E and HLA-F molecules are important ligands for natural killer (NK) cell inhibitory receptors. HLA-G is unique among the MHC-related proteins in that it is mainly expressed on fetal trophoblast cells during the first trimester of pregnancy. Placental trophoblast cells represent points of direct contact between maternal and fetal tissue—a potential source of alloantigens inherited from the father. HLA-G molecules are thought to contribute to maternal immune tolerance of the fetus by protecting placental tissue from destruction by NK cells. HLA-G binds to NK-cell inhibitory receptors, preventing an NK-cell-driven cytotoxic response. (See Chapter 2 for more information on NK cells.)

Several *nonclassical* class II genes have also been identified—including HLA-DM and HLA-DO. The products of these genes have been shown to play a regulatory role in antigen processing. HLA-DM helps to load peptides onto class II molecules, whereas HLA-DO modulates antigen binding.

The dramatic functional differences between class I and II MHC can largely be attributed to the mechanisms responsible for the processing and delivery of peptide antigen to the MHC molecules themselves. The following sections highlight the differences in the intracellular pathways that feed antigen into each MHC class.

The Class I MHC-Peptide Presentation Pathway

The class I MHC presentation pathway is sometimes referred to as the *endogenous* pathway of antigen presentation, because both the peptides and MHC molecules arise from inside the same cell. The endogenous peptide antigens presented by class I MHC represent a sampling of the many polypeptide chains composing the proteins found within the cytosol (fluid part of the cytoplasm). In a healthy cell, cytosolic peptides derive from host proteins. However, tumor cells or those infected with a virus or bacterium contain abnormal proteins that are unique to the tumor or are produced by the invading pathogen. The class I MHC presentation pathway provides cytotoxic T lymphocytes with a means of surveilling the interiors of cells throughout the body, allowing T cells to search for peptides associated with infection or malignancy.

Cytoplasmic proteins enter the class I pathway by undergoing proteolysis in an enzyme complex known as the *proteasome* **(Fig. 4–7).** This macromolecular structure contains dozens of enzymatic subunits arranged cylindrically to form a proteolytic tunnel. To generate peptide antigens, whole proteins are unfolded and threaded into the core of the proteasome. Catalytic sites within the proteasome cleave proteins into peptide fragments, which are then released into the cytosol.

MHC molecules are synthesized by ribosomes associated with the rough endoplasmic reticulum. As the class I α chain is being manufactured, several important *chaperone* proteins associate with it to ensure that the nascent molecule folds into the appropriate three-dimensional tertiary shape. One important chaperone, known as *calnexin,* stabilizes the α chain until it binds to β_2-microglobulin. When β_2-microglobulin binds, calnexin is released, and two additional chaperone molecules—calreticulin and tapasin—associate with the complex and help to stabilize it for peptide binding.

When synthesis of MHC molecules is complete, their antigen binding sites are oriented toward the interior of the endoplasmic reticulum, whereas the peptide antigens generated by proteasomal degradation are located within the cytoplasm. Two **transporters associated with antigen processing, TAP1** and **TAP2,** are essential for shuttling antigenic peptides into the lumen of the endoplasmic reticulum, allowing the peptides to interact with newly formed class I MHC molecules. TAP-driven translocation depends on adenosine triphosphate (ATP) and is most efficient for peptides of 8 to 16 amino acids in length. The TAP transporters are brought together with class I molecules by tapasin, a protein that bridges transporter and MHC, allowing peptides to be directly loaded. Once the α chain has bound the peptide, the class I MHC-peptide complex is rapidly transported to the cell surface (see Fig. 4–7).

As proteins are processed by the proteasome, thousands of peptides are generated, but only a small fraction of this overall peptide pool has the potential to serve as antigens for T cells. The binding of peptides to class I MHC is dictated by several variables, all of which must be met for successful presentation to occur. The first consideration in the binding of peptides to the MHC groove is the length of the peptide chain. As the class I MHC binding groove is closed at its ends, it can accommodate peptides of no longer than

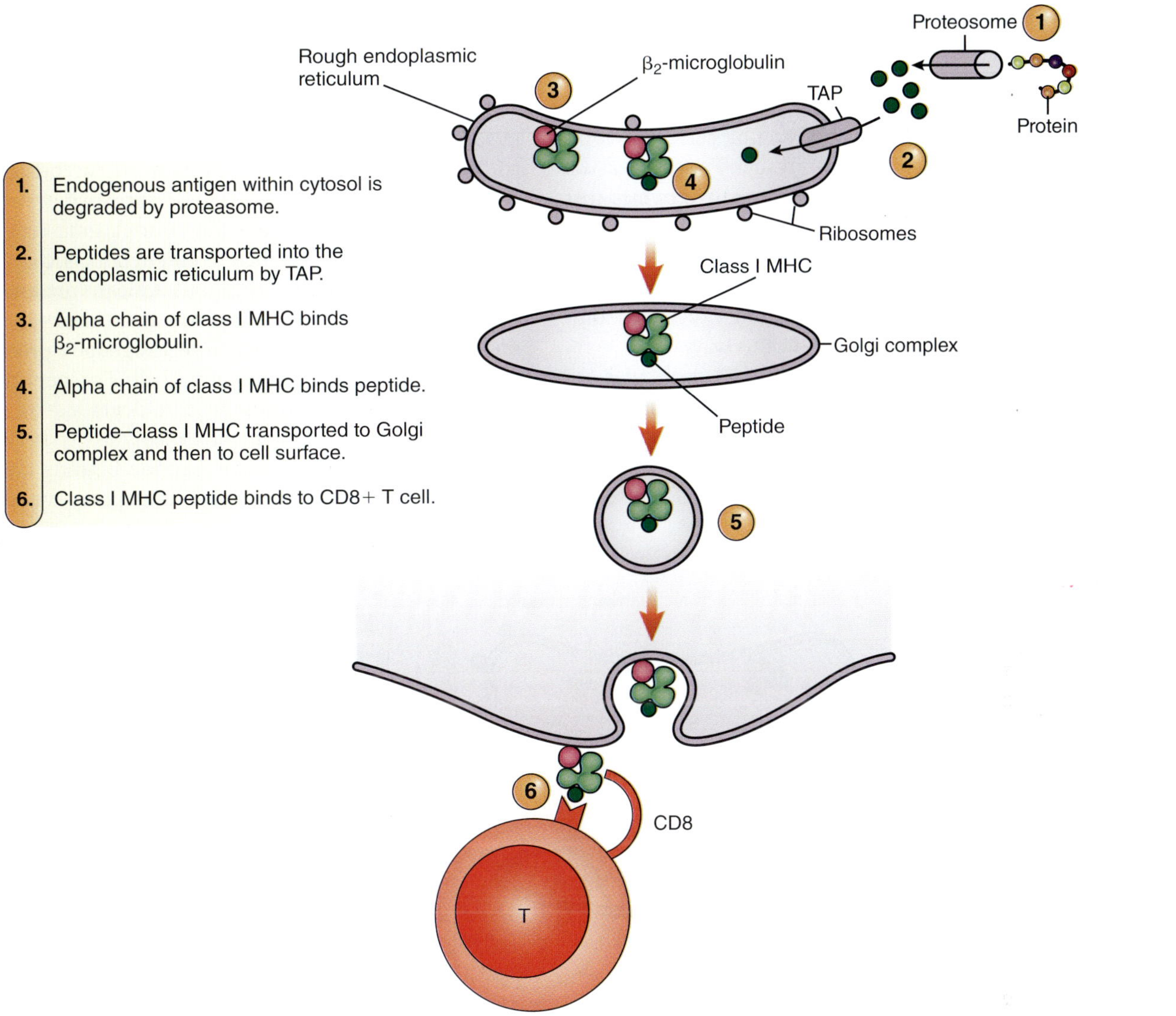

FIGURE 4–7 Antigen-processing pathway for endogenous antigens. Cytoplasmic proteins are degraded and fed into the MHC class I pathway for presentation to $CD8^+$ cytotoxic T cells.

11 amino acids. Peptide binding itself is determined by complementary noncovalent interactions between the peptide and the amino acids comprising the α helices that form the binding groove. In most cases, the interactions between peptide and MHC molecule are mediated by a few key intermolecular interactions.

It is estimated that a single cell may express between 100,000 and 200,000 copies of each class I molecule at its surface, meaning that countless different peptides are simultaneously displayed. As few as 10 to 100 class I MHC complexes bearing identical peptide antigen may be sufficient to induce a $CD8^+$ cytotoxic T-cell response. In healthy cells, all class I MHC molecules contain self-peptides that are ignored by patrolling T cells. In diseased cells, some of the peptides displayed originate from microbial proteins or proteins associated with cancer. If a cytotoxic T cell that recognizes a particular foreign peptide antigen in class I MHC makes contact with a cell presenting that antigen, the T cell may be triggered to lyse the infected cell **(Fig. 4–8)**.

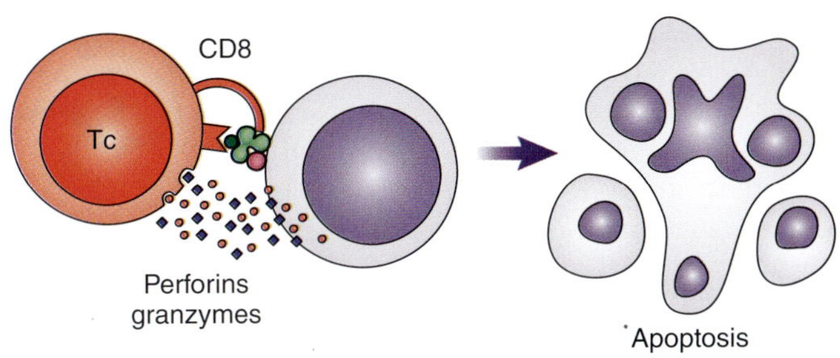

FIGURE 4–8 $CD8^+$ T cells recognize antigen in association with class I MHC. If endogenous antigens are recognized as being foreign by the T cell, cytotoxic molecules are released, resulting in destruction of the target cell.

The Class II MHC-Peptide Presentation Pathway

Class II MHC molecules function in the presentation of *exogenous* antigens to T cells. Exogenous peptide antigens are derived from proteins found *outside* of the presenting cell. For class II MHC presentation to occur, extracellular proteins must be taken up by means of either phagocytosis or endocytosis, processes by which cells ingest pathogens by enclosing them in a small portion of the plasma membrane that pinches off to form an intracellular vesicle containing the invader. Proteins that are captured in this way are digested by hydrolytic enzymes that accumulate within the vesicular lumen, resulting in peptide fragments of 13 to 18 amino acids in size. Dendritic cells, the immune cells considered to be the most potent activators of T cells, are excellent at capturing and digesting exogenous antigens from bacteria and other microbes in this way.

Similar to class I MHC molecules, class II molecules are synthesized in the rough endoplasmic reticulum **(Fig. 4–9).** Immediately after synthesis, class II molecules associate with a protein known as the **invariant chain (Ii),** a 31-kDa protein present in great excess of the number of class II molecules being synthesized. Ii is required during the production of class II MHC molecules to prevent endogenous peptides within the endoplasmic reticulum from binding to the class II peptide-binding groove. Thus, Ii serves as a placeholder, ensuring that only exogenous peptide antigens will be bound to MHC II molecules. Ii may also aid in bringing α and β chains together, a signal required for newly translated class II molecules to move from the endoplasmic reticulum into the Golgi complex, and then to enter endocytic or phagocytic vesicles where digested exogenous antigens are located.

Within endosomal compartments, class II molecules encounter peptides derived from exogenous proteins previously ingested by the presenting cell. For peptide antigens to bind to MHC II, Ii must first be degraded by a protease, leaving just a small fragment called *class II invariant chain peptide* (CLIP) attached to the peptide-binding cleft. CLIP is then exchanged for an exogenous peptide whose selective

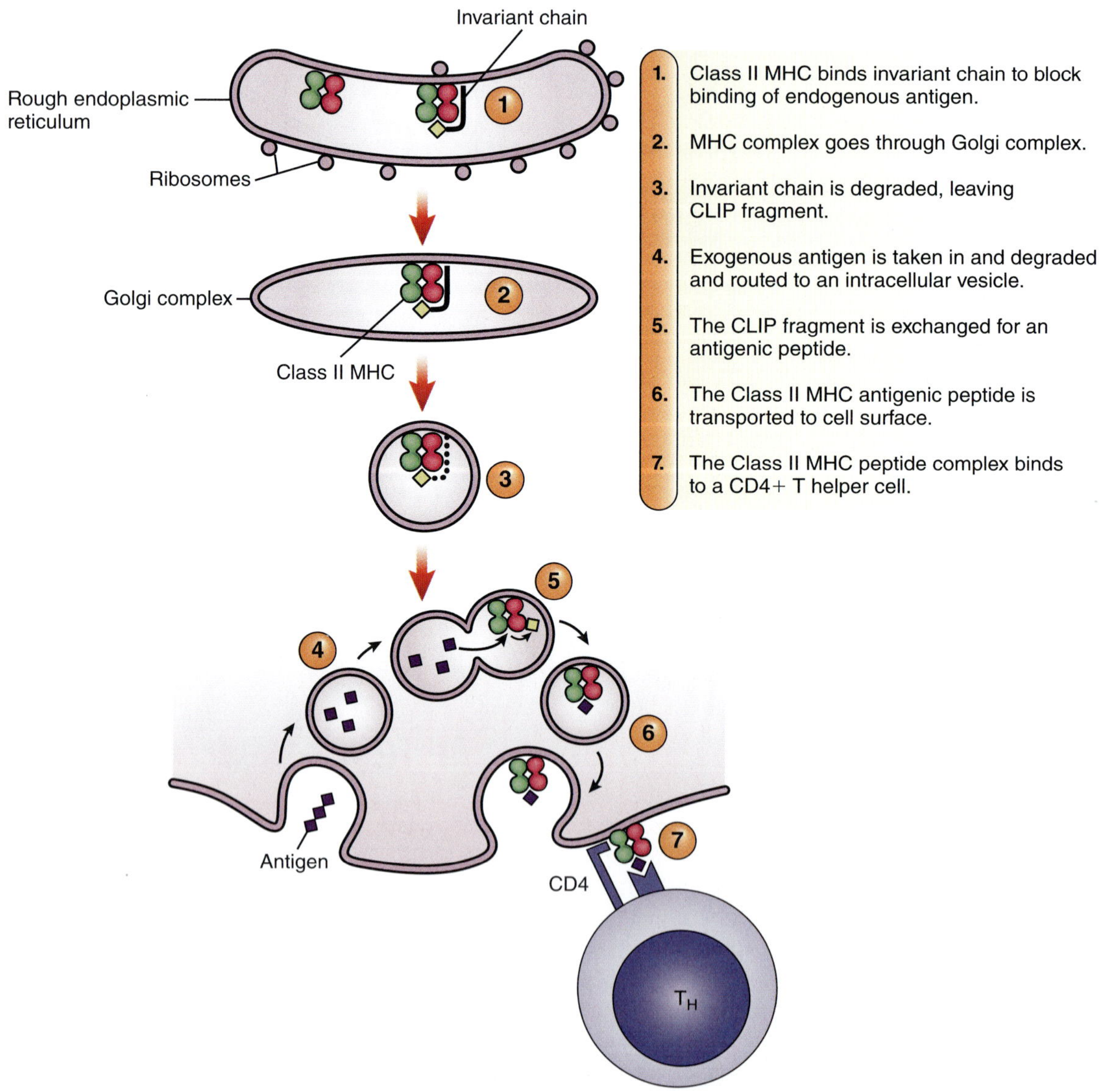

FIGURE 4–9 Antigen-processing pathway for exogenous antigen. The binding site of a class II MHC molecule is first occupied by an invariant chain (Ii). This is degraded and exchanged for short exogenous peptides in an endosomal compartment. The exogenous peptide class II MHC complex is then transported to the cell surface.

binding to the cleft is favored by the low pH of the endosomal compartment. Nonclassical class II MHC molecules such as HLA-DM assist with CLIP removal and guide exogenous peptides into the binding groove. Because the MHC II binding groove is open at both ends, the length of peptides that can be accommodated within it extends from 10 to nearly 30 amino acids (although the optimal size is between 12 and 16 amino acids). This contrasts with class I MHC molecules, which have closed ends, constraining the length of peptides that can bind.

With MHC class II molecules (as with class I molecules), only some of the amino acid residues composing the peptide antigen, perhaps 7 to 10, actually bind to the groove. For class II MHC, however, hydrogen bonding occurs along the length of the captured peptide, whereas binding of peptide to class I molecules occurs mostly at the amino and carboxy-terminal ends. The class II binding groove also features several pockets that can accommodate amino acids with large side chains, giving class II molecules greater flexibility than class I in the variety of peptides that can be bound.

Once peptide antigen has bound to an MHC II molecule, the class II protein-peptide complex is stabilized and transported to the cell surface (see Fig. 4–9). Once there, class II molecules bearing non-self-antigen serve as essential signals for the activation of CD4+ helper T cells. Helper T cells secrete proteins called *cytokines,* which influence the activities of other immune cells, including macrophages, cytotoxic T cells, and B cells. For example, **Fig. 4–10** shows how activated helper T cells affect B cells and antibody production. We discuss the important functions of helper T cells and the cytokines they secrete in Chapters 5 and 6.

Critical Thinking 4-3

In both class I and class II MHC molecules, the specific amino acids in the binding cleft that interacts with peptide antigens are not located sequentially in the amino acid chain (primary structure). Using your knowledge of protein structure, explain this fact.

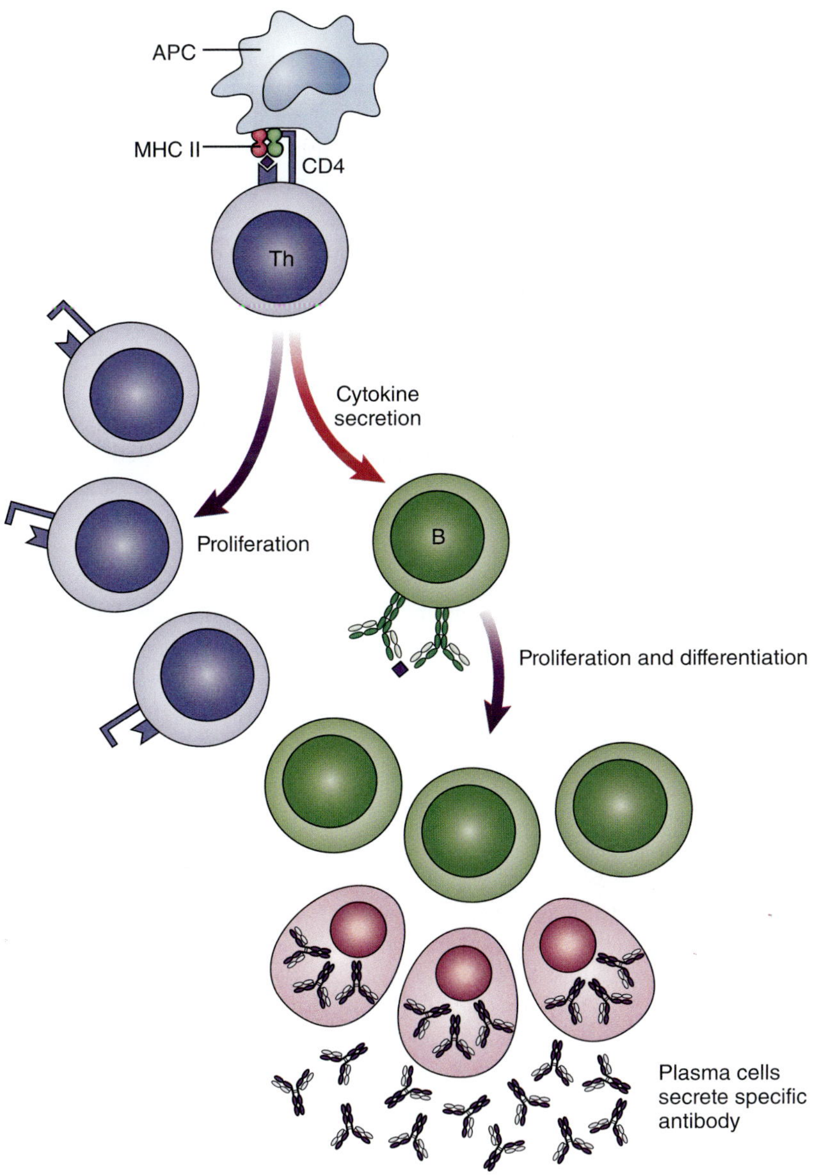

FIGURE 4–10 CD4+ T cells recognize exogenous antigen complexed with class II MHC on the surface of APCs such as macrophages. CD4+ helper T cells are stimulated by contact with antigen to proliferate and produce an identical clone of T cells that can respond to the antigen. These cells secrete cytokines that cause antigen-activated B cells to proliferate and differentiate into plasma cells, which make antibodies.

Table 4-1 Association of HLA Alleles and Disease

DISEASE	SYMPTOMS	HLA ALLELE	STRENGTH OF ASSOCIATION
Ankylosing spondylitis	Inflammation of the vertebrae of the spine	B-27	+++
Psoriasis	Patches of thick, red, sometimes scaly skin	C-w6	+++
Celiac disease	Diarrhea, weight loss, intolerance to gluten	DQB-1	+++
Rheumatoid arthritis	Inflammation of multiple joints	DRB-1	++
Type 1 diabetes	Increase in blood glucose caused by destruction of insulin-producing cells	DQB-1	+++

Clinical Significance of MHC

Because MHC molecules are expressed in nearly all body tissues and are critically important in immunity, identifying a person's MHC genotype and understanding its health implications is of considerable clinical importance. MHC testing in the laboratory is typically performed before tissue transplantation because an immune response against either class I or class II molecules can induce graft rejection. Modern transplant HLA testing involves molecular techniques to determine the MHC types of both donor and recipient and serological testing to detect antibodies in the recipient that target the MHC molecules of a potential donor (see Chapter 16).

Inheritance of certain HLA types may predispose individuals to developing an autoimmune disease. The closest association between MHC expression and autoimmunity is between the inheritance of the class I molecule HLA-B27 and a disease called *ankylosing spondylitis*—a progressive chronic inflammatory disorder affecting the vertebrae of the spine. See **Table 4–1** for other associations between specific HLA antigens and autoimmune diseases. This topic is discussed in more detail in Chapter 15. Certain drug hypersensitivities have also been linked to HLA alleles, and knowledge of one's HLA genes can be used to prevent severe reactions to these drugs.

In addition to their roles in transplantation and autoimmunity, class I and class II MHC molecules play a critical role in the immune response, as we discussed earlier. MHC molecules determine the types of peptide antigen to which an individual can mount an adaptive immune response, potentially defining a person's ability to overcome an infection. Although MHC molecules typically can bind a broad variety of peptides, small biochemical differences in the molecules can amount to large differences in the immune system's ability to react to a specific antigen. For instance, it is possible that individuals who do not respond to a particular vaccine lack the genetic capacity for an immune response to the vaccine antigen. On the other hand, the presence of a particular MHC protein may confer additional protection against an infection, as seen in the example of HLA B8 and increased resistance to HIV infection.

Research in this area has focused on the types of peptides that can be bound by specific MHC molecules to develop more effective vaccines and individualized treatments for diseases like cancer. Knowledge of a patient's MHC genotype and the variety of peptide antigens to which they can respond will likely continue to be important as more applications of *personalized medicine* are developed in the future.

KEY CONCEPTS

- Immunogens are substances that are capable of stimulating an adaptive immune response, in the form of either antibody production by B cells or the activation of T cells.
- The term *antigen* describes a substance recognized by the adaptive immune system but that may not necessarily elicit an adaptive response by itself (as in the case of haptens).

Factors Influencing the Immune Response

- The immunogenicity, or ability of a substance to stimulate an immune response, is influenced by factors such as age, health, route of inoculation, and genetic capacity.

Traits of Antigens and Immunogens

- Most immunogens are high molecular weight proteins (at least 100,000 Da) or glycoproteins that are foreign to the host.

Epitopes

- Although immunogens are fairly large molecules, the response of each B and T cell is directed against a small portion of the entire molecule, or *epitope*.
- B cells recognize epitopes found on the exterior of a protein—those regions that antibodies can reach. B cells can target linear epitopes, which are made of sequential amino acids in the peptide chain, or conformational epitopes produced by twisting and folding of the primary chain to bring distant amino acid residues together in the same epitope.
- T cells only recognize linear epitopes bound to MHC molecules. Unlike B-cell epitopes, T-cell peptides can come from any region of the protein antigen, even parts that are buried deeply inside the three-dimensional structure and are therefore hidden from antibodies.

Haptens

- Haptens are substances that are too small to provoke an adaptive immune response alone but stimulate a response when combined with a carrier.
- Once an antibody response is generated, haptens are capable of reacting with that antibody, but precipitation or agglutination reactions will not occur because the complexes formed are too small.

Adjuvants

- Adjuvants are substances that can be mixed with antigen to enhance an immune response.
- Adjuvants typically contain materials that simulate infection or prevent antigen from diffusing away from the site of inoculation.

Relationships of Antigens to the Host

- Antigens can be characterized by their relationship to the host. Autoantigens are those that belong to the host; alloantigens are from the same species as the host but are not identical to the host; heteroantigens are from other species.
- Heterophile antigens exist in unrelated species, but their structure is so similar that antibody formed to one antigen can cross-react with antigen from the unrelated species.

Major Histocompatibility Complex (MHC)

- The MHC/HLA genes encode class I and class II molecules, which play a major role in antigen presentation to T cells.
- Class I and class II MHC molecules bind peptides within cells and transport them to the plasma membrane, where the peptides can be recognized by T cells.

Genes Coding for MHC Molecules

- Class I MHC genes in humans are HLA-A, HLA-B, and HLA-C. Class II MHC genes are found in the HLA-D region, which can be divided into DR, DP, and DQ.
- So many different alleles are found in the human population for each MHC gene that the MHC system is considered the most polymorphic in the human genome.

Expression of Class I and Class II MHC Molecules

- Class I MHC molecules are found on all nucleated cells; these molecules associate with foreign antigens, such as viral proteins, synthesized within a host cell.
- Class II molecules are only found on APCs (B cells, monocytes, macrophages, dendritic cells, and thymic epithelium).

Structure of Class I MHC Molecules

- Class I MHC molecules consist of an α chain encoded by the MHC complex, and a second lighter chain called *β_2-microglobulin* encoded by a gene on chromosome 15.

Structure of Class II MHC Molecules

- Class II MHC molecules have an α and a β chain, both of which are encoded by genes in the MHC complex.

The Class I MHC-Peptide Presentation Pathway

- Class I MHC molecules present endogenous antigen to $CD8^+$ T cells, triggering a cytotoxic reaction.
- In the *endogenous pathway* for antigen presentation, cytosolic proteins are cleaved into peptide fragments that are transported into the endoplasmic reticulum and loaded onto MHC class I molecules.

The Class II MHC-Peptide Presentation Pathway

- Class II molecules present exogenous antigen to $CD4^+$ T cells, which are helper cells involved in antibody production.
- These molecules associate with foreign antigens taken into the cell from the outside, in the pathway known as *exogenous antigen presentation*. In this pathway, extracellular proteins are taken up by endocytosis or phagocytosed into antigen-presenting cells and degraded to peptides by proteolytic enzymes. Vesicles containing newly formed MHC II molecules merge with those containing peptide fragments, which bind within the peptide-binding groove.

Clinical Significance of MHC

- The widespread cellular expression and high degree of polymorphism of MHC molecules make them important alloantigens in transfusion and transplantation.
- MHC is important in connecting innate and adaptive immunity and thus affects the ability of an individual to respond appropriately to many infectious diseases and vaccinations.
- Specific HLA types are associated with various clinical conditions, including autoimmune diseases and hypersensitivities.

Study Guide: A Comparison of Class I and Class II MHC Molecules

CHARACTERISTIC	CLASS I MHC MOLECULES	CLASS II MHC MOLECULES
Cellular distribution	All nucleated cells	APCs: B cells, monocytes, macrophages, dendritic cells, thymic epithelial cells
Structure	One α chain and β_2-microglobulin	An α chain and a β chain
HLA proteins	A, B, C	DP, DQ, DR
Size of peptides bound	8 to 11 amino acids	10 to 30 amino acids (12 to 16 optimally)
Nature of peptide-binding cleft	Closed at both ends	Open at both ends
Interaction with T cells	Presents endogenous antigen to $CD8^+$ T cells	Presents exogenous antigen to $CD4^+$ T cells

CASE STUDIES

1. A 15-year-old teenager needs to have a kidney transplant because of the effects of severe diabetes. The family consists of a father, mother, and two sisters. All of them are willing to donate a kidney so that the patient can discontinue dialysis. The patient is also on a list for a cadaver kidney. The physician suggests that the family be tested first for the best HLA match.

Questions

a. How many alleles are shared by mother and the patient? Father and the patient?
b. What are the chances that one of the sisters would be an exact match?
c. Is there a possibility that a cadaver kidney might be a better match than any of the family members' kidneys?

2. A zombie plague is ravaging the world and destroying the human population. You are one of a few hundred million survivors. Chaos reigns. Although you have not yet completed your training in immunology, you are visited by government agents and recruited into designing a vaccine to protect against the plague. When you arrive at a secret military laboratory, you are told that the zombie pathogen has been identified and isolated. It is your mission to design an effective vaccine.

Questions

a. Other researchers have purified several different antigens from the plague virus: a lipid, a nucleic acid fragment, a polysaccharide, and a protein. Which of these plague antigens would make the most effective vaccine, and why?
b. Now that you have selected an antigen to use in the vaccine, what additional component might be required to make an effective zombie plague vaccine? What purpose does this additional component serve?

REVIEW QUESTIONS

1. All of the following are characteristics of an effective immunogen *except:*
   a. Composed of protein
   b. Large molecular weight
   c. The presence of numerous epitopes
   d. Found on host cells

2. Which of the following best describes a hapten?
   a. Cannot react with antibody
   b. Immunogenic only when coupled to a carrier
   c. Sufficient alone to activate B-cell receptors
   d. A large chemically complex molecule

3. Which would be the most effective immunogen?
   a. Protein with a molecular weight of 200,000
   b. Lipid with a molecular weight of 250,000
   c. Polysaccharide with a molecular weight of 220,000
   d. DNA with a molecular weight of 175,000

4. Which of the following individuals would likely respond most strongly to an immunogen?
   a. An adult who is 90 years of age
   b. A malnourished 40-year-old
   c. A weightlifter who is 35 years old
   d. A newborn baby

5. Which best describes an epitope?
   a. A peptide that must be at least 10,000 MW
   b. An area of an antigen recognized only by T cells
   c. A segment of sequential amino acids only
   d. A key portion of the antigen

6. Adjuvants act by which of the following methods?
   a. Activate innate immune cells
   b. Facilitate rapid diffusion of antigen from the tissues
   c. Inhibit presentation of peptide antigens to T cells
   d. Decrease recruitment of APCs

7. A heterophile antigen is one that:
   a. Is a self-antigen
   b. Is structurally similar to antigens found in other species
   c. Has been used previously to stimulate an antibody response
   d. Is from the same species but is different from the host

8. Which of the following is true of class II MHC (HLA) antigens?
   a. They are found on B cells and macrophages.
   b. They are found on all nucleated cells.
   c. They are also known as HLA-A, HLA-B, and HLA-C.
   d. They are coded for on chromosome 9.

9. If a person inherits unique alleles for all MHC genes, how many different HLA-DR molecules will be expressed on that individual's skin cells?
   a. 6
   b. 3
   c. 2
   d. 0

10. Class II MHC molecules are recognized by which of the following?
   a. $CD4^+$ T cells
   b. $CD8^+$ T cells
   c. NK cells
   d. Neutrophils

11. Which of the following best describes the role of TAP?
   a. Binds to class II molecules to help block the antigen binding site
   b. Binds to class I proteins in proteasomes
   c. Transports peptides into the lumen of the endoplasmic reticulum
   d. Helps cleave peptides for transport to endosomes

12. What is the purpose of the invariant chain in antigen processing associated with class II MHC molecules?
   a. Helps transport peptides into the endoplasmic reticulum
   b. Blocks binding of endogenous peptides
   c. Binds to $CD8^+$ T cells
   d. Cleaves peptides into the proper size for binding

13. A person is recovering from a bacterial infection and tests positive for antibodies to a protein on the surface of this bacterium. Which statement is true of this situation?
   a. Class I molecules have presented bacterial antigen to $CD8^+$ T cells.
   b. Class I molecules have presented bacterial antigen to $CD4^+$ T cells.
   c. Class II molecules have presented bacterial antigen to $CD4^+$ T cells.
   d. B cells have recognized bacterial antigen without help from T cells.

14. In relation to a human, alloantigens would need to be considered in which of the following events?
   a. Transplantation of a kidney from one individual to another
   b. Vaccination with the polysaccharide coat of a bacterial cell
   c. Oral administration of a live but heat-killed virus particle
   d. Grafting skin from one area of the body to another

15. Which is characteristic of class I MHC molecules?
   a. Consist of one α and one β chain
   b. Bind peptides made within the cell
   c. Able to bind whole protein antigens
   d. Coded for by HLA-DR, HLA-DP, and HLA-DQ genes

16. Which best explains the difference between immunogens and antigens?
   a. Only antigens are large enough to be recognized by T cells.
   b. Only immunogens can react with antibody.
   c. Only antigens are recognized as foreign.
   d. Only immunogens can trigger an immune response.

17. When a child inherits one set of six HLA genes together from one parent, this is called a(n):
   a. Genotype
   b. Phenotype
   c. Haplotype
   d. Allotype

18. HLA molecules A, B, and C belong to which MHC class?
   a. Class I
   b. Class II
   c. Class III
   d. Class IV

Chapter 4 Answer Key

Answers to Knowledge Checks

4.1 d 4.2 d 4.3 c 4.4 a

Answers to Review Questions

1. d	2. b	3. a	4. c	5. d	6. a	7. b
8. a	9. d	10. a	11. c	12. b	13. c	14. a
15. b	16. d	17. c	18. a			

5 Adaptive Immunity

Aaron Glass, PhD, MB^CM(ASCP)

LEARNING OUTCOMES

After finishing this chapter, you should be able to:

5.1 Compare and contrast adaptive immunity and innate immunity.

5.2 Differentiate between humoral and cell-mediated immune responses.

5.3 Discuss the stages of T-cell development in the thymus.

5.4 Describe the T-cell receptor (TCR).

5.5 Explain how positive and negative selection contribute to T-cell development.

5.6 List five different subsets of CD4 helper T (TH) cells and describe their roles in the immune response.

5.7 Describe the development of a B cell from the pro–B-cell stage to the plasma cell stage.

5.8 Contrast the antigen-independent and antigen-dependent phases of B-cell development.

5.9 Explain how cytotoxic T cells recognize and kill target cells.

5.10 Discuss the roles of class I major histocompatibility complex (MHC) and class II MHC molecules in the presentation of antigens to T cells.

5.11 Compare and contrast the immune response to T-dependent antigens with the response to T-independent antigens.

5.12 Discuss how TH cells influence the B-cell antibody response.

5.13 Indicate surface markers characteristic of T and B lymphocytes in various stages of development.

CHAPTER OUTLINE

You can go to **fadavis.com** keyword stevens for the laboratory exercises that accompany this text.

As you learned in Chapter 2, the concept of innate immunity encompasses the body's barrier defenses, such as the skin; preformed soluble factors, including complement proteins; and phagocytic cells, such as macrophages and neutrophils. Innate immunity is general in nature—entire classes of pathogens elicit nearly identical innate responses, and these responses are unchanging with time. In contrast, **adaptive immunity** is characterized by the following:

- Specificity for individual microbes and pathogens
- Memory of prior exposures to antigen
- Enhanced responses upon repeated exposures to the same antigen (i.e., memory)

When compared with innate immunity, adaptive immunity represents a more *tailored*, or pathogen-specific, response. One trade-off for this high degree of specificity is the time required after an initial pathogen exposure for an adaptive response to be mounted (often several days). Once under way, the adaptive response is highly effective and can often provide lifelong immunity against reinfection.

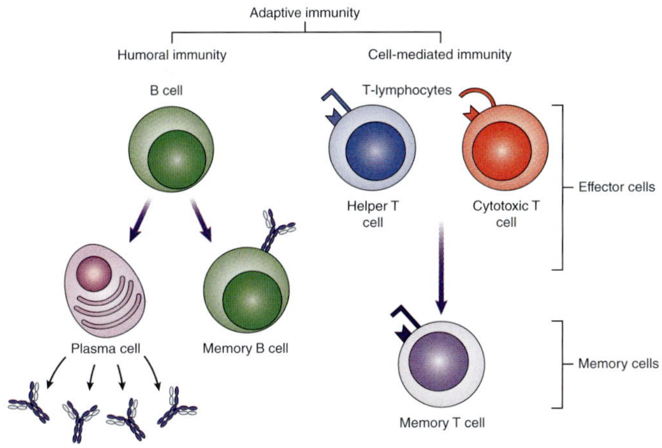

FIGURE 5-1 Adaptive immunity can be divided into the humoral and cellular arms. Humoral immunity is composed of immunoglobulins (antibodies), which are produced by B lymphocytes and plasma cells. Cell-mediated immunity is produced by T lymphocytes, which can be further classified into cytotoxic T (Tc) cells and helper T (TH) cells. Following a successful adaptive immune response, memory cells are often produced, conferring long-lasting immunity.

Cell-Mediated and Humoral Immunity

Adaptive immunity is traditionally divided into two main branches: (1) **cell-mediated immunity,** which is carried out by cells of the immune system, and (2) **humoral immunity,** which is mediated by soluble factors (antibodies) in body fluids **(Fig. 5–1).** T lymphocytes, or T cells, are responsible for the cell-mediated arm of adaptive immunity, whereas B lymphocytes (B cells) and plasma cells produce the immunoglobulins, or *antibodies,* that provide humoral immunity.

T lymphocytes can be classified into two broad groups: **cytotoxic T (Tc) cells** and **helper T (TH) cells.** The immune function of Tc cells is to kill target cells infected with intracellular pathogens, such as viruses and certain bacteria. Tc cells can also kill cancer cells. In contrast, TH cells do not directly kill cells, but instead, control the immune response through the secretion of *cytokines,* or signaling molecules that allow communication between immune cells (see Chapter 6). TH cells can be further divided into several subpopulations based on the types of cytokines they secrete.

The antibodies produced by B cells and plasma cells have many roles in immunity, such as (1) marking targets for ingestion by phagocytes, (2) rendering viruses and toxins inert through neutralization, and (3) blocking the adhesion of microbes to body tissues (see Chapter 3).

One key difference between the lymphocytes of adaptive immunity and the various cells of innate immunity is that the genes encoding the primary lymphocyte receptors undergo rearrangement during the early stages of T-cell or B-cell development. In theory, after gene rearrangement, each lymphocyte is equipped to respond to a unique antigen associated with a specific pathogen (see Chapter 3). Because each lymphocyte possesses a slightly different receptor specificity, the adaptive immune system represents an immune *army* that is theoretically capable of combating any conceivable infectious threat.

When infection occurs, only the lymphocytes responsive to antigens found on or in the invading pathogen(s) are activated and proliferate, a process known as **clonal selection.** Clonal selection is so named because proliferating lymphocytes give rise to cell populations with genetically identical receptors that are specific for the same antigen; therefore, these populations represent *clones* of each other.

The characteristic delay between an initial infection and an effective adaptive response arises because a handful of pathogen-responsive lymphocytes must undergo a massive clonal expansion before reaching the large number of effector cells needed to alter the course of an infection. Most of the progeny generated during clonal expansion are **effector cells** (i.e., T cells that secrete cytokines or are cytotoxic, or B cells that produce antibodies). However, a small proportion of the clones become **memory cells;** that is, they enter a long-lived quiescent (inactive) state and wait for antigen re-exposure. Memory cells are activated rapidly upon antigen encounter, providing a swift response without the lag period observed during the primary response.

Knowledge Check 5-1

Cell-mediated immunity refers to which of the following?

a. Any adaptive immune response
b. Production of antibody by B cells and plasma cells
c. Immune responses carried out by TH and Tc cells
d. Phagocytosis of antigen by macrophages

Lymphocyte Development

The body's production of lymphocytes begins very early in fetal life—a necessity because the rudiments of adaptive immunity must be in place at birth. T- and B-cell progenitors appear in the fetal liver as early as 8 weeks of pregnancy. Later, the bone marrow becomes the source of new lymphocytes and remains the primary producer of hematopoietic cells at birth and throughout adult life. The earliest precursors of T and B lymphocytes are generated by asymmetric division of lymphoid progenitor cells. *Asymmetry* in this context refers to the concept that when a progenitor cell divides into two, one of the resulting daughter cells begins to take on the characteristics of a lymphocyte, while the other daughter cell retains the stem cell–like plasticity of a lymphoid progenitor.

As we discussed in Chapter 1, lymphocytes mature in the bone marrow and thymus and become activated in the secondary lymphoid organs such as the lymph nodes and spleen. As T and B cells develop, they progress through a series of stages in which they undergo genetic changes, become antigen specific, and express certain cell surface markers. This process has often been referred to as *differentiation.* In the following sections, we provide a more detailed description of lymphocyte development and how these maturation processes prepare T and B cells for their roles in adaptive immune responses.

Critical Thinking 5-1

The response time following a first exposure to a pathogen is much slower for adaptive immunity than innate immunity. Based on your reading of the previous sections, explain this lag in the adaptive response.

T-Cell Development

Soon after their formation in the bone marrow, T-cell precursors enter the blood and are transported to the thymus. Thymic tissue can be divided into two histologically distinct regions: an outer cortex and inner medulla **(Fig. 5–2).**

Once in the thymus, T-cell precursors are known as **thymocytes.** Newly arriving thymocytes enter at the corticomedullary junction—the border between the medulla and cortex. Entering thymocytes immediately begin to migrate toward the thymic cortex under the direction of **chemokines,** or cytokines that control cellular movement. Over a 3-week period, thymocytes slowly migrate from the thymic cortex into the medulla. During this time, various developmental processes occur, including:

- Rearrangement of the **T-cell–receptor (TCR)** genes
- Changes in the expression of thymocyte cell surface markers
- Selection of thymocytes expressing functional receptors
- Deletion of thymocytes with self-reactive potential

Interactions with *stromal,* or supporting, cells within the thymus are critical for each of these developmental processes. Included among the types of thymic stromal cells are macrophages, dendritic cells, fibroblasts, and thymic epithelial cells. In the sections that follow, we discuss the major stages of T-cell development—the double-negative (DN) stage, double-positive (DP) stage, and mature, single-positive (SP) T cells. Key features of T cells in these stages are listed in **Table 5–1** and discussed in detail in the sections that follow.

Double-Negative Stage

TC cells and TH cells can be identified by their differential expression of two important cell surface markers, CD4 and CD8. CD4 is commonly used to identify TH cells, whereas CD8 is a reliable marker of TC cells. Because their fate has yet to be decided, early thymocytes lack both CD4 and CD8 and are therefore known as **double-negative (DN) thymocytes.** DN thymocytes aggregate in the outer cortex of the thymus, where they actively proliferate under the influence of cytokines such as interleukin-7 (IL-7).

During the DN stage of T-cell development, rearrangement of the genes coding for the TCR begins using a process that is similar to immunoglobulin gene rearrangement in B cells, which is we discussed in Chapter 3 **(Fig. 5–3).** Occurring at random, this shuffling and altering of the TCR genes results in the expression of a unique antigen receptor by each thymocyte—the underlying basis for a highly diverse population of T cells capable of responding to the myriad of antigens a person might encounter during a lifetime. The TCR is composed of two transmembrane proteins, the alpha (α) and beta (β) chains, each having an intracellular signaling domain, a membrane-spanning domain, and an extracellular domain containing a variable region. The variable regions of the α

Table 5-1 Stages of T-Cell Development

	DEVELOPMENTAL STAGE		
	DOUBLE NEGATIVE (DN)	**DOUBLE POSITIVE (DP)**	**SINGLE POSITIVE (SP)**
Key CD markers	CD3	CD3 CD4 CD8	CD3 *Either* CD4 or CD8
T-cell receptor (TCR)	—	TCR α/β	TCR α/β
Other features	TCR receptor gene rearrangement begins	Positive selection of thymocytes that can react with major histocompatibility complex molecules occurs in the cortex	Negative selection of thymocytes that strongly react with self-antigens occurs in the medulla and the interface between the cortex and the medulla

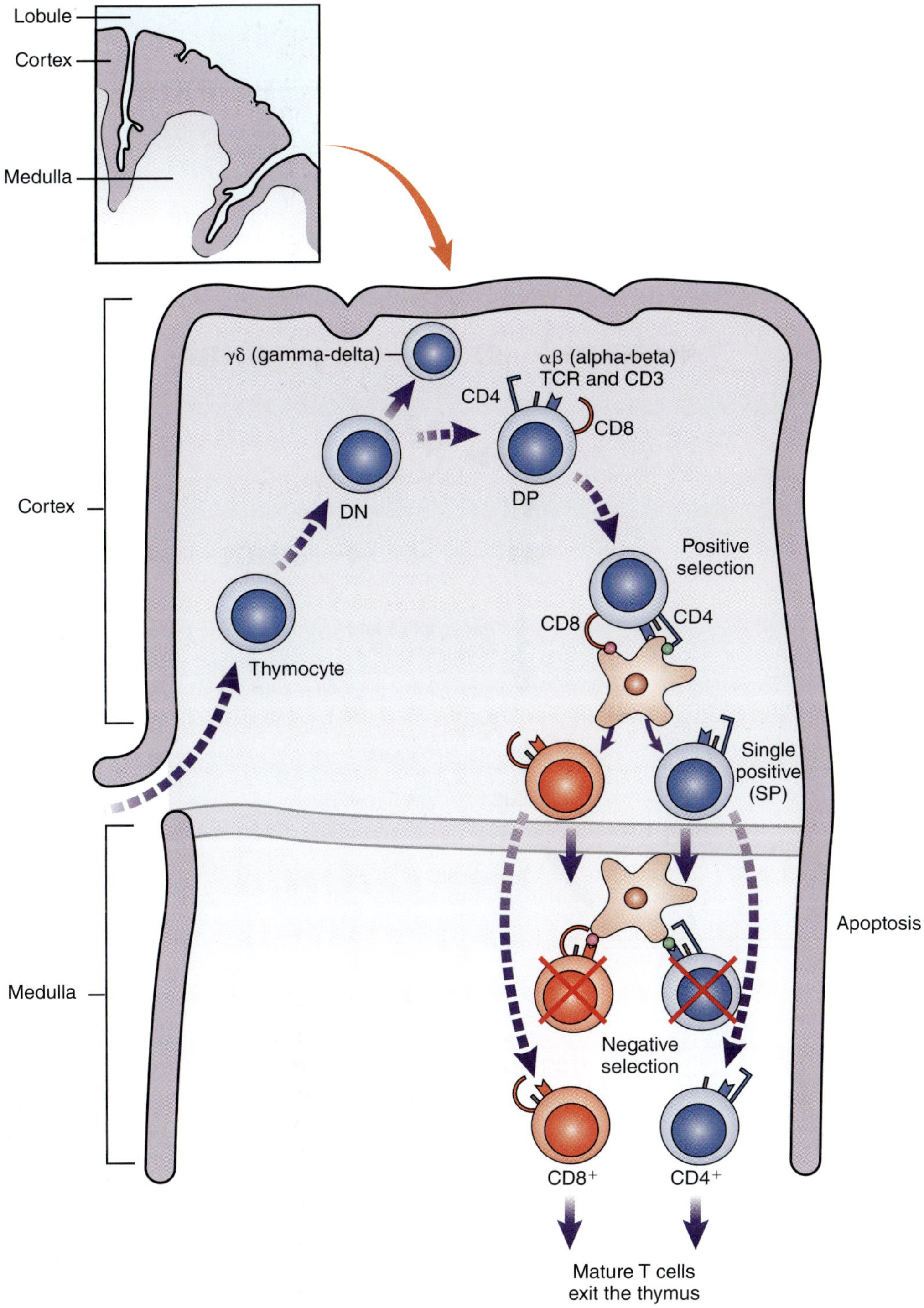

FIGURE 5–2 T-cell maturation in the thymus. T-lymphocyte precursors (thymocytes) enter the thymus at the corticomedullary junction and migrate into the cortex as *double-negative* (DN; lacking both CD4 and CD8) thymocytes. At this point, TCR rearrangement begins. A small percentage of DN thymocytes express gamma-delta (γδ) chains, whereas the majority develop alpha-beta (αβ) chains and become double-positive (DP) thymocytes. Positive selection occurs as DP thymocytes encounter thymic stromal cells, allowing interactions between major histocompatibility complex (MHC) molecules and newly formed TCRs. Positively selected thymocytes proceed to the single-positive (SP) stage and express either CD4 or CD8, depending on the type of MHC their TCR best interacts with. Further interactions with thymic macrophages or dendritic cells allow negative selection, where potentially autoreactive thymocytes are eliminated by a type of cell death called *apoptosis* before they can escape to the periphery. Thymocytes that successfully navigate these developmental hurdles exit the thymus as fully developed T_H and T_C cells.

and β chains are responsible for recognition of antigen and are therefore the only sections of the TCR genes that undergo rearrangement.

Before rearrangement, the genes encoding the variable region of the TCR β chain (found on chromosome 7) are divided into three large sections named *V*, *D*, and *J*, each containing multiple segments. During rearrangement, enzymes activated in DN thymocytes clip genomic DNA and begin stitching it back together in a way that randomly aligns one V segment, one D segment, one J segment, and a segment encoding the constant region. These enzymes are imprecise in the nucleotide positions at which DNA cleavage and ligation occur, a property that enhances TCR diversity but also introduces the possibility that some rearrangements will shift the translational frame of the gene in such a way as to result in a nonfunctional TCR. In cases where rearrangement leads to a faulty TCR β chain, developing T cells use two strategies aimed at generating a functional protein. First, because T cells are diploid, the β-chain genes on both copies of chromosome 7 simultaneously undergo rearrangement, doubling the probability of a functional β chain being produced. Second, the enzymes that mediate

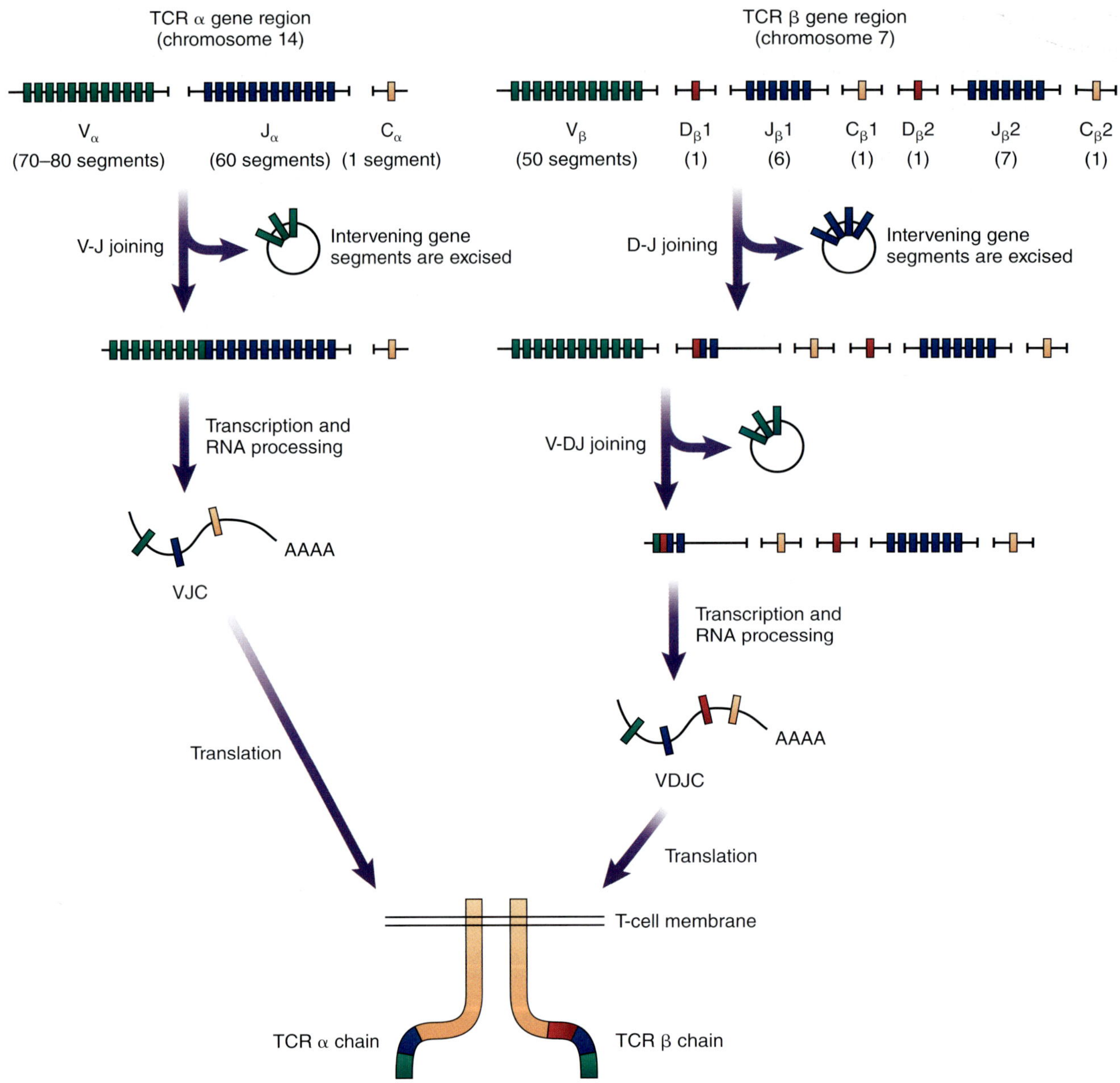

FIGURE 5–3 TCR gene organization and rearrangement. The TCR consists of two chains, α and β. The TCR α-chain genes are located on chromosome 14 and consist of a series of variable (Vα) gene segments, a series of joining (Jα) gene segments, and a single constant (Cα) gene segment. In contrast, the TCR β-chain genes are found on chromosome 7 and have a similar genetic structure to the TCR α genes except for the addition of diversity gene segments (Dβ) and duplicate regions of D (Dβ1 and Dβ2), J (Jβ1 and Jβ2), and C (Cβ1 and Cβ2) gene segments. During T-cell development in the thymus, the TCR genes undergo rearrangement, involving stepwise cleavage and joining. Thus, VJ and C are brought together in the TCR α chain, while VDJ and C are brought together in the TCR β chain. The variable region of each TCR chain, which interacts with MHCs and associated antigen peptides, is encoded by rearranged VD and J gene segments, whereas the C gene segments encode transmembrane and intracellular signaling domains.

TCR gene rearrangement continue clipping and stitching variable-region DNA until a functional TCR is generated (i.e., a TCR that can bind to an antigenic peptide bound to an MHC molecule).

To test the functionality of the TCR β chains produced by gene rearrangement, a surrogate α chain with no variable region is temporarily expressed and forms a *pre-TCR* with the newly rearranged β chain. If the DN thymocyte expresses a functional β chain, the pre-TCR provides survival signals to the T cell, ushering it into the next phase of T-cell differentiation, known as the *DP stage*.

Early on, some thymocytes, representing 10% or less of the total number, rearrange and express two distinct TCR chains—gamma (γ) and delta (δ)—when there is not a productive rearrangement of DNA coding for a β chain. Referred to as *gamma-delta* (γδ) *T cells*, this unique population of T lymphocytes proceeds down an alternate developmental pathway, typically remaining negative for both

CD4 and CD8. Interestingly, γδ T cells represent a significant proportion of the total T cells in some tissues, such as the intestinal and pulmonary epithelia, where they contribute to homeostasis of these delicate sites. In contrast to TH cells and Tc cells, γδ T cells do not require antigen presentation by MHC proteins, suggesting that γδ T cells represent an important bridge between innate and adaptive immunity.

Double-Positive Stage

In DN thymocytes, the presence of a functioning β chain provides signals to initiate TCR α-chain gene rearrangement. In contrast to the TCR β chain, α-chain gene variable regions are divided into only two sections, V and J (see Fig. 5–3). Excluding this fact, the process of α-chain gene rearrangement is identical to that of the β chains and similarly results in segments from the V and J regions being connected to a constant region. The appearance of a functional α chain on the cell surface sends a signal to suppress any further TCR gene rearrangements. Concurrently with α-chain rearrangement, thymocytes become both CD4-positive ($CD4^+$) and CD8-positive ($CD8^+$); in this stage of T-cell development, thymocytes are referred to as **double-positive (DP) thymocytes.**

The TCR α and β chains occur in a complex with six other molecules common to all T cells, known collectively as the *CD3/TCR complex.* The six chains of the CD3 portion of the complex assist in intracellular signaling when TCR binds to its specific peptide antigen in an MHC molecule. These chains occur in three pairs: delta-epsilon (δ-ε), gamma-epsilon (γ-ε), and a zeta-zeta (ζ-ζ) dimer found in the cytoplasm of the cell **(Fig. 5–4).**

T-cell receptors do not recognize peptide antigen alone (see Chapter 4). Instead, peptide antigen must be held in an MHC molecule, or "presented" to T cells, a requirement known as **MHC restriction.** This T-cell property is established during the DP stage of thymocyte development. Because gene rearrangement produces TCRs with nearly unlimited specificities, each newly formed receptor must be tested for its ability to interact with MHC through the process of **positive selection (Fig. 5–5).** During positive selection, thymocytes encounter stromal cells in the thymic cortex that express MHC class I and II proteins. These initial interactions between thymocyte TCRs and stromal cell MHC determine the thymocyte's fate: Thymocytes that have TCRs that bind to MHC survive, while those that fail to bind to MHC are induced to die by apoptosis. This selection step is crucial because T cells with receptors that do not bind to MHC cannot function as mature T cells.

Two important molecules for establishing the MHC restriction of T cells are CD4 and CD8, which bind to MHC class I and class II molecules, respectively. During the DP stage, thymocytes express both CD4 and CD8. As positive selection proceeds, a DP thymocyte whose TCR best interacts with a class I MHC molecule will stop expressing CD4 to become a $CD8^+$ "single-positive" (SP) thymocyte. Conversely, a thymocyte whose TCR interacts with class II MHC will cease CD8 expression to become a $CD4^+$ SP thymocyte. Stable expression of either CD4 or CD8 and loss of expression of the opposite marker signify the entrance of the thymocyte into the next phase of differentiation, the SP stage.

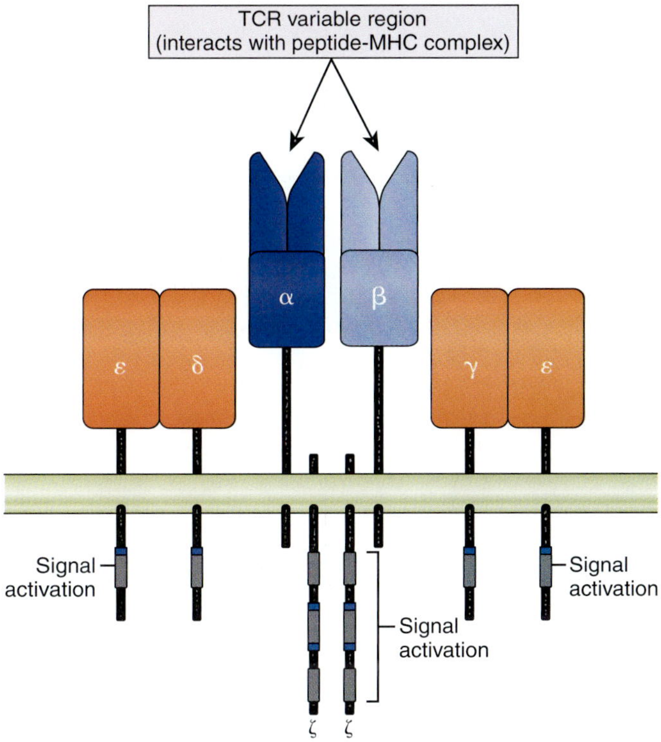

FIGURE 5–4 The TCR/CD3 complex. The main structures in the TCR are the α and β chains, which are responsible for binding to the peptide-MHC complex. Four other types of chains that associate with the α and β chains in the TCR complex are collectively known as *CD3*. These are the ε, γ, δ, and ζ molecules that are essential for transmitting a signal to the T cell's interior when antigen binding occurs. Note that the γ and δ proteins found here are different from the γδ chains of the γδ TCR.

Knowledge Check 5-2

Which phrase describes the structure of the T-cell receptor (TCR) for antigen?

a. Two α chains bound to two β chains
b. An α chain and β chain complexed with a CD3 molecule
c. An antibody complexed with a CD3 molecule
d. Two α chains complexed with a CD4 molecule

Single-Positive Stage

Thymocytes that survive positive selection must overcome one final developmental hurdle before exiting the thymus as mature T cells. A second selection process, called **negative selection,** occurs in the medullary and corticomedullary regions of the thymus. In negative selection, thymic stromal cells express a variety of self-antigens and present peptide fragments of these antigens to positively selected thymocytes **(Fig. 5–6).** A strong reaction between a thymocyte's TCR and any of the self-peptides presented by the thymic stroma

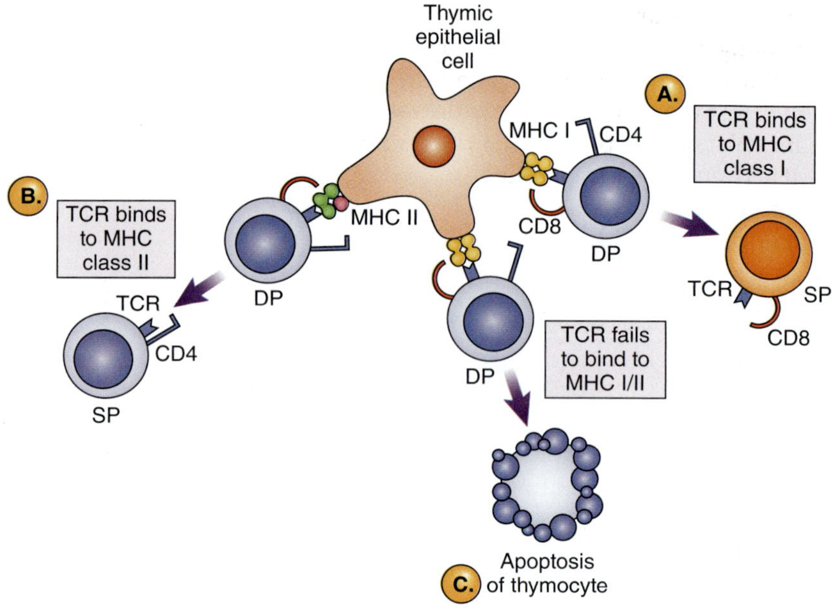

FIGURE 5–5 Positive selection of thymocytes in the thymic cortex. A. Double-positive (DP) thymocytes (expressing both CD4 and CD8) interact with thymic epithelial cells. B. DP thymocytes with TCRs that bind to MHC class I are positively selected as single-positive (SP) thymocytes expressing CD8. Thymocytes with TCRs that bind to MHC class II become SP cells expressing CD4. C. DP thymocytes with TCRs that do not interact with MHC undergo apoptosis.

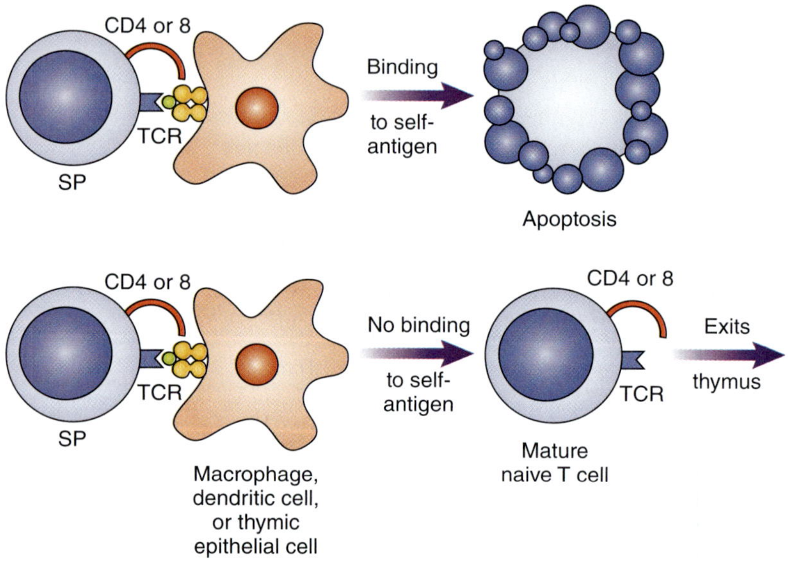

FIGURE 5–6 Negative selection of SP thymocytes in the thymic medulla. When self-antigen is presented in MHC I or II by thymic stromal cells to thymocyte TCRs, two fates are possible: *(top)* strong recognition of self-antigen signals autoreactive potential and results in thymocyte apoptosis; *(bottom)* low-affinity recognition of self-antigen indicates less autoreactive potential and results in thymocyte survival.

indicates a high potential for autoreactivity. To prevent potentially self-reactive T cells from leaving the thymus and subsequently attacking the body's own cells and tissues, thymocytes whose TCRs bind strongly to self-peptide antigens are negatively selected and undergo apoptosis.

To allow negative selection against antigens found in cells and tissues throughout the body, a specialized protein called **AIRE** (autoimmune regulator) is expressed in cells of the thymic medulla. AIRE is a *transcription factor*, a protein that controls gene expression. AIRE's role is to drive thymic expression of many peripheral genes, leading to translation of the encoded proteins, their processing into peptide antigen, and presentation on MHC molecules. One example of a gene whose expression is controlled by AIRE is the pancreatic hormone insulin. In the thymus, unlike in the pancreas, insulin is expressed not as a hormone to control blood glucose but as bait for potentially autoreactive developing T cells.

Critical Thinking 5-2

The pathogenesis of type 1 diabetes (T1D) involves an immune attack on pancreatic β cells, which control blood glucose levels by secreting insulin. Genetic studies have strongly linked the development of T1D to insulin gene mutations that alter the thymic expression of insulin. Using your knowledge of T-cell development, provide a possible mechanism linking insulin expression in the thymus to autoimmune destruction of pancreatic cells.

Mature T Cells

Once a T cell exits the thymus, it is considered *mature*. Mature T cells that have not yet encountered the specific peptide antigen recognized by their TCR are referred to as "naive." Mature naive T cells spend their lives circulating and recirculating between the blood and lymphatics to increase the probability of encountering antigen. During this time, each naive

T cell makes many contacts with MHC molecules on antigen-presenting cells (APCs) throughout the body. For an individual naive T cell, the journey to activation may last several years. Most will recirculate in vain, never uniting with an APC bearing the specific peptide antigen recognized by their TCR.

If antigen recognition occurs, naive T lymphocytes become *activated* and differentiate into functionally active cells. Activated CD4$^+$ TH cells immediately begin to proliferate and secrete cytokines. Signals in the environment where TH-cell activation occurs, such as cytokines secreted by nearby APCs, influence which cytokines the TH cells produce. CD8$^+$ TC cells are also activated by antigen recognition. Responsive to stimulation by APCs and cytokines produced by TH cells, TC cells proliferate and begin to seek and destroy cells displaying their specific antigen.

Knowledge Check 5-3

The most mature T cells possess:

a. Neither CD4 nor CD8
b. Both CD4 and CD8
c. CD4 or CD8
d. MHC II molecules

Stages in B-Cell Development

Like T cells, B cells are derived from early lymphocyte progenitor cells in the bone marrow. Unlike T cells, which arise in the bone marrow but develop in the thymus, B cells mature entirely within the bone marrow. There, stromal cells create special developmental niches, promoting the maturation of B-cell precursors. As with T cells, B-cell precursors undergo an ordered developmental process that prepares them for their role in antibody production and, simultaneously, restricts their antigen specificity.

The first phase of B-cell development, the **antigen-independent phase,** results in mature B cells that have not yet been exposed to antigen. This phase can be divided according to the formation of several distinct subpopulations: **pro-B cells** (progenitor B cells), **pre-B cells** (precursor B cells), **immature B cells,** and mature B cells. B cells that reach maturity and encounter their specific antigen begin an **antigen-dependent phase** of development that typically involves the generation of plasma cells and, in many cases, long-lived memory B cells. **Figure 5–7** depicts the changes that occur as B cells mature from the pro–B-cell stage to become memory cells or plasma cells. Key features of B cells in different developmental stages are listed in **Table 5–2** and discussed in detail in the sections that follow.

5-1 Clinical Correlations

Lymphocyte Surface Markers in Malignancies

Because the surface markers expressed by B cells and T cells change during their development, these markers are routinely used by the World Health Organization and the International Consensus Classification to classify leukemias and lymphomas into categories. Such grouping has allowed for more accurate diagnosis, determination of patient prognosis, and selection of the most effective therapies for individual patients (see Chapter 18).

Pro-B Cells

At the earliest developmental stage, B-cell progenitors receive signals from bone marrow stromal cells through cell-to-cell contact and soluble cytokines, such as IL-7. This signaling induces the expression of several transcription factors including E2A, early B-cell factor (EBF), interferon regulatory factor 8 (IFR8), and paired box protein 5 (PAX5). Working in concert, these factors drive the expression of genes that distinguish pro-B cells from progenitor cells. Such gene expression is required for continued survival and development of the pro-B cell.

One of the most important events of the pro–B-cell phase is rearrangement of the **B-cell–receptor (BCR)** genes. The BCR is simply a cell surface version of an *immunoglobulin,* or antibody molecule that can bind to a specific antigen (see Chapter 3). It is associated with transmembrane Igα and Igβ chains, which mediate signals to the B cell once an antigen is bound. Although structurally and functionally very different, BCRs share many similarities with T-cell receptors. For instance, both BCRs and TCRs:

- Are composed of two different chains (TCRs consist of α and β chains, whereas BCRs contain immunoglobulin *heavy* and *light* chains)
- Contain variable regions, which determine their antigen specificity
- Contain constant regions, which allow for intracellular signaling and activation
- Are encoded by genes with a similar *modular* structure (i.e., V, D, and J)
- Use similar mechanisms for gene rearrangement

BCR genes undergo rearrangement in a stepwise manner, beginning with the heavy chain genes. As with the TCR β chain, the heavy chain genes contain multiple V, D, and J segments. Enzymes bring together one V, one D, and one J segment by looping out intervening DNA. The enzyme terminal deoxynucleotidyl transferase incorporates random nucleotides into the joints between V-D and D-J. Because of this targeted gene rearrangement, pro-B cells generate unique BCR genes not found in the genome and (theoretically) not shared with any other B cell (see Chapter 3).

Because this process is random, certain BCR heavy chain rearrangements may shift the gene out of frame or result in a stop codon in the middle of the gene, leading to a nonfunctional heavy chain. In such cases, rearrangement continues for the heavy chain alleles on each chromosome 14 until a functional heavy chain can be produced. As with the TCR, once heavy chain rearrangement is completed successfully on one chromosome 14, allelic exclusion silences expression of the heavy chain gene on the opposite chromosome. For a pro-B cell to progress to the next phase of differentiation, at least one heavy chain gene must undergo successful rearrangement.

Pre-B Cells

Once production of successfully rearranged heavy chains begins, developing B cells enter the pre–B-cell developmental stage. During this stage, most translated heavy chains accumulate in the cytoplasm, while some travel to the cell surface and combine with a **surrogate light chain,** a complex of two

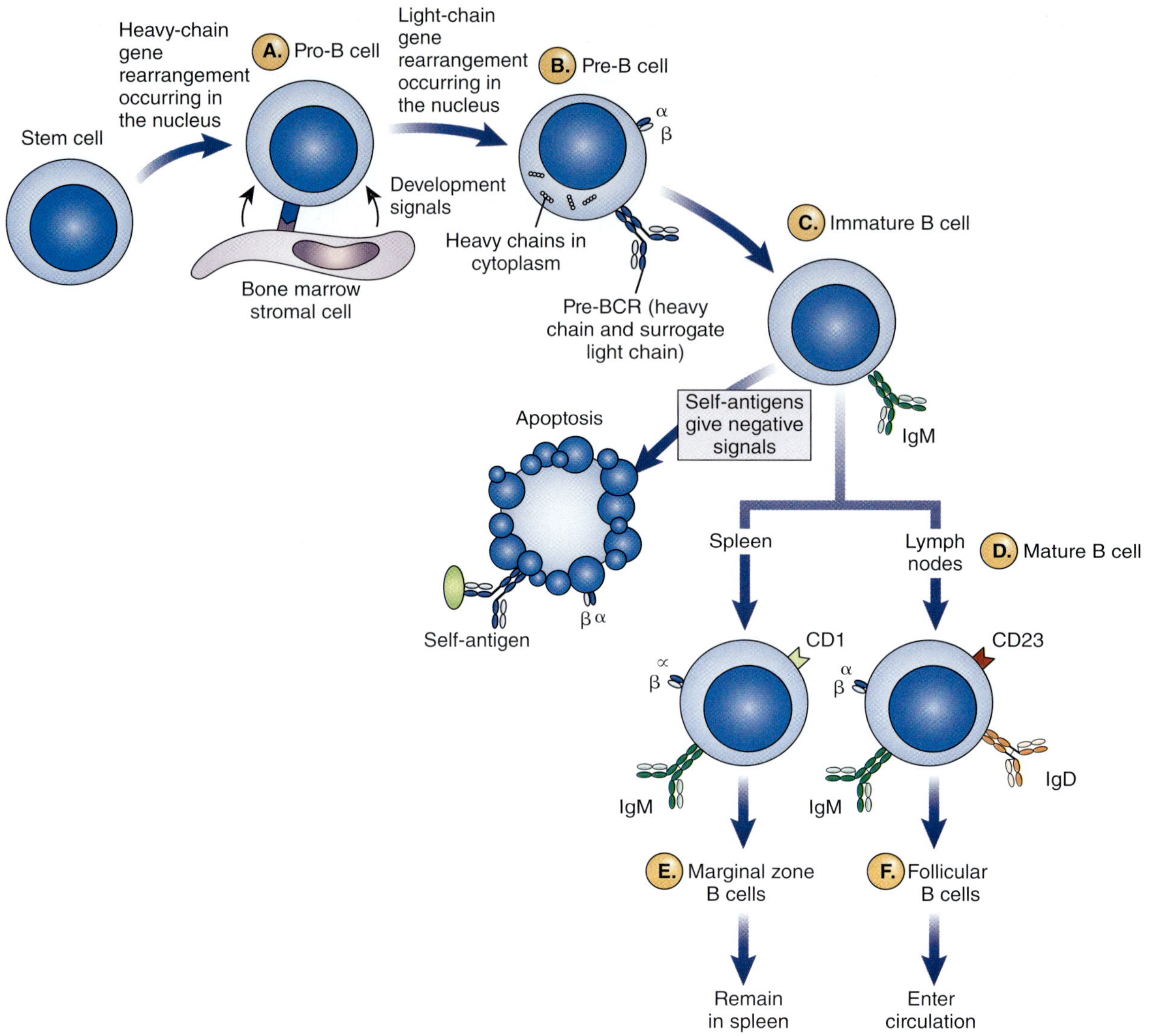

FIGURE 5–7 B-cell development. Selected markers are shown for the various stages in B-cell differentiation. (A) Pro-B cell. (B) Pre-B cell. (C) Immature B cell. (D) Mature B cell. (E) Marginal-zone B cell. (F) Follicular B cell. Stages A through C occur in the bone marrow, whereas stages E and F occur in the spleen and lymph nodes, respectively.

Table 5-2 Stages of B-Cell Development

	DEVELOPMENTAL STAGE				
	Pro-B Cell	**Pre-B cell**	**Immature B cell**	**Mature B cell**	**Plasma Cell**
Key CD markers	CD10 CD19	CD10 CD19 CD20	CD10 CD19 CD20 CD21 CD40	CD19 CD20 CD21 CD40	CD138
B-cell receptor	—	Pre-BCR: Immunoglobulin (Ig) heavy chain Surrogate light chain	Functional BCR: Immunoglobulin M (IgM) heavy chains and κ or λ light chains	Functional BCR: Immunoglobulin D (IgD) or IgM heavy chains and κ or λ light chains	—
MHC II	+	+	++	++	–

BCR = B-cell receptor; MHC = major histocompatibility complex.

proteins, which resembles the immunoglobulin light chain. The newly rearranged heavy chain and surrogate light chain combine with the signal transducing subunits Ig-α and Ig-β to form a structure known as the pre–B-cell receptor (pre-BCR). Pre-B cells that assemble the pre-BCR undergo several rounds of cell division, resulting in many clones of the original cell, all of which possess identical heavy chains.

Simultaneously with the appearance of the pre-BCR at the surface of the cell, light chain gene rearrangement begins. Humans, like most mammals, have two different types of light chain genes: κ and λ. Similar to the TCR α genes, the κ and λ light chain genes are composed of multiple V and J segments. During rearrangement, a V segment, J segment, and light chain constant region are stitched together. Successful rearrangement of either a κ or λ gene pauses gene rearrangement, allowing the gene product to be tested out.

Two light chains and two heavy chains are fastened together by disulfide bonds to form an immunoglobulin, which moves to the cell surface to replace the pre-BCR. Because the heavy chains made during the pre–B-cell stage incorporate the μ constant region, the first class of immunoglobulin produced is immunoglobulin M (IgM; see Chapter 3). The appearance of a functional BCR on the B-cell surface signifies entry of the cell into the next phase of development, the *immature B cell*.

Immature B Cells

The appearance of a functional IgM BCR on the cell surface indicates that rearrangement of the genes encoding the receptor is now complete, and that a new B cell exists with the potential to produce antibody for a specific and unique antigen. The immunoglobulin variable regions, found on both the light and heavy chains, determine the antigen specificity of the immature B cell and its IgM BCR.

Because gene rearrangement produces BCRs with random specificities, the likelihood is high that some newly formed BCRs may respond to self-antigens. Therefore, B cells (like T cells) require a process of negative selection. When antigen binds to the BCR, mature B cells respond by becoming activated, proliferating, and producing antibody. In contrast, immature B cells respond to the same signals by halting their development and undergoing apoptosis. Thus, most B cells capable of producing antibody to self-antigens (autoantibodies) are deleted before exiting the bone marrow. The elimination of B cells that bear self-reactive receptors is known as **central tolerance,** and it is estimated that more than 90% of B cells die in this manner (see Chapter 15).

Many surface markers other than IgM BCRs also begin to appear during the immature B-cell phase. CD21, CD40, and class II MHC molecules are just some of the proteins and glycoproteins that decorate the external membrane of the immature B cell. These markers are useful for laboratory identification of B cells and essential to the function of B cells, especially their role in antigen presentation to CD4⁺ TH cells. For instance, CD21 acts as a receptor for a breakdown product of the complement component C3, known as *C3d* (see Chapter 7). The CD21 receptor enhances the likelihood of contact between B cells and antigens because antigens often become coated with complement fragments during the immune response. CD40 and class II MHC are important for the interaction of B cells with TH cells.

A B cell that expresses a functional IgM BCR survives selection by not reacting to self-antigens, and begins to display certain B-cell markers (CD21, CD40, and MHC) is considered a mature B cell. B cells that have achieved these milestones exit the bone marrow and are carried in the blood to the spleen for the next stage in their development.

Mature B Cells

In the spleen, immature B cells develop into one of two types of mature B cells, *follicular B cells* and *marginal-zone B cells*. Follicular B cells constantly recirculate between the blood and secondary lymphoid organs in search of their specific antigens, whereas marginal-zone B cells remain in the spleen to respond quickly to bloodborne pathogens. Both marginal-zone and follicular B cells produce antibody, but the circumstances that trigger antibody production, the types of antibodies produced, and the duration of the response are very different between these two populations.

Most mature B cells are destined to become follicular B cells. *Follicular* refers to the lymph node region where this type of mature B cell tends to localize during its movements throughout the body (see Chapter 1). Lymphoid follicles represent dense clusters of naive B cells awaiting exposure to their specific antigens. When antigen recognition occurs, follicular B cells contact CD4⁺ follicular helper (Tfh) cells. Cooperation between antigen-activated B cells and Tfh cells is critical for many B-cell processes, including the formation of immunologic memory (see "Immune Response to T-Dependent Antigens").

Marginal-zone B cells receive their name from the anatomical site in which they are most concentrated, the marginal sinus of the spleen. Experimental evidence suggests that BCR specificity plays a role in determining which mature B cells come to reside in the spleen, because most marginal-zone B cells recognize polysaccharide antigens found on common bacterial pathogens. When marginal-zone B cells contact their specific antigens, they do not receive help from Tfh cells (see "Immune Response to T-Independent Antigens"). Instead, they differentiate into IgM-secreting plasma cells, each producing vast quantities of IgM and only stopping once the infection has been eliminated. Because Tfh cell help is essential for the formation of immunologic memory, the marginal-zone response must begin anew upon each exposure to a particular polysaccharide antigen.

In addition to an IgM BCR, most mature B cells also express an IgD form of the BCR. The IgM and IgD BCRs expressed on a particular B cell have the same antigenic specificity, although it is not clear what role IgD plays in sensing antigen or B-cell activation. Nevertheless, the presence of both IgM and IgD on the cell membrane signifies a mature B cell.

When a BCR binds its specific antigen, multiple BCR molecules are brought together, initiating an intracellular signaling cascade. These signals drive the B cell to enter a proliferative stage where it divides rapidly to produce both antibody-secreting plasma cells and, for follicular B cells, memory B cells **(Fig. 5–8).**

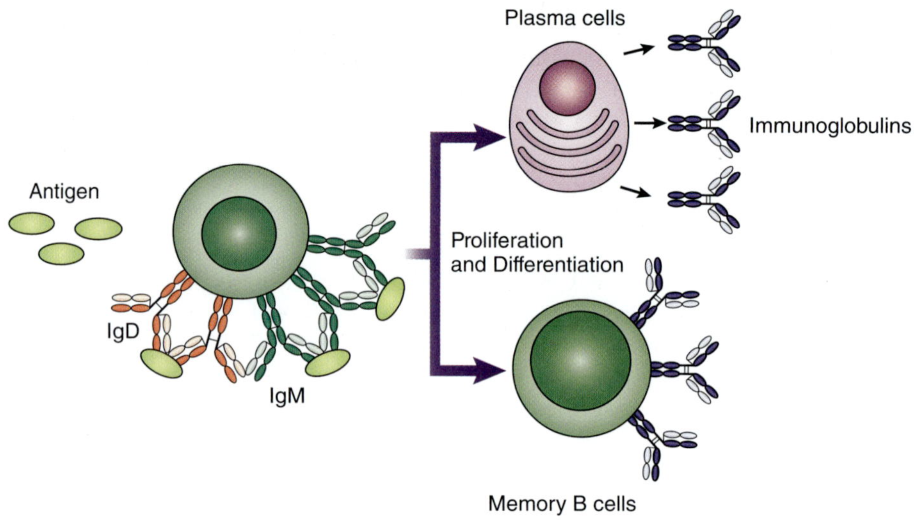

FIGURE 5–8 B-cell activation. B cells bind to antigen by means of immunoglobulin receptors (IgM and IgD). B cells activated by encountering antigen proliferate and may, upon receiving help from T cells, become antibody-secreting plasma cells or memory B cells capable of responding rapidly upon re-exposure to the same antigen.

Plasma Cells

The histological appearance of **plasma cells** reflects their role as fully differentiated antibody-production factories (see Fig. 1–9). Plasma cells express very little immunoglobulin on their surface membranes but have abundant cytoplasmic immunoglobulin. Because gene transcription in plasma cells is dominated by antibody-coding genes, their oval-shaped nuclei often contain heavily clumped, dark-staining chromatin signifying many silenced genes. To accommodate translation and post-translational processing of the large quantities of antibody being manufactured, plasma cells have ample endoplasmic reticulum and a well-defined Golgi apparatus. Resident plasma cells are a common feature of the bone marrow and the germinal centers found in peripheral lymphoid organs. Plasma cells survive in bone marrow niches surrounded by stromal cells, which provide stimulation to plasma cells via cytokines. Stromal cell support allows plasma cells to be long-lived and fosters their continual production of antibodies. In contrast, plasma cells located in tissues other than the bone marrow produce antibody for only a short time before dying. A key surface marker on plasma cells is CD138.

Knowledge Check 5-4

A peripheral blood sample from a patient with multiple myeloma, a plasma cell malignancy, is evaluated for treatment effectiveness by flow cytometry. If treatment is effective, which lymphocyte population would you expect to be most reduced?

a. $CD3^+$ $CD4^+$
b. $CD19^+$ $CD20^+$
c. $CD3^+$ $CD8^+$
d. $CD138^+$

The Roles of T Cells in the Adaptive Immune Response

When infection occurs, APCs such as macrophages and dendritic cells are among the first immune cells to respond. Sensing the presence of danger via innate receptors, such as toll-like receptors (see Chapter 2), APCs engulf pathogens and deliver antigens to local lymph nodes where APCs encounter naive T cells. Since each T cell has a TCR of a different specificity, very few circulating naive T cells (less than 1 in 10^5) are activated during a given infection. The continuous recirculation of naive T cells between the blood and lymph nodes greatly increases the likelihood of an APC connecting with the few T cells whose TCRs recognize the antigens associated with an infection.

Antigen Presentation

The primary mode of communication between T cells and APCs involves direct cell-to-cell contact (discussed in more detail in Chapter 4). Using a process known as *antigen presentation,* APCs display peptide antigens to T cells via MHC molecules, which cradle antigen peptides in a manner similar to a bun holding a hot dog. This linear presentation of the antigen peptide allows the TCR to bind along its entire length. Humans and related mammals express two different forms of MHC protein: MHC class I and MHC class II. The overall structures and functions of MHC class I and class II are similar. However, the source of the peptides presented by each type of MHC and the type of T cell each MHC class interacts with are quite different.

As we discussed in Chapter 4, class I MHC molecules present peptide antigens derived from cytoplasmic sources, such as endogenous peptides manufactured by healthy cells. In diseased cells, the antigens presented by class I MHC might include peptides associated with intracellular bacteria, viruses, or cancer cells. Class I MHC molecules present antigen to Tc cells, whose function is to destroy cells infected with intracellular pathogens and malignant cells. CD8 stabilizes the interaction between the Tc TCR and class I MHC.

In contrast, class II MHC molecules present peptides captured from the extracellular space, such as those derived from extracellular microbes. Class II MHC molecules allow APCs to present peptide antigens to TH cells. As with Tc cells, an additional protein is required to stabilize the interaction between class II MHC and the TH TCR, and this role is filled by CD4.

During the encounter between naive T cells and APCs in the lymph nodes, multiple contacts form between TCRs and the MHC molecules expressed by each APC. If the TCR recognizes one of the many peptide antigens simultaneously presented by an APC, the potential exists that the naive T cell will become activated. TCR recognition alone, however, is not sufficient to activate a naive T cell. For successful activation to occur, the APC must also provide costimulation by expressing CD80 or CD86 molecules, which bind to CD28 on the T-cell surface. This combination of signals initiates an intracellular signaling cascade within the T cell, leading to activation.

Knowledge Check 5-5

Which of the following terms are correctly paired?

a. Class I MHC–exogenous/extracellular peptide antigen
b. Class II MHC–CD8
c. Class I MHC–TH cell
d. Class II MHC–CD4

Actions of Helper T (TH) and Regulatory T (Treg) Cells

TH cells are instrumental in the adaptive immune response because of their role in secreting cytokines that drive the activities of other immune cells, including macrophages, granulocytes, TC cells, and B cells. When activated, some TH cells remain in the lymph node to direct the response of B cells and other T cells, while other activated TH cells travel to infected tissues to direct the responses of immune cells.

Several subsets of activated TH cells exist, each of which makes a distinct set of cytokines that influence the immune response in different ways. This topic is discussed in detail in Chapter 6. The most prominent TH subsets and their functions are as follows:

- **TH1 cells** activate CD8+ TC cells and macrophages to fight intracellular parasites.
- **TH2 cells** activate mast cells, B cells, and eosinophils to control the clearance of extracellular parasites, such as intestinal worms, and have a role in allergic responses.
- **TH17 cells** recruit neutrophils in response to extracellular bacterial and fungal infections and play a role in pathological autoimmune responses by enhancing inflammation.
- **Follicular helper T (Tfh) cells** reside in the lymph nodes and interact with B cells to assist in antibody production. They provide signals to B cells as they undergo activation, immunoglobulin class switching, affinity maturation, and the formation of B-cell memory (discussed later).
- **Regulatory T (Treg) cells** comprise about 5% of all CD4+ T cells. They suppress the responses of other TH subsets to self-antigens and harmless antigens, such as antigens present in common foods.

Polarizing cytokines direct the newly activated TH cells to differentiate into a selected subset, depending on the particular type of infection present. Each TH subset, in turn, produces a unique set of *effector cytokines* that carry out the type of immune response (cell-mediated or humoral) that will be most effective against the invading pathogen **(Fig. 5–9).**

During the many rounds of cell division that follow TH-cell activation, two distinct populations of cells are formed: *effector T cells* and *memory T cells*. Most of the TH cells become effector cells that secrete cytokines and possibly travel to infected tissues where their activities are most needed. A small percentage of the TH cells generated after activation will differentiate into memory cells. Memory TH cells enter a quiescent state and await re-exposure to their specific antigen. If contact with the same or similar antigens occurs again, memory lymphocytes respond rapidly by undergoing cell division and immediately secreting appropriate cytokines.

Action of Cytotoxic T (TC) Cells

CD8-expressing TC cells, also known as *cytotoxic T lymphocytes* (CTLs), play a different role than TH cells. Activated TC cells migrate to sites of infection and initiate apoptosis in cells infected with intracellular parasites and viruses, referred to as *target cells*. Unlike natural killer (NK) cells, which have a similar role but recognize infection through germline-encoded receptors, the activity of TC cells is driven by TCR recognition and is therefore antigen specific.

Upon recognition of peptide antigen in class I MHC on the surface of a target cell, TC cells kill their targets using two main strategies: (1) the release of cytotoxic granules from the T-cell cytoplasm or (2) ligation of death receptors on a target cell's surface. In either case, the target cell rapidly undergoes apoptosis **(Fig. 5–10).**

TC-cell granules contain two toxic substances: perforins and granzymes. Perforins are proteins that insert into target-cell membranes and polymerize to form pores. Granzymes are *serine proteases,* a class of enzymes that can initiate apoptosis in the target cell. TCR recognition of antigen by a TC cell causes accumulation of granules in the T-cell cytoplasm adjacent to the target cell. Subsequently, the granules are released by the T cell in the direction of the target cell. Almost immediately, perforin begins forming holes in the target-cell membrane, through which granzymes can enter. Once in the target cell, granzymes activate caspase enzymes that cleave DNA and disrupt mitochondria. With its genetic material shredded and energy levels dropping, the target cell quietly dies.

TC cells can also induce apoptosis in target cells by ligation of death receptors. In this situation, TCR recognition of antigen complexed with target-cell MHC leads to expression of the death-inducing protein Fas-ligand (FasL) by the T cell. When FasL binds to a Fas protein on the target-cell membrane, apoptotic pathways are set in motion.

The Role of B Cells in the Adaptive Immune Response

As we mentioned earlier, the function of B cells is to produce antibodies in the humoral immune response. The essential first step in the activation of a mature B cell is exposure of the IgM BCR to its specific antigen. Antigen recognition by the different types of mature B cells (follicular and marginal zone)

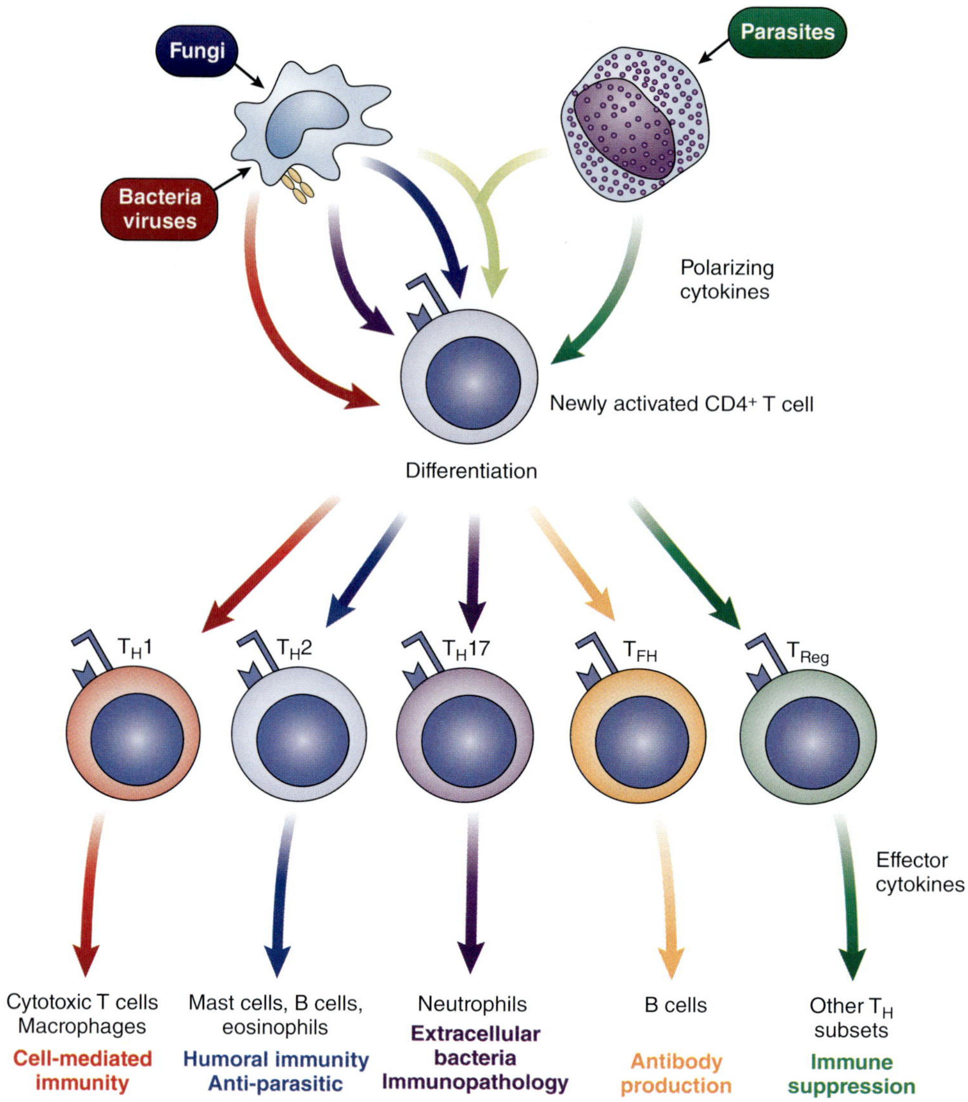

FIGURE 5–9 Helper T (TH) subsets. Depending on the type of pathogen encountered, APCs secrete a specific combination of polarizing cytokines that direct newly activated CD4⁺ TH cells to further differentiate into one type of TH (e.g., TH1, TH2, TH17, Tfh, or Treg). These specialized T cells release effector cytokines that coordinate an appropriate immune response against the pathogen.

occurs in different anatomical regions—the lymph nodes and the spleen, respectively. Because the follicular B-cell response depends heavily on the activity of Tfh cells to promote an effective antibody response, antigens that provoke this type of response are often referred to as **T-dependent antigens.** Correspondingly, as marginal-zone B cells do not require the help of Tfh cells, the antigens recognized by marginal-zone B cells are referred to as **T-independent antigens.**

Immune Response to T-Dependent Antigens

Because only protein-based antigens can stimulate a T-cell response, T-dependent antigens are almost always proteins or glycoproteins. For an adaptive response to occur, these antigens must travel from sites of infection to local lymph nodes, where mature naive follicular B cells and T cells reside. Protein antigens make this journey suspended in lymphatic fluid or carried by APCs (macrophages or dendritic cells).

The initial step in the T-dependent antibody response involves activation of antigen-specific CD4⁺ TH in the T-cell zones of the lymph nodes by contact with dendritic cells that have processed the antigen and combined it with an MHC II molecule (see **Fig. 5–11** and Chapter 4). Naive B cells in the follicles become activated by the same antigen through binding of the antigen to antigen-specific BCRs via surface immunoglobulin (see Fig. 5–8). In contrast to T-cell recognition of antigen, protein antigens bind to the BCRs in their *native* state (that is, not processed or denatured). BCR antigen recognition initiates a cascade of intracellular signaling within the B cell, driving the cell into an activated state. In response to BCR signaling, the B-cell cytoskeleton is mobilized to internalize the bound antigen using a process known as *endocytosis.* Antigen uptake allows for antigen processing and presentation of antigenic peptides on class II MHC molecules on the B-cell surface.

Following activation, the TH and B cells migrate toward each other by responding to *chemokines* (cytokines that induce lymphocyte migration) and begin to interact at the follicular edge. In this context, B cells act as APCs, presenting peptide fragments derived from internalized antigen to TH cells. If TCR recognition of the same antigenic peptide occurs, a T cell–B cell pair is formed (see Fig. 5–11). Some of the activated TH and B cells migrate into the lymph node follicles, where they form *germinal centers;* the TH are also induced to differentiate into Tfh.

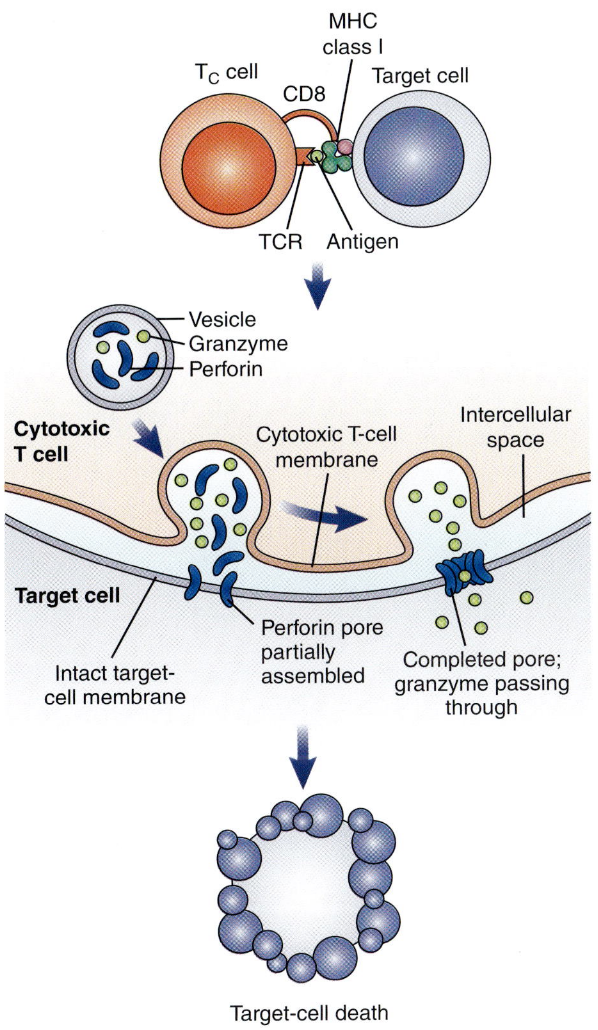

FIGURE 5–10 Activity of cytotoxic T cells. The $CD8^+$ Tc cell recognizes peptide antigen presented in class I MHC. When binding occurs, vesicles containing perforin and granzymes move toward the point of contact with the target cell. Granules fuse with the membrane and release their lytic contents into the space between the T cell and target cell. Perforin inserts itself into the target-cell membrane and polymerizes to form a pore. Granzymes enter the target cell and induce apoptosis.

After contact occurs, activated TH cells provide activated B cells with two additional signals that contribute to the B-cell response. One of these signals involves binding of the CD40 ligand (CD40L) on the TH to the CD40 molecule on B cells, which stimulates B-cell proliferation. The activated TH cells also secrete cytokines called *interleukins* that induce B-cell proliferation and differentiation into plasma cells. One of these cytokines, interleukin-2 (IL-2), stimulates proliferation of the antigen-specific TH.

Each B cell produced during this replicative explosion will inherit a BCR identical to that of the parent B cell and will therefore recognize the same antigen. Daughter B cells produced during the proliferative phase of the T-dependent response have two potential fates: Some remain in contact with T cells and differentiate into IgM-secreting plasma cells, whereas others form germinal centers within follicles.

In the germinal centers, three overlapping processes occur that enhance the antibody response over time: *immunoglobulin isotype switching, affinity maturation,* and *memory-cell generation.* These processes are described briefly here and discussed in detail in Chapter 3. Isotype switching involves immunoglobulin gene rearrangements occurring under the direction of TH cytokines, which results in a change of the immunoglobulin class produced from IgM to another class, such as IgA or IgG. Affinity maturation is a process caused by changes in the B-cell immunoglobulin genes that results in the ability of the antibodies to bind antigen more strongly (i.e., develop a higher affinity) over the course of the immune response. Plasma cells generated during the immune response exit lymph nodes and secrete large quantities of antibody of the isotype and affinity achieved.

Memory-cell generation results in the production of lymphocytes that can rapidly respond to a re-exposure to the same antigen by producing high-affinity, class-switched antibody. Memory cells may remain in the lymph nodes where they lie in wait for the antigen or travel to distal tissues.

5-2 Clinical Correlations

CD40 ligand deficiency

Some people fail to express the CD40 ligand protein on activated T cells, resulting in severe immunodeficiency. These patients are not capable of immunoglobulin class switching to IgG, do not exhibit affinity maturation during an adaptive response, and fail to generate substantial B-cell memory. They often have extremely high levels of circulating IgM antibody; hence, CD40 ligand-related immunodeficiencies are *hyper-IgM syndromes.*

Immune Response to T-Independent Antigens

Splenic marginal-zone B cells, which respond to polysaccharides, do not interact with T cells during their response to antigen. The presence of many repeating elements on these antigens causes cross-linking of multiple BCRs on a single B cell, inducing proliferation and antibody production **(Fig. 5–12).** Examples of T-independent antigens include plant lectins, polymerized proteins with repeating molecular patterns, and lipopolysaccharides in bacterial cell walls. Because T cells do not participate in this type of B-cell response, processes such as isotype switching, affinity maturation, and memory formation do not occur. Consequently, these antigens elicit IgM production only.

Knowledge Check 5-6

In contrast to T-dependent antibody responses, T-independent responses:

a. Require TH activity
b. Result in memory B-cell generation
c. Are characterized by affinity maturation
d. Are induced by polysaccharide antigens with repeating subunits

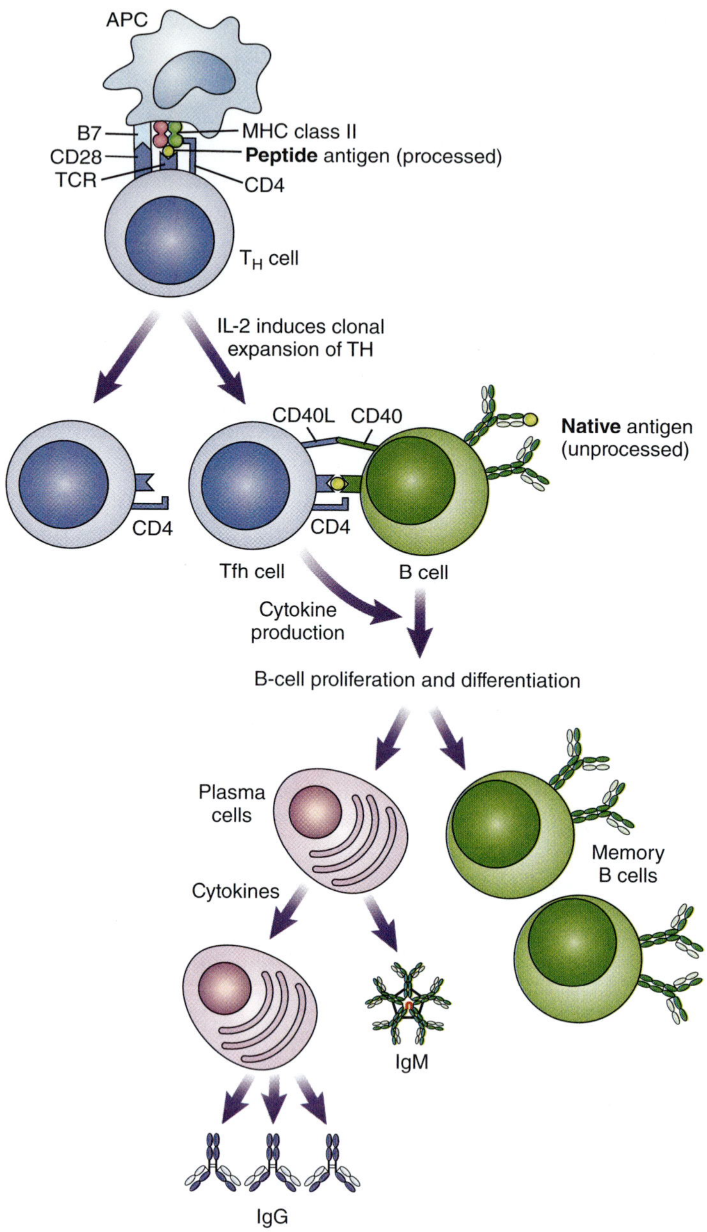

FIGURE 5–11 T- and B-cell cooperation in the immune response. CD4+ T cells recognize exogenous antigen on a macrophage, along with class II MHC. Binding between CD28 and B7 enhances interaction between the cells. TH cells go through clonal expansion and produce cytokines, including IL-2. B cells capable of responding to the same antigen present antigen to TH cells through the class II MHC receptor. The TCR binds antigen, and CD4 binds to class II MHC. CD40L binds to the costimulatory molecule CD40, enhancing the reaction. Cytokine production by the T cell causes B cells to proliferate and produce plasma cells, which secrete antibody.

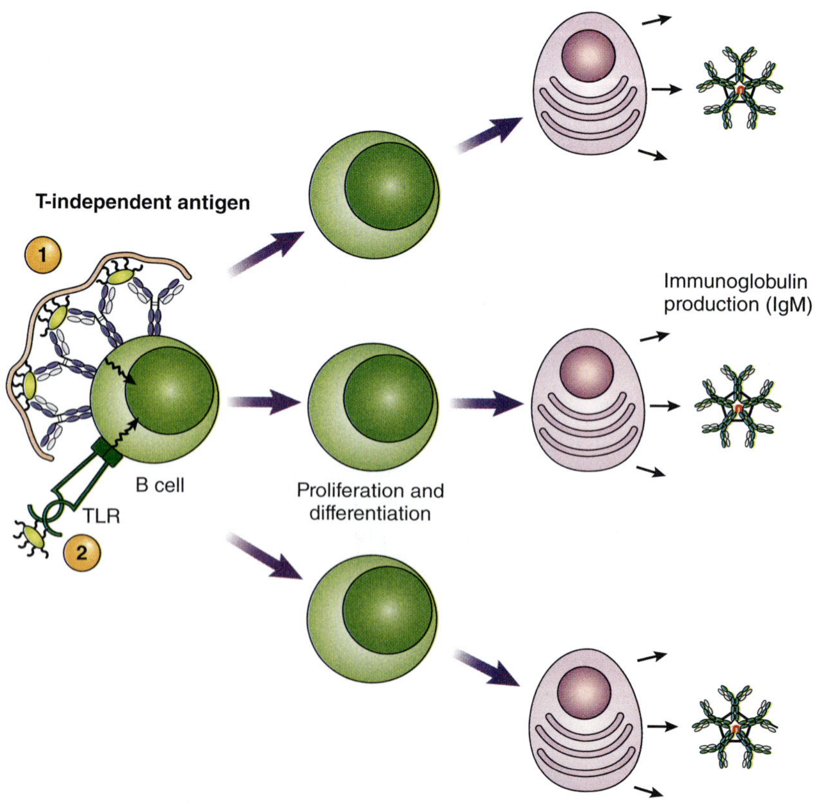

FIGURE 5–12 Activating signals for T-independent antigens. (1) T-independent antigens can bind to B cells through immunoglobulin receptors and trigger B-cell transformation directly. Several antigen receptors must be cross-linked to activate a B cell directly. (2) Antigens can also be bound to innate immune receptors on B cells, such as TLRs.

KEY CONCEPTS

Introduction

- Adaptive immunity is characterized by antigen specificity, memory, and enhancement upon repeated exposure to the same antigen.

Cell-Mediated and Humoral Immunity

- Adaptive immunity can be broadly divided into two branches: *cell-mediated* immunity, carried out by T cells, and *humoral* immunity, involving antibody production by B cells and plasma cells.
- The two major classes of T lymphocytes are helper T (TH) cells, which secrete cytokines, proteins that allow for cell communication in immune responses, and cytotoxic T (Tc) cells, which kill host cells infected with intracellular pathogens and tumor cells. The TH cells can be further divided into subpopulations based on their cytokine production and functions.
- Adaptive immune responses involve clonal selection, resulting in proliferation of antigen-specific lymphocytes (effector cells that mediate the immune response) and memory cells that can be activated quickly if re-exposure to the same antigen occurs.

Lymphocyte Development

- All lymphocytes arise in the bone marrow from hematopoietic stem cells (lymphoid progenitor cells), but T cells and B cells undergo different maturation processes.
- B lymphocytes remain in the bone marrow for most of their maturation, whereas T cells exit the bone marrow and continue their development in the thymus.
- The primary antigen receptors of the lymphocytes undergo genetic rearrangement so that each naive lymphocyte expresses a unique receptor with a different specificity than other lymphocytes. Taken as a whole, the body's lymphocyte population can respond to an almost unlimited variety of pathogens.
- The T-cell receptor (TCR) is composed of two protein chains called α and β. TCRs allow T cells to recognize peptide antigen, but the peptide must be presented by an MHC molecule on the surface of an APC.
- The BCR is composed primarily of an immunoglobulin molecule on the surface of the B cell. BCRs allow B cells to detect their antigen, which is usually exposed on the surface of an antigenic substance.
- In the thymus, T cells undergo several stages of development before becoming naive T cells capable of patrolling the body and responding to antigen: double negative (DN), double positive (DP), and single positive (SP). These stages are characterized by expression of the surface molecules CD4 and CD8.
- B-cell development can be divided into a series of *antigen-independent* stages, consisting of pro-, pre-, and immature B cells. B cells that survive antigen-independent development and encounter their specific antigens enter an *antigen-dependent* phase where they can become antibody-secreting plasma cells or memory cells.

The Role of T Cells in Adaptive Immune Responses

- Binding of a T cell to its specific antigen cannot occur until the antigen has been processed by a dendritic cell or macrophage (APCs) and displayed on the surface of the APC in combination with an MHC molecule.
- APCs present class I MHC-peptide complexes to the TCRs on antigen-specific Tc cells. The interaction is stabilized by the Tc marker, CD8.
- APCs present class II MHC-peptide complexes to the TCRs on antigen-specific TH cells. The interaction is stabilized by the TH marker, CD4.
- TH cells respond to extracellular antigens (e.g., from microbes outside of host cells) and are classified into subpopulations according to the cytokines they produce. Major subpopulations include TH1 cells, which activate cell-mediated immune responses; TH2 cells, which direct antibody responses; TH17 cells, which induce inflammation; Treg cells, which suppress harmful immune responses; and Tfh cells, which assist antibody production in the lymph nodes.
- After activation by APCs, TH cells travel to infected tissues, where they secrete cytokines that direct the immune response. Activated TH cells proliferate substantially, resulting in a large population of cells that respond to a particular antigen, and some develop into memory TH cells.
- Tc cells respond to intracellular antigens in diseased host cells. They induce apoptosis in cells infected with intracellular pathogens or in cancer cells by releasing perforins (pore-forming proteins) and granzymes (enzymes that cause DNA breakage and protein cleavage) from their cytotoxic granules in the direction of the target cell.

The Role of B Cells in the Adaptive Immune Response

- When they reach maturity, B cells become one of two populations, follicular B cells or marginal-zone B cells. Follicular B cells patrol and occupy B-cell follicles in lymph nodes, whereas marginal-zone B cells spend their lives in the marginal sinus of the spleen.
- Interaction between B cells and T cells in the lymph nodes is essential for T-dependent antibody responses. During this interaction, B cells that have bound native antigen via their BCR process the antigen and present it in combination with MHC II to antigen-specific TH that have been activated by APCs. The TH cells provide activating signals to these B cells through binding of their CD40L receptor to the CD40 molecule on the B cells, inducing the latter to proliferate. The TH cells also

release cytokines that enhance B-cell proliferation and differentiation into antibody-secreting plasma cells.

- Some of the activated TH cells in the T-dependent responses travel into the lymph node follicles and differentiate into Tfh cells, which interact with B cells to form germinal centers. In the germinal centers, three important events occur: immunoglobulin class switching (antibody production changes from IgM to IgG, IgA, or IgE), somatic hypermutation (antibody affinity increases during the response), and generation of memory B cells (allows rapid response upon reinfection with the same pathogen).
- Antibody responses to T-independent antigens, such as microbial polysaccharides that have repeating identical subunits, do not require T-cell help. Subunits from these antigens bind to multiple BCRs on the B-cell surface, cross-linking them to stimulate B-cell proliferation and differentiation. These responses are often IgM only, do not change throughout infection, and fail to generate immunologic memory.

Study Guide: Comparison of T and B Cells

T CELLS	B CELLS
Develop in the thymus	Develop in the bone marrow
Found in blood (majority of circulating lymphocytes), thoracic duct fluid, lymph nodes, thymus	Found in blood, bone marrow, spleen, lymph nodes
Principal cell in cell-mediated immune responses; assist or suppress antibody responses	Principal cell in humoral immunity
End products of helper T or cytotoxic T-cell activation are cytokines	End product of B-cell activation is antibody
Surface markers include CD2 (all T cells), CD3 (all T cells), CD4 (helper T and regulatory T cells), CD8 (cytotoxic T cells)	Surface markers include CD19, CD20, CD21, CD40, class II MHC
TCR consists of one α and one β chain associated with CD3	BCR consists of an IgM or IgD monomer associated with transmembrane Igα and Igβ chains

CASE STUDIES

1. A 2-year-old child is sent for immunologic testing because of recurring respiratory infections, including several bouts of pneumonia. The results show decreased immunoglobulin levels, especially of IgG. Although the white blood cell (WBC) count was within the normal range, the lymphocyte count was low. Flow cytometry was performed to determine the numbers of different types of lymphocytes. The results showed a decrease in $CD4^+$ cells and a normal $CD19^+$ lymphocyte count.

Questions

a. How can these findings be interpreted?
b. How can this account for the child's recurring infections?

2. During your immunology class, your instructor asks you to explain to a classmate why $CD8^+$ T cells are important to the immune response as well as antibodies.

Question

a. If $CD8^+$ T cells were not functioning properly, what effect would that have on a person's immunity?

REVIEW QUESTIONS

1. During which stage of T-cell development does the rearrangement of genes coding for the T-cell receptor (TCR) begin?
   a. Double-positive stage
   b. Single-positive stage
   c. Double-negative stage
   d. Gamma-delta ($\gamma\delta$) T-cell stage

2. Which MHC molecule is necessary for antigen recognition by $CD4^+$ T cells?
   a. Class I
   b. Class II
   c. Class III
   d. No MHC molecule is necessary.

3. Which statement is characteristic of an immune response to a T-independent antigen?
   a. IgG antibody is produced exclusively.
   b. Large numbers of memory cells are produced.
   c. Antigens bind only one receptor on B cells.
   d. Antigens are often polysaccharides.

4. *Humoral immunity* refers to which of the following?
   a. Production of antibody by plasma cells
   b. Production of cytokines by T cells
   c. Elimination of virally infected cells by cytotoxic cells
   d. Downregulation of the immune response

5. Where does antigen-independent maturation of B lymphocytes take place?
   a. Bone marrow
   b. Thymus
   c. Spleen
   d. Lymph nodes

6. In the thymus, positive selection of immature T cells is based on recognition of which of the following?
   a. Self-antigens
   b. Stress proteins
   c. MHC
   d. μ chains

7. Which of these are found on a mature B cell?
   a. IgG and IgD
   b. IgM and IgD
   c. α and β chains
   d. CD3 and CD4

8. How do cytotoxic T cells kill target cells?
   a. They produce antibodies that bind to the cell.
   b. They engulf the cell by phagocytosis.
   c. They stop protein synthesis in the target cell.
   d. They produce granzymes that induce apoptosis.

9. Which of the following can be directly attributed to antigen-stimulated T cells?
   a. Humoral response
   b. Plasma cells
   c. Cytokines
   d. Antibody

10. What is a distinguishing feature of a pre-B cell?
    a. Heavy chains in the cytoplasm
    b. Complete IgM on the surface
    c. Presence of CD21 antigen
    d. Presence of CD25 antigen

11. When does the initial rearrangement of genes coding for immunoglobulin light chains take place during B-cell development?
    a. Before the pro–B-cell stage
    b. During the pro–B-cell stage
    c. During the pre–B-cell stage
    d. During the immature B-cell stage

12. Which of the following antigens is found on "helper" T cells?
    a. CD4
    b. CD8
    c. CD11
    d. CD21

13. Which of the following represents a DN thymocyte?
    a. $CD3^+CD4^-CD8^+$
    b. $CD3^-CD4^+CD8^-$
    c. $CD3^+CD4^-CD8^-$
    d. $CD3^-CD4^-CD8^-$

14. Which of the following best applies to the TCR?
    a. It consists of IgM and IgD molecules.
    b. It is the same for all T cells.
    c. It is present in the DN stage.
    d. α and β chains are unique for each antigen.

15. Laboratory results belonging to a 3-year-old patient showed the following: normal $CD4^+$ T-cell count, normal $CD19^+$ B-cell count, low $CD8^+$ T-cell count. Which aspect of immunity would be affected?
   a. Production of antibody
   b. Formation of plasma cells
   c. Elimination of virally infected cells
   d. Downregulation of the immune response

16. Which of the following is a unique characteristic of adaptive immunity?
   a. Ability to fight infection
   b. Ability to remember a prior exposure to a pathogen
   c. A similar response to all pathogens encountered
   d. Process of phagocytosis to destroy a pathogen

17. Positive selection of T cells ideally achieves which of the following outcomes?
   a. Elimination of autoimmune responses
   b. Generation of $\gamma\delta$ T lymphocytes
   c. Allelic exclusion of chromosomes
   d. Elimination of T cells unable to bind to MHC antigens

18. Where are germinal centers found?
   a. In the thymus
   b. In the bone marrow
   c. In peripheral blood
   d. In lymph nodes

19. Which of the following TH-cell subsets is responsible for driving cell-mediated immunity against intracellular parasites, such as viruses and parasitic bacteria?
   a. TH1
   b. TH2
   c. TH3
   d. TH17

20. Which of the following processes could not occur in the absence of $CD4^+$ T-cell help to B cells?
   a. Immunoglobulin production
   b. Development of plasma cells
   c. Immunoglobulin class switching
   d. B-cell activation

Chapter 5 Answer Key

Answers to Knowledge Checks

5.1 c 5.2 b 5.3 c 5.4 d 5.5 d 5.6 d

Answers to Review Questions

1. c	2. b	3. d	4. a	5. a	6. c	7. b
8. d	9. c	10. a	11. c	12. a	13. c	14. d
15. c	16. b	17. d	18. d	19. a	20. c	

Cytokines 6

Linda E. Miller, PhD, I, MB(ASCP)[CM], SI

LEARNING OUTCOMES

After finishing this chapter, you should be able to:

6.1 Define *cytokine* and *chemokine*.

6.2 Distinguish between autocrine, paracrine, and endocrine effects of cytokines.

6.3 Recognize examples of pleiotropy and redundancy as they relate to cytokine activities.

6.4 Differentiate between a cytokine cascade and a cytokine network.

6.5 Describe the roles of pro- and anti-inflammatory cytokines in innate immune responses, providing examples of each type.

6.6 Associate subpopulations of helper T cells with their distinct cytokine profiles.

6.7 Describe the functions of the following cytokines: IL-1β, IL-1ra, IL-2, IL-4, IL-5, IL-6, IL-10, IL-13, IL-17, TNF-α, IFN-α, IFN-β, IFN-γ, TGF-β.

6.8 Discuss the roles of chemokines in the immune response and interpret the nomenclature used to name specific cytokines.

6.9 Discuss the biological roles of the hematopoietic growth factors.

6.10 Describe the condition known as *cytokine storm, hypercytokinemia,* or *cytokine release syndrome.*

6.11 Provide examples of cytokine and anti-cytokine therapies.

6.12 Discuss the clinical utility of cytokine profiling.

6.13 Differentiate between immunoassays and bioassays for cytokines, provide examples of each assay type, and discuss the advantages and limitations of each.

6.14 Describe the underlying principles of a sandwich immunoassay and the ELISpot for cytokine detection.

CHAPTER OUTLINE

You can go to **fadavis.com** keyword stevens for the laboratory exercises that accompany this text.

Immunity requires coordination between cells that may be widely dispersed throughout the body. Therefore, a form of intercellular communication between the cells is necessary to orchestrate a successful immune response. Cells of the immune system communicate with each other through chemical messengers called **cytokines,** which influence both innate and adaptive responses to infection.

Cytokine Characteristics and Functions

Cytokines are a diverse group of small proteins and glycoproteins that are produced by many types of immune and nonimmune cells in response to a variety of stimuli, including microorganisms, tissue injury, contact with other cells or cytokines, extranuclear DNA, and antigen-antibody complexes. Many cytokines are produced in response to infectious stimuli. For example, lipopolysaccharide (LPS), a component of gram-negative bacterial cell walls; flagellin; and other bacterial products cause innate immune cells to release several cytokines that promote inflammation. After their release, cytokines bind to receptors on target cells and activate intracellular signaling pathways that result in the expression of selected genes. Consequently, the target cells produce specific proteins that affect the growth, differentiation, function, and migration of other cells. For example, cytokines can activate or inhibit inflammation, induce proliferation and differentiation of lymphocytes in humoral and cell-mediated immune responses, regulate hematopoiesis, and recruit immune cells to tissues where they are needed. **Fig. 6–1** illustrates the general mechanism by which cytokines work.

Cytokine activity can be classified according to the distance traveled between the producing cell and its target cell(s). Some cytokines act locally, affecting only the producing cell or a few nearby cells, whereas other cytokines transmit their messages throughout the entire body. Cytokines that bind to receptors on the same cell from which they were secreted are said to signal in an **autocrine** manner. Cytokines that act on cells within the tissue region surrounding their cellular source transmit **paracrine** signals. Some cytokines diffuse into the bloodstream, allowing them to influence cells far from the cell or cells that produce them. In these cases, the cytokines are behaving as hormones, acting in an **endocrine** fashion **(Fig. 6–2).** Most cytokines are rapidly degraded in the extracellular environment, limiting their activity.

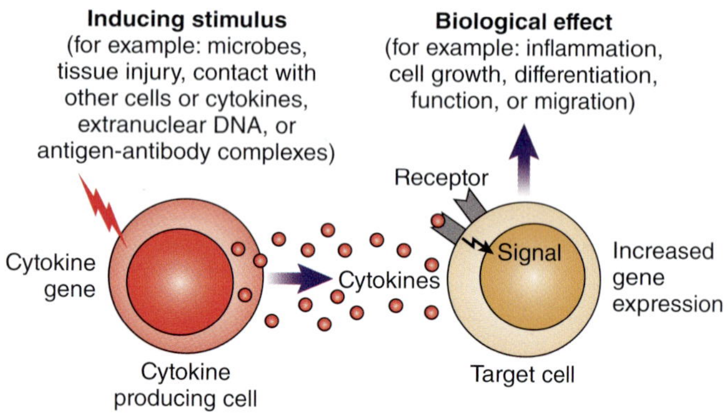

FIGURE 6–1 General mechanism of cytokine function.

Many cytokines exhibit the properties of pleiotropy and redundancy. **Pleiotropy** means that a single cytokine can have many different actions. For example, the cytokine interleukin-2 (IL-2) can stimulate proliferation of CD4+ helper T cells (TH), drive the differentiation of regulatory T cells (Treg), induce the differentiation of CD8+ cytotoxic T (TC) cells, and enhance the cytolytic activity of natural killer (NK) cells. **Redundancy** occurs when different cytokines activate some of the same pathways and genes. For example, the cytokines interleukin-4 (IL-4) and interleukin-13 (IL-13) can both induce B cells to switch their antibody production to IgE. Redundancy may be explained by the fact that many cytokines share receptor subunits. Thus, some cytokines may have overlapping effects and may alter the activity of many of the same genes.

Understanding the roles of individual cytokines in immunity is complicated by the fact that many do not act alone but, rather, in conjunction with other cytokines. If the effects of two different cytokines complement and enhance each other, the interaction is called **synergy (Fig. 6–3).** In contrast, if one cytokine counteracts the action of another, **antagonism** occurs (see Fig. 6–3). Synergy and antagonism may result when one cytokine induces changes in a receptor, a key signaling enzyme, or expression of mRNA for another cytokine. Furthermore, many cytokines induce the production of additional cytokines by target cells, resulting in a **cytokine cascade (Fig. 6–4).**

Successful immune responses often involve the expression of a complex network of cytokines, each influencing a different aspect of leukocyte activity and resulting in the elimination of an infection. In these networks, cytokines can act in several ways. **Figure 6–5** shows an example of a **cytokine network** involved in an immune response toward an antigen that causes an allergic reaction. Note the various cytokine effects shown in the figure. For example, IL-4 *synergizes* with IL-13 to activate B cells to produce IgE antibodies; IL-10 and TGF-β *antagonize* the action of IL-4; IL-6 and IL-23 induce TH cells to produce IL-17 in a *cytokine cascade*.

Knowledge Check 6-1

Interleukin-6 (IL-6) stimulates production of acute phase proteins by the liver, production and release of granulocytes from the bone marrow, and activation of B and T lymphocytes. This is an example of:

a. Synergy
b. Antagonism
c. Pleiotropy
d. Redundancy

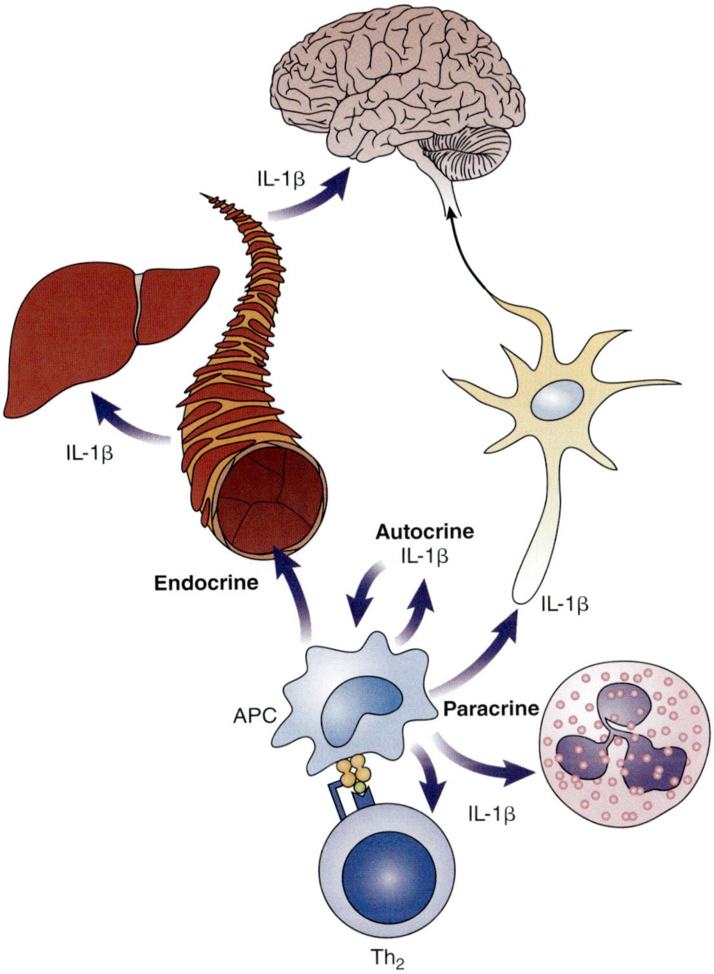

FIGURE 6–2 Range of cytokine activity. **Autocrine:** Cytokine acts on the cell that secreted it (e.g., IL-1β increases activation of an antigen-presenting cell [APC]). **Paracrine:** Cytokine acts on nearby cells (e.g., IL-1β stimulates T_H cells, activates neutrophils, and depolarizes neurons). **Endocrine:** Cytokine travels through blood vessels to distant cells (e.g., IL-1β stimulates acute phase protein synthesis in the liver and fever induction by the hypothalamus).

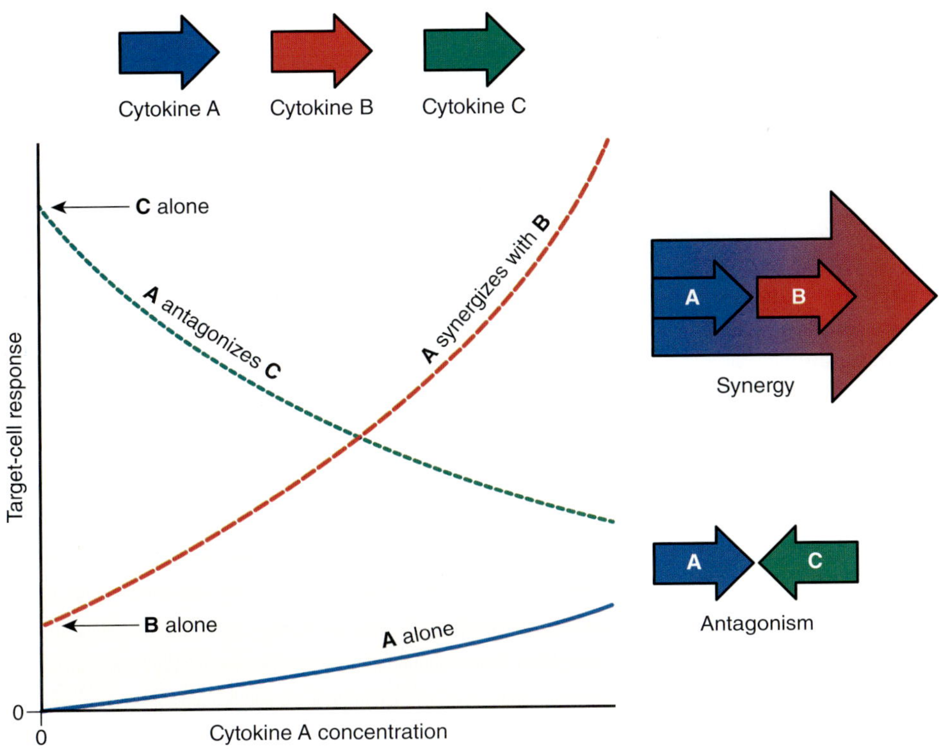

FIGURE 6–3 Cytokine characteristics of synergy and antagonism. **Synergy:** Neither cytokine A nor B induces a strong response individually; however, when combined, the net response is much greater than the sum of the individual responses. **Antagonism:** Individually, cytokine C induces a strong response, and cytokine A induces a weak (but positive) response. When combined, cytokine A diminishes the action of cytokine C. In this illustration, the concentrations of cytokines B and C are held constant, whereas cytokine A increases along the horizontal axis.

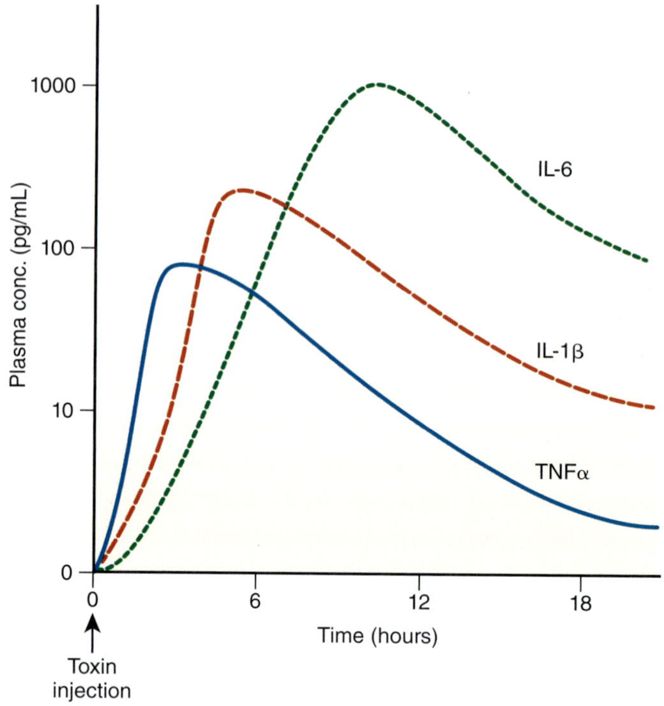

FIGURE 6–4 Cytokines can induce the release of other cytokines in an amplifying cascade. For example, following intravenous injection of a bacterial toxin, TNF-α is first released by monocytes and macrophages. Both the toxin and TNF-α induce the subsequent release of IL-1β by phagocytic cells. Then all three induce interleukin 6 (IL-6) release from a wide variety of cell types.

Cytokine Nomenclature

Initially, immunologists named cytokines based on their activities or on the immune cell population that produced them. Using this system, a cytokine that was observed to kill cancer cells was named "tumor necrosis factor," cytokines released from lymphocytes were called *lymphokines,* monocytes produced *monokines,* and leukocytes secreted *interleukins* that influenced other leukocytes. At times, the same cytokine was referred to by different names, leading to confusion.

Now, cytokines are grouped into families, based on similarities in their structure and amino acid sequence, rather than their function. Major cytokine families include tumor necrosis factor (TNF), interferon (IFN), chemokine, transforming growth factor (TGF), and hematopoietic growth factors. The **interleukins** are a diverse group of cytokines that were so named because of their involvement in communication between leukocytes. More than 40 interleukins have been discovered, and they are referred to by the prefix "IL-" followed by a number, designated according to the order of their discovery (e.g., IL-1, IL-2). While some of the interleukins have been classified into structurally similar families (e.g., the IL-1 family; see later section), others are included in some of the other groups. In this chapter, we discuss selected cytokines from each of these groups. Major cytokines and their functions are summarized in the Study Guides at the end of the chapter.

Importance of Cytokines in Immune Responses

Cytokines are a necessary component of both innate and adaptive immunity because they allow many different cells and molecules to cooperate in an organized manner to mount a successful immune response. We briefly introduce the important roles of cytokines in innate and adaptive responses in this section and describe them in more detail in the sections that follow.

Cytokines in Innate Immunity

For most species of pathogenic bacteria and fungi, infections begin once the body's skin and mucous membrane barriers have been breached. The first immune cells to encounter invading microorganisms are tissue-resident phagocytes, such as macrophages and dendritic cells (DCs). As we discussed in Chapter 2, these sentinel immune cells detect infection using pattern recognition receptors such as the toll-like receptors (TLRs) to recognize pathogen-associated molecular patterns (PAMPs) found on diverse types of microbes. Binding of these receptors to their corresponding PAMPs induces the production and secretion of **pro-inflammatory** cytokines, so named because they promote inflammation.

The major pro-inflammatory cytokines provoked by infection with extracellular microbes are interleukin-1 (IL-1), interleukin-6 (IL-6), and TNF-α. Once produced, these cytokines diffuse away from their sources to mediate important local (paracrine) effects, including the following:

- Increased capillary permeability, which allows soluble anti-microbial proteins such as complement and C-reactive protein to enter the tissues from blood plasma
- Increased platelet aggregation, which helps to seal off local blood vessels, preventing infection from disseminating into the blood
- Alteration of adhesion molecule expression on capillary endothelial cells, which enhances movement of leukocytes from the blood into inflamed tissues

Severe infections can stimulate the production of larger quantities of pro-inflammatory cytokines, causing systemic (endocrine) effects, including the following:

- An increase in body temperature, which may make the body less hospitable to invading microbes
- Increased production of immune cells by the bone marrow and acute phase reactants by the liver
- The subjective feeling of being ill

These effects are responsible for many of the physical symptoms of inflammation, including fever, swelling, pain, and infiltration of immune cells into damaged tissues. Perhaps the most important role of pro-inflammatory cytokines is the recruitment of effector cells, such as neutrophils and monocytes, into inflamed tissues. However, massive amounts of these cytokines can lead to hypotension, shock, and even death (see later section "Cytokines in Disease").

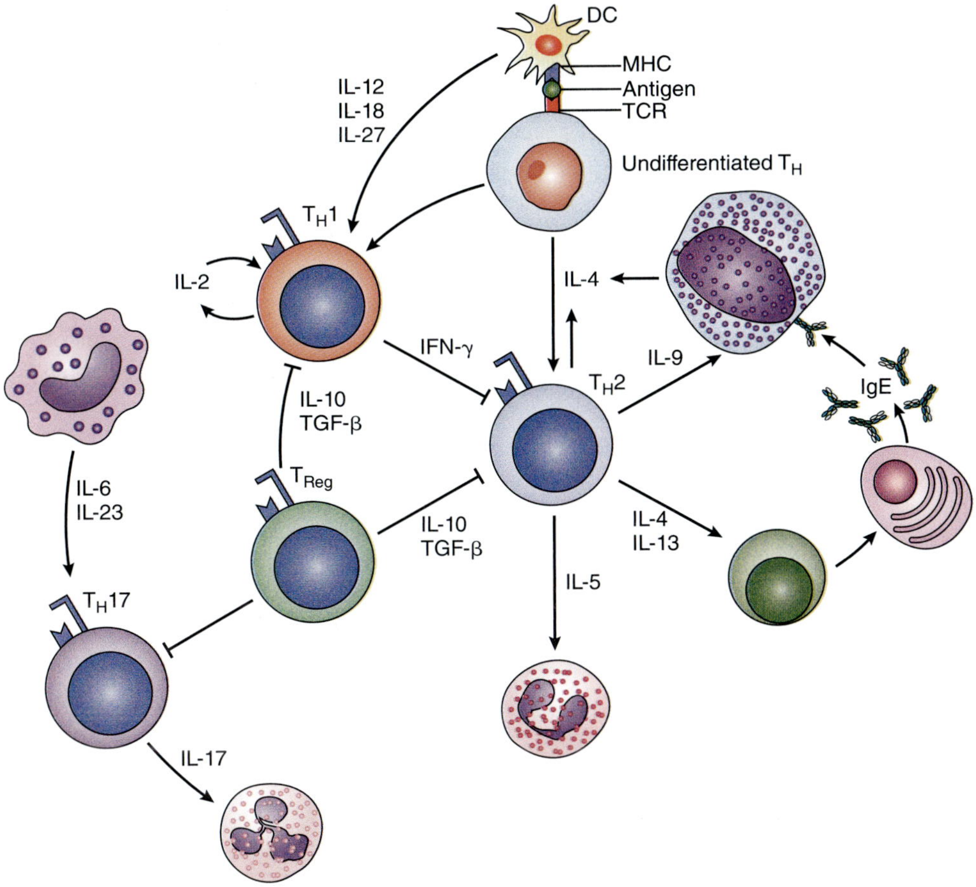

FIGURE 6–5 Example of a cytokine network. Activation responses are indicated by black arrows, and suppression is indicated by black bars. MHC = major histocompatibility antigen class II; TCR = T-cell receptor; TH = helper T cell; Treg = regulatory T cell.

Given the potentially harmful effects of cytokines, it is clear that the inflammatory response must be closely regulated to prevent damaging systemic inflammation. Anti-inflammatory cytokines antagonize the effects of TNF-α and IL-1β, thus resolving inflammation and limiting collateral damage to host cells. **Table 6–1** lists major pro-inflammatory and anti-inflammatory cytokines.

Cytokines in Adaptive Immunity

While innate defenses can prevent, successfully control, or eradicate many bacterial, fungal, and viral infections, overcoming infections with the most dangerous pathogens usually requires an adaptive immune response. As we discussed in Chapter 2, many of the cytokines produced during innate responses act in different ways to activate adaptive immunity.

Whereas cytokines involved in innate immunity are produced by many different cell types, the cytokines associated with adaptive responses are mainly secreted by T lymphocytes, especially CD4-positive ($CD4^+$) helper T (TH) cells and regulatory T (Treg) cells.

Helper T (TH) Cells

TH cells can be divided into several subpopulations, based on the profile of cytokines they produce. Immunologists have characterized at least four types of TH cells, each of which has a different immune function and produces a different array of cytokines. The four subpopulations are as follows:

- Helper T Type 1 (TH1) cells
- Helper T Type 2 (TH2) cells
- Helper T Type 17 (TH17) cells
- Follicular helper T (Tfh) cells

Table 6-1 Examples of Major Pro-Inflammatory and Anti-Inflammatory Cytokines

MAJOR PRO-INFLAMMATORY CYTOKINES	MAJOR ANTI-INFLAMMATORY CYTOKINES
TNF-α	TGF-β
IL-1	IL-1ra
IL-6	IL-10
IFN-γ	IL-13
Chemokines	IL-35

As we described in Chapters 4 and 5, initiation of an adaptive T-lymphocyte response begins when antigen-presenting cells (APCs), namely, dendritic cells and macrophages, arrive in the lymph nodes, carrying antigens gathered from an area of infection. APCs present fragments of pathogen-derived antigens to hundreds or thousands of TH cells in the lymph nodes, but T-cell activation occurs only after a specific T-cell receptor binds to its corresponding antigen fragment. Activation initiates proliferation of the antigen-specific TH cells, which, in larger numbers, will be more effective in attacking the infectious agent.

Following activation, TH cells undergo a process known as *differentiation,* during which they are transformed into TH1, TH2, TH17, or Tfh cells. The particular subset into which a TH cell differentiates is strongly influenced by the type of pathogen encountered by the host and the cytokines produced by the APCs and other cells in the lymphoid organ where the immune response began, such as natural killer (NK) cells, mast cells, innate lymphoid cells (ILCs), and epithelial cells. The differentiated TH cell subpopulations, in turn, release a characteristic set of effector cytokines that coordinate appropriate immune responses against the pathogen. These responses include recruitment of cells to the inflammation site, activation of macrophages to kill engulfed microorganisms and perform tissue repair, differentiation of B cells into antibody-producing plasma cells, and maturation of cytotoxic T (TC) cells with the capability of killing virus-infected host cells **(Table 6–2).**

For example, infections with viruses and intracellular bacteria such as *Mycobacterium tuberculosis* and *Listeria monocytogenes* induce production of IL-12 by dendritic cells and macrophages and IFN-γ by NK cells. These cytokines, in turn, stimulate undifferentiated TH to develop into TH1 cells, which drive cell-mediated immunity. The TH1 cells expand into a clone of cells that produce additional IFN-γ, which increases the microbicidal activity of the macrophages that have ingested the pathogens. TH1 cells also produce IL-2, which promotes differentiation of $CD8^+$ TC cells, which can destroy virus-infected host cells.

In contrast, TH2 cells are thought to be induced by IL-25 and IL-33 released by epithelial cells and IL-4 released by mast cells during initial responses to parasites such as helminths. The TH2 cells, in turn, produce IL-4, IL-5, and IL-13, which stimulate B cells to produce IgE antibodies and induce mast cells and eosinophils to degranulate and release enzymes that destroy extracellular parasites.

In a similar manner, IL-1 and other cytokines produced during the early immune response to extracellular bacteria and fungi promote differentiation of TH17 cells, which release IL-17 and IL-22. These cytokines stimulate the production of chemokines by other cells to recruit neutrophils and enhance inflammation at the site of infection.

Finally, IL-6 and other cytokines produced early in response to extracellular pathogens promote the development of Tfh cells in the lymph nodes. The Tfh cells, in turn, produce IL-4, IL-13, and IL-21, which induce the differentiation of B cells to promote an effective antibody-mediated immune response.

As these immune responses progress, they become more polarized, because each cytokine profile promotes the development of the particular TH subset that produced it and suppresses the development of the other TH subsets. This process ensures that the type of immune response that will be most effective against a particular pathogen dominates.

Regulatory T (Treg) Cells

As the host eliminates the pathogen, the specific immune response generated must be dampened; otherwise, immune hyper-reactivity can occur, resulting in harm to the host. $CD4^+$ regulatory T (Treg) cells play a major role in suppressing undesirable immune responses. These cells depend on the cytokines IL-2 and TGF-β for their development and are thought to suppress immune responses through multiple mechanisms, including production of the immunosuppressive cytokines, IL-10 and TGF-β (discussed in sections that follow).

Knowledge Check 6-2

Interferon gamma (IFN-γ) can be considered the signature cytokine of which helper T subpopulation?

a. TH1
b. TH2
c. TH17
d. Tfh

Table 6-2 Subpopulations of $CD4^+$ TH Cells and Their Cytokine Profiles

INDUCING PATHOGEN	CYTOKINES PRODUCED BY APCs AND OTHER CELLS AT THE SITE OF INITIAL INFECTION	TH SUBSET GENERATED	CYTOKINES RELEASED BY TH	MAJOR EFFECTS
Intracellular bacteria and viruses	IL-12, IFN-γ	TH1	IFN-γ, IL-2	Activation of macrophages, differentiation of TC
Parasites	IL-4, IL-25, IL-33	TH2	IL-4, IL-5, IL-13	Activation of eosinophils, mast cells, and B cells
Extracellular bacteria and fungi	IL-1, IL-6, IL-23, TGF-β	TH17	IL-17, IL-22	Recruitment and activation of neutrophils
Extracellular pathogens	IL-6, IL-12, IL-21, IL-23, TGF-β	Tfh	IL-4, IL-13, IL-21	Proliferation and differentiation of B cells; antibody production

APC = antigen-presenting cell; IFN = interferon; IL = interleukin; Tc = cytotoxic T; TH= helper T; Tfh = follicular T helper; TGF = transforming growth factor.

Functions of Specific Cytokines

As we mentioned earlier, it is current practice to classify cytokines based on their structural characteristics. However, in this section, we discuss selected cytokines from each of the major cytokine families based on their *major functions* to make it easier for you to better understand their roles in the immune response. The study guides at the end of this chapter provide a concise summary of the functions of selected cytokines.

Inflammatory Cytokines

Major cytokines involved in the inflammatory response include interleukin-1 (IL-1), interleukin-6 (IL-6), tumor necrosis factor (TNF-α), and chemokines. Next, we look at each of these cytokines in more detail.

The Interleukin-1 (IL-1) Cytokine Family

IL-1 is a family of 11 structurally and functionally related cytokines. The best characterized of the IL-1 cytokines are IL-1β, IL-1α, and IL-1 receptor antagonist (IL-1ra). IL-1β and IL-1ra are expressed in monocytes, macrophages, and DCs. In contrast, IL-1α is expressed in innate phagocytic cells and can also be detected in epithelial cells from the skin, lungs, and gastrointestinal tract.

Production of IL-1 is induced by many microbial components, such as lipopolysaccharide (LPS), lipoteichoic acid, and bacterial or viral nucleic acids. IL-1β mediates most of the local (paracrine) and systemic (hormonal) activity attributed to IL-1, including activation of phagocytes, fever, and production of acute phase proteins. IL-1β is released from macrophages and monocytes, but prior to secretion, it must be cleaved intracellularly to an active form (see Clinical Correlation "Inflammasomes Link Gout and Alum to Inflammation").

IL-1β

One of the most important paracrine effects of IL-1β is the recruitment of immune cells into inflamed tissues. Binding of IL-1β to IL-1 receptors on blood vessel endothelial cells alters adhesion molecule expression and stimulates the production of chemokines. These changes cause immune cells such as granulocytes and monocytes to stop moving through the blood and begin *diapedesis,* a process whereby blood leukocytes pass through vessel walls and enter inflamed tissues (see Chapter 2).

IL-1β is sometimes referred to as an "endogenous pyrogen" because of its ability to induce fever. IL-1 receptors on neurons of the hypothalamus allow this part of the brain to respond to the presence of systemic IL-1β by increasing body temperature. Fever serves several purposes during infection. For instance, higher body temperatures (1) inhibit the growth of many bacteria and fungi; (2) increase the microbicidal activities of macrophages and neutrophils; and (3) contribute to feelings of discomfort and fatigue, compelling sick individuals to reduce activity and conserve energy to combat the infection. IL-1β also induces the production of specific colony-stimulating factors (CSFs) in the bone marrow, spurring the production and release of additional immune cells into the circulation that can be recruited to serve as reinforcements in response to an infection or tissue damage.

IL-1α

IL-1α has similar biological effects to IL-1β, but IL-1α is retained within the cell cytoplasm and is released only after cell death. The presence of free IL-1α helps to attract inflammatory cells to areas where cells and tissues are being damaged or killed.

IL-1ra

In contrast to pro-inflammatory IL-1α and IL-1β, IL-1ra has an anti-inflammatory effect. This cytokine is so named because it *antagonizes,* or *works against,* the activity of other IL-1 cytokines. IL-1ra accomplishes this antagonism by binding to only one of the two transmembrane proteins that compose the IL-1 receptor. When ligated by pro-inflammatory IL-1α or IL-1β, these two receptor subunits are brought together, initiating an intracellular signaling cascade that alerts the target cell to the presence of IL-1. Because IL-1ra binds to only one IL-1 receptor subunit and repels the other, IL-1ra prevents receptor subunits from coming together to initiate signaling, even in the presence of IL-1α or IL-1β. In this way, IL-1ra helps to regulate the physiological response to IL-1 and turn off the response when it is no longer needed.

> **6-1 Clinical Correlations**
>
> **Inflammasomes Link Gout and Alum to Inflammation**
>
> Secretion of the biologically active form of IL-1β requires processing of the cytokine from an inactive pro–IL-1β to an active form. Processing is performed by multiprotein complexes known as *inflammasomes,* which assemble within the cytoplasm of innate immune cells in response to damage-associated molecular patterns (DAMPs; see Chapter 2). Central to the activity of inflammasomes is the enzyme caspase-1, which cleaves pro–IL-1β into active IL-1β. Following catalytic processing, active IL-1β is released from the cell, transmitting a powerful inflammatory signal.
>
> Inflammasome activation and IL-1β release occur in response to infection but can also occur in "sterile" inflammatory diseases such as gout. In gout, a surplus of uric acid leads to crystal deposition in the body's tissues. One specific type of uric acid crystal, monosodium urate, has been shown to act as a DAMP, causing inflammasome assembly. Drugs that block IL-1β signaling dramatically reduce the pain and inflammation associated with gout.
>
> Interestingly, the adjuvant alum has also been shown to cause inflammasome activation. Adjuvants are substances that enhance immune responses, and adjuvants such as alum are often incorporated into vaccines to help stimulate immunity to certain infections (see Chapter 25). In this case, the release of active IL-1β and the inflammatory signaling driven by the cytokine cause the immune system to associate the harmless molecules found in the vaccine with *danger,* leading to a strong immune response that provides protection against the harmful pathogens that the vaccine is intended to mimic.

Interleukin-6 (IL-6)

Another cytokine that is associated with the inflammatory response is IL-6. Structurally, IL-6 is related to many other cytokines, consisting of a single polypeptide chain that winds into four helices that fold on themselves to create a complicated tertiary structure. Two identical IL-6 polypeptide chains come together to form a homodimer, which represents the active form of the cytokine. Macrophages and monocytes are a common source of IL-6, but many other cell types are known to produce this cytokine, including endothelial cells, fibroblasts, some types of lymphocytes, and even skeletal muscle cells.

The activity of IL-6 is highly pleiotropic, influencing many biological systems. Functioning as an innate cytokine, IL-6 stimulates the production of acute phase proteins by liver hepatocytes and increases the production and release of granulocytes by the bone marrow. In adaptive immunity, IL-6 increases the activation of B and T lymphocytes and stimulates immunoglobulin synthesis by causing B cells to proliferate and differentiate into plasma cells.

The IL-6 receptor is composed of multiple subunits: one subunit specific to IL-6, known as the *IL-6 receptor* (IL-6R), and a signal-transducing subunit called *glycoprotein 130* (gp130). Binding of IL-6 causes a structural alteration in gp130 that allows its cytoplasmic domains to initiate intracellular signaling cascades. This change stimulates the expression of IL-6–mediated genes that code for products such as C-reactive protein, complement proteins, and fibrinogen.

Tumor Necrosis Factors

The cytokines that make up the **tumor necrosis factor (TNF)** superfamily were first identified in the laboratory as products of macrophages and lymphocytes. The name *tumor necrosis factor* emerged from the observation that these cytokines induce lysis of mouse tumor cells. In all, the TNF superfamily encompasses 19 proteins that induce diverse immunologic functions, including synthesis of inflammatory mediators, increased expression of adhesion molecules on vascular endothelial cells, cell proliferation, increased cell survival, tissue degeneration or regeneration, or apoptosis. TNF-α also enhances inflammation by inducing the production of IL-1.

The TNF superfamily members are manufactured as transmembrane proteins. Some TNFs remain cell bound, transmitting messages only when the producing cell and the target cell are in contact. An example of a surface-bound TNF discussed in Chapter 5 is CD40 ligand, which is essential for signaling between T and B lymphocytes. Other TNFs are released from the cell surface by enzymatic cleavage, after which they diffuse into the extracellular space, allowing signaling across a distance.

TNF-α

In regard to inflammation, the most important TNF is TNF-α. Microbial substances such as LPS are major inducers of TNF-α production. Innate immune receptor signaling in macrophages leads to the production of a TNF-α precursor protein, which migrates to the macrophage plasma membrane. At the cell surface, the transmembrane domains are enzymatically removed, and the resultant soluble polypeptide fragments reassemble in groups of three (called *homotrimers*), representing the active form of TNF-α.

TNF-α is a ligand for two receptors, TNF receptors 1 and 2 (TNFR1 and TNFR2). TNFR1 is constitutively expressed on many cells and tissues throughout the body, whereas the expression of TNFR2 is limited to cells of hematopoietic origin and endothelial cells. If levels of TNF-α near the membrane of the target cell reach a critical concentration, the TNF-α trimer draws together three TNF receptor molecules, resulting in downstream intracellular signaling. This results in activation of specific genes that cause the various effects of TNF described earlier.

TNF-β

TNF-β (or "lymphotoxin") is another soluble TNF. As its pseudonym suggests, TNF-β is produced by lymphocytes and causes cell death, or *cytotoxicity,* in many different types of cells. This cytokine also acts as an important signal during the development of lymphoid tissues in the gastrointestinal immune system. It is produced by a unique class of lymphocytes known as *lymphoid-tissue inducer cells.* Without these cells and the TNF-β they produce, secondary lymphoid tissues, such as the mesenteric lymph nodes and Peyer patches, fail to form.

Chemokines

Chemokines are a large family of cytokines that influence the motility and migration of their target cells. *Chemokine* is derived from the words *cytokine* and *chemotaxis,* the latter term meaning "movement of a cell toward a stimulus." Most immune cell movement arises from the activities of chemokines, including recruitment to and movement through areas of infection and inflammation and the continual migration of lymphocytes between the blood and lymphoid tissues. Directed migration of white blood cells (WBCs) is critical because these cells must be in the right place in the body at the right time so that their functions can be localized appropriately.

This special group of cytokines is produced by a variety of cell types, including leukocytes, endothelial cells, epithelial cells, fibroblasts, and stromal cells. Chemokines accomplish their function by binding to their corresponding receptors, which are present on all WBCs. Different types of leukocytes possess different combinations of chemokine receptors, and this influences their migration patterns.

Chemokines have been classified into four subfamilies based on the sequence of amino acids found in their N-termini, specifically, the positioning of cysteine residues, which play an important role in activating their receptors. The nomenclature of these groups contains a "C" for each N-terminal cysteine, and an "X" representing another amino acid.

- The CXC group of chemokines contains a single amino acid, "X," between the first and second cysteines.
- The CC group has cysteines that are adjacent to each other, with no intervening amino acid.
- The C chemokines have only a single cysteine.
- The CX3C chemokines have three amino acids between the cysteines.

Individual chemokines also contain an "L" for the ligand of the cysteine, and a number representing the order in which the chemokine was discovered. More than 40 chemokines and 19 chemokine receptors have been discovered. Examples of chemokines, their receptors, and major functions are shown in **Table 6–3.**

Many pro-inflammatory cytokines, including TNF-α and IL-6, induce the production of chemokines. In an inflammatory

Table 6-3 Examples of Chemokines, Their Receptors, and Major Functions

CHEMOKINE GROUP	CHEMOKINE NAME	CHEMOKINE RECEPTORS	FUNCTION
CC chemokines	CCL2	CCR2	Attraction of various WBCs
	CCL3	CCR1, CCR5	Attraction of various WBCs
	CCL4	CCR5	Attraction of monocytes, dendritic cells, T cells, and NK cells; coreceptor for HIV infection
	CCL5	CCR1, CCR3, CCR5	Attraction of various WBCs
CXC chemokines	CXCL1	CXCR2	Attraction of neutrophils
	CXCL8	CXCR1, CXCR2	Attraction of neutrophils
C chemokines	XCL1	XCR1	Attraction of dendritic cells
CX3C chemokines	CX3CL1	CX3CR1	Migration of T cells, NK cells, and monocytes

NK = natural killer; WBC = white blood cell.

context, one of the most important effects of chemokines is the recruitment of leukocytes from the blood into infected or damaged tissues. Chemokines recruit WBCs by facilitating the adhesion between leukocytes and the endothelial cells that line blood vessels. These interactions cause the leukocytes to *roll* along capillary walls, similar to a tennis ball rolling over a sheet of Velcro, and to subsequently exit the blood vessel and enter into the tissues (see Chapter 2).

Another important role of chemokines comes into play after leukocytes, such as neutrophils and monocytes, have entered inflamed tissues. Chemokine receptors allow these immune cells to detect chemokine gradients within inflamed tissues. Engagement of these receptors causes the immune cells' cytoskeletons to reorganize, increasing actin polymerization near the cell surface that faces the higher concentration of chemokine. Therefore, responding immune cells migrate in the direction of the chemokine source, allowing them to pinpoint the exact location of damaged or infected cells.

In many cases, the expression of chemokine receptors changes throughout an immune cell's life span. For example, DCs are responsible for initiating an adaptive immune response by presenting antigens to T and B lymphocytes (see Chapter 5). The activation of DCs by exposure to microbial substances causes them to express specific chemokine receptors, sensitizing them to chemokines produced by lymphatic endothelial cells. Following the gradient of these chemokines, DCs carrying microbial antigens journey into and through lymphatic capillaries. Eventually, the activated DCs arrive at local lymph nodes, where they interact with naive T and B lymphocytes.

Finally, chemokines play a role in development of the secondary lymphoid organs such as the lymph nodes. To accomplish this, chemokines bind to their corresponding receptors on T and B lymphocytes and direct their migration to specific locations in these organs, resulting in their anatomical structures, which we discussed in Chapter 1.

Interferons

The **interferons (IFNs)** were so named because they were identified as soluble substances produced by virally infected cells that *interfere* with the ability of viruses to replicate. IFNs are classified as type I, type II, and type III, according to the IFN receptor that they interact with. The type I IFNs, consisting of IFN-α and IFN-β, are perhaps the most important cytokines in innate responses to viral infection. Type II IFN, also known as IFN-γ, is primarily associated with the TH1 adaptive immune response, discussed in a later section of this chapter. The more recently described type III IFN, or IFN-λ, has anti-viral activity similar to the type I IFNs.

Interferon-α and Interferon-β (Type I Interferons)

Many cell types produce type I IFNs. IFN-α (which actually consists of 13 subtypes) is mainly the product of DCs and macrophages, whereas IFN-β can be produced by many types of virus-infected cells. Following viral infection of host cells, pattern recognition receptors (PRRs) in the cytosol bind to viral nucleic acids and initiate pathways of cell signaling that result in multiple effects (see Chapter 2). Importantly, these signals inhibit viral replication by blocking the synthesis of viral proteins and final virion assembly and by inducing the production of RNases that degrade viral RNAs. These changes also slow viral spread by preventing productive infection of neighboring host cells.

Type I IFNs also recruit innate lymphocytes, such as NK cells, to viral infection sites. When ligated by IFN-α or IFN-β, type I IFN receptors cause NK cells to become activated, traffic to virally infected tissues, and rapidly expand in number. The combination of IFN-α and IFN-β activity and NK cell killing constitutes the most important innate defense mechanism against viral infection.

To augment the activity of NK cells, type I IFNs also enhance the expression of class I major histocompatibility complex (MHC) proteins on target cells. As we discussed in Chapters 4 and 5, class I MHC molecules are important for the presentation of foreign (viral) peptide antigens to cytotoxic T cells. Increased expression of MHC I improves the likelihood that virus-specific T cells will recognize the presence of infection and induce apoptosis of the infected cell.

Interferon-γ (Type II Interferon)

IFN-γ is produced mainly by activated T cells and NK cells. Unlike IFN-α and IFN-β, IFN-γ does not have a potent anti-viral effect but is mainly involved in adaptive responses against intracellular microorganisms. It is the primary cytokine of the TH1 response, influencing the expression of more than 200 target-cell genes. Because TH1 cytokines are associated with cell-mediated immunity, IFN-γ tends to increase the expression of genes that shape the responses of T cells and macrophages. For example, a major function of IFN-γ is the enhancement of antigen presentation by class I and class II MHC molecules. Augmented expression of class I and II MHC molecules on antigen-presenting cells (APCs) increases the probability that peptide antigens will be presented to T lymphocytes capable of responding to the infection. IFN-γ is also a potent activator of macrophages, dramatically increasing their ability to kill ingested microbes. The resulting "super" macrophages possess enhanced phagocytic and cytotoxic abilities. IFN-γ also helps regulate and activate CD4⁺ TH1 cells, CD8⁺ cytotoxic T lymphocytes, and NK cells. Thus, IFN-γ influences the immune response in several key ways. Synthesis of IFN-γ is promoted by IL-12 and IL-18 and negatively regulated by IL-4 and IL-10.

Interferon-λ (Type III Interferon)

Discovered in 2003, the IFN-λ family contains four related proteins:

- IFN-λ1 (or IL-29)
- IFN-λ2 (or IL-28A)
- IFN-λ3 (or IL-28B)
- IFN-λ4

These proteins are mainly produced by dendritic cells but can also be made by other cell types. They have a primary role in defense against viral infections at the epithelial barriers of the gastrointestinal, respiratory, and reproductive tracts. IFN-λ also appears to have roles in modulating innate and adaptive immune responses, autoimmunity, and tumor growth.

Selected T-Cell Cytokines

T cells produce many cytokines that influence the immune response in various ways. T-cell cytokines can activate the adaptive immune response, stimulate innate immune defenses, or inhibit immune responses. The cytokines that perform these functions are too numerous to discuss completely in this chapter; thus, in the sections that follow, we discuss selected T-cell cytokines involved in the activation and suppression of immune responses.

T-Cell Cytokines That Activate Immune Responses

T-cell cytokines that activate immune responses are produced by CD4⁺ TH cells. Some of these cytokines were discussed briefly in a previous section and are listed in Table 6–2 according to the TH cell subset from which they were produced. In this section, we discuss the cytokines IL-2, IL-4, IL-5, IL-13, and IL-17 in more detail. IFN-γ, the signature cytokine of TH1 cells, was discussed previously in the section on Interferons.

Interleukin-2 (IL-2)

IL-2 is produced rapidly by CD4⁺ T cells following their activation by antigen and costimulatory signals (see Chapter 5). A major function of IL-2, originally termed *T-cell growth factor,* is to drive the proliferation and differentiation of antigen-activated T cells. This is accomplished through an autocrine mechanism, whereby IL-2 stimulates expression of the IL-2 receptor subunit, IL-2Rα (also known as CD25) and its combination with two other subunits (IL-2Rβ and IL-2Rγc) to form high-affinity receptors on the surface of the activated T cells. Binding of IL-2 to its receptors promotes dramatic proliferation of the T cells, resulting in up to a 1,000-fold expansion in antigen-specific CD4⁺ T cells and up to a 50,000-fold expansion of antigen-specific CD8+ T cells, greatly increasing the immune response toward the pathogen expressing the inducing antigen.

Under the influence of IL-2, many of the activated T cells develop into effector cells that have increased functional activities. CD8⁺ effector cells possess cytotoxic activity against host cells infected with intracellular pathogens, whereas CD4⁺ effector cells secrete additional cytokines such as IFN-γ and IL-4, which have a range of activities.

Another major function of IL-2 is to promote the development and survival of Treg cells, which are needed to suppress unwanted immune responses toward self- and other antigens. Additionally, IL-2 stimulates proliferation of NK cells, augments their ability to produce cytokines, and enhances their cytolytic activity.

6-2 Clinical Correlations

The Common Gamma Chain (γc) and Severe Combined Immunodeficiency

The IL-2R shares its γ subunit with the receptors for several other cytokines, including IL-4, IL-7, IL-9, IL-15, and IL-21. Given the structural similarities of these receptors and their incorporation of the γc, these cytokines comprise a family known as the *common γ-chain cytokines*.

Individuals who develop or inherit mutations in the γc gene exhibit severe impairment of immunity. Because the γc gene is carried on the X chromosome, the resultant immunodeficiency is referred to as *X-linked severe combined immunodeficiency disease*, or X-linked SCID (see Chapter 19). The effects of the disease on the immune system are so pronounced that without treatment, males who inherit a defective γc gene succumb to infection before their first birthday. In one famous case of X-linked SCID, David Vetter (known as the "Bubble Boy") was raised in a germ-free environment to protect him from the normally harmless microorganisms that can be lethal to such patients. Today, hematopoietic stem cell transplantation can be used to successfully treat SCID if a compatible donor is found and the patient is treated in the first year of life.

The severity of X-linked SCID is attributable to the fact that so many cytokine receptors incorporate the γc subunit. Among other immune irregularities, SCID results in a lack of functional T and B lymphocytes and disrupted NK cell development. Therefore, both innate and adaptive immunity are impacted.

Interleukin-4 (IL-4) and Interleukin-13 (IL-13)

IL-4 is produced mainly by the TH2 subset of $CD4^+$ T cells, but it can also be produced by Tfh cells, activated mast cells, and other tissue cells. It is one of the key cytokines regulating TH2 immune activities and helps drive antibody responses in a variety of diseases, notably allergies, autoimmune diseases, and parasitic infections. The IL-4 receptor is expressed on lymphocytes and on many nonhematopoietic cell types. IL-4 induces naive T cells to turn on the genes that generate TH2 cells and turn off the genes that promote TH1 cell differentiation.

IL-13 is made mainly by TH2 cells, but it can also be produced by innate lymphoid cells and other WBCs. It shares many structural and functional properties with IL-4. IL-4 and IL-13 are key cytokines involved in defense against helminths and in allergic responses. Together, these cytokines stimulate immunoglobulin class switching to IgE, recruitment of eosinophils, activation of macrophages, and increased peristalsis in the gastrointestinal tract, all of which are important in these immune responses (see Chapter 14). IL-13 also increases mucous secretion from cells in the respiratory tract and gut epithelium.

Interleukin-5 (IL-5)

$CD4^+$ TH2 cells and innate lymphoid cells are the primary sources of IL-5. Its main functions are to stimulate differentiation of eosinophils and to activate mature eosinophils in defense against helminths; eosinophils are also involved in allergic reactions.

Interleukin-17 (IL-17)

The TH17 subset secretes the IL-17 family of cytokines and plays critical roles in both innate and adaptive immune responses. Key cytokines that differentiate T cells to maintain them as TH17 cells are TGF-β and IL-6. Interleukin-23, produced by macrophages and DCs, also plays a role in finalizing the development of naive TH cells to TH17 cells.

IL-17A, the first IL-17 identified, is the most studied IL-17 cytokine. Other IL-17 family members include IL-17B, IL-17C, IL-17D, IL-17E, and IL-17F. Most of the IL-17 cytokine family members are potent pro-inflammatory cytokines that induce expression of TNF-α, IL-1β, and IL-6 in epithelial cells, endothelial cells, keratinocytes, fibroblasts, and macrophages.

TH17 cells play an important role in host defense against bacterial and fungal infections at mucosal surfaces. Upon an encounter with bacteria or fungi, APCs secrete cytokines that differentiate TH17 cell subsets. TH17 cells then invade the infected area and secrete IL-17 cytokines necessary for the continuous recruitment of neutrophils. IL-17A and IL-17F induce epithelial cells, endothelial cells, fibroblasts, and macrophages to produce the chemokine CXCL8, which is needed for the recruitment of neutrophils to the site of inflammation.

TH17 cells also secrete interleukin-21 (IL-21), which, along with IL-17, stimulates mucosal surfaces to secrete anti-microbial peptides such as the defensins. IL-21 also promotes regeneration of epithelial cells following tissue injury. Thus, TH17 cells in the tissues may be important for long-term maintenance of the anti-microbial response and for maintaining the integrity of the epithelial barriers during chronic bacterial infections.

T-Cell Cytokines That Inhibit Immune Responses

In order for the body to mount immune responses at an appropriate level, these responses must be tapered if they are directed against a self-antigen or if they persist after a foreign antigen has been successfully eliminated. If an immune response is allowed to continue inappropriately, it could intensify and lead to autoimmune disorders and other inflammatory conditions. Thus, the cellular events of the immune system must be carefully regulated to achieve a balance between effective immune responses for elimination of pathogens and prevention of hyper-responsiveness that could cause damage to the host. Two important components of immune regulation are **regulatory T cells (Tregs)** and inhibitory cytokines.

Tregs are a subclass of CD4-positive T cells that can be identified by the expression of CD4, CD25 (the IL-2Rα subunit), and the transcription factor FoxP3. Some Tregs are formed during thymic development, whereas others differentiate from naive T cells in the periphery, sometimes referred to as *induced Tregs (iTregs)*. Tregs are thought to exert their immune suppressive actions by multiple mechanisms, one of which is the production of inhibitory cytokines. Two major cytokines whose primary function is to suppress immune reactions are IL-10 and transforming growth factor-β (TGF-β).

Interleukin-10 (IL-10)

IL-10 is produced by Tregs and many other cell types, including activated macrophages and dendritic cells, TH1 and TH2 cells, and some B cells. The immunosuppressive actions of IL-10 arise from its ability to inhibit activated macrophages and DCs. A major effect of IL-10 is inhibition of IFN-γ production by suppressing IL-12 synthesis by these cells. Thus, IL-10 serves as an antagonist of IFN-γ, suppressing TH1 cells and promoting a TH2 cytokine pattern. IL-10 also suppresses antigen presentation to T cells by inhibiting the expression of class II MHC and costimulatory molecules on macrophages and DCs. By these mechanisms, IL-10 is able to prevent T-cell activation, suppress innate reactions, and terminate cell-mediated immune responses.

Transforming Growth Factor-β (TGF-β)

Transforming growth factor-β (TGF-β) is another important cytokine made by Tregs, but it can also be produced by macrophages and other cell types. Three isoforms of this cytokine, named TGF-β1, TGF-β2, and TGF-β3, exist and constitute the growth factor superfamily of the same name. TGF-β was originally characterized as a factor that induced growth arrest in tumor cells. Later, it was identified as a factor that induces anti-proliferative activity in a variety of cell types.

TGF-β is a pleiotropic cytokine that regulates cell growth, differentiation, apoptosis, migration, and inflammation. It downregulates inflammatory responses when they are no longer needed by inhibiting the activation of macrophages, neutrophils, and endothelial cells. Like IL-10, TGF-β blocks the production of IL-12 and therefore, IFN-γ production. It also hinders adaptive immune responses by inhibiting T- and B-cell proliferation.

TGF-β further exerts its immunosuppressive effects by regulating the differentiation of Treg cells. However, TGF-β also plays a role in the differentiation of TH17 cells. Additionally, TGF-β stimulates immunoglobulin class switching of B cells to IgA and promotes tissue repair by stimulating fibroblasts to synthesize collagen after inflammation subsides. Thus, TGF-β is a cytokine that affects the immune system in diverse, and sometimes opposing, ways.

Knowledge Check 6-3

Match each cytokine with its major function:

a. IL-1β	____ 1. Inhibits viral replication
b. IL-2	____ 2. Suppresses immune responses
c. IL-4	____ 3. Recruits neutrophils
d. IL-10	____ 4. Induces tumor cell lysis
e. IL-17	____ 5. Leads to chemotaxis of leukocytes
f. TNF-α	____ 6. Stimulates proliferation of T cells
g. IFN-α	____ 7. Induces fever
h. CCL3	____ 8. Simulates IgE production

Hematopoietic Growth Factors

An abundant supply of leukocytes is required to carry out the varied responses of the immune system. During innate and adaptive immune responses, several cytokines, called **hematopoietic growth factors,** are produced, which are involved in the renewal of the immune cell populations. Recall from Chapter 1 that this process is termed *hematopoiesis* and occurs in the bone marrow. The role of hematopoietic growth factors in hematopoiesis is to stimulate proliferation, differentiation, and maturation of the blood cell lineages from bone marrow progenitor cells. An important effect of hematopoietic cytokines is to increase WBC production in response to an ongoing inflammatory process.

Some hematopoietic growth factors are involved in the early stages of hematopoiesis, where they can affect multiple cell lineages. Fibroblasts in the bone marrow produce stem cell factor (SCF), also known as KIT-ligand (KIT-L). This cytokine acts in conjunction with other growth factors to promote survival and drive development and proliferation of undifferentiated hematopoietic stem cells (HSCs) and other cells in the early stages of hematopoiesis **(Fig. 6-6).**

As differentiation progresses, the cells become more committed to a particular lineage under the influence of cytokines whose effects are more directed toward specific cell population(s). IL-1, IL-3, IL-6, and IL-11 induce differentiation of pluripotent HSCs into common myeloid progenitors (CMPs), whereas IL-7 drives hematopoiesis in a different direction, forming common lymphoid progenitors (CLPs).

Several of the hematopoietic cytokines have been termed **colony-stimulating factors (CSFs)** because they stimulate the formation of colonies of cells in vitro and in the bone marrow. The various CSFs, their sources, and the cells whose development they influence are listed in **Table 6–4** and shown in Fig. 6–6.

Knowledge Check 6-4

All of the following are hematopoietic growth factors *except* for:

a. IL-3
b. SCF
c. GM-CSF
d. TGF-β

Cytokines in Disease

Cytokine interactions are powerful determinants of immunity, and the pattern of cytokines produced in response to a particular infection or other inflammatory event can impact the difference between an effective or inappropriate immune response. In extreme circumstances, dysregulation of cytokine production and massive overproduction of cytokines can result in hyperstimulation of the immune response or **hypercytokinemia,** a condition more commonly referred to as **cytokine release syndrome (CRS),** or **cytokine storm.** Instead of orchestrating an effective immune response against a pathogen, cytokine storms may lead to shock, multiorgan failure, or even death **(Fig. 6-7).**

Several human pathogens induce cytokine storms, including pathogenic viruses (e.g., influenza A, SARS-CoV-2, Ebola virus) and gram-positive and gram-negative bacteria (e.g., *Staphylococcus aureus, Escherichia coli*). Cytokine storms have been implicated in the lethality of the 1918 influenza pandemic and more recently, the COVID-19 pandemic. The scientific literature indicates that many of these deaths resulted not from the virus itself but from the production of extremely high levels of pro-inflammatory cytokines, such as TNF-α and IL-1β. When present in the blood at high concentrations, these cytokines cause severe symptoms, including hypotension, hypoxemia, fever, and edema, and can precipitate organ failure and death.

6-3 Clinical Correlations

The Role of Cytokine Storm in Ebola Virus Infection

The Ebola virus causes one of the most serious and fatal diseases known to humans. Ebola is a single-stranded RNA virus capable of infecting many different cell types throughout the body, including immune cells such as macrophages and DCs. Within a few days of exposure, symptoms become apparent. Infected individuals exhibit severe headache, fever, muscle pain, fatigue, diarrhea, vomiting, abdominal pain, and unexplained bruising or hemorrhaging. Ebola is extremely infectious and spreads quickly through a population, as evidenced by a major outbreak across West Africa in 2014.

In response to Ebola virus infection, immune cells release a massive amount of pro-inflammatory cytokines, including IL-1β, TNF-α, and IL-6. The cytokines produced and the magnitude of their concentrations in the blood have led immunologists to refer to this phenomenon as a "cytokine storm." Although infection with Ebola virus causes widespread cell death, many scientists have hypothesized that this aggressive cytokine response is the primary driver of Ebola pathogenesis. TNF-α, in particular, causes the blood vessels to become more permeable, resulting in dangerously low blood pressure. As the platelet count drops, excessive bleeding occurs from every orifice in the body. Death typically results in 1 to 2 weeks after infection. Interestingly, the virus inhibits the production of the anti-viral cytokines IFN-α and IFN-β by infected cells.

The cytokine storm associated with Ebola infection exemplifies the complicated role of cytokines in the immune

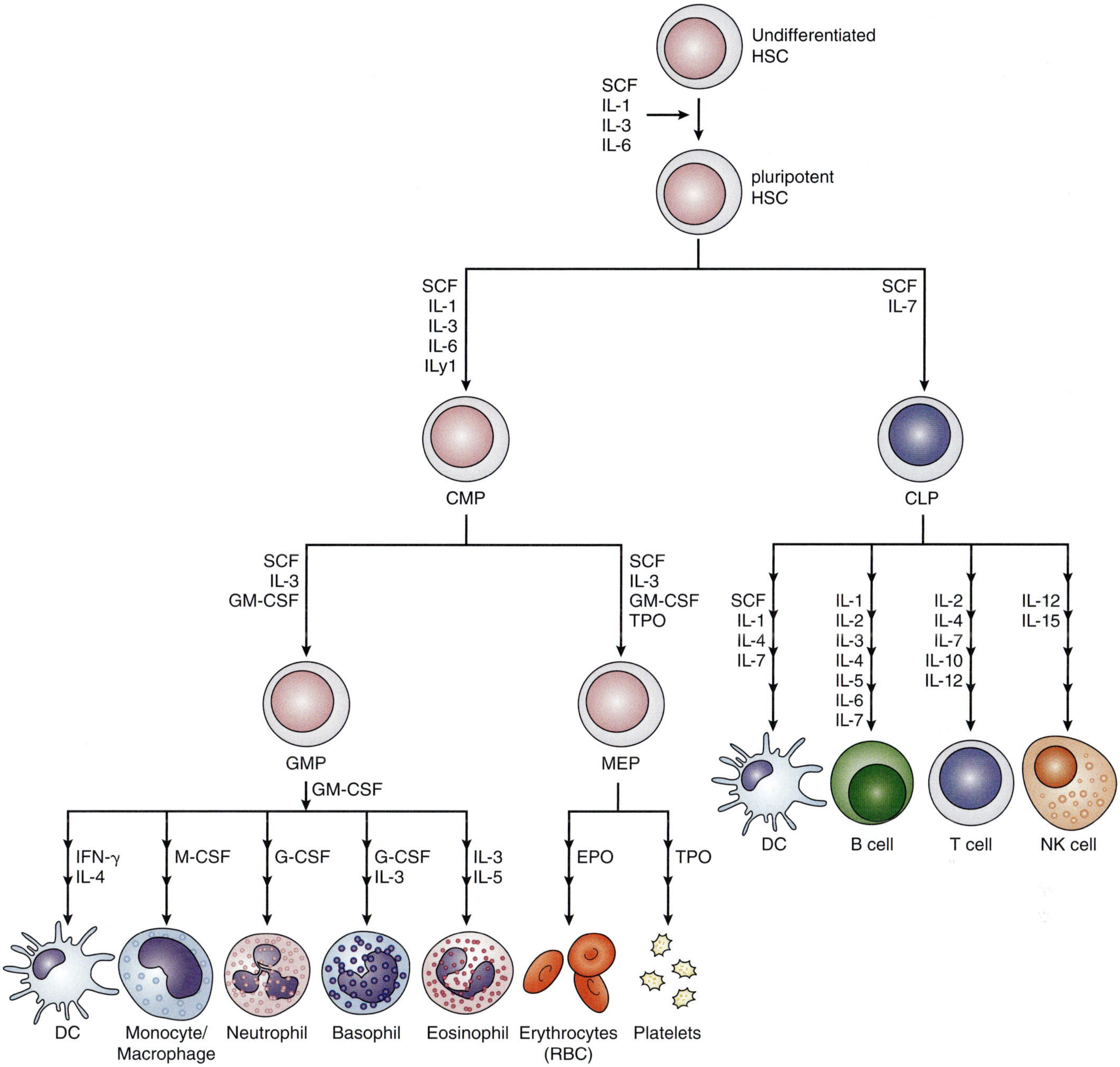

FIGURE 6–6 Influence of hematopoietic growth factors on development of blood cells. Multiple arrows indicate multiple steps. CLP = common lymphoid progenitor; CMP = common myeloid progenitor; EPO = erythropoietin; G-CSF = granulocyte colony-stimulating factor; GM-CSF = granulocyte-macrophage colony-stimulating factor; HSC = hematopoietic stem cell; IL = interleukin; M-CSF = macrophage colony-stimulating factor; MEP = megakaryocyte/erythrocyte progenitor; SCF = stem cell factor; TPO = thrombopoietin.

response. If regulation of these powerful immune mediators is lost, their benefits can be easily transformed into harmful and potentially lethal effects.

Dysregulation of TH cell subsets and Tregs and their secreted cytokines has also been implicated in the pathogenesis of multiple inflammatory diseases and several autoimmune conditions. Diseases associated with imbalances between pro-inflammatory and anti-inflammatory cytokines include rheumatoid arthritis (RA), systemic lupus erythematosus (SLE), multiple sclerosis, inflammatory bowel disease (IBD), psoriasis, and allergic asthma. We discuss the role of cytokines in the pathology of some of these diseases in Chapters 14 and 15.

Critical Thinking 6-1

Coronavirus disease 2019 (COVID-19), caused by the severe acute respiratory syndrome coronavirus-2 (SARS-CoV-2) has been responsible for millions of deaths around the world, especially before the development and administration of vaccines against the virus. In severe cases, patients develop potentially fatal symptoms, including acute respiratory distress, heart failure, hypotension, shock, hypercoagulation, and acute kidney injury. Based on your reading of this chapter, what is the underlying cause of these symptoms, and which cytokines would be most helpful to monitor the immune status of these patients?

Table 6-4 Hematopoietic Growth Factors

HEMATOPOIETIC GROWTH FACTOR	MAJOR SOURCE(S)	PRIMARY CELLS WHOSE DEVELOPMENT IS INDUCED
Granulocyte-macrophage colony-stimulating factor (GM-CSF)	Activated T cells, macrophages, vascular endothelial cells, fibroblasts	Myeloid cells (i.e., neutrophils, eosinophils, basophils, monocytes, and most dendritic cells), mast cells, megakaryocyte/erythrocyte progenitors (which develop into platelets and red blood cells)
Granulocyte colony-stimulating factor (G-CSF)	Macrophages, vascular endothelial cells, fibroblasts	Neutrophils, basophils
Macrophage colony-stimulating factor (M-CSF)	Macrophages, vascular endothelial cells, fibroblasts	Monocytes, macrophages
Erythropoietin (EPO)	Peritubular cells in kidneys	Erythrocytes (red blood cells)
Thrombopoietin (TPO)	Liver parenchymal cells	Platelets

Cytokine Therapies

Knowledge about the important functions of cytokines has prompted researchers to develop cytokine therapies to boost immune responses in patients with certain medical conditions. We discuss some examples of cytokine therapies here and in Chapters 15, 17, and 25.

Administration of hematopoietic growth factors has been one of the most successful types of cytokine treatments. Erythropoietin (EPO) is routinely administered to improve red blood cell (RBC) counts for patients with severe anemia induced by conditions such as chronic kidney disease or chemotherapy for cancer. Granulocyte-macrophage colony-stimulating factor (GM-CSF) and granulocyte colony-stimulating factor (G-CSF) are effective in correcting low neutrophil counts that may occur as a result of chemotherapy.

Another type of cytokine therapy is a modified form of IFN-α that is routinely used to boost anti-viral immunity in chronic hepatitis-B and hepatitis-C infections. The U.S. Food and Drug Administration (FDA) has approved several cytokines, including IFN-α, IL-2, IL-12, IL-15, IL-21, for clinical trials or treatment of various types of cancer with the goal of promoting lymphocyte infiltration into tumors and activating effective anti-tumor responses by NK cells and T cells.

It is important to recognize that development of cytokine therapies has been met with several challenges because of their short half-lives and ability to induce severe side effects due to their pleiotropic characteristics. Over the years, scientific advances have been making it possible for cytokine drugs to be used therapeutically with more effectiveness and reduced toxicity. These innovations include the following:

- Using recombinant (genetically engineered) cytokines
- Combining cytokines with polyethylene glycol (PEG; a process known as PEGylation) to increase their presence in the circulation
- Using computer-assisted protein engineering techniques to modify cytokine structure
- Fusing cytokines with antibodies to direct their localization in the body
- Attaching cytokines to nanoparticles to direct them to bind to their receptors
- Packaging mRNA that codes for a cytokine into nanoparticles and delivering them directly to tumor cells
- Genetically engineering cells to make certain cytokines

Anti-Cytokine Therapies

As we discussed previously, overproduction of cytokines can contribute to the pathology of many autoimmune and other inflammatory diseases. Anti-cytokine therapies aim to reduce inflammation by targeting the interactions between specific cytokines and their receptors. These therapies consist of either monoclonal antibodies that bind a particular cytokine or proteins that block specific cytokine receptors.

Development of anti-cytokine therapies has become a rapidly growing field that has had a great impact on clinical medicine. While these advancements are too numerous to discuss in detail, a few examples are listed here:

- Monoclonal antibodies that bind to TNF-α and a hybrid protein containing the binding domains of the TNF receptor for treatment of rheumatoid arthritis and other autoimmune diseases (see Chapter 15)
- Monoclonal antibodies that block IL-17 or the receptors for IL-17 or IL-23 for treatment of psoriasis
- Monoclonal antibodies that bind the IL-6 receptors for treatment of CRS

These and other anti-cytokine therapies provide symptomatic relief, and in some cases, improved survival, of patients with severe inflammatory conditions.

Knowledge Check 6-5

Rheumatoid arthritis is an autoimmune disease that involves inflammation of the joints. To reduce the inflammation, anti-cytokine therapies have been developed that target:

a. IL-3
b. TNF-α
c. EPO
d. IL-10

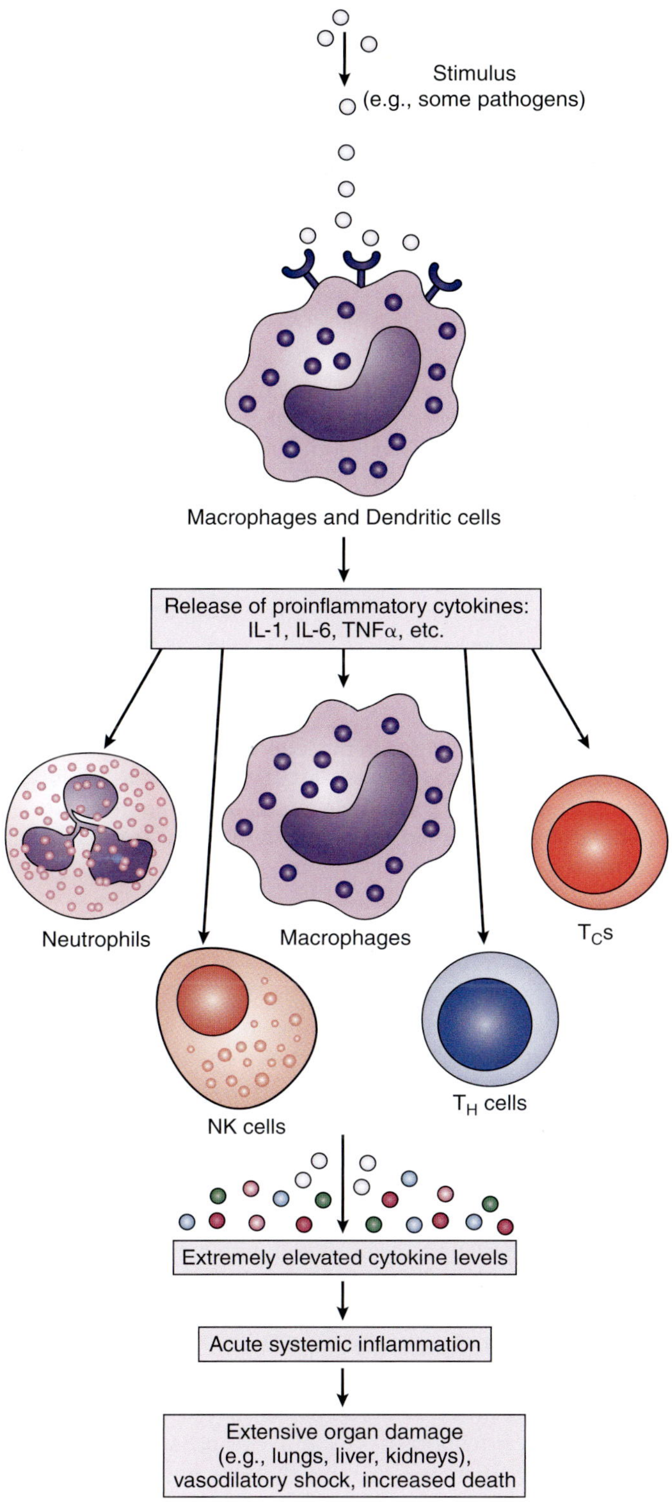

FIGURE 6–7 General principle of a cytokine storm. Macrophages and dendritic cells are initially activated in the innate immune response, and release proinflammatory cytokines such as IL-1, IL-6, and TNFα. These cytokines stimulate the production of chemokines, which recruit various WBCs to the site of inflammation. The recruited cells, in turn, secrete additional cytokines which exacerbate the inflammatory response. The massive cytokine release results in extensive organ damage and is associated with an increased risk for death. Exact mechanisms vary in specific situations.

Laboratory Methods for Cytokine Detection

Cytokine assays have been widely used in research laboratories for many years. More recently, expanding knowledge about the roles of cytokines in the pathology of various diseases and growing applications of cytokine and anti-cytokine therapies have increased the demand for cytokine assays in the clinical laboratory. Evaluation of cytokines in clinical samples can provide valuable information to physicians in assessing the diagnosis, stage, and prognosis of patients with inflammatory disorders, such as autoimmune diseases, allergies, cancer, sepsis, and CRS. Cytokine measurements can also be used to monitor the immune status of patients who are receiving cytokine-related treatments and adjust these therapies, if needed.

Different types of laboratory methods have been developed to measure cytokines in body fluids or cell culture supernatants. These can be broadly classified as (1) **immunoassays,** which measure the presence and quantities of cytokines, and (2) **bioassays,** which measure the biologic activities of cytokines. Specialized assays can detect cytokine production in cell populations, single cells, or tissue sections. Additionally, molecular methods such as polymerase chain reaction (PCR) can be used to detect RNA transcripts that code for specific cytokines or their receptors. Newer technologies, such as point-of-care biosensors that can detect changes in cytokine production in real time are being evaluated. This section presents information about two types of assays that have clinical applications: cytokine immunoassays and the ELISpot.

Cytokine Immunoassays

Clinical laboratories use commercially available sandwich immunoassays to measure cytokines in patient samples. They are based on the detection of a cytokine by its ability to bind simultaneously to a cytokine-specific capture antibody coated onto a solid phase (e.g., a membrane, microtiter well, microbead, or electrode) and a detection antibody linked to a reporter label, such as an enzyme, fluorescent, or chemiluminescent tag (discussed in detail in Chapter 11). **Figure 6–8** shows the basic principle of a sandwich immunoassay for cytokine detection.

Today, most cytokine immunoassays are multiplexed, meaning that they can detect multiple cytokines simultaneously, or determine a **cytokine profile.** Cytokine profiling is advantageous, because, as we discussed earlier, cytokines do not act alone but rather in concert with each other in complex networks to determine an immune response. Commercial cytokine assays can detect up to 30 cytokines in a sample, including pro- and anti-inflammatory cytokines, cytokines characteristically produced by TH1 and TH2 cells, and hematopoietic growth factors, providing a broader view of a patient's immune status than testing for a single cytokine.

Two types of immunoassays that have been developed for the measurement of cytokines are the enzyme-linked immunosorbent assay (ELISA) and the microbead assay.

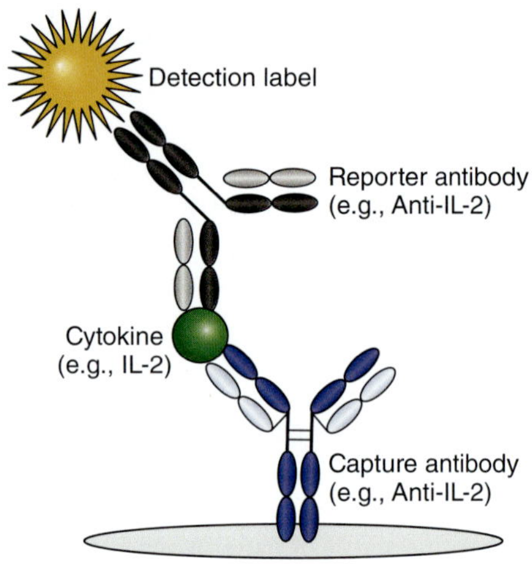

FIGURE 6–8 Basic components of a cytokine immunoassay.

Multiplexed ELISAs use different cytokine-specific capture antibodies bound to individual microwells or antibody microarrays and a panel of labeled detector antibodies, allowing for simultaneous identification of several cytokines from serum or plasma in a single test run. In the microarray format, each well on the slide contains a microarray of spotted antibodies, with "spots" for each of the cytokines plus additional "spots" for positive and negative controls. The replicate spots allow for the acquisition of reliable quantitative data from a single sample.

The widely used microbead assays use a collection of tiny beads that have been stained with a unique shade of red fluorescence for their identification. Each type of bead is linked to a capture antibody that is specific for a particular cytokine. Patient serum is incubated with the bead mixture, and the cytokines in the sample will bind to their corresponding beads. Cytokine binding is then detected by fluorescent-labeled detector antibodies, and the beads are counted by flow cytometry (see Chapter 13).

Multiplex immunoassays are advantageous for clinical laboratories for several reasons. They are automated, provide rapid results, and can detect many cytokines from a small volume of sample. In addition, they are highly sensitive, capable of detecting cytokines at the level of picograms/milliliter. Ultrasensitive assays, required for some conditions such as certain neurological disorders, can detect even lower concentrations (femtograms/milliliter).

However, several factors can influence the results of cytokine immunoassays. Delays in processing serum or plasma samples, prolonged sample storage at 4°C, or multiple freeze-thaw cycles can lead to rapid degradation of cytokines, creating falsely decreased concentrations. Falsely decreased levels can also result from the binding of soluble cytokine receptors that have been released from cell membranes to their corresponding cytokines. Immunoassays are also unable to detect cytokines that are located inside of cells or vesicles. In contrast, some anticoagulants, such as heparin, can induce cytokine release from WBCs, leading to falsely elevated results. Importantly, cytokine levels can change rapidly, as they can rise quickly after an immune stimulus, and most have a short half-life (minutes to hours), presenting a challenge for automated immunoassays, which detect cytokine concentrations at a single time point of sample collection. The use of biosensors that incorporate microfluidics and fluorescent or electrochemical detectors in point-of-care settings may facilitate monitoring of dynamic fluctuations in cytokine levels to quickly monitor changes in patient immune status in the future.

Critical Thinking 6-2

Suppose a laboratorian who was evaluating an immunoassay for IL-2 received serum samples from another laboratory that had already tested them with the same immunoassay for comparison. The IL-2 concentrations of the samples were as follows:

Sample Number	Results From Comparison Laboratory	Laboratorian's results
1	1.5 pg/mL	0.5 pg/mL
2	200 pg/mL	20 pg/mL
3	1,000 pg/mL	100 pg/mL

The controls provided in the laboratorian's test kit were within their expected ranges. Discuss possible reasons for the discrepancies in the sample results, assuming that both laboratories performed the test and recorded the results correctly.

ELISpot

ELISA and microbead assays allow for the quantitation of cytokine levels in a sample of plasma or cell culture supernatant but reveal no information about the cytokine source. In contrast, the **ELISpot** is a bioassay that is capable of detecting and enumerating individual cytokine-secreting cells. ELISpot assays accomplish this feat by using a modified ELISA technique on immune cells stimulated by an antigen in a cell culture microplate that has been coated with a cytokine-specific antibody. For example, IFN-γ ELISpot assays use capture antibodies that bind to an epitope of IFN-γ.

Figure 6–9 illustrates the steps of an ELISpot procedure to detect circulating T cells that secrete a specific cytokine in response to a peptide antigen. Recall that T cells are highly specific in their responses—each T cell possesses a unique T-cell receptor that recognizes a discrete polypeptide antigen. Adding a synthetic peptide antigen to T cells co-cultured with monocytes will elicit the production of cytokines by the T cells capable of reacting to that antigen. The monocytes in the sample act as antigen-presenting cells (APCs) to present the antigen to those T cells; most T cells in a given sample have receptor specificities that do not match epitopes found within the protein antigen and will not respond. A labeled detection antibody is then added to identify the cytokine-secreting cells, whose positions on the plate appear as dark spots. The spots can be counted with a microscope or with an automated ELISpot instrument.

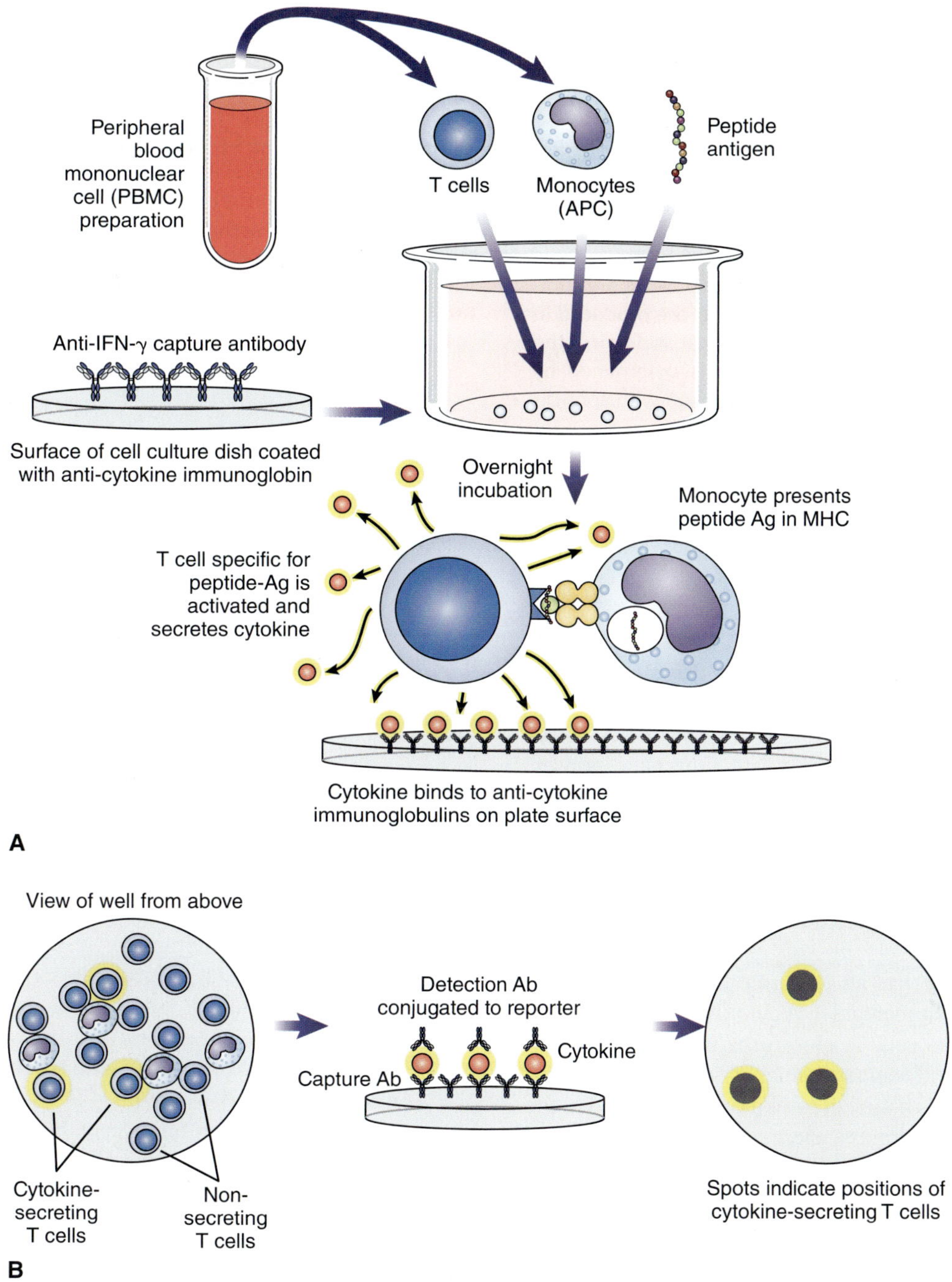

FIGURE 6–9 The ELISpot assay. (A) Peripheral blood mononuclear cells (PBMCs; which contain lymphocytes and monocytes) are prepared from a whole blood sample and added to a plate precoated with capture antibody specific to the target cytokine (IFN-γ in this example). The PBMCs are incubated overnight with a synthetic peptide antigen, which is processed by the monocytes and presented to antigen-specific T cells. T cells responsive to the peptide antigen are stimulated to secrete cytokines, including IFN-γ. (B) Target cytokine binds to the capture antibody and remains fixed to the plate even after the cells are washed away. A labeled detection antibody is added to the plate and binds to the target cytokine (IFN-γ), if present. After excess detection antibody is removed, "spots" indicate the positions where responsive T cells formerly rested on the microplate bottom. These spots can be quantified to assess the number of T cells in a given volume of sample that produce IFN-γ in response to the peptide antigen. *(Figure courtesy of Dr. Aaron Glass.)*

The ELISpot is commonly used in research laboratories to monitor immune responses in vaccine development and to study cytokine or antibody responses in cancer, allergies, and autoimmune diseases. A clinical application of ELISpot is the assessment of cell-mediated immune responses to *M tuberculosis* in people being screened for the infection. While the ELISpot is a sensitive assay that provides information about the cell source of cytokines, it is a complex method that can only be performed by specialized laboratories. Also, it is only capable of detecting the particular cytokine(s) being tested for.

6-4 Clinical Correlations

T-SPOT.TB Test

The T-SPOT.TB Test is an ELISpot method used to evaluate the cell-mediated immune response to *Mycobacterium tuberculosis*. In this test, PBMCs from a patient are incubated in microtiter wells that have been coated with antibody to IFN-γ. *M. tuberculosis*–specific antigens are added to the wells, and the plate is incubated for 16 to 20 hr. T cells from patients who have been exposed to *M. tuberculosis* are stimulated to release IFN-γ, and dark blue spots are produced in the locations of the IFN-γ–secreting cells after addition of the detection antibody. Clinical significance is determined by the number of spots produced, in comparison with controls (see Chapter 14).

Knowledge Check 6-6

In the clinical laboratory, cytokines are most often measured by what type of assay?

a. ELISpot
b. Bioassay
c. Multiplex immunoassay
d. Molecular methods

KEY CONCEPTS

Cytokine Characteristics and Functions

- Cytokines are small, soluble proteins secreted by immune cells and various other cells. They act as chemical messengers to regulate immune responses.
- Cytokine production is induced in response to specific stimuli such as bacterial LPS, flagellin, or other bacterial products.
- Cytokines regulate growth, differentiation, gene expression, and function of many different cell types.
- If a cytokine has an *autocrine* effect, it affects the same cell that secreted it. A cytokine with a *paracrine* effect targets cells in close proximity. Occasionally, cytokines will exert systemic, or *endocrine,* activities.
- The *pleiotropic* nature of cytokine activity relates to the ability of a cytokine to affect several different types of cells. *Redundancy* refers to the ability of several different cytokines to activate some of the same cells.
- Individual cytokines do not act alone but in conjunction with many other cytokines that are induced during the process of immune activation. In these complex *cytokine networks,* some cytokines act with synergy and others with antagonism. Sometimes, a cytokine can induce the production of other cytokines in a *cytokine cascade.*

Cytokine Nomenclature

- Cytokines are grouped into families based on similar structures and amino acid sequence.
- Major cytokine families include tumor necrosis factor (TNF), interferon (IFN), chemokine, T-cell growth factor (TGF), and hematopoietic growth factor.
- Interleukins are a large group of cytokines with diverse functions. They are designated by the prefix "IL-."

Functions of Specific Cytokines

- The major cytokines involved in the initial stages of the inflammatory response are IL-1, IL-6, TNF-α, and the chemokines. They are responsible for many of the physical symptoms of inflammation, such as fever, swelling, and pain, as well as movement of cellular infiltrates into damaged tissues.
- The primary sources of cytokines in adaptive immune responses are helper T cells. The TH subpopulations, TH1, TH2, TH17, and Tfh each produce a distinct set of cytokines that induce inflammatory, humoral, or cell-mediated immune responses that are most effective against a particular type of pathogen.
- The interleukins, so named because they are involved in communications between WBCs, are a large group of cytokines with diverse activities.
- Tumor necrosis factors (TNFs) were originally observed to lyse tumor cells but were later discovered to have a variety of effects, including inducing synthesis of inflammatory mediators.
- Chemokines are cytokines that stimulate migration of WBCs to inflamed tissues and to specific locations in secondary lymphoid organs during their development.
- Type I interferons (IFN-α and IFN-β) have potent anti-viral activity in innate immunity, whereas type II IFN (IFN-γ) is mostly involved in adaptive immune responses against intracellular pathogens.
- Hematopoietic growth factors are responsible for stimulating proliferation, differentiation, growth, and maturation of RBCs, platelets, and all WBC types derived from bone marrow progenitor cells.
- While many cytokines activate immune responses, the Treg-derived cytokines, IL-10 and TGF-β, have inhibitory effects to keep immune responses at an appropriate level.

Cytokines in Disease

- A *cytokine storm,* also known as *cytokine release syndrome (CRS)* or *hypercytokinemia,* is a severe, often fatal condition resulting from dysregulation of cytokine synthesis and massive overproduction of cytokines.

Cytokine Therapies

- Hematopoietic growth factors have been used to treat patients with low RBC or WBC counts caused by different conditions. Other cytokines have been used to treat viral hepatitis and cancer.

Anti-Cytokine Therapies

- Anti-cytokine therapies are aimed at disrupting the interaction between cytokines and their specific receptors in autoimmune and other inflammatory diseases.

Laboratory Methods for Cytokine Detection

- Multiplexed ELISAs and microbead assays can simultaneously detect several cytokines in a sample to determine a *cytokine profile.*
- ELISpot is a bioassay that quantitates the number of T cells that secrete specific cytokines in response to a protein antigen.

Study Guide: Inflammatory Cytokines

CYTOKINE	SECRETED BY	ACTIONS
Interleukin-1 β (IL-1β)	Monocytes, macrophages, DCs	Inflammation, fever, initiation of the acute phase response, induces production of chemokines and CSFs
Interleukin-6 (IL-6)	Monocytes, macrophages, endothelial cells, DCs, T cells	Initiation of the acute phase response, B- and T-cell activation, B-cell proliferation and differentiation
Tumor necrosis factor-alpha (TNF-α)	Monocytes, macrophages, NK cells, activated T cells	Inflammation, initiation of the acute phase response, death of tumor cells, induces IL-1 production
Chemokines (e.g., CCL2, CCL5)	WBCs, endothelial cells, epithelial cells, fibroblasts, stromal cells	Motility and migration of immune cells (chemotaxis); see also Table 6–3

CSF = colony-stimulating factor; DC = dendritic cell; NK = natural killer; WBC = white blood cell.

Study Guide: Interferons

CYTOKINE(S)	SECRETED BY	ACTIONS
Type I: Interferon-alpha (IFN-α), Interferon-beta (IFN-β)	Macrophages, DCs, virally infected cells	Protect host cells against viruses, increase class I MHC expression, activate NK cells
Type II: Interferon-gamma (IFN-γ)	Activated TH1 cells, NK cells	Activation of macrophages, increased expression of class I and II MHC molecules, increased antigen presentation, cell-mediated immunity against intracellular pathogens
Type III: Interferon-lambda (IFN-λ)	DCs	Defense against viral infections at epithelial barriers

DC = dendritic cell; MHC = major histocompatibility complex; NK = natural killer.

Study Guide: T-Cell Cytokines That Activate Immune Responses

CYTOKINE	SECRETED BY	ACTIONS
Interleukin-2 (IL-2)	$CD4^+$ T cells	Proliferation and differentiation of activated T cells, NK cell activation and proliferation, development and survival of Tregs
Interleukin-4 (IL-4)	TH2 cells, Tfh cells, mast cells, other tissue cells	Promotes TH2 differentiation, stimulates B cells to switch to IgE production, recruitment of eosinophils, macrophage activation
Interleukin-5 (IL-5)	TH2 cells, innate lymphoid cells	Eosinophil generation and activation
Interleukin-13 (IL-13)	TH2 cells, Tfh cells, mast cells, innate lymphoid cells	Stimulates B cells to switch to IgE production, recruitment of eosinophils, macrophage activation, stimulates increased mucous secretion by respiratory and gastrointestinal epithelia
Interleukin-17 (IL-17)	TH17 cells	Inflammation, defense against bacterial and fungal infections, induces production of chemokines and neutrophil recruitment, induces production of IL-1β, IL-6, and TNF-α

NK = natural killer; TNF = tumor necrosis factor.

Study Guide: T-Cell Cytokines That Suppress Immune Responses

CYTOKINE	SECRETED BY	ACTIONS
Interleukin-10 (IL-10)	Tregs, activated macrophages, DCs	Suppression of TH1 cells, inhibition of class I and class II MHC expression and antigen presentation, inhibition of IL-12 and IFN-γ production
Transforming growth factor-beta (TGF-β)	Tregs, macrophages, other cell types	Inhibits T- and B-cell proliferation, inhibits macrophage activation, inhibits IL-12 and IFN-γ production, induces IgA production, promotes tissue repair

DC = dendritic cell; MHC = major histocompatibility complex.

Study Guide: Hematopoietic Growth Factors

CYTOKINES	SECRETED BY	ACTIONS
Stem cell factor (SCF), IL-3, IL-7, GM-CSF, G-CSF, M-CSF, EPO, TPO	Fibroblasts, T cells, macrophages, vascular endothelial cells, others	Renewal of immune cell populations derived from hematopoietic stem cells and progenitors in the bone marrow (see also Table 6–4 and Figure 6-6)

EPO = erythropoietin; G-CSF = granulocyte colony-stimulating factor; GM-CSF = granulocyte-macrophage colony-stimulating factor; M-CSF = macrophage colony-stimulating factor; TPO = thrombopoietin.

CASE STUDY

1. A 55-year-old patient being treated for acute lymphocytic leukemia (ALL) was not responding well to chemotherapy. Physicians felt that increasing the dosage of chemotherapy drugs was necessary to eliminate the cancer. However, laboratory results showed the patient was severely neutropenic (477 neutrophils/µL) because of the drugs. The medical team could not risk further lowering of the neutrophil count because of the increased risk of infection. Therefore, it was necessary to treat the patient for neutropenia in order to continue with chemotherapy. The patient was also enrolled in a research study designed to look at cytokine expression in ALL patients with neutropenia. The study used a liquid bead array to detect the CSFs and the cytokines typically seen in the innate immune response and in TH1 and TH2 responses.

Questions

a. What CSF should the physicians prescribe to overcome the neutropenia?
b. What are some of the cytokines that might be detected in a TH1-type response?
c. What are some of the cytokines that might be detected in a TH2-type response?

REVIEW QUESTIONS

1. The ability of a single cytokine to alter the expression of several genes is called:
   a. Redundancy
   b. Pleiotropy
   c. Autocrine stimulation
   d. The endocrine effect

2. Which of the following effects can be attributed to IL-1?
   a. Mediation of the innate immune response
   b. Differentiation of stem cells
   c. Halted growth of virally infected cells
   d. Stimulation of mast cells

3. Which of the following precursors is a target cell for IL-3?
   a. Monocyte precursors
   b. Granulocyte precursors
   c. Erythroid precursors
   d. All of the above

4. A lack of IL-4 may result in which of the following effects?
   a. Inability to fight off viral infections
   b. Increased risk of tumors
   c. Lack of IgM
   d. Decreased eosinophil function

5. Which of the following cytokines is also known as the *T-cell growth factor?*
   a. IFN-γ
   b. IL-12
   c. IL-2
   d. IL-10

6. Which of the following represents an autocrine effect of IL-2?
   a. Increased IL-2 receptor expression by the TH cell producing IL-2
   b. Macrophages signaled to the area of antigen stimulation
   c. Proliferation of antigen-stimulated B cells
   d. Increased synthesis of acute phase proteins throughout the body

7. IFN-α and IFN-β differ in which way from IFN-γ?
   a. IFN-α and IFN-β are called *immune IFNs,* and IFN-γ is not.
   b. IFN-α and IFN-β primarily activate macrophages, whereas IFN-γ halts viral activity.
   c. IFN-α and IFN-β are made mainly by activated T cells, whereas IFN-γ is made by fibroblasts.
   d. IFN-α and IFN-β inhibit viral replication, whereas IFN-γ stimulates antigen presentation by class II MHC molecules.

8. A patient in septic shock caused by a gram-negative bacterial infection exhibits the following symptoms: high fever, very low blood pressure, and disseminated intravascular coagulation. Which cytokine is the most likely contributor to these symptoms?
   a. IL-2
   b. TNF-α
   c. IL-12
   d. IL-7

9. IL-10 acts as an antagonist to what cytokine?
   a. IL-4
   b. TNF-α
   c. IFN-γ
   d. TGF-β

10. Which would be the best assay to measure a cytokine profile?
    a. Blast formation
    b. T-cell proliferation
    c. ELISpot
    d. Microbead immunoassay

11. Destruction of TH1 cells by the HIV virus would contribute to immune suppression by which means?
    a. Decrease in IL-1
    b. Decrease in IL-2
    c. Decrease in IL-8
    d. Decrease in IL-10

12. Why might a CSF be given to a patient with cancer?
    a. Stimulate activity of NK cells
    b. Increase the production of certain types of leukocytes
    c. Decrease the production of TNF
    d. Increase the production of mast cells

13. Which of the following would result from a lack of TNF-α?
    a. Decreased ability to fight bacterial infections
    b. Increased expression of class II MHC molecules
    c. Decreased survival of cancer cells
    d. Increased risk of septic shock

14. Which cytokine acts to promote differentiation of T cells to the TH1 subclass?
    a. IL-1
    b. IL-4
    c. IL-12
    d. IL-10

15. What is the major function of Treg cells?
    a. Suppression of the immune response by inducing IL-12
    b. Suppression of the immune response by producing IL-10
    c. Proliferation of immune cells by producing IL-2
    d. Proliferation of immune cells by inducing IL-4

16. TH17 cells affect the innate immune response by producing which cytokines?
    a. IFN-γ and IL-2
    b. IL-4 and IL-13
    c. IL-17 and IL-21
    d. TNF-α and IL-6

17. TNF-α induces the production of IL-1 from macrophages. This is an example of:
    a. A cytokine cascade
    b. A cytokine network
    c. Synergism
    d. Pleiotropy

18. Which cytokine does not promote inflammation?
    a. IL-1β
    b. IL-6
    c. TGF-β
    d. TNF-α

19. In the cytokine CXCL1, the C's represent the term:
    a. Cytokine
    b. Chemokine
    c. Cascade
    d. Cysteine

20. Which cytokine is a major contributor to the condition known as cytokine storm?
    a. IL-4
    b. IL-6
    c. IL-10
    d. IFN-α

Chapter 6 Answer Key

Answers to Knowledge Checks

6-1 c 6-2 a 6-3 1-g; 2-d; 3-e; 4-f; 5-h; 6-b; 7-a; 8-c
6-4 d 6-5 b 6-6 c

Answers to Review Questions

1. b	2. a	3. d	4. d	5. c	6. a	7. d
8. b	9. c	10. d	11. b	12. b	13. a	14. c
15. b	16. c	17. a	18. c	19. d	20. b	

7 The Complement System

Ashley Frazer-Abel, PhD, D(ABMLI), and Bradley P. Dixon, MD, FASN

LEARNING OUTCOMES

After finishing this chapter, you should be able to:

7.1 Describe the characteristics and functions of the complement system.

7.2 Explain the steps of the classical, alternative, and lectin pathways, indicating the proteins and activators involved in each.

7.3 Discuss the formation of the three principal units of the classical pathway: recognition, activation, and membrane attack units.

7.4 Explain how C3 plays a key role in complement activation and identify the C3 convertase in all three pathways.

7.5 Discuss regulators of the complement system and their roles in inhibiting the complement pathways.

7.6 Describe deficiencies of complement components and the diseases they cause.

7.7 Describe the biological roles of specific complement receptors.

7.8 Describe potential disease manifestations of improper complement regulation.

7.9 Differentiate tests for functional activity of complement from measurement of individual complement components.

7.10 Discuss the requirements for sample collection and handling for the different types of complement tests and predict the consequences of improper specimen processing.

7.11 Analyze laboratory findings to indicate disease implications associated with complement abnormalities.

7.12 Discuss clinical applications of complement therapeutics and their effects on laboratory tests for complement.

CHAPTER OUTLINE

You can go to **fadavis.com** keyword stevens for the laboratory exercises that accompany this text.

The complement system is a complex group of more than 50 soluble and cell-bound proteins. Present in normal serum, complement is part of the innate immune system. However, as we discussed in previous chapters, the complement proteins have important roles in both innate and adaptive immune responses: Complement can lyse foreign cells, opsonize and tag foreign invaders for clearance, and direct leukocytes to the site of infection. Complement activation can also have strong pro-inflammatory effects because of its ability to increase vascular permeability, recruit monocytes and neutrophils to the area of antigen concentration, and trigger secretion of immunoregulatory molecules that amplify the immune response. In their pro-inflammatory roles, complement proteins serve as an important link between innate and adaptive immunity. However, dysregulation of complement activity plays a significant role in a growing list of disease pathologies. In such circumstances, complement activates the host's immune system but directs it at the host, leading to outcomes with harmful effects.

The interplay of complement with disease is also seen when complement's important "housekeeping" roles are lost. Complement recognizes cellular debris, such as apoptotic cells and immune complexes, tagging them for removal by innate immune cells. The loss of these functions is part of the link between complement and autoimmune rheumatic diseases, which affect the joints and supporting structures (see Chapter 15). Clearly, with such far-reaching and potentially deleterious effects, complement activation needs to be carefully regulated. The need for regaining tight control has been recognized by medical scientists, who have developed an increasing number of therapies directed at regulating various components of the complement system.

Pathways of the Complement System

The complement system can be activated three different ways. The **classical pathway** involves nine proteins that are triggered primarily by antigen-antibody complexes. The other two pathways, the alternative and lectin pathways, are antibody independent and play a major role as a natural defense system. The **alternative pathway** is directly activated by components of bacteria, yeast, fungi, viruses, and parasites that are not found in humans (e.g., lipopolysaccharide [LPS] in the cell walls of gram-negative bacteria). The **lectin pathway** is likely the oldest of the three pathways. In this pathway, **mannose-** (or mannan-) **binding lectin (MBL)** in the serum binds to mannose sugar in the cell walls or outer coating of bacteria, viruses, yeast, and protozoa. Similarly, proteins of the innate immune system called *ficolins* and *collectins* bind to pathogen-associated molecular patterns to activate the lectin pathway. Although we consider each of these pathways separately in this chapter, activation typically involves more than one pathway.

Most plasma complement proteins are synthesized in the liver, except for the C1 components, which are mainly produced by intestinal epithelial cells, and factor D, which is made in adipose tissue. Other hematopoietic cells, such as monocytes and macrophages, are additional sources of complement production. Many of these proteins are produced as inactive precursors, or *zymogens,* which are converted to active enzymes in a precise order. **Table 7–1** lists the characteristics of the main complement proteins. Note that while the early steps of each pathway involve unique proteins, the final steps of the pathways share the same proteins, which interact to cause inflammation and to form a complex that can lyse foreign cells.

The Classical Pathway

The classical pathway is the main antibody-directed mechanism for triggering complement activation. However, not all immunoglobulins can activate this pathway. The immunoglobulin (Ig) classes that can activate the classical pathway are IgM, IgG1, IgG2, and IgG3, but not IgG4, IgA, or IgE. Within the IgG group, IgG3 is the most effective, followed by IgG1 and then IgG2. IgM is the most effective of the activating immunoglobulins because it has multiple binding sites for complement; thus, it takes only one molecule attached to two adjacent antigenic determinants to initiate the cascade **(Fig. 7–1).** Two IgG molecules must attach to the antigen within 30 to 40 nm of each other before complement can bind; it may take at least 1,000 IgG molecules to ensure that there are two close enough to initiate such binding. A raft of six IgG molecules is ideal for interacting with C1q to initiate the classical pathway. Some epitopes, notably the Rh group on red blood cells (RBCs), are too far apart on the cell for this to occur; therefore, they are unable to fix complement.

In addition to antibodies, a few substances can bind complement directly to initiate the classical cascade. These include C-reactive protein (CRP), several viruses, mycoplasmas, some protozoa, and certain gram-negative bacteria such as *Escherichia coli.* However, most infectious agents can directly activate only the alternative or lectin pathways.

Complement activation can be divided into three main stages, each involving a combination of specific complement components to form a functional complex. The first stage involves the formation of the **recognition unit,** which, in the

Table 7-1 Proteins of the Complement System

SERUM PROTEIN (molecular weight)	CONCENTRATION (μg/mL)	FUNCTION	DISEASE ASSOCIATION
Classical Pathway			
C1q (410 kDa)	150	Binds to Fc region of IgM and IgG, synaptic pruning (elimination of neurons that are rarely or never used)	SLE; recurrent infections
C1r (85 kDa)	50	Activates C1s	
C1s (85 kDa)	50	Cleaves C4 and C2	
C4 (205 kDa)	300–600	Part of C3 convertase (C4b)	Often asymptomatic; RA, SLE, or recurrent infections
C2 (102 kDa)	25	Binds to C4b—forms C3 convertase	SLE, recurrent infections, may be asymptomatic
Lectin Pathway			
MBL (200–600 kDa)	0.0002–10	Binds to mannose	Mostly asymptomatic, bacterial infections, some autoimmune disorders
MASP-1 (93 kDa)	1.5–12	Activates MASP-2 and MASP-3	3MC syndrome
MASP-2 (76 kDa)	400–500 ng/mL	Cleaves C4 and C2	Mostly asymptomatic, respiratory infections
MASP-3 (94 kDa)	2.0–12.0	Cleaves Factor D precursor to its active form	3MC syndrome
C4 (205 kDa)	See Classical Pathway		
C2 (102 kDa)	See Classical Pathway		
Alternative Pathway			
Factor B (93 kDa)	200	Binds to C3b to form C3 convertase	*Neisseria* and pneumococcal infections; aHUS with gain of function
Factor D (24 kDa)	2	Cleaves factor B	Bacterial infection
Properdin (55 kDa)	15–25	Stabilizes C3bBb (C3 convertase)	Severe recurrent infection
Terminal Pathway Proteins (proteins common to the final steps of all three pathways)			
C3 (190 kDa)	1, 200	Key intermediate in all pathways	Severe recurrent infection; aHUS, C3G, AMD with gain of function
C5 (190 kDa)	80	Initiates formation of the MAC	*Neisseria* infection
C6 (110 kDa)	45	Binds to C5b in the MAC	
C7 (100 kDa)	90	Binds to C5bC6 in the MAC	
C8 (150 kDa)	55	Starts pore formation on cell membrane	
C9 (70 kDa)	60	Polymerizes to cause cell lysis	No known disease association

aHUS = atypical hemolytic uremic syndrome; AMD = age-related macular degeneration; C1-INH = C1 inhibitor; C3G = C3 glomerulopathy; DAF = decay-accelerating factor; Fc = crystallizable fragment; Ig = immunoglobulin; MAC = membrane attack complex; MASP-1 -2 and -3 = MBL-associated serine proteases; MBL = mannose-binding lectin; RA = rheumatoid arthritis; SLE = systemic lupus erythematosus.

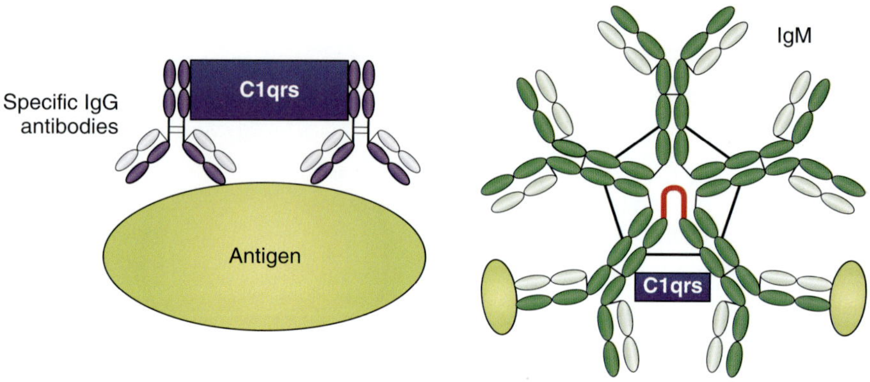

FIGURE 7.1 Binding of C1q to IgG (two molecules required) and IgM (one molecule required).

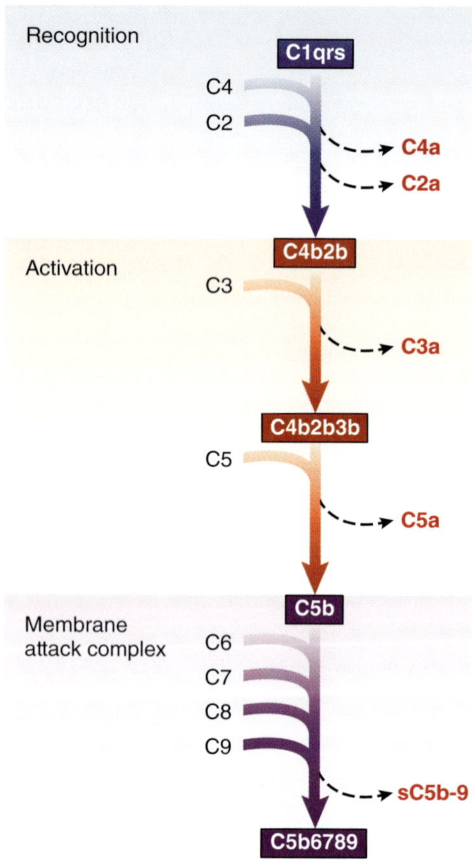

FIGURE 7.2 The basic steps of the complement cascade: recognition, activation, and membrane attack.

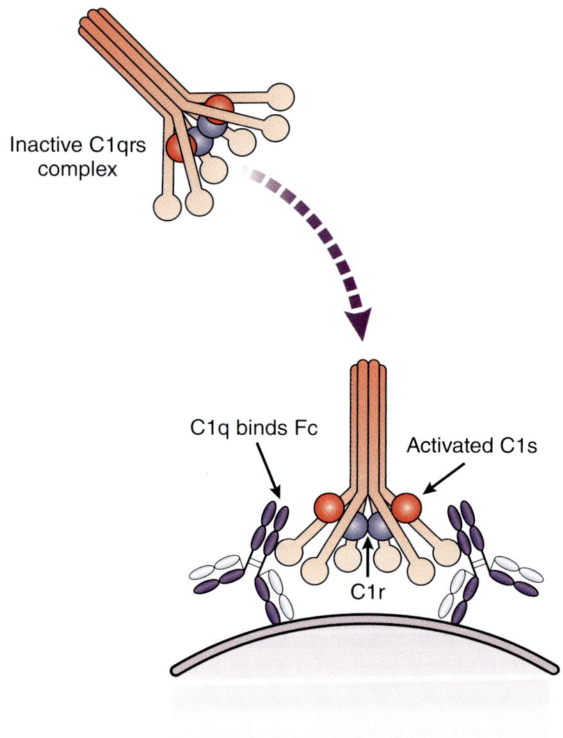

FIGURE 7.3 Structure of C1qr2s2. When two or more globular heads of C1q attach to bound immunoglobulin molecules, the collagen-like stalks change their configuration. The resulting shape change causes C1r to become a serine protease, which cleaves a small fragment of C1s, uncovering the C1s protease, whose only targets are C4 and C2.

case of the classical pathway, is C1. Once C1 is bound, the next components activated are C4, C2, and C3, known collectively as the **activation unit** of the classical pathway (and the lectin pathway). C5 through C9 make up the **membrane attack complex (MAC);** this last unit completes the lysis of foreign particles. We discuss each of these stages in detail in the following sections. **Figure 7–2** depicts a simplified scheme of the entire classical pathway. Note that the complement proteins were named as they were discovered before the sequence of activation was known; therefore, the numbering system does not correspond completely with the order in which the proteins are activated in the pathway.

Formation of the Recognition Unit

The first complement component of the classical pathway to bind is C1, a molecular complex of 740 kDa consisting of three subunits—C1q, C1r, and C1s. C1q is composed of six globular heads with a collagen-like tail portion. This structure has been likened to a bouquet of tulips with six blossoms extending outward. The C1 complex is made up of one C1q subunit, two C1r subunits, and two C1s subunits **(Fig. 7–3).** As long as calcium is present in the serum, C1r and C1s remain associated with C1q. Although the C1q unit is the component that binds to antibody molecules, the C1r and C1s subunits generate enzyme activity to begin the cascade.

C1q binds to the Fc regions from two (or ideally six) adjacent antibody molecules, and at least two of the globular heads of C1q must be bound to initiate the classical pathway. C1r and C1s are serine protease proenzymes, or zymogens. As binding of C1q occurs, both are converted into active enzymes. Autoactivation of C1r results from a conformational change that takes place as C1q is bound. Once activated, C1r cleaves a thioester bond on C1s which, in turn, activates it. Activated C1r is extremely specific because its only known substrate is C1s. Likewise, C1s has a limited specificity, with its only substrates being C4 and C2. Once C1s is activated, the recognition stage ends.

Formation of the Activation Unit

Phase two, the activation phase, begins when C1s cleaves C4 and ends with the production of the enzyme C3 convertase **(Fig. 7–4).** C4 is the second most abundant complement protein, with a serum concentration of approximately 600 μg/mL. C1s cleaves C4 to release a 77-amino acid fragment called C4a. In the process, it opens a thioester-containing active site on the remaining part, C4b. C4b must bind to protein or carbohydrate within a few seconds, or it will react with water molecules to form iC4b, which is rapidly degraded. Thus, C4b binds mainly to antigen in clusters that are within a 40-nm radius of C1. This represents the first amplification step in the cascade because for every C1 molecule attached, approximately 30 molecules of C4 are split and attached.

C2 is the next component to be activated. When combined with C4b in the presence of magnesium ions, C2 is cleaved by C1s to form the fragments, C2b (molecular weight, 70 kDa) and C2a (molecular weight, 34 kDa; see Fig. 7–4A). It is important to note that in 2019, the names of the C2 fragments were switched to mirror that of the other fragments because C2a is the smaller fragment and C2b is the larger fragment. Because of this more recent change, uses of both fragment names will be seen in the literature. This is the only case in which the letter "a" has been designated for the larger cleavage piece with enzyme activity. The short life of these reactive species serves as a mechanism of control, keeping the reaction localized.

The combination of C4b and C2b is known as *C3 convertase* because the C4bC2b complex is an active enzyme that acts on C3 (see Fig. 7–4B). This complex is not very stable. The half-life is estimated to be between 15 seconds and 3 minutes, so C3 must be bound quickly. If binding does occur, C3 is cleaved into two fragments, C3a and C3b.

C3, the major and central constituent of the complement system, is present in the plasma in a concentration of 1 mg/mL to 1.5 mg/mL. It serves as the pivotal point of convergence of all three complement pathways of activation. The cleavage of C3 to C3b represents the most significant step in the entire process of complement activation. The C3 molecule has a molecular weight of 190 kDa and consists of two polypeptide chains, alpha (α) and beta (β). The α chain contains a highly reactive thioester group. When C3a is removed by cleavage of a single bond in the α chain, the thioester is exposed; the remaining piece, C3b, is then capable of binding to hydroxyl groups on carbohydrates and proteins in the

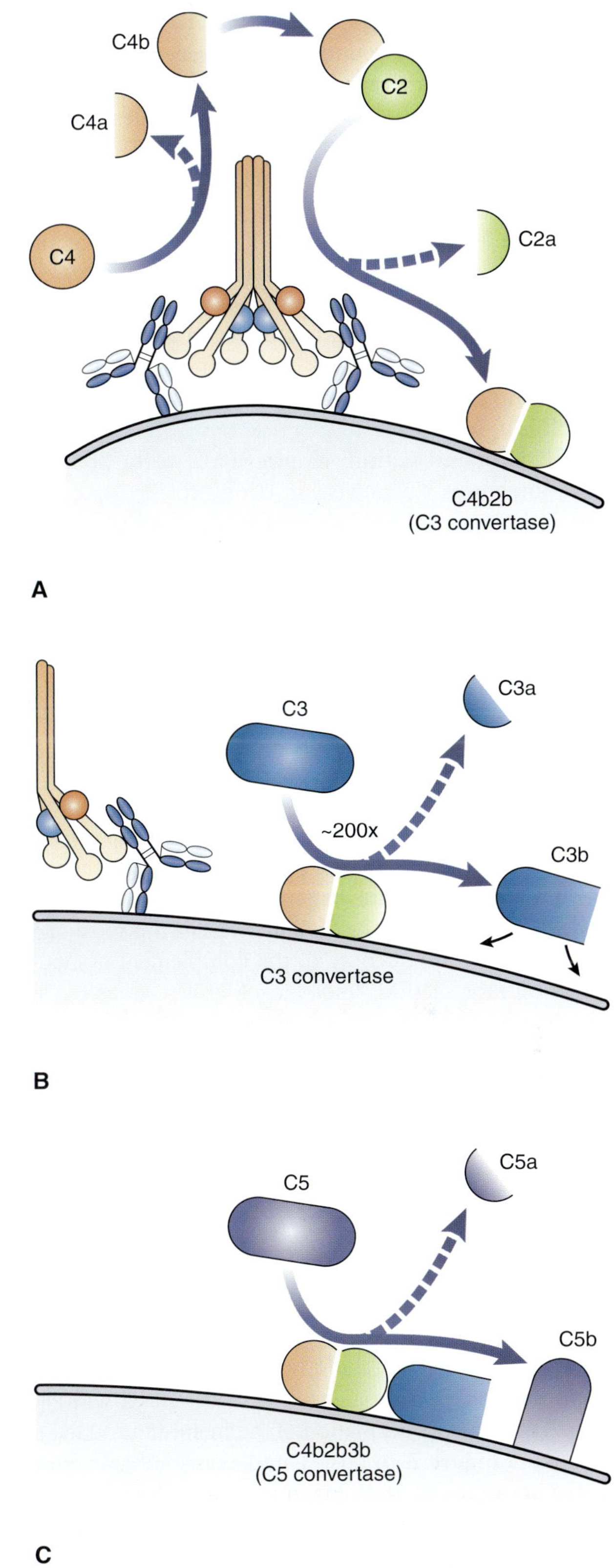

FIGURE 7.4 Formation of the activation unit. (A) Activated C1qrs cleaves C4 and C2, with the pieces C4b and C2b, binding to the target-cell surface and forming the enzyme C3 convertase. (B) Each C3 convertase cleaves ~200 C3 molecules into C3a and C3b. C3b is a powerful opsonin that binds to the target in many places. (C) Some C3b associates with C4bC2b, forming C4bC2bC3b, also known as C5 convertase. This convertase cleaves C5 into the anaphylatoxin, C5a, and C5b, which binds to the target cell.

immediate vicinity. C3b is estimated to have a half-life of 60 microseconds if not bound to an antigen. Therefore, only a small percentage of cleaved C3 molecules bind to adjacent surfaces; most are hydrolyzed by water molecules and decay in the fluid phase.

The cleavage of C3 represents a second and major amplification step because about 200 C3 molecules are split for every molecule of C4bC2b. In addition to being required for the activation of the terminal pathway, C3b serves as a powerful opsonin. Macrophages have specific receptors for C3b (discussed later in the chapter) and are primed to phagocytize antigen that has bound C3b. Large numbers of molecules are needed for this to occur, and hence the need for amplification.

If C3b is bound within 40 nm of the C4bC2b, a new enzyme known as *C5 convertase* (C4bC2bC3b) is created. Figure 7–4C depicts this last step in the formation of the activation unit. The cleaving of C5 with deposition of C5b at another site on the cell membrane constitutes the beginning of the MAC.

The Membrane Attack Complex (MAC)

C5 consists of two polypeptide chains, α and β, which are linked by disulfide bonds to form a molecule with a molecular weight of about 190 kDa. C5 convertase of the classical and lectin pathways, consisting of C4bC2bC3b, splits C5 into two fragments: a 74-amino acid fragment known as C5a, which is released into the circulation, and C5b, which attaches to the cell membrane, forming the beginning of the MAC. The splitting of C5 and the cleavage of C3 represent the most significant biological consequences of the complement system, as we explain in the section, "Biological Manifestations of Complement Activation." However, C5b is extremely labile and is rapidly inactivated unless binding to C6 occurs.

Once C6 is bound to C5b, subsequent binding of C7, C8, and multiple molecules of C9 occurs. The complex of C5b-C6-C7-C8 and C9 is known as *C5b-9* or the *membrane attack complex* (MAC). None of these proteins have enzymatic activity; they are all present in much smaller amounts in serum than the preceding components. C6 and C7 have similar physical and chemical properties. C8 is made up of three dissimilar chains, α, β, and γ, joined by disulfide bonds. C9 is a single polypeptide chain. The carboxy-terminal end of C9 is hydrophobic, whereas the amino-terminal end is hydrophilic. The hydrophobic part serves to anchor the MAC within the target cell membrane. Formation of the membrane attack unit is pictured in **Figure 7–5.** If the complex is soluble in circulation, it is known as **sC5b-9**. Measurement of the sC5b-9 concentration is an indicator of the amount of activation that is occurring in the terminal steps of the complement pathways.

When formed, the MAC produces a pore of 70 to 100 Å that allows ions to pass in and out of the cell membrane. Destruction of target cells occurs through an influx of water and a corresponding loss of electrolytes. The presence of C9 greatly accelerates lysis. However, sufficient disruption of the membrane can occur in the absence of C9 so that deficiencies in C9 appear largely benign.

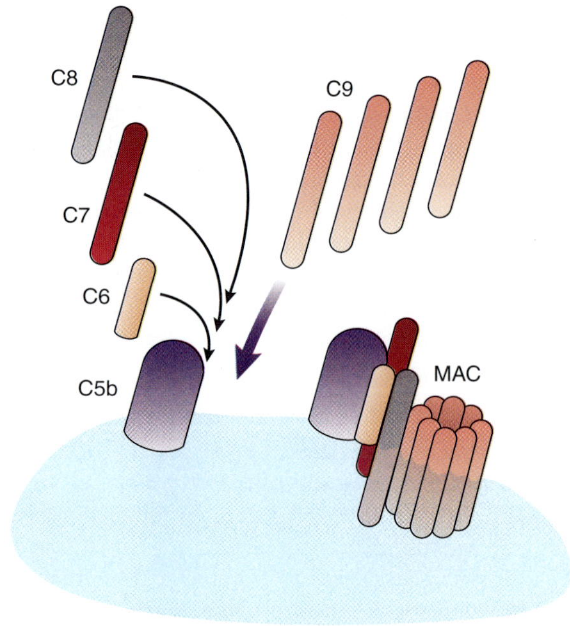

FIGURE 7.5 Formation of the MAC. C5b binds to the target cell, and C6 and C7 attach to C5b. C8 binds to these associated molecules and, along with C7, begins to penetrate the cell membrane. Multiple C9 molecules bind to C5bC6C7C8 and polymerize to form a transmembrane channel, the MAC, which causes lysis of the cell.

Knowledge Check 7-1

What is the key recognition component of the classical pathway?
a. C5
b. C4a
c. C1q
d. MAC

Knowledge Check 7-2

Which of the following is part of the membrane attack complex?
a. C5b
b. C6
c. C7
d. C9
e. All of the above
f. None of the above

The Lectin Pathway

The lectin pathway is another means of activating complement. Instead of activation through antibody binding, the lectin pathway is triggered by direct recognition of surface molecules on pathogens. This pathway allows for nonspecific recognition of carbohydrates that are common constituents of microbial cell walls and that are distinct from those found on human cell surfaces. The lectin pathway also plays an important role as a defense mechanism in infancy, during the interval between the loss of maternal antibody and the acquisition of a mature antibody response to pathogens.

The lectin pathway has some similarities to the classical pathway: proteins activated early in the lectin pathway are structurally similar to those of the classical pathway, and the lectin pathway also involves C4 and C2. The role C1q serves in the classical pathway is filled by three structurally similar classes of recognition molecules in the lectin pathway: lectins, ficolins, and collectins. One key protein, called **mannose-binding lectin (MBL)**, binds to mannose or related sugars in a calcium-dependent manner to initiate this pathway. These sugars are found in glycoproteins or carbohydrates in various microorganisms, such as bacteria, yeasts, viruses, and some parasites. MBL is considered an acute phase protein because it is produced in the liver and is normally present in the serum but increases during an initial inflammatory response.

After MBL binds to mannose on the surface of microorganisms, serine proteases called *MBL-associated serine proteases* (MASPs) associate with the complex. The enzymatic function of the MASPs is triggered, resembling the roles of C1r and C1s in the classical pathway. Three MASPs have been identified: MASP-1, MASP-2, and MASP-3. Although the recognition molecules are different for the lectin pathway, activation soon converges on the same C4 and C2 molecules that are involved in the classical pathway. Once C4 and C2 are cleaved, the rest of the pathway is identical to the classical pathway. However, there is mounting evidence for a possible bypass for the lectin pathway, in which C3 is activated in the absence of C4 and C2 activation.

The Alternative Pathway

First described by Pillemer and his associates in the early 1950s, the alternative pathway was originally named for the protein **properdin**, the only described positive regulator of complement. Properdin in normal serum has a concentration of approximately 5 to 15 µg/mL. Although the alternative pathway can be activated on its own, it appears that it functions largely as an amplification loop for activation started from the classical or lectin pathways. In addition to properdin, two other serum proteins, factor B and factor D, are unique to the alternative pathway. The alternative pathway is summarized in **Figure 7–6.**

Activation of the pathway begins with C3. Triggering substances for the alternative pathway include bacterial cell walls, especially those containing lipopolysaccharide; fungal cell walls; yeast; viruses; virally infected cells; tumor cell lines; and some parasites, especially trypanosomes. All these can serve as sites for binding the complex C3bBb, one of the key products of this pathway.

The alternative pathway also acts as a monitoring system, with a continual baseline level of activation, which must be kept in check. This continual low-level activation occurs because native C3 is not stable in plasma. Water can hydrolyze the C3 thioester bond, thus spontaneously activating a small number of these molecules. A C3b-like molecule, often referred to as $C3_{H2O}$, is formed by spontaneous hydrolysis and can start activation of the alternative pathway, as can C3b originating from the classical or lectin pathways. C3b or $C3_{H2O}$ then binds to factor B, which has a molecular weight of 93 kDa and is fairly abundant in the serum, at a level of around 200 µg/mL. The role of factor B is analogous to that of C2 in the classical pathway because it will form an integral part of the C3 convertase of the alternative pathway.

Once bound to C3b, factor B can be cleaved by factor D, a plasma protein that goes through a conformational change when it binds to factor B. The concentration of factor D in the plasma is the lowest of all the complement proteins, approximately 2 µg/mL. Factor D is a serine protease that cleaves factor B into two pieces: Ba (with a molecular weight of 33 kDa) and Bb (with a molecular weight of approximately 60 kDa). Bb remains attached to C3b, forming the initial *C3 convertase* of the alternative pathway. Bb is rapidly inactivated unless it binds to a site on one of the triggering cellular antigens.

As the alternative pathway convertase, C3bBb is then capable of cleaving additional C3 into C3a and C3b. Some C3b attaches to cellular surfaces and acts as a binding site for more factor B, resulting in an amplification loop that increases activation initiated by the classical or lectin pathways to levels of biological consequence. All C3 in plasma would be rapidly converted by this method were it not for the fact that the enzyme C3bBb is extremely unstable unless properdin binds to the complex. Binding of properdin increases the half-life of C3bBb from 90 seconds to several minutes. In this manner, optimal rates of alternative pathway activation are achieved.

C3bBb can also cleave C5, but it is much more efficient at cleaving C3. If, however, some of the C3b produced remains bound to the C3 convertase in combination with properdin, the complex is stabilized. The resulting enzyme, C3bBbC3bP, has a high affinity for C5 and exhibits C5 convertase activity. Thus, C5 is cleaved to produce C5b, the first part of the MAC. From this point on, the alternative, lectin, and classical pathways are identical. **Figure 7–7** shows the convergence of all three pathways.

Knowledge Check 7-3

Which of the following is known as the C3 convertase of the alternative pathway?

a. sC5b-9
b. C2b
c. C3bBb
d. None of the above

System Controls

Uncontrolled activation of complement could cause tissue damage and have devastating systemic effects. To ensure that infectious agents and not self-antigens are destroyed and that the reaction remains localized, several plasma proteins act as system regulators. Specific receptors on certain

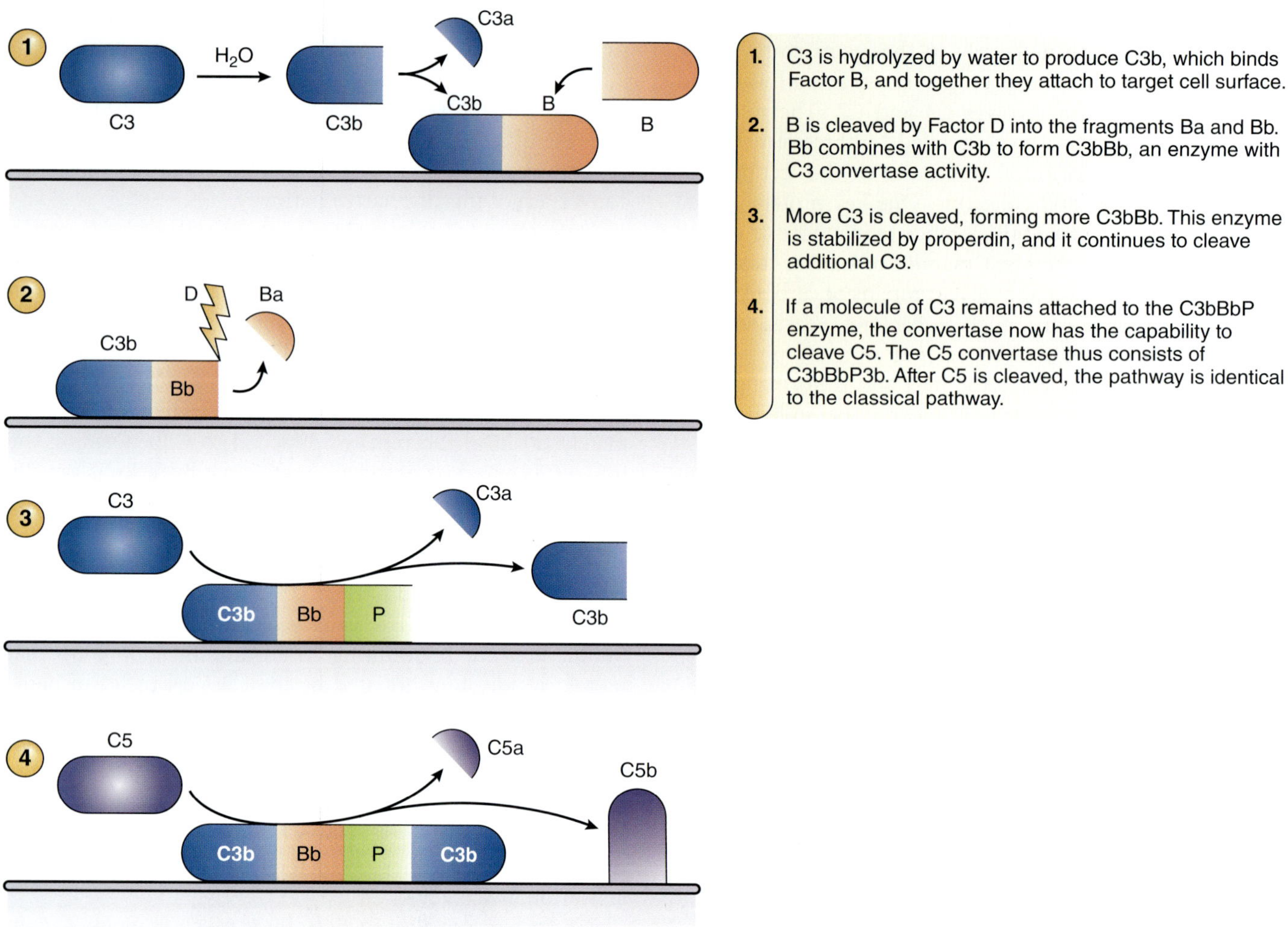

FIGURE 7.6 The alternative pathway. (1) The pathway starts when C3 interacts with water in the circulation to form 'C3b-like' molecules. The pathway can also be initiated by C3b created from activation of the classical or lectin pathways. The C3b or $C3_{H2O}$ is recognized by factor B, and the complex attaches to the cell surface. (2) Factor B is then cleaved by factor D into the fragments Ba and Bb. Bb combines with C3b to form a C3 convertase. (3) When properdin (P) is added to the complex, the half-life of the convertase is extended. (4) With more cleavage, an additional C3b is added, forming a C5 convertase (C3bBbC3bP) that cleaves C5 into C5a and C5b.

cells also exert a controlling influence on the activation process. In fact, about one-half of the complement components serve as controls for critical steps in the activation process. Because activation of C3 is the pivotal step in all pathways, most control proteins are aimed at halting accumulation of C3b. However, controls exist at all crucial steps of the three pathways.

Regulation of the Classical and Lectin Pathways

In this section, we discuss the major plasma and cell-bound regulators of the classical and lectin pathways according to their order of appearance.

Plasma Regulators

Major plasma regulators of the classical and lectin pathways are listed in **Table 7–2** and described as follows:

- **C1 inhibitor (C1-INH)** inhibits activation at the first stages of the classical and lectin pathways. Its main role is to inactivate C1 by binding to the active sites of C1r and C1s. Therefore, Clr and Cls become instantly and irreversibly dissociated from C1q. C1q remains bound to antibody, but all enzymatic activity ceases. C1-INH also inactivates MASP-2, blocking activity of the MBL-MASP complex and halting the lectin pathway. Like most of the other complement proteins, it is mainly synthesized in the liver; however, monocytes also may be involved to some extent in its production. One C1-INH molecule can

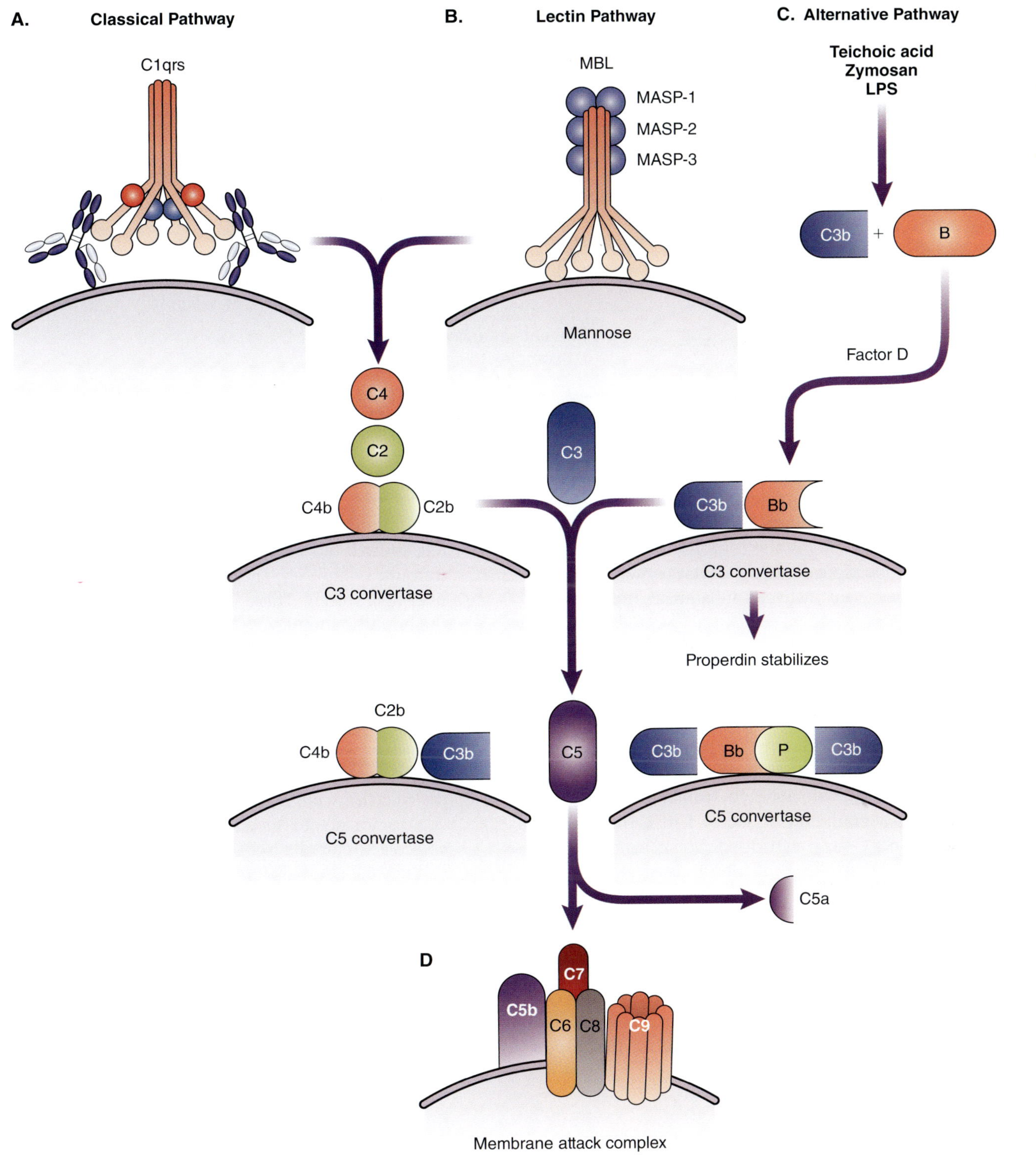

FIGURE 7.7 Convergence of the classical, alternative, and lectin pathways. Note that C3 is a key component in each pathway. (A) The binding of C1qrs to two IgG antibody molecules activates the classical pathway. Activation of C1s leads to the production of C4b2b, a C3 convertase that cleaves C3 into C3a and C3b. C3b combines with C4b2b to produce a C5 convertase, which cleaves C5 into C5a and C5b. (B) The lectin pathway is triggered by binding of MBL to mannose on bacterial cell walls. MASP-1, MASP-2, and MASP-3 bind to form an activated C1-like complex. MASP-2 cleaves C2 and C4, then the lectin pathway proceeds like the classical pathway. (C) The alternative pathway is started by hydrolysis of C3 to produce C3b in the presence of activating substances from microorganisms, such as lipopolysaccharides (LPS). C3b reacts with factor B and factor D to produce a C3 convertase, C3bBb. Properdin stabilizes the complex, producing a C5 convertase that consists of C3bBbC3bP. (D) After C5 is cleaved, the remaining steps are common to all three pathways, resulting in sequential binding of C6, C7, C8, and C9 to form the MAC (C5b6789).

Table 7-2 Plasma Complement Regulators

SERUM PROTEIN	CONCENTRATION (mg/mL)	FUNCTION	DISEASE ASSOCIATION
C1 inhibitor (C1-INH)	240	Dissociates C1r and C1s from C1q Inactivates MASP-2	Hereditary angioedema
Factor I	35	Cleaves C3b and C4b	aHUS, C3G, AMD
Factor H	300–450	Cofactor with Factor I to inactivate C3b; prevents binding of B to C3b	
C4-binding protein (C4BP)	250	Acts as a cofactor with Factor I to inactivate C4b	Atypical morbus, Behçet disease, angioedema, protein S deficit
S protein (vitronectin)	500	Prevents attachment of the C5b67 complex to cell membranes	

aHUS = atypical hemolytic uremic syndrome; AMD = age-related macular degeneration; C3G = C3 glomerulopathy.

only inhibit one serine protease and cannot be reused. Importantly for hereditary angioedema (HAE), as we describe later, C1-INH is also responsible for the control of several serine proteases of the contact system, a plasma protease cascade that activates inflammation and coagulation.

- Soluble **C4-binding protein (C4BP)** inhibits further formation of C3 convertase in the classical and lectin pathways. This inhibitor is a cofactor for **factor I,** a serine protease that inactivates C3b and C4b when bound. C4BP is abundant in the plasma and is capable of combining with either fluid-phase or cell-bound C4b. Thus, C4BP blocks C4b from binding to C2b and directs degradation by factor I. If C4BP attaches to cell-bound C4b, it can dissociate it from C4bC2b complexes, controlling further classical pathway activation.
- *MAp19,* a splice variant of MASP-1, and *Map44,* a splice variant of MASP-2, are rare regulators for just the lectin pathway. Genetic polymorphisms in *MAp19* have been associated with changes in mortality in patients receiving kidney transplants, largely because of infection. Research is still needed to fully elucidate the importance of *Map44.*

Cell-Bound Regulators

Major cell-bound regulators of the classical and lectin pathways and other complement receptors are listed in **Table 7–3** and described as follows:

- **Complement receptor type 1 (CR1),** also known as *CD35,* is a large polymorphic glycoprotein found mainly on the cell surface of peripheral blood cells, including neutrophils, monocytes, macrophages, erythrocytes, eosinophils, B lymphocytes, some T lymphocytes, and follicular dendritic cells. It binds C3b and C4b but has the greatest affinity for C3b. Once bound to CR1, both C4b and C3b can then be degraded by factor I.
- Importantly, CR1 also plays a key role in the clearance of immune complexes. CR1 is a key receptor on platelets and red blood cells (RBCs), which bind C3b-coated immune complexes, and facilitate their trafficking to the liver and spleen. There, fixed tissue macrophages strip the immune complexes from the RBCs, process the complexes, and return the RBCs intact to the circulation. The ability of cells to bind complement-coated particles is referred to as **immune adherence.**
- **Membrane cofactor protein (MCP),** or CD46, has a molecular weight of between 50 and 70 kDa and is found on the cell membrane of virtually all epithelial and endothelial cells except erythrocytes. MCP is the most efficient cofactor for factor I–mediated cleavage of C3b. It can serve as a cofactor for cleavage of C4b, but it is not as effective as C4BP. MCP also helps to control the alternative pathway because binding of factor B to C3b is inhibited.
- **Decay-accelerating factor (DAF)** or *CD55,* is a membrane glycoprotein with a wide tissue distribution. It is found on peripheral blood cells, endothelial cells, fibroblasts, and many types of epithelial cells. DAF can dissociate the C3 convertases of all three complement pathways. It can bind to both C3b and C4b in a manner similar to CR1. It does not prevent initial binding of either C2 or factor B to the cell but can rapidly dissociate both from their binding sites, thus preventing the assembly of an active C3 convertase. The carboxy-terminal portion of DAF is covalently attached to a glycophospholipid anchor that is inserted into the outer layer of the membrane lipid bilayer. This arrangement allows DAF mobility within the membrane so that it can reach C3 convertase sites that are not immediately adjacent to it **(Fig. 7–8).** DAF's presence on host cells protects them from **bystander lysis.** It is one of the main mechanisms used in discrimination of self from nonself because foreign cells do not possess this substance. However, it does not permanently modify C3b or C4b; they are capable of re-forming elsewhere as active convertases.

Table 7-3 Cell-Surface Complement Regulators/Receptors

RECEPTOR	LIGAND	CELL TYPE	FUNCTION	DISEASE ASSOCIATION
CR1 (CD35)	C3b, iC3b, C4b	RBCs, neutrophils, monocytes, macrophages, eosinophils, B and T cells, follicular dendritic cells	Cofactor for factor I; mediates transport of immune complexes	SLE
CR2 (CD21)	C3dg, C3d, iC3b	B cells, follicular dendritic cells, epithelial cells	B-cell coreceptor for antigen with CD19	Infections, connected to CVID
CR3 (CD11b/CD18)	iC3b, C3d, C3b	Monocytes, macrophages, neutrophils, NK cells	Adhesion and increased activity of phagocytic cells	LAD
CR4 (CD11c/CD18)	iC3b, C3b	Monocytes, macrophages, neutrophils, NK cells, activated T and B cells, dendritic cells	Adhesion and increased activity of phagocytic cells	
Collectin receptors	C1q	Neutrophils, monocytes, macrophages, B cells, platelets, endothelial cells	Enhance binding of C1q to Fc receptors	Individual deficiency can lead to infection. Double deficiency of collectins 10 and 11 leads to 3MC syndrome.
DAF (CD55)	C3b, C4b	RBCs, neutrophils, platelets, monocytes, endothelial cells, fibroblasts, T cells, B cells, epithelial cells	Dissociates C2b or Bb from binding sites, thus preventing formation of C3 convertase	PNH; protein-losing enteropathy
MIRL (CD59)	C8 and C9	RBCs, neutrophils, platelets, monocytes, endothelial cells, epithelial cells	Prevents insertion of C9 into the cell membrane	PNH; polyneuropathy
MCP (CD46)	C3b, C4b	Neutrophils, monocytes, macrophages, platelets, T cells, B cells, endothelial cells	Cofactor for factor I cleavage of C3b and C4b	aHUS

aHUS = atypical hemolytic uremic syndrome; C1-INH = C1 inhibitor; CVID = common variable immune deficiency; DAF = decay-accelerating factor; LAD = leukocyte adhesion deficiency; MASP-2 = mannose-associated serine protease; MBL = mannose-binding lectin; 3MC syndrome = group of rare autosomal recessive disorders previously designated as Carnevale, Mingarelli, Malpuech, and Michels syndromes; MIRL = membrane inhibitor of reactive lysis; NK = natural killer; PNH = paroxysmal nocturnal hemoglobinuria; RBC = red blood cell; SLE = systemic lupus erythematosus.

Regulation of the Alternative Pathway

The main soluble regulator of the alternative pathway is **factor H,** which acts by binding to C3b to prevent the binding of factor B. C3b in the fluid phase has a 100-fold greater affinity for factor H than for factor B, but on cell surfaces, C3b preferentially binds to factor B. Factor H also accelerates the dissociation of the C3bBb complex on cell surfaces. When factor H binds to C3bBb, Bb becomes displaced. In this manner, C3 convertase activity is curtailed in the plasma and on cell surfaces.

Factor H also acts as a cofactor that facilitates the degradation of C3b by factor I. It appears that only those molecules with tightly bound factor H acquire high-affinity binding sites for factor I. When factor I binds, a conformational change takes place that allows it to cleave C3b. On cellular surfaces, C3b is cleaved into C3f, which is released into the plasma, and iC3b, which remains attached but is no longer an active enzyme. Then, iC3b is further broken down to C3c and C3dg by factor I in conjunction with another cofactor, the CR1 receptor **(Fig. 7–9).** With this key role in complement regulation, factor H has been shown to play a role in a variety of disorders (discussed in the text that follows).

Regulation of Terminal Components

Formation of the MAC in the terminal steps of the complement pathways is inhibited primarily by one soluble regulatory protein and one cell-surface protein, as we describe next.

The **S protein** is a soluble control protein that acts at a deeper level of complement activation. Also known as *vitronectin,* S protein interacts with the C5b-7 complex as it forms in the fluid phase and prevents it from binding to cell membranes. Binding of C8 and C9 still proceeds, but polymerization of C9 does not occur; therefore, the complex is unable to insert itself into the cell membrane or produce lysis.

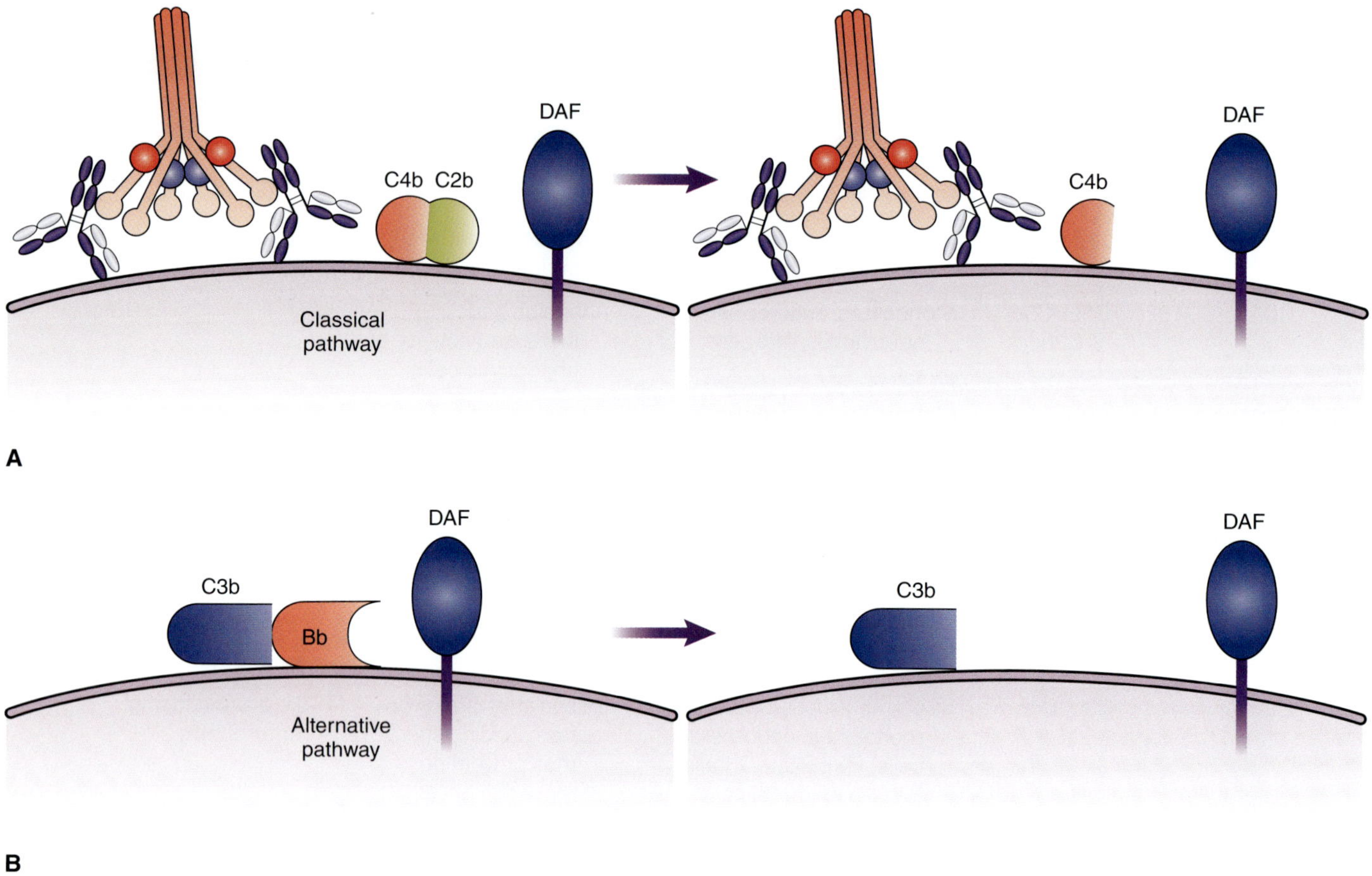

FIGURE 7.8 Inhibitory effects of DAF. (A) In the classical pathway, DAF dissociates C2b from C4b. (B) In the alternative pathway, DAF helps dissociate Bb from C3b.

In addition, a receptor, known by various terms, including **membrane inhibitor of reactive lysis (MIRL)** or *CD59*, blocks formation of the MAC by preventing C9 from inserting into the cell membrane. CD59 is widely distributed on the cell membranes of all circulating blood cells, including RBCs, endothelial cells, epithelial cells, and many other cell types.

Knowledge Check 7-4

Which pathway(s) is (are) controlled by C1-INH?

a. Classical pathway
b. Lectin pathway
c. Alternative pathway
d. Terminal pathway
e. a and b
f. a, b, and c

Complement Receptors and Their Biological Roles

Some complement receptors on host cells amplify the immune response by enhancing phagocytosis and stimulating accessory cells rather than acting as regulators (see Table 7–3). We discussed one of these receptors, CR1, in the previous section. A second receptor, CR2 (or CD21), is found mainly on B lymphocytes and follicular dendritic cells. Ligands for CR2 include degradation products of C3b, such as C3dg, C3d, and iC3b. The Epstein-Barr virus gains entry to B cells by binding to this receptor. CR2 is present only on mature B cells and is lost when differentiation to plasma cells occurs. CR2 plays an important role as part of the B-cell coreceptor for antigen. Acting in concert with CD19, it binds complement-coated antigen and cross-links it to membrane immunoglobulin to activate B cells. In this manner, immune complexes are more effective at enhancing B-cell differentiation and producing memory cells than is antigen by itself.

Another receptor, CR3 (CD11b/CD18), found on monocytes, macrophages, neutrophils, and natural killer (NK) cells, specifically binds particles opsonized with iC3b, a C3b degradation product. It does this in a calcium-dependent manner. The CR3 receptor plays a key role in mediating phagocytosis of particles coated with these complement fragments **(Fig. 7–10).** These proteins trigger surface adhesion and increased activity of phagocytic cells. Patients whose white blood cells (WBCs) lack these receptors fail to exhibit functions such as chemotaxis, surface adherence, phagocytosis, and aggregation. These individuals have an impaired capacity to bind iC3b-coated particles and are subject to recurrent infections.

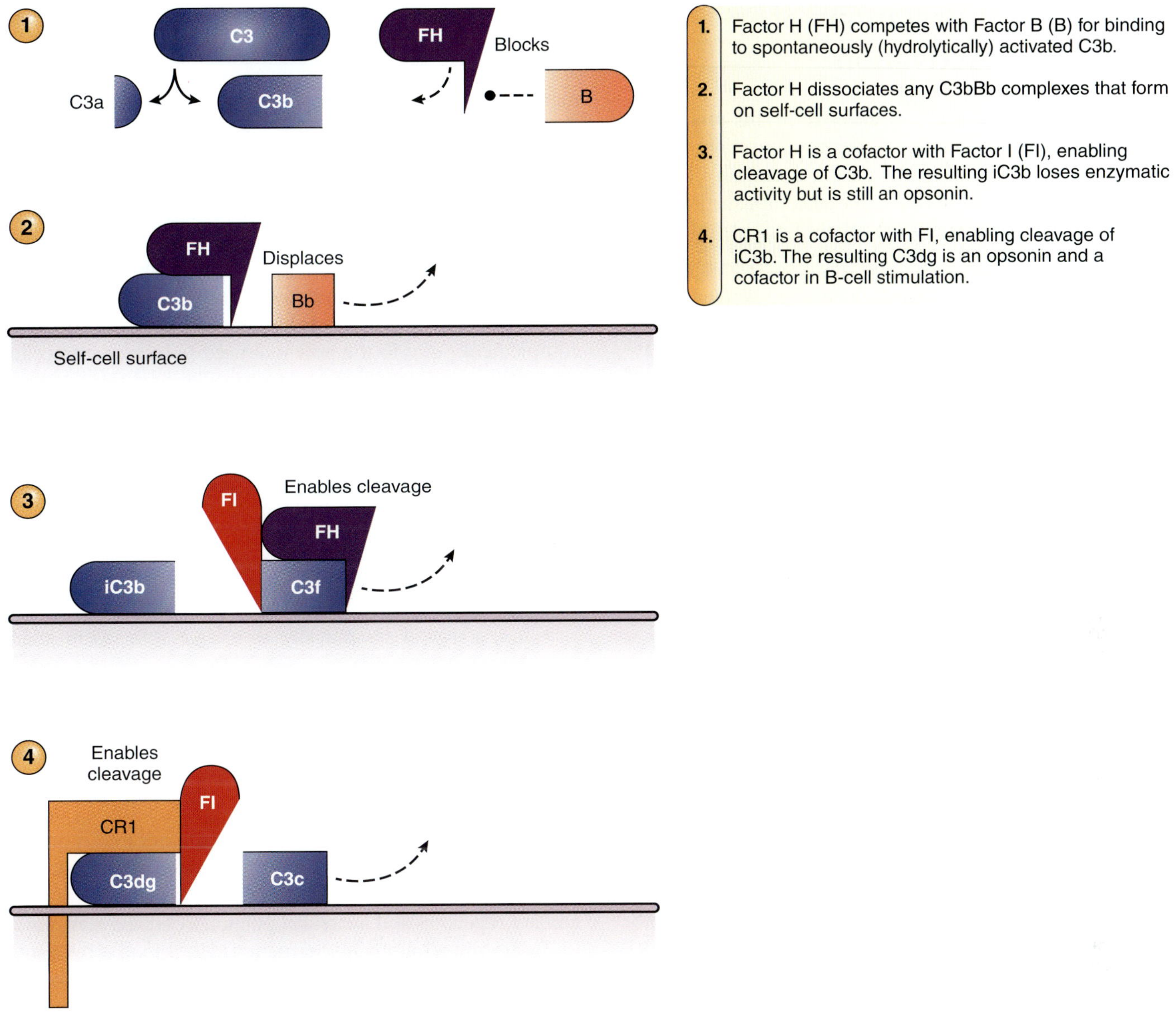

FIGURE 7.9 Complement controls. The CR1 receptor acts as a cofactor in the inactivation of C3b. Factor I cleaves C3b to form C3dg and C3c. C3dg is not an effective opsonin and is not capable of further participation in the complement cascade.

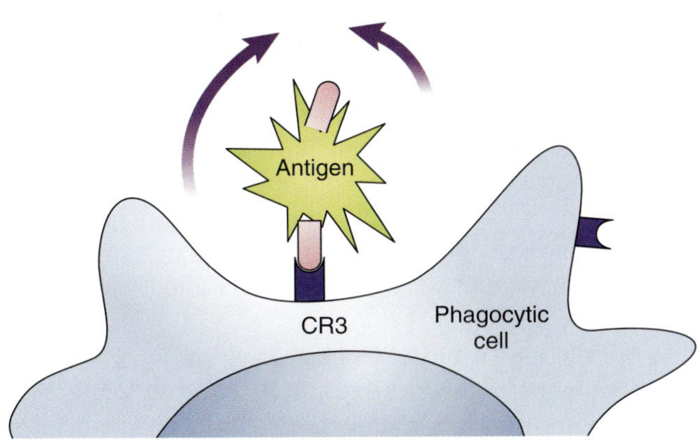

FIGURE 7.10 Role of C3b in opsonization. C3b is an important opsonin that coats antigens to enhance phagocytosis. Receptors for C3b (CR3) on the membrane of a phagocytic cell, such as a neutrophil or macrophage, bind C3b and pull the membrane around to envelop the antigen.

The CR4 (CD11c/CD18) receptor is similar to CR3 in that it also binds iC3b fragments in a calcium-dependent fashion. CR4 proteins are found on neutrophils, monocytes, tissue macrophages, activated T cells, dendritic cells, NK cells, and activated B cells. Neutrophils and monocytes, however, have smaller amounts of CR4 than CR3. The function of CR4 appears to be similar to that of CR3, and it may assist neutrophil adhesion to the endothelium during inflammation.

Receptors specific for C1q are found on neutrophils, monocytes, macrophages, B cells, platelets, and endothelial cells. These receptors, known as *collectin receptors*, bind the collagen portion of C1q and generally enhance the binding of C1q to Fc receptors. Interacting only with bound C1q, the receptors appear to increase uptake of immune complexes opsonized with C1q by phagocytic cells. C1q receptors may also act to enhance the respiratory burst triggered by IgG binding to Fc receptors on neutrophils.

Biological Manifestations of Complement Activation

Complement activation is a very effective means of amplifying the inflammatory response to destroy and clear foreign antigens. The complement pathways do not always have to proceed to completion for this to be accomplished; hence, some of the initiating proteins are much more plentiful than proteins that form the MAC. Complement proteins also serve as a means of linking innate and adaptive immunity. They act as opsonins to facilitate recognition and subsequent destruction by phagocytic cells; they also play a major role in the uptake and presentation of antigens so that a specific immune response can occur. Complement can also facilitate B-cell activation and is necessary for maintaining immunologic memory. Some of the complement proteins generated earlier in the cascade play a major role in all these areas. These proteins can be classified into three main categories:

- Anaphylatoxins
- Chemotaxins
- Opsonins

An **anaphylatoxin** is a small pro-inflammatory peptide that causes increased vascular permeability, contraction of smooth muscle, and release of histamine from basophils and mast cells. The activation products C3a and C5a are anaphylatoxins. Both have molecular weights between 9 and 11 kDa and are formed as cleavage products from larger complement components. Of these molecules, C5a is the most potent; it is at least 200 times more powerful than C3a.

C3a and C5a attach to specific receptors on neutrophils, basophils, mast cells, eosinophils, smooth muscle cells, and vascular endothelium. C3a attaches to the C3a receptor (C3aR), whereas C5a attaches to the C5a receptor (C5aR). When binding occurs on basophils and mast cells, histamine is released, increasing vascular permeability and causing smooth muscle contractions. C5a causes neutrophils to release proteolytic enzymes, oxygen radicals, and prostaglandins, which aid in the destruction of foreign antigens.

C5a also serves as a **chemotaxin** for neutrophils, basophils, eosinophils, mast cells, monocytes, and dendritic cells. In this manner, these cells are directed to the source of antigen concentration. Because of increased vascular permeability, neutrophils migrate from the blood vessels to the tissues and tend to aggregate.

Binding of C5a to monocytes causes them to undergo an oxidative burst that includes increased production of proteolytic enzymes, neutrophil chemotactic factor, platelet-activating factors, interleukin-1 (IL-1), and toxic oxygen metabolites. IL-1 is a member of the pro-inflammatory cytokine family that enhances T-cell activation. Activation may produce fever and lead to an increase in acute phase reactants, both of which are characteristic of an inflammatory response.

Another important function of complement is opsonization. As complement activation proceeds, the peptides C4b, C3b, iC3b, and C3dg are generated and accumulate on cell membranes. These peptides serve as **opsonins** by binding to specific receptors on erythrocytes, neutrophils, monocytes, macrophages, and dendritic cells to facilitate phagocytosis and clearance of foreign substances or cellular debris. Attachment of C3 products to an antigen has been found to enhance the B-cell response to the antigen.

Complement was historically considered only as a cascade of circulating proteins important in innate immunity. However, there is growing evidence of important roles for complement outside this narrow perspective, particularly in neural development (synaptic pruning) and in intracellular regulation. It remains to be seen how intracellular complement, or its deficiencies, manifests in human disease. These roles of complement point to the potential need to test for intracellular complement activation and to consider how the release of intracellular complement affects plasma testing in the future.

Complement and Disease States

Although complement acts as a powerful weapon to combat infection, in some cases it can contribute to tissue damage or death. For example, complement can be harmful if

- It is activated systemically on a large scale, as in gram-negative septicemia.
- It is activated by tissue necrosis, such as myocardial infarction (heart attack).
- It is involved in hypersensitivity reactions.
- There is complement-directed damage to the kidney basement membrane.

In the case of septicemia caused by a gram-negative organism, large quantities of C3a and C5a are generated, leading to neutrophil aggregation and blood clotting. Damage to the tiny pulmonary capillaries and interstitial pulmonary edema may result.

Tissue injury following obstruction of the blood supply, such as occurs in a myocardial infarction, can cause complement activation and deposition of MACs on cell surfaces. Receptors for C3a and C5a have been found in coronary plaques, indicating that complement components may increase damage to heart tissue.

As we discussed in Chapter 14, complement activation plays a major role in hypersensitivity types II and III. For example, in hemolytic anemias, autoantibodies bind to RBCs, and complement fixation results in lysis. In other autoimmune disorders such as systemic lupus erythematosus (SLE), immune complex formation results in complement activation and creation of C3a and C5a; these complement proteins induce chemotaxis of neutrophils, which, in turn, release lysosomal enzymes that damage surrounding tissues (see Chapters 14 and 15).

As we discuss in more detail in later sections, the basement membrane of the kidneys and the eyes are particularly susceptible to off-target complement attack. This is believed to be due to the reliance of these membranes on complement control by factor H. The failure of factor H and factor I directed control of complement on these membranes has been connected with certain rare kidney diseases and age-related macular degeneration.

Deficiencies in Major Pathway Complement Components

Although excess activation of the complement system can result in disease states, the lack of individual components also has a deleterious effect. Hereditary deficiency of any complement protein, except for C9, usually manifests itself in increased susceptibility to infection and delayed clearance of immune complexes. Most of these conditions are inherited with an autosomal recessive pattern and are quite rare, occurring in much less than 1% of the general population. A lack of C2 is the most common deficiency. C2-deficient individuals are more prone to recurrent streptococcal and staphylococcal infections. Because the factor B gene is near the C2 gene, C2-deficient persons often have decreases in factor B also. Although rare, deficiencies of early components of the classical pathway, including C1q, C4, and C2, also cause a lupus-like syndrome because of failure to clear immune complexes from the circulation.

A second deficiency that occurs with some frequency is that of MBL. Deficiencies and polymorphisms in MBL occur in about 30% of the population. The health consequences of such variation in MBL levels remain unclear. Lack of MBL has been associated with pneumonia, sepsis, and meningococcal disease in infants; however, most individuals deficient in MBL appear to have no deleterious effects.

The most serious deficiency is that of C3 because it is the key mediator in all three activation pathways. C3 deficiencies are, however, extremely rare. People with a C3 deficiency are prone to developing severe, recurrent, life-threatening infections with encapsulated bacteria such as *Streptococcus pneumoniae* and may also be subject to immune complex diseases like SLE. The complexes can be deposited in the kidneys and result in glomerulonephritis.

A deficiency of the terminal components of the complement cascade, C5–C8, has been associated with increased susceptibility to systemic *Neisseria* infections, including meningococcal meningitis and disseminated gonococcal disease.

Deficiencies in Regulatory Complement Components

A growing number of diseases have been associated with a missing or defective regulatory component, including paroxysmal nocturnal hemoglobinuria, hereditary angioedema, atypical hemolytic uremic syndrome, and C3 glomerulopathy.

Paroxysmal Nocturnal Hemoglobinuria (PNH)

Patients with **paroxysmal nocturnal hemoglobinuria (PNH)** have RBCs that are deficient in CD55 and CD59. The loss of these important complement control proteins is caused by a genetic defect in the ability to make the glycophospholipid anchor that attaches CD55 and CD59 to the cell membrane. With the loss of these cell-surface proteins, the RBCs are subject to lysis by means of the bystander effect once the complement system has been triggered. When C3b is deposited on RBCs through activation of any of the pathways, the result is complement-mediated intravascular and extravascular hemolysis, resulting in a chronic hemolytic anemia. This occurs because, as we mentioned previously, CD55 dissociates cell-surface C3 convertases and CD59 prevents formation of the MAC.

Hereditary Angioedema (HAE)

Another complement deficiency disorder that involves a regulatory protein is **hereditary angioedema (HAE).** HAE is characterized by recurrent attacks of swelling that affect the extremities, skin, gastrointestinal tract, and other mucosal surfaces. HAE is caused by a deficiency or lack of C1-INH. Although C1-INH was named for its role in controlling complement, the function of C1-INH in controlling the contact pathway of the coagulation system is critical in this disease. C1-INH is a serpin (serine protease inhibitor) that controls many of the serine proteases on contact. The lack of C1-INH reduces control of the production of the inflammatory protein *bradykinin,* resulting in localized swelling that can occur under the skin or within the gastrointestinal or upper respiratory tracts. Normally, the swelling spontaneously subsides in 48 to 72 hours, but if edema occurs in the area of the oropharynx, life-threatening upper-airway obstruction may develop. These attacks can be quite debilitating, even when they are not life threatening, so there is a need for proper diagnosis.

Most cases of HAE are classified into one of two types. Type I HAE is characterized by a decrease in the C1-INH protein. In type II HAE, the C1-INH level is normal, but its function is decreased. The genetic cause of either type is a heterozygous mutation in the *SERPING1* gene that codes for a dysfunctional or an inactive C1-INH protein and is inherited in an autosomal dominant pattern. In addition to the hereditary forms of the disorder, there are acquired forms that result from consumption of C1-INH or from autoantibodies blocking the function of C1-INH. To differentiate the acquired and hereditary forms, measurement of C1q can be helpful; C1q will be low in the acquired forms but not in the hereditary forms. Measurement of C4 or C2 can also be a very helpful test for HAE, particularly during an attack, because patients usually show a decrease in C4 and C2 at that time.

There is a third class of HAE in which patients have normal C1-INH levels and function, but the clinical presentation is largely identical to the type I and type II forms. The exact cause of this third type is yet to be conclusively determined but it is expected to be heterogeneous.

Atypical Hemolytic Uremic Syndrome (aHUS) or Complement-Mediated Thrombotic Microangiopathy (TMA)

As we mentioned previously, the kidney is particularly impacted by poor complement control. **Figure 7–11** shows an example of how this can occur. Key among the diseases associated

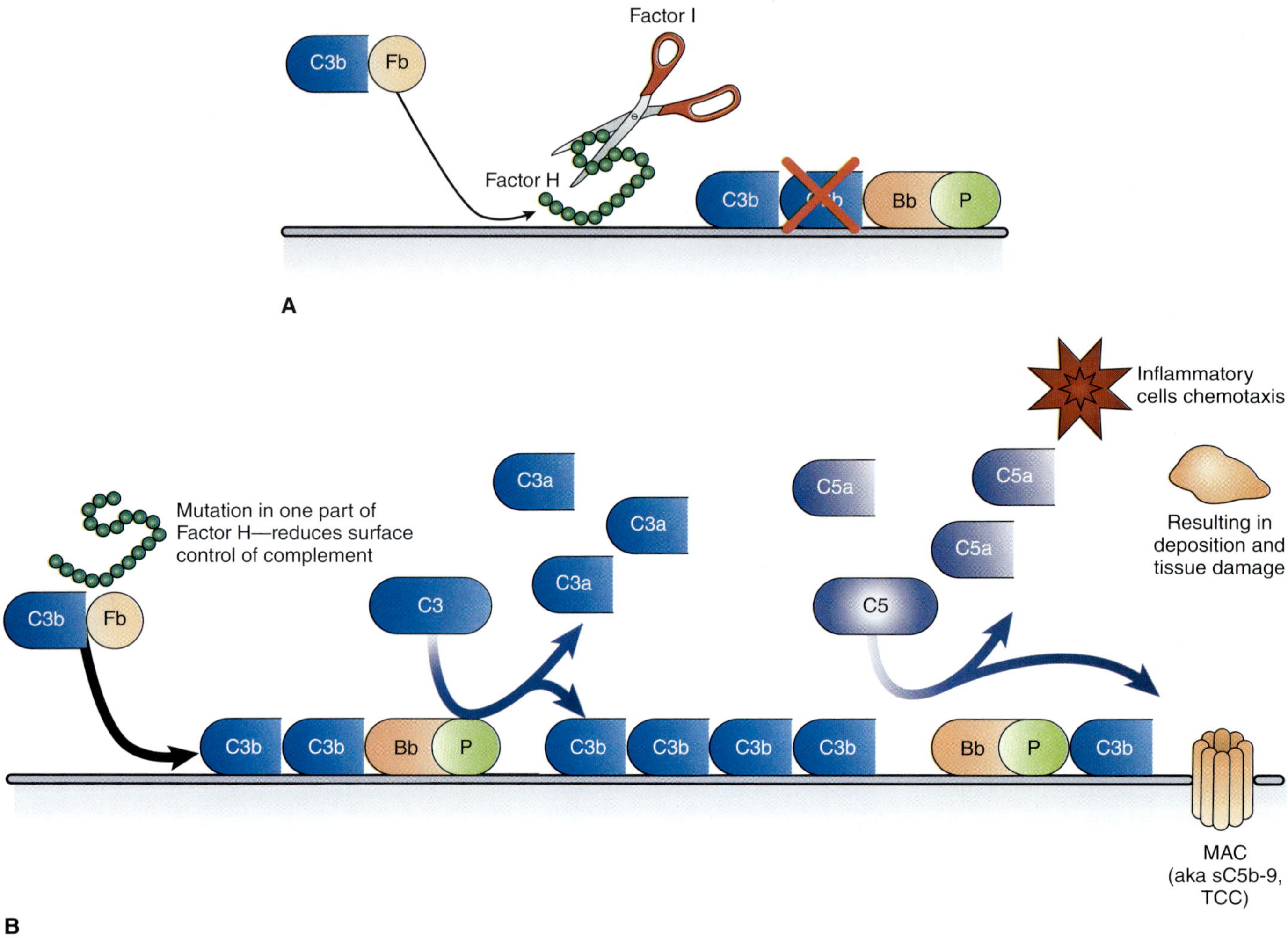

FIGURE 7.11 Control of complement by factor H and factor I in the kidney: (A) When factor H and factor I are functioning correctly, they control the assembly of the alternative pathway convertases on the surface of the kidney basement membrane. (B) If factor H is not able to properly bind to the membrane, or if factor I is not able to correctly cleave C3b, then the complement activation can occur off target and lead to inflammation and immune cell infiltration.

with abnormalities in regulatory complement proteins is a group of rare kidney disorders, referred to as **atypical hemolytic uremic syndrome (aHUS)** or **complement-mediated thrombotic microangiopathy (TMA).** TMAs are a group of disorders characterized by RBC destruction, decreased platelets, and organ damage caused by formation of tiny blood clots in the capillaries and small arteries. The main disorders in this group are aHUS and thrombotic thrombocytopenic purpura (TTP).

Hemolytic uremic syndrome (HUS) is one of the most common causes of acute renal failure in children worldwide. It is characterized by hemolytic anemia, low platelet count, and acute renal failure. Its primary cause in most cases is exposure to a Shiga toxin from an acute diarrheal illness, most commonly caused by Shiga-toxin–producing strains of *Escherichia coli.* In about 5% of cases, HUS occurs in the absence of Shiga-toxin exposure and is caused by mutations in complement regulatory proteins, a condition known as *aHUS*. The causes of aHUS include mutations in the genes coding for factor H, MCP, factor I, factor B, C3, and thrombomodulin, and inactivating autoantibodies against factor H. aHUS may have an acute or gradual onset; otherwise, the clinical presentation is similar to Shiga-toxin–associated HUS. Genetic testing for mutations in the aforementioned complement regulators can be performed to differentiate aHUS from other forms of HUS and TTP, in which similar symptoms can occur. In contrast, TTP is caused by mutations in the *ADAMTS13* gene or autoantibodies against the ADAMTS13 protein (a disintegrin and metalloproteinase).

C3 Glomerulopathy (C3G)

Dysregulation of complement has also been implicated in **C3 glomerulopathy (C3G)**, a disease that causes inflammation of the glomeruli of the kidneys, leading to hematuria, proteinuria, hypertension, and gradual decline of kidney function. The two forms of C3 glomerulopathy, called *dense deposit disease* (DDD) and *C3 glomerulonephritis* (C3GN), have recently been reclassified from an older description of these diseases known as *membranoproliferative glomerulonephritis (MPGN)*, based on isolated or dominant presence of C3 by immunofluorescence on a kidney biopsy. A minority of patients (10% to 15%) with C3G have mutations or polymorphisms in complement proteins, specifically C3, factor B, factor H, or factor I. Most patients (up to 60% of patients with C3GN and up to 80% of patients with DDD) have acquired autoantibodies that cause complement dysregulation, known as **C3 nephritic factors (C3NeFs).**

A C3NeF is an antibody that binds the C3-convertase from the alternative pathway, C3bBb, holding the complex together and making it resistant to the normal control mechanisms. In this way, a C3NeF leads to uncontrolled cleavage of C3 and uncontrolled deposition of C3 in the renal glomeruli. C3G caused by C3NeF is clinically indistinguishable from hereditary deficiency of complement regulators such as factor H, and laboratory testing to determine the presence or absence of a C3NeF is required to differentiate these disorders.

Laboratory Detection of Complement Abnormalities

Determining the levels of complement components can be useful in diagnosing disease. Hereditary deficiencies can be identified, and much can be learned about inflammatory or autoimmune states by monitoring the consumption of complement proteins from activation by antigen-antibody complexes. Techniques to determine complement abnormalities generally fall into two categories: (1) measurement of individual complement proteins as antigens in serum and (2) assays for functional complement pathway activity. Many assays that are unavailable in routine clinical laboratories are performed in specialized laboratories. We discuss some of the more common assays in the text that follows.

Specimen Collection and Handling

As we previously discussed, the complement cascade is inherently unstable, ready to react to a threat. Complement can be activated soon after a blood specimen is collected, simply by how it is handled. Therefore, serum or plasma samples for complement testing must be processed quickly and tested within 2 hours of blood draw or stored at –80°C if testing is to be performed later. A delay in processing or storage at –20°C can lead to artificial decreases in complement values. Thawing should be performed on ice, and repeated freeze/thaw cycles should be avoided. This is especially important for the complement function assays but is less critical for measuring intact parent components such as C3 and C4. If shipment to a reference lab is needed, the sample should be transported on dry ice.

Tests for complement activation fragments such as C5a require the use of ethylenediaminetetraacetic acid (EDTA) plasma to chelate the calcium needed for classical and lectin pathway activation and to avoid cross-pathway cleavage of complement during the clotting process. The use of serum instead of plasma in these assays would result in dramatic increases in measured levels of complement activation fragments and affect interpretation of test results.

Immunologic Assays of Individual Components

Some of the most common methods of measuring complement protein concentrations are based on the principle of antigen-antibody equivalence (see Chapter 10). For these tests, the amount of reagent antibody to the component is kept constant; when the antibody and antigen (i.e., the complement protein measured) are in equilibrium, immune complexes will form that can be detected. The most common methods for measuring individual complement proteins are nephelometry and immunoturbidimetry. Historically, radial immunodiffusion (RID) was also used, but this technique has become less common in favor of automated methods. C3 and C4 levels are routinely measured in most clinical laboratories by automated nephelometry or immunoturbidimetry. Measurement of these and other complement proteins relies on the precipitation of immune complexes produced when the patient sample (i.e., the source of complement) is incubated with a reagent antibody directed against the corresponding complement component. Nephelometry measures the concentration of an individual complement protein according to the amount of light scattered by the antigen-antibody mixture, whereas immunoturbidimetry is based on the reduction in light transmission resulting from immune complex formation (refer to Chapter 10 for more details).

None of the precipitation techniques are able to distinguish whether the molecules are functionally active or have been cleaved during activation of the complement cascade. Thus, although these assays give quantitative results and are relatively easy to perform, test results must be interpreted carefully. Therefore, it may be important to use other methods, such as enzyme-linked immunosorbent assay (ELISA), for measurement of the activation fragments, particularly in relation to testing for diseases involving improper complement control.

Assays for Classical Pathway Function

Assays that measure lysis, the endpoint of complement activation, are functional tests that are frequently run in conjunction with measuring individual components and have become more important with the advent of complement-blocking therapies. The **hemolytic titration (CH50) assay** was the original assay used for this purpose. This assay measures the amount of patient serum required to lyse 50% of a standardized concentration of antibody-sensitized sheep erythrocytes. Because all proteins from C1 to C9 are necessary for this to occur, functional or quantitative absence of any one component will result in an abnormal CH50, essentially reducing this number to zero.

The titer is expressed in CH50 units, or the reciprocal of the dilution that can lyse 50% of the sensitized RBCs. The 50% point is used because this is when the maximum change in lytic activity per unit change in complement occurs **(Fig. 7–12).**

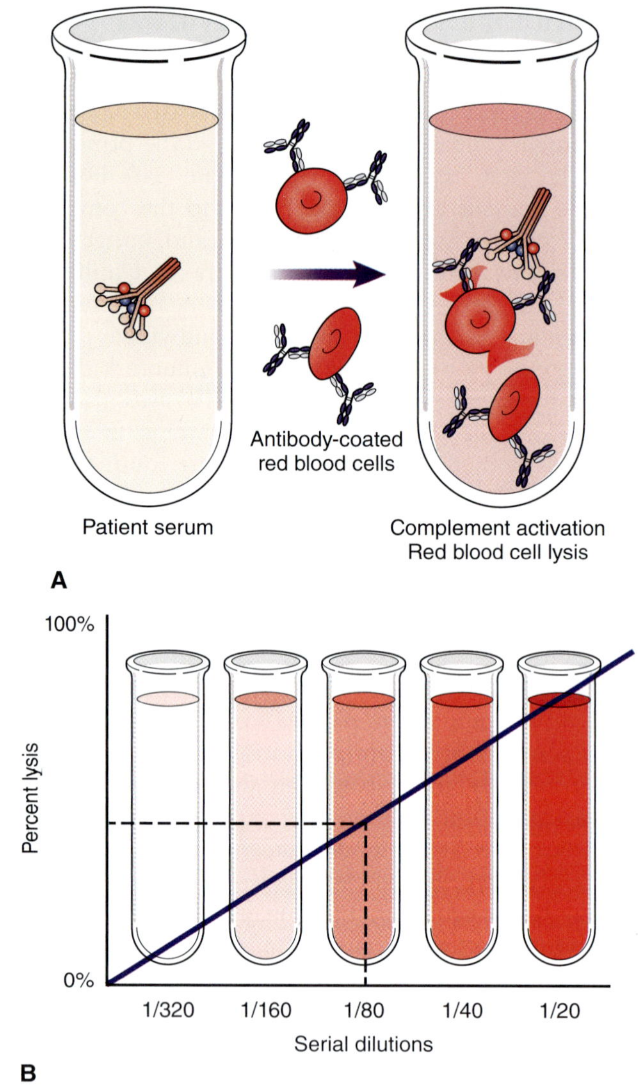

FIGURE 7.12 Traditional CH50 test. (A) Antibody-coated RBCs are added to dilutions of patient serum, leading to complement activation and RBC lysis Although only C1qrs is shown for simplicity, this test requires C1 through C9 to be present for lysis to occur. The degree of lysis indicates the functional capacity of the complete classical pathway. (B) After incubation at 37°C, the reciprocal of the serum dilution required to lyse 50% of the RBCs is determined. In this example, the CH50 value is about 80 units/ml.

The newer and more common version of this test is based on the ability of complement in the patient sample to lyse antibody-coated liposomes that release the enzyme, glucose-6-phosphate dehydrogenase (G6PD; see **Figure 7-13**). The enzyme reacts with a substrate solution (nicotinamide adenine dinucleotide [NAD] plus glucose-6-phosphate [G6P]) to produce NADH (a reduced form of NAD). The resulting change in absorbance can be measured by many laboratory analyzers, most commonly immunoturbidimetric or nephelometers, and is proportional to the complement activity in the sample. The test is simpler to perform than traditional CH50 testing and is more reproducible for the standard laboratory. However, this form of classical pathway function testing, although well suited for immunodeficiency diagnosis, may not be ideal for following the effectiveness of complement inhibition therapies. One reason for the discrepancy is that the liposomal assays involve testing at an acidic pH, whereas the ELISA and hemolytic methods involve physiological pH. Regardless of which assay is used, individual laboratories must establish their own normal values.

More recently, 96-well ELISA assays have been developed to test complement function. These assays rely on activation of complement at the surface of the plate, followed by detection of newly formed epitopes on C9 that are only present when the component is part of the **terminal complement complex (TCC,** also known as the *MAC*). The assays can be easily adapted by the routine clinical laboratory.

The ability to accurately follow the effectiveness of complement blockade therapies requires a method to provide a high level of sensitivity to detect low levels of specific complement products. All the methods for measuring classical pathway function were originally developed to evaluate patients for inborn errors of the complement system, testing that did not require the same level of sensitivity.

Critical Thinking 7-1

A 32-year-old patient presented with lupus-like symptoms but with no history of autoimmunity. The physician ordered complement and rheumatology tests, and the following results were obtained: Autoantibodies against nuclear antigens and DNA were negative; CH50 was low, C3 was at the lower end of the normal range, C4 was low. What additional complement test could be useful in diagnosing this patient and why?

Alternative-Pathway (AP) and Lectin-Pathway (LP) Assays

Alternative pathway activation can be measured by several different means. Hemolytic tests for alternative pathway activation, referred to as AH50, can be performed in the same manner as the CH50, except magnesium chloride and ethylene glycol tetraacetic acid (EGTA) are added to the buffer, and calcium is left out. This buffer chelates calcium, blocking classical pathway activation. Rabbit RBCs are used as the indicator because they provide an ideal surface for alternative pathway activation.

Another assay to test for alternative pathway function is ELISA. For example, ELISA can detect C3bBbP or C3bP complexes in very small quantities. Microtiter wells are typically coated with bacterial LPS to trigger activation of the alternative pathway.

One test system has been developed that can determine the activity of all three pathways. Strips used for the classical pathway are coated with IgM, strips for the alternative pathway are coated with LPS, and strips for the MBL pathway are coated with mannose. Deficiencies can be detected using the combined test results. The test is easy to perform as it does not depend on the use of animal erythrocytes, which may be hard to obtain.

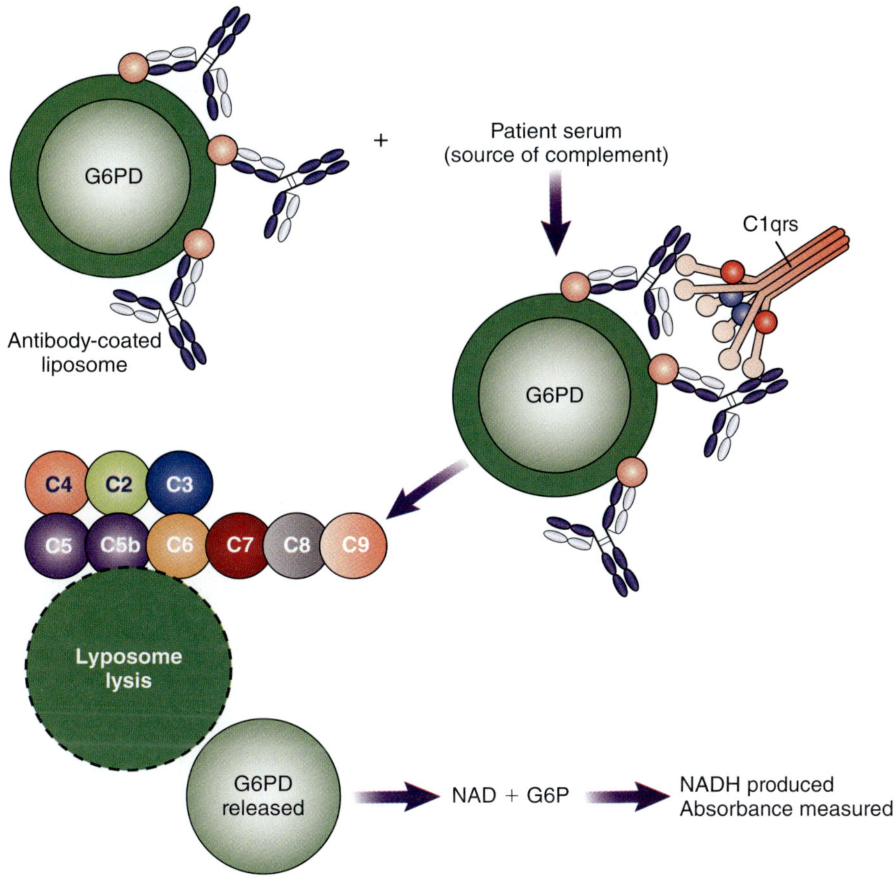

FIGURE 7.13 Liposomal CH50 test. Patient serum is incubated with antibody-coated liposomes filled with glucose-6-phosphate dehydrogenase (G6PD). Complement in the serum lyses the liposomes, releasing G6PD, which then reacts with nicotinamide adenine dinucleotide (NAD) and glucose-6-phosphate (G6P) to produce NADH. The change in absorbance is proportional to the complement activity in the sample.

Testing Levels of Complement Activation

With increased recognition of the role that improper complement control plays in a growing list of diseases, there is considerable interest in monitoring the balance of complement activation and control. Measurement of C3 and C4 levels has been used for monitoring autoimmune-mediated diseases, but such measurements of the parent complement components are not as sensitive as those that measure the fragments formed upon activation. Assays that test for complement activation are generally ELISA or multiplex versions of immunoassays (see Chapter 11).

Measuring complement fragments has several potential benefits. First, these tests are more sensitive to any complement activation, so they can more easily separate a change from baseline. Second, measuring anaphylatoxin (C3a and C5a) levels directly can be informative about the degree of inflammation that is being driven by complement. Third, by measuring individual fragments, it is possible to determine which pathway or pathways are activated and where any control is achieved in the cascade of complement activation. Specifically, measuring C4a will reflect classical/lectin pathway activation, and Bb or Ba will demonstrate the level of alternative pathway activation. Measuring the soluble version of the MAC, sC5b-9, also known as **sMAC** or the TCC, can provide information about the level of activation reaching the terminal pathway, which has the greatest biological effects.

Unfortunately, there are also challenges with measuring the fragments. As many of these fragments are strongly proinflammatory, the body has developed mechanisms to control their action; therefore, most have very short half-lives in the circulation. C5a has the shortest half-life, less than 1 minute. Additionally, dramatic increases in measured levels of complement activation fragments can occur if there is a delay in sample processing, if the sample is not collected in an EDTA tube, or if the sample is not stored at the proper temperature (–80°C) prior to testing.

Knowledge Check 7-5

What could be measured to determine the level of terminal pathway activation in a sample of patient serum?

a. C1-INH function
b. C4 levels
c. sC5b-9 levels
d. Bb levels

Interpretation of Laboratory Findings

In complement-function tests, decreased levels of complement components or activity may be caused by several factors:

- In vitro consumption from post–blood draw handling
- Decreased production by the patient
- Consumption of components (i.e., increased usage and depletion) because of certain diseases
- Inhibition by certain therapies

Effects of Post–Blood Draw Handling

Interpretation of complement laboratory testing can be complex and complicated by the effects of post-draw handling. As we discussed previously, specimen handling is extremely important. The tube should be centrifuged, and the serum or plasma should be frozen at –80°C or placed on dry ice if it is not tested within 2 hours. If a sample is left at room temperature, stored at –20°C, or subjected to multiple freeze-and-thaw cycles, artificially low complement function may be measured. In such situations, results may be invalid, and the test needs to be repeated with a fresh sample. It is important to keep in mind that improper post-draw handling of a sample would cause the test to return a falsely low functional value. (It is very unlikely for improper preanalytical handling to lead to a false-normal result.)

Specimen handling is also critical when testing for activation markers, such as C3a or sC5b-9. These tests require an EDTA plasma tube to chelate calcium and help control post-draw complement activation. If a serum tube is used by mistake, the clotting process will produce a large increase in these fragments post-draw that may obscure any activation occurring in the patient. Failure to freeze the sample promptly at the correct temperature will also lead to an artificially elevated result. Assays for standard measurements of C3 and C4 have been developed so as not to be as sensitive to specimen handling; however, they cannot distinguish between intact C3 or C4 and their activation fragments.

Decreased Production or Consumption of Complement

If a complement deficiency is suspected, it is possible to narrow down the possible candidate components with CH50 and AH50 assays.

- If the CH50 is low but the AH50 is normal, the components unique to the classical pathway should be investigated.
- If the CH50 is normal but the AH50 is low, the alternative pathway components need to be investigated.
- If both the CH50 and AH50 are low, suspicion should be on C3 and the components of the terminal pathway because those components are shared by both the classical and alternative pathways.

Although this analysis will be true for most patients, it is also possible, if there is sufficient activation of complement by any one pathway, that enough components could be consumed to lower the function of the other pathways. As we previously stated, complement activation is rarely limited to just one pathway. Consumption can result from the loss of a control protein, the presence of an autoantibody, an ongoing infection, or other activation circumstances.

Once the CH50 and AH50 assays have been performed, it is appropriate to determine the levels or function of individual complement components based on the test results. For many of the components, an antigen level is sufficient to determine where the deficiency lies; however, there are a few instances in which measurement of the function would be more informative. For example, it is necessary to measure the function of C8 because it is a three-subunit protein. The loss of one of the three subunits would not put the level of C8 out of normal range, but it would render the remaining two subunits nonfunctional. In addition, type II C2 deficiency results from a genetic mutation in C2 that renders the protein nonfunctional but does not decrease the level of expression. In type II HAE, C1-INH may be present in normal levels but be nonfunctional.

A typical screening procedure for complement abnormalities usually includes the CH50 and quantitation of C3 and C4. Testing for products of complement activation such as C3a, C4a, C5a, Bb, and Ba, and breakdown products, such as iC3b and C4d, can also be performed to monitor inflammatory processes such as rheumatoid arthritis and SLE. **Table 7–4** presents possible examples of screening results and correlates these with deficiencies of individual factors. An understanding of these patterns may be helpful in differentiating hereditary deficiencies from activation states that consume available complement components. Additional testing is necessary, however, to precisely determine hereditary deficiencies.

Therapeutic Inhibition of Complement

With the advent of complement-targeted therapeutics, there is more demand to measure complement and a need to appreciate the effect of complement-inhibiting drugs on the complement assays. This would be reflected in a low CH50 or AH50 measurement. This is also expected to lead to lower levels of activation markers but only those downstream of the point of inhibition. For example, a C5 inhibitor would reduce levels of sC5b-9 but not C3a.

Complement Therapeutics

With increased recognition of complement's role in the pathogenesis of many diseases, several complement-targeted therapeutic agents have been developed for clinical use or are under investigation in human clinical trials. These drugs include monoclonal antibodies, small molecules, and peptides that affect complement activity. The agents specifically target key points in the complement pathways, so determining the specific laboratory tests best suited to monitor the treatment response and disease activity in patients receiving these therapies is important.

The first complement therapy approved by the U.S. Food and Drug Administration (FDA) for clinical use was a recombinant protein that targeted the classical pathway to restore C1-INH function in patients with HAE. Such treatment during an HAE crisis would be expected to restore activity of the classical pathway to normal, and this would be evident by an increase in C4 and C2 levels and normalization of low classical pathway function.

Table 7-4 Diagnostic Testing for Complement Deficiencies or Therapeutic Inhibition

	FUNCTIONS			COMPONENTS				ACTIVATION MARKERS			
Complement component affected (deficient or target of inhibition)	CP	LP	AP	CP[b]	LP[c]	AP[d]	TP[e]	CP (C4a, C4d)	LP (C4a, C4d)	AP (Bb, Ba)	TP (C3a, C3d, sC5b-9)
C1q, C1r, C1s	Low	Normal	Normal	Low	Normal	Normal	Normal	Normal	Normal	Normal	Normal
C4, C2	Low	Low	Normal	Low	Low	Normal	Normal	Low/absent[a]	Low/absent[a]	Normal	Normal
MBL, MASP-1, MASP-2	Normal	Low	Normal	Normal	Low	Normal	Normal	Normal	Low/absent	Normal	Normal
Factor B, Factor D, and properdin	Normal	Normal	Low	Normal	Normal	Low	Normal	Normal	Normal	Low/absent[a]	Normal
C3, C5, C6, C7, C8, C9	Low	Low	Low	Normal	Normal	Normal	Low/normal	Normal	Normal	Normal	Normal/low/absent[a]
C1-INH	Low	Low	Normal	Low	Low	Normal	Normal	High	High	Normal	Normal
Factor H and factor I	Low	Low	Low	Normal	Normal	Low/normal	Low/normal	Normal	Normal	High	Low/normal
Improperly handled sample	Low	Low	Low	Normal	Normal	Normal	Normal	High	High	High	High

AP = alternative pathway; CP = classical pathway; LP = lectin pathway; TP = terminal pathway.

[a]Whether the component or activation fragment would be low or absent will depend on the component that is deficient or inhibited.

[b]Classical pathway components: C1q, C1s, C1r, C2, C4, C1-INH.

[c]Lectin pathway components: MBL, MASP1, MASP2, MASP3, C2, C4, C1-INH.

[d]Alternative pathway components: factor B, factor D, factor H, factor I.

[e]Terminal pathway components: C3, C5, C6, C7, C8, C9.

Complement therapeutics now reach well beyond the treatment of HAE. An example of a complement-inhibiting drug is eculizumab, a monoclonal antibody directed against C5, which is routinely used to treat PNH and aHUS. Other diseases for which complement therapies have been FDA approved include TMA, cold agglutinins disease, neuromyelitis optica spectrum disorder (a rare inflammatory disease affecting the optic nerves and spinal cord), geographic atrophy secondary to age-related macular degeneration (a progressive disorder involving retinal cell death and irreversible vision loss), ANCA-associated vasculitis (see Chapter 15), myasthenia gravis (an autoimmune disease involving muscle weakness; see Chapter 15), and coronavirus disease of 2019 (COVID-19; see Chapter 23).

Future developments include a monoclonal antibody targeting C1s for treatment of cold agglutinin autoimmune hemolytic anemia (see Chapter 14), which is expected to decrease complement function by blocking classical pathway activation. The lectin pathway is also a target for therapeutic agents in clinical development, specifically a monoclonal antibody targeting MASP-2 for IgA nephropathy, a kidney disease in which the lectin pathway has been implicated. Because agents that inhibit complement have a large potential to counteract the inflammatory effects of complement dysregulation, this is an area of active research, and more therapies are likely to be approved for treatment of many other disorders in the future.

Laboratory Testing

Because the development and approval of complement therapeutics has moved very quickly, the recommendations for complement testing are still in development. With some of the early drug approvals, measuring complement function was used to assess if appropriate levels of complement inhibition have been achieved. With the advent of new-generation, long-acting forms of drug therapy, measuring classical pathway function has proven less consistent with the level of inhibition in patients. This, together with varied targets of therapeutic inhibition in the complement pathway for the different drugs, has led to evaluation of drug effectiveness being focused on the patient's clinical presentation.

However, research in this area continues, because complement measurements have the potential to predict which patients would benefit from complement therapeutics and to determine if the appropriate level of inhibition has been achieved. Studies are focusing on the measurement of complement activation products such as C3a, C5a, and sC5b-9. The utility of this testing will be determined in the future.

Critical Thinking 7-2

You are reviewing results for a young patient with aHUS who has been treated with a C5 inhibitor. You have samples from before the patient was given their first dose of the inhibitor and a sample from the day after the dose. The post-dose sample has a very low CH50 and low sC5b-9. You expected these results because the inhibitor blocks terminal pathway activity and the C5 cleavage needed to form the sC5b-9. However, the pre-dose sample has a very low CH50 and high sC5b-9. What could be the reasons for the results of the predose sample?

KEY CONCEPTS

- The complement system is a series of more than 50 soluble and cell-bound proteins that participate in innate and adaptive immune defenses against infection.
- Activities of complement include lysis of foreign or damaged cells, opsonization, increase in vascular permeability, and attraction of neutrophils and monocytes to areas where they are needed. Thus, complement activation can influence the inflammatory state of the host.

Pathways of the Complement System

- The classical complement pathway is triggered by IgG or IgM binding to the surface of pathogens. Nine major proteins (C1-C9) are involved in this pathway.
- Three distinct units are formed in the classical pathway. They are the recognition unit consisting of C1qrs; the activation unit consisting of C2, C4, and C3; and the MAC, consisting of C5, C6, C7, C8, and C9.
- The lectin pathway is activated by carbohydrates present in microbial cell walls and serves as an important link between the innate and adaptive immune responses. Proteins unique to the lectin pathway include MBL, MASP-1, MASP-2, and MASP-3.
- The alternative pathway can be triggered by bacterial and fungal cell walls, yeast, viruses, tumor cells, and certain parasites. Factors unique to the alternative pathway include factor B, factor D, and properdin.
- The alternative pathway has an important role in amplifying activation that starts with the classical or lectin pathway.
- Complement activation that is clinically important usually involves more than one pathway.
- All three pathways terminate with the formation of the MAC.

System Controls

- Plasma protein regulators of the complement system play a very important role because, if uncontrolled, complement activation could have devastating systemic effects.
- Soluble regulators include C1-INH, C4BP, factor H, factor I, and S protein.
- Examples of cell-bound regulators are CR1, MCP, and DAF.

Complement Receptors and Their Biological Roles

- Specific complement receptors on host cells amplify the immune response by enhancing phagocytosis and stimulating WBCs. Some of these receptors include CR1, CR2, CR3, CR4, and collectin receptors.

Biological Manifestations of Complement Activation

- Effector molecules generated during complement activation play a major role in inflammation, recognition and presentation of antigens, activation of B cells, and maintenance of immunologic memory. Some are classified as anaphylatoxins, chemotaxins, and opsonins.
- Anaphylatoxins (C3a, C5a) increase vascular permeability, whereas chemotaxins (C5a) attract phagocytic cells to a specific area, and opsonins (C3b, C4b, iC3b, C3dg) coat damaged or foreign cells to enhance phagocytosis.

Complement and Disease States

- Complement can cause harm to the host if it is activated systemically, activated by tissue necrosis, causes RBC lysis, or causes damage to the kidney basement membrane.

Deficiencies in Major Pathway Complement Components

- Hereditary deficiencies of complement components can place an individual at risk for severe, recurrent infections.
- Deficiencies in C1q, C4, C2, or C3 can cause a lupus-like syndrome due to delayed ability to clear immune complexes.
- Deficiencies in the terminal complement components (C5-C8) are associated with susceptibility to systemic *Neisseria* infections.

Deficiencies in Regulatory Complement Components

- Missing or deficient regulators are the cause of diseases such as PNH and HAE.
- Improper control of complement can lead to several diseases related to inflammation, such as aHUS, C3G, and age-related macular degeneration. This list continues to grow as complement-driven inflammation is found to play a role in more diseases.
- The aHUS, also known as complement-mediated TMA, is a thrombotic microvascular disease that is rooted in improper control of the alternative pathway of complement caused by genetic mutations in the complement system.

Laboratory Detection of Complement Abnormalities

- Techniques to determine complement abnormalities can be classified into two groups: (1) tests measuring individual complement components and (2) assays for functional complement pathway activity.
- Serum or plasma samples for complement testing must be processed quickly and tested within 2 hours of blood draw or stored at –80°C because a delay in processing or storage at –20°C can cause artificial decreases in complement values, especially in tests for complement function.
- The original method for testing complement function is the hemolytic titration or CH50 assay. CH50 detects lysis of antibody-coated RBCs to measure the endpoint of complement activation in the classical pathway. The AH50 assay is a similar test for measuring the activity of the alternative pathway.
- The liposomal CH50 test is the newer method for classical pathway function. In this method, complement in patient serum lyses antibody-coated liposomes filled with G6PD, which reacts with NAD and G6P to produce NADH. The change in absorbance is proportional to the complement activity in the sample.
- Complement proteins such as C3 and C4 in patient serum are quantitated routinely using automated nephelometry or immunoturbidimetry. Complement activation fragments are measured in plasma samples by ELISA.
- Complement levels may vary between different assays and laboratories, so it is important to compare results to the laboratory's established reference range.

Complement Therapeutics

- Recombinant C1-INH is used to restore C1-INH function in patients with HAE.
- Overactivation of complement can have unwanted inflammatory effects, leading to pathology in many diseases.
- Therapeutic agents to reduce complement activity include monoclonal antibodies, small molecules, and peptides that specifically target key proteins in the complement pathways (e.g., C5). These drugs are being developed for a growing number of diseases.
- Studies are focused on identifying appropriate laboratory tests to determine the effectiveness of complement therapies.

Study Guide: Complement Pathways

PATHWAY	CLASSICAL	LECTIN	ALTERNATIVE	TERMINAL
Key pathway initiators	Antigen-antibody complexes (IgM > IgG) C-reactive protein bound to ligand	Mannose and related sugars on pathogens	Components of bacterial cell walls (e.g., LPS, teichoic acid) and yeast cells (e.g., zymosan) $C3_{H2O}$ C3b (from classical or lectin pathways)	Effector pathway; initiated by any of the three pathways after cleaving C3
Recognition unit	C1qrs	Mannose-binding lectin (MBL) bound to mannose or related sugars	C3bBb bound to one of the key pathogen components initiating the pathway	
Key enzymes	C1r, C1s C4bC2b C4bC2bC3b	MBL-associated serine proteases (MASPs) C4bC2b (C3 convertase) C4bC2bC3b (C5 convertase)	Factor D C3bBb (C3 convertase) C3bBbC3bP (C5 convertase)	

Study Guide: Biologic Functions of Selected Complement Activation Products

FUNCTION	DEFINITION	COMPLEMENT PRODUCTS INVOLVED
Membrane attack complex	Product generated in the terminal steps of complement activation that creates a pore in the membrane of the target cell, leading to cell lysis	C5b6789
Anaphylatoxin activity	Release of histamine from mast cells and basophils, producing increased vascular permeability and contraction of smooth muscle	C5a, C3a
Chemotaxis	Migration of white blood cells toward the site of antigen concentration	C5a
Opsonization	Coating of an antigen to facilitate phagocytosis	C3b, C4b, iC3b, C3dg

CASE STUDIES

1. A 3-year-old child with a history of serious infections is currently hospitalized with meningitis. The doctor suspects that the child may have a complement deficiency and orders testing. The following results are obtained: decreased classical pathway and alternative pathway function, and normal C4 and C3 levels.

Questions

a. Which component(s) is (are) likely to be lacking?
b. What follow-up testing would be recommended?

2. A young adult appeared at the local hospital emergency department with symptoms of abdominal pain, severe vomiting, and swelling of the legs and hands. The patient has had these symptoms on several previous occasions. After ruling out appendicitis, the physician ordered a battery of tests, including some for abnormalities of complement components. The following results were obtained: RBC and WBC count normal, total serum protein normal, classical pathway function decreased, alternative pathway function normal, C3 and C1q levels normal, and C4 and C2 levels decreased.

Questions

a. What symptoms led physicians to consider a possible complement abnormality?
b. What are possible reasons for a decrease in both C4 and C2? What information does the normal C1q add?
c. What other testing would confirm your suspicions?

REVIEW QUESTIONS

1. The classical complement pathway is activated primarily by:
   a. Most viruses
   b. Antigen-antibody complexes
   c. Fungal cell walls
   d. Mannose in bacterial cell walls
2. Which of the following is characteristic of complement components?
   a. Normally present in serum
   b. Mainly synthesized by B cells
   c. Present as active enzymes
   d. Heat stable
3. All of the following are true of the classical pathway recognition unit *except:*
   a. It consists of C1q, C1r, and C1s.
   b. The subunits require calcium for binding together.
   c. Binding occurs at the Fc region of antibody molecules.
   d. C1q becomes an active esterase.
4. Which of the following is (are) referred to as *C3 convertase*?
   a. C1qrs
   b. C4bC2b3b
   c. C3bBb
   d. Only b and c
5. Mannose-binding lectin (MBL) in the lectin pathway is most similar to which classical pathway component?
   a. C3
   b. C1rs
   c. C1q
   d. C4
6. Which of the following describes the role of properdin in the alternative pathway?
   a. Stabilization of C3 convertase
   b. Conversion of B to Bb
   c. Inhibition of C3 convertase formation
   d. Binding and cleavage of factor B
7. Which best characterizes the MAC?
   a. Each pathway uses different factors to form it.
   b. C5 through C9 are not added in any particular order.
   c. One MAC unit is sufficient to lyse any type of cell.
   d. C9 polymerizes to form the transmembrane channel.
8. All of the following represent functions of the complement system *except:*
   a. Decreased clearance of antigen-antibody complexes
   b. Lysis of foreign cells
   c. Increase in vascular permeability
   d. Migration of neutrophils to the tissues
9. Which of the following diseases are associated with complement deficiencies or improper control?
   a. Paroxysmal nocturnal hemoglobinuria (PNH)
   b. Atypical hemolytic uremic syndrome
   c. C3 glomerulopathy
   d. All of the above
10. Which of the following is *not* true of the amplification loop in the alternative pathway of complement activation?
    a. Improper control can lead to disease.
    b. It can amplify activation that is initiated by the classical pathway.
    c. C3b is the product that is increased.
    d. Increasing amounts of C1qrs are produced.
11. Which disease is associated with lack of proper factor H function?
    a. PNH
    b. aHUS
    c. HAE
    d. SLE
12. Which best describes the role of CR2 on cell membranes?
    a. Binds C1qrs to inactivate it
    b. Acts as coreceptor on B cells for antigen
    c. Increases clearance of immune complexes
    d. Binds particles opsonized with C3b
13. Which of the following would be expected to be true for the testing of a patient who is on a complement C5 inhibitor?
    a. Low classical pathway function
    b. Low alternative pathway function
    c. High sC5b-9
    d. a and b are true
14. Which of the following best characterizes HUS?
    a. It is a common cause of renal failure in children.
    b. It never has neurological manifestations.
    c. It is associated with a high platelet count.
    d. It is associated with antibody to C3 convertase.
15. The CH50 test measures which of the following?
    a. Complement in patient serum required to lyse 50% of sensitized sheep RBCs
    b. Functioning of both the classical and alternative pathways
    c. Genetic deficiencies of any of the complement components
    d. Functioning of the lectin pathway only

16. A decreased CH50 level and a normal AH50 level indicate which deficiency?
    a. Decrease in components in the lectin pathway only
    b. Decrease in components in the alternative pathway only
    c. Decrease in components of both classical and alternative pathways
    d. Decrease in components of the classical pathway only

17. Which best describes the role of an anaphylatoxin?
    a. Coats cells to increase phagocytosis
    b. Increases antibody production
    c. Increases C1q levels
    d. Causes increased vascular permeability

18. Which of the following is *not* a cofactor for factor I?
    a. Factor H
    b. C4-binding protein
    c. Membrane cofactor protein (MCP, CD46)
    d. C3bBbC3b

19. **A lack of C1-INH has been associated with which of the following conditions?**
    a. Paroxysmal nocturnal hemoglobinuria
    b. Hemolytic uremic syndrome
    c. Hereditary angioedema
    d. Increased bacterial infections

20. If a specimen for complement testing was left on a laboratory bench overnight and not properly frozen, which of the following would be true?
    a. The classical pathway function level would be falsely low.
    b. The alternative pathway function level would be falsely high.
    c. A measure of C3a would be falsely low.
    d. A C3 level by nephelometry would be changed.

Chapter 7 Answer Key

Answers to Knowledge Checks

7.1 c 7.2 e 7.3 c 7.4 e 7.5 c

Answers to Review Questions

1. b	2. a	3. d	4. c	5. c	6. a	7. d
8. a	9. d	10. d	11. b	12. b	13. d	14. a
15. a	16. d	17. d	18. d	19. c	20. a	

II

Basic Immunologic Procedures

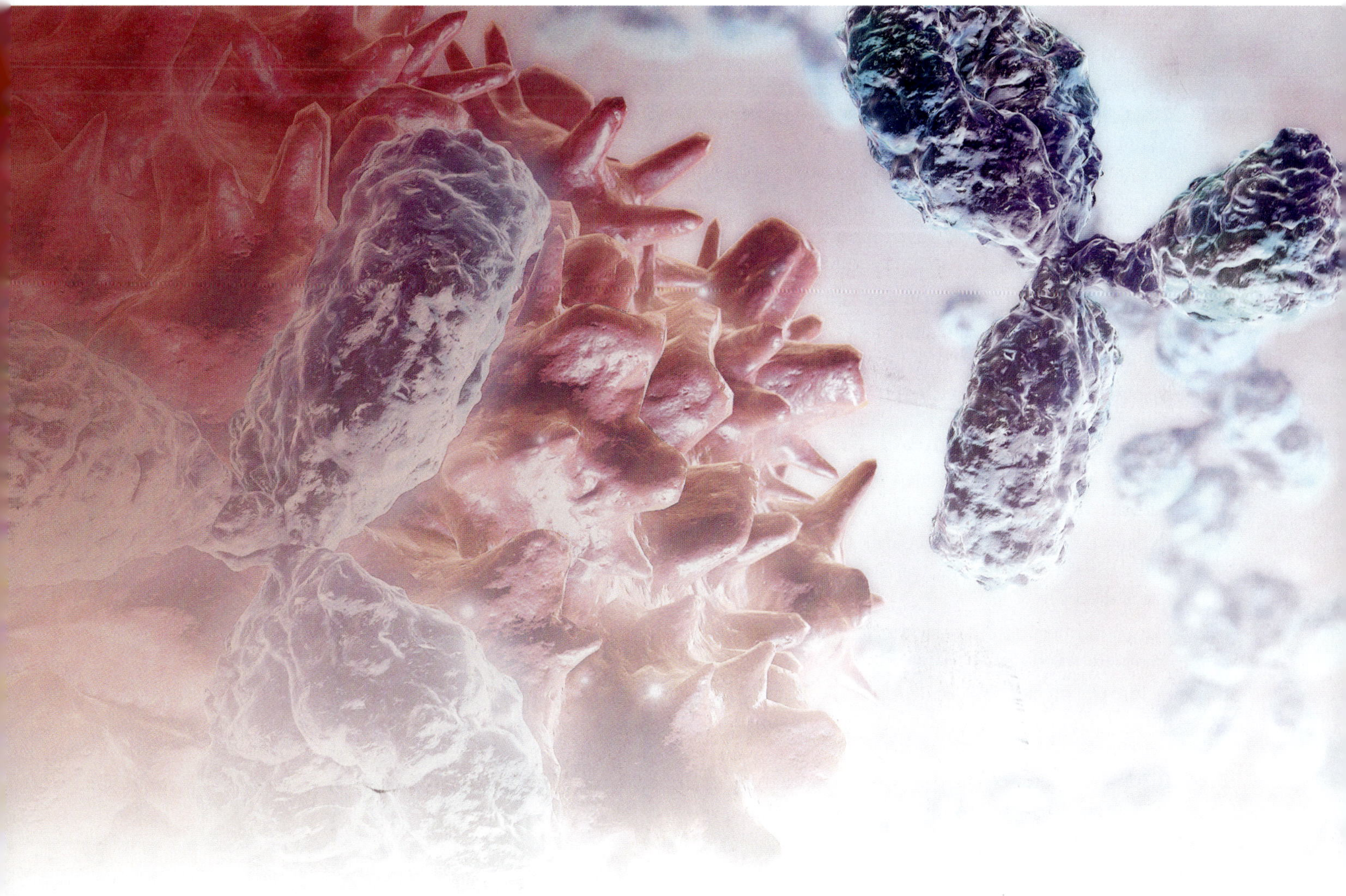

8 Safety and Quality Management

Marjorie Schaub Di Lorenzo, MLS(ASCP)SH

LEARNING OUTCOMES

After finishing this chapter, you should be able to:

8.1 Define and give an example of the types of safety hazards encountered in the laboratory.

8.2 Describe the six components of the chain of infection and the safety precautions that will break the chain.

8.3 Correctly perform hand hygiene procedures following Centers for Disease Control and Prevention (CDC) guidelines.

8.4 Describe the types of personal protective equipment (PPE) used by laboratory personnel.

8.5 Define Standard Precautions (SPs) and state their purpose.

8.6 State the acceptable procedures for disposal, decontamination, and spill control of biological waste in the laboratory.

8.7 Discuss the federal regulations and guidelines for preparing and shipping patient samples from the laboratory.

8.8 Explain the requirements mandated by the Occupational Exposure to Bloodborne Pathogens compliance directive.

8.9 Discuss the purpose of a Chemical Hygiene Plan, the information contained in a Safety Data Sheet (SDS), and the use of the Globally Harmonized System (GHS).

8.10 Describe precautions that laboratory personnel should take when radioactive, electrical, fire, and physical hazards are encountered.

8.11 Explain the RACE (Rescue, Alarm, Contain, Extinguish or Evacuate) and PASS (Pull, Aim, Squeeze, Sweep) actions to be taken when a fire is discovered.

8.12 State and interpret the components of the National Fire Protection Association (NFPA) hazardous material labeling system.

8.13 Define the preexamination (preanalytical), examination (analytical), and postexamination (postanalytical) components of quality management (QM).

8.14 Distinguish between the components of internal, external, and electronic quality control (QC), and external quality assessment (EQA; proficiency testing).

CHAPTER OUTLINE

You can go to **fadavis.com** keyword stevens for the laboratory exercises that accompany this text.

8.15 Discuss the roles of the Clinical Laboratory Improvement Amendments (CLIA), Clinical and Laboratory Standards Institute (CLSI), The Joint Commission (TJC), College of American Pathologists (CAP), and the Commission on Laboratory Accreditation (COLA) in the regulation of health care.

8.16 State and describe the 12 quality system essentials (QSEs) used in a quality management system (QMS).

8.17 Describe the purpose of quality indicators.

8.18 List the six areas of the Lean system and describe how it can benefit the laboratory.

8.19 State the purpose of the Six Sigma methodology in a QMS.

8.20 Demonstrate knowledge of root cause analysis (RCA) as it relates to laboratory testing.

To work safely in the clinical laboratory, laboratorians must learn what hazards exist and apply basic safety precautions to reduce the risks associated with them. Laboratories must also guarantee excellent patient care by adhering to quality management principles and systems and health care regulations. In this chapter, we discuss the major classes of hazards encountered in the laboratory, the precautions that must be taken by laboratory personnel, and the regulations laboratories must follow to ensure employee safety and quality laboratory results.

Laboratory Hazards

The clinical laboratory contains a wide variety of safety hazards, many capable of producing serious injury or life-threatening disease. Some hazards are unique to the health care environment, and others are encountered routinely throughout life **(Table 8–1).** It is essential that laboratory personnel know where all safety equipment is located and be trained in all aspects of its use on a yearly basis.

Biological Hazards

In the clinical laboratory, the most significant hazard exists in obtaining and testing patient specimens. Understanding how microorganisms are transmitted **(chain of infection)** is necessary to prevent infection. The chain of infection requires a continuous link between six elements: (1) an infectious agent, (2) a reservoir, (3) a portal of exit, (4) a means of transmission, (5) a portal of entry, and (6) a susceptible host. **Figure 8–1** shows the chain of infection, the universal symbol for **biohazardous** material, and the prescribed safety practices that can break the chain of infection. In the sections that follow, we discuss these concepts in more detail.

Chain of Infection Components

The chain of infection has six components.

Infectious agent (pathogen). Infectious agents include bacteria, fungi, parasites, and viruses. The chain of infection is broken by early detection of one of these agents. The treatment of infectious agents can reduce their opportunity for growth.

Reservoir. The reservoir is a place, such as a contaminated clinical specimen or an infected patient, where the infectious agent can live and multiply. Humans, animals, or contaminated inanimate objects, called **fomites,** can serve as reservoirs, particularly when they contain blood, urine, or other

Table 8-1 Types of Safety Hazards

TYPE	SOURCE	POSSIBLE INJURY
Biological	Infectious agents	Bacterial, fungal, viral, or parasitic infections
Sharps	Needles, lancets, and broken glass	Cuts, punctures, or bloodborne pathogen exposure
Chemical	Preservatives and reagents	Exposure to toxic, carcinogenic, or caustic agents
Radioactive	Equipment and radioisotopes	Damage to a fetus or generalized overexposure to radiation
Electrical	Ungrounded or wet equipment and frayed cords	Burns or shock
Fire or explosive	Open flames and organic chemicals	Burns or dismemberment
Physical	Wet floors, heavy boxes, and patients	Falls, sprains, or strains

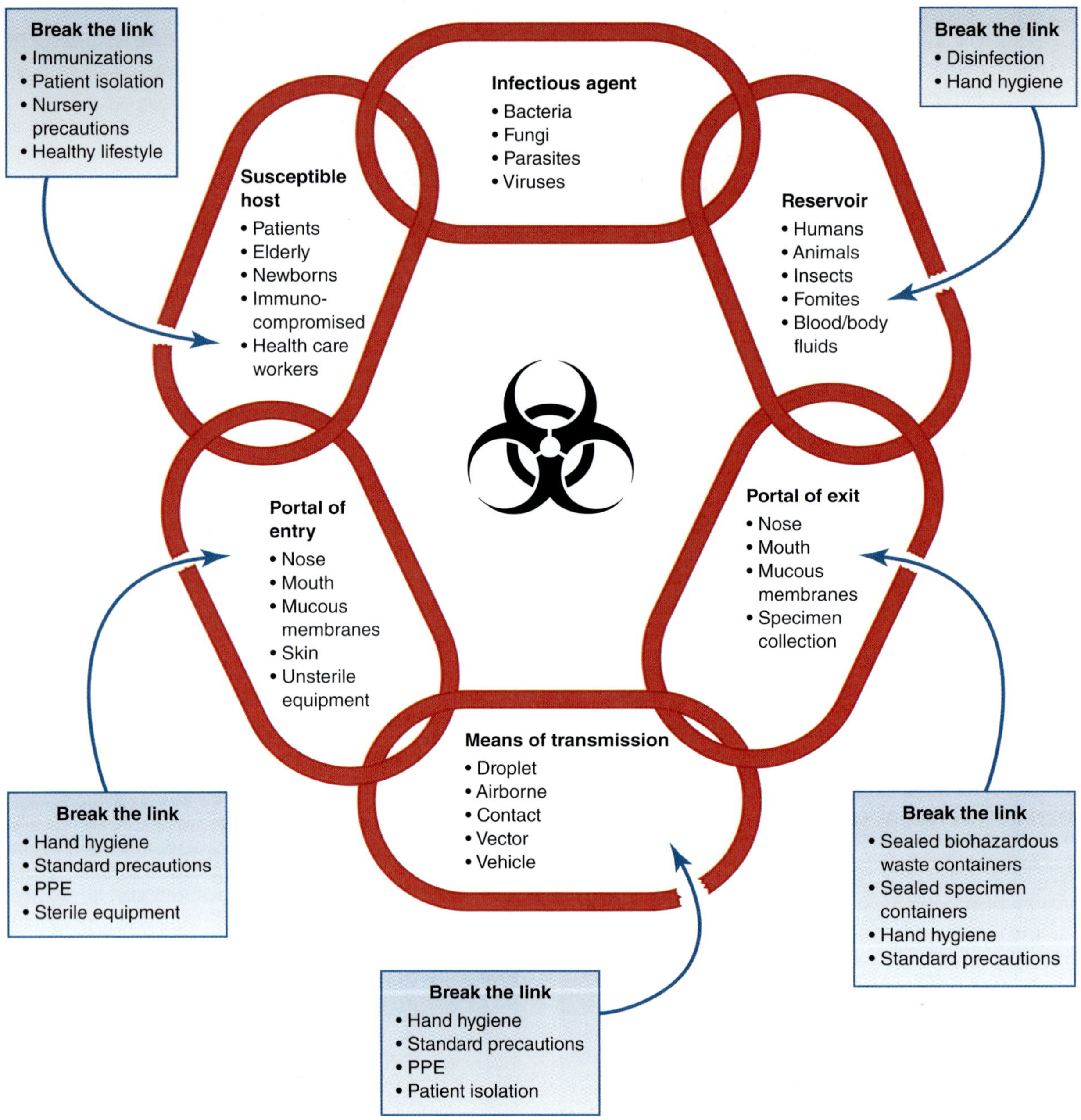

FIGURE 8–1 Chain of infection and safety practices related to the biohazard symbol.

body fluids. Some microorganisms form spores or become inactive when conditions are not ideal, such as in dried blood, and wait until a suitable reservoir is available. Disinfecting the work area kills the infectious agent and eliminates the reservoir, thereby breaking the chain of infection.

Portal of exit. The infectious agent must have a way to exit the reservoir to continue the chain of infection. This can be through the mucous membranes of the reservoir's nose, mouth, and eyes as well as in the blood or other body fluids. The chain of infection is broken when contaminated materials are placed in biohazard containers and when tubes and specimen containers are sealed. When contaminated materials are in the appropriate containers that remain sealed, the infectious agent still has a reservoir but no means of exit.

Means of transmission. Once an infectious agent has left the reservoir, it must have a way to reach a susceptible host. Means of transmission include the following:

- Direct contact: the unprotected host touches or is touched by the reservoir (a patient, specimen, or a contaminated object)
- Droplet: the host inhales infected aerosol droplets from the reservoir (e.g., aerosol droplets from a patient or an uncapped tube or when specimens are aliquoted or spilled)
- Airborne: the host inhales dried aerosol particles circulating on air currents or attached to dust particles
- Vehicle: the host ingests contaminated food or water
- Vector: from an animal or insect bite

Hand sanitizing and adhering to **Standard Precautions (SPs)**, safety guidelines developed by the Centers for Disease Control and Prevention (CDC) to protect personnel, are methods to break the chain of infection (see section that follows).

Portal of entry. After the infectious agent has been transmitted to a new reservoir, it must have a means to enter the reservoir. The portal of entry can be the same as the portal of exit, which includes the mucous membranes of the reservoir's nose, mouth, and eyes; breaks in the skin; and open wounds. Disinfection, sterilization, and strict adherence to SPs block the portal of entry, breaking the chain of infection.

Susceptible host. In the health care environment, there are several people who are at increased risk of infection. The susceptible host can be another patient during invasive procedures, visitors, and health care personnel exposed to infectious specimens. Patients receiving chemotherapy and immunocompromised patients are often more susceptible hosts. The immune system is still developing in newborns and infants and begins to weaken as people age, making these groups of patients more susceptible to infection. The immune system also is depressed by stress, fatigue, and lack of proper nutrition, factors that can contribute to the susceptibility of patients and health care personnel. Once the chain of infection is complete, the infected host becomes another source able to transmit the microorganisms to others. To break the chain of infection, health care personnel must sanitize hands often, wear gloves, stay current with the required immunizations and tests for immunity, and maintain a healthy lifestyle.

The most likely source of infection in serological testing is through contact with patient specimens and exposure to viruses such as the hepatitis viruses and HIV. Preventing completion of the chain of infection is the primary objective of biological safety. The **infection control** team develops procedures to control and monitor infections occurring in health care facilities.

Preventing transmission of microorganisms from infected sources to susceptible hosts is critical in controlling the spread of infection. Procedures used to prevent microorganism transmission include hand hygiene, wearing **personal protective equipment (PPE)**, isolating highly infective or highly susceptible patients, and properly disposing of contaminated materials. We discuss these procedures in the sections that follow. Strict adherence to guidelines published by the CDC and the **Occupational Safety and Health Administration (OSHA)** is essential.

Hand Hygiene

Hand contact represents the number one method of infection transmission. Personnel should always sanitize their hands before patient contact; after gloves are removed; before leaving the work area; whenever the hands have been knowingly contaminated; before going to designated break areas; before and after using bathroom facilities; and after nose blowing, coughing, or sneezing. Hand hygiene includes both handwashing and using alcohol-based antiseptic cleansers. Alcohol-based cleansers are not recommended after contact with spore-forming bacteria, including *Clostridioides difficile* and *Bacillus* species, because they do not destroy the spores.

The CDC's guidelines for the correct handwashing technique are pictured in **Figure 8–2.** When using alcohol-based cleansers, apply the cleanser to the palm of one hand. Rub your hands together and over the entire cleansing area, including between the fingers and thumbs. Continue rubbing until the alcohol dries.

1. Remove your jewelry. Wet your hands with warm water. Do not allow parts of the body to touch the sink.
2. Apply soap, preferably anti-microbial.
3. Rub to form a lather, create friction, and loosen debris. Thoroughly clean between your fingers and under your fingernails for at least 20 seconds; include thumbs and wrists in the cleaning.
4. Rinse your hands in a downward position to prevent recontamination of hands and wrists.
5. Dry your hands with a paper towel.
6. Turn off the faucets with a clean paper towel to prevent contamination.

Personal Protective Equipment (PPE)

PPE used in the laboratory includes gloves, face shields, and Plexiglas countertop shields.

Gloves. Gloves are worn to protect the health care worker's hands from contamination by patient body substances and to protect the patient from possible microorganisms on the health care worker's hands. Gloves must be worn when working with patients, when processing specimens and performing testing procedures, and when cleaning equipment and work areas. However, wearing gloves is not a substitute for hand sanitizing. Hands must always be sanitized when gloves are removed. Gloves used in the laboratory should be removed when noticeably contaminated or damaged and before leaving the laboratory. A variety of gloves are available, including sterile and nonsterile, powdered and unpowdered, and latex and nonlatex.

Laboratory personnel should be alert for symptoms of reactions associated with latex contact. Reactions to latex include irritant contact dermatitis, which produces patches of dry, itchy rash on the hands; delayed hypersensitivity reactions resembling poison ivy appearing 24 to 48 hours after exposure; and immediate hypersensitivity reactions characterized by facial flushing and respiratory difficulty (see Chapter 14). Hand sanitizing immediately after removing gloves and avoiding powdered gloves may help prevent the development of latex allergy. Any signs of a latex reaction should be reported to a supervisor because a true latex allergy can be life threatening. Fortunately, allergy to latex has decreased among health care workers because of the availability of other types of gloves.

Critical Thinking 8-1

A laboratorian noticed a dry itchy red rash on their hands after removing their gloves. What could be the cause of this rash? What other reactions could occur? How can this situation be resolved?

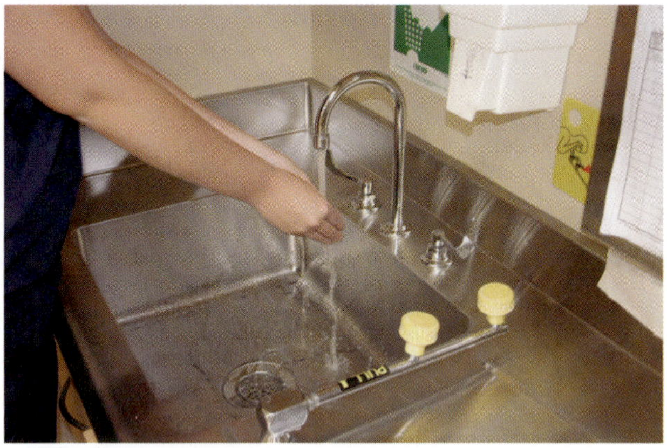

1. Remove your jewelry. Wet your hands with warm water. Do not allow parts of the body to touch the sink.

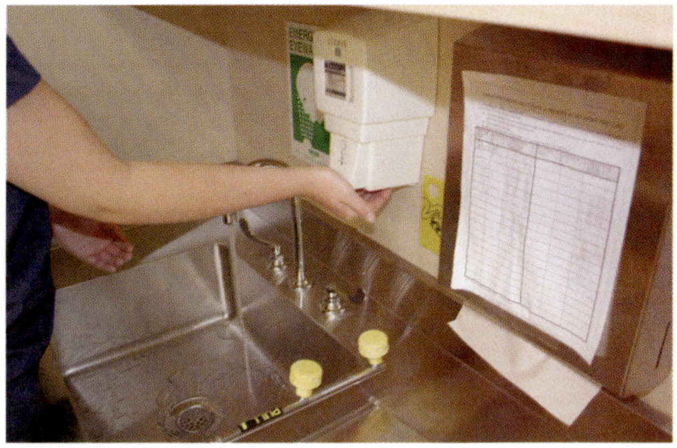

2. Apply soap, preferably antimicrobial.

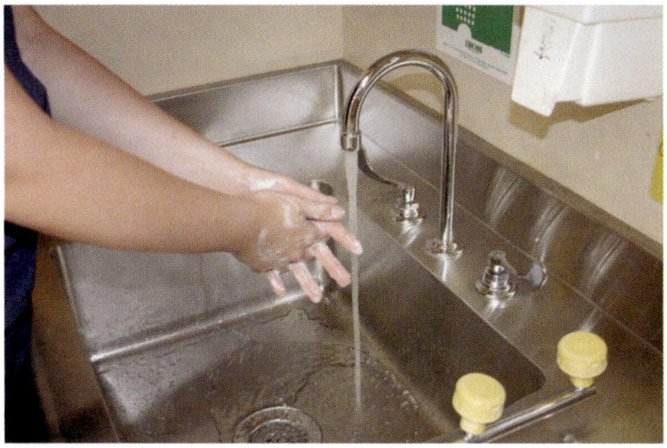

3. Rub to form a lather, create friction, and loosen debris. Thoroughly clean between your fingers and under your fingernails for at least 20 seconds; include thumbs and wrists in the cleaning.

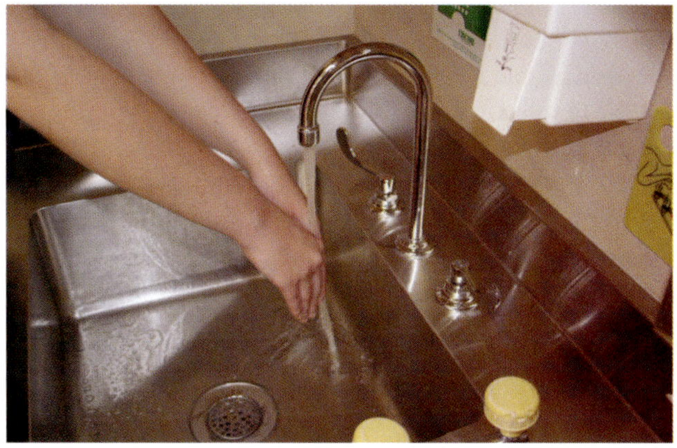

4. Rinse your hands in a downward position to prevent recontamination of hands and wrists.

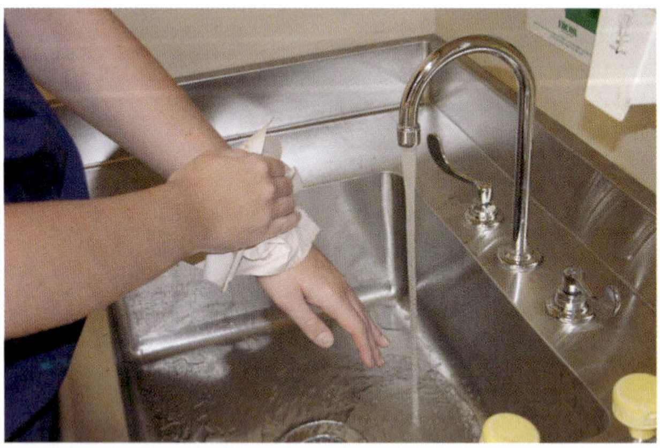

5. Dry your hands with a paper towel.

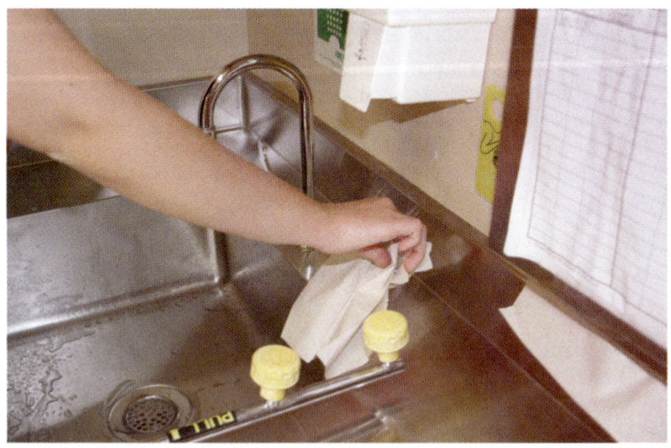

6. Turn off the faucets with a clean paper towel to prevent contamination.

FIGURE 8–2 Hand hygiene.

Laboratory coats. In the immunology laboratory, fluid-resistant laboratory coats with wrist cuffs are always worn to protect skin and clothing from contamination by patient specimens. They must be completely buttoned, with gloves pulled over the cuffs. Both gloves and laboratory coats should be changed as soon as possible if they become visibly soiled and must be removed when leaving the laboratory.

Masks, goggles, and face shields. The mucous membranes of the eyes, nose, and mouth must be protected from specimen splashes and aerosols. A variety of protective equipment is available, including goggles, full-face plastic shields, and Plexiglas countertop shields **(Fig. 8–3).** To avoid splashes and aerosols, remove specimen caps under a Plexiglas shield or with gauze. Transfer pipettes should be used when aliquoting samples from a specimen

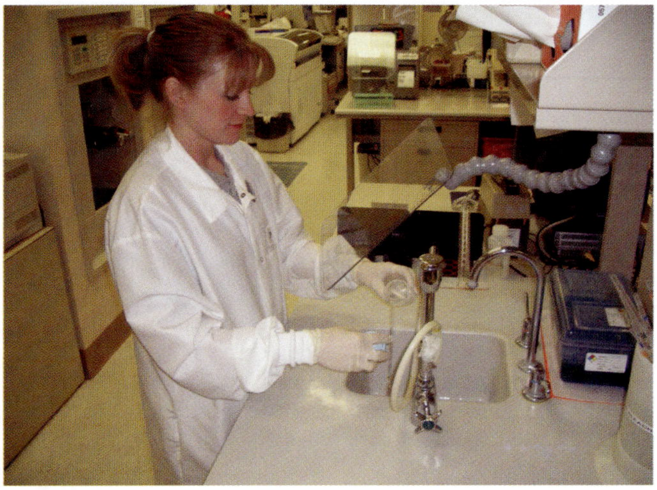

FIGURE 8–3 PPE using a plastic shield.

container. Never centrifuge specimens in uncapped tubes or in uncovered centrifuges. When specimens are received in containers with contaminated exteriors, the exterior of the container must be disinfected; if necessary, a new specimen may be requested.

Standard Precautions (SPs)

The CDC developed SPs by combining recommendations of Universal Precautions (UPs) and Body Substance Isolation (BSI) procedures. Under UPs, all patients were assumed to be potential carriers of **bloodborne pathogens (BBPs).** The BSI modified UPs by requiring that gloves be worn when encountering blood or any other body substance. The CDC continually modifies SPs as changes occur in the health care environment. SPs assume every person in the health care setting is potentially infected or colonized by an organism that could be transmitted. SPs apply to blood, all body fluids, mucous membranes, and nonintact skin and emphasize hand sanitizing.

SPs that apply directly to the laboratory are as follows:

- **Hand hygiene:** Hand hygiene includes both handwashing and the use of alcohol-based antiseptic cleansers. Sanitize hands with soap and water or alcohol-based antiseptic cleansers after touching blood, body fluids, secretions, excretions, and contaminated items, whether or not gloves are worn. Sanitize hands immediately after removing gloves, between patient contacts, and when otherwise indicated to avoid transfer of microorganisms to other environments.
- **Gloves:** Wear gloves (clean, nonsterile, latex-free gloves are adequate) when touching blood, body fluids, secretions, excretions, and contaminated items. Remove gloves promptly after use, before touching noncontaminated items and environmental surfaces, and before going to another patient. Sanitize hands immediately to avoid transfer of microorganisms to other patients or environments.
- **Mouth, nose, and eye protection:** Wear a mask and eye protection or a face shield to protect mucous membranes of the eyes, nose, and mouth during procedures and patient-care activities that are likely to generate splashes or sprays of blood, body fluids, secretions, and excretions.
- **Gown:** Wear a gown (a clean, nonsterile gown is adequate) to protect skin and to prevent soiling of clothing during procedures that are likely to generate splashes of blood, body fluids, secretions, or excretions. Select a gown that is appropriate for the activity and amount of fluid likely to be encountered (e.g., fluid-resistant gown). Remove a soiled gown before leaving the laboratory environment and sanitize hands to avoid transfer of microorganisms to other environments.
- **Respiratory hygiene and cough etiquette:** Educate health care personnel, patients, and visitors to contain respiratory secretions to prevent droplet and fomite transmission of respiratory pathogens. Offer masks to coughing patients, distance symptomatic patients from others, and practice good hand hygiene to prevent transmission of respiratory pathogens.
- **Needles:** Never recap used needles or otherwise manipulate them using both hands. Never use any technique that involves directing the point of a needle toward any part of the body; rather, use self-sheathing needles or a mechanical device designed to conceal the needle. Do not remove unsheathed needles from disposable syringes by hand; use a mechanical device. Do not bend, break, or otherwise manipulate used needles by hand. Place used disposable syringes and needles, scalpel blades, and other sharp items in appropriate puncture-resistant containers. Place reusable syringes and needles in a puncture-resistant container for transport to the reprocessing area. (See *Sharps Hazards* later for additional information.)

Knowledge Check 8-1

All of the following are examples of PPE *except:*

a. Gloves
b. Lab coats
c. Anti-bacterial soap
d. Countertop shields

Occupational Exposure to Bloodborne Pathogens

The federal government has enacted regulations to protect health care workers from exposure to BBPs. These regulations are monitored and enforced by OSHA. The Occupational Exposure to Bloodborne Pathogens Standard requires all employers to have a written Bloodborne Pathogen Exposure Control Plan and to provide necessary protection, free of charge, for employees. A later compliance directive called *Enforcement Procedures for the Occupational Exposure to Bloodborne Pathogens Standard* places more emphasis on using engineering controls to prevent accidental exposure to BBPs. The components of the current Bloodborne Pathogens Exposure Control Plan that is required of all institutions are shown in **Box 8-1.** Each health care facility is responsible for designing and implementing its own exposure control plan.

Any accidental exposure to blood through needlestick, mucous membranes, or nonintact skin must be reported to a supervisor, and a confidential medical examination must be immediately started. Evaluation of the incident must begin right away to ensure that appropriate **postexposure prophy-**

8-1 In the Laboratory

Components of the OSHA Bloodborne Pathogen Exposure Control Plan

Engineering Controls

1. Providing sharps disposal containers and needles with safety devices
2. Requiring discarding of needles with the safety device activated and the holder attached
3. Labeling all biohazardous materials and containers

Work Practice Controls

1. Requiring all employees to practice SPs and documenting training on an annual basis
2. Prohibiting eating, drinking, smoking, and applying cosmetics in the work area
3. Establishing a daily work surface disinfection protocol

Personal Protective Equipment

1. Providing laboratory coats, gowns, face shields, and gloves to employees and laundry facilities for nondisposable protective clothing

Medical

1. Providing immunization for the hepatitis B virus free of charge
2. Providing medical follow-up to employees who have been accidentally exposed to BBPs

Documentation

1. Documenting annual training of employees in safety standards
2. Documenting evaluations and implementation of safer needle devices
3. Involving employees in the selection and evaluation of new devices and maintaining a list of those employees and the evaluations
4. Maintaining a sharps injury log, including the type and brand of safety device, location, and description of the incident, and confidential employee follow-up

8-2 In the Laboratory

Postexposure Prophylaxis (PEP)

1. Draw a baseline blood specimen from the employee and test it for HBV, HCV, and HIV.
2. If possible, identify the source patient; collect a blood specimen; and test it for HBV, HCV, and HIV. Patients must usually give informed consent for these tests, and they do not become part of the patient's record. In some states, a physician's order or court order can replace patient consent because a needlestick is considered a significant exposure.
3. Testing must be completed within 24 hours for maximum benefit from PEP.

Source Patient Tests Positive for HIV

1. Employee is counseled about receiving PEP using anti-retroviral medications.
2. Medications are started within 24 hours.
3. Employee is retested at intervals of 6 weeks, 12 weeks, and 6 months.
4. Additional evaluation and counseling are needed if the source patient is unidentified or untested.

Source Patient Tests Positive for HBV

1. Unvaccinated employees can be given hepatitis B immune globulin (HBIG) and HBV vaccine.
2. Vaccinated employees are tested for immunity and receive PEP, if necessary.

Source Patient Tests Positive for HCV

1. No PEP is available.
2. Employee is monitored for early detection of HCV infection and treated appropriately.
3. Any exposed employee should be counseled to report any symptoms related to viral infection that occur within 12 weeks of the exposure.

laxis (PEP) is initiated within 24 hours. Needlesticks are the most frequently encountered exposure and place laboratory personnel in danger of contracting bloodborne infections with HIV, hepatitis B virus (HBV), and hepatitis C virus (HCV). The CDC has recommended procedures to prevent these infections (see **Box 8-2**).

Biological Waste Disposal

All biological waste, except urine, must be placed in appropriate leakproof containers labeled with the **biohazard** symbol and decontaminated, usually by incineration, autoclaving, or pick up by a certified hazardous waste company before disposal. This includes specimens and the materials with which the specimens came in contact. Any supplies contaminated with blood and body fluids must also be disposed of in containers clearly marked with the biohazard symbol or with red or yellow color coding. These supplies include alcohol pads, gauze, bandages, disposable tourniquets, gloves, masks, gowns, and plastic tubes and pipettes. Urine can be discarded down the sink. The sink should be rinsed well with water and cleaned daily with a 1:10 sodium hypochlorite solution (bleach). Disposal of needles and other sharp objects is discussed in the section, *Sharps Hazards.*

Decontamination

Contaminated nondisposable equipment, blood spills, and blood and body fluid processing areas must be disinfected regularly. Laboratory countertops should be disinfected after every work shift and after any spill occurs. The CDC recommends the use of a 1:10 dilution of sodium hypochlorite (household bleach) prepared weekly and stored in a plastic, not glass, bottle. The solution should be allowed to air-dry on the contaminated area. Other products are commercially available in prefilled spray bottles or single-use wipes. However, it must be confirmed that the product is effective enough to eliminate most bacteria, including *Mycobacterium tuberculosis,* fungi, and viruses. It is also important to know the contact time needed for disinfectant chemical products to work effectively on laboratory surfaces as prescribed by the manufacturer.

When spills occur, do not mop or wipe the fluid; instead, use absorbent powder (e.g., Zorbitrol) or paper towels to remove as much fluid as possible before disinfecting. When using an absorbent powder, the liquid will solidify and can be scooped up. If paper towels are used to absorb the liquid, pour bleach over the towels. Dispose of the absorbent material and paper towels used for disinfection in the appropriate biohazard container. Disinfect the spill area with bleach or a phenol solution.

Transporting Patient Specimens

When a laboratory accepts specimens from other health care institutions, it is important to know the regulations for packaging, transporting, and receiving these specimens. The U.S. Department of Transportation (DOT) and the International Air Transport Association (IATA) have designated two classifications for infectious substances, and they regulate the interstate shipping of these infectious substances and diagnostic specimens.

Category A infectious substances can cause permanent disability or life-threatening disease in otherwise healthy humans or animals upon exposure. A culture of *Bacillus anthracis* is an example of a category A infectious substance.

Category B infectious substances are not generally capable of causing permanent disability or life-threatening or fatal disease in otherwise healthy humans or animals upon exposure. A blood specimen to be transported to a reference laboratory for cholesterol testing represents a category B classification.

DOT and IATA Specimen Transport. The DOT stipulates strict guidelines for specimen packaging and labeling. Under DOT and IATA regulations, all diagnostic specimens require triple packaging **(Fig. 8–4)** that includes the following:

- The primary container (glass, metal, or plastic) must be watertight with a positive (screw-on) cap.
- The primary container is enclosed in a secondary container with sufficient absorbent material capable of absorbing all its contents in case of leakage or breakage. Multiple specimens must be wrapped individually before placing them in the leakproof secondary container, such as a biohazard bag.
- The secondary container must be placed in a sturdy outer container made of corrugated fiberboard, wood, metal, or rigid plastic. An itemized list of contents in a sealed plastic bag is also placed in the outer container. Ensure that specimens are kept cool by transporting them in Styrofoam containers using plastic refrigerant packs. Do not place refrigerant packs directly on or against the specimen containers. Place them between the secondary and the outer container. Additional measures must be taken when using ice and dry ice. Specimens that must remain frozen should be packaged in CO_2-permeable containers with dry ice. Add a class 9 miscellaneous label when the package contains dry ice.

Courier-Delivered Specimen Transport. Specimens transported by a hospital courier among clinics, physicians' offices, and the hospital laboratory are exempt from most DOT rules, unless they are suspected of containing an infectious substance. If specimens may contain an infectious substance, then all DOT rules apply. The transport vehicle should be used exclusively for transporting specimens and should be equipped to secure the transport containers. Minimum shipping standards for this type of transportation include the following:

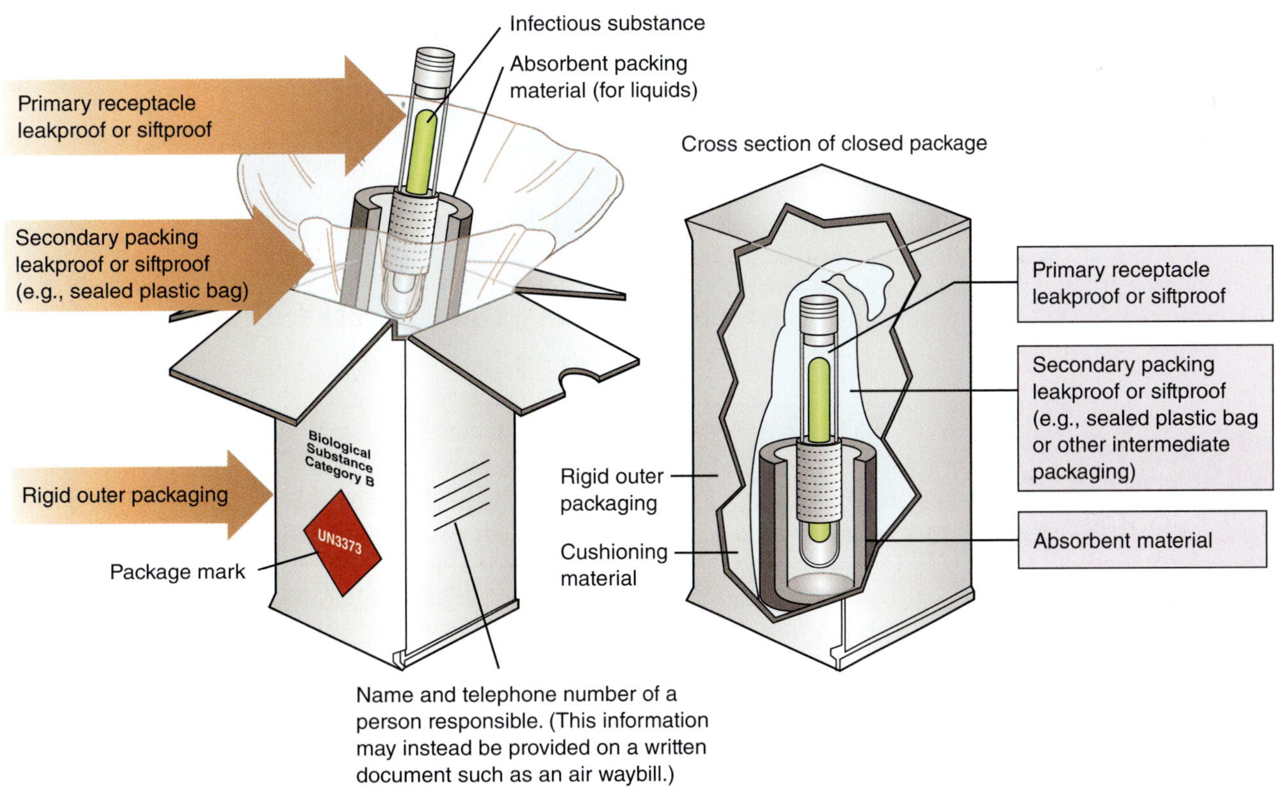

FIGURE 8–4 Packing and labeling of category B infectious substances. If multiple fragile primary receptacles are placed in a single secondary package, they must be either individually wrapped or separated to prevent contact. *(Adapted from Transporting Infectious Substances Safely, U.S. Department of Transportation. Pipeline and Hazardous Materials Safety Administration, 2006.)*

- Leakproof, watertight specimen containers
- Tightly capped tubes placed in a rack to maintain an upright position
- Leakproof inner packaging surrounded by enough absorbent material to completely absorb all the liquid present
- A leakproof plastic or metal transport box with a secure, tight-fitting cover
- Properly labeled transport boxes accompanied by specimen data and identification forms

Specimens picked up by a courier that are to be shipped to an out-of-the-area laboratory, such as a reference laboratory, must follow DOT regulations. Many of these laboratories supply shipping containers to their clients.

Critical Thinking 8-2

A medical laboratory professional places tightly capped potentially infectious serum tubes in a rack and places the rack and the specimen data in a labeled, leakproof metal courier box. Is there anything wrong with this scenario?

Sharps Hazards

Sharp objects in the laboratory, including needles, lancets, and broken glassware, present a serious biological hazard for possible exposure to BBPs caused by accidental puncture. Although BBPs are also transmitted through contact with mucous membranes and nonintact skin, a needle or lancet used to collect blood can produce a significant exposure to BBPs. It is essential that safety precautions always be followed when sharp hazards are present.

The number one personal safety rule when handling needles is to *never* recap a needle. Many types of safety devices are available for needle disposal that provide a variety of safeguards. These include needle holders that become a sheath, needles that automatically resheath or become blunt, and needles with attached sheaths. All sharps must be disposed of in puncture-resistant, leakproof containers labeled with the biohazard symbol **(Fig. 8–5).** Containers should be near the work area. The biohazard sharp containers should not be more than three-fourths full and must always be replaced when the waste level inside reaches the safe capacity mark. Never use any technique that involves directing the point of a needle toward any part of the body.

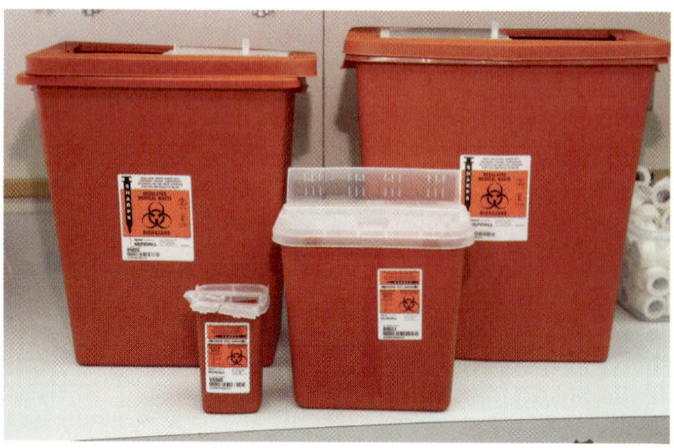

FIGURE 8–5 Examples of puncture-resistant containers.

Chemical Hazards

Serological testing may involve the use of chemical reagents that must be handled in a safe manner to avoid injury. The general rules for safe handling of chemicals include taking precautions to avoid getting chemicals on the body, clothes, and work area; wearing PPE such as safety goggles when pouring chemicals; preparing reagents under a fume hood, observing strict labeling practices; and following instructions carefully. Chemicals should never be mixed together unless specific instructions are followed, and they must be added in the order specified. This is particularly important when combining acid and water because acid should always be added to water, rather than adding water to acid, to avoid the possibility of sudden splashing. Chemicals should be in containers that are of an easily manageable size. Pipetting by mouth is unacceptable in the laboratory.

When skin or eye contact with chemicals occurs, the best first aid is to immediately flush the area with large amounts of water for at least 15 minutes and then seek medical attention. For this reason, laboratory personnel should know the location and proper use of the emergency shower and eyewash station. No attempt should be made to neutralize chemicals that come in contact with the skin.

Knowledge Check 8-2

When combining acid and water:

a. Acid is added to water.
b. Water is added to acid.
c. Water is slowly added to acid.
d. Both solutions are combined simultaneously.

Safety Data Sheets (SDSs)

The OSHA Federal Hazard Communication Standard requires that all employees have a right to know about all chemical hazards present in their workplace. All chemicals and reagents containing hazardous ingredients in a concentration greater than 1% are required by OSHA to have a **Safety Data Sheet (SDS)** on file in the workplace. By law, vendors must provide these sheets to purchasers; however, the facility itself is responsible for obtaining and making SDSs available to employees. Information contained in an SDS includes the following:

- Physical and chemical characteristics
- Fire and explosion potential
- Reactivity
- Health hazards and emergency first aid procedures
- Methods for safe handling and disposal
- Primary routes of entry
- Exposure limits and carcinogenic potential

State and federal regulations should be consulted for the disposal of chemicals. Containers of chemicals that pose a high risk must be labeled with a chemical hazard symbol representing the possible hazard, such as flammable, poison, corrosive, and so on **(Fig. 8–6)**.

The Globally Harmonized System (GHS) of Classification and Labeling of Chemicals

The **Globally Harmonized System (GHS)** is an international effort to standardize both the classification of hazardous chemicals and the symbols used to communicate these hazards on labels and in SDS documentation. It includes criteria for the classification of health, physical, and environmental hazards. The standard label elements include GHS pictograms, signal words, and a GHS hazard statement **(Fig. 8–7)**. The SDS under GHS provides a clear description of the data used to identify hazards and has 16 sections in a specified order.

OSHA aligned its Hazard Communication Standard with the GHS and requires that all employees be trained on the new label elements and SDS format. Adoption of the GHS in the United States has increased awareness and understanding of hazards in the workplace.

FIGURE 8–6 Chemical hazard symbols.

Chemical Hygiene Plan

OSHA requires that all facilities that use hazardous chemicals have a written **Chemical Hygiene Plan** available to employees. The purpose of the plan is to detail the following:

- Individual chemical hygiene responsibilities
- Standard operating procedures
- PPE
- Engineering controls, such as fume hoods and inflammable safety cabinets
- Laboratory equipment
- Safety equipment
- Chemical management

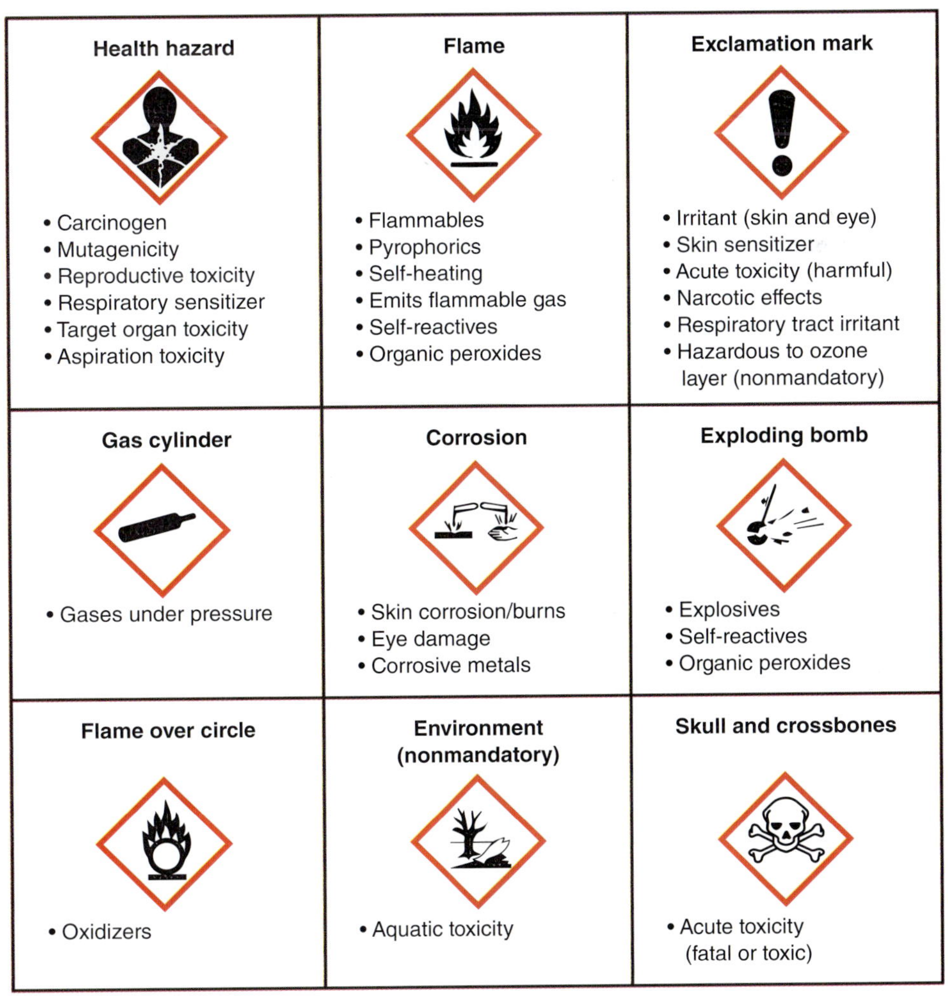

FIGURE 8–7 GHS pictograms and hazards chart. *(Courtesy of U.S. Department of Labor.)*

- Housekeeping
- Emergency procedures for accidents and spills
- Chemical waste
- Employee training
- Safety rules and regulations
- Laboratory design and ventilation
- Exposure monitoring
- Compressed gas safety
- Medical consultation guidelines

Each facility must appoint a chemical hygiene officer who is responsible for implementing and documenting compliance with the plan.

Chemical Spills

The SDS gives specific information for the appropriate action to be taken for a chemical spill. Chemical spill kits containing protective apparel, nonreactive absorbent material, and disposable bags and waste tags for disposing of contaminated materials should be available for cleaning up spills. Liquids are absorbed using a neutralizer, such as sodium bicarbonate, and a sand mixture or ground clay. After the liquid is absorbed, it is scooped up and placed into a waste bag and labeled appropriately for disposal. The area is then cleaned thoroughly.

Chemical Waste Disposal

Any hazardous chemical waste should be disposed of per current Environmental Protection Agency (EPA) regulations. Most reagents used in the laboratory come with an SDS that gives specific information for disposal of chemicals. All chemicals used should be disposed of by following the SDS directions. Many kits used in immunologic testing often contain sodium azide as a preservative, which can be disposed of by flushing it down the drain with plenty of water. Sinks and drains should be flushed with large amounts of water after disposal of chemical waste to avoid buildup in plumbing.

Radioactive Hazards

Radioactivity may be encountered in the clinical laboratory when procedures using radioisotopes for tests such as radioimmunoassay are performed. The amount of radioactivity present in most medical situations is very small and represents little danger; however, the effects of radiation are cumulative related to the length of exposure. The amount of radiation exposure is related to a combination of time, distance, and shielding. People working in a radioactive environment are required to wear measuring devices to determine the amount of radiation exposure that they are accumulating.

Laboratory personnel should be familiar with the radioactive symbol shown in **Figure 8–8.** This symbol must be displayed on the doors of all areas where radioactive material is present. Exposure to radiation during pregnancy presents a danger to the fetus; personnel who are or who think they may be pregnant should avoid areas with this symbol.

Medical Radioactive Waste Disposal

Disposal of medical radioactive waste is regulated by the Nuclear Regulatory Commission (NRC) and is also subject to local regulations. Such waste must be separated from other waste materials in the laboratory and placed in containers marked with the radioactive symbol. Disposal varies with the type of material (solid, liquid, or volatile chemical) and depends on the amount of radioactivity present. Very few clinical laboratories use radioactivity in testing anymore, mainly because of the problem of waste disposal. If radioactivity is used, the laboratory typically contracts with a waste disposal service that picks up the radioactive waste material.

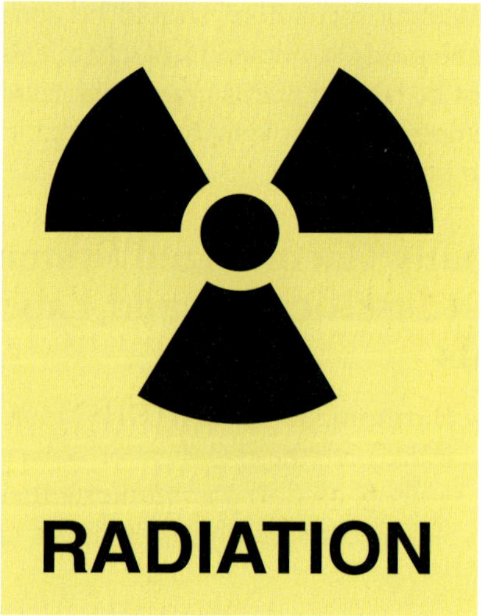

FIGURE 8–8 Radioactive symbol.

Electrical Hazards

The laboratory setting contains electrical equipment with which workers have frequent contact. The same general rules of electrical safety observed outside the workplace apply in the laboratory. The danger of water or fluid coming in contact with equipment is greater in the laboratory setting. Equipment should not be operated with wet hands. Designated hospital personnel monitor electrical equipment closely; however, laboratory personnel should continually observe for any dangerous conditions, such as frayed cords or overloaded circuits, and report them to the supervisor. Equipment that has become wet should be unplugged and allowed to dry completely before reusing. Equipment also should be unplugged before cleaning. All electrical equipment must be grounded with three-pronged plugs.

When an accident involving electrical shock occurs, the electrical source must be removed immediately. This must be done without touching the person or the equipment involved to avoid transferring the current. Turning off the circuit breaker, unplugging the equipment, or moving the equipment using a nonconductive glass or wood object are safe procedures to follow. The victim should receive immediate medical assistance following discontinuation of the electricity. Cardiopulmonary resuscitation (CPR) may be necessary.

Fire and Explosive Hazards

Clinical laboratory work involves the use of potentially volatile or explosive chemicals that require special procedures for handling and storage. Flammable chemicals should be stored in safety cabinets and explosion-proof refrigerators. Cylinders of compressed gas should be located away from heat and securely fastened to a stationary device to prevent accidental tipping. Fire blankets should be present in the laboratory. Persons with burning clothes should be wrapped in the blanket to smother the flames.

The Joint Commission (TJC), an independent body that certifies and accredits health care organizations in the United States, requires that all health care facilities post evacuation routes and detailed plans to follow in the event of a fire. Laboratory personnel should be familiar with these procedures. When a fire is discovered, all employees are expected to take the actions described by the acronym RACE **(Box 8-3).**

8-3 In the Laboratory

RACE

1. Rescue—rescue anyone in immediate danger.
2. Alarm—activate the institutional fire alarm system.
3. Contain—close all doors to potentially affected areas.
4. Extinguish or Evacuate—attempt to extinguish the fire if possible, or evacuate, closing the door.

The National Fire Protection Association (NFPA) classifies fires with regard to the type of burning material and classifies the type of fire extinguisher that is used to control them. The multipurpose ABC fire extinguishers are the most common, but always check the label before using the extinguisher. The code word PASS can be used to remember the steps in operating a fire extinguisher **(Box 8-4).**

8-4 In the Laboratory

PASS

1. Pull pin.
2. Aim at the base of the fire.
3. Squeeze handles.
4. Sweep nozzle side to side.

The Standard System for the Identification of the Fire Hazard of Materials, NFPA 704, is a symbol system used to inform firefighters of the hazards they may encounter when fighting a fire in a particular area. The color-coded areas contain information relating to health, flammability, reactivity, use of water, and personal protection. These symbols are placed on doors, cabinets, and reagent bottles. Examples of hazardous material symbols and information are shown in **Figure 8–9.**

Physical Hazards

Physical hazards are not unique to the laboratory; routine precautions observed outside the workplace apply. General pre-

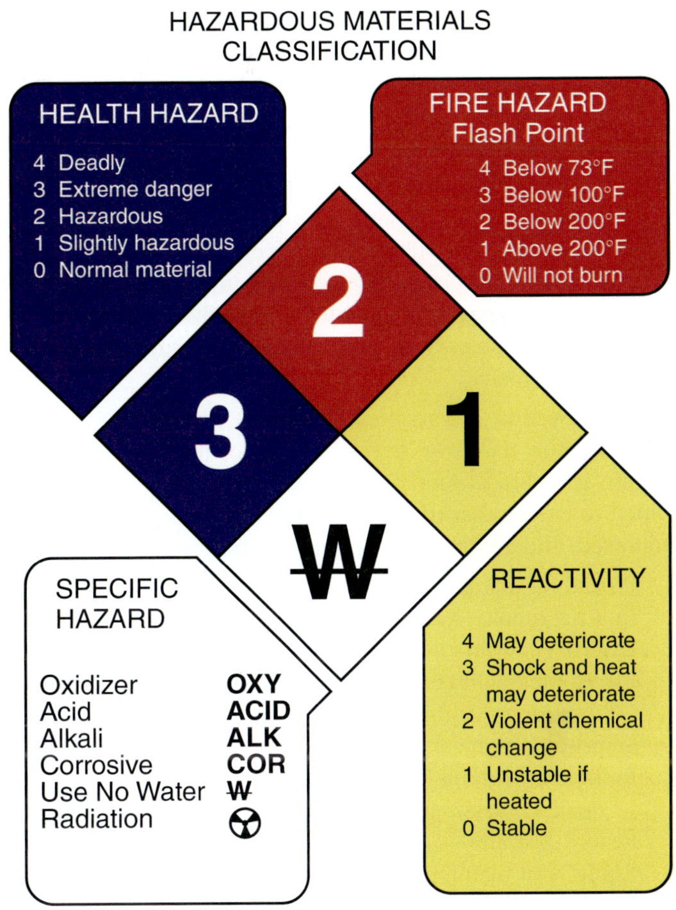

FIGURE 8–9 NFPA hazardous material symbol and classification.

cautions to consider are to avoid running in rooms and hallways, watch for wet floors, bend the knees when lifting heavy objects, keep long hair pulled back, avoid dangling jewelry, and maintain a clean, organized work area. Closed-toed shoes that provide maximum support are essential for safety and comfort.

Quality Management

The term **quality management (QM)** refers to the overall process of guaranteeing quality patient care, and it is regulated throughout the total testing system. QM is the continual monitoring of the entire test process, from test ordering and specimen collection through reporting and interpreting results. Written policies and documented actions as they pertain to the patient, the laboratory, ancillary personnel, and the health care provider are required. Written remedial actions mandating the steps to take when any part of the system fails are also essential to a QM program. QM in the clinical laboratory is an integration of many factors used to monitor, evaluate, and improve the quality of laboratory services through all three phases of patient testing.

A quality management system (QMS) refers to all the laboratory's policies, processes, procedures, and resources needed to achieve quality testing. Several factors, or **variables,** if changed or altered, can affect test results. Therefore, a QMS includes not only testing controls, referred to as *quality control* (QC), but also encompasses the following variables:

- **Preexamination variables** (formerly referred to as *preanalytical* variables; include specimen collection, handling, and storage)
- **Examination variables** (formerly called *analytical* variables; e.g., reagent and test performance, instrument calibration and maintenance, personnel requirements, technical competence, review, and interpretation)
- **Postexamination variables** (formerly called *postanalytical* variables; e.g., reporting of results and specimen management)

Identification of variables throughout the testing process provides the basis for developing procedures and policies within the clinical laboratory. Documentation must be provided to ensure that the QMS program is being meticulously followed, and all the following must be included:

Procedure manuals
Internal quality control
External control
Electronic quality control
Calibration or calibration verification
Standardization
Proficiency testing (PT), more formally known as external quality assessment (EQA)
Record-keeping
Equipment maintenance
Safety programs
Training
Education and competency assessment of personnel
A review process that is scheduled and documented

The **Clinical Laboratory Improvement Amendments (CLIA)** are regulations that specify required components for QM, including patient test management assessment, quality control (QC) assessment, proficiency testing assessment, comparison of test results, relationship of patient information to patient test results, patient confidentiality, specimen identification and integrity, personnel competency, personnel qualifications and evaluations, communication protocols, complaint investigations, review with staff, and maintenance of records for 2 years.

Documentation of QM procedures is required by all laboratory **accreditation** agencies, including TJC, the College of American Pathologists (CAP), the Association for the Advancement of Blood and Biotherapies (AABB), the American Osteopathic Association (AOA), the American Society for Histocompatibility and Immunogenetics (ASHI), the American Association for Laboratory Accreditation (A2LA), and the **Commission on Laboratory Accreditation (COLA);** it is also required for Medicare and Medicaid reimbursement. Guidelines published by CAP and the **Clinical and Laboratory Standards Institute (CLSI)** provide complete instructions for documentation and are used as a reference for our discussion of the specific areas of immunology QM and QC that follows. Documentation in the form of a procedure manual is required in all laboratories. This format is used as the basis for the following discussion.

Immunology Procedure Manual

A procedure manual (paper or digital) containing all the procedures performed in the immunology section of the laboratory must be available for reference in the working area and must comply with the CLSI guidelines. The following information is included for each procedure:

- Principle and purpose
- Clinical significance
- Patient identification and preparation
- Specimen type and method of collection
- Specimen labeling
- Specimen preservation
- Conditions of transport and storage before testing
- Specimen acceptability and criteria for rejection
- Reagents
- Standards and controls acceptability and expiration policy
- Instrument calibration and maintenance protocols and schedules
- Step-by-step procedure
- Calculations
- Frequency and tolerance limits for controls and corrective actions
- Reference values and critical values
- Interpretation of results
- Common interferences
- Specific procedure notes
- Limitations of the method
- Method validation
- Confirmatory testing
- Recording of results
- References
- Effective date
- Author
- Review schedule

Current package inserts for all test kits should be reviewed and available at the workplace. The laboratory must also have a documented procedure for the correction of erroneous results.

The printed procedural manuals and electronic procedural manuals are subject to proper document control. Only authorized persons may make changes, and these changes must be dated and signed (manually or digitally). The manuals must undergo periodic review; documentation of the review is included in the manual.

Evaluating procedures and adopting new methods is an ongoing process in the clinical laboratory. Whenever changes are made, a person with designated authority, such as the laboratory director or section supervisor, should review and reference the procedure, and then sign off on the change. Personnel should be notified of the changes. There must be documentation of an annual review of all procedures by the designated authority.

The procedure manual provides the basis for all testing in the clinical laboratory. Quality care in testing relies on strictly following procedures as written. Documentation includes every step, from specimen collection to the reporting of results. A well-documented QM program ensures quality test results and patient care.

Preexamination Variables

Preexamination (preanalytical) variables occur before the actual testing of the specimen and include test requests, patient preparation, timing, specimen collection, handling and transport, and storage. Health care personnel outside of the laboratory control many of these factors, such as ordering tests and specimen collection. Communication between departments and adequate training on the correct procedures for ordering a test (test utilization), collecting, and transporting the specimen improve the **turnaround time (TAT)** of results, avoid duplication of test orders, and ensure a high-quality specimen. TAT is the amount of time required between the point at which a test is ordered by the health care provider until the time results are reported to the health care provider. Laboratories determine the TAT for tests, including both stat and routine tests, as appropriate. Then the laboratory can monitor the TATs to determine areas in the process that need improvement.

Specimen Collection and Documentation

The beginning of each procedure listed in the manual should state specific information on specimen collection and handling. Requisition forms and electronic entry forms should designate the type of specimen to be collected and the time and date of collection. The form should include space for documenting (1) the patient's first and last name, (2) the patient's identification number, (3) the patient's sex, (4) the patient's age or date of birth, (5) the name of the person requesting the test, (6) the name of the person to contact with critical results, (7) the name of the test ordered, (8) any special handling requirements, (9) the time and date of specimen collection, (10) the time the specimen was delivered to the laboratory, and (11) any additional information pertinent to laboratory interpretation. Information regarding patient preparation (e.g., fasting or elimination of interfering medications) and the type and volume of specimen required must be included in the specific procedure.

Criteria for specimen rejection for both physical characteristics and labeling errors must be present. When a specimen is rejected, the criteria for rejecting that specimen must be documented and available to the health care provider and nursing staff. Laboratory personnel must determine the suitability of a specimen and document any problems and corrective actions taken. This enables the laboratory director to capture the information to determine a **root cause analysis (RCA)** and develop a preventive or corrective action plan. Laboratory information systems are able to electronically generate these forms for review. An acceptable specimen requires verification of the patient's identification information on the requisition form and the tube label, proper collection and processing procedures, and timely transport to the laboratory.

8-1 Clinical Correlations

The Importance of Biological Sex

Test requisition forms include much information so that a patient sample can be correctly identified. In addition to being an identifier, the patient's sex is also important to know because factors like hormones and hormone treatment, body size, and sex chromosomes/genes and can affect the results of many laboratory tests (e.g., hemoglobin, iron levels, cardiac troponin, creatinine concentration, cytogenetics). For such tests, laboratories have established different reference ranges based on sex to ensure correct interpretation of results.

Examination Variables

The examination (analytical) variables are the processes that directly affect the testing of specimens. They include reagents, instrumentation, and equipment, testing procedure, QC, access to procedure manuals, review and interpretation of results, and the competency of personnel performing the tests. Also included is **preventive maintenance (PM)** (i.e., regular, scheduled maintenance performed proactively to ensure optimal test performance by keeping laboratory instruments in excellent condition); this includes cleaning, lubrication, inspection, and parts replacement.

Reagents

The procedure manual should state the name and chemical formula of each reagent used, instructions for preparation, when necessary, or company source of prepared materials, storage requirements, and procedures for reagent QC. The type of water used for preparing reagents and controls must be specified. Distilled or deionized water or clinical laboratory reagent water (CLRW) must be available. CLRW quality must be monitored regularly for microbial contamination as well as ionic and organic impurities. A written policy must be available with the procedures to follow when the CLRW quality is not within the tolerance limits. A bold-type statement of any safety or health precautions associated with reagents should be present.

All reagents must be properly labeled with the date of preparation or opening, purchase and received date, expiration date, and appropriate safety information. Reagents should be checked against two levels of commercial control solutions on each shift, or at a minimum of once a day and whenever a new reagent is opened. Results of all reagent checks are properly recorded.

Instrumentation and Equipment

The procedure manual should clearly state the instructions for the operation, performance, and frequency of calibration; the limitations of the instrumentation and equipment; and the procedures to follow when limitations or linearity are exceeded (e.g., preparation of dilutions). Instructions detailing the appropriate recording procedures must be included.

Two levels of commercial controls must be run and recorded. There must be documentation of showing evidence of corrective action for any failed QC tests. No testing of patient samples may be performed until QC is acceptable. As mandated by the TJC or CAP guidelines, a routine PM schedule for instruments and equipment should be prepared and records kept of all routine and nonroutine maintenance performed.

Deionized water used for reagent preparation is quality controlled by checking its pH and purity meter resistance on a weekly basis, and the bacterial count on a monthly schedule. All results must be recorded on the appropriate forms.

Testing Procedures

Detailed and concise testing instructions are written in a step-by-step manner. Instructions should begin with specimen preparation, such as time and speed of centrifugation, and include types of glassware needed, time limitations and stability of specimens and reagents, calculation formulas and a sample calculation, health and safety precautions, QC checks, reference ranges, and procedures. Additional procedural information, including reasons for special precautions, sources of error and interfering substances, helpful hints, clinical situations that influence the test, alternative procedures, and acceptable TATs for stat tests are listed under the title of Procedure Notes following the step-by-step procedure.

Reference sources should be listed. The manufacturer's package inserts may be included but cannot replace the written procedure. The laboratory director must sign and date new procedures and all procedure modifications before they are used.

Quality Control

Quality control (QC) refers to the materials, procedures, and techniques that monitor the *accuracy, precision,* and *reliability* of a laboratory test. **Accuracy** is the ability to obtain the expected result, and **precision** is the ability to obtain the same result on the same specimen during duplicate or repeated testing. **Reliability** is the ability to maintain both precision and accuracy.

QC procedures are performed to ensure that acceptable standards are met during the process of patient testing. The step-by-step instructions for each test should include specific QC information regarding the type of control specimen, preparation and handling, frequency of use, tolerance levels, and methods of recording. QC is performed at scheduled times, such as at the beginning of each shift or before testing patient specimens, and it must always be performed if reagents are changed, an instrument malfunction has occurred, or test results are questioned by the health care provider. Control results must be recorded in a paper or electronic log. Patient test results may not be reported until the QC is verified.

External Controls. External controls are used to verify the accuracy and precision of a test, and they are exposed to the same conditions as the patient specimens. Analysis of at least two levels of control material is required. One of these is a high-level control, and the other is a low-level control. The concentrations of the controls should be at medically significant levels and should be as similar to human specimens as possible. Documentation of QC includes dating and initialing the material when it is first opened and recording the manufacturer's lot number and the expiration date each time a control is tested and the test result is obtained. Food and Drug Administration (FDA) standards require that control material test negative for HIV and HBV. The same person who is performing testing on patient samples should perform the testing and interpretation of external controls in the laboratory.

Control data are evaluated before releasing patient results. Data obtained from repeated measurements have a Gaussian distribution or spread in the values that indicate the ability to repeat the analysis and obtain the same value. The laboratory, after repeated testing, establishes the value for each analyte and calculates the **control mean** (the average of all data points) and the **standard deviation (SD)** (a measurement statistic that describes the average distance each data point in a normal distribution is from the mean). The **coefficient of variation (CV)** is the SD expressed as a percentage of the mean. The CV indicates whether the distribution of values around the mean is in a narrow range vs a broad range; an acceptable CV should be less than 5%. *Confidence intervals* are the limits between which the specified proportion or percentage of results will lie. Control ranges are determined by setting confidence limits that are within ±2 SD or ±3 SD of the mean, indicating that 95.5% to 99.7% of the values are expected to be within that range.

Values are plotted on Levey-Jennings control charts to visually monitor control values. Immediate decisions about patient results are based on the ability of control values to remain within a preestablished limit. Changes in the accuracy of results are indicated by either a *trend* or a *shift*. A **trend** is a *gradual* change in the mean in one direction that may be caused by a *gradual* deterioration of reagents, controls, or instrument performance, whereas a **shift** is an *abrupt* change in the mean that may be caused by a malfunction of the instrument, loss of calibration, or a new lot number of reagents **(Fig. 8–10).** Changes in precision are shown by a large amount of scatter around the mean and an uneven distribution above and below the mean that are most often caused by errors in technique.

Corrective action, including the use of new reagents or controls and the verification of lot numbers and expiration dates, must be taken when control values are outside the tolerance limits. All correction actions taken are documented. A protocol for corrective action is shown in **Figure 8–11.** A designated supervisor reviews all the QC results.

Knowledge Check 8-3

Would a control sample that has accidentally become diluted produce a trend or a shift in the Levey-Jennings chart plot?

a. Trend
b. Shift

Laboratories may participate in a commercial QC program. Participating laboratories return results from the same lot of QC material sent by the manufacturer back to the manufacturer for statistical analysis and comparison with other laboratories using the same methodology.

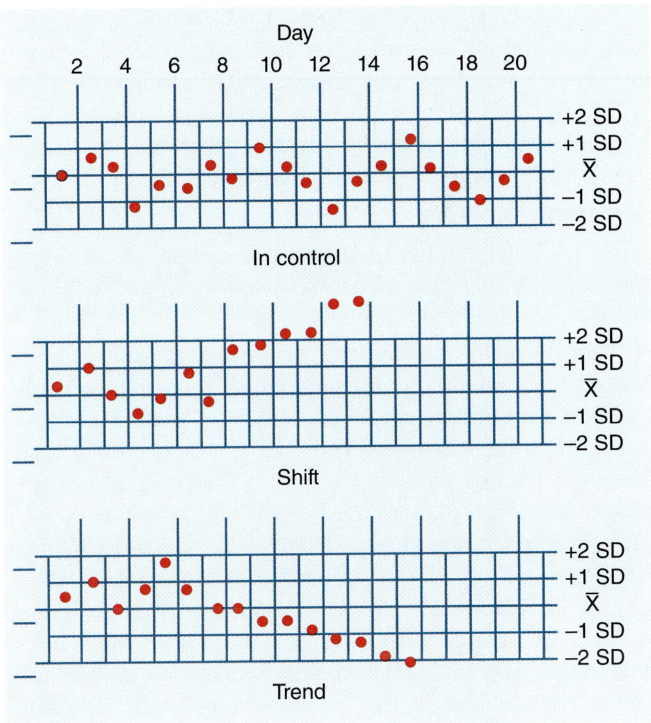

FIGURE 8–10 Levey-Jennings charts showing in-control, shift, and trend results.

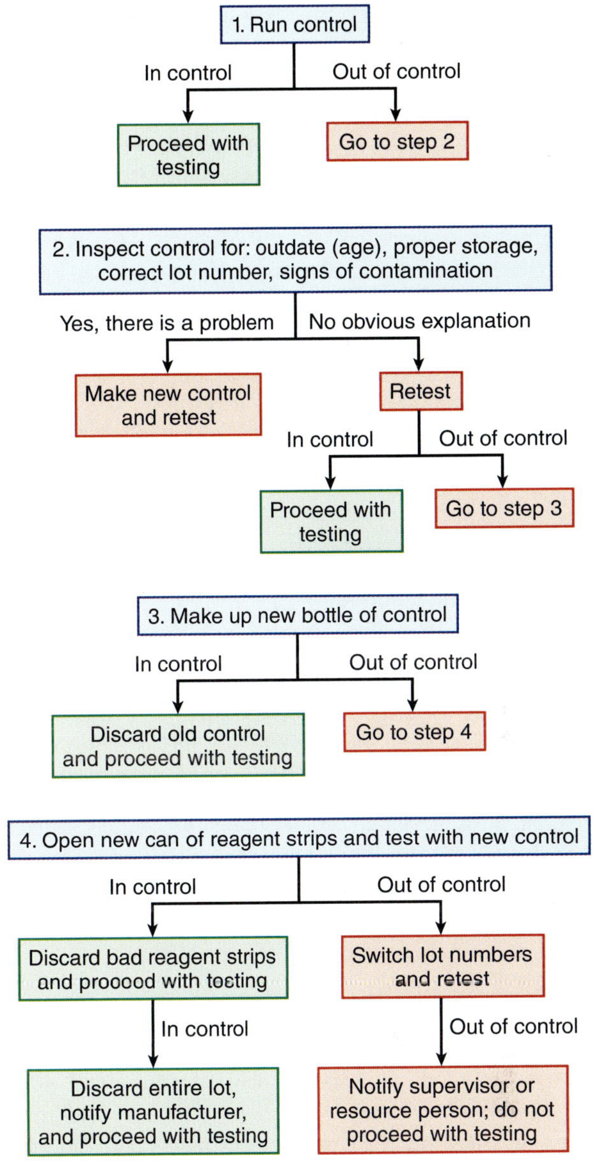

FIGURE 8–11 Procedure for "out of control" results. *(Adapted from Schweitzer SC, Schumann JL, Schumann GB. Quality assurance guidelines for the urinalysis laboratory.* J Med Technol. *1986;3(11):567-572.)*

Internal Controls. Internal controls, also called *procedural controls,* consist of internal monitoring systems built into the test system. Internal controls monitor the sufficient addition of a patient sample or reagent, the interaction between the instrument and reagent, and for lateral flow test methods, whether the sample migrated through the test strip properly (see Chapter 11).

Electronic Controls. Electronic controls use a mechanical or electrical device in place of a liquid QC specimen. This type of QC can be an internal or an external component inserted into a point-of-care (POC) instrument. Electronic controls verify the functional ability of a testing device but do not verify the integrity of the testing supplies. Many test systems use a combination of external and internal controls to verify that the entire test system is working properly.

Proficiency Testing (External Quality Assessment). Proficiency testing, or **external quality assessment (EQA),** is the testing of unknown specimens received from an outside agency. It provides unbiased validation of the accuracy of patient test results. Several commercial vendors, such as the CAP, provide proficiency testing programs. Laboratories subscribing to these programs receive lyophilized or ready-to-use specimens. The results are returned to the proficiency testing vendors, where they are statistically analyzed along with those from all participating laboratories. The laboratory director receives a report from the vendor, which enables the director to evaluate the laboratory's accuracy and compare it with other laboratories using the same method of analysis. The director ensures that the laboratory takes action to correct unacceptable results. The CLIA mandate comparison testing for laboratory accreditation.

Critical Thinking 8-3

The mean value for the level 2 liquid C-reactive protein control was 90 mg/L. While documenting the daily controls, the laboratorian noticed that for the last 6 days, the results for level 2 were trending up with values of 91, 92, 93, 94, 95, and 96 mg/L. What could be the cause of the upward trend in values and how can this be resolved?

Individualized Quality Control Plan. An individualized quality control plan (IQCP) is an alternative CLIA QC option that provides equivalent quality testing to meet the CLIA regulations for moderate- and high-complexity tests and provider-performed microscopy procedures (PPMP). IQCP considers the entire testing process—preexamination, examination, and postexamination—to ensure quality testing, not just the frequency of QC and number of QC materials. With this option, the laboratory can determine the frequency of QC testing based on information about the test, the risk assessment, and the accreditation agencies' requirements.

An IQCP requires risk assessment (RA), a quality control plan (QCP), and quality assessment (QA). RA identifies and evaluates potential problems that may occur in the entire testing process from preexamination through the examination and postexamination processes. Components that are assessed for potential errors are the specimen, test system, reagents, environment, and testing personnel. A QCP establishes control procedures to reduce the possibility of reporting an inaccurate patient test result. It must include the number, type, and frequency of testing, as well as criteria for acceptable results of the QCs. An IQCP QA involves selecting quality monitors that include the following:

- QC records
- Proficiency testing records
- Review of patient results
- Specimen rejection logs
- TAT reports
- Records of preventive measures, corrective actions, and follow-up
- Personnel competency records

Knowledge Check 8-4

What steps are taken when the results of the QC testing are outside of the stated confidence limits?

a. Check the expiration date of the control material.
b. Retest the control.
c. Open a new control bottle.
d. All of the above

Personnel and Facilities

QC is only as good as the personnel performing and monitoring it. Personnel assessment includes education and training, continuing education (CE), competency assessment, and performance appraisals. Each new employee must have documentation of training during their orientation to the laboratory. This is a checklist of procedures, and it must include the date and initials of the person doing the training and of the employee being trained. Up-to-date reference materials and atlases should be readily available, and documentation of CE must be maintained.

An adequate, uncluttered, safe working area is also essential for quality work and personnel morale. SPs for handling body fluids must be followed at all times.

Postexamination Variables

Postexamination variables are processes that affect the reporting of results and correct interpretation of data. Reporting of results to the appropriate health care provider in an efficient and accurate manner is essential to quality patient care. Laboratory reports must be present in the patient record. Required information includes the following:

- Patient's first and last name
- Patient's unique identification number
- Specimen collection date and time
- Specimen source (if pertinent to the test)
- Condition of unsatisfactory specimen
- Tests performed, the results, and the reference ranges of the tests
- Date and time of the final results generated
- Facility where the test was performed

Reporting Results

Reports may be handwritten or instrument printouts. Reports may be delivered by phone or fax or transmitted electronically to the requesting health care provider.

Written Reports. Standardized reporting methods minimize health care provider confusion when interpreting results. Forms for reporting results should provide adequate space for writing and should present the information in a logical sequence. Each procedure covered in the procedure manual should include a standardized reporting format and, when applicable, reference ranges. There must be a written procedure for reporting, reviewing, and correcting errors.

Electronic Results. Electronic transmission is the most common method for reporting results. Many automated instruments have the capability for the operator to electronically transmit results directly from the instrument to the designated health care provider. It is essential that the operator carefully review results before transmittal. The operator may also enter the results manually into the laboratory computer system and then transmit them to the health care provider.

Telephone (Verbal) Results. The telephone is frequently used to convey results of stat tests and critical values. Personnel on hospital units and from health care providers' offices often call requesting additional results. When telephoning results, the laboratorian must confirm that the results are being reported to the appropriate person. The time of the call and the name of the person receiving the results must be documented according to the facility's policy.

Critical Results. There should be written procedures available for the reporting of critical values. *Critical values* are test results that are significantly higher or lower than the normal reference range. They may be life-threatening and must be relayed to the health care provider immediately, following the facility's policy.

Result Errors

Errors may be discovered in the laboratory through a QM procedure known as the **delta check** that compares a patient's test results with their previous results. Variation outside the established parameters alerts laboratory personnel to the possibility of an error that occurred during the testing procedure or in patient identification. Many laboratory analyzers now have **autoverification,** an automated comparison of patient results with predetermined, preapproved criteria programmed into them.

Erroneous results must be corrected in a timely manner to ensure that the patient does not receive treatment based on incorrect results. Errors can occur in patient identification, specimen labeling, or result transcription. The patient's record should be corrected as soon as the error is detected. However, the original result must not be erased if the health care provider treated the patient based on the erroneous results. An incident (variance) report documenting the problem and corrective action may need to be submitted. Appropriate documentation of erroneous results should follow facility protocol. The procedure manual must contain a written procedure for reporting, reviewing, and correcting errors.

Documentation of the reporting of results is essential and required by accrediting agencies. Permanent records of all reported results must also be available. A method to verify the actual reporting of results also must be available and used by all employees.

Interpreting Results

The analytical specificity and sensitivity for each test should be included in the procedure manual for correct interpretation of results. **Analytical sensitivity** (the lowest level of an analyte that a test can detect) and **analytical specificity** (the likelihood of measuring the analyte desired) vary among manufacturers. The procedure manual should list all known interfering substances for evaluation of patient test data. A well-documented QM program ensures quality test results and patient-care data. **Box 8-5** summarizes QM errors in each phase of laboratory testing.

Regulatory Issues

QM is regulated throughout the total testing system. Health care regulation systems include both governmental and public agencies. All agencies have the same goal, which is to provide safe and effective health care.

8-5 In the Laboratory

Summary of Quality Management Errors

Preexamination

Patient misidentification
Wrong test ordered
Incorrect specimen type collected
Insufficient specimen volume
Delayed transport of specimen to the laboratory
Inadequate processing of specimen
Delayed separation of serum or plasma from cells
Incorrect storage of specimen

Examination

Sample misidentification
Erroneous instrument calibration
Reagent deterioration
Poor testing technique
Instrument malfunction
Interfering substances present
Misinterpretation of QC data

Postexamination

Patient misidentification
Poor handwriting
Transcription error
Poor quality of instrument printer
Failure to send report
Failure to call critical values
Inability to identify interfering substances

Clinical Laboratory Improvement Amendments (CLIA)

The CLIA are federal regulations administered by the Centers for Medicare and Medicaid Services (CMS) and the FDA. The regulations provide standards for patient test management, quality assurance, quality control, proficiency testing, personnel qualifications, complaint investigations, and periodic inspections. CLIA stipulates that all laboratories that perform testing on human specimens for the purpose of diagnosis, treatment, monitoring, or screening must be licensed and obtain a certificate from the CMS. Laboratories with CLIA certification are inspected every 2 years to document compliance with the regulations. The inspections may be performed by personnel of the CMS or an accrediting agency recognized by the CMS, such as the CAP, the TJC, COLA, AABB, A2LA, ASHI, or AOA.

The FDA classifies clinical laboratory tests by their complexity into four categories: (1) waived testing, (2) provider-performed microscopy procedures (PPMPs), (3) moderate-complexity testing, and (4) high-complexity testing (see **Box 8-6**). Laboratories must obtain the correct certification for the level of testing complexity performed. For each category, there is a description of the educational level necessary for personnel who may perform the test and the type of quality assessment procedures that must be in place.

Clinical and Laboratory Standards Institute (CLSI)

The CLSI is a global nonprofit organization that publishes recommendations by nationally recognized experts for the performance of laboratory testing. CLSI standards are considered

8-6 In the Laboratory

CLIA Test Classifications

Waived Testing

- Tests considered easy to perform by following the manufacturer's instructions. These tests have little risk of error. No special training or education is required.
- Example: Whole blood infectious mononucleosis rapid test (Monospot)

Provider-Performed Microscopy Procedures (PPMPs)

- Microscopy tests performed by a physician, midlevel practitioner, or dentist
- Example: Microscopic urinalysis

Nonwaived Tests

Moderate-complexity tests

- Tests that require documentation of training in test principles, instrument calibration, periodic proficiency testing, and on-site inspections
- Example: Automated immunoassays

High-complexity tests

- Tests that require sophisticated instrumentation and a high degree of interpretation
- Proficiency testing and on-site inspections are required.
- Example: Immunofixation electrophoresis (IFE)

the standard of care for laboratory procedures. The **standard of care** is the attention, caution, and prudence that a reasonable person in the same circumstances would exercise. In a legal situation, the CLSI standards would be considered the standard of care that should have been met.

The Joint Commission (TJC)

TJC is an independent, nonprofit organization that accredits and certifies more than 22,000 health care organizations and programs in the United States. The mission of TJC is to continuously improve the safety and quality of care provided to the public through the provision of health care accreditation and related services that support performance improvement in health care organizations. To maintain accreditation, organizations must pass an on-site inspection by a survey team every 3 years. Laboratories are inspected every 2 years.

TJC has published *National Patient Safety Goals.* It is essential that health care organizations adhere to these goals to maintain their accreditation. As of 2023, the *National Patient Safety Goals* pertaining to the laboratory are as follows:

- *Identify patients correctly.* Use at least two ways to identify patients who are using laboratory services. For example, use the patient's first and last name, an assigned identification number, and date of birth. The patient's room number or physical location is not used as an identifier. Label containers used for blood and other specimens in the presence of the patient.
- *Improve staff communication.* Get important test results to the right staff member on time. Report critical results of tests to the appropriate health care worker on a timely basis.
- *Prevent infection.* Use the current hand hygiene guidelines from the CDC or the World Health Organization (WHO). Set and use goals to improve hand cleaning.

College of American Pathologists (CAP)

The CAP is an organization of board-certified pathologists that advocates high-quality and cost-effective medical care. The CAP provides laboratory accreditation and proficiency testing for laboratories.

For accreditation purposes, CAP-trained pathologists, laboratory managers, and medical laboratory scientists perform on-site laboratory inspections on a biennial basis. Inspectors examine the laboratory's records and quality control of procedures for the preceding 2 years. Inspection also includes the qualifications of the laboratory personnel, including CE attendance; the laboratory's equipment, facilities, and safety program; and laboratory management. CAP accreditation is accepted by both the CMS and TJC and fulfills the requirements of Medicare and Medicaid.

Laboratories that subscribe to the proficiency program receive periodic samples to analyze and return their results to the CAP. The laboratory receives a report on how its results compared with those of other laboratories performing the procedures in a similar manner. Failure to perform satisfactorily on a proficiency test can result in a laboratory losing its CLIA certificate to perform the failed test.

The Commission on Laboratory Accreditation (COLA)

The COLA is a physician-directed accrediting agency popular with physician office laboratories (POLs) and independent laboratories. It enables laboratories and clinical personnel to meet CLIA and other regulatory requirements.

Knowledge Check 8-5

Which of the following organizations publishes guidelines that are considered the standard of care for laboratory procedures?

a. CLIA
b. CLSI
c. TJC
d. CAP

Quality Management Systems

A **quality management system (QMS)** incorporates many of the objectives of total QM and continuous quality improvement to ensure quality results, staff competence, patient and employee safety, and efficiency within an organization. In addition, a QMS also utilizes the concepts of the International Organization for Standardization (ISO 151189) and the Lean and Six Sigma methods. The requirements of TJC, the CAP, the CMS, and CLIA accreditation organizations are included in a QMS.

A QMS coordinates activities to direct and control an organization with regard to quality and the reduction of medical errors. The first step in a laboratory QMS is to determine the pathway of workflow through the laboratory, as we discussed previously under the preexamination, examination, and postexamination phases of testing. In each area of the pathway, all the processes and procedures that occur are determined and analyzed so that everyone knows what they are supposed to do, how they are supposed to do it, and when they are supposed to do it. Instructions must be available for each activity.

Quality System Essentials

Quality system essentials (QSEs) form the foundation of a QMS. The quality processes that are outlined in each QSE are not only part of providing quality patient care but are also mandates from regulatory, standard-setting, and accrediting agencies. Per the CLSI, the 12 QSEs are the management infrastructure that supports the workflow of the organization **(Table 8–2).** Quality **indicators** are the measurements developed by each laboratory to determine if the QSEs are being met. They may include the appropriateness of the testing, correct patient identification, timely reporting of laboratory results, and correct proficiency testing results.

As part of the QMS, facilities must develop a *nonconforming event (NCE)* management program based on the quality indicators. The purpose of an NCE program is to do the following:

- Identify problems with the processes in the laboratory's workflow path and within the supporting processes of the QMS.

Table 8-2 Description of the 12 Laboratory Quality System Essentials (QSEs)

QSE	PURPOSE	PROCESS EXAMPLES
Organization	Leadership responsibilities to meet requirements and maintain quality	Quality planning Management review
Customer focus	Determining customer expectations and designing processes to meet them	Customer feedback
Facilities and safety	Physical environment, safety, and maintenance programs	Disaster management Health risk assessment
Personnel	Obtaining and retaining qualified competent staff	Training Competency
Purchasing and inventory	Agreements with suppliers for products and services	Inventory management Supply ordering
Equipment	Selecting, installing, and maintaining equipment and instrumentation	Preventive maintenance
Process management	Processes related to the path of workflow	Method validation Plan development
Documents and records	Creating, managing, and retaining documentation of policies and procedures	Document review Document management
Information management	Managing confidential information generated or entered into information systems	Release of information Downtime procedures
Nonconforming event (NCE) management	Detecting and documenting occurrences that deviate from established laboratory standards	Investigation of NCEs
Assessments	Verifying that processes meet requirements	Proficiency testing Quality indicators
Continual improvement	Identifying areas for improvement	Lean Root cause analysis Six Sigma

- Improve the process quality and safety of patients and employees.
- Implement processes and procedural changes that support continual improvement.
- Work to remove the cause of NCEs.

The NCE process must complete the following:

- Document the NCE episode and associated actions.
- Classify the event type and its seriousness.
- Initiate remedial action, when possible.
- Begin an investigation and corrective action plan.

The Lean System

The **Lean system** originated with the automobile manufacturing industry in Japan. The concepts of Lean have been adopted by many American industries, including the health care industry. Lean focuses on the elimination of waste to allow a facility to do more with less while simultaneously increasing customer and employee satisfaction. In the health care environment, the ability to decrease costs while providing quality health care is of primary importance. Lean utilizes a tool called "6S," which stands for sort, straighten, scrub, safety, standardize, and sustain. The use of the Lean tools enhances efficiency and proficiency, as described in **Table 8–3.**

Table 8-3 Lean 6S in the Laboratory

LEAN S	TASK	BENEFIT
Sort	Identify items in the department that can be discarded	More space and less clutter
Straighten	Identify designated areas for equipment and supplies	Less time is spent searching for supplies
Scrub	Maintain the work area daily	Less time is spent on major cleanups
Safety	Identifying potential hazards that can be eliminated or reduced	Less chance of accidents
Standardize	All work areas are stocked in the same manner	Any work area can be restocked by anyone in the department
Sustain	Everyone maintains the five other Ss daily	Less employee frustration and better outcomes

Six Sigma

Six Sigma is a statistical modification of the original Plan-Do-Check-Act (PDCA) method adopted by TJC as a guideline for health care organizations. It focuses on minimizing variability in process outputs that lead to wasted time and resources. Reducing variation will potentially reduce costs, improve performance, and increase profitability. The primary goals of Six Sigma are to measure process performance and quantify errors, and then reduce variables and decrease errors to a level of 3.4 defects per 1 million opportunities. Attaining this goal indicates that the laboratory is addressing factors critical to customer satisfaction and quality care.

The Six Sigma methodology is represented by the acronym DMAIC:

Define goals and current processes.
Measure current processes and collect data.
Analyze the data for cause-and-effect information.
Improve the process using the data collected.
Control the correction of concerns displayed in the data.

Root Cause Analysis

Similar to Lean, **root cause analysis (RCA)** has roots in the manufacturing industry. RCA is a tool widely used in the investigation of adverse events in the health care setting. TJC mandates the use of RCA to investigate "sentinel events," which are defined as an unexpected occurrence involving death or serious physical or psychological injury or the risk thereof. An RCA protocol begins with the investigation and reconstruction of the adverse event to determine how the event occurred. RCA focuses on the process failures, not on the individual mistakes of personnel.

By instituting quality improvement methodologies, a health care institution can develop a structured, standardized format to systematically assess and document the quality of services to the customer.

KEY CONCEPTS

Biological Hazards and Sharps

- Transmission of biological hazards that are encountered when testing patient specimens requires a chain of infection consisting of an infectious agent, reservoir, portal of exit, mode of transmission, portal of entry, and susceptible host.
- Hand hygiene and wearing PPE are essential actions to prevent transmission of infectious organisms. Standard Precautions (SPs) should be followed at all times.
- Contaminated supplies and all specimen types except urine must be disposed of in a labeled biohazard container.
- All sharps, including needles and holders, must be disposed of in puncture-proof sharps containers. Recapping of needles is prohibited.
- The Occupational Exposure to Bloodborne Pathogens Standards are a means of providing protection from accidental exposure to BBPs through the use of engineering controls, work practice controls, and the use of PPE.
- When transporting biological specimens, the DOT and International Air Transit Association regulations must be followed. They include placing specimens in screw-cap containers; wrapping them in absorbent material; and placing them in a sturdy, leak-proof container.

Chemical Hazards

- Follow specific directions when mixing chemicals, and always add acid to water, rather than water to acid.
- When chemical contact with the skin or eyes occurs, immediately flush the area with water for 15 minutes.

Safety Data Sheets and Globally Harmonized System

- An SDS and a Chemical Hygiene Plan must be available to employees. Dispose of chemicals per EPA guidelines.
- The SDS contains information about the physical and chemical properties of a reagent, its flammability, explosion reactivity, health hazards, primary routes of entry, exposure limits, carcinogenic potential, precautions for safe handling, spill cleanup, and emergency first aid.
- The Globally Harmonized System (GHS) of Classification and Labelling of Chemicals is an international standardization for labeling and SDS formatting of hazards posed by chemicals.

Radioactive, Electrical, Fire, and Physical Hazards

- Dispose of radioactive material following NRC guidelines.
- Be observant for frayed cords, overloaded circuits, and improperly grounded equipment. Avoid working with electrical equipment when you are wet or the equipment is wet.
- Follow routine safety protocols and maintain a clean, organized work area to avoid physical hazards.
- The acronym RACE outlines the steps to follow when a fire is discovered: (R) rescue anyone in danger; (A) activate the fire alarm; (C) contain the fire; (E) extinguish the fire if possible or evacuate, closing the door.

Quality Management

- QM is the overall process of guaranteeing quality throughout the entire testing system.
- A QMS coordinates activities within a department and an organization to facilitate quality work and reduce medical errors.

- QC involves performing individual procedures using acceptable standards and control material at various medically significant levels.
- Documentation includes a procedure manual, policies to control and monitor procedure variables, and records of competency assessment and CE.
- Preexamination variables occur before sample testing. Examination variables occur during the specimen testing. Postexamination variables occur during reporting of test results.

Regulatory Issues

- Agencies and regulations regulating the laboratory include the following:
- CLIA—provides requirements for persons performing waived, PPMP, moderate-complexity, and high-complexity testing
- TJC—provides accreditation and certification of health care organizations
- CAP—provides laboratory accreditation and proficiency testing
- CLSI—develops written standards and guidelines for specimen collection, handling, and processing, and laboratory testing and reporting; considered the standard of care
- COLA—provides accreditation of POLs

Quality Management Systems

- The 12 quality essentials provide the management documentation needed to demonstrate quality work. Quality indicators are developed to monitor each phase of testing.
- The Lean system uses the "6S" tools (sort, straighten, scrub, safety, standardize, and sustain) to enhance efficiency and proficiency.
- The goal of the statistical Six Sigma method is to reduce variables and decrease errors to a level of 3.4 defects per 1 million opportunities.
- RCA focuses on process failures, not on the individual mistakes of personnel.

CASE STUDIES

1. An immunology supervisor is training a new employee. A dilution of a patient's serum must be made to run a particular test. The supervisor is having difficulty using a serological pipette, so they remove one glove. In uncapping the serum tube, a small amount of serum splashes onto the workbench. The supervisor cleans this up with a paper towel, which they discard in the regular paper trash. They also spill a small amount onto their disposable laboratory coat. They tell the new employee that because it is such a small amount, they aren't going to worry about it and continue to pipette the specimen. They then replace the glove onto their ungloved hand and say that because it is almost break time, they will wait to wash their hands until then.

Questions

a. Identify all the safety violations involved.
b. What component of the chain of infection is involved?
c. How can the chain of infection be broken?

2. As the supervisor of the immunology section, you encounter the following situations. Explain whether you would accept them or take corrective action.

Situations

a. You are told that only the supervisor performs the CAP proficiency survey.
b. QC is not performed daily on a laboratory instrument.
c. The reporting procedure for a laboratory test has been recently revised.
d. Opened, unlabeled commercial QC bottles are in the refrigerator.

3. The medical laboratory professional working in immunology is accused of failure to report a critical result to the patient's nurse.

Questions

a. What documentation is requested from the laboratorian assigned to make the call?
b. What agency requires this?

4. The immunology supervisor is conducting competency testing for the immunology personnel. Complete the assignment by indicating whether each of the following would be considered a (1) preexamination, (2) examination, or (3) postexamination variable by placing the appropriate number in the space.

______ Checking the reagent expiration date
______ Rejecting a hemolyzed specimen
______ Constructing a Levey-Jennings chart
______ Telephoning a critical result to the nurse
______ Calibrating the centrifuge
______ Pipetting the diluent

REVIEW QUESTIONS

1. Exposure to toxic, carcinogenic, or caustic agents is what type of laboratory safety hazard?
   a. Biological
   b. Sharps
   c. Chemical
   d. Fire/explosive

2. In the chain of infection, a contaminated work area would serve as which of the following?
   a. Reservoir
   b. Means of transmission
   c. Portal of entry
   d. Portal of exit

3. The only biological waste that does not have to be discarded in a container with a biohazard symbol is:
   a. Urine
   b. Serum
   c. Feces
   d. Used serum tubes

4. Centrifuging an uncapped specimen may produce a biological hazard in the form of:
   a. Vectors
   b. Sharps contamination
   c. Aerosols
   d. Specimen contamination

5. The current routine infection control policy developed by the CDC and followed in all health care settings is:
   a. Universal Precautions
   b. Isolation Precautions
   c. Blood and Body Fluid Precautions
   d. Standard Precautions

6. Hand hygiene is performed:
   a. Before putting on gloves
   b. After removing gloves
   c. When gloves are visibly soiled
   d. All of the above

7. Personnel in the immunology laboratory should wear laboratory coats that:
   a. Do not have buttons
   b. Are fluid resistant
   c. Have short sleeves
   d. Have full-length zippers

8. An acceptable disinfectant for decontamination of blood and body fluids is:
   a. Sodium hydroxide
   b. Anti-microbial soap
   c. Hydrogen peroxide
   d. Sodium hypochlorite

9. Patient specimens transported by the DOT must be labeled as a:
   a. Diagnostic specimen
   b. Clinical specimen
   c. Biological specimen, category b
   d. Laboratory specimen

10. The Occupational Exposure to Bloodborne Pathogens Standard developed by OSHA requires employers to provide all of the following *except:*
    a. Hepatitis B immunization
    b. Safety training
    c. Hepatitis C immunization
    d. Laundry facilities for nondisposable laboratory coats

11. An employee who is accidentally exposed to a possible pathogen should immediately:
    a. Apply sodium hypochlorite to the area.
    b. Notify a supervisor.
    c. Receive HIV prophylaxis.
    d. Receive a hepatitis B booster shot.

12. The first thing to do when acid is spilled on the skin is to:
    a. Notify a supervisor.
    b. Neutralize the area with a base.
    c. Apply burn ointment.
    d. Flush the area with water.

13. To determine the chemical characteristics of sodium azide, an employee would consult the:
    a. Chemical Hygiene Plan
    b. *Merck Manual*
    c. SDS
    d. NRC guidelines

14. The GHS requires which of the following on a chemical label?
    a. Biohazard symbol, warning sign, environmental impact
    b. Hazard pictogram, signal words, hazard statement
    c. Biological symbol, hazard pictogram, long-term effects
    d. Signal words, hazard statement, biological symbol

15. Laboratory personnel who are pregnant should avoid working with:
    a. Organic chemicals
    b. Radioisotopes
    c. HIV-positive serum
    d. Needles and lancets

16. The acronym RACE should be followed when:
   a. Determining the type of fire extinguisher to use
   b. Operating a fire extinguisher
   c. Classifying fires and fire extinguishers
   d. Discovering a fire

17. The NPFA classification symbol contains information on all of the following, *except:*
   a. Fire hazards
   b. Biohazards
   c. Reactivity
   d. Health hazards

18. Which of the following laboratory regulatory agencies classifies laboratory tests by their complexity?
   a. OSHA
   b. CAP
   c. TJC
   d. FDA

19. "QM" refers to:
   a. Performance of two levels of testing controls
   b. Reliable control results
   c. Increased productivity
   d. Quality of specimens and patient care

20. An error in correctly reporting a patient's test result is considered a/an:
   a. Preexamination error
   b. Examination error
   c. Postexamination error
   d. Analytical error

21. When external QC is run, what information must be documented?
   a. The reagent lot number
   b. Expiration date of the control
   c. Date the control was run
   d. All of the above

22. When a new bottle of QC material is opened, what information is placed on the label?
   a. The date and the laboratory worker's initials
   b. The supervisor's initials
   c. The lot number
   d. The time the bottle was opened

23. The testing of a specimen from an outside agency and the comparison of results with participating laboratories is called:
   a. External QC
   b. Electronic QC
   c. Internal QC
   d. Proficiency testing

24. What is the primary goal of QMS?
   a. Precise test results
   b. Increased laboratory productivity
   c. Improved patient outcomes and reduced medical errors
   d. Reproducible test results

25. A recommended way to measure and assess QSEs is to establish:
   a. QC
   b. Quality indicators
   c. Preventive maintenance
   d. Quality management

26. Quality indicators in the immunology department measure:
   a. Appropriateness of the testing
   b. Timely reporting of laboratory results
   c. Correct proficiency testing results
   d. All of the above

27. The basic principle of the Lean system is to increase efficiency and proficiency through:
   a. Customized work shifts
   b. Continuous quality improvement
   c. Elimination of waste
   d. Development of quality indicators

28. Six Sigma is a:
   a. Departmental evaluation of variables
   b. Departmental assessment of errors and quality
   c. QC method
   d. Statistical determination of variable and error reduction

29. What is the focus of RCA?
   a. Patient errors
   b. Health care provider errors
   c. Process errors
   d. Personnel errors

Chapter 8 Answer Key

Answers to Knowledge Check

8.1 c 8.2 a 8.3 b 8.4 d 8.5 b

Answers to Review Questions

1. c	2. a	3. a	4. c	5. d	6. d	7. b
8. d	9. c	10. c	11. b	12. d	13. c	14. b
15. b	16. d	17. b	18. d	19. d	20. c	21. d
22. a	23. d	24. c	25. b	26. d	27. c	28. d
29. c						

9

Principles of Serological Testing

Linda E. Miller, PhD, I, MB^{CM}(ASCP) SI, Christine Dorresteyn Stevens, EdD, MT(ASCP), and Marnie Imhoff, MA, MBA, MLS(ASCP)^{CM}

LEARNING OUTCOMES

After finishing this chapter, you should be able to:

9.1 Describe how whole blood is processed to obtain serum for serological testing.

9.2 List other body specimen types that can be used in serological testing.

9.3 Explain the difference between a volumetric pipette and a graduated pipette.

9.4 Explain the difference between to contain (TC) and to deliver (TD) pipettes.

9.5 Define the following: serial dilution, solute, diluent, and compound dilution.

9.6 Describe how accurate measurements are made using volumetric and graduated pipettes.

9.7 Given the volumes of diluent and solute, calculate the dilution obtained.

9.8 Calculate the amount of diluent or solute needed to prepare a specific dilution of a serum sample.

9.9 Explain how an antibody titer is determined.

9.10 Calculate the dilution factor required to change a given dilution to a specified new dilution.

9.11 Given a starting dilution and a dilution factor, determine the new dilution obtained.

9.12 Calculate the final dilution of a sample, given the initial dilution and all subsequent dilutions.

9.13 Determine how to make a specific percentage solution from a concentrate.

9.14 Define analytical sensitivity and specificity.

9.15 Calculate the diagnostic sensitivity and specificity of a serological test and discuss the significance of these parameters.

9.16 Discuss the clinical significance of positive and negative predictive values.

9.17 Explain how complement inactivation is achieved.

CHAPTER OUTLINE

You can go to **fadavis.com** keyword stevens for the laboratory exercises that accompany this text.

Serology is the study of the fluid components in the blood, especially antibodies. **Serum,** the liquid portion of the blood minus the coagulation factors, is the most frequently encountered specimen in immunologic testing. Knowing how to collect specimens and prepare dilutions is essential to understanding all serological testing in the clinical laboratory.

Specimen Preparation and Storage

It is necessary to consult test protocols to accurately collect, process, and store the correct specimen type. The most common patient sample used in serologic testing is serum. Blood is collected aseptically by venipuncture into a sterile tube that does not contain an anticoagulant (i.e., a red-top, gold-top, or serum separator tube). Care must be taken to avoid hemolysis, as this may produce a false-positive test. The blood specimen is allowed to clot at room temperature or 4°C, depending upon the protocol for the specific procedure. It is then centrifuged, after which serum should be promptly separated into another tube without transferring any cellular elements **(Fig. 9–1).** Fresh serum that has not been inactivated by heating is usually recommended for testing. However, complement must be inactivated prior to some tests because it interferes with test results. In this case, the serum is heated to 56°C for 30 minutes to destroy complement proteins. In either situation, if testing cannot be performed immediately, serum may be stored between 2°C and 8°C for up to 72 hours. If there is an additional delay in testing, the serum should be frozen at –20°C or colder.

In addition to serum, other types of body fluids, including cerebral spinal fluid (CSF), urine, synovial fluid, and plasma, may be used for immunologic testing. The type of specimen required often depends on the principle of the test being performed. You can consult individual laboratory procedures for the specimen type, processing, and storage required.

Knowledge Check 9-1

The type of specimen most commonly used in serologic testing is:

a. plasma
b. serum
c. urine
d. synovial fluid

Pipettes and Measuring

Pipettes are commonly used to measure serum for testing and liquids for making reagents and dilutions. Pipettes are classified as either *to deliver* (TD) or *to contain* (TC). Manufacturers often print these designations near the top of the pipette. TD pipettes dispense the exact volume indicated. TC pipettes are designed to hold a specific volume but they do not deliver that exact volume, as a small amount of residual fluid will remain in the pipette following drainage of the liquid under the force of gravity alone.

The two main types of pipettes used in the laboratory are volumetric or graduated. **Volumetric pipettes** are a type of TD pipette that is marked and calibrated to deliver only one volume of a specified liquid. These pipettes have a very high degree of accuracy, enabling the user to dispense the exact amount of liquid with a small drop left behind. The volumetric pipettes have an oval bulb in the center and a tapered dispensing end **(Fig. 9–2).** Volumetric pipettes are used with a suctioning device such as a rubber bulb; recall from Chapter 8 that mouth pipetting is not allowed to prevent contact with hazardous biologic and chemical materials. The bulb is squeezed to draw the measured amount of liquid into the pipette. Excess fluid is wiped off the outside of the pipette, and then the pipette is held vertically, with the tip against the surface of a container. The suction is released, and the liquid is allowed to flow by gravity into the container.

Graduated pipettes or measuring pipettes have markings at regular increments all along their length that allow for varying amounts of liquid to be measured. They can either be TC or TD. If it is a **serological pipette,** the marks go all the way down to the tip. Some serological pipettes are called *blowout pipettes* because the last drop of liquid must be forced out using a pipette bulb or other device to deliver an accurate volume. These TC pipettes have a frosted band or two small rings near the top to identify them.

Alternately, a specified amount of liquid can be measured from point to point in the pipette. Keep in mind that the graduated markings may start from the top of the pipette and increase to the bottom. For example, 3 mL can be measured

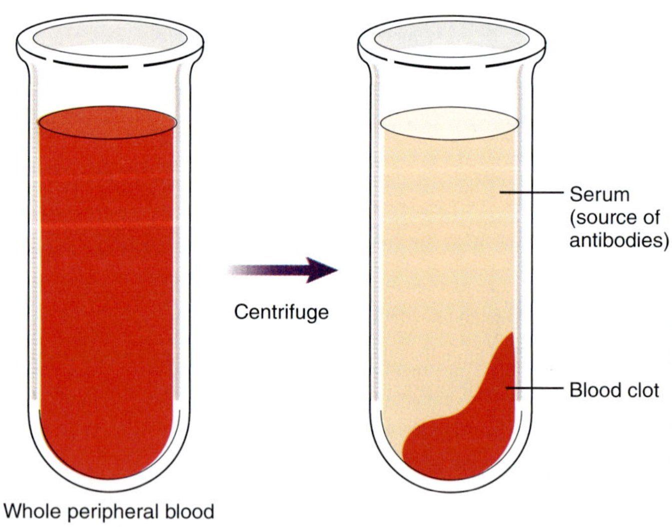

FIGURE 9–1 Serum collection.

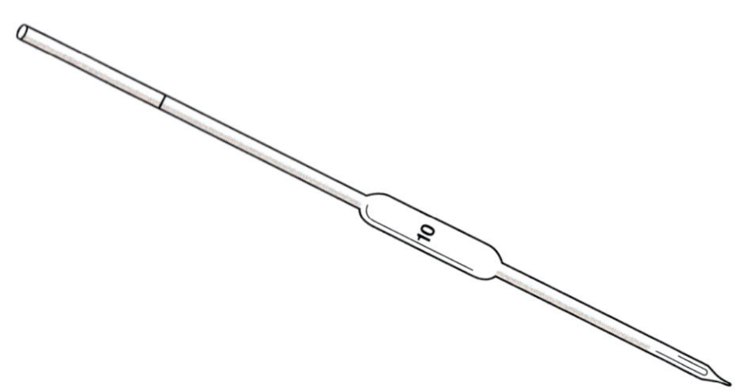

FIGURE 9–2 Volumetric pipette.

with a 10-mL TC pipette by filling the pipette to the 7-mL mark and dispensing down to the end rather than filling it to the 0-mL mark and allowing the liquid to flow to the 3-mL mark **(Fig. 9–3)**.

Generally, a measuring pipette is held in a vertical position when drawing up a liquid **(Fig. 9–4)**. The bottom of the meniscus (curve in the surface liquid caused by surface tension) should be level with the calibration line on the pipette. This is observed at eye level (see **Fig. 9–5**). Often, an automatic pipette filler is used with measuring pipettes to increase accuracy **(Fig. 9–6)**.

In practice, volumetric and graduated pipettes are more often used to prepare reagents rather than to measure patient

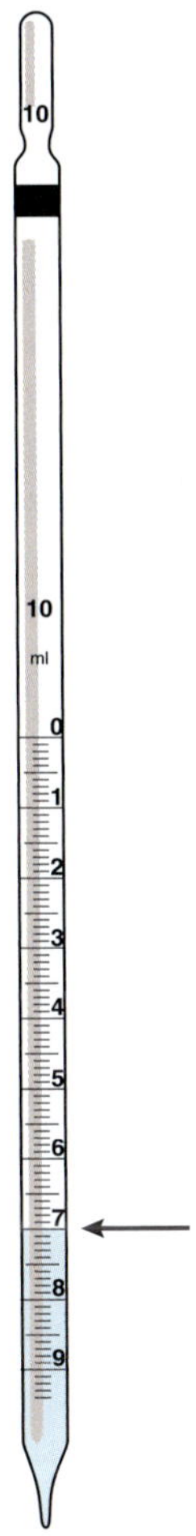

FIGURE 9–3 Graduated pipette prepared to deliver 3 mL.

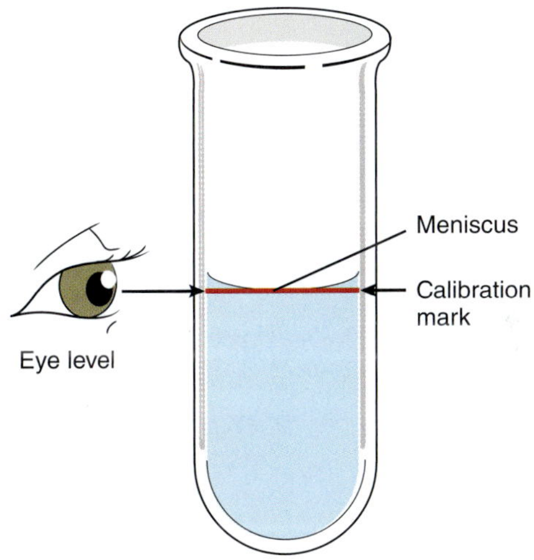

FIGURE 9–5 How to read a meniscus.

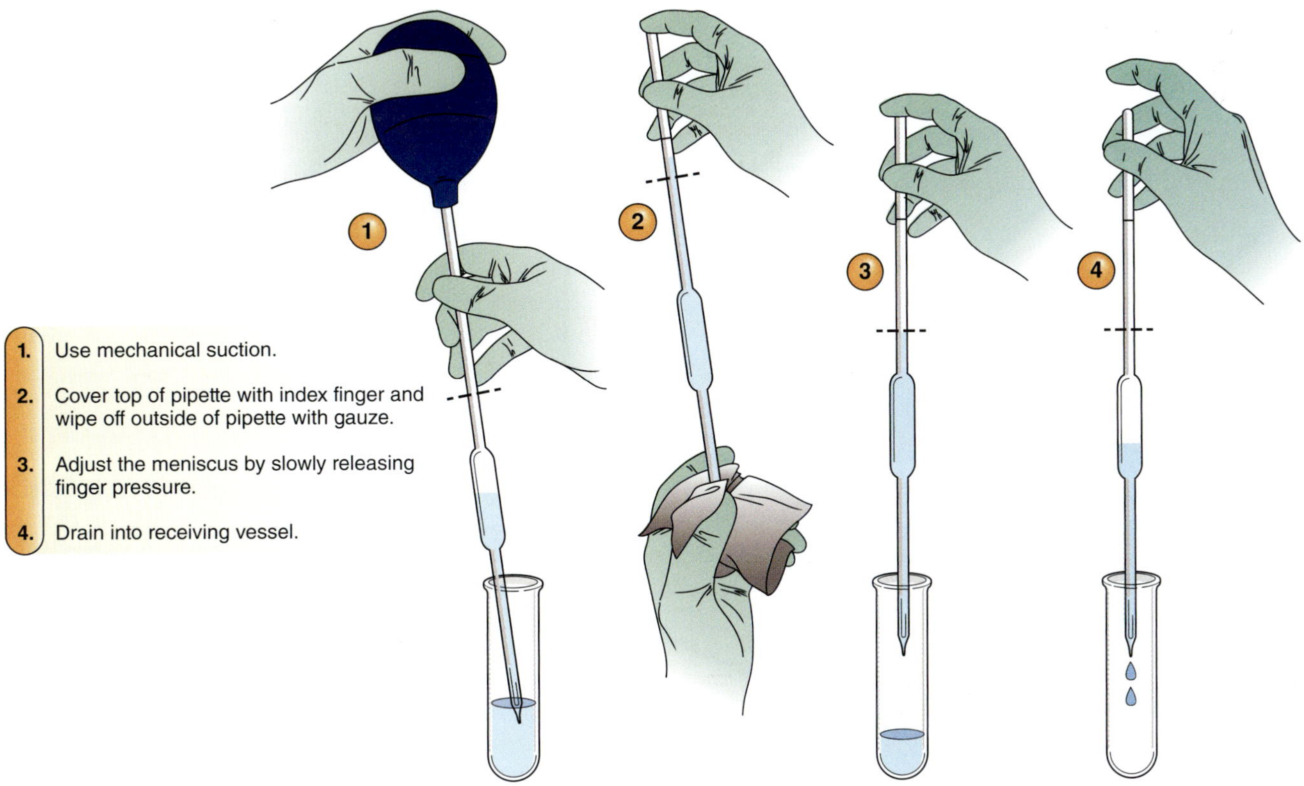

FIGURE 9–4 Steps in accurately measuring a liquid with a serological pipette.

specimens and controls. **Micropipettes** are much more accurate for patient specimens, controls, and calibrators because they deliver volumes in the microliter (μL) range and can be used when very small volumes are needed. Micropipettes are mechanical pipettes that draw up and then release a specific volume by depressing a plunger **(Fig. 9–7).** Different single-use disposable tips are used for each specimen. Some micropipettes are adjustable and can hold a range of volumes, whereas others only hold a fixed volume.

Micropipettes must be calibrated regularly to ensure they deliver the correct volume(s). A common technique for calibrating micropipettes is the gravimetric method. When using this method, the temperature and humidity of the room are documented and considered during calculations. The gravimetric method involves aliquoting a set volume of distilled water into a container and weighing the aliquot with a calibrated analytical balance. The measured volume is calculated by subtracting the weight of the empty container from the weight recorded after dispensing the water into the container. The accuracy of the pipetted volume is determined by dividing the weight of the dispensed distilled water by the density of water at the known temperature. The calculated volume is compared to the desired calibration volume to assess accuracy. If the measured volume significantly deviates from the desired volume, the pipette manufacturer's guidelines are consulted for directions on adjusting the pipette. If the micropipette can dispense different volumes, the calibration procedure should be repeated at different volume settings within the micropipette's range. Maintaining a detailed record of the calibration process, including all measurements and adjustments for each pipette, is essential.

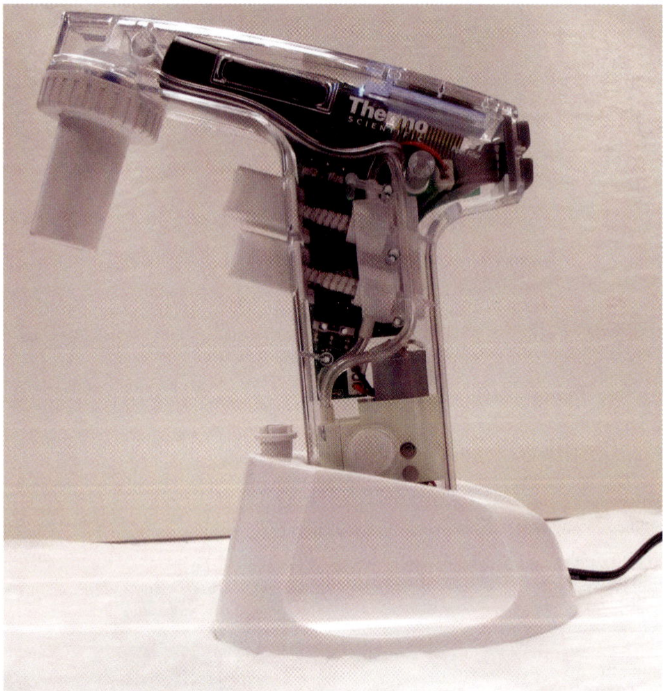

FIGURE 9–6 A pipette filler for use with serological pipettes ranging in size from 1 mL to 100 mL.

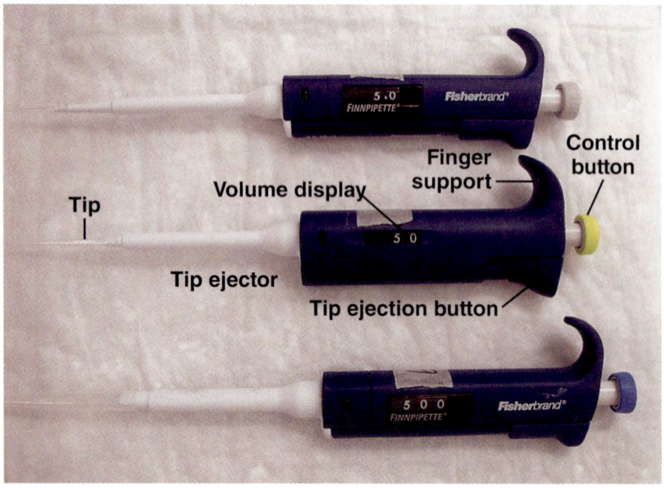

FIGURE 9–7 Micropipettes calibrated to deliver different volumes.

Knowledge Check 9-2

Which of the following is a TD pipette that is designed to deliver one volume of liquid?

a. Blowout pipette
b. Graduated pipette
c. Serological pipette
d. Volumetric pipette

Dilutions

In the clinical laboratory, it is often necessary to make a less concentrated solution from a reagent, such as an acid or a buffer, to be able to use the reagent in a particular procedure. In this case, either water or buffer is mixed with the concentrate to make the reagent the proper strength for testing. For many serology tests, diluting patient serum with saline may be necessary for a visible reaction to occur. If the relative proportions of antigen and antibody are not similar, the reaction cannot be detected (see Chapter 10).

A reaction endpoint may not be reached when too much antibody is present. In this case, the serum that contains antibody must be diluted. Therefore, knowledge about dilution preparation is essential to understanding all serological testing. Accurate preparation of simple and compound dilutions and interpretation of serial dilutions are skills that are necessary for quality analysis in the clinical laboratory.

Simple Dilutions

A dilution involves two entities: the **solute**, which is the substance being diluted, and the **diluent**, which is the liquid making up the rest of the solution. The relationship between solute and diluent is a ratio that can also be expressed as a fraction. For example, a 1:20 dilution can be expressed as the fraction 1/20. This dilution implies 1 part of solute and 19 parts of diluent. The number on the bottom of the fraction is the total volume, calculated by adding the volumes of the solute and diluent together.

To create a certain volume of a specified dilution, it is necessary to know how to adjust the volumes of solute and diluent appropriately. Using the following equation, an algebraic calculation can be set up to find the total volume, the amount of solute, or the amount of diluent needed to make a dilution:

$$\frac{1}{\text{Dilution}} = \frac{\text{Amount of Solute (Often the Serum)}}{\text{Total Volume (Solute + Diluent)}}$$

Let's see how this equation can be applied by considering the following examples:

Example 1

- Suppose 2 mL of a 1:20 dilution of serum is needed to run a specific serological test. What volumes of serum and diluent are needed to make this dilution?

This problem can be solved by placing the appropriate numbers into the corresponding places in the preceding equation as follows:

$$\frac{1}{20} = \frac{X}{2\text{ mL}}$$

Note that 20 represents the total number of parts in the solution and that 2 mL is the total volume desired.

Solving this equation for x gives 0.1 mL for the amount of serum needed to make this dilution. The amount of diluent is obtained by subtracting 0.1 mL from the total volume of 2.0 mL to give 1.9 mL of diluent. To check the answer, one can set up a proportion between the amount of solute calculated over the total volume. This should equal the dilution desired. By doing this for the preceding problem, you can see that the correct answer has been obtained:

$$\frac{0.1\text{ mL}}{(1.9\text{ mL Diluent} + 0.1\text{ mL Serum})} = \frac{1}{20}$$

Example 2

In this example, the amount of serum to be used is known, and the amount of diluent needed to make a specific dilution must be determined:

- Suppose a 1:5 dilution of patient serum is needed to run a serological test. Using 0.1 mL of serum, what amount of diluent is necessary to make this dilution?

The solution to this problem can be set up in the following manner:

$$\frac{1}{5} = \frac{0.1}{(x + 0.1)}$$

Cross-multiply to get: $x + 0.1 = 0.5$

$$x = 0.4\text{ mL of diluent}$$

Note that the final volume is obtained by adding 0.1 mL of solute to 0.4 mL of diluent. Dividing the volume of the solute by the total volume of 0.5 mL yields the desired 1:5 ratio.

Example 3

- Instructions coming with a reagent bottle of concentrated buffer indicate that 1 part of buffer must be mixed with 19 parts of water for use in a serological test. What is the desired dilution, and how much water should be added to 50 mL of buffer concentrate to obtain this dilution?
- The desired dilution would be: 1/(1 + 19) = 1/20

To determine the volume of water needed, set up the equation as follows:

$$\frac{1}{20} = \frac{50}{(50 + x)}$$

Cross-multiply to get: $50 + x = 1{,}000$

$$x = 950\text{ mL of diluent}$$

Therefore, to make the dilution, you would add 50 mL of buffer concentrate to 950 mL of water to get 1,000 mL total.

Sometimes it is necessary to dilute a concentrate to a specific percentage. A percentage is simply a different way of expressing a dilution. For instance, a 10% solution can also be expressed as 1/10. In dealing with liquids, the relationship between the solute and diluent is volume/volume. If a solid is to be dissolved in a liquid, the relationship is expressed as weight/volume. Let's look at another example to see how this type of problem would be solved:

Example 4

- Suppose you wish to dilute concentrated glacial acetic acid in water to make 500 mL of a 10% solution for a testing procedure. How much glacial acetic acid and water are needed to make the dilution?

Because the final volume and the percentage are known, we can solve for the amount of the concentrated acetic acid needed, as follows:

$$\frac{1}{10} = \frac{x}{500\text{ mL}}$$

Cross-multiplying and solving for x gives us 50 mL of glacial acetic acid. Alternatively, 500 mL could be multiplied by 10%, or 0.10 to get 50 mL. The amount of water is determined by taking the total volume and subtracting the volume of concentrate: 500 mL – 50 mL = 450 mL of water to make up the 10% solution.

Additional problems that give more practice with dilution calculations can be found in the Review Questions at the end of this chapter.

Knowledge Check 9-3

In a serological assay to determine an antibody titer, the substance being diluted would be:

a. Diluent
b. Saline
c. Patient serum
d. An antigen

Compound Dilutions

The previous examples represent simple dilutions. Sometimes it is necessary to make a *compound dilution,* which involves preparing a larger dilution from a previously prepared smaller dilution. To solve this type of problem, use the formula:

$$C1V1 = C2V2$$

In this equation, C1 is the starting concentration, C2 is the final concentration, V1 is the starting volume, and V2 is the ending volume. Let's look at an example to see how this equation would be used:

Example 1

- Suppose you wish to prepare 2 mL of a 1:20 dilution from an already-prepared 1:5 dilution of a solute. What volumes of the 1:5 dilution and diluent would be required?

To solve this problem, we can place the numbers into the equation, C1V1 = C2V2, to get:

$$\left(\frac{1}{5}\right)\mathrm{V1}=\left(\frac{1}{20}\right)2$$

Solving for V1, we get 0.5 mL. The volume of diluent = 2 – 0.5 = 1.5 mL. Thus, we have made a 1:4 dilution of the original 1:5 dilution to get a 1:20 dilution [0.5/(0.5 + 1.5)].

Occasionally, it is necessary to make a very large dilution; if so, it is more accurate and less costly to do this in several steps rather than all at once. The same approach is used as in the previous example, but several dilutions are made in sequence. Consider the following example:

Example 2

Suppose a 1:500 dilution is needed. To make this dilution in a single step, you could mix 49.9 mL of diluent with 0.1 mL of serum. If only a small amount of solution is needed to run the test, this is wasteful. Furthermore, inaccuracy may occur if the solution is not properly mixed. Therefore, it is helpful to make several smaller dilutions.

The first step to solving a problem such as this one is to plan the number and sizes of simple dilutions necessary to reach the desired endpoint. In the preceding example, a 1:500 dilution can be made by making a 1:5 dilution of the undiluted serum, followed by a 1:10 dilution from the first dilution and a 1:10 dilution of the second dilution, as shown here:
Serum Dilutions:

1:5 dilution →	*1:10 dilution →*	*1:10 dilution*
0.1 mL serum	0.1 mL of 1:5 dilution	0.1 mL of 1:10 dilution
0.4 mL diluent	0.9 mL diluent	0.9 mL diluent

Multiplying 1/5 × 1/10 × 1/10 equals 1/500, or the total dilution. Each of the simple dilutions is calculated individually by doing mental arithmetic or by using the formula given for simple dilutions. In this example, the 1:500 dilution was made using very little diluent in a series of test tubes, rather than having to use a larger volume in a flask. The volumes were kept small enough so that mixing could take place easily. The final volume of 1.0 mL is all that is needed to perform the test.

Serial Dilutions

If the dilution factor is exactly the same in each dilution step, this is known as a **serial dilution.** A **dilution factor** is a numerical value representing the extent to which a solution has been diluted. The dilution factor is often expressed as a fraction or ratio. To prepare a serial dilution, a series of test tubes is set up with exactly the same amount of diluent in each. Each tube in the series contains 1/*n* the concentration of the preceding sample.

The series of tubes illustrated in **Figure 9–8** is an example of a 2-fold serial dilution system, in which each tube is one-half as concentrated as the tube before it. The series, 1:5, 1:25, 1:125, 1:625, 1:3125, is an example of a 5-fold serial dilution system, in which each tube is diluted five times as much as the preceding tube. Serial dilutions are often used to obtain an antibody **titer,** an indicator of the amount of antibody in the original serum sample. Once the serum has been serially diluted, a constant amount of the corresponding antigen is added to each tube, and the tubes are observed for an antigen–antibody reaction (e.g. agglutination of red blood cells; see Chapter 10). The antibody titer is the reciprocal of the last dilution in the series that demonstrates the desired reaction. For example, if the last tube to show a visible reaction contained a 1:125 dilution, the titer would be stated as 125.

The antibody dilutions in each tube of a serial dilution system can be calculated by using a series of four steps. It is also helpful to visualize the problem by making a drawing of the setup before performing the calculations. Let's proceed to solve the following example by using this process.

Example: Serial Dilution

Suppose you set up a series of 10 tubes. You pipet 0.8 mL of saline into tube 1 and 0.4 mL of saline into tubes 2 to 10. Next, 0.2 mL of a serum sample is added to tube 1. The tube is mixed, and 0.4 mL is serially transferred through tube 10. Finally, 0.1 mL of antigen is added to all the tubes. What is the final titer of tube 4?

A drawing illustrating the set-up for this problem is shown in **Figure 9-9**.

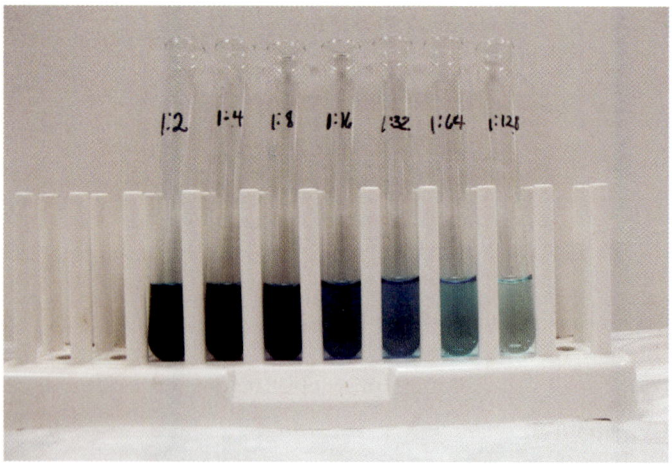

FIGURE 9–8 Serial dilution. Each tube contains the same amount of diluent and a blue dye. Each time a dilution is made, the amount of dye is cut in half in each successive tube. The final volume in each tube should be exactly the same. The color becomes visibly lighter with each dilution.

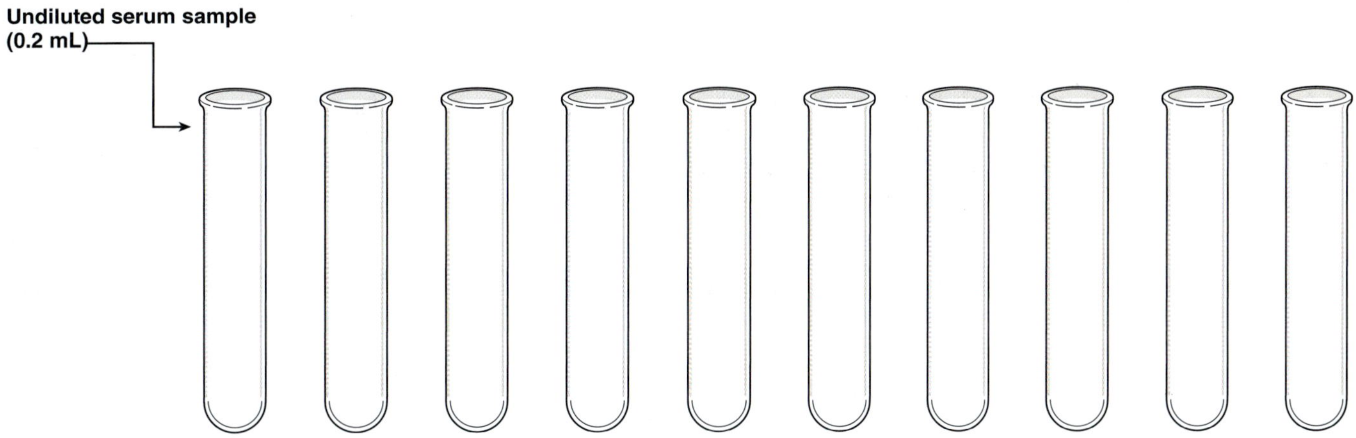

Tube number	1	2	3	4	5	6	7	8	9	10
Saline (diluent)	0.8 mL	0.4 mL	0.4 mL	0.4 mL	0.4 mL	0.4 mL	0.4 mL	0.4 mL	0.4 mL	0.4 mL
Volume transferred from previous tube	------	0.4 mL	0.4 mL	0.4 mL	0.4 mL	0.4 mL	0.4 mL	0.4 mL	0.4 mL	0.4 mL
Amount of antigen added	0.1 mL	0.1 mL	0.1 mL	0.1 mL	0.1 mL	0.1 mL	0.1 mL	0.1 mL	0.1 mL	0.1 mL
Dilutions before antigen addition	1:5	1:10	1:20	1:40	1:80	1:160	1:320	1:640	1:1280	1:2560
Dilutions after antigen addition	1:6.25	1:12.5	1:25	1:50	1:100	1:200	1:400	1:800	1:1600	1:3200

FIGURE 9–9 Sample serial dilution problem.

Step 1

The first step to solving such a problem is to determine the dilution of serum in tube 1. This is equal to

$$\frac{0.2}{(0.2+0.8)} = \frac{1}{5}$$

Step 2

The second step in such a problem is to determine the dilution fold, which can be calculated using the following formula:

$$\frac{1}{\text{Dilution Fold (df)}} = \frac{\text{Volume Transferred}}{\text{Total Volume}}$$

The total volume is equal to the volume transferred from one tube to the next in the series plus the volume of diluent in the tube. To determine the dilution fold, it is best to use the volumes in any tube except tube 1, which may sometimes have a different volume of diluent than the other tubes.

In this example, the 1/df is equal to

$$\frac{0.4}{(0.4+0.4)} = \frac{1}{2}$$

Step 3

Once the dilution of tube 1 and the dilution fold are determined, these numbers can be used to calculate the dilutions in the remaining tubes before the addition of antigen. The dilution of each tube can be determined using the following formula:

$$\text{Dilution of Tube } n = \text{Dilution of Tube } 1 \times \left(\frac{1}{\text{Dilution Fold}}\right)^{(n-1)}$$

By placing the numbers in this example into this formula, the dilution of tube 4 would be calculated as follows: $1/5 \times [1/2]^{(4-1)} = 1/5 \times \frac{1}{2} \times \frac{1}{2} \times \frac{1}{2} = 1/40$

Step 4

The final titer is then calculated by incorporating the amount of antigen added to the tube, using the equation $C1V1 = C2V2$, where C1 and V1 refer to the tube before the addition of antigen, and C2 and V2 refer to the tube after the addition of antigen. V1 is the volume in the tube after the serial dilution has been performed (i.e., volume of diluent plus volume transferred from the previous tube, minus volume transferred to the next tube). In this example, C1 = 1/40, V1 = 0.4 mL, and V2 = 0.5 mL. The final dilution of tube 4 (C2) can be calculated as follows:

$$1/40 \times 0.4 = C2 \times 0.5$$

$$C2 = 1/40 \times 0.4/0.5 = 1/50$$

The antibody titer in tube 4 is the reciprocal of this number, or 50. This titer would be reported by the laboratory if tube 4 was the last tube demonstrating a visible antigen–antibody reaction.

Critical Thinking 9-1

A 2-fold serial dilution is made of a patient sample. The first tube is a 1:2 dilution. What would be the dilution in tube 3?

Test Parameters

A question sometimes arises as to whether a patient actually has the condition or disease being tested for when the results are obtained from a laboratory test. Knowing the ***diagnostic sensitivity*** and ***diagnostic specificity*** of a particular test can help answer those questions. When assessing these parameters, it is important to understand what true positive, false positive, true negative, and a false negative test results mean.

- A **true positive** result occurs when a person has a medical condition, and a test accurately identifies them as having that condition.
- In contrast, the result is a **false positive** when a person does not have a certain condition, but the test for the condition is positive.
- A **true negative** result means that the test is negative when a person does not have a specified condition.
- In contrast, a **false negative** result occurs when a person has a condition, but the test for that condition is negative.

Diagnostic sensitivity is the proportion of people who have a specific disease or condition and also have a positive test result. Diagnostic sensitivity is a measure of the true-positive results and can be calculated using the following formula:

$$\text{Diagnostic Sensitivity (\%)} = \frac{\text{True Positives}}{\text{True Positives} + \text{False Negatives}} \times 100$$

The diagnostic sensitivity refers to the ability of a laboratory test to identify individuals with a given disease or condition. This is not to be confused with the **analytic sensitivity,** which is the lower limit of detection for the analyte measured by a laboratory test (see Chapter 11).

Diagnostic specificity is the proportion of people who do not have a disease or condition and who have a negative test. Diagnostic specificity is a measure of the true-negative results and can be calculated using the following formula:

$$\text{Diagnostic Specificity (\%)} = \frac{\text{True Negatives}}{\text{True Negatives} + \text{False Positives}} \times 100$$

The diagnostic specificity refers to the ability of a laboratory test to correctly identify individuals in whom a particular disease or condition is absent. This is not to be confused with the **analytic specificity,** which refers to the ability of a laboratory method to only detect the analyte it is designed to measure, without detecting other related (i.e., cross-reacting) substances.

Let's look at an example of test results to see how the diagnostic sensitivity and specificity are calculated.

Example

Suppose a new laboratory test was used with a particular population. The following results were obtained after 200 patients were tested: Among the patients with the disease, 160 gave a positive test result (true positives), and 1 gave a negative result (false negative); among the patients without the disease, 14 gave a positive test result (false positives), and 25 gave a negative result (true negatives). Calculate the diagnostic sensitivity and specificity of the test.

Solution

To help clarify the problem, a table containing the given results can be constructed:

	Number of Patients With Disease	Number of Patients Without Disease
Positive test result	160 (true positives)	14 (false positives)
Negative test result	1 (false negative)	25 (true negatives)

The diagnostic sensitivity and specificity can then be calculated by placing these numbers into the formulas we previously discussed:

$$\text{Diagnostic Sensitivity (\%)} = [160 \div (160 + 1)] \times 100 = 99.4\%$$

$$\text{Diagnostic Specificity (\%)} = [25 \div (25 + 14)] \times 100 = 64.1\%$$

This particular test is highly sensitive, detecting 99.4% of people who have the disease being tested for. However, the test is not very specific because it gives true-negative results in only 64.1% of people without the disease, and the remaining 35.9% without the disease have false-positive results.

Sensitivity and specificity are characteristics of the test itself. However, to determine the probability that a person with a particular test result actually has the disease or not, it is important to consider how often the disease occurs in the population being tested. The parameters used to make this determination are called *predictive values.* The **positive predictive value** is the probability that a person with a positive test actually has the disease being tested for. The positive predictive value is determined by dividing the true-positive results by the true-positive and the false-positive results added together:

$$\text{Positive Predictive Value (\%)} = \frac{\text{True Positives}}{\text{True Positives} + \text{False Positives}} \times 100$$

In the example given earlier, out of 200 patients, 160 were truly positive and 14 were falsely positive. Using these values in the equation gives us:

$$\text{Positive Predictive Value (\%)} = [160 \div (160 + 14)] \times 100 = 91.95\%$$

Thus, in this case, if an individual tests positive for a certain disease, there is approximately a 92% probability that the individual has that disease.

Likewise, the **negative predictive value** is the probability that a person with a negative screening test does not have the disease. It can be determined using the following formula:

$$\text{Negative Predictive Value (\%)} = \frac{\text{True Negatives}}{\text{True Negatives} + \text{False Negatives}} \times 100$$

Now let's use this formula to calculate the negative predictive value for the test results discussed in the previous example:

$$\text{Negative Predictive Value (\%)} = [25 \div (25 + 1)] \times 100 = 96.2\%$$

In this case, there is a 96.2% probability that a person with a negative test result does not have the disease in question. These values can help clinicians make a decision about an individual patient based on their test results and the prevalence of the disease in the population being tested.

Knowledge Check 9-4

The test parameter that is a measure of the true negative result is known as:

a. Diagnostic sensitivity
b. Diagnostic specificity
c. Positive predictive value
d. Negative predictive value

Critical Thinking 9-2

In a population of 200 people, 175 who were known to have a disease tested positive with a new laboratory assay, and 25 tested negative. Of the 200 people known not to have the condition, 167 tested negative, and 33 tested positive. Calculate the diagnostic specificity of this assay.

KEY CONCEPTS

Specimen Preparation and Storage

- Serum for serological testing is obtained by allowing a sterile tube of blood to clot at either room temperature or 4°C and then carefully removing the serum from the clot after centrifugation has taken place.
- For some serology tests, plasma, CSF, urine, or synovial fluid may be used and should be processed according to manufacturer's instructions.

Pipettes and Measuring

- Volumetric pipettes hold a specified amount of liquid and are calibrated to deliver (TD) that exact amount.
- Serological pipettes are calibrated all the way to the bottom of the pipette. The liquid remaining in such a pipette must be blown out to deliver the exact amount of liquid required. These pipettes are labeled "TC" (to contain).
- Micropipettes are calibrated to deliver an exact volume. They are commonly used for patient samples due to their accuracy with smaller volumes.

Dilutions

- A dilution is prepared by adding either a reagent or a sample of patient serum (the solute) to a liquid (called the *diluent*) to make a weaker solution. It is often necessary to make a dilution for a visible endpoint to occur in antigen–antibody reactions.
- In serological testing, an antibody in a sample of patient serum can be made less concentrated by adding it to a diluent. The resulting dilution can be expressed as a ratio (e.g., 1:20) or as a fraction—for example, 1/20.
- In a *serial dilution*, a series of dilutions is made using a constant dilution factor.
- Serial dilutions are used to determine the titer, or strength, of an antibody. The last tube in which a visible reaction is seen is considered the endpoint.

Test Parameters

- *Diagnostic sensitivity* is defined as the proportion of people who have a specific disease or condition and have a positive test result for that disease or condition.
- *Diagnostic specificity* refers to the proportion of people who do not have the disease or condition and who have a negative test result for that disease or condition.
- These terms are not to be confused with *analytic sensitivity* (the lower limit of detection for an analyte) and *analytic specificity* (the ability of a test to detect only a specific analyte).
- If a test is highly sensitive and highly specific, it is a good indicator that a patient has the disease or condition if positive results are obtained.
- The positive predictive value is the likelihood that a person with a positive screening test actually has the disease.
- The negative predictive value is the probability that a person with a negative screening test does not have the disease.
- Positive and negative predictive values help clinicians determine whether a positive or a negative test is likely to be a true result based on a specific test population.

CASE STUDIES

1. A serology supervisor who has worked for the last 20 years in a clinical laboratory is training a new employee. A dilution of a patient's serum must be made to run a particular test. The supervisor is showing the new employee how to pipet the serum specimen. The amount needed is 0.1 mL. Using a serological pipette, the supervisor draws up the patient specimen to the 0.9-mL mark and then lets it drain out. There is a tiny drop left in the pipette, but the supervisor explains to the new person that this is close enough. The supervisor then adds 1.9 mL of diluent to the tube with the serum. A 1:40 dilution of the serum is needed to run the test.

Questions

a. Explain any mistakes the supervisor may have made during the demonstration.
b. Was the dilution prepared correctly? If not, indicate how the dilution should be prepared, showing your calculations.

2. A serology supervisor is considering implementing a new method for detecting condition A in the laboratory. To validate the new assay, 200 samples were tested:

- 100 samples were from patients known to have condition A and the remaining 100 samples were from people known not to have condition A.
- Of the 100 samples from patients known to be positive for condition A, 80 samples tested positive and 20 samples tested negative.
- Of the 100 samples from patients known to be negative for condition A, 95 samples tested negative and 5 samples tested positive.

Questions

a. How many of the samples are true positives?
b. How many of the samples are false positives?
c. How many of the samples are true negatives?
d. How many of the samples are false negatives?
e. Calculate the diagnostic sensitivity of the assay.
f. Calculate the diagnostic specificity of the assay.
g. Calculate the positive predictive value of the assay.
h. Calculate the negative predictive value of the assay.
i. What can you conclude about the likelihood that a patient in this population who has a positive test result truly has condition A?

REVIEW QUESTIONS

1. If serum is not tested immediately, how should it be treated?
   a. It can be left at room temperature for 24 hours.
   b. It can be stored in the refrigerator for up to 72 hours.
   c. It can be stored in the refrigerator for up to 48 hours.
   d. It needs to be frozen immediately.

2. A 1:750 dilution of serum is needed to perform a serological test. Which of the following series of dilutions would be correct to use in this situation?
   a. 1:5, 1:15, 1:10
   b. 1:5, 1:10, 1:5
   c. 1:15, 1:10, 1:3
   d. 1:15, 1:3, 1:5

3. How much diluent needs to be added to 0.2 mL of serum to make a 1:20 dilution?
   a. 19.8 mL
   b. 4 mL
   c. 3.8 mL
   d. 10 mL

4. If glacial acetic acid needs to be diluted in water to make a 10% solution, what does the glacial acetic acid represent?
   a. Solute
   b. Diluent
   c. Titer
   d. Serial dilution

5. A pipette that has markings all the way down to its tip is called a
   a. Volumetric pipette
   b. Serial pipette
   c. Graduated pipette
   d. Micropipette

6. A serological test requires 5 mL of a 1:50 dilution. How much serum is required to make this dilution?
   a. 0.5 mL
   b. 0.01 mL
   c. 1 mL
   d. 0.1 mL

7. If 0.02 mL of serum is diluted with 0.08 mL of diluent, what dilution of serum does this represent?
   a. 1:4
   b. 1:5
   c. 1:10
   d. 1:20

8. A tube containing a 1:40 dilution is accidentally dropped. A 1:2 dilution of the specimen is still available. A volume of 4 mL is needed to run the test. How much of the 1:2 dilution is needed to remake 4 mL of a 1:40 dilution?
   a. 0.2 mL
   b. 0.4 mL
   c. 0.5 mL
   d. 1.0 mL

9. If 0.4 mL of serum is mixed with 15.6 mL of diluent, what dilution of serum does this represent?
   a. 1:4
   b. 1:40
   c. 2:70
   d. 1:80

10. How much diluent needs to be added to 0.1 mL of serum to make a 1:15 dilution?
    a. 1.4 mL
    b. 1.5 mL
    c. 5 mL
    d. 15 mL

11. Which of the following choices would be considered a serial dilution?
    a. 1:5, 1:15, 1:20
    b. 1:2, 1:10, 1:25
    c. 1:15, 1:30, 1:40
    d. 1:5, 1:15, 1:45

12. Dilutions were set up to titer an antibody. The following results were obtained: 1:4 +, 1:8 +, 1:16 +, 1:32 +, 1:64 –. How should the titer be reported?
    a. 4
    b. 16
    c. 32
    d. 64

13. If a serological test is positive for an individual who does not have a particular disease, the result was caused by a problem with
    a. sensitivity.
    b. specificity.
    c. accuracy.
    d. poor pipetting.

14. Which of the following would be the correct way to make a 5% solution of hydrochloric acid from concentrated hydrochloric acid?
    a. 0.5 mL of acid and 9.5 mL of water
    b. 0.5 mL of acid and 95 mL of water
    c. 0.1 mL of acid and 9.9 mL of water
    d. 0.1 mL of acid and 4.9 mL of water

15. What is the final dilution of serum obtained from the following serial dilutions: 1:4, 1:4, 1:4, 1:4, 1:4, 1:4?
    a. 1:24
    b. 1:256
    c. 1:1,024
    d. 1:4,096

16. Suppose you set up a row of 10 tubes. You pipet 0.4 mL of saline into tube 1 and 0.6 mL of saline into tubes 2 to 10. Next, you add 0.4 mL of patient serum to tube 1. Then, you serially transfer 0.2 mL from one tube to the next, discarding 0.2 mL from tube 10. What is the dilution of tube 4?
    a. 1:16
    b. 1:54
    c. 1:128
    d. 1:256

17. Suppose you set up a row of 10 tubes. You pipet 0.8 mL of saline in tube 1 and 0.9 mL of saline in tubes 2 to 10. You add 0.2 mL of patient serum to tube 1, and serially transfer 0.1 mL through tube 10. Finally, you add 0.9 mL of antigen to each tube. What is the final titer of tube 3?
    a. 1:500
    b. 1:1,000
    c. 1:5,000
    d. 1:10,000

18. A new laboratory assay gave the following results: number of patients tested = 100; number of true positives = 54, number of true negatives = 42; number of false positives = 2; number of false negatives = 2. What is the specificity of this assay in whole numbers?
    a. 75%
    b. 85%
    c. 95%
    d. 98%

19. What is the sensitivity of the assay in Question 18?
    a. 84%
    b. 90%
    c. 92%
    d. 96%

20. A screening test gave the following results: number of patients tested = 150; number of true positives = 50; number of true negatives = 85; number of false positives = 5; number of false negatives = 10. What is the positive predictive value rounded off to a whole number for a patient whose test is positive?
    a. 91%
    b. 83%
    c. 89%
    d. 56%

Chapter 9 Answer Key

Answers to Knowledge Checks

9.1 b 9.2 d 9.3 c 9.4 b

Answers to Review Questions

1. b	2. a	3. c	4. a	5. c	6. d	7. b
8. a	9. b	10. a	11. d	12. c	13. b	14. a
15. d	16. c	17. b	18. c	19. d	20. a	

10

Precipitation and Agglutination Reactions

Christine Dorresteyn Stevens, EdD, MT(ASCP), Linda E. Miller, PhD, I, MB[CM](ASCP)SI, and Marnie Imhoff, MA, MBA, MLS(ASCP)[CM]

LEARNING OUTCOMES

After finishing this chapter, you should be able to:

10.1 Discuss affinity and avidity and their influence on antigen-antibody reactions.

10.2 Describe how the law of mass action relates to antigen-antibody binding.

10.3 Define *precipitation* and *agglutination* and differentiate between the two types of reactions.

10.4 Describe the relative concentrations of antigen and antibody in the three zones of the precipitin curve and discuss why optimal precipitation occurs in the zone of equivalence.

10.5 Define *prozone* and *postzone* and discuss their clinical significance.

10.6 Differentiate between immunoturbidimetry and nephelometry and discuss the role of each in the measurement of precipitation reactions.

10.7 Contrast single immunodiffusion and double immunodiffusion.

10.8 Summarize the principle of the endpoint method of radial immunodiffusion (RID).

10.9 Deduce the relationship between two antigens by looking at the pattern of precipitation resulting from Ouchterlony immunodiffusion.

10.10 Describe the principle of immunofixation electrophoresis (IFE).

10.11 Describe the principle of flocculation.

10.12 Recognize how immunoglobulin M (IgM) and immunoglobulin G (IgG) differ in their ability to participate in agglutination reactions.

10.13 Describe physiological conditions that can be altered to enhance agglutination.

10.14 Explain the principle and give an example of each of the following: (a) direct agglutination, (b) passive agglutination, (c) reverse passive agglutination, (d) agglutination inhibition, (e) hemagglutination inhibition, and (f) coagglutination.

10.15 Describe the principle of the particle-enhanced turbidimetric inhibition immunoassay (PETINIA), the particle counting immunoassay (PACIA), and the kinetic interaction of microparticles in a solution (KIMS).

10.16 Identify conditions that must be met for optimal results in agglutination testing.

CHAPTER OUTLINE

You can go to **fadavis.com** keyword stevens for the laboratory exercises that accompany this text.

Combining an antigen with a specific antibody plays an important role in the laboratory in diagnosing many diseases. Immunoassays have been developed to detect either antigen or antibody and vary from easily performed manual tests to highly complex automated assays. The first such assays were based on the principles of precipitation or agglutination. **Precipitation** involves combining soluble antigen with soluble antibody to produce visible insoluble complexes. **Agglutination** is the aggregation of particulate antigens to form larger visible complexes when a specific antibody is present. Examples of particles used in agglutination tests are red blood cells (RBCs), bacterial cells, and inert particles such as latex or charcoal coated with antigen. Precipitation and agglutination are considered *unlabeled immunoassays* because a marker label is not needed to detect the reaction. We consider *labeled immunoassays,* which were developed much later, in Chapter 11.

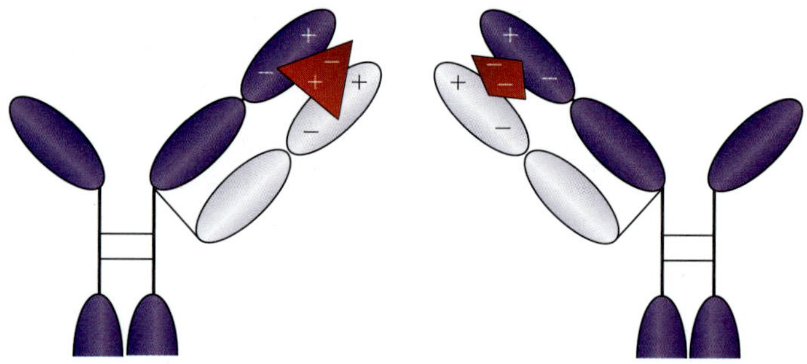

FIGURE 10–1 Affinity is determined by the three-dimensional fit and molecular attractions between one antigenic determinant and one antibody binding site. The antigenic determinant on the left has a better fit and charge distribution than the epitope on the right and, hence, will have a higher affinity for the antibody.

Antigen-Antibody Binding

The union of binding sites on an antibody with specific epitopes on an antigen depends on two antibody characteristics: *affinity* and *avidity.* These characteristics are important because they affect the sensitivity and specificity of clinical laboratory testing.

Affinity

Affinity is the initial force of attraction between a single Fab site on an antibody molecule and a single epitope or determinant site on the corresponding antigen. As the epitope and binding site come near each other, they are held together by weak bonds occurring over a short distance (about 1×10^{-7} mm).

The strength of attraction depends on the specificity of an antibody for a particular antigen. One antibody molecule may initially attract many different antigens, but the epitope's shape and the way it fits together with the binding sites on an antibody molecule determine whether the bonding will be stable. Antibodies can also react with antigens that are structurally similar to the original antigen that induced antibody production, a phenomenon known as **cross-reactivity.** The more the cross-reacting antigen resembles the original antigen, the stronger the bond between the antigen and the binding site will be. However, if the epitope and the binding site have a perfect lock-and-key fit, as is the case with the original antigen, the affinity will be maximal **(Fig. 10–1).** The assay reaction is more sensitive when the affinity is higher because more antigen-antibody complexes are formed and more easily detected.

Avidity

Avidity represents the overall strength of antigen-antibody binding and is the sum of the affinities of all the individual antibody-antigen combining sites. It involves the binding of a multivalent antibody to a multivalent antigen and is a measure of the overall stability of an antigen-antibody complex, or the force that keeps the molecules bound together. A high avidity can compensate for a low affinity. Different classes of antibodies differ in their avidities. The more bonds that form between antigen and antibody, the higher the avidity is and the less likely the reaction is to be reversed. Immunoglobulin M (IgM), for instance, has a higher avidity than IgG because IgM has a valence of 10 (i.e., 10 antigen binding sites), whereas IgG has just 2 **(Fig. 10–2;** also see Chapter 3 for a comparison of IgG and IgM**).** Both affinity and avidity contribute to the stability of the antigen-antibody complexes, which is essential to detect the presence of an unknown, whether it is antigen or antibody.

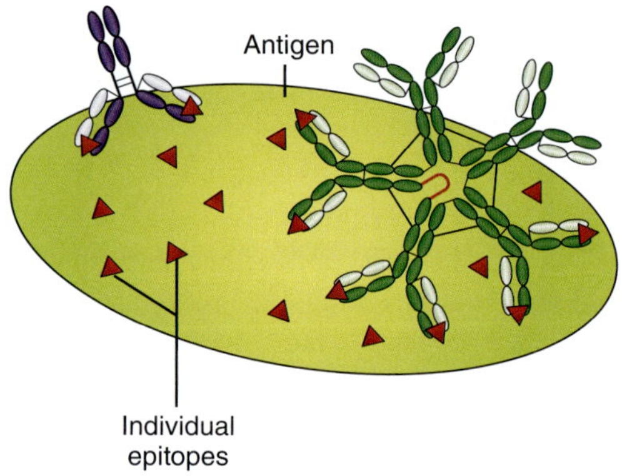

FIGURE 10–2 Avidity is the sum of the forces binding multivalent antigens to multivalent antibodies. IgM has a higher avidity than IgG because it has more potential binding sites for antigen (10 vs 2). The monomer subunits in IgM can swing up or down to bind antigen more effectively.

Law of Mass Action

All antigen-antibody binding is reversible, as represented by the following reaction:

$$\text{Antigen} + \text{Antibody} \leftrightarrow \text{Antigen-Antibody complex}$$

This reaction is governed by the **law of mass action.** According to this law, the concentrations of bound reactants (antigen-antibody complex) and free reactants (antigen and antibody) are constant when the reaction reaches equilibrium. The equilibrium constant *K* represents the difference in the rates of the forward and reverse reactions according to the following equation:

$$K = [AgAb]/[Ab][Ag]$$

where [*AgAb*] is the concentration of the antigen-antibody complex (mol/L), [*Ab*] is the concentration of free antibody (mol/L), and [*Ag*] is the concentration of free antigen (mol/L).

The value of *K* depends on the strength of binding between antibody and antigen. As the binding becomes stronger, the tendency of the antigen-antibody complexes to dissociate decreases, thus increasing the value of *K*. When the value of *K* is higher, the amount of antigen-antibody complex is larger, and the assay reaction is more visible or easily detectable. The ideal conditions for a laboratory test would be to have an antibody with a high affinity, or initial force of attraction, and a high avidity, or strength of binding. The higher the values are for both affinity and avidity, the more antigen-antibody complexes are formed, and the more sensitive is the test.

Knowledge Check 10-1

According to the law of mass action, the rate of antigen-antibody binding is directly proportional to the:

a. Temperature at which the reaction is occurring
b. Molecular size of the antigen and antibody
c. Concentrations of the bound reactants and unbound reactants
d. pH of the reaction solution

Principles of Precipitation Reactions

Precipitation was first noted in 1897 by Kraus, who found that culture filtrates of enteric bacteria would precipitate when mixed with specific antibodies. **Precipitation reactions result from** soluble antigens combining with soluble antibodies to produce visible insoluble complexes. Antibodies that participate in a precipitation reaction are called **precipitins.** For precipitation reactions to occur, both the antigen and antibody must have multiple binding sites for one another, and the relative concentration of each must be equal.

Precipitation Curve

In addition to the affinity and avidity of the antibody, precipitation depends on the relative proportions of antigen and antibody present. Optimal precipitation occurs when the relative amounts of antigen and antibody binding sites are equivalent, and neither is in excess compared to the other. This relationship was discovered in 1932 by Heidelberger and Kendall, who set up a series of tubes containing a constant amount of antibody and increasing amounts of the corresponding antigen. As you can see in **Figure 10–3,** when the concentration of antigen is plotted on the *x*-axis of a graph and the number of antigen-antibody complexes is plotted on the *y*-axis, a bell-shaped curve results. The curve can be divided into three zones: (1) the zone of antibody excess (prozone), (2) the zone of antigen excess (postzone), and (3) the zone of equivalence.

Three Zones of the Precipitation Reaction

In the *zone of antibody excess,* the concentration of antibody molecules is greater than the concentration of antigen molecules. This results in the formation of small immune complexes, with little or no precipitation. Likewise, in the *zone of antigen excess,* the concentration of antigen molecules is greater than the concentration of antibody molecules. Again, little or no precipitation results, and the reaction is less than optimal.

In the **zone of equivalence** seen in the middle of the curve, the number of multivalent sites of antigen and antibody are approximately equal. In this zone, precipitation is the result of random, reversible reactions whereby each antibody binds to more than one antigen, and vice versa, forming a stable network or **lattice.** The concept of lattice formation, as formulated by Philippa Marrack, is based on the assumptions that each antibody molecule must have at least two binding sites, and the antigen must be multivalent. As antigen and antibody combine, a multimolecular lattice forms that increases in size until it precipitates out of solution.

As you can see in Figure 10–3, when increasing amounts of soluble antigen are added to a constant amount of antibody,

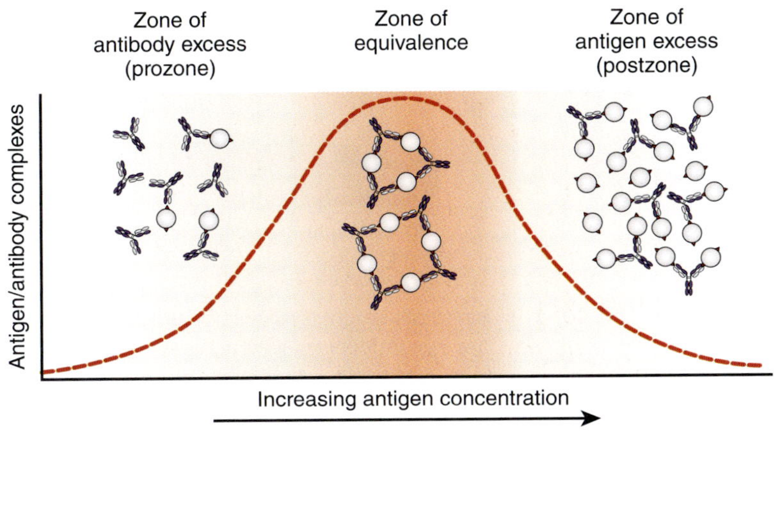

FIGURE 10–3 Precipitin curve. The precipitin curve shows how the amount of precipitation varies with increasing antigen concentrations when the amount of antibody is kept constant. Optimal precipitation occurs in the zone of equivalence. A large excess of antibody results in a prozone, whereas a large excess of antigen creates a postzone.

the number of antigen-antibody complexes (and thus, the amount of precipitation) increases until the zone of equivalence is reached. When the amount of antigen becomes greater than the number of antibody binding sites present, precipitation begins to decline because fewer lattice networks are formed. Thus, optimal precipitation occurs in the zone of equivalence. (The same type of curve would result if the antibody concentration is changed and the amount of antigen is kept constant.) It is important to note that the relationship between the amounts of antigen and antibody and the formation of immune complexes also applies to immunologic reactions other than precipitation and is the basis for all serological testing.

Prozone and Postzone

As you can see in the precipitin curve, precipitation declines on either side of the equivalence zone because of an excess of either antigen or antibody. When antibody excess is extreme, a **prozone** occurs, in which antigen combines with only one or two antibody molecules, and no cross-linkages are formed (see left side of the curve in Fig. 10-3). In the prozone, only one site on an antibody molecule is usually used, many free antibody molecules remain in solution, and precipitation is undetectable.

At the right side of the curve, where there is an area of extreme antigen excess, a **postzone** occurs in which small aggregates are surrounded by excess antigen. In this case, every available antibody site is bound to a single antigen, and no cross-links are formed. Again, no lattice network is formed, and precipitation does not occur (see Fig. 10–3).

The clinical laboratory must consider the prozone and postzone phenomena because negative reactions occur in both. A false-negative reaction may occur in the prozone because of a high antibody concentration in the unknown sample, such as patient serum. If the reaction is suspected to be a false negative, diluting the antibody until equivalence is reached and then performing the test again can produce a positive result.

In the postzone, excess antigen may obscure the presence of a small amount of antibody. If the antigen to be detected is in the patient sample, the sample can be diluted to reach equivalence with the antibody reagent. If the antigen is a reagent in the test, the test may be repeated with another sample from the patient collected about a week later. The extra time may allow for the further production of antibody by the patient. If the repeated test is negative, the patient is unlikely to have that particular antibody.

Critical Thinking 10-1

A patient displays the classic symptoms of measles; however, the measles IgM antibody test is negative. Based on what you have learned about the precipitation curve, what could explain the test results, and how might this discrepancy be resolved?

Immunoturbidimetry and Nephelometry

Precipitation is one of the simplest methods of detecting antigen-antibody reactions because most antigens are multivalent and, therefore, capable of forming aggregates in the presence of the corresponding antibody. When antigen and antibody solutions are mixed, the antigen cross-links with numerous antibody molecules, and the lattice networks become so large that they precipitate out of solution. Although the oldest methods to measure precipitation were manual, in today's clinical laboratory, precipitation reactions are most commonly measured by automated methods based on immunoturbidimetry or nephelometry.

Immunoturbidimetry involves the optical measurement of the *turbidity* or cloudiness of a solution. The turbidity is a result of antigen-antibody complexes precipitating out of solution. A spectrophotometer or an automated analyzer is used to measure the turbidity of the solution with a photodetector. The photodetector is placed 180 degrees from an incident light, collecting the light after it has passed through the solution **(Fig. 10–4).** This device measures the reduction in light intensity caused by reflection, absorption, or scatter of light as immune complexes are formed. The result is recorded in absorbance units, a measure of the ratio of incident light to transmitted light. As the concentration of immune complexes increases, the amount of light absorbed increases, and light transmission decreases.

Nephelometry measures the light that is scattered at a particular angle from the incident beam as it passes through a suspension (see Fig. 10–4). Scattering occurs when a beam of light passes through a solution, encounters molecules in its path, and bounces off the molecules. The light travels

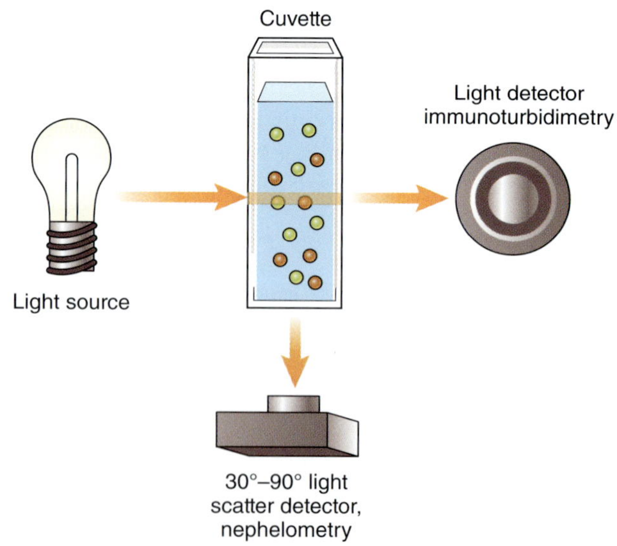

FIGURE 10–4 Principles of immunoturbidimetry and nephelometry. In immunoturbidimetry, light rays passing directly through the solution are measured, in contrast to nephelometry, which measures light scatter with a light-detection device located at an angle to the incident light.

in all directions and is measured by an instrument called a *nephelometer,* which contains a photodetector between 30 and 90 degrees from the light source. The amount of light scatter is proportional to the size, shape, and concentration of molecules in solution, in this case, free antigen, free antibody, and antigen-antibody complexes. Thus, light scatter increases as the number of immune complexes increases and is an indication of the concentration of antigen or antibody in solution.

Clinical instruments use a technique called **rate nephelometry** to measure serum proteins. In this instance, patient serum contains the antigen, and a reagent containing the corresponding antibody is added to the reaction cuvette. For example, to measure C-reactive protein (CRP) in patient serum, an anti-CRP reagent is added. The rate of light scatter increase is measured immediately after adding the reagent antibody; thus, several samples can be assayed in just a few minutes. The antibody concentration is kept constant, and the rate of light scatter increase is directly related to the antigen concentration in the patient serum. A computer extrapolates light scatter to give the concentration of antigen in the patient sample in milligrams per deciliter (mg/dL) or international units per milliliter (IU/mL), based on established values of standards.

Rate nephelometry and immunoturbidimetry are commonly used to quantify the immunoglobulins IgG, IgA, IgM, and IgE, and kappa and lambda light chains. Other serum proteins measured by these methods include complement components such as C3 and C4, CRP, haptoglobin, and ceruloplasmin. Nephelometry and immunoturbidimetry provide accurate and precise quantitation of serum proteins, and because of automation, the cost per test is typically lower than manual methods. Additionally, very small sample volumes can be analyzed. Both rate nephelometry and immunoturbidity can be subject to postzone phenomenon; therefore, dilutions may be necessary to screen for antigen excess. In general, nephelometry is more sensitive than immunoturbidimetry, with a lower limit of detection of 1 to 10 mg/L, although the sensitivity of immunoturbidimetry methods has increased.

Passive Immunodiffusion Techniques

The precipitation of antigen-antibody complexes can also be detected by manual methods that use a support medium, such as a gel. Agarose, a purified high molecular weight complex polysaccharide derived from seaweed, is used for this purpose. When antigen and antibody diffuse toward one another in a gel matrix, visible lines of precipitation will form. Agarose stabilizes the diffusion process and allows visualization of the precipitin bands.

Antigen and antibody are added to wells cut into the gel, diffuse through the gel medium, and combine with each other. This process is known as **passive immunodiffusion** when no electrical current is used to speed up the migration of the reactants. The rate of diffusion is affected by several factors, including the size of the particles (larger particles migrate slower than smaller ones), temperature (warmer temperatures speed up the reaction), and gel viscosity (molecules travel slower when the gel is more viscous and less hydrated). The reactions can be classified as single or double immunodiffusion based on the number of reactants diffusing in the gel and the direction of diffusion.

Radial Immunodiffusion

Radial immunodiffusion (RID) is a quantitative single-diffusion technique involving migration of antigen only. In this method, reagent antibody is uniformly mixed into the support gel in a flat plate, and antigen contained in commercial standards or patient samples is applied to wells cut into the gel. During incubation, the antigen diffuses out from each well and combines with specific antibody in the agarose to form rings of precipitation around the wells. The rings expand in size until the zone of equivalence is reached, and a stable lattice network is formed. The diameter of the ring obtained is a measure of the antigen concentration in a particular well. The antigen concentration within a patient sample can be derived from a standard curve obtained by using antigens of known concentrations. **Figure 10–5** depicts typical RID results. The absence of a ring indicates absence of the antigen in the patient sample. The larger the precipitation ring, the greater is the antigen concentration in the patient sample.

The **endpoint method** is one RID technique developed by Mancini. In this technique, antigen is allowed to diffuse to completion; when equivalence is reached, there is no further change in the ring diameter. Equivalence occurs between 24 and 72 hours of incubation. The square of the ring diameter is directly proportional to the concentration of the antigen. When concentrations of antigen standards are plotted on the *x*-axis and their corresponding ring diameters are squared and plotted on the *y*-axis, a linear graph connecting the points

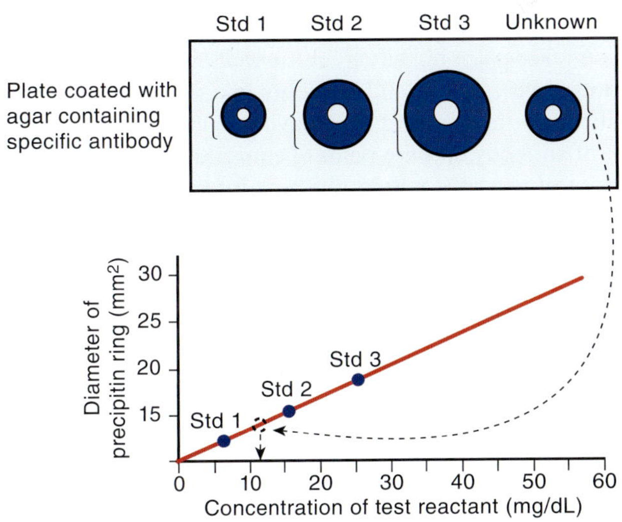

FIGURE 10–5 Radial immunodiffusion. The amount of precipitate formed is in proportion to the amount of antigen in the sample. In the Mancini endpoint method, the antigen concentration is in proportion to the diameter squared. The concentration of the test reactant in the unknown sample can be determined from a curve generated from standards with known concentrations of the reactant.

is created. The major drawback to this method is the time it takes to obtain results. Another method, the kinetic or Fahey method, uses ring-diameter readings taken at about 19 hours before equivalence is reached. In this case, the ring diameter is proportional to the log of the antigen concentration, and a graph is plotted using semilog paper. The diameter is plotted on the *x*-axis, and the antigen concentration is on the *y*-axis, automatically giving a log value. Commercial kits may also contain a chart provided by the manufacturer that indicates concentration relative to the ring diameter.

The precision of the assay is directly related to accurate measurement of samples and standards. Sources of error include overfilling or underfilling the wells with sample, nicking the side of the wells when filling, spilling sample outside the wells, improper incubation time and temperature, and incorrect measurement of ring diameters. Like nephelometry and immunoturbidimetry, RID has been used to measure immunoglobulin classes and subclasses, complement components, and other serum proteins. Immunodiffusion is simple to perform and requires no instrumentation but uses expensive reagents, has a long turnaround time to results, and is subject to technical artifacts. For these reasons, it has been largely replaced by automated techniques such as nephelometry in the clinical laboratory.

Ouchterlony Double Diffusion

One of the older, classic immunochemical techniques is **Ouchterlony double diffusion.** In this technique, antigen and antibody diffuse independently through a semisolid medium in two dimensions, horizontally and vertically. Wells are cut into a gel, and reactants are added to the wells. Most Ouchterlony plates are set up with a central well surrounded by four to six equidistant outer wells. Antibodies are placed in the central well, and different antigens are placed in the surrounding wells to determine if the antigens share identical epitopes. Diffusion takes place radially from the wells. After an incubation period of between 12 and 48 hours in a moist chamber, precipitin lines form where the moving front of antigen meets that of antibody and the point of equivalence is reached. The density of the lines reflects the amount of immune complex formed.

The position of the precipitin bands between wells allows for the antigens to be compared with one another. Three patterns of precipitation are possible **(Fig. 10–6):**

1. *Identity:* The two precipitin lines fuse together at their junction to form an arc representing serological identity or the presence of a common epitope on the antigens.
2. *Nonidentity:* A pattern of crossed lines demonstrates two separate reactions and indicates that the compared antigens share no common epitopes.
3. *Partial identity:* Indicated by fusion of two continuous lines with a spur. In the case of partial identity, the two antigens share a common epitope, but one of the antigens is more complex and contains additional epitopes. Some antibody molecules are not captured by the simpler antigen and travel through the initial precipitin line to combine with additional epitopes found in the more complex antigen. Therefore, the spur always points to the simpler antigen.

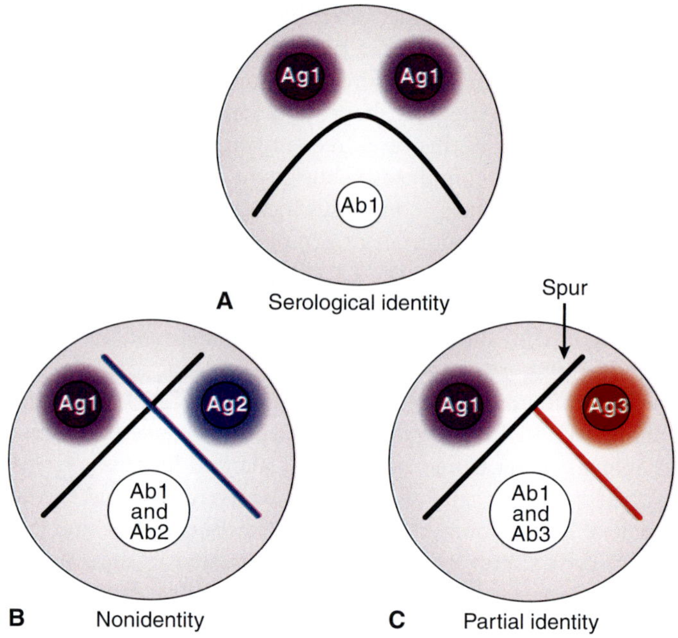

FIGURE 10–6 The three Ouchterlony diffusion patterns. An antibody mixture is placed in the central well of a gel. Unknown antigens are placed in the outside wells. The antibodies (Ab) and antigens (Ag) diffuse radially out of the wells. (A) Serological identity. If the antigens are identical, they will react with the same antibody, and the precipitate line forms a continuous arc. (B) Nonidentity. If the antigens share no identical determinants, they react with different antibodies, forming two crossed lines. (C) Partial identity. Antibodies react with two similar antigens, forming two lines and a spur that points toward the simpler antigen (the antigen that reacts least with the antibody). For example, suppose antigen 3 has an epitope in common with antigen 1, and there are two antibodies in the center well (anti-1 and anti-3). Antibody 3 reacts with the epitope common to both antigens. Antibody 1 reacts with an epitope on antigen 1 that is absent on antigen 3. Two precipitin lines form, with a spur pointing toward antigen 3.

Although Ouchterlony double diffusion is of limited use because it is labor intensive, requires experience to read, and takes time for results to develop, it is still used to identify antibodies to some fungal organisms, such as *Aspergillus, Blastomyces, Coccidioides,* and *Candida.*

Knowledge Check 10-2

In an Ouchterlony double-diffusion immunoassay, the formation of a fused precipitation line between two antigen wells and an antibody well indicates:

a. Reactivity of the antibody with identical antigens of interest
b. Reactivity of the antibody with only one of the two antigens
c. A false negative due to the prozone phenomenon
d. A false positive due to the prozone phenomenon

Flocculation

Flocculation is a variation of precipitation reactions. In a flocculation reaction, immune complex formation happens over a narrow range of antigen concentrations, resulting in fine particulate precipitants. The nontreponemal tests for syphilis, rapid plasma reagin, and Venereal Disease Research Laboratories assay are based on the principle of flocculation (see Chapter 21).

Electrophoretic Techniques

Diffusion can be combined with electrophoresis to speed up or sharpen the results. **Electrophoresis** separates molecules according to their size and electrical charge differences when placed in an electric field. Electrophoresis uses tightly controlled test parameters and a buffer that gives antigens and antibodies a net negative charge. A direct electrical current is applied to the gel using electrodes. One electrode is a cathode, which is negatively charged, and the other is a positively charged anode. When the electrical current is applied to the gel, the negatively charged antigens and antibodies migrate toward the anode **(Fig. 10-7).** Antigens and antibodies carry different negative charge levels, allowing them to separate out on a gel. As diffusion takes place, distinct precipitin bands are formed based on the charge and molecular weight of the proteins. The expected results from electrophoresis of a normal serum sample are shown in Fig. 3–1.

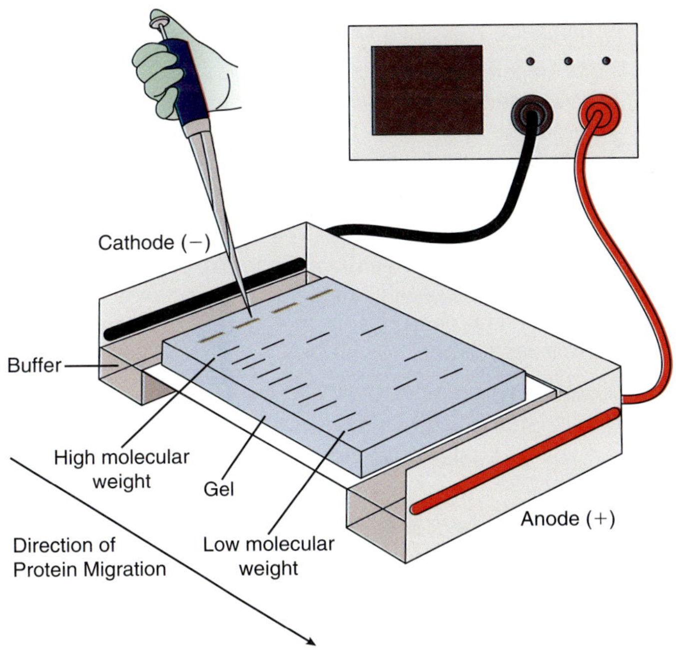

FIGURE 10–7 Electrophoresis. A sample containing antigens or antibodies is loaded into wells in a gel, and the gel is exposed to an electrical current. When a special buffer is used (typically, pH 8.6), the proteins in the sample acquire a negative charge and migrate toward the positively charged anode.

Several precipitation techniques have been combined with electrophoresis, including immunoelectrophoresis, counter-immunoelectrophoresis, rocket immunoelectrophoresis, and immunofixation electrophoresis. One of the more common techniques used in the laboratory is immunofixation electrophoresis.

Immunofixation electrophoresis (IFE), a technique first described by Alper and Johnson, is typically a follow-up test to a serum or urine protein electrophoresis (see Chapter 18). In this method, patient serum is applied to six lanes of an agarose or cellulose acetate gel and electrophoresed to separate the proteins in the sample. Because diffusion occurs across a thin gel (approximately 1 mm), separation occurs in less than 1 hour. After electrophoresis, the five lanes are overlaid with one of the following reagent antibodies: antibody to γ, α, or μ heavy chains and κ or λ light chains. The sixth lane is overlaid with antibodies to all serum proteins and serves as the reference lane. Reactions in each of the five lanes are compared with the reference lane. Immunoprecipitates form only where a specific antigen-antibody combination has taken place and the complexes have become trapped in the gel. The gel is washed to remove any nonprecipitating proteins and can then be stained for easier visibility.

IFE is a qualitative technique used to visualize increases or decreases in immunoglobulin production and to differentiate monoclonal from polyclonal immunoglobulins. IFE is commonly used to detect monoclonal gammopathies such as multiple myeloma (a plasma cell malignancy) or antibody deficiency disorders (see Chapters 18 and 19). Hypogammaglobulinemias, which are characterized by low antibody production, exhibit faintly staining bands, whereas polyclonal hypergammaglobulinemias (overproduction of antibody) show darkly staining bands in the gamma region. The presence of monoclonal antibody, such as that found in B-cell and plasma cell malignancies, results in dark, narrow bands in specific lanes **(Fig. 10–8).**

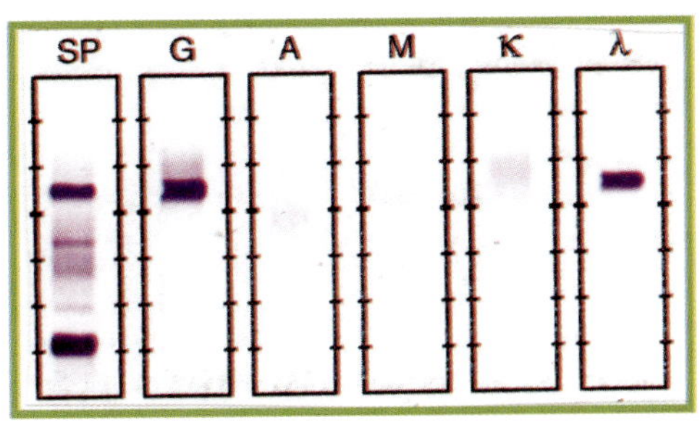

FIGURE 10–8 Immunofixation electrophoresis (IFE). A complex antigen mixture such as proteins in a serum sample is separated by electrophoresis. An antiserum template is aligned over the gel. Then a protein fixative and monospecific antisera to IgG, IgA, IgM, κ, and λ are applied to different sections of the gel. After an incubation, the gel is stained and examined for the presence of abnormal immunoglobulins. Precipitates form where a specific antigen-antibody combination has taken place. In this case, the patient has an IgG monoclonal antibody with λ chains. *(Courtesy of Helena Laboratories, Beaumont, TX.)*

10-1 Clinical Correlations

Immunoproliferative Diseases

Normally, the immune system produces polyclonal immunoglobulins, generated by many clones of B cells as they respond to different antigens in our environment. Patients with cancers involving B cells or plasma cells produce high levels of a monoclonal antibody that originate from the single malignant clone. These conditions are referred to as *immunoproliferative diseases* and include multiple myeloma, which is most commonly characterized by the production of monoclonal IgG, IgA, or free light chains, and Waldenström macroglobulinemia, in which patients produce monoclonal IgM. See Chapter 18 for details.

Comparison of Precipitation Techniques

Each type of precipitation technique has distinct advantages and disadvantages. Manual techniques are simple to perform but have a longer turn-around time to results, whereas automated methods are more expensive but provide faster and more accurate results. Each type of precipitation testing has particular applications for which it is best suited. **Table 10–1** presents a comparison of the precipitation techniques we discussed in this chapter.

Principles of Agglutination Reactions

Whereas precipitation reactions involve soluble antigens, agglutination is the visible aggregation of particles or cells caused by combination with specific antibody. Antibodies that produce these reactions are often called **agglutinins.** Because the reaction takes place on the surface of the particle or cell, the antigen must be exposed and be able to bind with antibody. Types of cells and particles participating in agglutination reactions include erythrocytes, bacteria, and inert carriers such as latex beads. Each cell/particle must have multiple antigenic determinant sites, which are cross-linked to sites on other particles through the formation of antibody bridges. Agglutination occurs when one antibody binds to multiple antigens, creating large immune complexes that can be visualized.

In 1896, Gruber and Durham published the first report about the ability of antibody to clump cells, based on observations of agglutination of bacteria by serum. This finding gave rise to the use of serology as a tool in the diagnosis of disease and led to the discovery of the ABO blood groups. Widal and Sicard developed one of the earliest diagnostic tests in 1896 to detect antibodies occurring in typhoid fever, brucellosis, and tularemia. Agglutination reactions have had a variety of applications in detecting both antigens and antibodies over the years. Such testing is simple to perform, and the endpoints can be easily visualized.

Agglutination, similar to precipitation, is a two-step process that results in the formation of a stable lattice network.

Table 10-1 Comparison of Precipitation Techniques

TECHNIQUE	APPLICATIONS	PRINCIPLE
Immunoturbidimetry	Quantitation of immunoglobulins, complement, CRP, other serum proteins	Light transmitted through the solution is measured with a detector that is in direct alignment with the light source Transmission decreases as antigen concentration increases and makes the solution more turbid
Nephelometry	Quantitation of immunoglobulins, complement, CRP, other serum proteins	Light scattered by particles (free antigen, free antibody, and antigen-antibody complexes) is measured at a specific angle from the incident beam and is proportional to the number of immune complexes formed
Radial immunodiffusion (RID)	Quantitation of immunoglobulins, complement	Antigen is placed in a well and diffuses out into a gel that is infused with antibody. Measurement of the precipitin ring diameter indicates the concentration of the antigen.
Ouchterlony double diffusion	Identification of antibodies to complex antigens, such as fungal antigens	Both antigen and antibody diffuse out from wells in a gel. The patterns of precipitate lines formed indicate the relationship of the antigens or antibodies.
Immunofixation electrophoresis (IFE)	Detects over- or underproduction of immunoglobulins; presence of monoclonal antibody	Antibodies are identified by electrophoresis of serum followed by direct application of reagent antisera to the gel.
Flocculation	Nontreponemal assays for syphilis	Formation of fine precipitins over a narrow range of antigen concentrations

The first step, called **sensitization,** involves antigen-antibody combination through single antigenic determinants on the cell/particle. Sensitization is rapid and reversible. The formation of immune complexes is not visible at this time. The second step, *lattice formation,* involves the development of cross-links that form visible aggregates. Lattice formation represents the stabilization of antigen-antibody complexes with multiple antigenic determinants binding together **(Fig. 10–9).**

Sensitization is affected by the nature of the antigens on the agglutinating particles. If epitopes are sparse or obscured by other surface molecules, they are less likely to interact with antibody. Lattice formation is influenced by antibody class and environmental conditions, including temperature, pH, ionic strength of the test solution, and electrical charge. For example, RBCs and bacterial cells have a slightly negative surface charge; because like charges tend to repel one another, it is sometimes difficult to bring such cells together into a lattice formation.

Antibodies must be able to bridge the distance between two particles for a lattice to form, making the class of immunoglobulin important. Because IgM is a pentamer with a potential valence of 10, it is more than 700 times more efficient in agglutination than IgG, which has a valence of 2 (see Fig. 10–2 and Chapter 3). Antibodies of the IgG class often cannot bridge the distance between particles because their small size, and restricted flexibility at the hinge region may prohibit multivalent binding. IgM antibodies, on the other hand, are strong agglutinins because of their larger size.

Achieving visible reactions with IgG often requires the use of enhancement techniques that vary physicochemical conditions, such as the ionic strength of the solution, the pH, and the temperature. Antibodies belonging to the IgG class agglutinate best at 30°C to 37°C and are referred to as *warm-reacting antibodies,* whereas IgM antibodies are *cold-reacting,* working best at temperatures between 4°C and 27°C. Because naturally occurring antibodies against the ABO blood groups belong to the IgM class, these reactions are best run at room temperature. Antibodies to other human blood groups usually belong to the IgG class, so tests for these must be run at 37°C. Warm-reacting IgG reactions are the most important to consider in selecting compatible blood for a transfusion because they can actually occur in the body.

Knowledge Check 10-3

In agglutination assays, the sensitization step is affected by:

a. Epitopes being obscured by other molecules on the cell surface
b. Ionic strength of the test solution
c. The temperature of the reaction
d. pH of the test solution

10-2 Clinical Correlations

Coombs Reagent

In addition to temperature considerations, detection of IgG antibodies often requires the use of a second antibody, anti-human immunoglobulin, to visualize the reaction. Anti-human immunoglobulin is also known as *Coombs reagent* and is used frequently in blood bank testing. Coombs reagent attaches to the Fc portion of IgG and helps to bridge the gap between RBCs so that a visible agglutination reaction can occur. **Figure 14–9** (Chapter 14) demonstrates how Coombs reagent works.

Types of Agglutination Reactions

Agglutination tests are easy to perform, require no complicated equipment, and can be done as needed in the laboratory without having to batch specimens. Agglutination assays can be performed in test tubes, in microtiter wells, or on slides. Many kits are available for standard testing, so reagent preparation is minimal. Agglutination reactions can be used to iden-

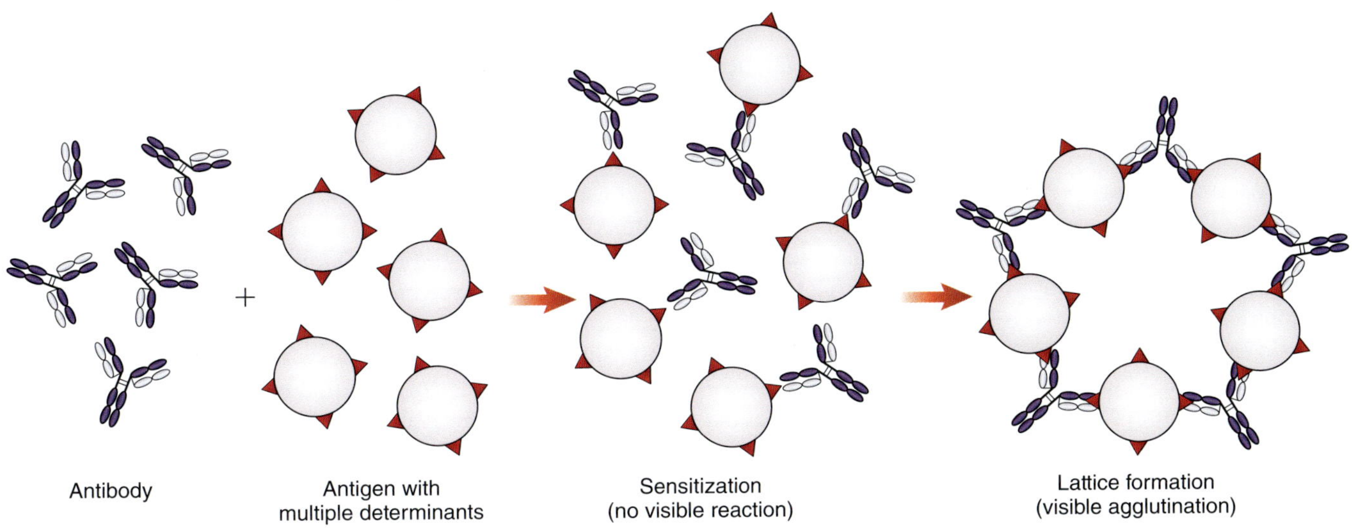

FIGURE 10–9 Phases of agglutination. Sensitization: Single epitopes on the antigen bind to antibody. Lattice formation: Multiple antigen and antibody molecules bind together to form a stable lattice.

tify either antigen or antibody. Typically, most agglutination tests are qualitative, simply indicating the absence or presence of antigen or antibody, but dilutions of the test sample can be made to obtain semiquantitative results. Many variations exist that can be categorized according to the type of particle used in the reaction and whether the antigen or antibody is attached. The main types of agglutination reactions are direct agglutination, passive agglutination, reverse passive agglutination, and agglutination inhibition. We discuss these reactions in the sections that follow and summarize their principles in the Study Guide at the end of this chapter.

Direct Agglutination

Direct agglutination occurs when antigens are found naturally on a particle, such as an RBC or bacterial cell. One of the earliest types of direct agglutination tests developed uses known bacterial antigens to detect bacterial antibodies in a patient. Typically, patient serum is diluted in a series of tubes or wells on a slide and reacted with bacterial antigens specific for the suspected disease. Refer to Chapter 9 for detailed information about serial dilutions. Detection of antibodies is mainly used in the diagnosis of diseases for which the bacterial agents are extremely difficult to culture. One such example is the Widal test, a rapid screening test for antibodies to *Salmonella typhi* antigens, which has been used to help detect typhoid fever. A significant finding is a fourfold increase in antibody titer over time when paired dilutions of serum samples are tested with these antigens. More specific tests are now available, but the Widal test is still considered useful in diagnosing typhoid fever in developing countries and remains in use in some areas of the world because of its low cost.

An agglutination reaction involving RBCs is called **hemagglutination (Fig. 10–10).** This type of agglutination reaction is simple to perform, relatively sensitive, and easy to read. The best example of hemagglutination is ABO blood group typing of human RBCs, one of the world's most frequently used immunoassays. Patient RBCs are mixed with antisera of the IgM type to determine the presence or absence of the A and B antigens; this reaction is usually performed at room temperature, without the need for any enhancement techniques. Group A RBCs will agglutinate with anti-A antibody, and group B RBCs will agglutinate with anti-B antibody.

Other examples of direct hemagglutination tests are some versions of the Monospot and cold agglutinins tests (see Chapters 14 and 23). The Monospot test is used to detect the heterophile antibody characteristic of infectious mononucleosis by its ability to agglutinate horse or bovine RBCs. Cold agglutinins, produced by patients with certain autoimmune disorders, malignancies, or infections, are antibodies that agglutinate human type O RBCs when incubated at cold temperatures.

An antibody titer in a patient sample can be determined by making serial dilutions of the sample in test tubes or microtiter plates. Semiquantitative results are obtained, and the reciprocal of the last dilution still exhibiting a visible reaction is the titer, indicating the antibody's strength. Test interpretation is based on the cell sedimentation pattern. If the test is performed in a microtiter plate, a dark red, smooth button at the bottom of the microtiter well indicates that the result is negative. A positive result will have cells spread across the bottom of the well because of the formation of an antigen-antibody lattice, which may be smooth or have a jagged pattern with an irregular edge. Test tubes can be centrifuged and gently shaken to see if the cell button can be evenly resuspended. If it is resuspended with no visible clumping, then the result is negative. Positive reactions can be graded to indicate the strength of the reaction **(Fig. 10–11).**

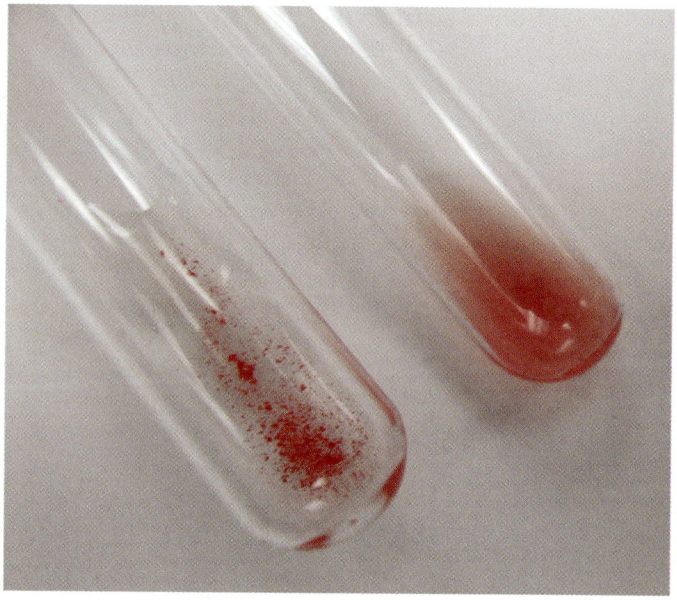

FIGURE 10–10 RBC agglutination. The tube on the left is a positive test for RBC agglutination, whereas the tube on the right is a negative test showing that the unbound RBCs have remained in a smooth suspension. *(Courtesy Linda Miller.)*

Passive Agglutination

Passive, or indirect, **agglutination** uses inert carrier particles that are coated with antigens not normally found on their surfaces. Various particles, including erythrocytes, latex, and gelatin, are used for passive agglutination. Synthetic beads or particles provide the advantages of consistency and uniformity. Reactions are easy to read visually and give rapid results. Many antigens, especially polysaccharides, adsorb to RBCs spontaneously, so they are also relatively easy to manipulate. Particle sizes vary from 7 mm for RBCs to 0.8 mm for fine latex particles.

In 1955, Singer and Plotz found by happenstance that IgG was naturally adsorbed to the surface of polystyrene latex particles. Latex particles are inexpensive, relatively stable, and not subject to cross-reactivity with other antibodies. Many antibody molecules can be bound to the surface of latex particles, so the number of antigen binding sites is large. Additionally, the large particle size facilitates reading of the test. Passive latex agglutination tests have been used to detect many antibodies, including rheumatoid factor (an anti-IgG found in some autoimmune disorders), antibodies to group A *Streptococcus* antigens, and antibodies to viruses such as cytomegalovirus and rubella.

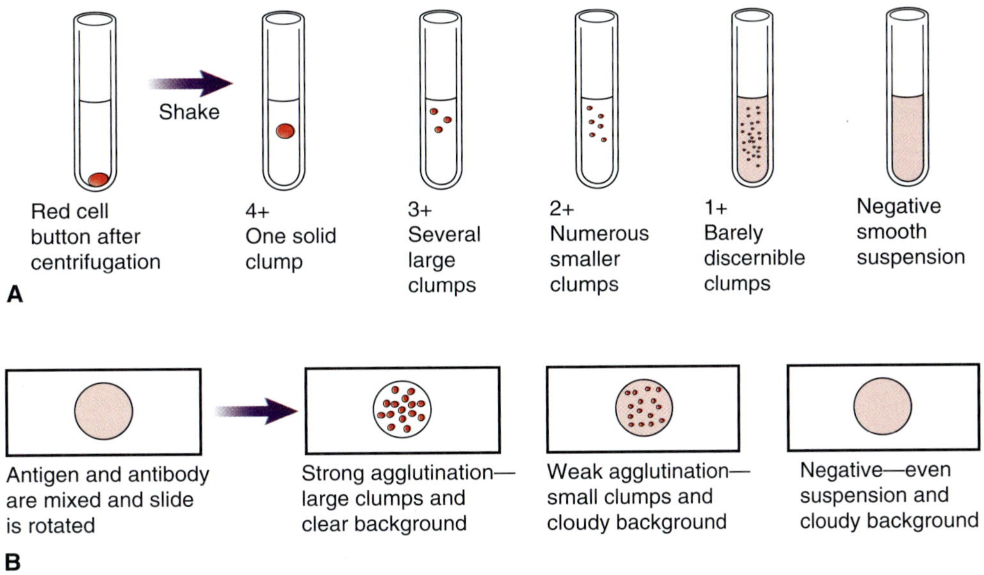

FIGURE 10–11 Grading of agglutination reactions: (A) Tube method. If tubes are centrifuged and shaken to resuspend the button, reactions can be graded from negative to 4+, depending on the size of the clumps observed. (B) Rapid slide method and results.

Because many of these kits are designed to detect IgM antibody, there is a risk of nonspecific agglutination caused by the presence of other IgM antibodies, and reactions must be carefully controlled and interpreted. Commercial tests are usually performed on disposable plastic slide cards or glass slides. Kits contain positive and negative controls; if the controls do not give the expected results, the test is not valid. Such tests are typically used as screening tools, which are followed by more extensive testing if the results are positive.

10-3 Clinical Correlations

Passive Agglutination Tests for Syphilis

A hemagglutination test called the *microhemagglutination assay for Treponema pallidum antibodies* (MHA-TP) was developed to detect antibodies to *T. pallidum*, the cause of syphilis, but has been replaced by a more sensitive gel particle agglutination method, the TP-PA. In this test, patient serum is incubated with gel particles coated with *T. pallidum* antigen in microtiter plate wells. A positive test is indicated by a smooth mat of particles (lattice) covering the well and is seen in patients who currently have syphilis or had syphilis in the past (see Chapter 21).

Reverse Passive Agglutination

In **reverse passive agglutination**, antibody rather than antigen is attached to a carrier particle. The antibody is attached with its active sites facing outward. Adsorption may be spontaneous, or it may require some of the same treatments used for antigen attachment. This type of testing is often used to detect microbial antigens. **Figure 10–12** shows the differences between passive and reverse passive agglutination.

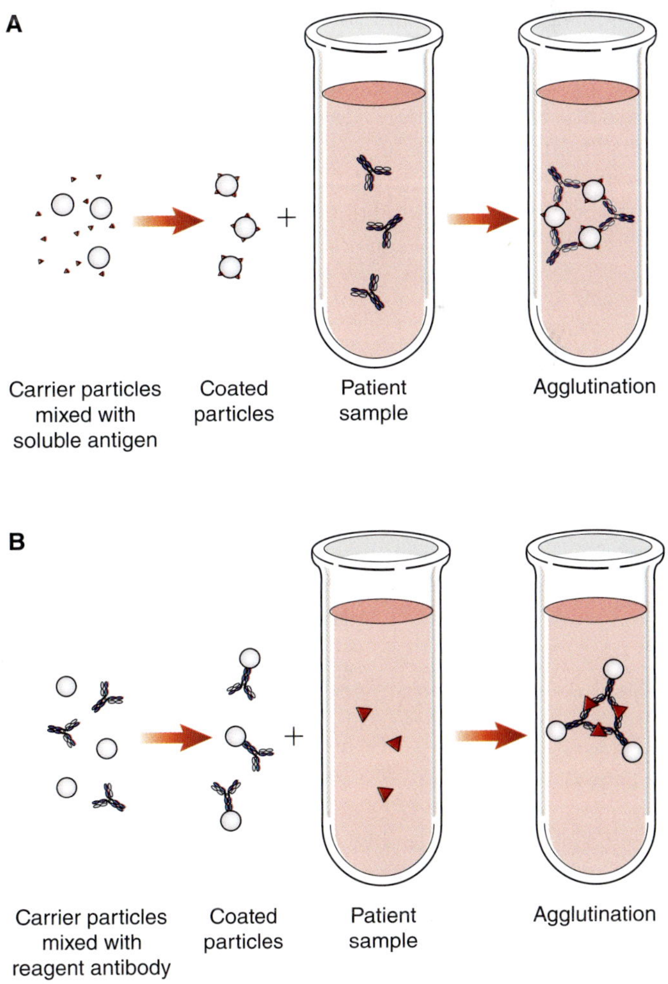

FIGURE 10–12 (A) Passive agglutination. Antigen is attached to carrier particles; agglutination occurs if patient antibody is present. (B) Reverse passive agglutination. Antibody is attached to carrier particles; agglutination occurs if patient antigen is present.

Many kits are available for the rapid identification of antigens from infectious agents such as group A *Streptococcus,* group B *Streptococcus, Staphylococcus aureus,* rotavirus, and *Cryptococcus neoformans.* Rapid agglutination tests have found the widest application in detecting soluble antigens in urine, spinal fluid, and serum. The principle is the same for all these tests: Latex particles coated with antibody are reacted with a patient sample containing the suspected antigen. In some cases, an extraction step is necessary to isolate antigen before the reagent latex particles are added. Organisms can be identified in a few minutes with fairly high sensitivity and specificity, although this varies for different tests. The use of monoclonal antibodies has greatly reduced cross-reactivity, but there is still the possibility of interference or nonspecific agglutination.

Such tests are most often used to detect infections with organisms that are difficult to grow in the laboratory or for instances when rapid identification will allow treatment to be initiated more promptly. Reverse passive agglutination testing has also been used to measure levels of certain therapeutic drugs, hormones, and plasma proteins such as haptoglobin and CRP.

Coagglutination reactions are a type of reverse passive agglutination. In coagglutination, bacteria serve as the inert particle to which antibodies are attached. *Staphylococcus aureus* is one of the most common bacteria used in coagglutination assays due to the presence of protein A on its surface. Protein A readily attaches to the Fc region of antibodies, leaving the Fab region of antibodies available to react with antigens in the patient sample. Coagglutination techniques are often used to enhance the visibility of agglutination.

Agglutination Inhibition

Agglutination inhibition reactions are based on competition between particulate and soluble antigens for limited antibody-combining sites. Typically, this type of reaction involves haptens that are complexed to proteins; the hapten-protein conjugate is then attached to a carrier particle. The patient sample is first reacted with a limited amount of reagent antibody that is specific for the hapten being tested. Indicator particles that contain the same hapten one wishes to measure in the sample are then added. If the patient sample has no free hapten, the reagent antibody can combine with the carrier particles and produce visible agglutination.

In this method, agglutination is a negative reaction, indicating that the patient did not have sufficient hapten to inhibit the secondary reaction **(Fig. 10–13).** In contrast, if the patient sample contains a significant concentration of hapten, it will bind to the reagent antibody and inhibit agglutination; thus, a lack of agglutination indicates a positive reaction.

Either antigen or antibody can be attached to the particles. The sensitivity of the reaction is governed by the avidity of the antibody. Sensitive assays are capable of detecting small quantities of antigen. Tests used to detect illicit drugs such as cocaine or heroin are examples of agglutination inhibition tests.

Hemagglutination inhibition reactions use the same principle, except RBCs are the indicator particles. This type of testing has been used to detect antibodies to certain viruses, such as rubella, influenza, and respiratory syncytial virus (RSV). RBCs have naturally occurring receptors for these viruses. When virus is not bound to antibody, spontaneous agglutination occurs because the virus particles link the RBCs together.

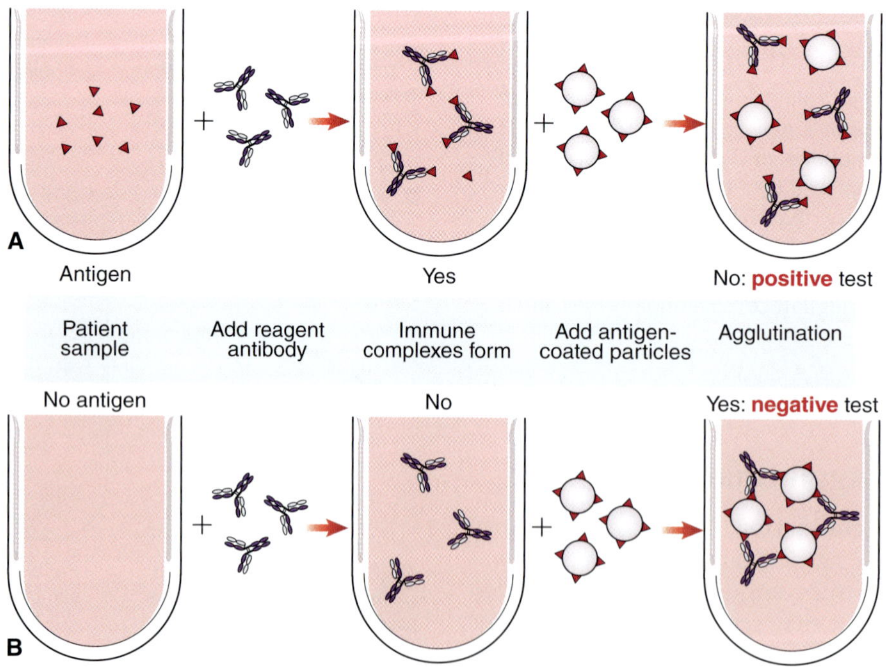

FIGURE 10–13 Agglutination inhibition. Reagent antibody is added to the patient sample. (A) If antigen is present in the patient sample, antigen-antibody combination results. When antigen-coated particles are added, no agglutination occurs, indicating a positive test. (B) If antigen is not in the patient sample, the reagent antibody combines with the particles to produce agglutination, indicating a negative test.

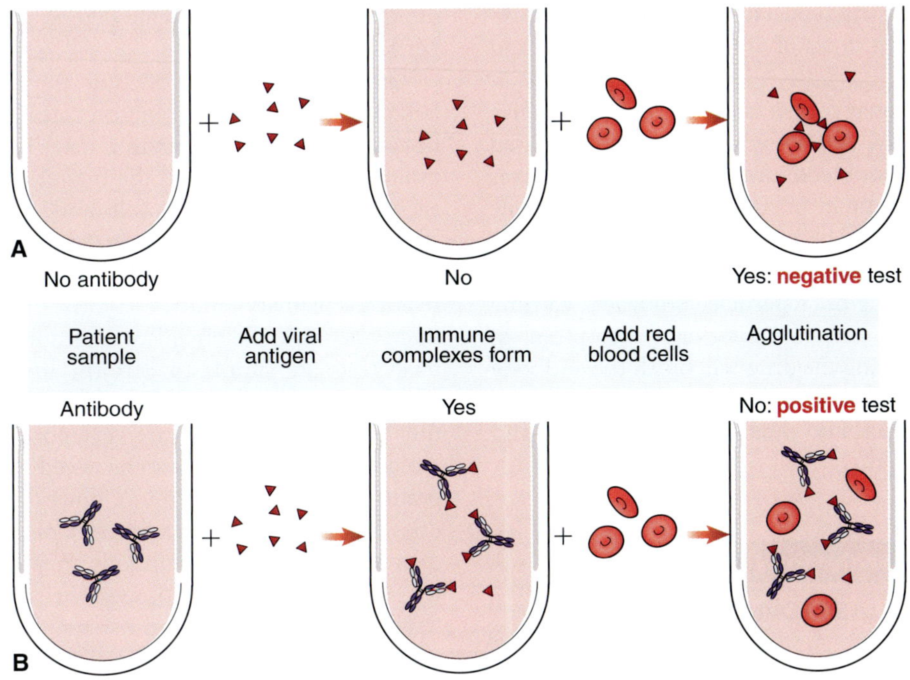

FIGURE 10–14 Hemagglutination inhibition. (A) In the presence of certain viruses, RBCs spontaneously agglutinate. (B) However, if patient antibody is present, then agglutination is inhibited. Thus, a lack of agglutination indicates the presence of antibody.

The presence of patient antibody inhibits the agglutination reaction **(Fig. 10–14)**.

To perform a hemagglutination inhibition test, dilutions of the patient's serum are incubated with a viral preparation. Then RBCs that the virus is known to agglutinate are added to the mixture. If antibody is present, it will attach to the viral particles and prevent agglutination, so a lack of or reduction in agglutination indicates the presence of patient antibody. Controls are necessary because there may be a factor in the serum that causes agglutination, or the virus may have lost its ability to agglutinate RBCs.

Knowledge Check 10-4

What is the key difference between direct agglutination and indirect agglutination assays?

a. Direct agglutination is faster, while indirect agglutination is more sensitive.
b. Direct agglutination is used for viral infections, while indirect agglutination is used for bacterial infections.
c. Direct agglutination requires a secondary antibody, while indirect agglutination does not.
d. Direct agglutination relies on antigens that are naturally occurring on a particle, while indirect agglutination uses carrier particles coated with antigens that are not naturally found on the particles.

Instrumentation

Although agglutination reactions do not require complicated instrumentation, several chemistry analyzers have been developed using automation to increase sensitivity. Nephelometry and immunoturbidimetry have been applied to the reading of agglutination reactions, and the term *particle-enhanced immunoassay* is used to describe such reactions. When particles are used, the sensitivity can be increased to nanograms per milliliter. For this type of reaction, latex particles with a diameter smaller than 1 mm are used. The latex particles are coated with antigen, whole antibody molecules, or $F(ab')_2$ fragments. Use of the latter reduces interference and nonspecific agglutination.

One type of assay involving automated measurement of agglutinated particles is a homogeneous competitive immunoassay called *PETINIA (particle-enhanced turbidimetric inhibition immunoassay)*. In this method, the specimen is incubated with latex beads coated with the analyte of interest and a reagent antibody to the analyte. If a low amount of analyte is present in the sample, the reagent antibody will bind to the latex beads, resulting in aggregate formation and a high level of turbidity. In contrast, when the concentration of the analyte in the patient sample is high, the analyte will bind to the reagent antibody and prevent it from binding to the latex beads, resulting in less turbidity. This method is commonly used to measure small analytes, such as therapeutic drugs (e.g., digoxin), in a sample. The amount of turbidity is inversely proportional to the concentration of the drug analyte in the sample.

Another type of automated assay that assesses agglutination is called a *particle counting immunoassay (PACIA)*. The principle of PACIA is based on using a cell counter to count the number of free particles instead of the particles that have agglutinated. The method provides an inverse measure of the analyte concentration in the patient sample since the more agglutination there is, the fewer free particles remain. PACIA is used for determining the concentration of various substances, such as different types of antibodies, antigens, and haptens.

Another automated assay format is the *kinetic interaction of microparticles in a solution (KIMS),* which is commonly used for drug testing of urine or blood samples. This test measures light transmission following incubation of the patient sample with microparticles that have been conjugated to the test drug. When the sample has no drug present, an anti-drug reagent can bind freely to the drug-microparticle conjugates, causing the particles to aggregate and increasing light absorption. In contrast, samples containing the drug will block the antibody from binding to the drug-microparticle conjugates, resulting in less particle aggregation and thus reducing turbidity and sample absorbance.

10-4 Clinical Correlations

Anti-Streptolysin O (ASO) Detection by Nephelometry

ASO is an antibody that is measured in the laboratory to detect acute rheumatic fever or poststreptococcal glomerulonephritis, sequelae of group A *streptococcal* infections (see Chapter 20). ASO is routinely measured by a nephelometric method in which patient serum is mixed with streptolysin O antigen that has been attached to particles made from a synthetic polymer. The rate of light scatter increases with the formation of immune complexes during the antigen-antibody reaction and is an indication of the concentration of ASO in the patient sample.

Critical Thinking 10-2

C-reactive protein (CRP) is an acute phase reactant produced and released by liver cells into the bloodstream. Increased levels of CRP in the blood indicate inflammation resulting from injury, infection, or a chronic disease. Testing for CRP helps detect and monitor inflammation in patients. Based on your reading about agglutination assays, what type of agglutination assay might be used to detect CRP in a patient's blood sample?

Quality Control and Result Interpretation

Although agglutination reactions are simple to perform, the results must be carefully interpreted. Techniques must be standardized regarding the antigen concentration, incubation time, temperature, diluent, and reading method. The possibility of cross-reactivity and interfering antibody should always be considered. Cross-reactivity is caused by antigenic determinants that resemble one another so closely that antibodies formed against one will react with the other. Cross-reactivity can usually be avoided by using monoclonal antibody reagents directed against an antigenic determinant that is unique to a particular antigen.

Other considerations include proper storage of reagents and close attention to expiration dates. Reagents should never be used beyond the expiration date. Each new lot should be evaluated before use, and the manufacturer's instructions for each kit should always be followed. Also, the sensitivity and specificity of different kits may vary and must be considered.

Advantages of agglutination reactions include rapidity; relative sensitivity; and the fact that if the sample contains a microorganism, the organism does not need to be viable. Also, most tests are simple to perform and require no expensive equipment. Tests are conducted on cards, tubes, and microtiter plates, all of which are very portable. A wide variety of antigens and antibodies can be tested for in this manner. Laboratorians must keep in mind, however, that a negative result does not rule out the presence of a disease or an antigen. The quantity of antigen or antibody may be below the sensitivity of the test system. Although the number of agglutination tests has decreased in recent years, they continue to play an important role in the identification of rare pathogens such as *Francisella* and *Brucella* and more common organisms such as rotavirus and *Cryptococcus,* for which other testing is complex or unavailable.

Knowledge Check 10-5

To help prevent cross-reactivity, what type of reagent antibody is recommended?

a. Interfering antibody
b. Monoclonal antibody
c. Monovalent antibody
d. Polyclonal antibody

KEY CONCEPTS

Antigen-Antibody Binding

- Precipitation involves the combination of soluble antigen with soluble antibody to produce insoluble complexes that are visible.
- The initial union of antigen and antibody depends on *affinity,* or the force of attraction that exists between one antibody binding site and a single epitope on an antigen.
- *Avidity* is the sum of all attractive forces between multiple binding sites on antigen and antibody and determines the stability of the complexes formed.

Principles of Precipitation Reactions

- Maximum binding of antigen and antibody occurs when the aggregate number of multivalent sites of antigen and antibody are approximately equal. The concentrations of antigen and antibody that yield maximum binding represent the zone of equivalence.

- In the prozone, antibody is in excess as compared with antigen, and manifestations of antigen-antibody combination, such as precipitation or agglutination, cannot be detected.
- In the postzone, antigen is in excess compared with the concentration of antibody, so precipitation and agglutination are undetectable.

Immunoturbidimetry and Nephelometry

- Immunoturbidimetry is an automated method that measures the reduction in light transmission that occurs during the formation of immune complexes.
- Nephelometry is an automated technique that measures, at a particular angle from an incident beam, the amount of light scattered from free antigen or antibody molecules and from antigen-antibody complexes in solution.

Passive Immunodiffusion Techniques

- RID is a single-diffusion technique in which antibody is incorporated into a gel. Antigen placed in wells cut into the gel diffuses out and reacts with the antibody, forming rings of precipitation around the wells. The diameter of each precipitate ring is directly related to the amount of antigen in the well.
- In Ouchterlony double diffusion, both antigen and antibody diffuse from wells in a gel and migrate toward each other. Precipitin lines may indicate identity, nonidentity, or partial identity, depending on the pattern formed between a known antigen or antibody and an unknown antigen or antibody.

Flocculation

- In a flocculation reaction, immune complexes form over a narrow range of antigen concentrations, resulting in fine particulate precipitants. This is the basis for nontreponemal tests for syphilis.

Electrophoretic Techniques

- In IFE, antibody is applied directly to a gel after electrophoresis of antigens has taken place. IFE is commonly used to detect monoclonal immunoglobulins produced by patients with immunoproliferative diseases such as multiple myeloma.

Comparison of Precipitation Techniques

- See Table 10–1 for test principles, sensitivity, and applications of the various precipitation techniques discussed in this chapter.

Principles of Agglutination Reactions

- Agglutination is the process by which particulate antigens, such as latex beads, RBCs, or gel particles, react with specific antibody to form large aggregates or clumps.
- The process of agglutination can be divided into two steps: (1) *sensitization*, or initial binding of antigen and antibody, which depends on the nature of the antibody and the antigen-bearing surface, and (2) *lattice formation*, which is governed by factors such as pH, ionic strength, and temperature.
- Because of its larger size, IgM is usually able to mediate lattice formation with antigen without additional enhancement. In contrast, agglutination methods involving IgG require enhancement techniques that vary physicochemical conditions and the addition of an anti-human immunoglobulin (Coombs reagent) to see a visible reaction.

Types of Agglutination Reactions

- In direct agglutination tests, patient serum is incubated with antigens that are found naturally on the indicator particles.
- In passive agglutination tests, patient serum is reacted with antigens that are artificially attached to such particles.
- Reverse passive agglutination is so called because antibody, rather than antigen, is attached to the indicator particles.
- Coagglutination is a type of reverse passive agglutination that uses antibody-coated bacteria as the particles.
- Agglutination inhibition is based on competition between antigen-coated particles and soluble patient antigen for a limited number of antibody sites. It is the only type of method in which agglutination represents a negative test.
- Agglutination inhibition tests using RBCs are called hemagglutination inhibition. These tests can be used to detect patient antibodies to certain viruses.
- Agglutination reactions are typically used as rapid screening tests. They are sensitive and can yield valuable information when interpreted correctly.
- *Particle-enhanced immunoassays such as PETINIA* use automated analyzers to measure agglutination, resulting in enhanced sensitivity.

Quality Control and Result Interpretation

- Several factors must be taken into consideration when conducting precipitation and agglutination tests, including proper storage of reagents, close attention to reagent expiration dates, and the possibility of cross-reactivity caused by closely related antigens.
- Using monoclonal antibody reagents directed against unique antigenic determinants can eliminate cross-reactivity and reduce false-positive results.
- The diagnostic and analytical sensitivity and specificity of agglutination assays must be considered when interpreting results. A false-negative result may occur if the antigen or antibody concentration falls below the test limits of the assay.

Study Guide: Comparison of Agglutination Reactions

TYPE OF REACTION	PRINCIPLE	RESULTS
Direct agglutination	Patient serum is reacted with antigen that is naturally found on a cell or particle (e.g., RBCs, bacteria).	Agglutination indicates the presence of patient antibody to a natural antigen.
Indirect (passive) agglutination	Patient sample is reacted with particles (e.g., latex beads) coated with antigens not normally found on their surfaces.	Agglutination indicates the presence of patient antibody to an artificially attached antigen.
Reverse passive agglutination	Patient sample is reacted with particles that are coated with reagent antibody.	Agglutination indicates the presence of specific antigen in the patient sample.
Coagglutination	Bacteria serve as the inert carrier of antibodies. Patient sample is reacted with the carrier to detect antigen.	Agglutination indicates the presence of a specific antigen in the patient sample.
Agglutination inhibition	Haptens are attached to carrier particles. Particles compete with patient antigens for a limited number of antibody sites.	Lack of agglutination is a positive test, indicating the presence of antigen in the patient sample.
Hemagglutination inhibition	RBCs spontaneously agglutinate in the presence of viral particles.	Lack of agglutination is a positive test, indicating the presence of patient antibody, which binds to the viral particles, preventing RBC agglutination.

CASE STUDIES

1. A patient stool culture has grown a suspected *Shigella* species. The clinical laboratory performed a *Shigella* serogrouping slide agglutination test to identify the species of *Shigella*. The test uses reagent antibodies directed against specific O antigens that *Shigella* strains naturally possess. The different O antigens are used to classify *Shigella* into four species. The following results were obtained from the test.

Antiserum	Result
Shigella flexneri	No agglutination
Shigella sonnei	Agglutination
Shigella dysenteriae	No agglutination
Shigella boydii	No agglutination

a. Based on the results, what is the *Shigella* species?
b. Based on the assay information, what type of agglutination test is being used? Explain your answer.

2. A 30-year-old patient visits a physician because of a generalized skin rash, malaise, and fatigue. The doctor notes that the patient had an active sexual history. Among other tests, the doctor orders a *T. pallidum* particle agglutination assay (TP-PA) test to check for syphilis. The test result showed the presence of a smooth mat of particles covering the well of the microtiter plate when a 1:80 dilution of patient serum was used.

Questions

a. Does the smooth mat of particles indicate a positive or negative test result? Explain your answer.
b. Suppose a 1:40 dilution of patient serum was used, and the result was negative. How can the discrepancy between the 1:40 and 1:80 results be explained?
c. Does the test result mean that the patient has an active case of syphilis?

REVIEW QUESTIONS

1. In a precipitation reaction, how can the ideal antibody be characterized?
   a. Low affinity and low avidity
   b. High affinity and low avidity
   c. High affinity and high avidity
   d. Low affinity and high avidity

2. Precipitation differs from agglutination in which way?
   a. Precipitation can only be measured by an automated instrument.
   b. Precipitation occurs with univalent antigen, whereas agglutination requires a multivalent antigen.
   c. Precipitation does not readily occur because few antibodies can form aggregates with antigen.
   d. Precipitation involves a soluble antigen, whereas agglutination involves a particulate antigen.

3. When soluble antigens diffuse in a gel that contains antibody, in which zone does optimal precipitation occur?
   a. Prozone
   b. Zone of equivalence
   c. Postzone
   d. Prezone

4. Which of the following statements applies to rate nephelometry?
   a. Readings are taken before equivalence is reached.
   b. It is more sensitive than immunoturbidimetry.
   c. Measurements are time dependent.
   d. All of the above apply.

5. Which of the following is characteristic of the endpoint method of RID?
   a. Readings are taken before equivalence.
   b. The antigen concentration is directly in proportion to the square of the ring diameter.
   c. The ring diameter is plotted against the log of the concentration.
   d. It is primarily a qualitative rather than a quantitative method.

6. In which zone might an antibody-screening test be false negative?
   a. Prozone
   b. Zone of equivalence
   c. Postzone
   d. None of the above

7. How does immunoturbidimetry differ from nephelometry?
   a. Immunoturbidimetry measures light that is scattered at an angle.
   b. Immunoturbidimetry measures the decrease in light after it passes through a solution.
   c. Immunoturbidimetry deals with univalent antigens only.
   d. Nephelometry is not affected by large particles falling out of solution.

8. Which of the following refers to the force of attraction between an antibody and a single antigenic determinant?
   a. Affinity
   b. Avidity
   c. Van der Waals attraction
   d. Covalence

9. If crossed lines result in an Ouchterlony immunodiffusion reaction with antigens 1 and 2, what does this indicate?
   a. Antigens 1 and 2 are identical.
   b. Antigen 2 is simpler than antigen 1.
   c. Antigen 2 is more complex than antigen 1.
   d. The two antigens are unrelated.

10. Which technique represents a single-diffusion reaction?
    a. Radial immunodiffusion
    b. Ouchterlony diffusion
    c. Counter-immunoelectrophoresis
    d. Immunofixation electrophoresis

11. Which best describes the law of mass action?
    a. Once antigen-antibody binding takes place, it is irreversible.
    b. The equilibrium constant depends only on the forward reaction.
    c. The equilibrium constant is related to the strength of antigen-antibody binding.
    d. If an antibody has a high avidity, it will dissociate from antigen easily.

12. Agglutination of dyed bacterial cells represents which type of reaction?
    a. Direct agglutination
    b. Passive agglutination
    c. Reverse passive agglutination
    d. Agglutination inhibition

13. If a single IgM molecule can bind many more antigens than a molecule of IgG, which of the following is higher?
    a. Affinity
    b. Initial force of attraction
    c. Avidity
    d. Initial sensitization

14. Agglutination inhibition could best be used for which of the following types of antigens?
    a. Large cellular antigens, such as erythrocytes
    b. Soluble haptens
    c. Bacterial cells
    d. Coated latex particles

15. Which of the following correctly describes reverse passive agglutination?
    a. It is a negative test.
    b. It can be used to detect autoantibodies.
    c. It is used for identification of antigens.
    d. It is used to detect sensitization of RBCs.

16. Reactions involving IgG may need to be enhanced for which reason?
    a. IgG is only active at 25°C.
    b. IgG may be too small to produce lattice formation.
    c. IgG has only one antigen binding site.
    d. IgG is only able to produce visible precipitation reactions.

17. For which of the following tests is a lack of agglutination a positive reaction?
    a. Hemagglutination
    b. Passive agglutination
    c. Reverse passive agglutination
    d. Agglutination inhibition

18. Typing of RBCs with reagent antiserum represents which type of reaction?
    a. Direct hemagglutination
    b. Passive hemagglutination
    c. Hemagglutination inhibition
    d. Reverse passive hemagglutination

19. Consider the following test principle: separation of proteins based on charge and size, followed by specific antibody identification. What precipitation technique does this describe?
    a. Immunoturbidity
    b. Immunofixation electrophoresis
    c. Nephelometry
    d. Ouchterlony double diffusion

20. Which of the following describes the principle of a flocculation immunoassay?
    a. Agglutination of antibody-coated latex particles by antigens in the patient sample
    b. Electrophoretic separation of molecules based on charge and size, followed by identification of the specific antibodies present
    c. Formation of immune complex that occurs over a narrow range of antigen concentrations, resulting in fine particulate precipitants
    d. Precipitation of antigens by a known concentration of antibodies in a gel matrix

21. Which of the following best describes the principle of coagglutination?
    a. Fine particulate precipitants form over a narrow range of antigen concentrations.
    b. It involves the use of inert particles, such as *Staphylococcus aureus*, coated with antibodies that bind the corresponding antigen in a sample to produce agglutination.
    c. Naturally occurring antigens on a particle bind to antibodies in the patient sample to form visible clumps.
    d. Precipitation of antigens by antibodies occurs in a gel matrix.

Chapter 10 Answer Key

Answers to Knowledge Checks

10.1 c 10.2 a 10.3 a 10.4 d 10.5 b

Answers to Review Questions

1. c	2. d	3. b	4. d	5. b	6. a	7. b
8. a	9. d	10. a	11. c	12. a	13. c	14. b
15. c	16. b	17. d	18. a	19. b	20. c	21. b

Labeled Immunoassays

11

Paul R. Johnson, PhD, MBA, MT (ASCP), DABCC

LEARNING OUTCOMES

After finishing this chapter, you should be able to:

11.1 Explain the principles of competitive and noncompetitive immunoassays.

11.2 Distinguish between heterogeneous and homogeneous immunoassays.

11.3 Describe major characteristics of colorimetric, chemiluminescent, radioactive, and fluorescent labels, and recognize examples of each type.

11.4 Explain the principle of biotin-streptavidin labeling and its applications in immunoassays.

11.5 Outline the steps of a noncompetitive indirect enzyme-linked immunosorbent assay (ELISA) to detect an antibody in a patient sample.

11.6 Outline the steps of a sandwich, capture, or immunometric assay to detect an antigen in a patient sample.

11.7 Cite clinical applications for homogeneous enzyme immunoassays (EIAs).

11.8 Describe basic principles and clinical uses for rapid immunoassays.

11.9 Compare and contrast the differences between direct and indirect immunofluorescence techniques in terms of their methodology and applications.

11.10 Discuss the principles and applications of the enzyme-multiplied immunoassay technique (EMIT), cloned enzyme donor immunoassay (CEDIA), multiplex immunoassay (MIA), particle-based multi-analyte technology (PMAT), Western blot, and isoelectric focusing (IEF).

11.11 Discuss advantages and disadvantages of immunoassays, based on each method design.

11.12 Choose an appropriate immunoassay for a particular analyte.

11.13 Discuss interfering factors and other technical concerns that may contribute to false-positive or false-negative immunoassay results, and any corrective actions that can be taken when such results are suspected.

CHAPTER OUTLINE

You can go to **fadavis.com** keyword stevens for the laboratory exercises that accompany this text.

The unlabeled immunoassays, such as the precipitation and agglutination reactions we discussed in Chapter 10, are fairly simple techniques that are often performed without sophisticated equipment. However, these techniques have a relatively poor analytical sensitivity because visualizing a macroscopic reaction (large enough to be viewed without the aid of an instrument) requires that the sample have a sufficiently high concentration of the biomarker analyte. In contrast, labeled immunoassays are designed to improve analytical sensitivity by using instrumentation equipped with sensitive detectors to measure substances at much lower concentrations. Labeled immunoassay techniques are commonly used in the clinical laboratory to measure a variety of substances in blood, urine, and tissues. The substance measured is often called the **analyte** (or biomarker). Biological analytes measured by immunoassay techniques include proteins, peptides, hormones, tumor markers, immunoglobulins, and microbial antigens. Small-molecule antigens, or haptens, can also be measured with immunoassays. In certain clinical situations, it may be of interest to detect and quantify antibody levels rather than antigen levels to support a clinical diagnosis. The methods by which antigens or antibodies are measured vary extensively, depending on individual immunoassay techniques developed across different in vitro diagnostic (IVD) test manufacturers.

The analyte of interest is usually a protein. It can be either antigen or antibody, depending on clinical need. An anti-human immunoglobulin reagent is used to react specifically with the analyte if the protein being detected is an antibody from patient serum. The anti-human immunoglobulin in such a test system is derived from another species (mouse, rabbit, or goat). One reactant, either antigen or antibody, will contain a label as a detection marker so that the amount of binding can be monitored.

Affinity and avidity (binding strength) of the antigen-antibody pair are important to achieve optimal reaction conditions, and this largely influences the reaction's specificity. High **analytical specificity** implies that only the analyte of interest is detected and measured, while **analytical sensitivity** defines the lowest measurable concentration of analyte, usually described as the *lower limit of detection (LoD)*. The detection limits of immunoassays are determined by several variables, including the type of label as well as the antigen-antibody affinity and avidity. As a general rule, analytical sensitivity is optimal when using a chemiluminescent substrate, followed by a fluorophore. A colorimetric product is the least sensitive. Radioisotopes generally have sensitivity close to that achieved by fluorescent labels. In principle, each label may be coupled to any assay design.

The development of rapid, specific, and sensitive immunoassays to determine the presence of important biological molecules has ushered in a new era of testing in the clinical laboratory. The ability to detect very small quantities of antigen or antibody has revolutionized the diagnosis and monitoring of many diseases, leading to earlier treatment.

Immunoassay Labels

Labeled immunoassays differ from unlabeled techniques by including a detection molecule (label) in the test system. Most current techniques use nonisotopic labels to generate a light signal. Depending on manufacturer design, labels may include a colorimetric substrate, fluorescent compound (fluorophore), or luminescent molecule. Earlier generation immunoassays used radioactive isotope elements as the label, but these techniques are now less commonly used in clinical laboratories. Generation of the detection signal also varies across manufacturers. Labels are sometimes referred to as "tracer" molecules because they can trace the detection signal. One technique common to many labeled immunoassay methods is enzyme-mediated catalysis of a reagent substrate to generate a light signal.

Different manufacturers have developed a variety of test designs, and selection of the label is aimed at the testing needs for measuring the analyte of interest. Each of these labels is described in detail as we discuss each immunoassay format.

General Immunoassay Formats

All immunoassay designs require separation of the bound and free tracer labels before the signal is measured. The approaches to achieve separation are broadly categorized as *heterogeneous* or *homogeneous*. Additional subclassifications are made to describe whether immunoassay method designs are *competitive* or *noncompetitive*, based on the principle of the test reaction. We present various immunoassay formats, along with their classification, in **Table 11–1** and discuss them in detail in the sections that follow.

Heterogeneous vs Homogeneous Immunoassays

Heterogeneous immunoassays require physical separation of bound and free components; this can be achieved by different methods, including centrifugation, binding to solid-phase material, or magnetic separation. Solid-phase materials are the most common means of separation and include polystyrene reaction wells, microparticle beads, latex beads, and plastic tubes.

Homogeneous immunoassays are immunoassay methods that do not require a physical separation step. Although all homogeneous immunoassay designs have this property in common, the methods by which they measure the detection signal and patient analyte concentration can vary extensively across manufacturers.

Table 11–1 Homogeneous and Heterogeneous Immunoassay Formats

HOMOGENEOUS	HETEROGENEOUS	OTHER (TISSUE/CELL BASED)
Enzyme-multiplied immunoassay technique (EMIT)	Enzyme immunoassay (EIA)	Direct immunofluorescence assay
Cloned enzyme donor immunoassay (CEDIA)	Enzyme-linked immunosorbent assay (ELISA)	Indirect immunofluorescence assay
	Chemiluminescent microparticle immunoassay (CMIA)	Multiplex immunoassay (MIA)
	Radioimmunoassay (RIA)	
	Fluorescence immunoassay (FIA)	
	Rapid immunoassay (immunochromatography)	

Knowledge Check 11-1

Which of the following is a characteristic of homogeneous immunoassays?

a. Antigen and antibody molecules remain in solution.
b. Free antigen is separated from antigen bound to antibody.
c. A solid phase, such as microparticle beads, is used.
d. A single common design is used by all immunoassay manufacturers.

Competitive vs Noncompetitive Immunoassays

As we mentioned earlier, labeled immunoassays can also be categorized as competitive or noncompetitive. In competitive immunoassays, the analyte in the patient sample competes with a labeled analyte of the same type for binding to a corresponding antibody reagent. In noncompetitive immunoassays, all the analyte in the patient sample can bind freely to the corresponding reagent antibodies, which are provided in excess. In the following sections, we discuss the principles of both assay types in detail.

Competitive Immunoassays

In **competitive immunoassays,** the test system reagents consist of a limited amount of reagent antibody (Ab), tracer or labeled antigen (Ag*), and reagent substrate. The only variable in the reaction is the concentration of patient antigen (Ag), which is the analyte of interest. All the reactants are mixed together simultaneously; labeled tracer antigen (Ag*) competes with unlabeled patient antigen (Ag) for a limited number of binding sites on the antibody (Ab). The concentration of the labeled analyte (Ag*) is in excess to ensure all binding sites on the antibody will be occupied whether or not sample antigen is present.

After washing to remove unbound label, the amount of antibody-bound label (Ag*Ab) is measured and used to determine the amount of patient antigen present. If patient antigen is present, some binding sites will be occupied with unlabeled analyte, thus decreasing the amount of bound label detected **(Fig. 11–1).** Therefore, the amount of bound label is inversely proportional to the concentration of the labeled antigen, meaning that the more labeled antigen detected, the less antigen is present in the patient sample.

We can illustrate this relationship by considering the ratio of tracer-bound antigen to sample antigen (analyte) in the example that follows **(Fig. 11–2).**

Suppose labeled antigen (Ag*) and unlabeled antigen (Ag) occur in three different ratios: 2:1, 1:1, and 1:2. Binding of Ag* and Ag to a limited number of antibody sites will take place. The reaction between the antigens and their corresponding antibody (Ab) can be depicted in an equation where the reactants are listed on the left side of the arrow and the products on the right:

$$Ag^* + Ag + Ab = Ag^*Ab + AgAb$$

In our example, labeled antigen and reagent antibody are held constant, at 100 units and 50 units, respectively. As you can see in the table in Figure 11–2, the amount of labeled antigen bound to antibody will change according to the patient antigen concentration. Thus, on the right side of the equation, one-third (33%) of binding sites are occupied by labeled antigen (Ag*Ab) when the Ag*:Ag ratio is 2:1; 25% of binding sites are occupied at a 1:1 ratio, and 17% at a 1:2 ratio.

Additional ratio values of labeled antigen (Ag*) to patient antigen (Ag) help to further illustrate this relationship, as shown in the graph in Figure 11–2. You can see that the detection signal is inversely proportional to the patient antigen concentration on a nonlinear scale. The relationship can be mathematically linearized to generate a standard curve, using calibrators with known amounts of antigen, to extrapolate the signal to the concentration of antigen in the patient sample. Alternatively, a nonlinear method for standard curve analysis can be generated by instrument software, often for competitive immunoassays.

Noncompetitive Immunoassays

In a standard **noncompetitive immunoassay,** reagent antibody *(capture antibody)* is first passively adsorbed onto a solid-phase material, such as microtiter plates, nitrocellulose membranes, or

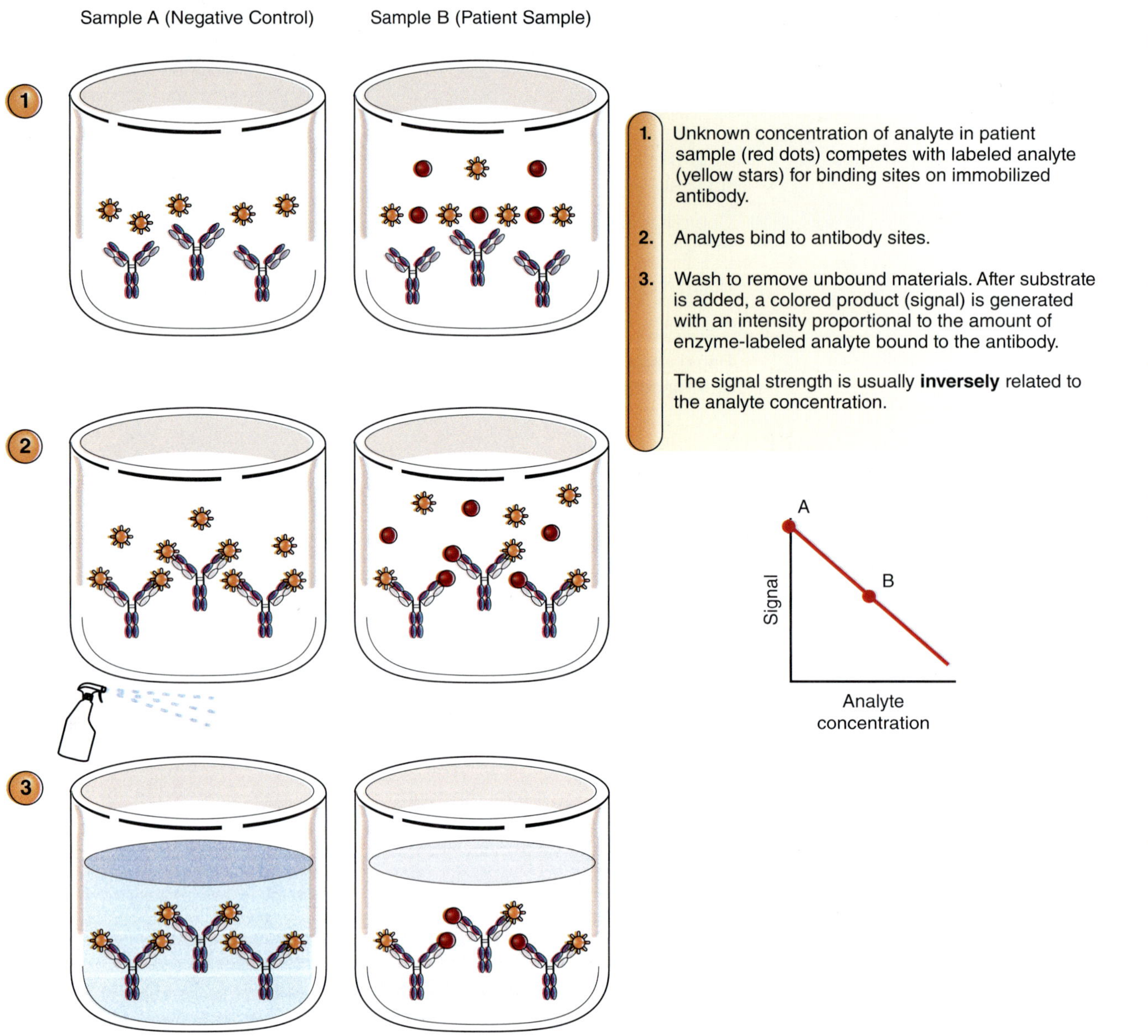

FIGURE 11–1 Principle of a competitive immunoassay.

plastic beads. Excess capture antibody is present to ensure that any antigen present in the patient sample will be bound. Unknown patient antigen reacts with (i.e., is captured by) the solid-phase antibody. After washing to physically remove unbound constituents in the sample, a labeled antibody, directed against a different epitope on the antigen of interest, is added to the reaction **(Fig. 11–3)**. The amount of label measured is directly proportional to the amount of patient antigen present and is represented by a mathematical linear relationship.

Knowledge Check 11-2

In a competitive immunoassay:

a. The amount of label detected is directly proportional to the concentration of antigen in the patient sample.
b. The amount of label detected decreases as the patient antigen concentration increases.
c. Separation of free antigen from antigen bound to antibody is not required.
d. The antigen is located in between a capture antibody and a labeled detector antibody.

Radioimmunoassay (RIA)

The original immunoassay was based on a competitive principle using a radioisotope label. Rosalyn Yalow and Solomon Berson developed this technique, called **radioimmunoassay (RIA)**, in the late 1950s, to measure insulin hormone levels in humans. Yalow was honored with the 1977 Nobel Prize in Physiology or Medicine for her groundbreaking work. The success of this original immunoassay design ultimately led researchers to develop additional RIA methods to measure other clinical analytes, including several hormones

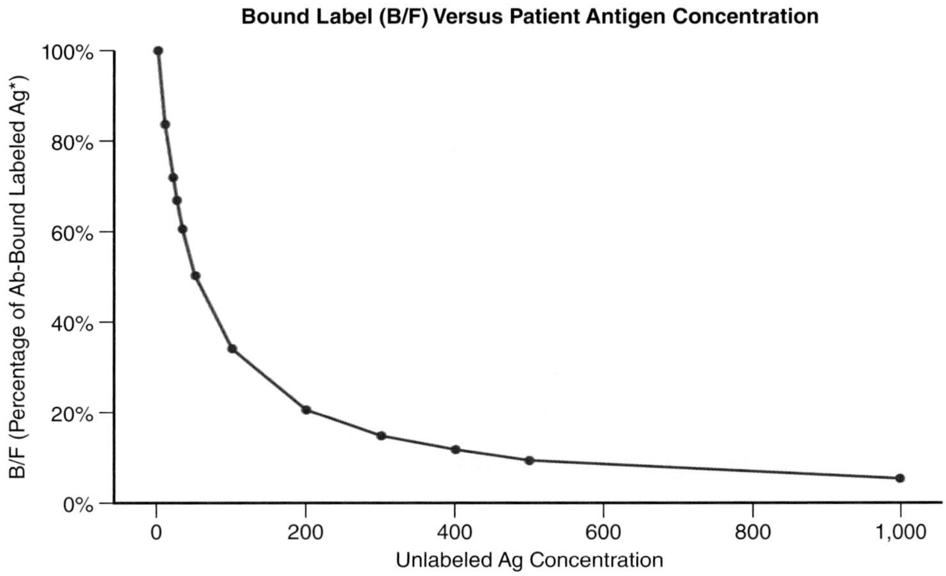

C1	C2	C3	C4	C5	C6	C7	C8	C9
Ratio of Labeled Ag*/Patient Ag	Patient Ag Concentration	Labeled Ag* Concentration	Ab	AgAb	Ag*Ab	% Bound (C6/C3)	Free Ag* (C3–C6)	B/F C6/C8
2:1	50	100	50	17	33	33%	67	49%
1:1	100	100	50	25	25	25%	75	33%
1:2	200	100	50	33	17	17%	83	20%

FIGURE 11–2 Example of the effect of the ratio of labeled antigen to unlabeled antigen on the percentage of labeled antigen bound to antibody in a competitive immunoassay. *(Figure courtesy of Dr. Paul Johnson.)*

(e.g., aldosterone, cortisol), serum proteins, drugs, viral antigens, and immunoglobulins.

Radioactive elements have nuclei that decay spontaneously into other elements and, in the process, release energy, which is measured by radiation detectors. Depending on the immunoassay design, radiolabeled antigens can be tagged with various radioactive elements, most commonly iodine (^{125}I or ^{131}I), which emit beta particles, and gamma rays, tritium (^{3}H) or carbon (^{14}C), which emit beta particles. Detectors can measure very low quantities of radioactivity, giving these immunoassays extremely high analytical sensitivity.

However, the chief disadvantages of RIA methods include health hazards from working with radioactive substances (especially those producing beta particles and gamma rays, which can cause damage to tissues and DNA when in direct contact), radioactive waste disposal problems, and the limited shelf life of some elements (e.g., ^{125}I has a half-life of about 60 days). For these reasons, RIA testing in clinical laboratories has become limited.

Enzyme Immunoassays (EIAs)

Enzyme immunoassays (EIAs), using enzymes as labels, were developed as alternatives to RIA. **Enzymes** are naturally occurring molecules that catalyze biochemical reactions. When used in a test system, they convert reagent substrates into chemically modified products that can be detected. Substances produced and detected in this method emit colored or visible light, ultraviolet (UV) light, fluorescent light, or luminescence. These methods have sufficient analytical sensitivity for many clinical tests and eliminate the disposal problems and health hazards associated with radioactive isotopes. Because one molecule of enzyme can generate many molecules of product, addition of an enzyme label further improves analytical sensitivity.

Enzyme labels for immunoassays are chosen according to their physical properties, including the number of substrate molecules converted per molecule of enzyme, ease and speed of detection, and stability. The availability and cost of the enzyme and substrate may factor into the design of a particular enzyme reagent. An example of a common substrate is TMB (3,3′,5,5′-tetramethylbenzidine) when a peroxidase enzyme label is used. A "stop solution" of sulfuric acid stops the enzymatic reaction by acidifying the TMB, changing the color from blue to yellow for reading at 450 nm. Common enzymes used as labels in EIAs include horseradish peroxidase (HRP), alkaline phosphatase (ALP), β-D-galactosidase, and glucose-6-phosphate dehydrogenase (G6PDH). EIAs can be classified as either heterogeneous or homogeneous based on whether a separation step is necessary, as we previously mentioned.

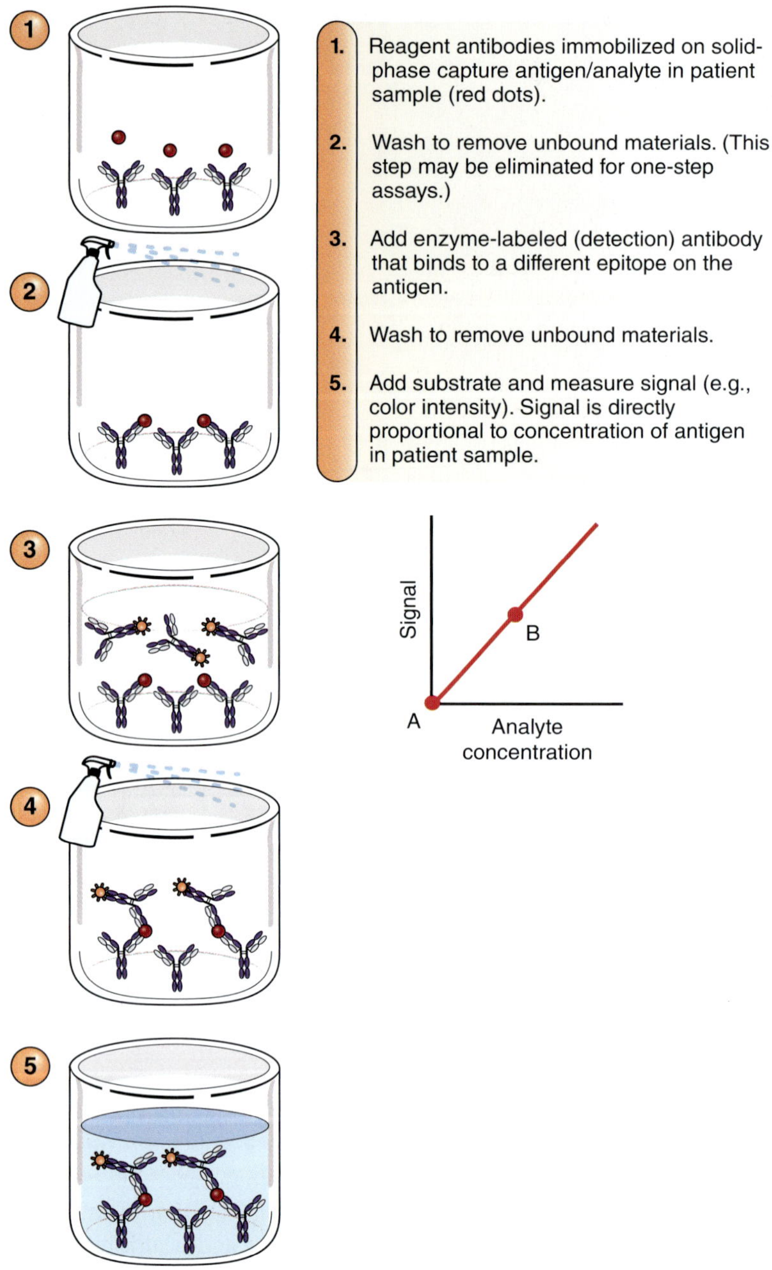

FIGURE 11–3 Principle of a noncompetitive immunoassay (capture, sandwich, or immunometric assay) to detect patient antigen.

Heterogeneous Enzyme Immunoassays

Heterogeneous EIAs involve a physical means of separating bound from free labeled components. They include competitive EIAs, noncompetitive EIAs, and capture immunoassays. Some of these assays use biotin-avidin labeling to increase sensitivity.

Competitive Enzyme Immunoassays

The first EIAs, developed by Eva Engvall and Peter Perlmann in 1971, were based on the competitive principles of RIA. Capture antibodies were adsorbed onto plastic tubes, leading these investigators to name this new method **enzyme-linked immunosorbent assay (ELISA).** Alkaline phosphatase (enzyme) was conjugated to the antigen of interest. In competitive ELISAs, antigen in the test sample competes with enzyme-conjugated reagent antigen for a limited number of binding sites on antibody molecules attached to a solid phase, such as plastic tubes or microtiter plate wells. After careful washing to remove unbound antigen, enzyme activity present in the final reaction catalyzes the conversion of the substrate to a detectable product. The product signal is inversely proportional to the concentration of the test substance, as seen in **Fig. 11–4.**

In the original ELISA method, sample antigen was accurately detected at a concentration as low as 1 ng/mL, achieving comparable analytical sensitivity to RIA. Since the time that ELISA methods were introduced, they have dramatically increased in popularity and have become a mainstay of testing in research and clinical laboratories. In practice, an ELISA is an EIA, so these terms may be used interchangeably.

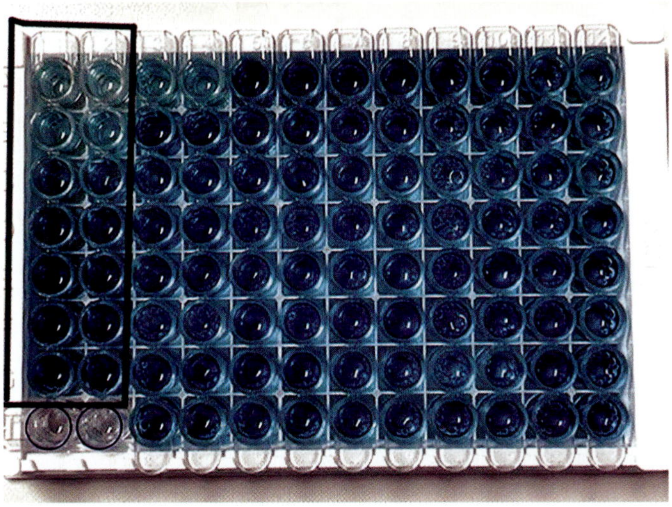

FIGURE 11–4 Sample wells from a competitive ELISA. Decreasing concentrations of analyte, from highest to lowest, were placed in wells A1 through F1, respectively, and duplicated in wells A2 through F2. Note the increasing intensity of blue color formed after reaction of the substrate tetramethylbenzidine with peroxidase enzyme as the analyte concentration decreases. Wells G1 and G2 contain no analyte. *(Courtesy of Dr. Paul Johnson).*

Noncompetitive Enzyme Immunoassays

Alternately, ELISA/EIA methodology may be based on a noncompetitive design. Noncompetitive immunoassay formats can be used to detect the presence of either an antigen or an antibody in the test sample. Immunoassays that detect antibody are most commonly called **indirect ELISAs**, whereas those that detect antigen are termed "capture immunoassays." ELISA test kit procedures often use 96-well microtiter plates as the solid phase. In addition to microtiter plates, other solid-phase supports have been developed, including plastic reaction tubes, plastic beads, magnetic particles, and latex particles. Today, most automated immunoassays are designed on similar noncompetitive principles. Clinical laboratories use this type of immunoassay most frequently because of its sensitivity, specificity, and ease of use.

Indirect ELISAs

Indirect ELISAs are most commonly used to detect a patient antibody of interest. They are termed "indirect" because the enzyme-labeled reagent does not participate in the initial antigen-antibody reaction. In these immunoassays, the associated antigen is bound to the solid phase, and patient serum with an unknown antibody concentration is added. Incubation time allows for specific interaction between solid-phase antigen and patient antibody. After a wash step, an enzyme-labeled anti-globulin, or secondary antibody, is added. This second antibody reacts with any patient antibody that is bound to the solid phase. If no patient antibody is bound to the solid phase, the second labeled antibody will not be bound and will be removed during a second wash step. This is followed by incubation with the enzyme substrate, and finally, a stop solution to cease enzyme activity after a specified period of time. The amount of color, fluorescence, or luminescence generated by action of the enzyme label on the substrate is measured using a detection device and is compared with calibrators containing known amounts of antibody according to a standard curve. In the noncompetitive format, signal detection is directly proportional to the amount of antibody in the specimen (**Figs. 11–5** and **11–6**).

Clinical applications include measurement of antibody to infectious agents that are difficult to isolate in the laboratory; for example, this technique is useful in detecting patient antibodies to viruses such as HIV, hepatitis B, and hepatitis C. Another clinical application is identification of autoantibodies produced in autoimmune diseases (i.e., antibodies directed against self-antigens); for example, detection of autoantibodies to insulin and glutamate decarboxylase helps to support a diagnosis of type 1 diabetes mellitus.

> **Critical Thinking 11-1**
>
> In an indirect ELISA to detect antibody to the rubella antigen in patient serum, what would the enzyme label be attached to?

Capture (Sandwich) Immunoassays

When antigen is the analyte of interest, antibody is bound to the solid phase. These immunoassays are termed **sandwich immunoassays, capture immunoassays,** or **immunometric assays.** The antigens captured in these immunoassays must have multiple epitopes. Excess antibody attached to the solid phase is allowed to combine with the test sample to capture any antigen present. After an incubation period, enzyme-labeled antibody is added. This secondary antibody recognizes a different epitope or binding site than the solid-phase antibody. The final complex formed with sample antigen in between the two reagent antibodies creates the "sandwich." Depending on the particular enzyme and substrate used, a colored, fluorescent, or chemiluminescent reaction product is detected. Product formation is directly proportional to the amount of antigen in the test sample (see Fig. 11–3). The use of monoclonal antibodies has made this a very specific test system.

Capture immunoassays are best suited to antigens that have multiple determinants, such as cytokines, proteins, tumor markers, and microorganism antigens. If detecting microorganisms, the epitope must be unique to the organism being tested and, ideally, must be present in all strains of that organism. Capture immunoassays are also used to measure immunoglobulins, especially those of certain classes. For instance, the presence of IgM can help indicate a recent infection. When measuring immunoglobulins, the specific immunoglobulin class being detected is technically acting as the antigen, and the reagent antibody is anti-human immunoglobulin.

Biotin-Avidin Labeling

Biotin-avidin labeling is used in some labeled immunoassays to increase analytical sensitivity, especially for detection of analytes present in very low amounts. Avidin, a protein enriched

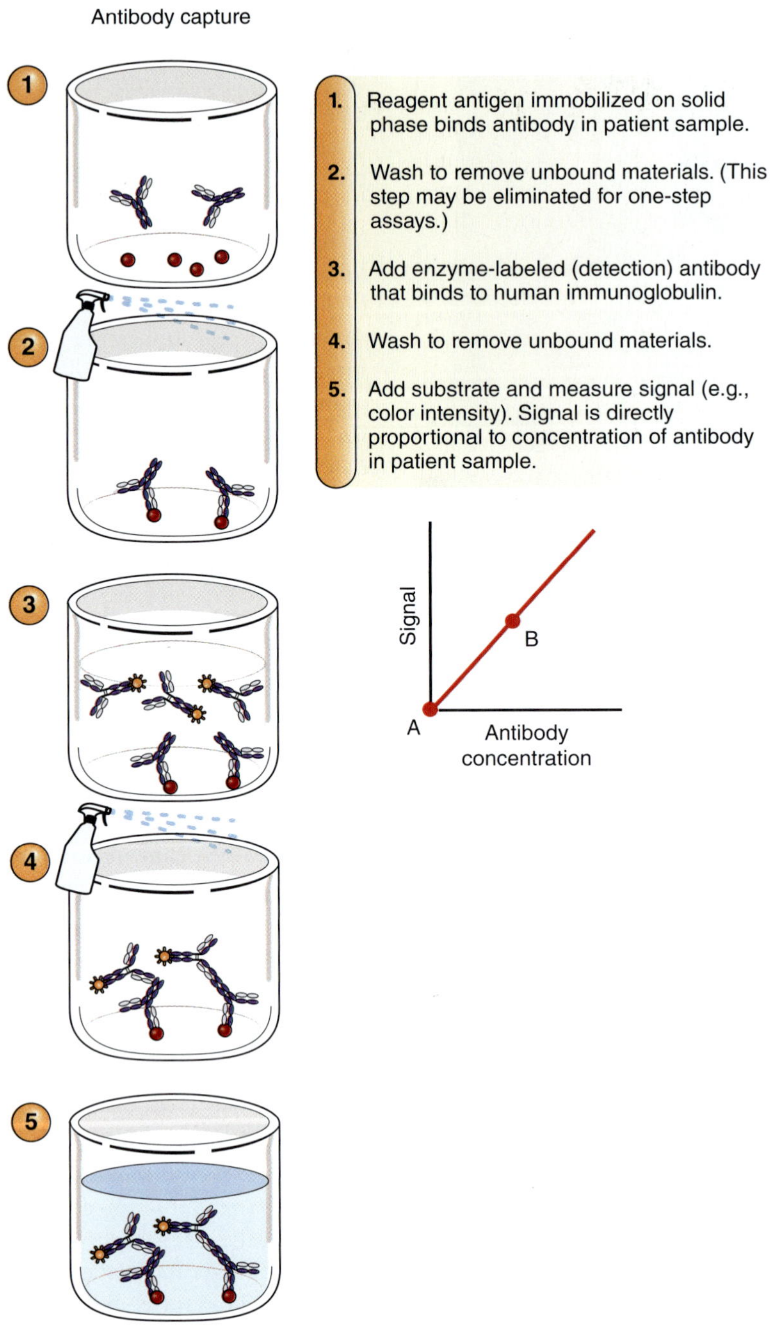

FIGURE 11–5 Noncompetitive, indirect immunoassay to detect patient antibody.

in egg whites, has four binding sites for **biotin,** a vitamin of the B-complex family also known as vitamin B_7 or vitamin H **(Fig. 11-7).** The discovery of this interaction led researchers to isolate another version of avidin from the bacterium *Streptomyces avidinii,* called **streptavidin (SAv),** which has a stronger binding affinity for biotin.

The formation of biotin-SAv complexes is the rationale for using these molecules in immunoassays, especially as each molecule of SAv has multiple high-affinity binding sites for biotin. The end result is signal amplification with enhanced detection when coupled to one of the previously discussed nonisotopic labels. Biotin-SAv labeling can be used in both indirect ELISAs and capture immunoassays. Depending on the immunoassay design, biotin is complexed to either the capture antibody or the detection antibody, and SAv is bound to either the solid phase or the enzyme label. When a biotin-SAv design is used in a capture immunoassay, it is sometimes referred to as a *delayed capture immunoassay* because the final incubation step includes binding of the sandwich complex to SAv on the solid phase (see Fig. 11–7).

Although all these immunoassay formats are useful in measuring antigen or antibody levels in patients, clinical laboratorians must be aware of certain limitations; in the subsequent section, we describe commonly encountered immunoassay test interferences in detail.

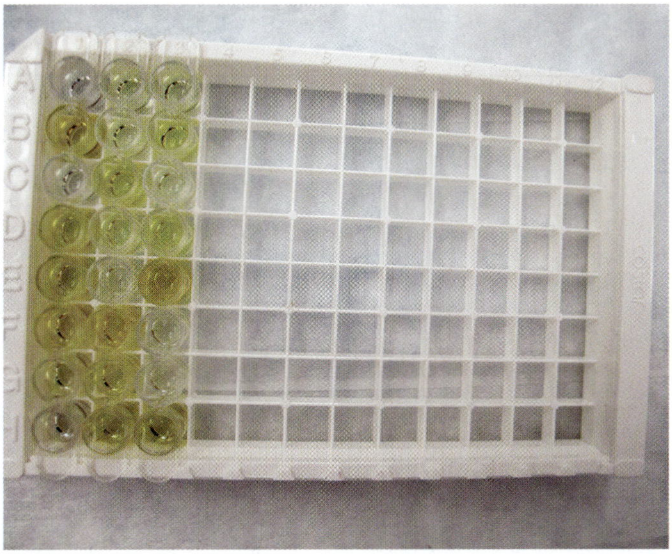

FIGURE 11–6 Sample wells from an indirect ELISA to detect patient antibody (in this example, antibody to the rubella virus). Well A1 is the reagent blank; well B1 is the positive control; well C1 is the negative control; and wells D1, E1, and F1 are calibrators run in triplicate. The remaining wells are individual patient samples. Note that the negative wells remain colorless, whereas wells containing samples that are positive for the antibody produce a yellow color after addition of the stop solution. Absorbance values are read on a spectrophotometer. *(Figure courtesy of Dr. Linda Miller.)*

Interferences in Immunoassays

False-positive or false-negative results in immunoassays may occur for a variety of reasons. In some cases, they are produced because of certain physical properties of the specimen itself; for example, some biological substances in urine or plasma can cause quenching of light emission or exhibit background fluorescence. Additional test interferences may occur for several different reasons related to immunoassay design. Most of the interferences described are mainly observed when heterogeneous methods are used to measure the test analyte, rather than homogeneous methods.

Antigen Interference

The improved turnaround time, speed, and sensitivity of capture immunoassays have made them excellent tools for measuring several biological substances. However, they are subject to certain limitations. The most commonly observed of these is the **high-dose hook effect**, or *postzone* effect, where excess patient antigen causes falsely decreased detection, leading to an analyte concentration that appears to be low or normal. This effect is illustrated in **Figure 11–8.** Note that the curve that depicts the relationship between the analyte and the intensity of the reaction signal takes on the shape of a "hook." The high-dose hook effect occurs mainly when there are not enough capture antibody sites for antigen binding because most binding sites are filled, so the remainder of patient antigen has no place to bind and gets removed during the wash step. When a hook effect is suspected, the laboratory professional should dilute the sample to the point where the concentration is within the analytical measuring range (calibration range). An increased antigen concentration reading after dilution provides evidence that a hook effect was present in the original undiluted sample.

Antibody Interference

Antibodies made by the patient may interfere with immunoassays if they are able to bind to the test kit reagents. Examples of such antibodies include autoantibodies and heterophile antibodies.

Autoantibodies

Production of autoantibodies by individuals with an autoimmune disease is one possible source of interference. A clinical example is rheumatoid factor (RF), an autoantibody directed against IgG produced by patients with rheumatoid arthritis and other autoimmune disorders (see Chapter 15). If present, RF can cause false-positive results (or, less commonly, false-negative results) in clinical tests that use immunoglobulin G (IgG) antibodies. If this is suspected, serum can be pretreated with a blocking reagent to avoid this problem. For example, animal IgG antibodies may be added to the patient sample to bind RF before testing. Importantly, these "blocking antibodies" must be of a different species than the capture and detection antibodies used in the immunoassay test. Other blocking reagents include polyethylene glycol, which precipitates RF, and pronase, an enzyme that destroys RF.

Heterophile Antibodies

Similar interference mechanisms may occur in individuals who have **heterophile antibodies** that react with animal proteins because the detection antibodies used in the test reagents are generated in nonhuman species (mouse, rabbit, goat). Heterophile antibodies may be produced by patients with certain infections, patients who have received therapeutic animal globulins, or patients who have frequent contact with animals.

11-1 Clinical Correlations

Rheumatoid Factor (RF)

RF is an antibody directed against the Fc portion of IgG molecules. It is produced by many patients with systemic autoimmune diseases that affect the joints, although it can be found in some individuals who do not have these conditions (see Chapter 15). Most commonly, the RF is an IgM antibody. The IgM anti-IgG can bind to IgG reagents in immunoassays and produce false-positive or false-negative results. In sandwich immunoassays, RF can cause false-negative results by blocking the capture antibody or false-positive results by bridging the capture antibody and the labeled antibody. In competitive immunoassays, RF can produce false-positive results by binding to the antibody reagent and preventing it from reacting with the labeled antigen through steric hindrance.

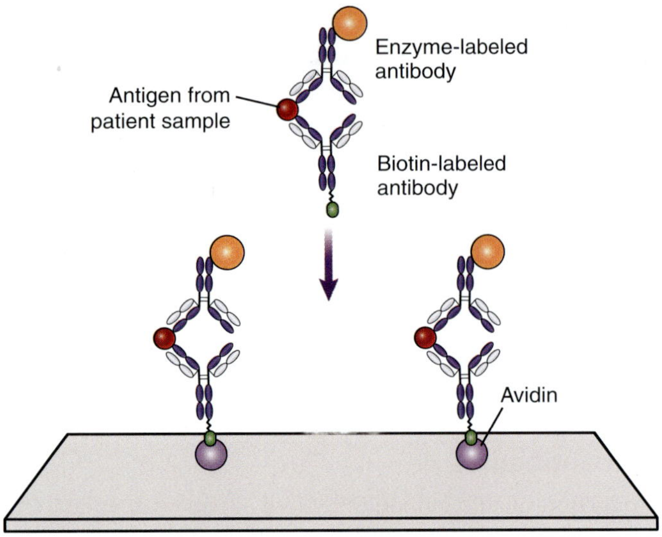

FIGURE 11–7 Biotin-streptavidin labeling in a delayed capture immunoassay. Antigen in patient serum binds in between an enzyme-labeled detection antibody and a biotinylated capture antibody, forming a sandwich in solution. The complex then binds to a streptavidin-coated solid phase. (Only one of the four binding sites is shown on each avidin molecule for easier visualization.)

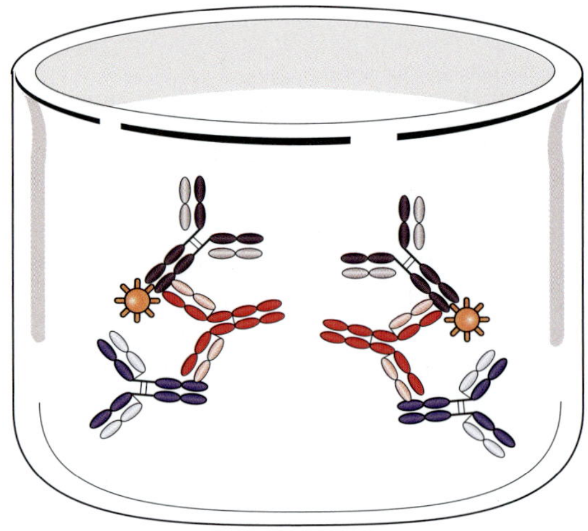

FIGURE 11–9 Interference by heterophile or anti-animal antibodies. Heterophile or anti-animal antibodies (red) can cause both false decreases and false increases, depending on their reactivity against the antibody species used in an immunoassay. However, false increases caused by linking the capture antibodies (blue) and the detection antibodies (black) together are most likely, as shown.

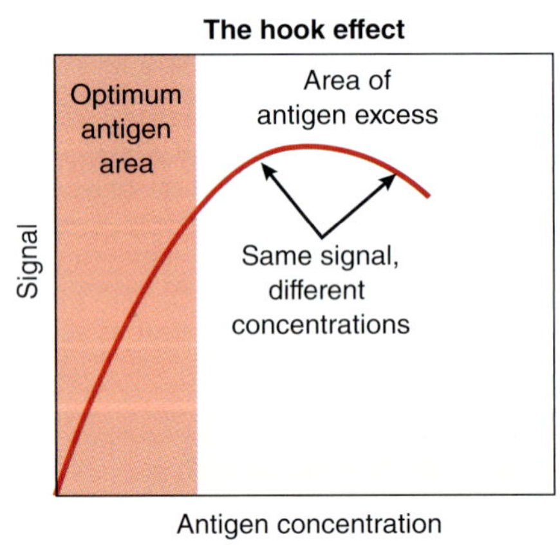

FIGURE 11–8 The high-dose hook effect. Antigen excess can saturate capture antibodies, and the intended "sandwich" configurations cannot form, leading to a false decrease in signal.

Heterophile interference occurs when antibodies produced by the patient are similar to reagents used in the test kit, such as anti-mouse, -rabbit, or -goat antibodies. Heterophile antibodies will often cross-link reagent capture and detection antibodies in the absence of antigen (test analyte) to produce a falsely increased test signal **(Fig. 11–9).** In rarer cases, heterophile antibodies can cause a falsely decreased test result by binding to the antigen of interest or by binding to the labeled detector antibody, preventing the formation of an immune complex.

11-2 Clinical Correlations

Human–Anti-Mouse Antibodies (HAMAs)

Human–anti-mouse antibodies (HAMAs) are a type of heterophile antibody that commonly causes interference in immunoassays. These antibodies are often produced by patients who receive mouse monoclonal antibodies as therapeutic agents for diseases such as cancer and autoimmune disorders (see Chapter 25).

Biotin Interference

When test reagent kits also use a biotin-SAv complex, even more unpredictable interferences can occur. The most pressing concern facing clinical laboratorians using this immunoassay format occurs when the person being tested has recently taken high-dose biotin as a nutritional supplement or medication (usually 1 mg/1,000 mcg or greater). The ingested biotin causes interference by binding to the SAv reagent in the immunoassay. Depending on the immunoassay design, test results may be falsely increased (competitive design) or decreased (noncompetitive immunoassay). Such interference is usually discovered when reported test results are found to be inconsistent with the patient's clinical picture. For example, a markedly abnormal thyroid-stimulating hormone (TSH) test result may be observed in a person with no other evidence of pituitary or thyroid disease. Fortunately, having the patient refrain from taking biotin for 8 to 48 hours before blood sample collection corrects or prevents this problem. Alternatively, measuring the same analyte by a different method that does not use the biotin-SAv reaction could be performed on the sample to obtain reliable results. Biotin interference in the original test result would be suspected if the result on the retested sample normalizes when the alternative method is used.

Spectral Interference

Labeled immunoassays that are designed to detect UV/visible light by spectrophotometry have the potential to detect background color from the sample depending on the enzyme (e.g., horseradish peroxidase) and chromogenic substrate (color indicator) used in the reaction. For example, detection of an immunoassay label that transmits light in the 405 to 450 nm range also corresponds to the peak absorbance for yellow-colored substances. Clinical samples, calibration standards, and quality control (QC) materials are often yellow in color. Measuring in the near UV range (340 nm) can also detect some of the yellow color in patient and control samples. For this reason, a background correction may be needed to reduce any spectral interference that can occur in such situations.

Other Technical Concerns

Cross-reactivity describes detection of a substance other than the analyte of interest. This often occurs because the substance has a similar structure to the analyte(s) used to calibrate the test method. When cross-reactivity occurs, it is typically observed as a false-positive result. Multiple cases of cross-reactivity in drug immunoassays have been reported in the literature. One example was a false-positive opiate immunoassay screen result in which naloxone (an opiate antagonist) was detected as an opiate by a homogeneous EIA method (CEDIA, described in a later section). In such instances, an alternative method must be used to confirm the initial result obtained by the immunoassay. It should be noted, however, that *intentional* cross-reactivity for drugs of abuse is commonly incorporated in immunoassay screens so that drugs in the same class can be detected. For instance, the "opiate" immunoassay screen uses morphine as the calibration standard. Any compound related structurally, or metabolized to morphine, will produce a positive test result. Key examples include codeine and heroin. Distinguishing between these different drugs is not possible with the opiate screen immunoassay, and follow-up with a confirmatory method for exact identification is necessary.

Finally, clinical laboratorians must be cautious whenever interpreting immunoassay results across different manufacturers, as direct comparisons may not be possible. Because test manufacturers often develop capture and detection antibodies to slightly different epitopes, the reference interval (normal range) established for an immunoassay can vary widely across manufacturers, even for the same clinical test. This is especially critical when serial measurements of tumor marker proteins are being performed to monitor medical treatment of patients with cancer (see Chapter 17).

Critical Thinking 11-2

A patient with relapsing fever, caused by the bacterium *Borrelia miyamotoi,* tested positive in an EIA test for antibodies to *Borrelia burgdorferi,* the cause of Lyme disease. What is the likely reason for this result?

Techniques Involving Electrophoresis

Some techniques involve separation of proteins by electrophoresis and their subsequent identification by incubation with a labeled detector antibody. Examples include immunofixation electrophoresis (IFE), the Western blot, and isoelectric focusing. We discuss the latter two methods in this section and IFE in Chapters 10 and 18.

Western Blot

The **Western blot** test, also known as **immunoblotting,** separates and identifies specific proteins found in a complex mixture of proteins extracted from a sample. In this method, proteins are first separated according to their size by polyacrylamide gel electrophoresis. Protein antigens of a low molecular weight migrate easily through the pores of the gel and move toward the bottom, whereas antigens of high molecular weight remain closer to the top of the gel because they become trapped in the gel matrix.

The separated proteins are then blotted onto a durable test membrane such as nitrocellulose or polyvinylidene difluoride (PVDF) to allow binding of detector antibodies. Protein transfer is performed by various methods including capillary diffusion, vacuum pressure, and electroelution. In this way, the proteins are immobilized on the membrane at positions corresponding to those on the electrophoresis gel. The membrane is then treated with a blocking solution such as nonfat milk or bovine serum albumin, which binds to areas of the membrane to which the proteins have not attached to block nonspecific binding of antibodies and reduce background staining.

After the blocking step and a wash step to remove excess protein, the membrane is incubated with antibodies, most commonly using an indirect immunoassay. In this method, the membrane is first incubated with an unlabeled primary antibody, which binds to the protein of interest. Excess primary antibody is removed with a wash step. The next step involves addition of a secondary antibody conjugated to an enzyme, chemiluminescent, or fluorescent label. The secondary antibody binds to the primary antibody, and after another wash and addition of the appropriate substrate, a detection signal is visible as a band at the position of the migrated protein **(Fig. 11–10).** The band position provides information about the size of the protein, while its thickness is an indicator of protein quantity, which can be measured by instrumentation.

The Western blot has been an important technique in research laboratories to identify antigens or analyze changes in the quantity of known proteins from samples treated under different experimental conditions. Clinical laboratories have also used it to detect specific antibodies when patient serum, the source of primary antibody, is incubated with test membranes to which antigens from pathogens have been bound. Examples include detection of antibodies to *B. burgdorferi* as a confirmatory test for the diagnosis of Lyme disease (see Chapter 21) and the former confirmatory test for HIV infection (see Chapter 24).

The Western blot is more technically demanding than ELISA or other immunoassays but provides an antibody

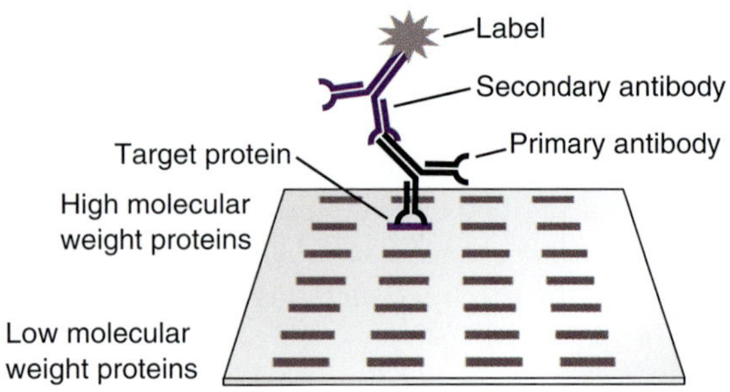

FIGURE 11–10 Western blot principle. A complex mixture of proteins is electrophoresed on a gel to separate the proteins based on their molecular weights. The separated proteins are blotted onto a membrane. Western blots that detect patient antibodies to a target protein involve binding of the primary antibody in patient serum to its target antigen on a membrane, followed by binding of a labeled secondary antibody (anti-human Ig).

profile of the sample that reveals the specificities to individual antigens. Patients can also be followed over time to determine whether there is a change in the antibody pattern. Because Western blot testing is highly dependent on the laboratorian's technical skill and subjective interpretation, it is generally performed only in specialized reference or research laboratories. Positive and negative control sera must be included in the test run to provide quality control.

Isoelectric Focusing (IEF)

In **isoelectric focusing (IEF),** proteins are separated based on differences in their isoelectric point (pI). The pI is the pH at which a molecule has no net electrical charge (i.e., is electrically neutral). Protein separation is achieved in IEF by conducting electrophoresis within a narrow pH gradient. At first, proteins move in the gel toward the electrode of opposite charge. As they migrate, they either acquire or lose protons, slowing their mobility. Eventually, they acquire a net zero charge and stop migrating once they arrive at their pI. After electrophoresis, immunoblotting can be performed, allowing protein bands to be visualized after incubation with a detection antibody conjugated to an enzyme label, commonly peroxidase.

IEF combined with immunoblotting provides better resolution (i.e., more protein bands are visible due to better separation) than traditional electrophoresis and is an important tool in research laboratories to purify and analyze proteins, and for proteomics studies. In clinical laboratories, it has become the gold standard to identify oligoclonal banding in the CSF of patients with multiple sclerosis (see Chapter 15) and genetic variants of α_1-antitrypsin deficiency (see Chapter 2). IEF has also been used to identify variant hemoglobins in prenatal screening and polymorphic proteins in forensic serology.

Homogeneous Enzyme Immunoassays

The main use of homogeneous immunoassays has been in the measurement of low molecular weight analytes (haptens), such as hormones, therapeutic drugs, and drugs of abuse, in both serum and urine. Homogeneous immunoassays **(Fig. 11–11)** may provide faster test results because wash steps are not required, and as we mentioned, these immunoassays tend to be less prone to analytical interferences. Despite the advantages of homogeneous immunoassays, their analytical sensitivity is not as robust as heterogeneous immunoassays.

The original homogeneous immunoassay design, which is still used today on multiple platforms, is the **enzyme-multiplied immunoassay technique (EMIT),** first developed by the Syva Corporation (now part of Siemens). The EMIT immunoassay is based on the principle of change in enzyme activity as specific antigen-antibody interaction occurs in solution. Reagent antigen is bound to an enzyme tag, commonly G6PDH. When reagent antibody binds to spe-

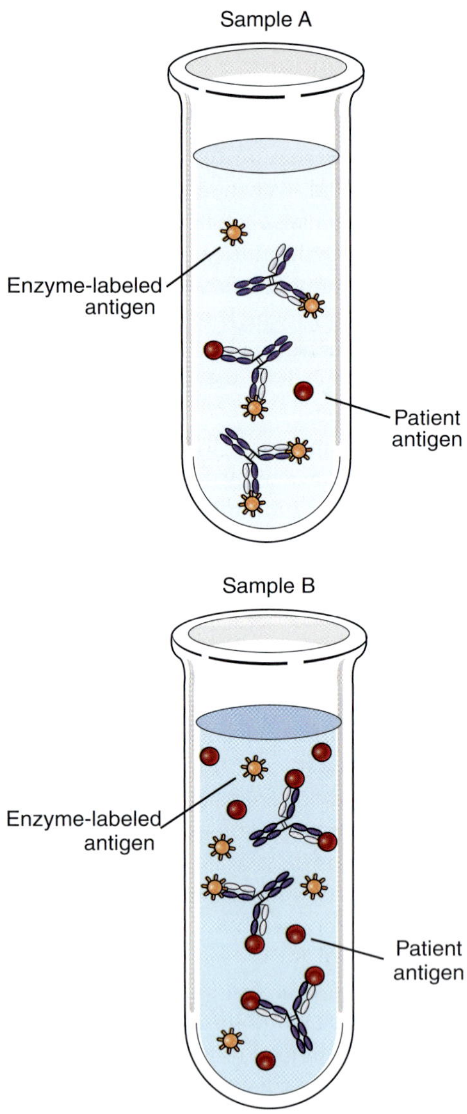

FIGURE 11–11 Homogeneous immunoassay. Reagent antibody is in solution. Patient antigen and enzyme-labeled antigen are added to the test tube, where they compete for a limited number of binding sites on the antibodies. When patient antigen is present, the enzyme-labeled reagent antigen is not blocked by the antibodies, so color development is observed. Sample A has a low concentration of patient antigen, whereas Sample B contains more patient antigen and has stronger color development.

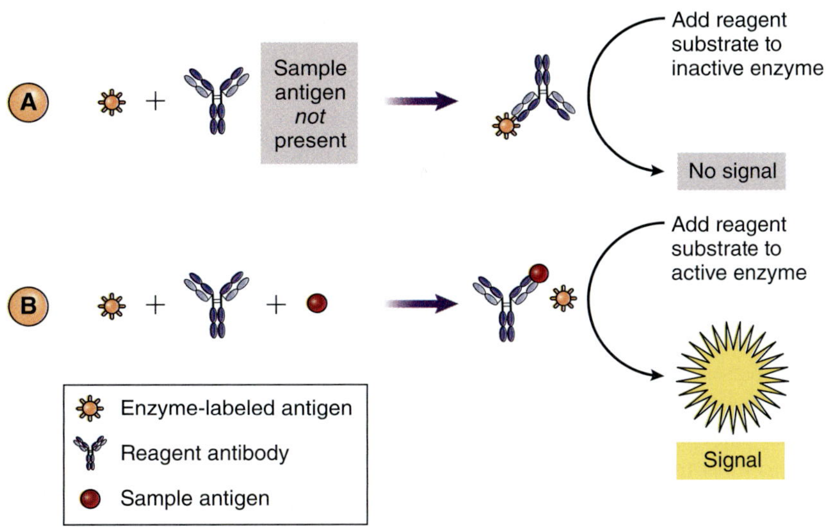

FIGURE 11–12 EMIT immunoassay design. *(Figure courtesy of Dr. Paul Johnson.)*

cific determinant sites on the enzyme-antigen pair, the active site on the enzyme is blocked, resulting in a measurable loss of activity. Free analyte (antigen in the patient sample) competes with enzyme-labeled analyte for a limited number of antibody binding sites. G6PDH catalyzes the reduction of NAD^+ (nicotinamide adenine dinucleotide) to NADH (NAD-hydrogen), leading to increased absorbance in the peak UV-wavelength measurement of NADH (340 nm). The resulting enzyme activity and signal generated are directly proportional to the concentration of patient antigen in the test solution **(Fig. 11–12).**

The **cloned enzyme donor immunoassay (CEDIA)** is another example of a homogeneous immunoassay. CEDIA was developed using genetic engineering techniques to produce the β-galactosidase enzyme in two parts: acceptor and donor. When separated, the enzyme is not fully formed, and there is no enzymatic activity; when the acceptor-donor pair combine, enzymatic activity is restored, and reagent substrate is catalyzed to generate a product signal that is measured by photometry. To achieve this reaction, the hapten antigen (Ag) is attached to the enzyme donor piece. The enzyme donor Ag competes with patient Ag (analyte) for limited antibody binding sites. As patient Ag binds to reagent Ab, it leaves the enzyme donor free to bind with the enzyme-acceptor molecule. Therefore, enzymatic activity and signal are directly proportional to patient Ag concentration. This reaction occurs in solution without need of a solid-phase material, making it a homogeneous immunoassay. Its most common clinical use is to detect or quantitate levels of therapeutic and abused drugs.

Another homogeneous format in common use is an unlabeled immunoassay, *kinetic interaction of microparticles in a solution* (KIMS; see Chapter 10).

Chemiluminescent Immunoassays

Most available immunometric assays are based on chemiluminescent label detection and collectively called **chemiluminescent immunoassays. Chemiluminescence** is the emission of light caused by a chemical reaction, typically an oxidation reaction, producing an excited molecule that releases light during return to its original ground state. The reaction may be triggered by different means, such as an enzyme label or electrode. Large numbers of molecules are capable of chemiluminescence, and some of the most common substances used in test systems are luminol, acridinium esters, ruthenium derivatives, and nitrophenyl oxalates. When these substances are oxidized, intermediates are produced that are of a higher energy state. These intermediates spontaneously return to their original ground state, emitting photon energy (light) in the process. Light emissions range from a rapid flash of light to a continuous glow that can last for hours. For example, when acridinium esters are oxidized by hydrogen peroxide under alkaline conditions, they emit a quick flash of light. When luminol is used in the reaction, the light signal remains for a longer time period.

Chemiluminescent technology is the basis for several types of automated immunoassays, which are used to detect a wide variety of clinical analytes, including antigens and antibodies. The design can be applied to heterogeneous or homogeneous immunoassay formats. Haptens such as therapeutic drugs and steroid hormones are measured using competitive immunoassays, whereas the sandwich or capture format is used for larger analytes such as protein hormones. These immunoassays also demonstrate excellent analytical properties for measuring serum antibodies produced in several infectious diseases and autoimmune disorders.

Chemiluminescent immunoassays have superior analytical sensitivity and a wide dynamic range, the latter implying that the immunoassay performs well at both very low and very high analyte concentrations. This provides excellent sensitivity to detect very low levels and reduces the need for sample dilution because extremely elevated results can be accurately measured. Detecting high antigen concentration without need for sample dilution can be especially useful when measuring tumor markers or autoantibodies in diseased patients, where concentration levels can be 10-fold or greater than the upper limit of the normal cutoff value.

Chemiluminescent Microparticle Immunoassay

In the **chemiluminescent microparticle immunoassay (CMIA),** antibody-coated microparticles are used in the reagent. In this method, patient antigen competes with a hapten (Ag) labeled with an acridinium ester for binding to the antibody **(Fig. 11–13).** Magnets are used to attract the microparticles for physical separation and allow for unbound substances to be washed off. As such, CMIA is a heterogeneous immunoassay because the particles are physically separated by magnets.

As antigen concentration increases in the patient sample, it prevents labeled Ag molecules from binding to the Ab-coated microparticles. Conversely, a low concentration of patient antigen enables more labeled Ag to bind to the microparticles. A final test signal is generated by adding hydrogen peroxide to the alkaline solution, which destabilizes the acridinium ester, resulting in a flash of light (chemiluminescence). The resulting signal is indirectly proportional to the antigen concentration in the patient sample. CMIA technology has been largely applied for use in drug measurements, for example, phenytoin, a common anti-epileptic drug measured in therapeutic drug monitoring (TDM), to ensure the patient's drug levels are within the effective dose range and are not at toxic or subtherapeutic levels.

Electrochemiluminescence Immunoassay

A newer modification of the traditional chemiluminescent immunoassay is the **electrochemiluminescence immunoassay (ECLIA).** The assay uses ruthenium, a chemical indicator, conjugated to an antibody in a capture immunoassay. It undergoes an electrochemiluminescent reaction with another chemical substance, tripropylamine (TPA), at the surface of an electrode. When ruthenium is oxidized and then returned to its reduced state through interaction with TPA, it emits light that can be measured by a photomultiplier tube. Magnetic beads or microparticles are often used as the solid phase to capture the labeled antibody.

Fluorescent Immunoassays

In 1941, Albert Coons demonstrated that antibodies could be labeled with molecules that fluoresce. These fluorescent compounds, called **fluorophores** or **fluorochromes,** can absorb energy from an incident light source and convert it into light of a longer wavelength and lower energy as the excited electrons return to the ground state. Fluorophores are typically organic molecules with a ring structure; each has a characteristic optimal absorption range. The time interval between energy absorption and fluorescence emission is very short and can be measured in nanoseconds.

Ideally, a fluorescent probe should exhibit high intensity, remain stable in solution, and be distinguished from sample background fluorescence. The two compounds most often used are fluorescein and rhodamine, usually in the form of isothiocyanates, because these can be readily coupled to antigen or antibody. Fluorescein absorbs maximally at 490

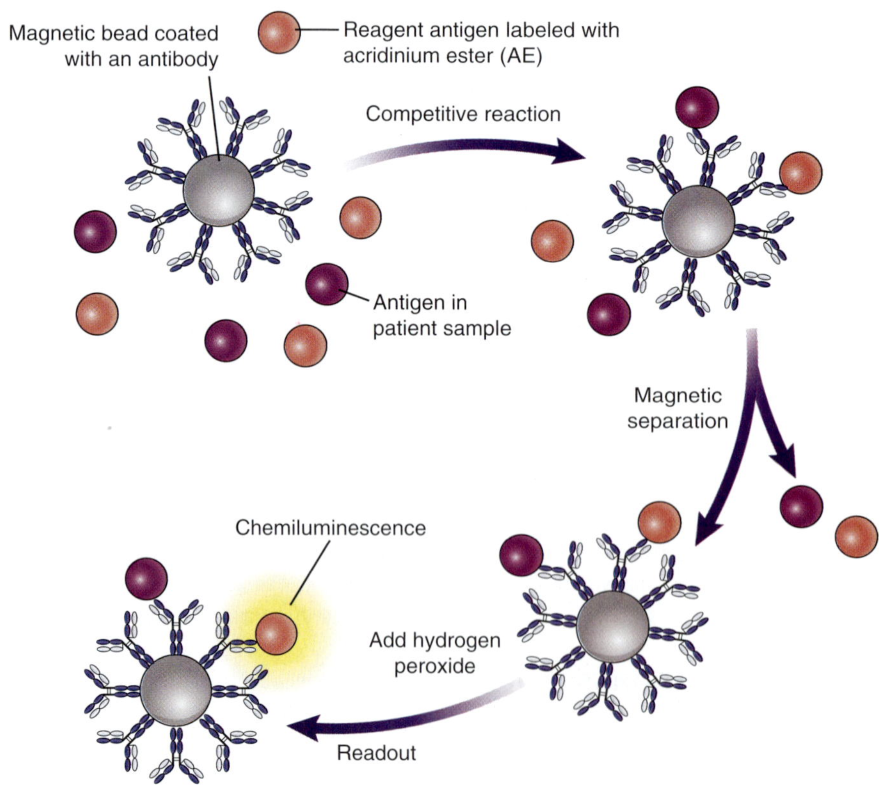

FIGURE 11–13 Chemiluminescent microparticle immunoassay (CMIA) principle. Antigen in patient sample competes with a reagent antigen conjugated to a chemiluminescent label for an antibody coated onto microparticles. In this example, an enzyme (hydrogen peroxide) is used to trigger the reaction. AE = acridinium ester.

to 495 nm and emits a green color at 520 nm. It has high intensity, good photostability, and a high quantum yield. Tetramethylrhodamine absorbs at 550 nm and emits red light at 585 nm. Because their absorbance and emission patterns differ, fluorescein and rhodamine can be used together.

Fluorescent-labeled antibodies or antigens have been used in a variety of immunoassays, including direct and indirect immunofluorescence assays, and multiplex immunoassays (MIAs). Many fluorescent immunoassays take place on a microscope slide or on the surface of live cells. These techniques are called **immunofluorescence assays (IFAs).** In the text that follows, we present the principles of laboratory methods that use fluorescent labels and examples of their clinical applications.

Knowledge Check 11-3

In contrast to fluorochromes, chemiluminescent substances:

a. Produce a colored product after reaction with an enzyme.
b. Require hazardous waste removal.
c. Release light of a higher wavelength than they absorbed.
d. Emit light after an oxidation reaction.

Direct Immunofluorescence Assays

Fluorescent staining methods can be categorized as either direct or indirect, depending on whether the antibody specific for the antigen has a fluorescent tag attached to it. **Figure 11–14** depicts the difference between the two techniques.

Direct immunofluorescence assays may be used to detect antigens on tissue sections fixed onto a microscopic slide or in live cell suspensions. In a direct IFA performed on a microscope slide, antibody that is conjugated with a fluorescent tag is added directly to sample antigen fixed onto the slide (Fig. 11–14). After incubation and a wash step to remove unbound antibody, the slide is read using a fluorescence microscope. The bound fluorescent probe is detected after excitation by a high-intensity light source. In this manner, multiple antigens can be detected with a high degree of sensitivity and specificity. Antigens are typically visualized as bright-apple-green or orange-yellow objects against a dark background. Examples of antigens detected by direct IFA methods include bacterial pathogens (e.g., *Legionella pneumophila, Chlamydia trachomatis*), viruses (e.g., herpes simplex), and parasites (e.g., *Toxoplasma gondii, Giardia lamblia*) **(Fig. 11–15).**

Cell-based direct IFA methods combine the principles of hematology cell counters with fluorescent-labeled antibodies to better classify cells. An important application of direct IFA is to differentiate cell populations of the immune system, such as T and B lymphocytes, based on their cluster of differentiation (CD) antigens by incubating the cells with fluorescent-labeled antibodies specific for those markers. For example, direct IFA assay is very useful in the detection and quantitation of abnormal cell populations observed in leukemias. The results are analyzed by automated **flow cytometry** (see Chapter 13).

More recent advances in flow cytometry include *mass cytometry* profiling of cells based on CD marker identification.

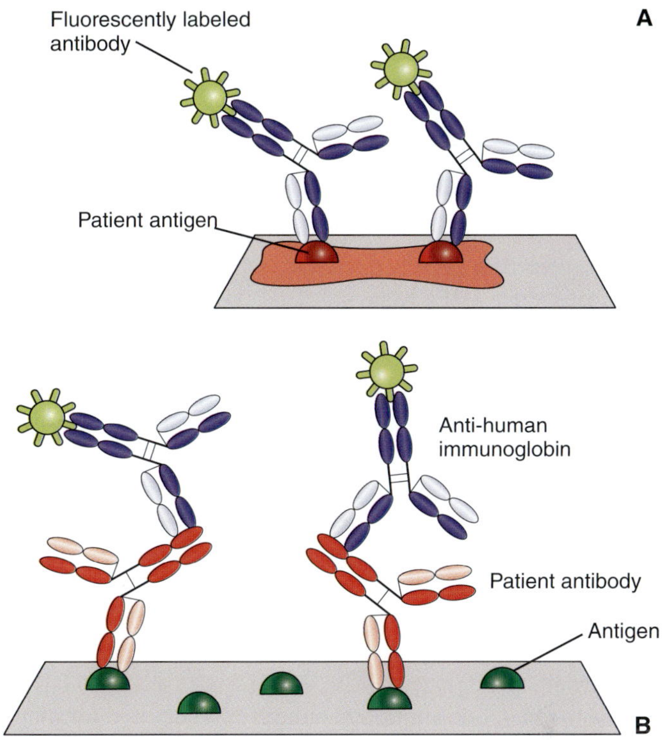

FIGURE 11–14 Direct versus indirect immunofluorescent assays. (A) In a direct fluorescent immunoassay, the patient antigen is fixed to a microscope slide and incubated directly with a fluorescent-labeled antibody. The slide is washed to remove unbound antibody. If specific antigen is present in the patient sample, fluorescence will be observed. Alternately, patient cells can be incubated with a fluorescent-labeled antibody in suspension. (B) In indirect immunofluorescence, well-characterized tissues or cells are fixed to slides. Specific antibody in patient serum (red) binds to the antigens on the slides. A wash step is performed, and a labeled anti-human immunoglobulin is added. After a second wash step to remove any uncombined anti-human immunoglobulin, the fluorescence of the sample is determined. The amount of fluorescence is directly in proportion to the amount of patient antibody present.

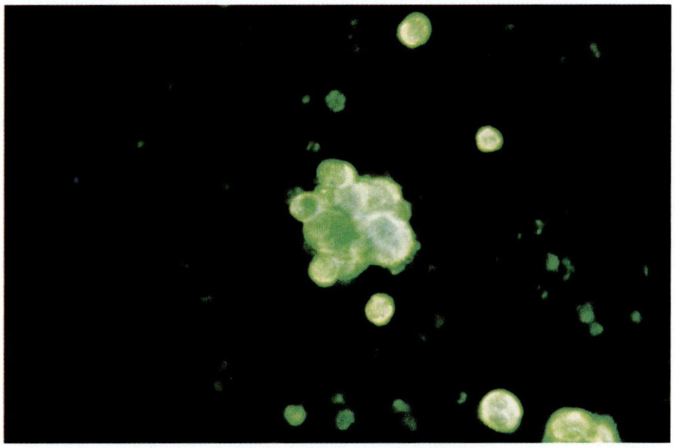

FIGURE 11–15 Direct IFA example. Using a fluorescein isothiocyanate (FITC) conjugated immunoglobulin staining technique, and under direct immunofluorescence (DIF), this tissue sample extracted from a vesicle and ulcer reveals the presence of herpes simplex antigen in a patient determined to have a herpes simplex virus type-2 (HSV-2) infection. *(CDC/Courtesy of Dr. Craig Yerla).*

In this method, fluorescent labels are replaced with metal isotope labels for detection. Metal isotopes can simultaneously detect a greater number of cellular markers as compared with traditional fluorescent labels.

Indirect Immunofluorescence Assays

In general, a direct immunofluorescence assay is used for only antigen detection in cells or tissues, whereas **indirect immunofluorescence (IIF) assays** can be used for either antigen or antibody identification, depending on the intended clinical application. IIF assays involve two steps, in a manner similar to reagent-based capture immunoassays. In the first step of IIF assays to detect antibody in patient serum (the *primary* antibody), the serum is incubated on a microscope slide to which a known antigen has been attached. Tissue antigens are usually affixed to the slide; for example, human epithelial cells are used for anti-nuclear antibody (ANA) testing. The slide is then washed, and an anti-human immunoglobulin containing a fluorescent tag is added. This labeled immunoglobulin, or *secondary* antibody, combines with the first antibody to form a sandwich, which localizes the fluorescence (see Fig. 11–14). In this manner, one antibody conjugate can be used for many different types of reactions, eliminating the need for numerous purified, labeled reagent antibodies.

IIF assays generate increased staining because multiple labeled antibodies can bind to each primary antibody, making this a more sensitive technique. IIF is especially useful in antibody identification and has been used to detect treponemal antibodies in syphilis, viral antibodies, and autoantibodies such as ANAs and anti-neutrophil cytoplasmic antibodies (ANCAs; see Chapters 15 and 21). Interpreting immunofluorescent slides is partly subjective because the laboratorian reports results based on the visual presence or absence of a fluorescent signal and the signal intensity in positive samples. Technical experience is essential for accurate and reliable reporting of slide test results.

Knowledge Check 11-4

Which of the following describes an immunofluorescence assay to detect patient antibody?

a. Patient serum is labeled with fluorescein and incubated with cells in suspension.
b. Patient serum is labeled with fluorescein and incubated with antigen attached to a microscope slide.
c. First, patient serum is incubated with antigen attached to a microscope slide; after a wash step, fluorescein-labeled anti-human IgG is added.
d. Patient serum is captured onto a microscope slide coated with an anti-human IgG antibody; after a wash step, fluorescein-labeled antigen is added.

Multiplex Microparticle Fluorescent Immunoassays

More recently developed formats of IIF assays use microparticles as the solid phase instead of a microscope slide. One such method is the **multiplex immunoassay (MIA)**, or *fluorescent microbead immunoassay.* This high-throughput, automated method has improved ease of clinical testing, especially in testing for autoimmune diseases. Polystyrene beads are used as the solid phase. When the technique is used to detect antibodies in patient serum, beads conjugated to different antigens are used. The beads can be distinguished by their unique shade of red, created by a specific combination of infrared and fluorescent dyes. Patient sample is added to the bead mixture, and antibodies in the sample are detected with a fluorescent-tagged anti-human immunoglobulin. The beads containing the immune complexes are identified by flow cytometry (see Chapter 13). A benefit of MIA technology is that it allows for multiple antibodies to be detected simultaneously. Clinical applications of MIA include ANA testing (see Chapter 15) and detection of antibodies in transplant patients to donor antigens (see Chapter 16 and Fig. 16–8). MIA can also be used to simultaneously detect multiple antigens in a test sample when the polystyrene beads are coated with the corresponding antibodies. For example, MIA can detect multiple cytokines in the serum of patients with inflammatory disorders (see Chapter 6) and cytokines produced by cells cultured under different conditions.

Like MIA, the **particle-based multi-analyte technology (PMAT)** is a recently developed automated immunoassay that uses microparticles and fluorescence to simultaneously detect multiple antibodies. This technique uses paramagnetic particles coupled to different antigens. The particles have a unique proprietary signature that allows them to be differentiated from each other through use of a specialized optical module. During incubation with a mixture of different particles, antibodies in patient serum bind to their corresponding antigens on selected particles. After a wash step to remove unbound antibodies, a red-protein pigment complex, phycoerythrin (PE), conjugated to the secondary antibody is added and binds to any patient antibody on the particles. Following a second wash to remove unbound labeled antibody, the particles are aligned with magnets and placed in a chamber where they are exposed to two spectrally distinct light-emitting diodes (LEDs). A camera then captures high-resolution digital images that are used to identify the specific antigen-coated particles and quantify antibody isotypes (IgA, IgG, IgM) based on the amount of bound PE. The main clinical application of PMAT is detection of antibodies found in autoimmune diseases (see Chapter 15).

Rapid Immunoassays

Rapid immunoassays are membrane-based tests that are easy to perform and give reproducible results. Although designed mainly for point-of-care testing, many have found use in clinical laboratories because of their faster result turnaround time, ease of use, and little space needed for setup. These assays test urine or serum samples and are designed as single-use, disposable immunoassays in a plastic cartridge. Given this design, it is important to recognize that both internal and external quality controls (QC) are used. Internal QC is represented by the "control" line on each test cartridge to ensure that the volume added is adequate to flow through the membrane, as we describe in the paragraphs that follow. External QC is performed by testing the positive and negative controls that are supplied with the reagent kit and must be done at least every 24 hours when patient samples are tested.

The original rapid immunoassays are based on a flow-through design. The membrane and its large surface area enhance immunofiltration of the sample to provide speed and a high level of sensitivity. This method is a two-step immunoassay in which antigen or antibody in the patient sample is first absorbed onto the membrane containing the corresponding antibody or antigen. After a wash step to remove unbound sample components, a detection reagent is added. The reaction is then read by looking for the presence of a colored reaction product.

Newer **immunochromatography** methods combine all the previously mentioned steps into one step. The analyte is applied at one end of the strip and migrates toward the distal end, where there is an absorbent pad to maintain a constant capillary flow rate. The labeling and detection zones are set between the two ends. Sample is added to an application point; the application point also contains a labeled antigen or antibody conjugated to colored latex or colloidal gold particles. The sample reconstitutes the conjugate, where the two form a complex that migrates across the membrane. An antigen or antibody immobilized in the detection zone captures the immune complex and forms a colored line for a positive test when the immunoassay is of a noncompetitive format **(Fig. 11–16).** This type of test device has been used to detect diverse analytes of interest. Clinical applications of rapid immunoassays include detecting the human chorionic gonadotropin (hCG) hormone as an indicator of pregnancy **(Fig. 11–17)**; identifying microorganisms such as *Streptococcus pyogenes*, the cause of streptococcal pharyngitis (see Fig. 20–13); detecting cardiac troponin to diagnose a heart attack; testing nasopharyngeal swabs or saliva for coronavirus disease 2019 (COVID-19); and detecting HIV antibody (see Chapter 24).

The immunochromatographic design illustrated in Figure 11–16 is based on a capture or noncompetitive design. Some newer test systems, which use similar materials, are based on a competitive format. These results must be carefully interpreted because the line observed in competitive tests indicates a negative result, and absence of the line is a positive result. Rapid screening tests to detect drugs of abuse are one example of this format.

A **single-step, competitive, immunochromatographic method** contains detection antibody adsorbed onto colloidal gold particles and dried onto the entire membrane surface. Drug conjugates (drug bound to bovine serum albumin) are made for each drug to be detected, all of which are immobilized to a unique test-line position on the membrane. When the sample (urine) is added, it wicks along the entire surface of the white membrane. As it passes along each test lane, drug-free urine sample dissolves the antibody–gold particle complex at each lane, resulting in observation of purple-red

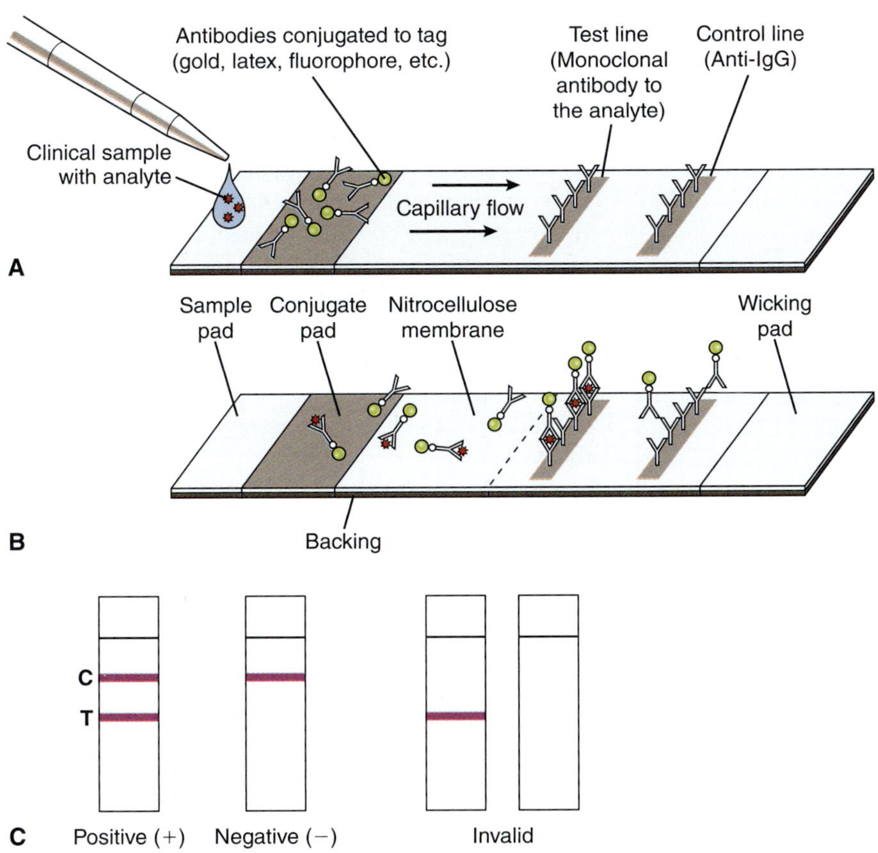

FIGURE 11–16 Noncompetitive immunochromatographic assay for patient antigen. (A) Patient sample is added to a cassette containing antibody labeled with colloidal gold. (B) Antigen in the sample combines with antibody on the gold nanoparticles, and the complexes are moved along by capillary flow. Monoclonal antibody to the analyte captures the patient antigen attached to gold-labeled antibody in the test zone, producing a colored line. Anti-IgG embedded in the membrane captures the colloidal gold-labeled antibody in the control zone and produces a colored line. (C) Test results seen for a patient sample containing the antigen (positive result) and a patient sample without the antigen (negative result). Note that if a control line is not seen, the test is considered invalid, regardless of the patient result.

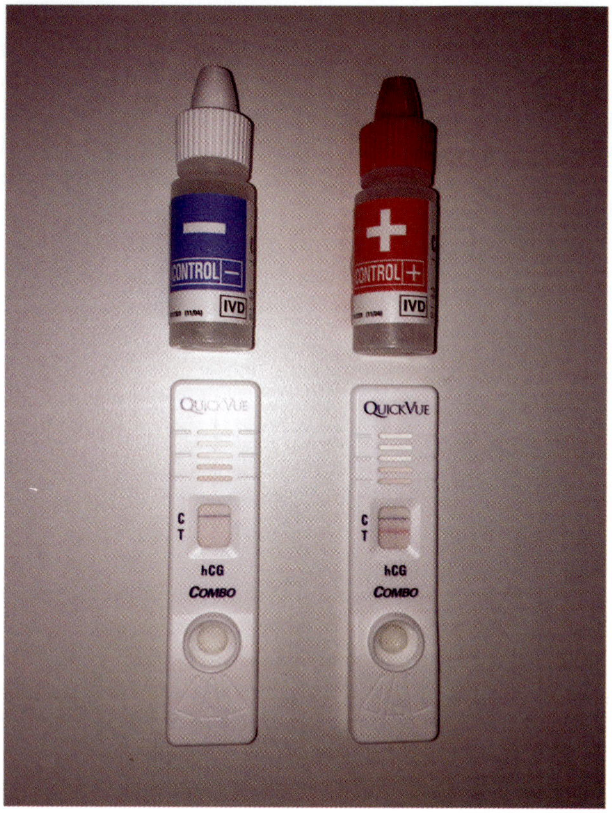

FIGURE 11–17 Rapid immunoassay for human chorionic gonadotropin (hCG). The negative control (left) has a line in the control region only. The positive control (right) has lines in both the control (C) region and the test (T) region. The control line must be present for the results to be valid, regardless of the test result. *(Photo courtesy of Dr. Paul Johnson.)*

colored lines. Any drug present in the sample will inhibit that reaction, so that no line will be observed on the white membrane background. As this method is based on a competitive design, it may lead to initial confusion when interpreting test results. This is because the color line indicator is observed only when there is no antigen or drug present in the sample (negative result), while the absence of the line indicator is a positive result. The test system may include a strip-reading device, which aids the laboratorian in interpreting the final results. All single-use immunoassays include a control line to ensure proper functioning of the cartridge in the test kit before reporting results (see Figs. 11-16 and 11–17).

Knowledge Check 11-5

Most rapid immunoassays are based on the principle of:
a. Chemiluminescence
b. Fluorescence
c. Precipitation
d. Immunochromatography

KEY CONCEPTS

Introduction

- Labeled immunoassays were developed to improve measurement of antigens and antibodies that may be small in size or present in very low concentrations.
- The substance being measured is called the *analyte,* or biomarker.
- Antibodies used in immunoassays must be very specific and have a high affinity for the antigen in question. Specificity helps to reduce cross-reactivity, and the antibody affinity determines how stable the binding is between antigen and antibody. These two factors help to determine the specificity and sensitivity of immunoassay methods.

Immunoassay Labels

- Labeling techniques include the use of radioactivity, enzymes, fluorescence, chemiluminescence, and chromatography.

General Immunoassay Formats

- The two major formats of immunoassays are heterogeneous and homogeneous. In heterogeneous immunoassays, physical separation of bound and free components is required. Homogeneous immunoassays do not require a physical separation step.
- Additional subclassifications describe whether immunoassay method designs are competitive or noncompetitive. In competitive immunoassays, all the reactants are added at the same time, and labeled antigen competes with patient antigen for a limited number of antibody binding sites.
- In competitive immunoassays, the amount of bound label is inversely proportional to the concentration of the labeled antigen. In other words, the greater the amount of labeled antigen detected, the less antigen is present in the patient sample.
- In noncompetitive immunoassays for antigen, reagent antibody is passively absorbed onto a solid-phase material. Excess capture antibody is present to ensure that any patient antigen will be bound. A labeled antibody, directed against a different epitope of the antigen, is added.
- In noncompetitive immunoassays, the amount of the label detected is directly proportional to the amount of patient antigen present.

Radioimmunoassay (RIA)

- Radioimmunoassays (RIAs) are based on a competitive principle, using a radioisotope label. These assays have extremely high analytical sensitivity but have disadvantages associated with handling radioactive substances.

Enzyme Immunoassays (EIAs)

- Enzyme immunoassays (EIAs) use enzymes that catalyze biochemical reactions. They convert reagent substrates to produce chemically modified products that can be detected.

Heterogeneous Enzyme Immunoassays

- In competitive enzyme-linked immunosorbent assays (ELISAs), antigen in the sample competes with enzyme-conjugated antigen for a limited number of binding sites on antibody molecules attached to a solid phase. Enzyme activity present in the final reaction catalyzes the conversion of a substrate to a detectable product.
- Indirect ELISAs are a type of noncompetitive immunoassay used to detect patient antibody. These immunoassays are termed *indirect* because the enzyme-labeled reagent does not participate in the initial antigen-antibody reaction. The associated antigen is bound to the solid phase. Patient serum with an unknown antibody concentration is added. A second antibody reacts with any patient antibody that is bound to the solid phase.
- Immunoassays that detect antigen are termed *capture immunoassays*. In capture or sandwich immunoassays, the antibody is bound to a solid phase, and any patient antigen is allowed to bind or be captured. A second enzyme-labeled antibody is added. The final complex formed with sample antigen in between the two reagent antibodies creates the "sandwich."
- Increased analytical sensitivity of labeled immunoassays can be achieved by complexing biotin to the capture antibody and streptavidin to the solid-phase material. Biotin-SAv labeling can be used in both indirect ELISAs and capture immunoassays.

Interferences in Enzyme Immunoassays

- The most commonly observed limitation of capture immunoassays is the high-dose hook effect, or *postzone* effect. Excess patient antigen causes falsely decreased detection, leading to an analyte concentration that appears to be low or normal.
- Antibodies produced in vivo, notably autoantibodies and heterophile antibodies, may interfere with immunoassays. Rheumatoid factor (anti-IgG) can cause false-positive results in tests that use IgG antibody reagents. Heterophile antibody interference occurs when the patient produces anti-animal antibodies that bind to reagent antibodies used in the test kit.
- Test kits using a biotin-SAv complex can have unpredictable interferences when using samples from patients who have taken high-dose biotin supplements or medications.
- *Cross-reactivity* describes detection of a substance other than the analyte of interest. It is typically observed as a false-positive result. The exception can occur with drug immunoassay screens that are often designed to detect a class of drugs rather than a single drug.

Homogeneous Enzyme Immunoassays

- Homogeneous enzyme immunoassays require no separation step. They are based on the principle that enzyme activity changes as specific antigen-antibody binding occurs. When antibody binds to enzyme-labeled antigen, steric hindrance results in a loss of enzyme activity.
- Homogeneous immunoassays are used for the detection of low molecular weight analytes, such as hormones, therapeutic drugs, and drugs of abuse.
- The enzyme-multiplied immunoassay technique (EMIT) and the cloned enzyme donor immunoassay (CEDIA) are examples of homogeneous immunoassays.

Chemiluminescent Immunoassays

- Most immunometric assays are based on chemiluminescent label detection. Chemiluminescence (light emission) is produced by the oxidation of certain compounds, such as luminol, acridinium esters, and ruthenium derivatives.
- Chemiluminescent microparticle immunoassays (CMIA) use antibody-coated microparticles. Electrochemiluminescence immunoassays (ECLIA) measure the reaction at the surface of an electrode.

Fluorescent Immunoassays

- Fluorochromes are fluorescent compounds that absorb energy from an incident light source and convert that energy to light of a longer wavelength.
- Direct immunofluorescence assays involve antigen detection with a specific antibody that is labeled with a fluorescent tag. Fluorescence is detected with a fluorescent microscope that uses a high-intensity light source.
- In indirect immunofluorescent assays, the primary antibody is unlabeled. Incubation with antigen is followed by addition of a second fluorescent-labeled anti-immunoglobulin that detects antigen-antibody complexes.
- Multiplex immunoassays (MIAs) use polystyrene beads conjugated to different antigens as the solid phase. Patient serum is incubated with the beads, and antibodies to the corresponding antigens are detected with a fluorescent-tagged anti-human Ig reagent. MIA technology allows multiple antibodies or antigens to be detected simultaneously.

Rapid Immunoassays

- Rapid immunoassays use test devices that capture antigen or antibody from a patient sample as it migrates to a specific location on a membrane.
- These single-use disposable immunoassays are based on immunochromatography, easy to use, and provide results within minutes.
- Rapid immunoassays can be used in point-of-care settings, clinical laboratories, or home test kits to detect analytes such as hCG and drugs in urine and COVID-19 virus in nasopharyngeal swabs or saliva.

Study Guide: Labeled Immunoassays

TYPE OF IMMUNOASSAY	PRINCIPLE	RESULTS
Homogeneous enzyme immunoassay	No physical separation step of bound and labeled antigens is required. Patient antigen and labeled antigen react with reagent antibody in solution. Enzyme label is inactivated when reagent antigen binds to antibody.	Patient antigen concentration is directly proportional to the signal.
Heterogeneous	Requires solid-phase material to allow for antigen or antibody binding. Includes both competitive and noncompetitive immunoassay designs.	In a noncompetitive immunoassay, the concentration of patient antigen is directly proportional to the signal. In a competitive immunoassay, the patient antigen concentration is inversely proportional to the signal.
Competitive immunoassay for antigen	Patient antigen (Ag) competes with labeled antigen (Ag*) for limited antibody binding (Ab) sites. Final detected signal is Ag*Ab (labeled antigen bound to antibody), as shown in the reaction: $Ag + Ag^* + Ab \rightarrow Ag^*Ab + AgAb$	Inverse ratio: The more patient antigen present, the less label is detected.
Noncompetitive, indirect ELISA for antibody detection	Excess solid-phase antigen binds patient antibody, and a second labeled antibody (anti-human immunoglobulin) is added.	All patient antibody is allowed to bind. Amount of label is directly proportional to the amount of patient antibody present.
Capture or sandwich (immunometric)	Excess solid-phase antibody binds patient antigen, and a second labeled antibody (to the antigen) is added after a wash step.	All patient antigen is allowed to bind. Amount of label is directly proportional to the amount of patient antigen present.
Western blot (immunoblotting)	A complex mixture of antigens is electrophoresed on a gel and blotted onto a membrane. Unlabeled primary antibody binds to its corresponding antigen. After a wash step, secondary labeled antibody is added and binds to the primary antibody.	The label is visualized as bands that correspond to the detected antigens in the positions to which they have migrated, based on their size.
Isoelectric focusing (IEF)	Proteins are separated by electrophoresis in a pH gradient according to differences in their isoelectric point (pI). After electrophoresis, a detection antibody conjugated to an enzyme label can be added to visualize the bands.	Bands representing the antigens are visualized.
Enzyme-multiplied immunoassay technique (EMIT)	Reagent antigen is bound to an enzyme tag. Change in enzyme activity is observed as specific antigen-antibody interaction occurs in solution. If reagent antibody binds to the enzyme-antigen pair, enzyme activity is blocked. Otherwise, enzyme is active. Active enzyme (commonly glucose-6-phosphate dehydrogenase) catalyzes the reduction of NAD^+ to NADH, leading to increased absorbance in the UV-wavelength region.	All patient antigen is allowed to bind. Amount of signal generated is directly proportional to the amount of patient antigen present.
Direct immunofluorescence	Patient sample (e.g., tissue) is attached to a slide. Specific fluorescent-labeled antibody is added. In cell-based immunoassays, patient cells are incubated with fluorescent-labeled antibody to a cell surface antigen.	If fluorescence is detected, patient sample is positive for the antigen. Fluorescence on cell surface indicates that the cell is positive for the antigen.

Indirect immunofluorescence	To detect patient antibody, reagent antigen is attached to a slide and incubated with the patient sample. A second fluorescent-labeled antibody (anti-human immunoglobulin) is added. To detect antigen, patient sample is fixed to a slide and incubated with antibody to the antigen (primary antibody), followed by labeled secondary antibody, directed against the primary antibody.	If fluorescence is detected, antibody or antigen is present in the sample, and the test is positive.
Rapid immunochromatographic assays	Patient sample migrates through a test membrane to interact with its corresponding antibody or antigen. When detecting patient antigen, the antigen in the sample complexes to antibody-labeled particles or competes with antigen-labeled particles across individual test lanes at unique detection zones. When detecting patient antibody, antibody in the sample binds to antigen on the test membrane and is detected with a labeled reagent.	Presence of a test line may indicate either positive or negative result, depending on manufacturer design.

CASE STUDIES

1. A 60-year-old adult presented to a primary care physician with fatigue, loss of appetite, weight loss, and abdominal pain. The urine was dark in color. The physician suspected the patient may have pancreatic cancer based on family history of the disease. Ultrasonography of the abdominal region identified a large mass, which appeared localized to the pancreas. A computed tomography (CT) scan confirmed the presence of a mass and supported a diagnosis of pancreatic cancer. Before initiating chemotherapy and radiation therapy treatments, the physician ordered a serum CA 19-9 tumor marker immunoassay to establish a baseline value, then reordered the test at the patient's follow-up visit 3 months later. The baseline sample was sent to a hospital laboratory that uses an Instrument from Manufacturer "A." The test result at the patient's 3-month office visit was sent to the regional testing laboratory, which uses an Instrument from Manufacturer "B."

Questions

a. Based on the patient's baseline test value, what technical concern should the laboratorian have upon seeing the most recent test result (at 3 months' post-treatment)?

b. What procedure could the laboratorian perform to verify that the test result is correct?

c. What is the disadvantage of monitoring a patient's tumor marker immunoassay test result when immunoassays developed by different manufacturers are used?

d. If the need to send the patient's blood sample to another clinical laboratory using a different immunoassay instrument could not be avoided, what is the best course of action to interpret the test result?

Test results are included in the table that follows.

CA 19-9 Test Result	Testing Notes	Reference Interval Cutoff	Date of Result	Instrument Used
1,250 U/mL	Final result reported after sample dilution	Less than 38 U/mL	Just before initiation of treatment regimen	"A"
110 U/mL	Undiluted sample result	Less than 55 U/mL	3 months after treatment was initiated	"B"
950 U/mL	Instrument result of 95 U/mL after 1:10 dilution of sample	Less than 55 U/mL	3 months after treatment was initiated	"B"

REVIEW QUESTIONS

1. Which statement accurately describes heterogeneous competitive binding immunoassays?
   a. Excess binding sites for the analyte are provided.
   b. Test signal is generated in solution without the need of a solid-phase support material.
   c. The concentration of patient analyte is inversely proportional to bound label.
   d. All the patient analyte is bound in the reaction.

2. How do heterogeneous immunoassays differ from homogeneous immunoassays?
   a. Heterogeneous immunoassays require a separation step.
   b. Heterogeneous immunoassays require less technical skill to perform than homogeneous immunoassays.
   c. For noncompetitive immunoassays, the concentration of patient analyte is indirectly proportional to bound label in heterogeneous immunoassays.
   d. Homogeneous immunoassays have better analytical sensitivity compared with heterogeneous immunoassays.

3. Which of the following responses characterizes a capture or sandwich enzyme immunoassay?
   a. Less analytically sensitive than competitive enzyme immunoassays
   b. Labeled antigen attached to a solid phase
   c. Best for small antigens with a single epitope determinant
   d. Excess number of antibody sites on solid-phase material

4. What advantage do enzyme immunoassays have over radioimmunoassays?
   a. Decrease in hazardous waste
   b. Shorter shelf life of kit reagents
   c. No interference by biological inhibitors
   d. Must be read manually

5. Which of the following is characteristic of direct fluorescence immunoassays?
   a. The anti-immunoglobulin has the fluorescent tag.
   b. Antibody is attached to a solid phase.
   c. This method can be used for identification of cellular antigens.
   d. The amount of color is inversely proportional to the amount of antigen present.

6. Which of the following is true of the enzyme-multiplied immunoassay technique (EMIT)?
   a. It is classified as a heterogeneous method.
   b. Nicotinamide adenine dinucleotide (NAD^+) is a substrate used in the test reaction.
   c. When the patient sample antigen concentration is high, the final test signal will be low.
   d. Patient sample antigen blocks the enzyme active site in the test reaction.

7. A fluorescent substance is best described as one in which:
   a. Light energy is absorbed and converted to a longer wavelength.
   b. The emitted wavelength can be seen under normal white light.
   c. There is a long time between the absorption and emission of light.
   d. It spontaneously decays and emits light.

8. In a noncompetitive ELISA, if a negative control shows the presence of signal, which of the following might be a possible explanation?
   a. No reagent was added.
   b. Washing steps were incomplete.
   c. The enzyme was inactivated.
   d. No substrate was present.

9. Which of the following best characterizes chemiluminescent immunoassays?
   a. Only the antigen can be labeled.
   b. Tests can be read manually.
   c. These are only homogeneous immunoassays.
   d. A chemical is oxidized to produce light.

10. Immunofluorescence assays may be difficult to interpret for which reason?
    a. Autofluorescence of substances in serum
    b. Nonspecific binding to serum proteins
    c. Subjectivity in reading results
    d. Any of the above

11. Which statement best describes rapid immunochromatographic assays?
    a. Test results are always reported as quantitative values.
    b. They are designed primarily for point-of-care testing.
    c. Urine is the only acceptable sample type.
    d. Formation of a colored line always indicates a positive result.

12. Which of the following is characteristic of an indirect enzyme immunoassay?
    a. The primary antibody has the enzyme label.
    b. Only one antibody is required.
    c. Color is directly proportional to the amount of patient antibody present.
    d. Enzyme specificity is not needed.

13. In an indirect ELISA, what would be the outcome of an improper wash after the antibody-enzyme conjugate is added?
    a. Results will be falsely decreased.
    b. Results will be falsely increased.
    c. Results will be unaffected.
    d. No wash step is required in the ELISA procedure.

14. In a heterogeneous enzyme immunoassay, if the patient sample produces more signal than the highest positive control, what action should be taken?
    a. Report the results as determined.
    b. Dilute the patient sample.
    c. Repeat the immunoassay using one-half the volume of the patient sample.
    d. Report the results as falsely positive.

15. Which of the following can uniquely cause interferences in immunoassays designed with streptavidin bound to the solid-phase surface?
    a. Elevated concentration of biotin in the patient test sample can cause falsely increased results.
    b. Heterophile antibodies present in the patient sample cause falsely decreased results.
    c. Antibody excess in the patient sample leads to a hook effect.
    d. Solid-phase particles will dissolve easily if the reaction temperature is increased.

16. Which type of assay is best suited for quantitation of therapeutic drug levels?
    a. Direct immunofluorescence assay
    b. Indirect ELISA
    c. Homogeneous enzyme immunoassay
    d. Rapid immunoassay

Chapter 11 Answer Key

Answers to Knowledge Checks

11.1 a 11.2 b 11.3 d 11.4 c 11.5 d

Answers to Review Questions

1. c 2. a 3. d 4. a 5. c 6. b 7. a
8. b 9. d 10. d 11. b 12. c 13. b 14. b
15. a 16. c

12 Molecular Diagnostic Techniques

Lela Buckingham, PhD, MB (ASCP), DLM (ASCP)

LEARNING OUTCOMES

After finishing this chapter, you should be able to:

12.1 Describe the structure of deoxyribonucleic acid (DNA) and ribonucleic acid (RNA).

12.2 Identify complementary nucleic acid sequences.

12.3 Describe nucleic acid isolation by solid-phase and in-solution methods and explain how the quality and quantity of the isolated DNA or RNA are analyzed.

12.4 Define hybridization.

12.5 Interpret results from gel or capillary electrophoresis.

12.6 Indicate the use of restriction enzymes for DNA analysis.

12.7 Describe the principle of CRISPR-Cas.

12.8 Describe array hybridization analysis.

12.9 Discuss the principles of the polymerase chain reaction (PCR).

12.10 Describe methods by which products of PCR, qPCR, and dPCR are analyzed.

12.11 Distinguish absolute and relative template quantity by dPCR and qPCR.

12.12 Discuss isothermal DNA and RNA amplification methods.

12.13 Describe chain termination and pyrosequencing technologies.

12.14 Characterize next-generation sequencing libraries.

12.15 Describe next-generation sequencing technologies.

12.16 Define *coverage*, *filtering*, and *annotation* in sequence analysis.

CHAPTER OUTLINE

You can go to **fadavis.com** keyword stevens for the laboratory exercises that accompany this text.

Nucleic acids carry genetic information for protein structure. Primary characteristics of nucleic acids, such as nucleic acid complementarity and melting temperature, form the basis of specificity for almost all nucleic-acid–based tests, as we discuss in this chapter. Methods of analysis are under continual development among laboratories, with gel and capillary electrophoresis, spectrophotometry, and fluorescence methods in common use. Molecular diagnostics make important contributions to therapeutic decisions, transplant selection, drug efficacy, forensics, genetics, infectious diseases, and disease prognosis.

Deoxyribonucleic Acid (DNA) and Ribonucleic Acid (RNA)

Deoxyribonucleic acid (DNA) and **ribonucleic acid (RNA)** are macromolecules composed of nucleotides. A **nucleotide** is a phosphorylated ribose sugar carrying a nitrogen base. In the absence of a phosphate group, the structure is called a **nucleoside.** The five nitrogen bases that make up most nucleic acids found in nature are adenine (A), cytosine (C), guanine (G), thymine (T; found in DNA), and uracil (U). Uracil is found only in RNA and has a structure similar to thymine except that it lacks the methyl group (CH3) bound to the 5′ carbon. A and G have a double-ring structure and are classified as *purines;* whereas C, T, and U, which have a single ring, are *pyrimidines* **(Fig. 12-1).**

Positions in the deoxyribose and nitrogen base rings are numbered as shown in **Figure 12–2.** In DNA, the nitrogen base of a nucleotide, either G, A, C, or T, is attached to the 1′ carbon of the deoxyribose sugar. The 3′ carbon of the sugar carries a hydroxyl group (OH), and the 5′ carbon is mono-, di-, or tri-phosphorylated.

In contrast to the deoxyribose sugar in DNA, nitrogen bases are attached to a ribose sugar in ribonucleic acid (RNA). Also, RNA has uracil nucleotides instead of thymine. While deoxyribonucleotides are hydroxylated on the 3′ carbon, the phosphorylated ribose sugar in RNA carries hydroxyl groups on carbons 2′ and 3′ **(Fig. 12–3).**

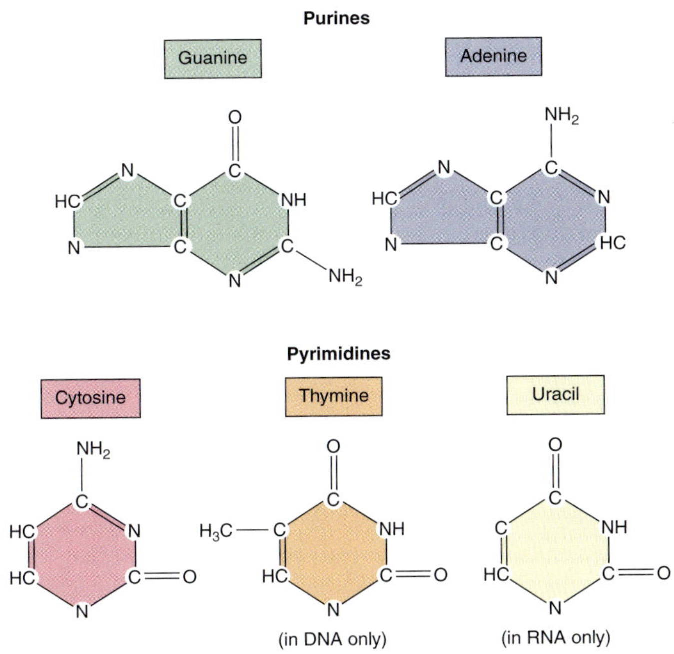

FIGURE 12–1 The nitrogen bases found in nucleic acids are adenine (A), cytosine (C), guanine (G), thymine (T; only in DNA), and Uracil (U; only in RNA). A and G have a double-ring structure and are classified as *purines;* whereas C, T, and U, which have a single ring, are *pyrimidines*.

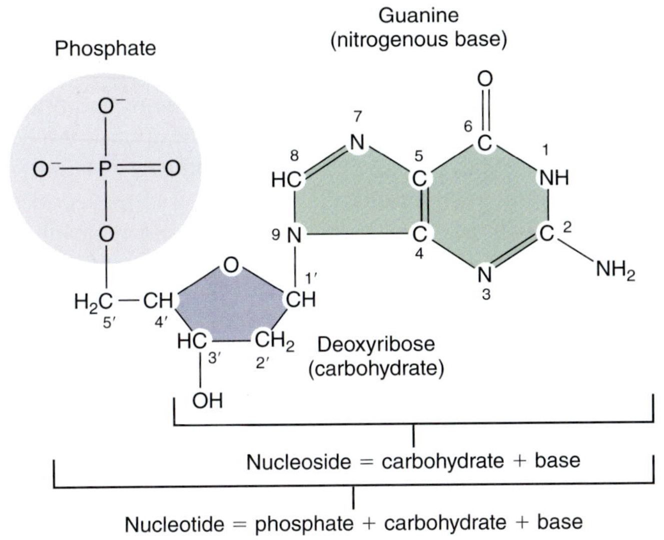

FIGURE 12–2 Nucleoside and nucleotide structure. A nucleoside is an unphosphorylated (deoxy) ribose sugar carrying a nitrogen base, whereas a nucleotide is composed of a (deoxy) ribose sugar bound to a nitrogen base and a phosphate group. Nitrogen base ring positions are numbered ordinally, and the ribose ring positions are numbered with prime numbers.

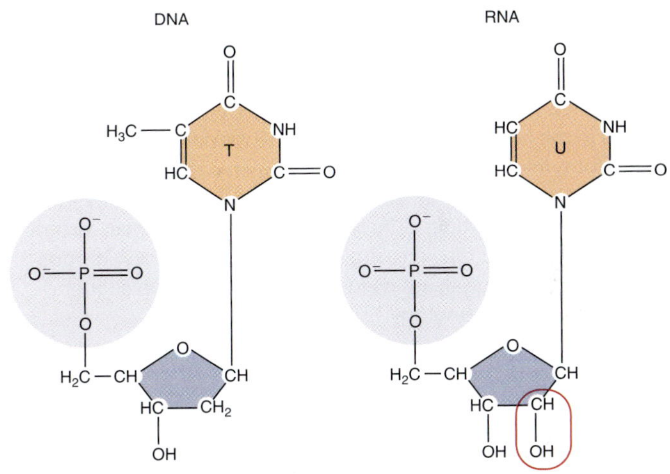

FIGURE 12–3 The ribose sugar in RNA is hydroxylated on the 2′ and 3′ carbons (right), whereas in DNA, it is only hydroxylated at the 3′ carbon (left). The nitrogen base uracil, found in RNA (right), is similar to thymine found in DNA (left).

Modified Nucleotides

Natural modifications of the nucleotide structure include methylation, deamination, additions, substitutions, and other chemical modifications. These natural modifications may be enzymatically catalyzed in the cell or products of spontaneous reactions. Such modifications can result in nucleotides with new properties. For example, addition and removal of methyl groups (CH_3) to cytosines in DNA affect gene function. Deamination, or removal of NH_2 groups, can result in double-stranded DNA breaks.

Nucleotide base modifications are also caused by environmental insults such as chemicals or radiation. These changes can lead to undesirable effects such as dysregulated cell proliferation, seen in cancer.

Gram-negative bacteria use modified nucleotides in a type of immune system, the restriction modification (rm) system. The bacterium adds methyl groups to its own DNA to distinguish it from that of invaders, such as bacterial viruses. Recognizing its own DNA in this way, the bacterium can target the invader's DNA for enzymatic degradation. Bacteria can also copy invading nucleic acid sequences for degradation by the Cas9 enzyme in another type of defense called *clustered regularly interspaced short palindromic repeats* or *CRISPR-Cas9*.

Clinical Correlations

Modified Nucleotides

Modified nucleotides and nucleosides are used in the clinic and in the laboratory. For example, the modified nucleosides azidothymidine and acyclovir are antiviral agents that have been used against HIV and herpes viruses, respectively. The modified nucleotide, 5-fluorouracil, is an anticancer drug. Dideoxynucleotides, missing the 2′ and 3′ hydroxyl groups on the ribose sugar, are used in chain termination sequencing and array technology.

The Nucleic Acid Polymer

Nucleotides are joined together to create a nucleic acid polymer. This occurs through the formation of *phosphodiester bonds*, which are made by attaching the 3′ hydroxyl group on the sugar molecule of each nucleotide to the 5′ phosphate group on an adjacent nucleotide. A chain of ribonucleotides or deoxyribonucleotides makes up one strand of RNA or DNA, respectively **(Fig. 12-4A)**.

While most (but not all) RNA exists without a partner strand (single-stranded), DNA is mostly double-stranded. The two DNA chains are held together by hydrogen bonds between their nucleotide bases, which are found in the center of the molecule **(Fig. 12-4B)**. The sugar-phosphate groups are on the outer sides of the molecule, forming its backbone. The hydroxyl groups on the 3′ carbons of deoxyribose and the phosphate groups on the 5′ carbons give DNA strands *polarity:* that is, a 5′ phosphate end and a 3′ hydroxyl end. By convention, sequences are ordered in the 5′ to 3′ direction. The two strands are connected in an *antiparallel* arrangement, with the 5′ phosphates of the two strands at opposite ends of the molecule. In its three-dimensional form, the two DNA chains are wrapped around each other to form a double helix, with alternating sugar and phosphate groups on the outside of the structure **(Fig. 12-4C)**.

There is a **complementary** relationship between the bases in the two strands of the DNA double helix, meaning that only certain bases can bond with each other. In DNA, cytosines (Cs) can only pair with guanines (Gs) in the partner strand and do so through three hydrogen bonds. Adenines (As) can only pair with thymines (Ts), attaching through two hydrogen bonds. Thus, by knowing the nucleotide sequence of the original strand, you can deduce the nucleotide sequence on the partner strand **(Fig. 12-5)**.

Two bases paired together in this way are called a base pair (bp). The length of a double-stranded DNA macromolecule is measured in bp. The length of a single strand of RNA (or DNA) is measured in bases (b). Metric prefixes are used to describe long strands of DNA or RNA, for example, one thousand bp or b compose a ***kilobase pair*** (kbp) or ***kilobase*** (kb), respectively. One million bp or b constitute a ***megabase pair*** (Mbp) or ***megabase*** (Mb), respectively.

Most microorganisms contain one double helix in circular or linear form, which is a few Mbp in size. Viruses may carry a double- or single-stranded DNA or RNA molecule of a few to 100 kb in size. In plants and animals, DNA is separated into multiple chromosomes per cell. Each chromosome is a double helix of DNA that can be hundreds of Mbp long.

In humans, there are 46 chromosomes contained in the cell nucleus, two copies of each of the 22 autosomes (non–sex chromosomes 1 to 22) and two copies of the X chromosome in females (designated 46, XX) or one copy each of the X and Y chromosome in males (designated 46, XY). The autosomes are numbered according to size from the largest (chromosome 1; 246 Mbp), to the smallest (chromosome 22; 47 Mbp). The X chromosome, 154 Mbp, is much larger than the Y chromosome (57 Mbp).

Genes are regions in chromosomes that carry nucleotide sequence information for either protein or noncoding RNA. Humans have less than 30,000 protein coding genes carried on the 23 chromosomes, with two copies of each chromosome per somatic cell. In diploid animals, sperm and egg cells contain half the number of chromosomes. In addition to the nuclear chromosomes, mitochondria, energy-producing organelles located in the cytoplasm of eukaryotic cells, carry their own genome. The mitochondrial genome is circular, containing about 16,500 bp in human cells. Bacterial and animal cells may also carry extra-chromosomal DNA in the form of small, usually circular plasmids, several thousands of bp in size.

With the development of array and sequencing technology, it is possible to investigate the entirety of DNA in the cell **(genome)** or a population of microorganisms in a host **(microbiome)**. In contrast to testing one gene at a time, these *-omic* studies are designed to analyze whole microbial populations, multiple genes, gene regions, or all the genes in the genome to assess the status of an organism or population of organisms.

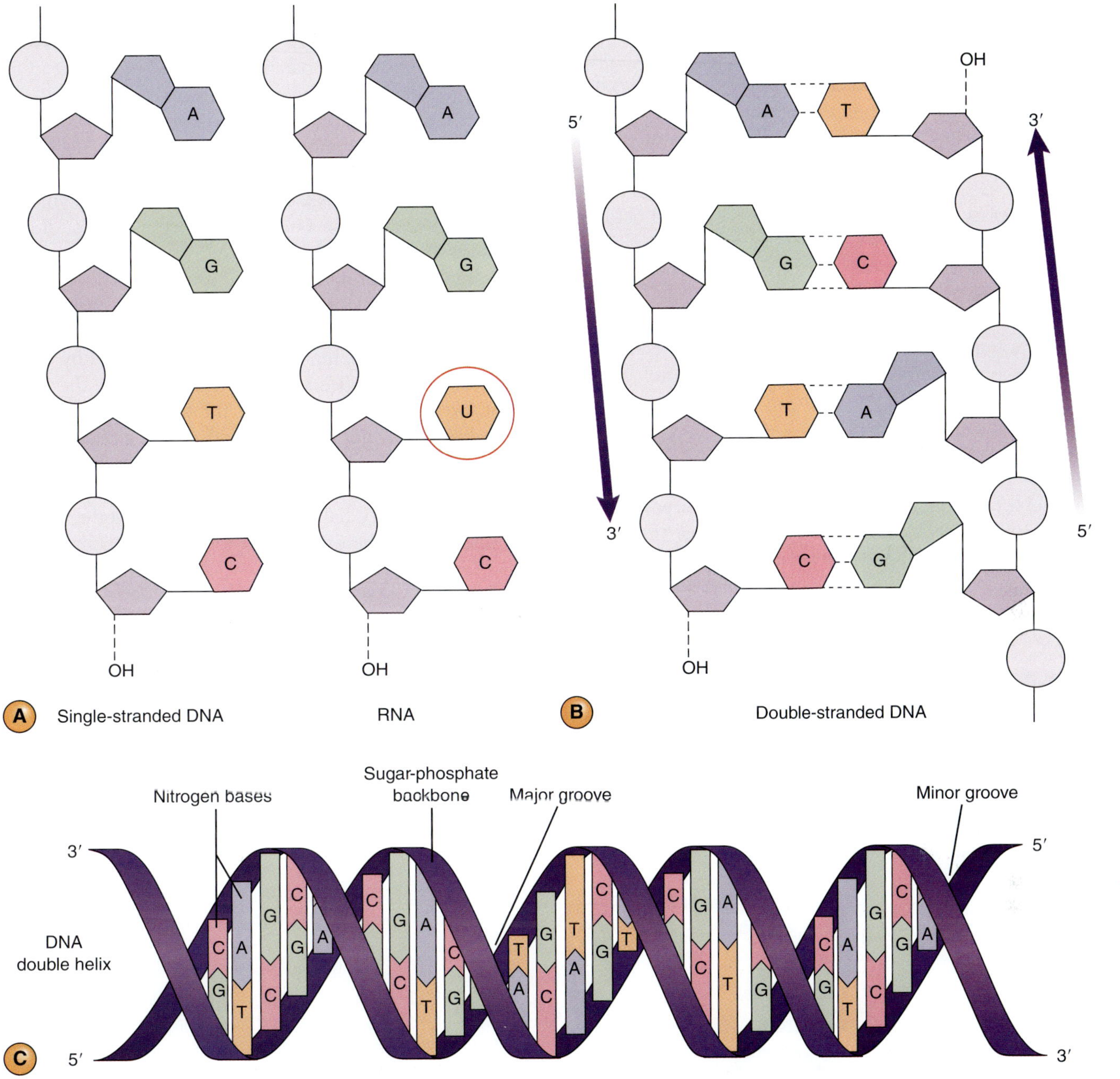

FIGURE 12–4 (A) Nucleic acids are composed of a sequence of covalently attached nucleotides. The sugar-phosphate groups of adjacent nucleotides form the backbone of the molecule. RNA is single stranded and has uracil rather than thymine. (B) DNA is usually double stranded, consisting of two antiparallel chains. The base pairs are in the center of the two strands, which are held together by hydrogen bonds (indicated by dotted lines). The two strands are complementary, since the A's in one strand always pair with T's on the opposite strand, and C's always pair with G's. (C) The DNA double helix. The major and minor grooves of the helix are sites that interact with proteins, dyes, or other DNA binding molecules.

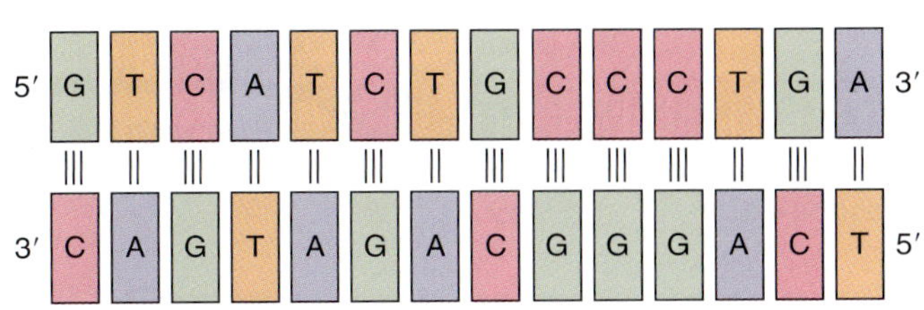

FIGURE 12–5 The order of nucleotides of a single nucleic acid strand can be deduced from its complementary strand. Complementary strands of DNA are also anti-parallel so that the 5′ ends of the molecules are on opposite ends of the double-stranded DNA. A:T base pairs are held together by two hydrogen bonds (vertical lines), and G:C base pairs are held together by three hydrogen bonds.

DNA Replication

In bacteria, the single circular chromosome is attached to the cell membrane and replicated prior to binary fission. Plasmids and viruses replicate by continuously using host cell machinery. The division cycle in eukaryotic cells has four phases: G1 (gap 1), S (DNA synthesis), G2 (gap 2), and M (mitosis) **(Fig. 12–6).** DNA replication takes place during the S phase, so that the DNA complement of the cell is doubled before it enters the G2 phase. One set of chromosomes will be divided into each of two daughter cells during mitosis. Each daughter cell will then be in the G1 phase. Movement of the cell cycle from G1 to S is strictly regulated, as is movement from G2 to M. Checkpoints allow the cell to repair damaged DNA before proceeding to replication and mitosis. Loss of control at these "checkpoints" can result in uncontrolled cell division or damaged DNA as is seen in cancer.

Replication of DNA is semiconservative; that is, the two strands of the DNA duplex are separated, and each single strand serves as a template for a newly synthesized complementary strand. DNA replication proceeds with the formation of phosphodiester bonds between the 5′ phosphate of an incoming nucleotide with the 3′ hydroxyl of the previously added nucleotide **(Fig. 12-7).** This reaction is catalyzed by DNA polymerases. The parental template strand is read from the 3′ to 5′ direction, while synthesis proceeds 5′ to 3′, making the completely replicated strands antiparallel.

DNA synthesis cannot begin without a preexisting 3′ hydroxyl group. To begin synthesis in vivo, a primer of RNA is synthesized by an RNA polymerase (primase) enzyme. This aspect of DNA synthesis is useful in the laboratory for directing synthesis to a specific place in DNA. Synthetic single-stranded DNA fragments (primers) are used routinely to direct copying of specific regions of DNA by the polymerase chain reaction (PCR) and other nucleic acid amplification methods.

DNA undergoing replication can be observed by electron microscopy as a ***replication fork***. This is because the requirement for DNA synthesis to read the template strand in a 3′ to 5′ direction is not consistent with copying of both strands simultaneously in the same direction. To accommodate this arrangement, one strand is copied discontinuously away from the replication fork (lagging strand) while the other is copied continuously in the direction of replication (leading strand).

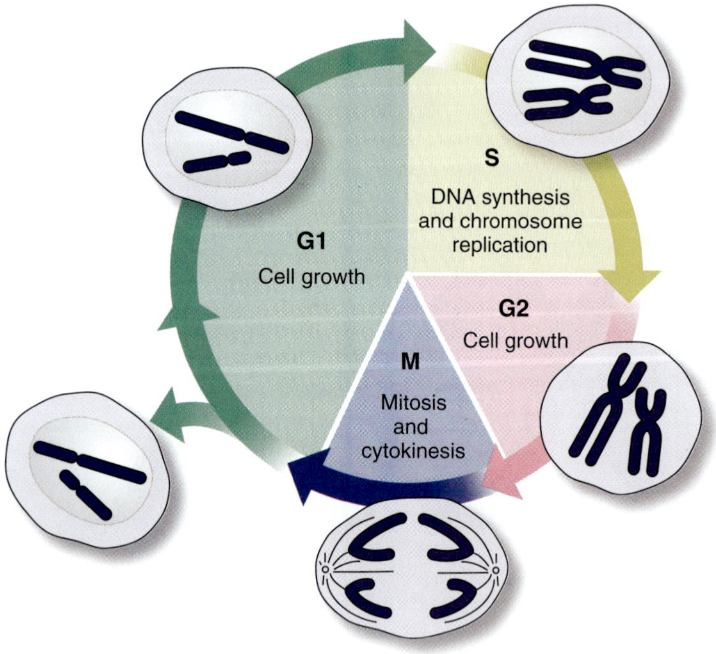

FIGURE 12–6 The cell cycle consists of four phases: G1, S, G2, and M. G1 and G2 are stages that prepare the cell to divide. DNA replication takes place during the S phase of the cell cycle in diploid organisms. In mitosis (M), the cell divides, and one chromosome set moves to each daughter cell. Mitosis has four main stages: prophase, metaphase, anaphase, and telophase. Before and after mitosis, cells are said to be in interphase.

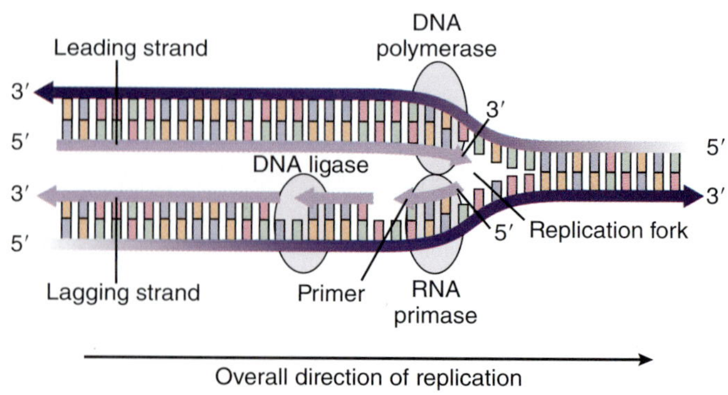

FIGURE 12–7 DNA is replicated in a semiconservative manner where each parent strand serves as a template or guide for addition of nucleotides to its newly synthesized complementary strand. DNA polymerase forms a phosphodiester bond between the 3′ hydroxyl group of the previously added nucleotide to the 5′ phosphate of the incoming nucleotide, releasing two phosphate molecules. To maintain the 5′ to 3′ direction, synthesis proceeds in a continuous manner on the leading strand and discontinuously on the lagging strand, forming a replication fork.

The short strands made on the lagging strand are then bound together with the help of the DNA ligase enzyme.

Knowledge Check 12-1

This component of the nucleotide ribose sugar is required for formation of a phosphodiester bond by DNA polymerase.

a. 1′ NH_2
b. 2′ OH
c. 3′ OH
d. 4′ H

RNA Types and Synthesis

Several types of RNA are found in cells. About 80% to 90% of the total RNA is **ribosomal RNA (rRNA)**, an important component of the ribosomes, organelles where protein synthesis takes place. A second type is **messenger RNA (mRNA)**, a complementary copy of DNA that carries the genetic information for the amino acid sequence of a protein. The process by which the genetic code in DNA is converted to mRNA is called **transcription (Fig. 12-8).** Small **transfer RNA (tRNA)** molecules carry the amino acids specified by mRNA to the ribosome during protein synthesis. Other types of RNA, including microRNA and long noncoding RNA, are involved in regulating protein synthesis.

RNA synthesis proceeds in a manner that is chemically similar to that of DNA synthesis, with some exceptions. RNA synthesis is catalyzed by RNA polymerase, which begins the process by binding to its recognition start site in DNA (called a *promoter*). Unlike DNA synthesis, RNA synthesis can start de novo (from the beginning) without a primer. RNA synthesis is catalyzed by RNA polymerases, which are more error prone and slower (50 to 100 bases/sec) than DNA polymerases (1,000 bases/sec). There are more start sites in the genome for RNA polymerization than for DNA synthesis. The bulk of DNA synthesis occurs in the S phase of the cell cycle, while RNA synthesis occurs throughout the cell cycle and varies depending on the cell's requirements.

RNA is copied from almost all of the genome; however, only about 2% of the RNA-encoding regions produce messenger RNA that is translated into protein. These coding sequences, also called open reading frames, are continuous in prokaryotes. In eukaryotes, the protein coding sequences **(exons)** are interrupted by noncoding sequences **(introns).** The initial copy of DNA into RNA (heteronuclear RNA, hnRNA) contains introns. The introns are removed or spliced out of the hnRNA to make mRNA. Some genes do not code for proteins but code for tRNA and rRNA. Large portions of the genome are occupied by retrotransposons, DNA elements that can move from one location to another through an RNA intermediate.

Noncoding RNA, along with methylated nucleotides and modified histone proteins associated with DNA, are components of **epigenetic** mechanisms. In contrast to genetics, which is based on the order or sequence of nucleotides, these mechanisms can affect *phenotype* (an observable trait in an individual) independent of the nucleotide sequence in the DNA.

Protein Synthesis

After DNA is transcribed by RNA polymerase into mRNA, the transcripts are converted into amino acid sequences by a process called **translation.** RNA to be translated into protein is marked by a guanidine nucleotide, covalently attached to its 5′ end in an unusual 5′-5′ bond (cap), and 2 to 20 adenines at the 3′ end (polyadenylation). These structures maintain the stability of the mRNA and allow it to be recognized by ribosomes in the cell cytoplasm. Prokaryotic and eukaryotic ribosomes are composed of ribosomal proteins and rRNA. Ribosomes assemble on the mRNA for protein synthesis.

The language held in the sequence of the four nucleotides in the DNA chains must be translated into the order or sequence of the 20 amino acids making up a protein chain. The nucleotide sequence of mRNA contains the genetic code in a 3-base recognition sequence, or **codon**, for each of the 20 amino acids **(Table 12–1).** The codons are carried from the nucleus to the cytoplasm in mRNA to be translated into protein.

tRNA serves as an adaptor molecule between the nucleotide sequence in mRNA and the amino acid sequence in proteins. There are distinct tRNAs for each of the 20 amino acids. Distinct aminoacyl-tRNA synthetase enzymes covalently attach amino acids with their specific tRNA. Each tRNA, folded into a structure that resembles the Greek letter Γ, carries an amino acid at the 3′ end and a three-base sequence, or ***anti-codon,***

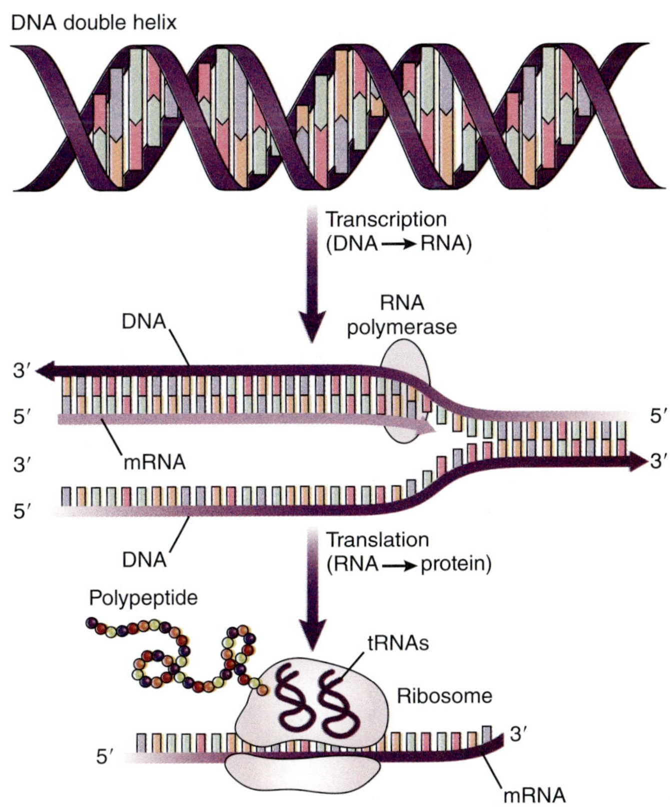

FIGURE 12–8 mRNA is transcribed from DNA using RNA polymerase. The mRNA delivers the information to ribosomes, where protein synthesis takes place. As each amino acid is added, the peptide chain continues to grow. This process, known as ***translation,*** is accomplished with the help of tRNAs, which carry individual amino acids to the site.

which is complementary to the codon of that amino acid. The anti-codon hydrogen bonds to the complementary codon on mRNA within the ribosome, holding the amino acid in place to be covalently attached to the growing peptide by peptidyl transferase activity in the ribosome (Fig. 12–8).

The tRNA covalently attached to its amino acid (charged tRNA) assembles with the ribosome subunit and mRNA to initiate protein synthesis. Synthesis proceeds as the ribosome moves in three-base steps along the mRNA as each charged tRNA binds. Synthesis terminates when the ribosome encounters a three-base *stop codon* in the mRNA (see Table 12–1). Multiple initiation, elongation, and termination factors participate in this process. Newly synthesized proteins are directed through the endoplasmic reticulum of the cell to their final destination.

Mutations and Variants

A **mutation** or **variant** is a change in the nucleotide sequence in DNA. Depending on its frequency of occurrence, a nucleotide sequence change may also be referred to as a *polymorphism*. The term "variant" is recommended for nucleotide sequence changes that are inherited (germline), while "mutation" is a more general term for spontaneous or environmentally caused changes in DNA that are not inherited (somatic). These alterations may range in size from single base pairs up to millions of base pairs, as seen in chromosomal structural abnormalities. Point mutations that involve one or a few base pairs result in a change in the corresponding mRNA codon and are classified by their effect on the amino acid sequence **(Table 12–2).** Conservative and silent mutations are changes that do not directly affect phenotype, while nonconservative, nonsense, and frameshift mutations will likely affect protein structure and/or function, depending on their location in the protein sequence. Alterations early in the gene sequence will likely have a greater effect on protein function than mutations that occur toward the end of the protein coding sequence.

There is a recommended nomenclature for naming nucleotide changes in clinical reports. In nucleic acid, mutations are indicated by the location of the change in the nucleotide sequence, the original nucleotide, followed by an arrow, and then the replacement nucleotide. For example, a mutation that replaces a guanidine with an adenosine nucleotide at position 2,175 in the gene sequence would be expressed as:

Table 12-1 mRNA Codons for the 20 Amino Acids[a]

AMINO ACID	ABBREVIATION	SINGLE-LETTER CODE	CODONS
Alanine	Ala	A	GCU, GCG, GCC, GCA
Arginine	Arg	R	AGA, AGG, CGA, CGC, CGG, CGU
Asparagine	Asn	N	AAC, AAU
Aspartic acid	Asp	D	GAU, GAC
Cysteine	Cys	C	UGU, UGC
Glutamine	Gln	Q	CAA, CAG
Glutamic acid	Glu	E	GAA, GAG
Glycine	Gly	G	GGU, GGA, GGC, GGG
Histidine	His	H	CAU, CAC
Isoleucine	Ile	I	AUU, AUC, AUA
Leucine	Leu	L	UUA, UUG, CUA, CUC, CUG, CUU
Lysine	Lys	K	AAA, AAG
Methionine	Met	M	AUG
Phenylalanine	Phe	F	UUU, UUC
Proline	Pro	P	CCU, CCA, CCC, CCG
Serine	Ser	S	AGU, AGC, UCU, UCC, UCA, UCG
Threonine	Thr	T	ACU, ACA, ACG, ACC
Tryptophan	Trp	W	UGG
Tyrosine	Tyr	Y	UAU, UAC
Valine	Val	V	GUU, GUA, GUC, GUG
Stop codons		X	UAA, UAG, UGA

[a] *The genetic code connects the four-base nucleotide sequence to the 20 amino acids. Each amino acid has at least one associated three-base sequence (codon) carried in messenger RNA. Stop codons direct mRNA synthesis to stop.*

Table 12-2 DNA Changes Affect Codons and Amino Acid Sequences

TYPE	EXAMPLE CODON (mRNA) CHANGE	EXAMPLE AMINO ACID CHANGE
Conservative substitution	AUC→CUC	Isoleucine → Leucine
Nonconservative substitution	CAU → CCU	Histidine → Proline
Silent	UAU → UAC	Tyrosine → Tyrosine
Nonsense	CAA → UAA	Glutamine → Stop
Frameshift	UGU AAC CAG → UGU AAA CCA G . . .	Cys Asn Gln → Cys Lys Pro . . .

2175G→A. The term may be preceded by further notations (g., c., r.) to indicate whether the alteration is in genomic DNA, complementary DNA derived from an RNA sequence, or RNA, respectively. In large databases, the original nucleotide followed by the location and the substituted nucleotide may be used with the prefix (e.g., c.G2175A).

Changes in the amino acid sequence are indicated by the original amino acid, followed by the location in the protein, and then, the substituted amino acid. For example, a replacement of a glycine with a valine at the 339th amino acid in a protein would be expressed as G339V, or p.G339V, using the single-letter code for the amino acid (Table 12–1). These expressions are designed to avoid confusion when referring to amino acid or nucleotide changes, since the letters A, C, G, and T are also used in the single-letter amino acid codes. The nomenclature for DNA, RNA, and protein sequence variants has been globally standardized by the Human Genome Variation Society (HGVS), under the auspices of the Human Genome Organization (HUGO).

Knowledge Check 12-2

Which alteration in an mRNA codon will result in premature termination of a protein?

a. UUC → UUA
b. UAU → UUU
c. UGU → AGU
d. UUG → UAG

Polymorphisms

Structurally, mutations, variants, and polymorphisms are the same thing, changes from a reference amino acid or nucleotide sequence. Alterations in DNA and/or protein sequences shared by at least 2% of a population are **polymorphisms.** The different versions of the affected sequences are referred to as **alleles.** Polymorphisms can involve a single base pair (referred to as **single nucleotide polymorphisms [SNPs]**) or millions of base pairs (structural variants). Inherited SNPs may be referred to as **single nucleotide variants (SNVs).**

Polymorphic changes may or may not have phenotypic effects. Deleterious phenotypic changes are usually limited so that they do not reach the required frequency in a population; however, there are balanced polymorphisms that are maintained by an association with a beneficial phenotypic effect. A well-known balanced polymorphism in humans is the A to T base substitution in the β-globin gene on chromosome 11 that causes sickle cell anemia. This DNA substitution results in the replacement of glutamic acid (E) with valine (V) at position 6 in the protein sequence (E6V). The mutation results in abnormal red blood cells (RBCs) that do not circulate efficiently. The deleterious effect is balanced by a beneficial phenotype of resistance to *Plasmodium* species that cause malaria. This DNA alteration is maintained in human populations due to this beneficial selective effect.

A highly polymorphic region in the human genome is the major histocompatibility complex (MHC) locus on chromosome 6. The different nucleotide sequences result in multiple versions or alleles of the human leukocyte antigen (HLA) genes in the human population (see Chapter 16). These alleles differ by nucleotide sequence at the DNA level and by amino acid sequence. Every person has a particular set of HLA alleles that are inherited from their parents. "Nonself" proteins are identified by the differences in the HLA alleles.

Other highly polymorphic areas of the genome include the genes coding for the antibody proteins and antigen receptor proteins in B cells and T cells, respectively (see Chapters 3 and 5). These polymorphisms are not in the germline (inherited from parents) as are those in the MHC locus. They are introduced in each cell through gene rearrangements followed by enzymatically catalyzed sequence changes called *somatic hypermutations.* Thus, these sequences differ from cell to cell, allowing for the generation of a large repertoire of antibodies and antigen receptors to better match any foreign antigen.

Polymorphisms are found all over the genome. SNPs occur every thousand bp in the human genome. Larger polymorphic differences are found less frequently in the genome. Individual polymorphic differences in humans are the basis for familial ancestry testing.

Polymorphisms can create, destroy, or otherwise affect DNA sequences that are naturally recognized and degraded by nuclease enzymes isolated from bacteria. These changes are detected in the laboratory as **restriction fragment length polymorphisms (RFLPs)** when the DNA is cut into specific sizes by restriction enzymes. Repeat sequence polymorphisms, such as *short tandem repeats (STRs)* and *variable number tandem repeats (VNTRs),* are consecutive nucleotide repeats consisting of a single bp to over 100 bp repeat units. STRs and VNTRs can be detected as RFLPs or by using amplification procedures. STR analysis is used for human identification (DNA fingerprinting) and for parentage testing. STR and VNTR are also commonly used markers for engraftment monitoring after allogeneic bone marrow transplantation.

Polymorphisms are also frequently found in two regions of mitochondrial DNA sequences called ***hypervariable regions.*** These polymorphisms are not transcribed into RNA and do not affect protein structure. They can be followed for maternal lineage testing as all maternal relatives share the same mitochondria and so have the same mitochondrial polymorphisms.

Nucleic Acid Isolation

Extraction of nucleic acids from fluids or tissues is required to release and collect the target molecules for most nucleic acid procedures. Ideally, the target nucleic acid should be free of contamination with protein, carbohydrate, lipids, or other nucleic acid (i.e., DNA free of RNA or RNA free of DNA). Some applications require particular strand lengths.

Microbial and human nucleic acids are primarily contained in cells. Nucleic acids are also found in the blood, outside of cells. The presence of circulating cell-free DNA or RNA in humans has clinical applications in oncology and genetic studies.

Since nucleic acid in human blood or bone marrow comes mostly from leukocytes, anticoagulants are added to the sample during collection to prevent trapping of nucleated cells in a clot. Serum from clotted blood is a rich source of proteins, lipids, or other molecules. Plasma carries nucleated cells, microorganisms, and cell-free nucleic acids. In the laboratory, white blood cells (WBCs) can be purified of red blood cells (RBCs) and other blood components by simple settling, differential density gradient centrifugation, or differential lysis of the RBCs. Following separation, the WBCs form a "buffy coat" above the RBCs, which settles below them in anticoagulated blood or bone marrow.

Fresh or frozen tissue samples must be dissociated before DNA isolation. This is achieved by grinding the frozen tissue in liquid nitrogen, homogenizing the tissue, or mincing the tissue using a scalpel. Tissues may also be fixed with preservatives such as formalin for analysis by the pathology laboratory at a later date. To isolate nucleic acids from fixed, paraffin-embedded tissue, the sample must first be deparaffinized by soaking in xylene or less toxic alternatives and then rehydrated by soaking in decreasing concentrations of ethanol. For some protocols, nucleic acid may be isolated without dewaxing. While fixation preserves tissue morphology, the fixatives can damage the nucleic acid chains, resulting in false negatives or other artifacts. Longer chains will be affected to a larger extent than shorter chains. In general, products less than 1 kbp can be obtained from fixed tissue.

Solid tissues, particularly tumors and transplanted organs, release cells, exosomes, and nucleic acid into the bloodstream. The cells and the nucleic acid they have released have the molecular characteristics of the shedding tissue or organ. Exosomes are small vesicles, 30 to 100 nm in diameter, secreted by living cells. They contain proteins, lipids, and nucleic acid and can be collected by centrifugation. Cells, exosomes, and cell-free nucleic acids in blood samples are analytes for diagnostic and prognostic testing. Such a test is called a *liquid biopsy*. Liquid biopsies are a less invasive approach to cancer diagnosis than tissue biopsies. They also allow serial biopsy testing. Analysis of cell-free nucleic acid requires procedures to concentrate the target nucleic acid before isolation. These procedures include solid-phase collection of nucleic acid on beads or columns. Circulating tumor cells can be collected on special columns and filters that will selectively bind to these cells and eliminate other circulating nucleated cells.

Nucleic acid isolation can be performed either in solution or using solid-phase methods. Clinical laboratories commonly use commercial reagents, which are often combined in testing kits.

Nucleic Acid Isolation in Solution

The initial steps in nucleic acid isolation depend on the nature of the starting material and the test method. Some test systems include sample collection vessels and reagents that begin the nucleic isolation in transport to the laboratory. Details of sample collection are important because of the diversity of sample types and nucleic acid sources (viruses, bacteria, nucleated cells, cell free). Viral nucleic acid from free viruses or viruses integrated into the host genome is isolated along with host nucleic acid. Some procedures use cell-free specimens, such as plasma for viral detection. Others may require concentration of viroids by centrifugation.

The first step in nucleic acid isolation involves breaking open the cell and nuclear membranes to release the nucleic acids. For bacteria, the cell wall must be broken. Nucleic acids must be protected from degradation during this process. The presence of the chelating agent, ethylenediaminetetraacetic acid (EDTA), protects the DNA from damage by DNAse enzymes. Guanidinium isothiocyanate (GITC) is a strong denaturant of RNAse enzymes that can destroy RNA. Other buffers and inhibitors of nucleases may be included in commercial isolation systems.

After cell lysis, any debris is removed by centrifugation, and the nucleic acid is present in the supernatant. The supernatant is then treated with organic or enzymatic reagents to remove contaminating molecules such as sugars, proteins, and lipids. Many laboratories use an inorganic method called "salting out" to isolate DNA. In this method, a low pH and high salt solution is used to precipitate contaminating proteins, and the DNA remains in solution **(Fig. 12–9).**

Following removal of contaminants, the solution is treated with an alcohol, either isopropanol or ethanol, which precipitates the nucleic acid. The nucleic acid is further purified by centrifugation and washing the pellet in alcohol. The pellet is then resuspended in buffer to a volume that brings the sample to the optimal concentration for the subsequent procedures.

Solid-Phase Isolation

Manual and most automated solid-phase nucleic acid extractions are performed using solid matrices to bind and hold the nucleic acid. Silica-based products effectively bind nucleic acid in high salt conditions. These solid matrices are in the form of columns or beads.

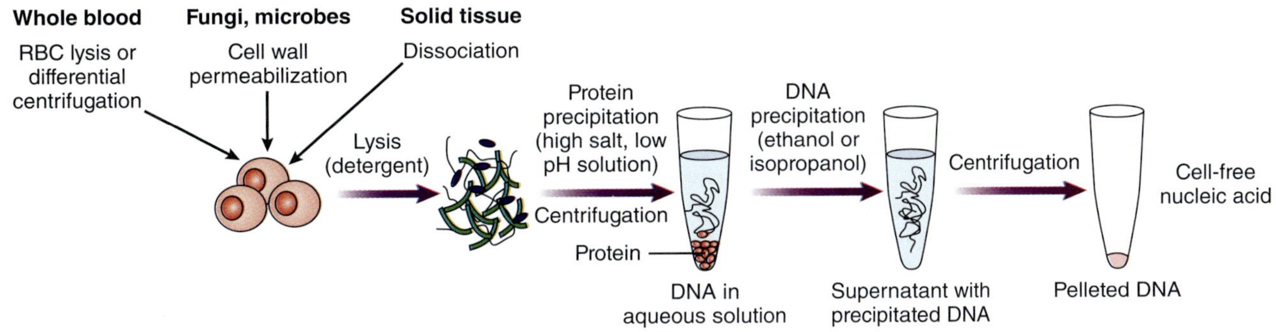

FIGURE 12–9 Isolation of DNA in solution starts with single-cell suspensions. Cell walls must be permeabilized and solid tissue dissociated to generate suspensions of membrane-bound single cells. For DNA analysis from whole blood, RBCs can be removed by lysis or differential centrifugation. After detergent lysis, proteins are precipitated from the solution in a high salt buffer. After pelleting the precipitated proteins and cell debris, the DNA in the supernatant can be precipitated with ethanol or isopropanol and resuspended to the working concentration.

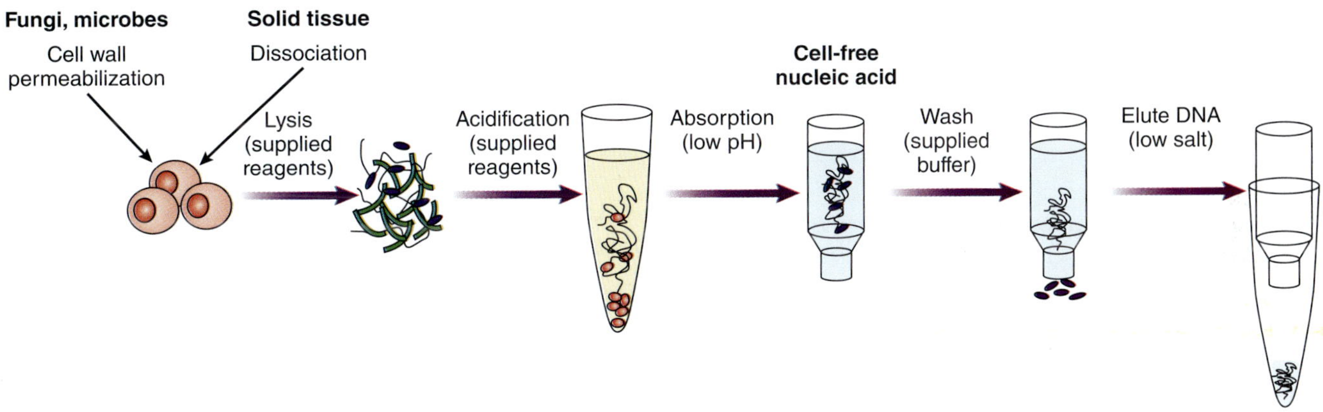

FIGURE 12–10 Solid-phase isolation workflow starts with single-cell suspensions. Cell walls must be permeabilized and solid tissue dissociated to generate suspensions of membrane-bound single cells. After release by detergent lysis, the nucleic acid is collected on the solid support, which can be a column as shown or beads coated with the silica material. The adherent nucleic acid is cleaned of contaminating molecules by column flow-through or pelleting of the beads. Finally, nucleic acid is eluted with a low-salt buffer.

Preparation of samples for solid-phase isolation starts with cell lysis and release of nucleic acids, like procedures performed in solution. Buffer systems designed for specific applications (e.g., bacterial cell lysis or human cell lysis) are commercially available. Lysis buffers may have pH levels incompatible with efficient binding of the DNA to the solid phase. Acidification buffers with lower pH precipitate contaminating proteins and enhance nucleic acid binding. Once adhered to the matrix, the nucleic acid is purified by flowing buffers through the column or rinsing beads followed by centrifugation. Finally, the nucleic acid is released using low-salt buffers at volumes to produce the desired nucleic acid concentration **(Fig. 12–10)**.

Coated beads are supplied in suspensions for use in amounts appropriate for the sample nucleic acid quantity. Columns come in various sizes, depending on the amount of nucleic acid to be isolated. Small "spin columns" that fit inside microcentrifuge tubes are commonly used to isolate viral and bacterial nucleic acid from serum, plasma, or cerebrospinal fluid. They are also used routinely to isolate nucleic acid for HLA testing, forensics, genetic testing, and oncology.

Solid-phase systems have facilitated the development of automated nucleic acid isolation. Body fluid or tissue samples are processed by instruments that provide cleaned nucleic acid solutions. Some instruments are networked to downstream processes such as the polymerase chain reaction and associated bioinformatics to provide the test results in electronic text or tabular form.

Knowledge Check 12-3

In solid-phase isolation systems, nucleic acid binds to:

a. Silica
b. Cotton
c. Plastic
d. Paraffin

Analysis of Nucleic Acid Quality and Quantity

After isolating the nucleic acid, the laboratory must analyze the sample to determine if it is of high integrity (i.e., intact) and of sufficient concentration to be used in molecular tests. Analysis of nucleic acid quantity and quality can be performed by a variety of methods, including spectrophotometry, fluorometry, and gel or capillary electrophoresis.

Spectrophotometry measures absorption of light at 260 nm by nucleotides. An absorbance of 1 unit at 260 nm corresponds to 50 µg/mL of DNA or 40 µg/mL of RNA. Proteins absorb light at 280 nm. DNA is considered pure if the 260-nm:280-nm absorbance ratio is 1.8 or greater. A ratio of 2.0 to 2.3 is considered pure for RNA. Other contaminants, including GITC, EDTA, detergents, phenol, and polysaccharides, absorb light at 230 nm. A 260-nm:230-nm absorbance ratio of 2.0 to 2.2 is acceptable for DNA or RNA.

Fluorometry measures DNA concentration by binding of a DNA-specific dye (Hoechst 33258 or PicoGreen). An internal standard is required to determine the DNA concentration, which is reported by the instrument. This method is more accurate than spectrophotometry for measurement of intact DNA. While spectrophotometry measures natural absorbance from individual nucleotides, which could include degraded DNA, the dyes used in fluorometry signal only from intact double helices.

Electrophoresis of Nucleic Acids

Electrophoresis can be used to observe the sizes or amounts of nucleic acid. **Electrophoresis** is the movement of particles under the force of an electric current. Particles can move through gas, liquid, or even solid-phase matrices. Under the force of the electric current, nucleic acids, which are negatively charged, will move from the negative pole (cathode) to the positive pole (anode). Smaller (shorter) nucleic acid chains will move faster through the matrix than larger ones.

Gel Electrophoresis

In gel electrophoresis, nucleic acid polymers are sieved through a semisolid matrix or gel. There are two types of gels used for nucleic acid analysis: agarose and polyacrylamide. Agarose gels are natural polymers of agarobiose, a disaccharide found in plants. Polyacrylamide gels are synthetic polymers of acrylamide and bis-acrylamide. The synthetic polymers are more precisely designed for high-resolution separation, distinguishing differences in nucleic acid size as small as one nucleotide. Polyacrylamide gels are also used for protein resolution by size or charge. In contrast, agarose gels do not have such high resolution but are less expensive and less toxic to prepare than acrylamide. Agarose gels are useful for standard laboratory separations of nucleic acids of 50 bp or more. Gels with agarose in low concentrations can resolve very large nucleic acids of tens of thousands bp.

Agarose gels are prepared from powdered agarose or agarose tablets dissolved and melted in a buffer solution (running buffer) that will carry the electric current. The concentration of agarose used for electrophoresis depends on the expected size of the products because smaller products will be able to migrate more easily between the small spaces of a highly concentrated agarose solution, whereas larger products will not be able to fit through the pores. High agarose concentrations (2% to 5%) resolve fragments less than 500 bp in length. Low concentrations (0.5% to 1%) resolve large fragments up to tens of thousands of bp. Polyacrylamide gels are prepared from mixtures of acrylamide plus N,N′-methyl bis-acrylamide and running buffer in proportions to generate a matrix of desired resolution capability. Because powdered acrylamide is toxic, most laboratories purchase predissolved acrylamide solutions or polymerized gels.

Different types of running buffers are used for different types of nucleic acids and different gel types. Tris-borate-EDTA (TBE) or tris-acetate-EDTA (TAE) buffers carry current for separating short or long DNA fragments, respectively. Specialized buffers containing denaturing agents, such as glyoxal or formamide, are used to separate RNA fragments. Denaturation is required to break the hydrogen bonds that hold single-stranded RNA in a folded secondary structure. Folded RNA will not accurately separate according to size.

To form the gel, the agarose suspension is heated to a clear liquid, poured into a mold, and allowed to cool and polymerize. Liquid acrylamide in solution solidifies at room temperature upon addition of a nucleating agent (tetramethyl-ethylene-diamine [TEMED]) and a catalyst (ammonium persulfate [APS]). For both agarose and polyacrylamide gels, a plastic comb is placed in the liquid gel before polymerization to form wells at one end of the gel for loading of the samples **(Fig. 12–11).**

After solidifying, the gels are placed in a bath of running buffer. To detect the nucleic acid, a fluorescent stain

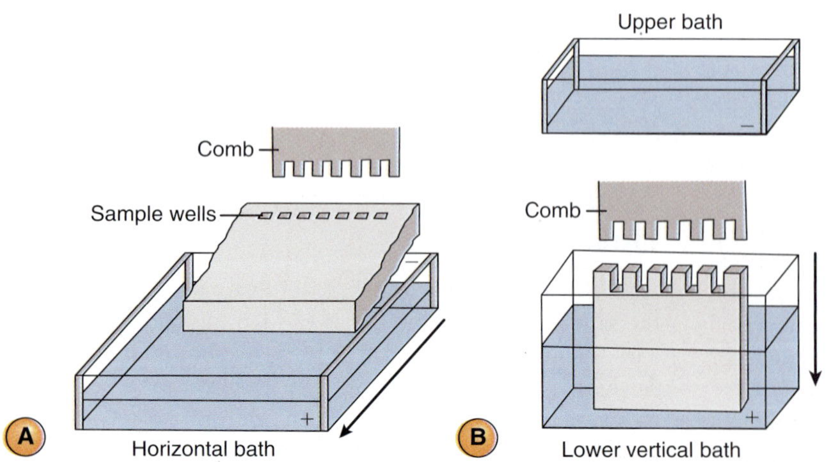

FIGURE 12–11 Gel electrophoresis systems are designed in (A) horizontal or (B) vertical formats. In both orientations, the gels are polymerized around a comb to create wells for sample loading. The combs are removed, the gels are submerged in the running buffer, and samples are pipetted into the wells. In the horizontal system, an electric field is applied between platinum electrodes at either end of the gel bath. For vertical gels, the field is applied from the upper to the lower bath. In both cases, negatively charged nucleic acids will migrate through the gel to the positive electrode (+) as indicated by the arrows.

(ethidium bromide, SYBR Green, or others) can be mixed with the gel solution or placed in the gel bath. Alternatively, the gel can be soaked in the stain solution after electrophoresis is complete.

The nucleic acid sample to be separated is mixed with a loading solution that contains a density agent (glycerol or Ficoll-Paque) and a visual dye, such as bromophenol blue. The density agent allows loading of the sample into the wells of the gel as it is submerged in the running buffer. The visual dye aids in seeing the sample while loading it into the well and during electrophoresis. The dye will also mark the progress of migration, as the stain moves faster through the gel matrix than the nucleic acids. The gel bath is connected to a power supply that will establish a current between platinum wires at the top (negative pole) and bottom (positive pole) of the electrophoresis unit. The negatively charged nucleic acids will move under the force of the current toward the positive pole, working their way through the gel matrix at a speed that depends on their size.

After electrophoresis, the nucleic acids can be visualized through excitation of the fluorescent stain by ultraviolet light. Nucleic acid chains of identical or similar sizes will merge to form lines or bands on the gel, as shown in **Figure 12–12A.** The distance from the loading well to the band will be inversely proportional to the size of the nucleic acid. Shorter chains will appear below longer ones because smaller nucleic acids can travel faster through the gel. A standard molecular weight marker of nucleic acid chains of known sizes run with the test samples allows estimation of the size of the test nucleic acids in bases or bp.

Gel electrophoresis may also be used to estimate the quality of the isolated nucleic acids. **(Fig. 12–13A).** Intact nucleic acids will have a high molecular weight, and appear as bands close to the application well, whereas DNA that has been degraded into fragments will appear as multiple smaller bands that may fuse together to form a smudge. The distribution of fragments across the size range of isolated DNA is used to determine a DNA Integrity Number (DIN). DIN is calculated on a scale of 1 to 10. A high DIN indicates highly intact DNA, and a low DIN a strongly degraded DNA sample. Similarly, an RNA integrity number (RIN), ranging from 1 to 10, is calculated from electrophoresis of large and small ribosomal RNAs, the most abundant RNA in cells.

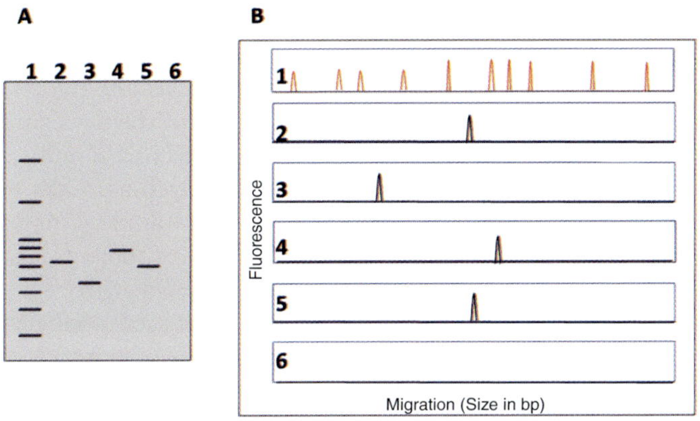

FIGURE 12–12 After gel electrophoresis, nucleic acids are visualized by detection of a nucleic-acid–specific fluorescent dye such as ethidium bromide or SYBR Green (A). The agarose gel shown has six lanes, where samples and controls were loaded. The first lane (1) shows the molecular weight standard. Lanes 2 through 5 show sample DNA. The size of the DNA fragments can be estimated by observing how far they migrated in the gel compared to the molecular weight standard. For example, the fragment in lane 4 is of higher molecular weight than that of lane 3. A negative (blank) control is in lane 6. (B) In capillary electrophoresis, the gel is replaced by an electropherogram. Instead of bands, peaks appear representing the nucleic acid fragments (rows 2 through 5). The first row on the electropherogram shown is the molecular weight standard. From it, the instrument computes and displays the lengths of the nucleic acid fragments (rows 2 through 5) in bp. Row 6 is the blank or negative control (no DNA). All the fragments shown and the molecular weight marker were run simultaneously through a single capillary.

Capillary Electrophoresis

Capillary electrophoresis is a semiautomated separation system moving particles through a gas, liquid, or gel. Because nucleic acids do not resolve in solution, a gel or polymer is inserted into the capillary to sieve the nucleic acids; this method is called capillary *gel* electrophoresis. Instruments for capillary gel electrophoresis may have a single capillary or up to 96 capillaries that run simultaneously. Ampules of premixed polymer solution and buffers are automatically injected into the capillary or capillaries of the instrument.

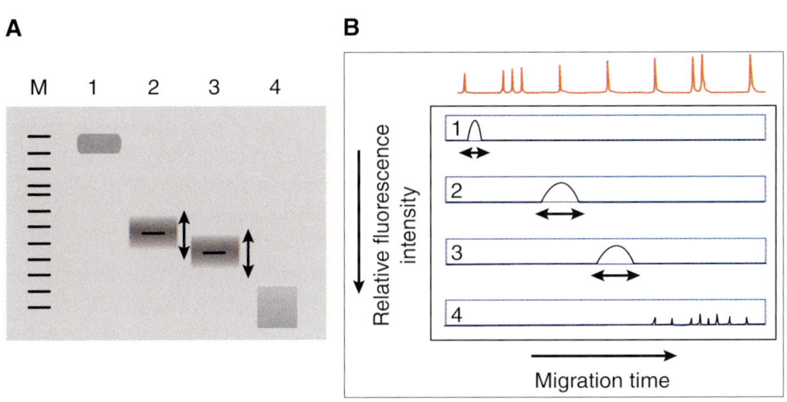

FIGURE 12–13 Good quality high molecular weight DNA measured by (A) gel or (B) capillary electrophoresis resolves as a thick band (A. lane 1) or peak (B. scan 1) near the point of application. DNA fragmentation, immunoglobulin gene rearrangements, or other methods may produce populations of products within specific size ranges (lanes/scans 2,3). The mean size of the fragment population should be optimal for its intended use. Low-quality nucleic acid will resolve as smears to the bottom of the gel or short peak populations trending to the right of the electropherogram (lane/scan 4). The arrows indicate the (A) direction or (B) time of migration.

For detection, DNA chains must carry a label consisting of a covalently attached molecule that emits fluorescence. A laser inside of the capillary instrument excites the fluorescent labels as they move through the capillary. The dyes emit fluorescence, which is detected and transferred to a computer as an electrical signal. The signals are displayed as peaks of fluorescence **(Figs. 12–12B and 12–13B)**. Multiple samples can run through a single capillary, as the instruments can detect fluorescent signals at more than one wavelength.

Prior to loading onto the instrument, fluorescently labeled nucleic acid samples are diluted in formamide, and a molecular weight standard is added directly to the sample. Formamide denatures the double-stranded nucleic acid for efficient migration and accurate sizing of the single strands. The samples are placed into the instrument either in separate tubes or in a plate format. The samples enter the capillary by an electrokinetic process that attracts the negatively charged DNA to the end of the capillary, which is submerged into the tube or plate well containing the sample. During electrophoresis, the nucleic acids sieve through the capillary as they would in a gel. The shorter fragments move faster than the longer ones **(Fig. 12–14)**. As each labeled nucleic acid chain passes by the detector, a peak of fluorescence is generated by the computer (Fig. 12–14). The molecular weight markers move through the same capillary with the sample, enabling the instrument to automatically assess the size of the fragments in bp.

Applications of capillary gel electrophoresis include Sanger sequencing, human identification using STR polymorphisms, and assessing template library fragment sizes for next-generation sequencing (see "DNA Sequencing" section).

Knowledge Check 12-4

The speed that nucleic acid travels through a gel matrix under the force of an electric current is inversely proportional to which characteristic?

a. Charge
b. Size
c. Solubility
d. Sequence

Molecular Analysis

Nucleic acid tests are designed to detect changes in the DNA sequence or to measure differences in amounts of DNA present or RNA synthesized. There are four main approaches to nucleic acid analysis: strand cleavage methods, hybridization methods, amplification methods, and sequencing.

Strand Cleavage Methods

Strand cleavage methods involve the use of enzymes to cut the DNA into smaller fragments for analysis. These methods include restriction enzyme digestion and CRISPR-Cas.

Restriction Enzyme Digestion

Restriction endonucleases are microbial enzymes that separate the phosphodiester bonds between specific DNA nucleotides. They are named for the bacteria from which they were isolated. For example, *Eco*R1 is the first enzyme to be isolated from ***Escherichia coli***, strain R, and ***Hind*III** is the third enzyme isolated from ***Haemophilus influenzae***, strain d.

These endonucleases recognize and bind to specific nucleotide sequences in DNA so that they will only cut the DNA at those locations. Restriction enzymes are classified as type I, II, III, or IV based on their recognition site structure and additional enzymatic functions such as DNA methylation. Type II restriction enzymes used in clinical laboratory applications recognize palindromic sites—that is, nucleotide sequences that read the same 5′ to 3′ on both strands of the DNA. For example, *Eco*R1 recognizes the following palindrome sequence and cuts both DNA strands between the 5′ G and A:

5′G^AATTC3′

3′CTTAA^G5′

There are hundreds of restriction enzymes with unique binding and cleavage sites. DNA can be characterized by the pattern of fragments produced after incubation with restriction enzymes and electrophoresis. DNA samples with different

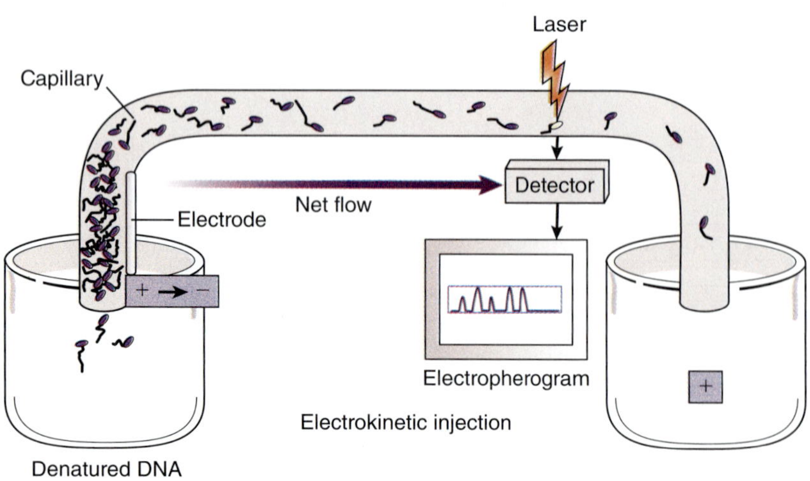

FIGURE 12–14 In capillary electrophoresis, nucleic acids enter the capillary by electrokinetic injection where they are attracted by a transitory positive charge induced by the electrode. The positive charge then moves to the far end of the capillary, and the nucleic acids travel at different speeds, according to their size. Small fragments travel faster and reach the detector first. Each fragment has a fluorescent label that is excited by a laser to emit fluorescence for the detector. The signals are imaged as peaks of fluorescence on the electropherogram.

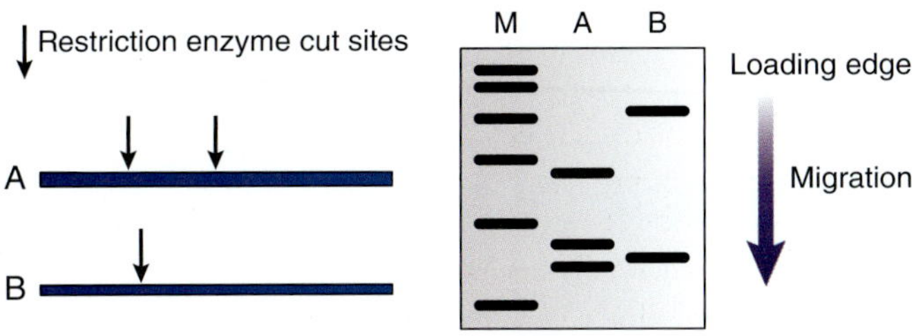

FIGURE 12–15 Restriction enzyme mapping characterizes DNA by the pattern of fragments generated when the DNA is cut with restriction enzymes. DNA double helix A has two restriction sites (arrows), while the DNA B has only one. When these two DNAs are digested with the restriction enzyme, DNA A will yield three fragments, and DNA B will yield two. These band patterns are a characteristic of these DNAs. M = molecular weight standard, used for sizing the DNA fragments.

nucleotide sequences will yield different sizes and numbers of bands characteristic of that DNA. **Figure 12–15** shows results from digestion of different bacterial plasmids or cloned linear fragments of DNA with the same enzymes. Restriction fragment length polymorphism (RFLP) analysis has been applied to epidemiological studies of microorganisms and identification of resistance factors carried on bacterial plasmids.

CRISPR-Cas9

DNA analysis using restriction enzymes is limited to the sequences recognized by the enzymes. Another type of restriction system found in archaea and gram-positive bacteria, called CRISPR/Cas9, uses a common enzyme guided by short fragments of RNA to specific sites in DNA. **Clustered regularly interspaced short palindromic repeats (CRISPRs)** are classes of repeated DNA sequences found in microbial DNA. The repeated sequences are interrupted by spacer sequences matching regions extracted from invading plasmids or viruses. In bacteria, these spacer sequences serve as adaptive immunity with memory of the invading DNA. The locus also contains sequences encoding the CRISPR-associated protein (Cas) enzyme. To fend off an invader, short RNA sequences transcribed from the CRISPR spacer regions guide the Cas enzyme to the matching sequences in the invading DNA **(Fig. 12–16).**

CRISPR/Cas9 has been used in the laboratory to alter DNA at user-defined locations. To perform CRISPR methods, a short RNA that is complementary to a desired DNA sequence is made in the laboratory. The RNA and the Cas9 enzyme are introduced into living cells by bacterial plasmids or viral vectors. The synthetic RNA guides the Cas9 endonuclease to the site of choice, providing the specificity of restriction enzymes and the versatility of guiding cuts to any sequence site.

In research laboratories, CRISPR has been used for DNA analysis and genome editing. Clinical applications of CRISPR that are being studied include gene therapy, engineering T cells for cancer therapy, and treatments for genetic diseases involving administration of lipid particles that contain the guide RNA and mRNA that codes for the Cas9 enzyme.

Hybridization Methods

Restriction enzyme cleavage methods are highly informative for investigating small genomes, such as those of microorganisms or plasmids. For complex genomes, such as human DNA, such analyses were initially not practical as the DNA is too large and complex to generate readable fragment patterns. The development of hybridization methods has facilitated

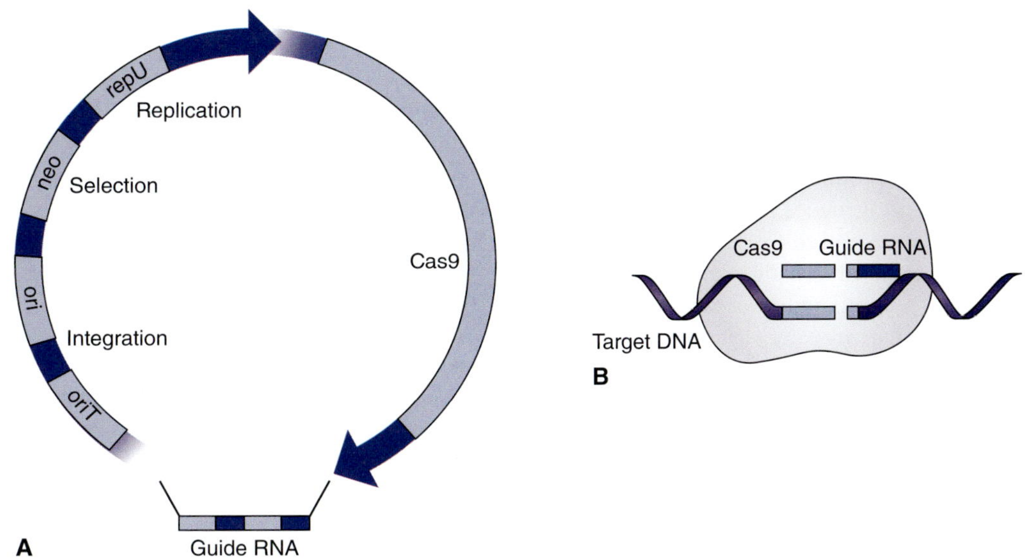

FIGURE 12–16 Clustered regularly interspaced short palindromic repeats (CRISPR) can be used in the laboratory to target specific regions of DNA for enzymatic restriction or gene editing. (A) User-defined guide RNA is ligated into a vector encoding the *Cas9* gene. This vector also carries genes for selection of successfully transfected cells, initiation of its replication, and integration into the host genome following transfection or transduction into cells. Once inside the cell, *Cas9* and guide RNA are expressed from constitutive promoters (arrows). (B) The guide RNA then leads the Cas9 enzyme to complementary sites to enzymatically act on the target DNA.

analysis of large fragments. **Hybridization,** as related to molecular techniques, involves the binding of two strands of nucleic acids, the template strand, and a complementary *probe*. Hybridization procedures include blotting methods, arrays, and in situ hybridization.

Blotting Techniques

The first hybridization procedure to be developed was the *Southern blot*, invented by Edwin Southern in the 1970s. The Southern blot was performed by incubating test genomic DNA with restriction enzymes, separating the millions of resulting fragments by gel electrophoresis, and then transferring or blotting them from the gel to a membrane for detection. The presence or size of specific fragments is revealed with a probe, a complementary single strand of nucleic acid carrying a detectable label. A variation of the Southern blot, called the *Northern blot,* was subsequently developed to analyze RNA structure and expression. *Western blots* are used to detect proteins and protein modifications by hybridization with antibodies specific for the proteins of interest (see Chapter 11).

Arrays

An *array* is a reverse dot blot hybridization, that is, hybridization of a labeled sample to an unlabeled immobilized probe. There are three basic types of arrays: *comparative genomic arrays, RNA expression arrays,* and *high-density oligonucleotide arrays,* including bead arrays. Comparative genomic hybridization arrays are used to detect DNA amplifications or deletions. Gene expression is measured with expression arrays that detect RNA synthesis; in these methods, labeled RNA from the test material is hybridized to the probes. High-density arrays have single nucleotide resolution and can even be used to determine a DNA nucleotide sequence.

Microarrays use thousands of highly specific unlabeled probes attached directly to a very small area on a solid support. The support can be a glass microscope slide, quartz, or beads (bead arrays). The test sample, nucleic acids or proteins isolated from cultures, cells, or body fluids, is labeled and hybridized to the many immobilized probes. Some bead arrays and bead chip arrays use secondary labels that are not attached directly to the sample molecules. Microarrays have various applications. In cytogenetics, *comparative genomic hybridization (CGH) arrays* are used for virtual karyotyping, to detect tiny losses or gains of genetic material at specific chromosomal locations as compared to a normal reference sample. In *gene expression arrays*, the levels of RNA transcribed from thousands of genes are compared to normal reference samples to look for up- or down-regulation of gene transcription.

Standard microarrays are manufactured by printing single-stranded DNA probes onto glass slides. After hybridization of the fluorescently labeled sample DNA, the signals are read in a scanner and analyzed for the color and amount of fluorescence. Fluorescent sample labeling allows simultaneous detection of the test samples and/or reference samples hybridized to the array for relative measurement of the amounts of test material **(Fig. 12–17).**

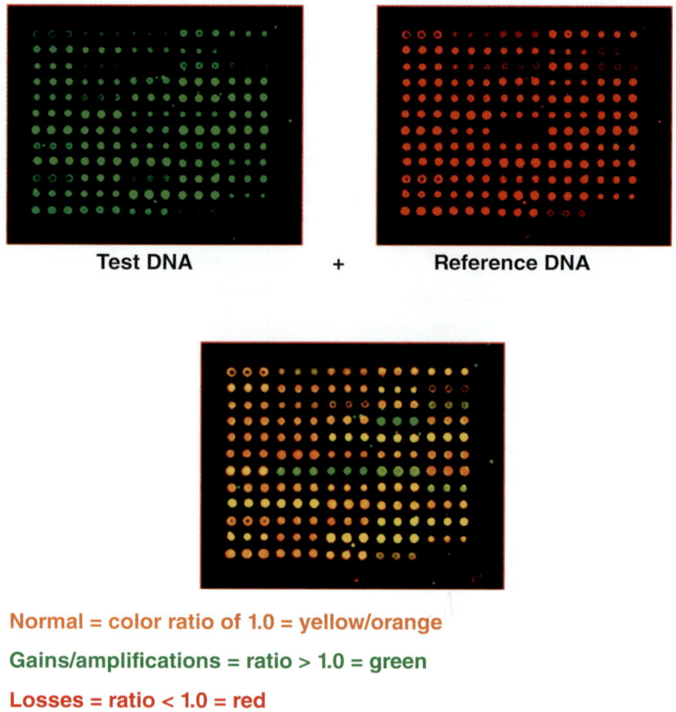

FIGURE 12–17 For array analysis, labeled sample fragments (green) are hybridized to unlabeled immobilized probes. A reference material (red) is hybridized to the same array. The results of the array are relative test:reference colors. In this example, a green color indicates amplified gene regions, and the neutral yellow colors indicate no amplification nor deletion of those regions. Red color would indicate deletion of a gene region.

High-density arrays are manufactured by synthesizing short probes (10 to 30 bases long) directly on a quartz support. In this way, many more probes per unit area can be placed on the array. While standard microarrays carry hundreds to thousands of probes, high-density microarrays carry tens of thousands of probes within the same unit area. The short probes will only hybridize efficiently with their exact complement in the sample sequences. Even a single noncomplementary base will destabilize hybridization of sample nucleic acid to the probe. This results in single nucleotide resolution, or the ability to detect nucleotide sequences that differ by one base. As with standard arrays, sample DNA is fragmented, denatured, labeled with fluorescent molecules, and then hybridized to the probes on the array.

Suspension bead array assays are based on preparations of beads of 100 to 400 different fluorescent "colors." Each colored bead is attached to a nucleic acid probe or an antibody that will bind specifically to the target molecules or sequences **(Fig. 12–18).** The sample nucleic acid molecules may be directly labeled, or for protein targets, a secondary antibody conjugated to a fluorescent signal may be used to detect the presence of the bound target. Because many beads are used, each bound to a different antibody or probe, multiple targets can be simultaneously detected in a single assay run; in other words, a *multiplex* assay is performed. Applications include HLA typing and respiratory virus panels.

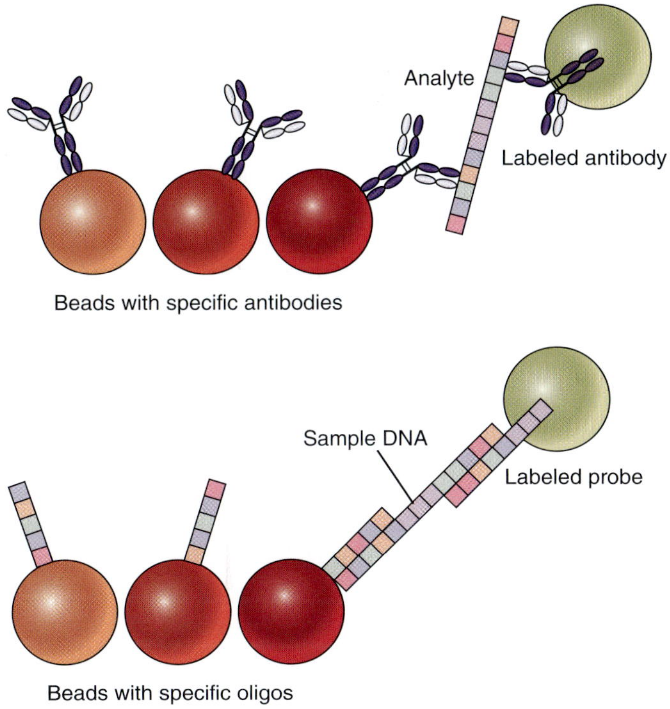

FIGURE 12–18 In suspension bead analysis, antibody probes are attached to beads identified by bead color. (A) The illustration shows three of 100 to 400 bead colors, each with antibody to a different analyte. Multiple targets can be detected by the colors of the beads that have associated fluorescence from the secondary antibody. Flow cytometry is used to assay each bead separately for associated fluorescence. (B) For nucleic acid analysis in suspension arrays, bead array antibodies are replaced with single-stranded oligonucleotide probes complementary to the test nucleic acid. If present, biotinylated sample DNA will hybridize to the sequences, and the biotin-specific conjugate will generate a signal.

The *bead chip array* is a type of high-density array designed to detect single nucleotide DNA alterations. In these arrays, probes are bound to beads, and the beads are randomly immobilized on a silica chip. The silica wafer is etched to form millions of tiny wells, each accommodating a single bead.

Probes in bead chip arrays are longer than those in other array types. Each probe includes about 50 bases complementary to the test DNA plus a 20- to 30-base *address sequence* to identify the location of the probe on the array **(Fig. 12–19A).** The complementary component of the probe ends one base 5′ to the base to be identified in the sample DNA. Thousands of copies of the same probe are attached to each bead. Beads with the same probe sequence are called a *bead type*. A mixture of thousands of suspensions of different bead types is randomly applied to the etched silica chip to make the array **(Fig. 12–19B).** Bead chip arrays accommodate over a million probes.

For the bead chip array assay, DNA samples fragmented to 300 to 600 bp length pieces are denatured but not labeled. The fragmented denatured sample DNA is then hybridized to the probes on the array. A single base extension catalyzed by DNA polymerase adds a labeled dideoxynucleotide triphosphate (ddNTP) to the probe using the sample DNA as a template. A ddNTP is a DNA nucleotide in which the sugar lacks a 3′-OH group, preventing further elongation of the probe. The fluorescent label colors indicate which nucleotide has been attached to the probe. The sample DNA is removed for scanning of the single base extended probes. Array scanners and software detect and analyze the fluorescent signals from the array.

This assay produces high-dimensional data (hundreds of thousands of results per sample). A data reduction process may be used to interpret the results. High-density oligonucleotide

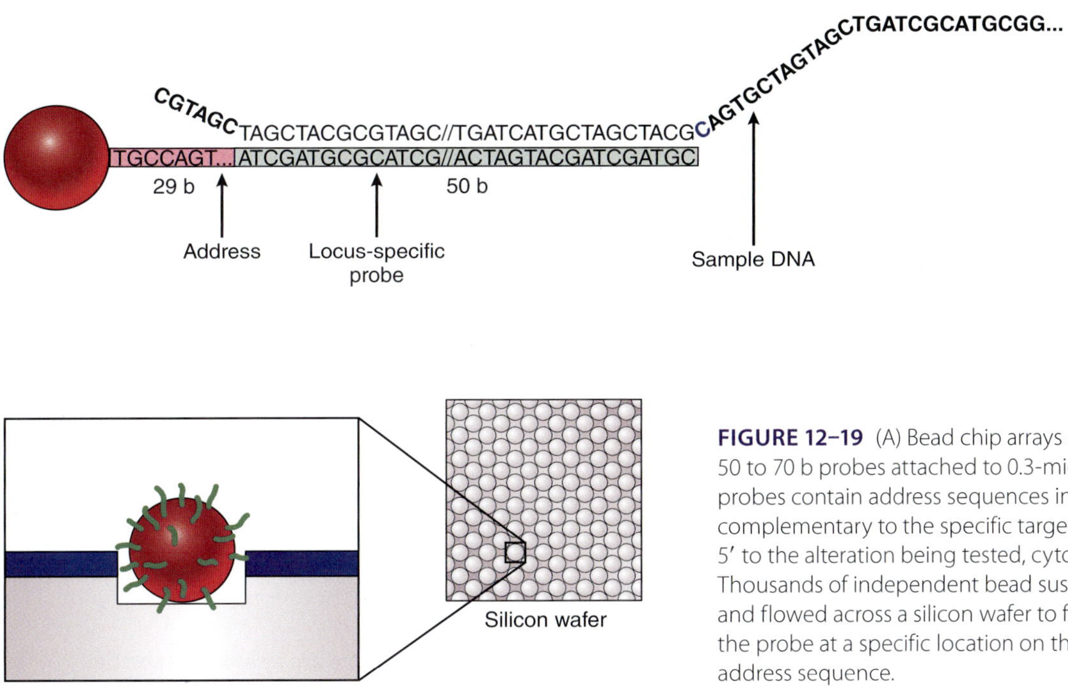

FIGURE 12–19 (A) Bead chip arrays are manufactured with 50 to 70 b probes attached to 0.3-micron diameter beads. The probes contain address sequences in addition to sequences complementary to the specific target. The probe ends one base 5′ to the alteration being tested, cytosine in this example. (B) Thousands of independent bead suspensions are prepared, mixed, and flowed across a silicon wafer to form the array. The identity of the probe at a specific location on the array is determined by the address sequence.

arrays, also called *SNP arrays*, are used for studies of the genome, RNA transcripts, and epigenetics (DNA methylation). Applications of bead chip arrays include genome-wide association studies and ancestry testing.

Knowledge Check 12-5

Probes in microarrays are:
a. Fluorescently labeled
b. Double stranded
c. Phosphorylated
d. Unlabeled

In Situ Hybridization

In situ hybridization (ISH) refers to detection of targets *in place* as they appear in tissues, cells, or subcellular structures. Labeled probes are designed to bind or hybridize to the targets. In situ hybridization is a critical component of pathology studies of tissues and cell suspensions. **Immunohistochemistry** (IHC) is a type of in situ hybridization where chromogenically labeled antibodies bind to clinically significant protein targets expressed in some tumor cells (see Chapter 17). Probes for these studies are monoclonal antibodies linked to enzymes, such as horseradish peroxidase, that produce colorimetric or visible signals from chromogenic substrates. Binding of enzyme-linked secondary antibodies to the unlabeled primary antibody isotype is an alternative labeling approach.

IHC is frequently performed on tissue that has been soaked in a fixative to preserve tissue morphology. The most common fixative, 10% buffered formalin, can change protein structure and cause covalent attachment of unrelated proteins. Fixation can affect the ability of test antibodies to recognize epitopes. Protein cross-linking can be reversed by heating and treatment with proteolytic agents that break the cross-links and expose the antigenic sites.

Positive and negative controls must be included in ISH testing to ensure accuracy of the results. Normal tissue that expresses the protein target should serve as the positive control, whereas an adjacent section cut from the test tissue without the addition of the primary antibody and tumor tissues that do not express the antigen should serve as negative controls. Ideally, the control tissues are processed with the test tissue. Control tissues processed differently from the test tissue validate reagent performance but do not verify the tissue preparation. If staining of positive control tissue is not satisfactory, or if unwanted staining occurs in negative controls, all results with the patient specimen should be considered invalid.

Fluorescence In Situ Hybridization (FISH)

Fluorescence in situ hybridization (FISH) uses fluorescently labeled nucleic acid probes and requires specialized microscopes equipped to detect the different wavelengths of emitted fluorescent signals. FISH studies detect specific cytogenetic changes (gene rearrangements) directly on the chromosomes, including translocations (transfer of a chromosome fragment onto a different chromosome), deletions, or gene amplifications. FISH detects gene rearrangements that are not easily visualized by standard karyotyping.

In FISH methods, nucleic acid probes ranging in size from a few thousand to hundreds of thousands of bases in length are covalently attached to a fluorescent molecule. In interphase FISH, cells are deposited on glass slides. The cell membranes are permeabilized to allow entry of the probe. The probes hybridize to their complementary sequences directly in the cell nuclei. The resulting signals will show the state of the gene or region complementary to the probe. Target gene probes in combination with reference centromeric gene probes detect deletions or amplifications **(Fig. 12–20).** Interphase FISH offers higher resolution than karyotyping for specific targets but is limited to the regions complementary to the FISH probes. Specific probes are designed to hybridize to critical areas that are amplified, deleted, translocated, or otherwise rearranged in disease states.

In another approach, metaphase FISH, probes are bound to compacted chromosomes. Cells are incubated with a mitogen to stimulate movement through the cell cycle and then arrested in metaphase as done in karyotyping. FISH is then performed on the visible mitotic chromosomes. Metaphase FISH with multicolor probes can detect complex gene rearrangements involving multiple chromosomes. A specialty research procedure, spectral karyotyping, can detect different color probes for every chromosome.

FISH methods are sensitive to the buffer and temperature conditions of hybridization (stringency). Protocols must be strictly followed to avoid false-positive results caused by nonspecific binding of probes or false negatives caused by failure of the probe to bind. Comparative genome hybridization arrays complement FISH testing in cases of multiple or complex genetic abnormalities, gene amplifications, or microdeletions.

Amplification Methods

Methods in molecular diagnostics frequently involve some aspect of amplification, that is, copying of target nucleic acids. Historically performed in vivo using high copy number plasmid replication of cloned fragments in bacteria, the development of the in vitro polymerase chain reaction (PCR) greatly facilitated and broadened the potential applications of gene amplification. PCR was quickly followed by modifications of the method and by alternative target amplification methods, such as reverse transcriptase PCR (RT-PCR), transcription-mediated amplification (TMA), and loop-mediated isothermal amplification (LAMP).

Polymerase Chain Reaction (PCR)

The **polymerase chain reaction (PCR)** is an in vitro DNA replication procedure. A PCR reaction solution includes all the necessary components required for DNA replication: a sample containing the DNA template to be copied, deoxyribonucleotides, which will be joined together, oligonucleotide primers to prime the synthesis of the copies, DNA polymerase to covalently join the deoxyribonucleotides, and buffer containing monovalent and divalent cations with a pH optimal for the polymerase activity.

The oligonucleotide primers are key to the specificity of the PCR reaction. Primers are synthetic single-stranded nucleic

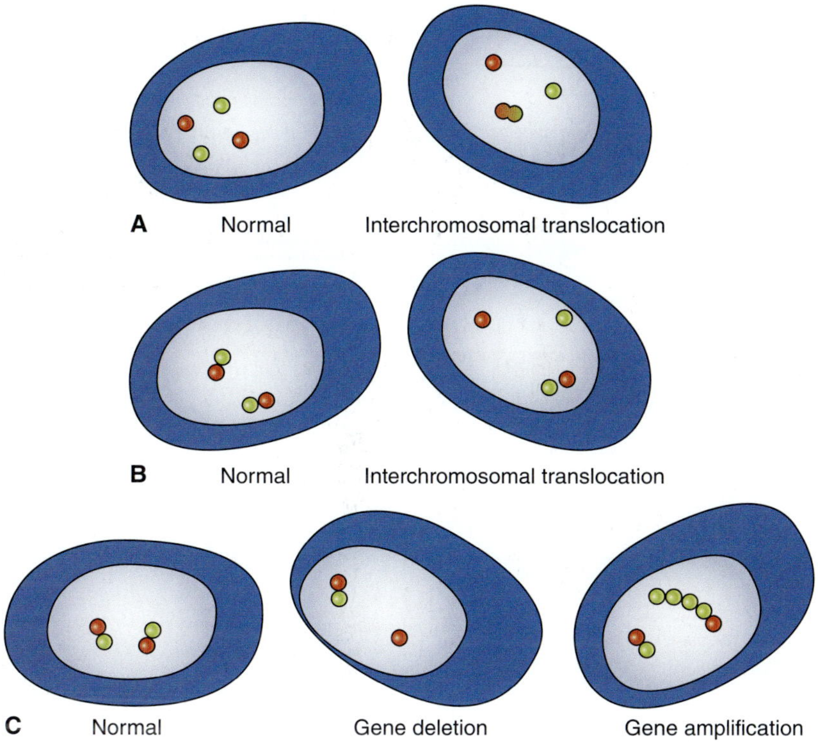

FIGURE 12–20 FISH analysis detects chromosomal abnormalities. (A) Fluorescent probes (orange and green) complementary to specific gene regions on different chromosomes in a diploid cell should show two copies of each region. If a translocation occurs between the probed regions, the two probes will be brought together. (B) Another way to detect interchromosomal translocations is to use breakaway probes. A translocation involving the probed region with any other chromosome will separate the two probes. (C) To detect amplifications or deletions, the probe specific for the target gene is labeled green, while a probe complementary to the centromere of the chromosome on which the gene is located is labeled orange. Normally there are two copies of each chromosome, each carrying one gene in each nucleus (normal). If a gene or the region of the gene is deleted, only one green probe will be present. Gene amplification will have multiple green signals associated with a single orange signal (amplified).

acids, usually 18 to 30 bases in length. They are complementary to sequences flanking the region of the template DNA to be copied **(Fig. 12–21).** Thus, primers determine the genetic location and size of the PCR product. Primer design (selecting sequences of the primers) is important for the success of the PCR reaction. Forward and reverse primer sequences, which bind to the 3′ ends of the two DNA template strands, must be of a similar melting temperature for even hybridization to the target sequences. The melting temperature (T_m) of the short primer sequences (the temperature at which 50% of the double-stranded DNA formed after binding of the primers to the template is denatured into single strands) can be estimated from the number of G:C and A:T bonds formed with the template using the following formula:

$$T_m = (4 \times \text{Number of G:C pairs}) + (2 \times \text{Number of A:T pairs})$$

Primer sequences must also be designed to avoid inter- and intramolecular self-complementarity, that is, hybridization within and between primer pair sequences. Primer pairs that hybridize at their 3′ ends will copy each other, producing *primer dimers*. Self-copying will lower the sensitivity of the reaction by using up reaction components. Intramolecular complementarity of primers will result in secondary structures or folding that may interfere with binding to the intended target. Primer design is especially challenging in multiplex PCR reactions where more than one target is copied in the same PCR reaction.

Primer sequences can be determined manually from the target sequence or with available software tools. In the latter case, target sequences, preferred product length, and other parameters are entered into the software program, yielding one or more suggested primer pairs. Once established, the primer sequences should be checked for specificity by searching in GenBank or other search tools for complementary sequences other than the intended target. The primer sequences are then submitted to a DNA synthesis facility for manufacture. Commercially prepared primers are also available for some target sequences.

The ingredients of a PCR reaction mix—primers, nucleotides, heat-stable DNA polymerase enzyme, and target template (sample DNA)—can be combined manually. Alternatively, premixed PCR reagents (deoxyribonucleotides, primers, and buffer) are supplied from manufacturers to which only the template DNA and, in some cases, enzyme are added. Universal reagent mixes also require the addition of primers. A blank control reaction with all ingredients except the template should be included in all PCR runs to check for contamination of the reaction components.

The PCR reaction mix is subjected to an amplification program consisting of a designated number of cycles. A cycle is composed of timed temperature changes. A standard three-step PCR cycle includes the following:

1. A denaturation step to break the hydrogen bonds between the two strands of the DNA helix, separating them so they can each be used as a template (94°C to 96°C)
2. An annealing step to allow for binding of the primers to the templates (50°C to 70°C)
3. An extension step to lengthen the bound primers by adding complementary nucleotides to the 3′ end (68°C to 72°C)

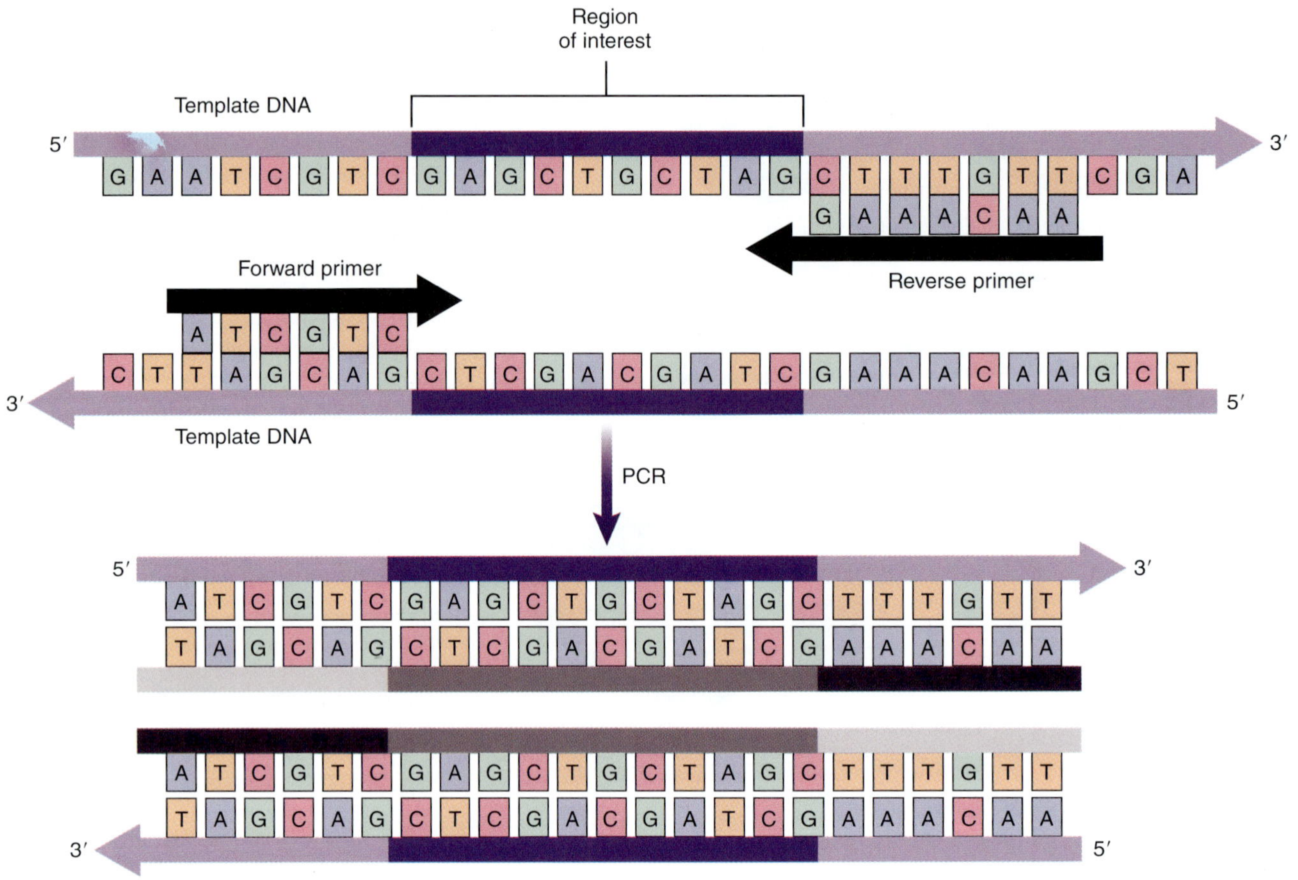

FIGURE 12–21 In the PCR reaction, short, single-stranded primers (black arrows) hydrogen bond to complementary sequences flanking the region of interest. The PCR reaction will produce millions of copies of the desired sequences. (Note that the sequence is shortened in the image). Primers are usually 18 to 30 bases long, and the PCR products range from 50 to more than 1,000 base pairs.

In a standard cycle, each of these temperatures will be held for 30 to 60 seconds. PCR cycles vary depending on the target DNA and the protocol. Two-step cycles and complex multi-step cycles are also often used. The target DNA region is copied once (doubled) in each cycle. Each cycle is repeated 20 to 50 times, depending on the assay. The set of repeated cycles makes up the PCR program. The program may also include an initial 5- to 15-minute incubation at the denaturation temperature to activate polymerases designed to remain inactive at room temperature. The program may end with a final 7- to 10-minute step at the extension temperature to allow complete copying of the products. To ensure stability of the product, a hold at 4°C may be added to the end of the amplification program. The products are stable at this temperature.

The instrument that carries out the PCR program is the *thermal cycler.* There are a variety of thermal cyclers configured for different applications. In general, thermal cyclers are either chamber or block based. In chamber-based cyclers, the sample tubes are subjected to the amplification program temperatures through the surrounding air in the chamber. In block cyclers, sample tubes are placed in a metal block that is heated and cooled according to the amplification program. Amplification programs may include the time it takes to achieve the different temperatures (ramp speed). Ramp speed affects the efficiency of the amplification and the time required to complete the program. Chamber cyclers allow faster ramp speeds than block cyclers; however, chamber cyclers have become less popular due to the risk of whole chamber contamination in the event of tube breakage.

PCR amplification produces millions of copies or ***amplicons*** of the region of interest. At 100% PCR efficiency (every target molecule is copied), the number of copies will be 2^n, where n is the number of cycles (20 to 50) in the amplification program. The products of the PCR reaction are visualized by gel or capillary gel electrophoresis, as the last part of a PCR procedure **(Fig. 12–22).** The gel image or electropherogram can be inspected for the presence of unintended products caused by mis-primes or primer dimers. The blank control reaction should demonstrate no product. For some applications, the presence, absence, or size of a PCR product is the test result. PCR products may be directly placed into subsequent reactions, such as restriction enzyme analysis or sequencing.

A variety of modifications have been made for different applications of the PCR reaction. These include multiplex PCR to simultaneously amplify multiple targets in the same reaction, nested PCR to increase the sensitivity of the reaction, and **reverse transcriptase PCR (RT-PCR).**

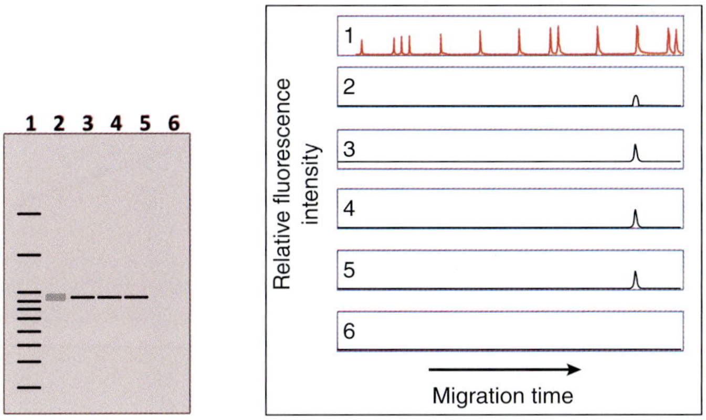

FIGURE 12–22 Detection of PCR products by (A) gel and (B) capillary gel electrophoresis. The first lane in the gel and the first scan in the electropherogram (top) contain molecular weight markers (fragments of known size). The next four lanes or scans are PCR products from different samples, followed by a reagent blank control for contamination (lane 6 and last scan). The fainter gel band or smaller peak in lane 2 may indicate lower amounts of target, or lower PCR efficiency, possibly resulting from PCR inhibiting substances in the sample.

RT-PCR starts with an RNA template. Complementary or copy DNA (cDNA) is synthesized from the RNA using reverse transcriptase, an RNA-dependent DNA polymerase. The cDNA serves as the template for the PCR reaction. Alternatively, enzymes that copy both RNA and DNA are included in simultaneous RT and PCR reactions that do not require a separate RT reaction. RT-PCR is a method of analysis for cellular RNA or qualitative detection of RNA viruses such as HIV, severe acute respiratory syndrome coronavirus 2 (SARS Co-V2), and HCV (hepatitis C virus).

PCR primer design introduces additional flexibility into the PCR protocol. In sequence-specific primer PCR (SSP-PCR, also called *amplification refractory mutation system PCR* or ARMS-PCR), primers are designed so that they will end on a potentially mutated or polymorphic base. Annealing of the last base at the 3′ end of the primer is critical for the polymerase activity. If the last 3′ base of the primer is not complementary to the template, DNA polymerase will not recognize the primer as a substrate for extension, and no PCR product will be made. SSP-PCR is a common approach to detect mutations and polymorphisms such as in HLA typing by SSP-PCR.

Unlike the 3′ end of primers, the 5′ end does not have to be complementary to the template. Noncomplementary sequences containing restriction enzyme recognition sites or RNA polymerase binding sites can be added to the 5′ end of the primers. The resulting PCR products will then carry these sequences. These amplicons can be conveniently inserted into plasmids for biological analyses or transcribed into RNA and translated to in vitro transcription/translation systems. Labels in the form of fluorescent molecules, biotin, or other molecules may also be covalently attached to the 5′ end of primers. This allows capture immobilization of the PCR products or detection in capillary electrophoresis systems (Fig. 12–22B).

Knowledge Check 12-6

Which type of DNA polymerase is used for PCR amplification?

a. Heat sensitive
b. Heat stable
c. RNA dependent
d. Sequence specific

Quantitative PCR (qPCR)

Standard or endpoint PCR results are interpreted as the presence, absence, or size of the PCR product, but the quantity of starting material is not easily measured. In 1993, scientists observed that target quantification could be achieved by following the accumulation of PCR products in real time during amplification. This is the basis for **quantitative PCR (qPCR).** Both DNA and RNA targets can be measured by qPCR. For RNA, complementary DNA made from the RNA using reverse transcriptase is the input material. Although originally termed ***real-time PCR*** (RT-PCR), the preferred term is *quantitative PCR (qPCR)* to avoid confusion with reverse transcriptase PCR (RT-PCR).

To be detected during amplification, the qPCR product was initially followed by photography and then by using a fluorescent dye specific for double-stranded DNA (ethidium bromide). Product labeling is currently performed using a less toxic DNA-specific dye, SYBR Green, or target-specific probes.

While primers determine the intended target, more specific detection of a product is achieved with probes. There are four types of probes in general use: fluorescence resonance energy transfer (FRET), TaqMan, molecular beacon, and Scorpion probes **(Fig. 12–23).** These probes hybridize because their sequence is complementary to the target sequence. Fluorescent signals from the accumulating PCR products are generated when the probes bind to their target. SYBR Green is not sequence-specific, so artifacts of the PCR reaction (misprimes and primer dimers) will also produce a signal. Since the probes are sequence-specific, they provide higher specificity than SYBR Green for the intended product.

Figure 12–24 shows PCR product accumulation detected with TaqMan probes through 50 PCR cycles. Depicted on the *y*-axis is the fluorescence signal from the dye or probe. The log of the fluorescence units plotted vs the cycle number on the *x*-axis generates a curve similar to a bacterial growth curve with a lag phase, log phase, linear phase, and stationary phase. The length of the lag phase is assessed by counting the number of PCR cycles required to reach a threshold level of fluorescence. The threshold is determined from the standard deviation of the background or baseline fluorescence levels. The cycle on the *x*-axis at which the fluorescence of each sample reaches this value is called the *threshold cycle* or *Ct*.

A relationship between the amount of target and the Ct values is established by generating a standard curve of dilutions of known target nucleic acid concentrations **(Fig. 12–25).** The molar concentration can be converted to number of molecules using Avogadro's number (6.022×10^{23} molecules/mole). Each test sample target is quantified by converting its

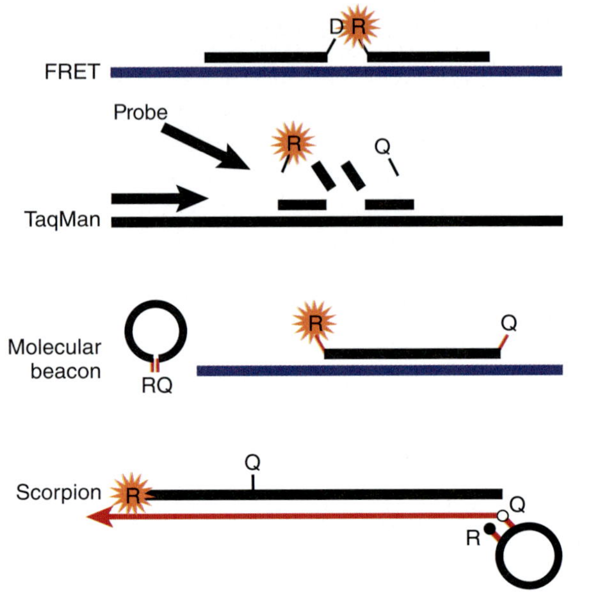

FIGURE 12–23 Probe systems for quantitative PCR. **FRET probes** generate signal when target (or copies of target) sequences are present. When the donor (D) and reporter (R) probes bind, energy provided to the reporter dye by the donor dye generates a fluorescent signal. **TaqMan probes** generate a signal as the target DNA is copied, resulting in the degradation of the probe, releasing the reporter dye (R) from a quencher (Q) and allowing the reporter dye to fluoresce. **Molecular beacons** also contain a reporter (R) and quencher (Q), which are separated upon probe hybridization to the target. **Scorpion probes** are molecular beacons covalently attached to the 5′ end of a primer. With each replication of target, the Scorpion probe is opened, separating the reporter from the quencher dye and generating signal.

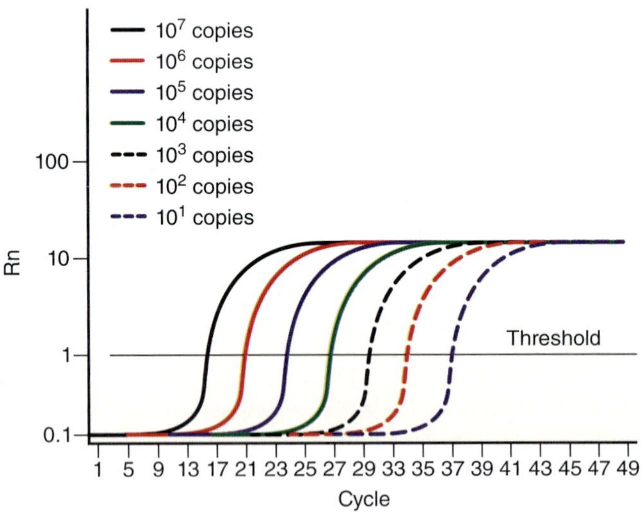

FIGURE 12–24 Real-time quantitative PCR signal generated from a TaqMan probe. The normalized fluorescence (ΔRn) is plotted against PCR cycles 1 to 50. The threshold level (the value at which fluorescence becomes detectable) is indicated by the black line. The number of PCR cycles required to reach the threshold (the Ct) is inversely correlated with the amount of starting material. For example, in this graph, the Ct value of the sample with 10^7 copies is 15, whereas the Ct value of the sample with 10^1 copies is 37.

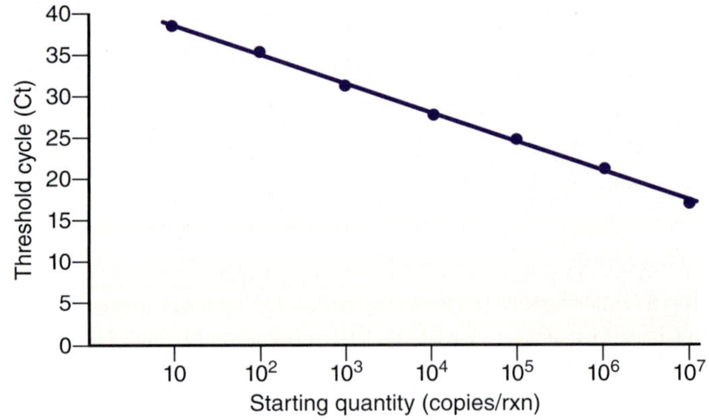

FIGURE 12–25 Ct values (*y*-axis) were determined for serial 10-fold dilutions of a synthetic target of known concentration (*x*-axis). The resulting standard curve is used to convert Ct values of a test sample to its concentration.

Ct to the concentration or number of molecules according to the standard curve.

To correct for differences in the amount of sample nucleic acid added to each reaction and reduce other variations from the test sample, an internal amplification control is included in each qPCR reaction. This control is a gene target that is always present at a constant level. For qPCR and RT-qPCR, internal controls also confirm negative results as true negatives and not PCR failure. The internal control can also be used as an alternate way to quantify the sample.

Internal comparison of test targets relative to control targets is known as the delta Ct (ΔCt) method. Genes that are constitutively expressed under diverse conditions such as β-actin and 18S rRNA, are common choices for reference or control genes. Quantification of the target gene relative to the control is determined by the difference (ΔCt) resulting from subtracting the threshold cycle of the control gene from that of the target gene in the test sample:

$$\Delta Ct = Ct_{\text{target gene}} - Ct_{\text{control gene}}$$

In RT-qPCR, the relative quantification of target gene transcripts in test samples may be normalized to that of control or reference samples. Normalization is determined by a second ΔCt, or ΔΔCt, the difference resulting from subtracting the gene's ΔCt in the reference sample from the gene's ΔC in the test sample:

$$\Delta\Delta Ct = \Delta Ct_{\text{target sample}} - \Delta Ct_{\text{reference sample}}$$

To determine the effect or state of gene expression in the test sample, $2^{-\Delta\Delta cT}$ is calculated by raising 2 to the negative ΔΔCt. This is the fold increase or decrease of relative target gene expression in the test sample relative to the reference sample.

These calculations assume optimal amplification efficiencies of the target and control genes in test and reference samples. If a control gene amplification efficiency is not optimal or dissimilar to that of the target gene, then the standard curve method may be used.

Frequent applications of qPCR and RT-qPCR include detecting microorganisms, especially viruses and other pathogens that are difficult or dangerous to culture in the laboratory, gene expression, and tissue typing. qPCR testing has also been applied to measurement of donor bone marrow in the recipient after a heterologous bone marrow transplant.

Digital PCR (dPCR)

Another type of quantitative PCR is **digital PCR (dPCR)**, which provides absolute quantification, that is, numerical expression of the number of molecules in the sample, in contrast to the concentration or the number of molecules relative to a control. Furthermore, digital PCR measurements are made after the amplification program has finished (at the endpoint); therefore, they are not affected by variations in PCR efficiencies.

Digital PCR is based on limiting dilution of sample template molecules and separate amplification of each molecule in separate picoliter- to nanoliter-volume reactions. Separate reactions occur in partitions on microfluidic chips or disks, microarrays, microdroplets in oil-water emulsions, or qPCR-like plates. In chamber-based dPCR, a microfluidic distribution system delivers PCR reagents to fixed microchambers **(Fig. 12–26A).** In droplet-based partitioning (droplet digital PCR [ddPCR]), microfluidic emulsification systems produce uniform droplets forming a water-in-oil emulsion that is stable under the PCR conditions **(Fig. 12–26B).** The number of separate reactions or partitions (over 20,000 in fixed array microchambers) must be large enough to achieve limiting dilution of sample target, where most partitions will have at least one or no target templates.

The partitioned reaction mixes are subjected to a PCR amplification program. DNA-specific fluorescent dyes or target-specific probes are used to detect the presence of product. After amplification, partitions that received at least one template molecule will contain product, and those without template will not. Therefore, only those reactions that have received at least one template will have a fluorescent signal. Instrument detection systems capture the fluorescence from fixed microchambers in the dPCR reactions. Droplets in oil emulsion are counted sequentially by a flow-cytometry–like analysis. Instrument software translates the positive:total droplet ratio to the absolute number of target molecules in the starting sample.

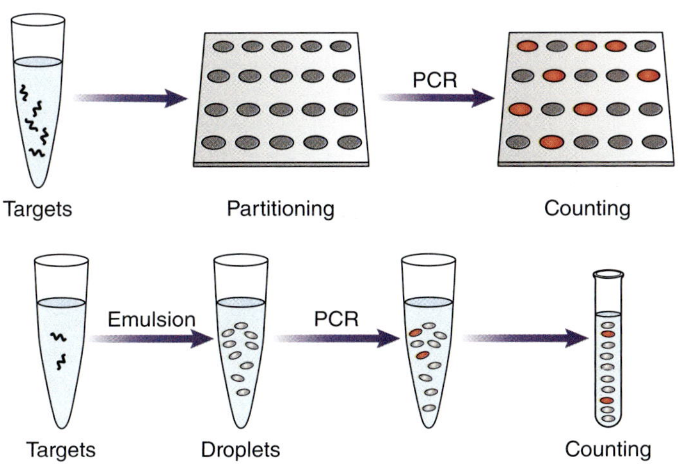

FIGURE 12–26 (A) Digital PCR requires partitioning of the sample such that any partition will receive one or no target templates. After PCR, the partitions are counted, and the ratio of positive wells:negative wells determines the absolute number of target molecules in the original sample. (B) Droplet digital PCR quantifies the absolute number of target molecules by limiting dilution into an emulsion of individual aqueous droplets, each containing one or no template molecule. After the PCR droplets with product are counted, the ratio of empty droplets to product-containing droplets determines the absolute number of molecules in the specimen.

The dynamic range of dPCR is less than that of qPCR, such that the starting concentration of target in dPCR must be sufficient for limiting dilution in the number of available partitions. The linear response of the digital PCR quantification, however, allows the resolution of small changes in target number that is not possible by qPCR. Digital PCR has been applied to analysis of gene copy number variation, detection of rare mutations, liquid biopsies, and infectious disease.

Knowledge Check 12-7

Unlike qPCR, dPCR detects:

a. Absolute quantity of product
b. Relative quantity of products
c. Relative quantity of template
d. Absolute quantity of template

Isothermal Amplification Methods

A variety of methods have been developed since the introduction of PCR that do not require temperature cycling. We discuss these methods in the sections that follow.

Transcription-Mediated Amplification (TMA)

Commercial versions of amplification through an RNA intermediate include transcription-mediated amplification (TMA), nucleic acid sequence–based amplification (NASBA), and self-sustaining sequence replication (3SR). These methods are similar, with variations in enzyme systems.

For transcription-based amplification systems, RNA is the target as well as the primary product. A complementary DNA copy (cDNA) is synthesized from the target RNA, and then transcription of the cDNA produces millions of copies of RNA products. The RNA products transcribed from the cDNA can also serve as target RNA for synthesis of more cDNA **(Fig. 12–27).** The RNA products are detected by chemiluminescence with acridinium ester or, in the case of NASBA, molecular beacon probes.

Targeting RNA allows for direct detection of RNA viruses, such as HCV and HIV. Targeting the RNA of organisms with DNA genomes, such as *Mycobacterium tuberculosis,* is more sensitive than targeting the DNA, because each microorganism makes multiple copies of RNA, whereas it has only one copy of DNA per cell. Detection of *Chlamydia trachomatis* in genital specimens, and cytomegalovirus (CMV) quantification in blood are additional applications for TMA. The high sensitivity of TMA is especially suitable for critical tests such as blood screening.

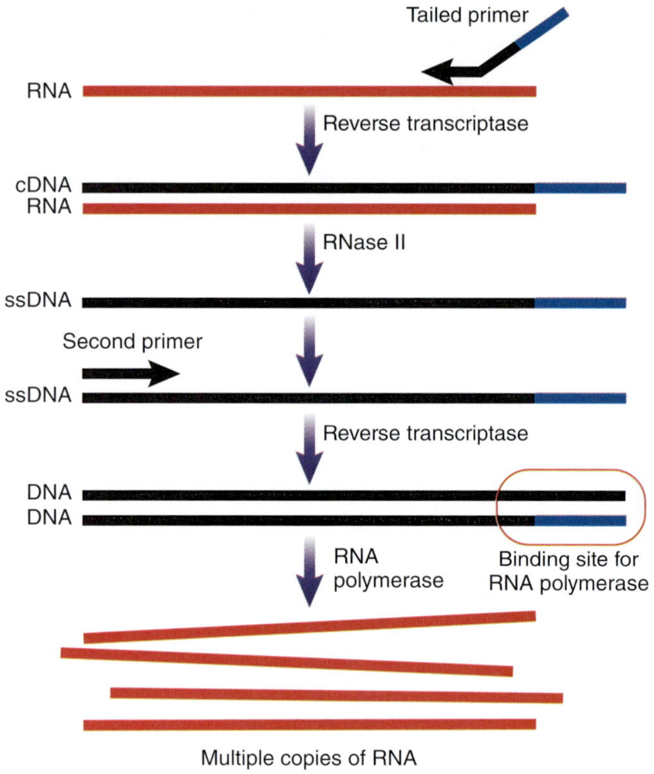

FIGURE 12–27 Transcription-mediated amplification (TMA) targets RNA. In the first step, a cDNA:RNA hybrid is synthesized by reverse transcriptase using a primer with a tail (that will ultimately form the binding site for a later enzyme). Hybridized (but not single-stranded) RNA is degraded by RNase II, leaving single-stranded DNA. This ssDNA serves as a template for reverse transcriptase to synthesize a complementary strand of DNA, including the primer tail, to complete the binding site for RNA polymerase. The RNA polymerase uses dsDNA as a template to synthesize many copies of RNA. This new RNA can cycle back to step one and repeat the process, resulting in a large amplification of product.

Loop-Mediated Amplification (LAMP)

In **loop-mediated amplification (LAMP)**, double-stranded DNA templates can be amplified without repeatedly raising the reaction temperature to denature them. Forward and reverse PCR primers carry sequences at the 5′ end to make products that will self-hybridize, forming loops. The single-stranded loops then serve as primer binding sites for further amplification without having to raise the reaction temperature for denaturation **(Fig. 12–28).** An advantage of this process is the shortened run time (less than 30 minutes). LAMP methods are used to detect CMV, *Staphylococcus aureus*, *E. coli*, and HIV.

Knowledge Check 12-8

Which of the following is an isothermal amplification mechanism?

a. Enzymatic probe dissociation
b. Repeated thermal denaturation of double-stranded DNA
c. Limiting template dilution
d. Primer binding sites on hairpin loops

Critical Thinking 12-1

DNA was isolated from formalin-fixed paraffin-embedded tumor tissue. A long (160 bp) and a short (90 bp) product were amplified from the isolated DNA. The laboratory assessed the integrity of the DNA by qPCR. The DNA integrity was calculated by subtracting the Ct of the short product from the Ct of the long product. If the difference between the Ct values of the 90 bp fragment and the 160 bp fragment was large (e.g., 50 cycles), how would this affect the molecular testing of the tumor DNA? What would a small difference in the Ct values of the two fragments (e.g., three cycles) mean?

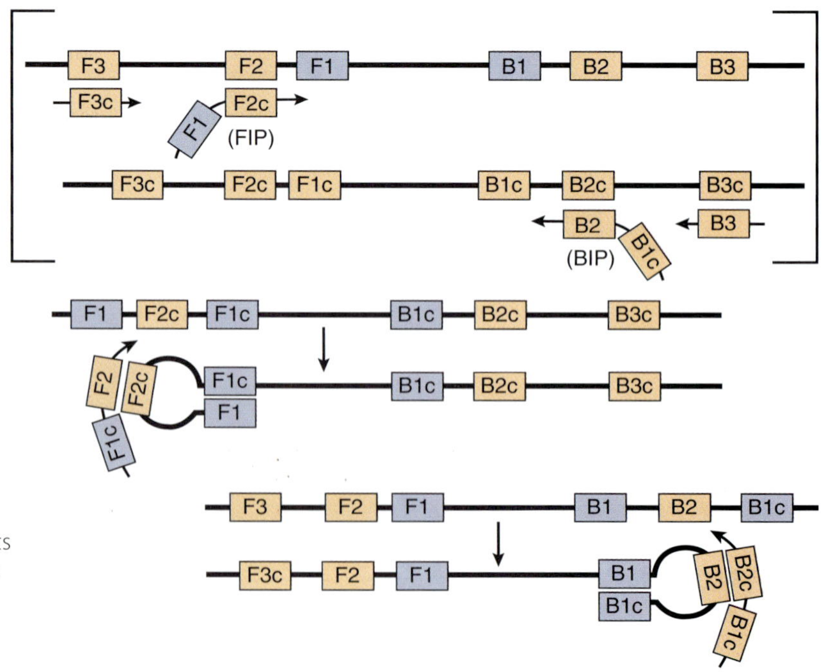

FIGURE 12–28 (A) In loop-mediated amplification (LAMP), the forward inner primer (FIP) and reverse or backward inner primer (BIP) are tailed with sequences complementary to sequences within the copied area (F1 and B1c). (B) Displacement of the copied DNA by extension of outer primers (F3c and B3) produces products that will form single-stranded loops. This system achieves isothermal amplification through repeated copying primed by FIP and BIP in the single-stranded looped sequences.

DNA Sequencing

Sequencing and resequencing of DNA and RNA are routine laboratory methods. Sequence alterations are not always in predicted locations in genes, requiring survey of most or all of the gene or transcript. Sequencing is used extensively in microbiology, genetics, and oncology for definitive identification of organisms or gene abnormalities. It is also used for high-resolution HLA typing of potential donors and recipients for bone marrow and tissue transplants.

Germline or inherited variations in the human DNA are readily detected, usually from blood specimens. Somatic (noninherited) mutations in clinical specimens, such as cancerous tumors, are sometimes difficult to detect as they may be diluted by normal sequences that mask the somatic change.

Chain Termination (Sanger) Sequencing

Chain termination sequencing, named after biochemist Frederick Sanger, is a modification of the DNA replication process that uses dideoxy nucleotide triphosphates (ddNTP), which lack a hydroxyl group on the 3′ carbon of the ribose sugar moiety, as we previously mentioned **(Fig. 12–29).**

In a standard sequencing reaction, a short, synthetic single-stranded DNA fragment (primer) complementary to sequences just 5′ to the region of DNA to be sequenced is needed to start DNA synthesis. All components required for DNA synthesis are added to the primer and template. This reaction would ordinarily result in polymerization of deoxyribonucleotides to make full-length copies of the DNA template. However, because fluorescently labeled ddNTPs are added to the reaction, DNA synthesis will stop upon incorporation of a ddNTP into the growing DNA chain (chain termination) because the 5′-3′ phosphodiester bond cannot be made. Therefore, the newly synthesized chains will terminate at different lengths when the ddNTP is added in different positions **(Fig. 12–30).**

To perform a manual dideoxy sequencing reaction, the region of the sample DNA to be sequenced is first amplified by PCR. The double-stranded PCR product is cleaned of residual PCR primers and other reaction components using an exonuclease enzyme and/or alcohol precipitation. The resulting cleaned product is the sequencing template. The template is mixed with ingredients of the sequencing reaction, which includes a sequencing primer, dNTPs, DNA polymerase, and the four ddNTPs. Each ddNTP is labeled with a different fluorescent wavelength molecule (ddATP green, ddCTP blue, ddGTP black or yellow, ddTTP red) so that the products of the sequencing reaction that compose the DNA ladder can be distinguished by color.

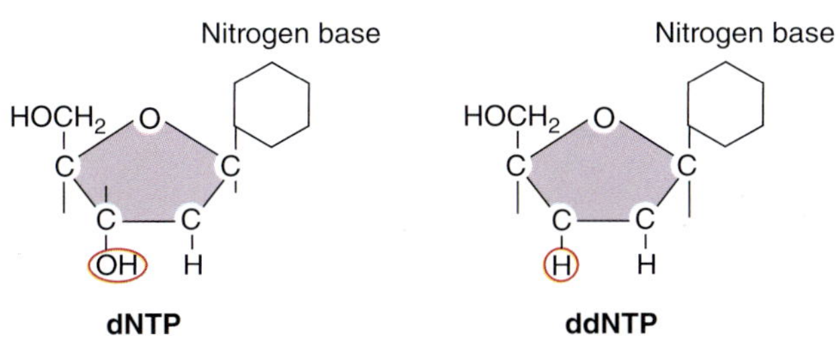

FIGURE 12–29 Dideoxyribonucleotides lack the 3′ hydroxyl group necessary for formation of the phosphodiester bond during DNA replication.

The sequencing reaction takes place in a thermal cycler programmed to copy one strand of the template primed by the single sequencing primer. Template copies will terminate whenever DNA polymerase inserts a ddNTP. Proper proportion of ddNTPs to dNTPs in the reaction ensures the even termination of copied strands throughout the template sequence. If the ddNTP:dNTP ratio is too high, only short fragments will be generated. If the ddNTP:dNTP ratio is too low, mostly full-length copies of the template will result. The product of a successful sequencing reaction is a DNA ladder with equal representation of long and short fragments, terminated by the four ddNTP.

The resulting fluorescently labeled DNA ladder is resolved by capillary gel electrophoresis. In contrast to fragment size analysis by gel electrophoresis, the sequencing image from capillary gel electrophoresis is an electropherogram of fluorescent peaks **(Fig. 12–31).** Sequences are read by color, left to right (smaller to larger fragments).

A Sanger sequencing reaction is performed on a single DNA strand of the double-stranded template. When a sequence change is detected, the alteration can be confirmed by sequencing the complementary strand of the DNA by priming the synthesis reaction on the strand complementary to the strand that was sequenced. Alterations affecting a single base pair may be subtle on an electropherogram, especially if the alteration is in the heterozygous form, or mixed with normal reference sequence, as is the case in hematological or solid tumor samples in oncology. Sanger sequencing with capillary electrophoresis was the method of choice for the introduction of high-resolution HLA typing.

Pyrosequencing

Pyrosequencing is an alternate sequencing method first developed in the 1980s. The procedure relies on the generation of light (luminescence) when nucleotides are added to a growing strand of DNA. With this system, there are no gels, fluorescent dyes, or ddNTPs. The sequencing is performed on a pyrosequencer. The pyrosequencer is a luminometer that delivers nucleotides (dNTPs) and detects emitted light.

The pyrosequencing reaction is performed on single-stranded DNA templates prepared from double-stranded PCR products by denaturation and bead capture of one strand. The beads carrying the templates are then mixed with a sequencing primer, enzymes, and reaction mix. In a predetermined order, the pyrosequencer introduces dNTPs sequentially to the reaction. If the introduced nucleotide is complementary to the base in the template strand next to the 3′ end of the primer, DNA polymerase forms a phosphodiester bond between the primer and the nucleotide, releasing pyrophosphate (PPi; **Fig. 12–32**). The released PPi enters

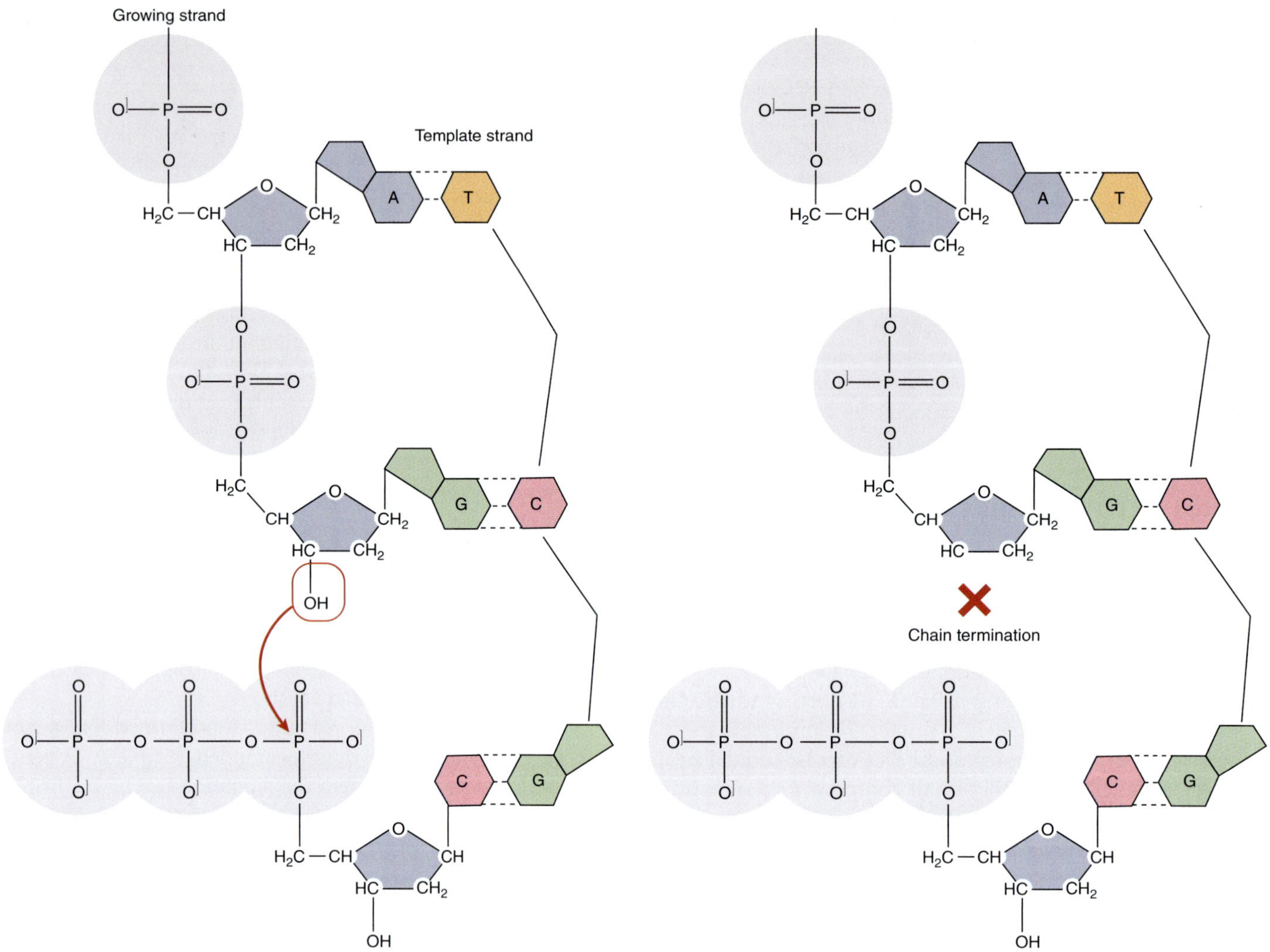

FIGURE 12–30 (A) DNA synthesis proceeds by formation of a phosphodiester bond between the ribose 3′OH of a previous nucleotide and the ribose 5′ phosphate group of the incoming nucleotide. (B) If the 3′OH is missing, as in ddNTP, synthesis terminates (right).

a reaction cascade that generates a luminescent signal. This signal indicates that the introduced nucleotide is the correct base in the sequence. The pyrosequencing reaction generates a pyrogram of luminescent peaks associated with the addition of the complementary nucleotides (Fig. 12–32).

Because pyrosequencing produces short- to moderate-length sequence information (up to 100 bases), it is not as versatile as Sanger sequencing, which can produce reads longer than 1,000 bases. However, two factors have kept pyrosequencing in use. With increasing identification of clinically important gene "hot spots" of variants and SNPs, it became necessary to sequence only targeted areas, the immediate regions around the nucleotide base change. Since pyrosequencing is less labor intensive than Sanger sequencing, it is more convenient for these types of short sequence analyses. Also, the first instruments developed with the introduction of genomic or next-generation sequencing used the pyrosequencing chemistry.

Knowledge Check 12-9

Which molecule will result in DNA synthesis chain termination?

a. Pyrophosphate
b. Dideoxynucleotide triphosphate
c. Adenosine 5′ phosphosulfate
d. Deoxynucleotide triphosphate

Next-Generation Sequencing

The highly informative, original sequencing methods were limited by the expense and labor required to analyze large genetic regions or microbial populations. **Next-generation sequencing (NGS)** methods now provide the ability to investigate whole genomes and microbiomes. There are two components of this technology: library preparation and sequencing.

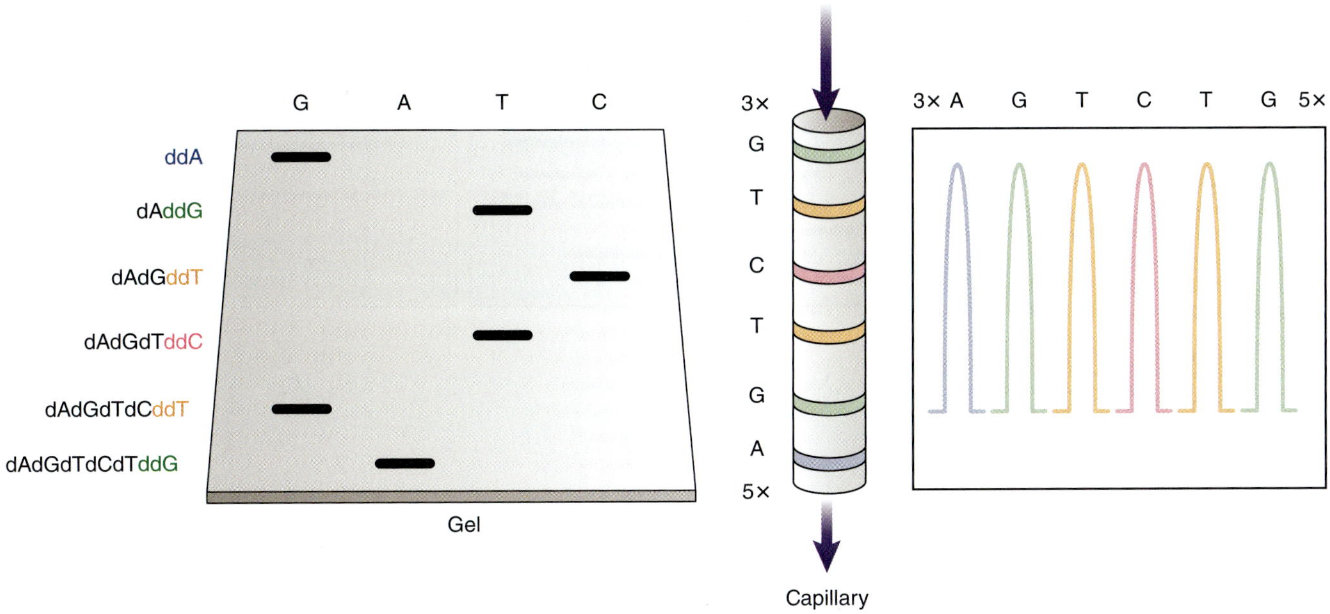

FIGURE 12–31 A DNA ladder (left) resolved by capillary gel electrophoresis is read from the bottom of the gel to the top of the gel (shortest fragment to the longest). The terminating base is determined by its presence of a band in the corresponding gel lane (G, A, T, or C). In dye terminator sequencing, the sequence is read automatically as fluorescently labeled fragments migrate through the gel or capillary. Each fragment passes a detector that will generate an electropherogram of fluorescent peaks (right). Sequencing software will produce a text report of the DNA sequence.

Step 1

$$(DNA)_n + dNTP \xrightarrow{\text{Polymerase}} (DNA)_{n+1} + PPi$$

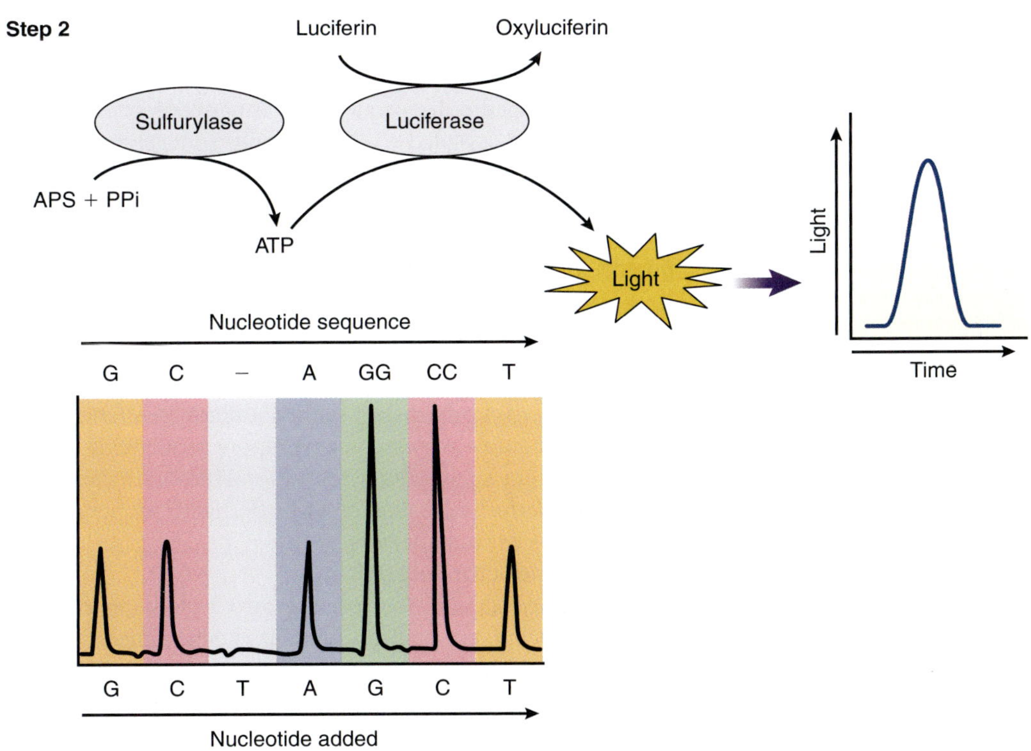

FIGURE 12–32 Pyrosequencing determines a nucleotide sequence by introducing dNTPs to the sequencing reaction in a predetermined order. If the nucleotide is not complementary to the template sequence, no reaction occurs, and the nucleotide is then degraded. If the nucleotide is complementary to the sequence, polymerase forms a phosphodiester bond extending the primer and releasing pyrophosphate (PPi, step 1). The pyrophosphate then goes through a series of reactions to ultimately produce a chemiluminescent signal (step 2). The pyrosequencing output is a pyrogram, as shown at the bottom.

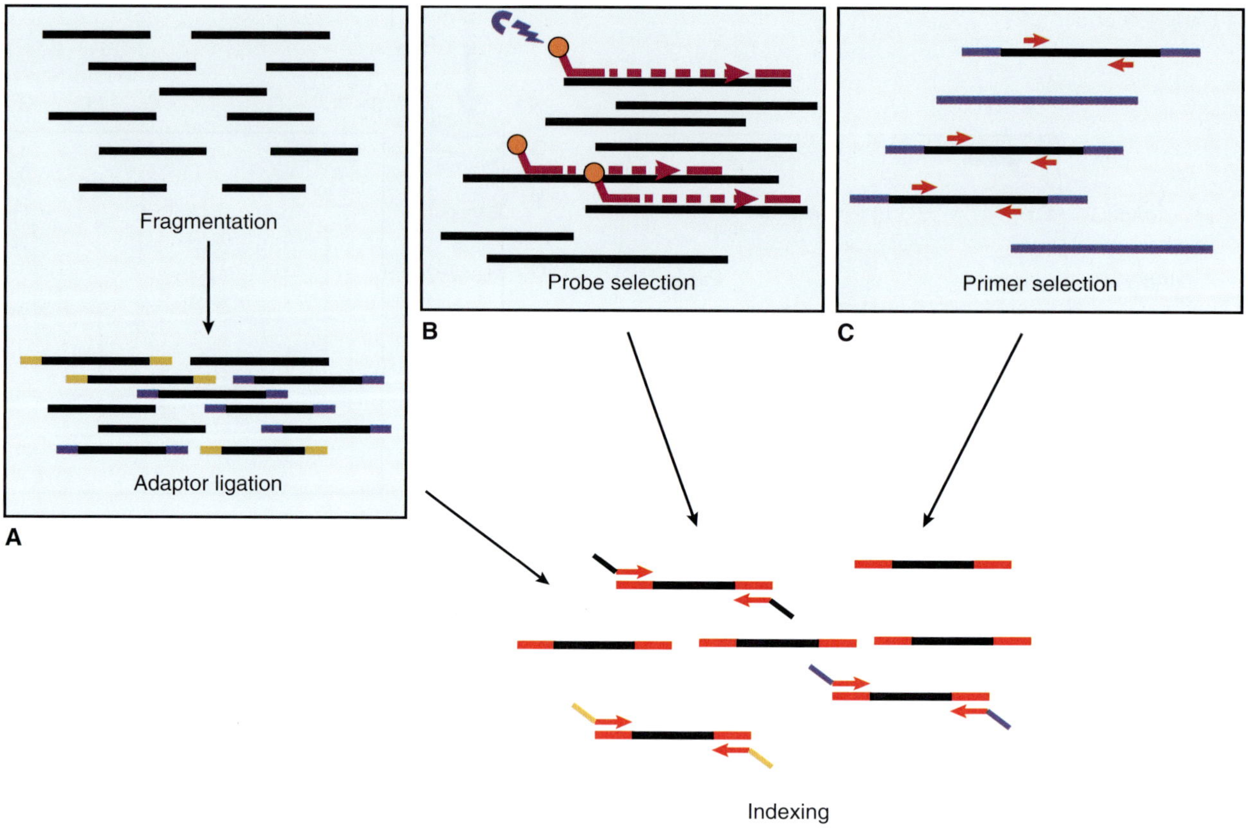

FIGURE 12–33 DNA libraries for NGS are prepared using fragmentation, probe enrichment, or primer selection of specific genes or gene regions. (A) Adapters carrying primer binding sites are ligated to the ends of fragmented DNA. These adapters carry primer binding sites as well as index sequences for direct amplification and sequencing. (B) The library can be enriched for selected regions using probes. Probes are attached to magnetic beads to capture the complementary DNA regions with magnets applied to the outside of tubes or plates. (C) Primer selection produces high coverage sequencing of specific genes. Primers may be tailed with binding sites for subsequent unbiased amplification of the selected regions. In a second PCR reaction, primers that carry short index DNA sequences identify each sample, as all samples in a run are pooled and sequenced simultaneously.

Library Preparation

In contrast to chain termination sequencing, most NGS is performed on short DNA templates, usually less than 1 kb. A set of fragments can be prepared from enzymatically digested or sonicated genomic DNA **(Fig. 12–33A).** Short sections of DNA can be selected from whole genomes or from larger fragments with probes **(Fig. 12–33B)** or primers **(Fig. 12–33C)** to further define the sequencing targets.

A collection of fragments generated by these methods comprises a *library.* A library can include selected genes or gene regions *(targeted libraries* or *gene panels),* all coding DNA or exons *(whole exome sequencing),* or whole genomes *(whole genome sequencing).* Targeted and exome sequencing are applied to clinical testing. For example, libraries for analysis of the MHC locus by NGS are constructed by PCR selection and amplification of the class I and class II genes.

After selection of regions to be sequenced, sequence adapters are added to the fragment ends by ligation or 5′ end tailed to primers. Adapters are synthetic oligonucleotides carrying PCR primer binding sites. These common primer binding sites allow secondary unbiased PCR amplification of all fragments in a sample. Indexing primers also carry short noncomplementary sequences or "bar codes" to identify samples pooled together for sequencing. A bar code or index is a short sequence assigned to each sample and gene region in the library. As multiple samples are sequenced together in a run, bar codes associate sequences with their samples. The PCR products are then cleaned of residual reaction products, pooled, and introduced to the sequencer.

Sequencing

Mass-marketed technologies of next-generation sequencing included array-based pyrosequencing, sequencing by synthesis with reversible dyes, ion semiconductor, sequencing by ligation, and single molecule or nanopore sequencing. Clinical applicaltions such as high-resolution HLA typing are most commonly performed using ion semiconductor sequencing or reversible dye terminator sequencing.

Ion Semiconductor Sequencing

In ion semiconductor sequencing, also called *ion conductance sequencing,* the nucleotide order is determined through release of hydrogen ions by DNA synthesis on a semiconductor or ion chip. The chip contains millions of wells covering an ion-sensitive layer.

DNA library fragments are attached to and amplified on millions of beads. The beads are then distributed across the chip into millions of wells. The chip is then flooded sequentially with each of the four nucleotides. When a nucleotide complementary to a template is introduced and incorporated, the release of a hydrogen ion is detected by a pH change in the reaction **(Fig. 12–34A).** Unattached dNTP molecules are washed away before introducing the next cycle of dNTP addition. The metal-oxide-semiconductor chip contains an ion-sensitive layer, which allows parallel, simultaneous detection of hundreds of thousands of independent sequencing reactions.

One limitation of ion semiconductor sequencing is potentially inaccurate detection of single base repeat sequences (homopolymers). In a template sequence with a long homopolymer stretch, a percentage of the pH change may be lost with each sequential repeating nucleotide incorporation. As a result, the detected change in pH is not exactly correlated with the number of hydrogen ions released per reaction. The sequence detected may therefore not have accuracy at these single base repeats. Another limitation of this method is the shorter read length (about 400 nucleotides per read), compared to other sequencing methods. An advantage of ion semiconductor sequencing is the use of nonmodified, nonlabeled nucleotides, which lowers the cost and increases the availability of the procedure. Another advantage is the more rapid sequencing speed compared to fluorescence-based sequencing.

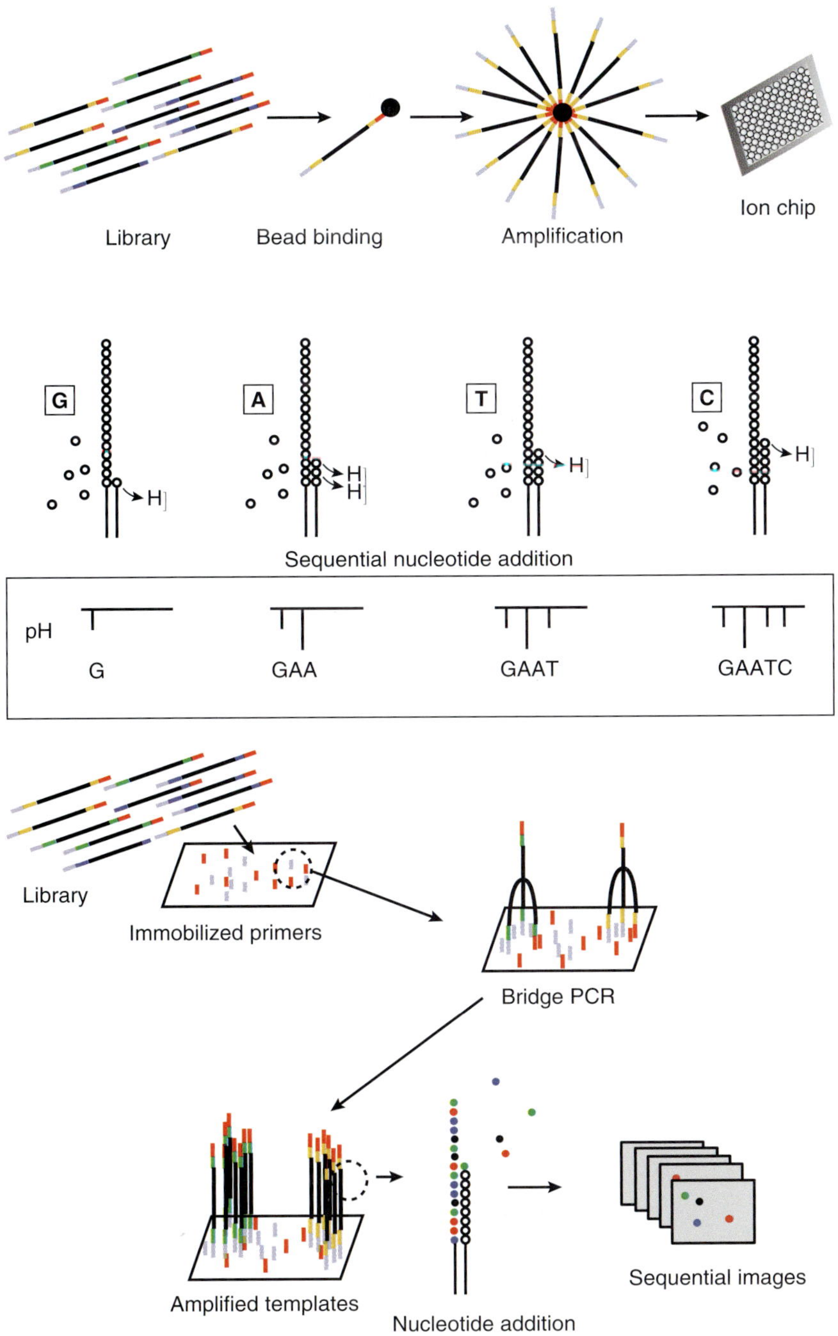

FIGURE 12–34 (Top) In ion chip sequencing, the pooled, indexed DNA libraries and sequencing primers are applied to an ion chip in individual micro-DNA synthesis reactions. Nucleotides are introduced sequentially to the chip, and if the introduced nucleotide is complementary to the template sequence, a phosphodiester bond is formed, releasing a hydrogen ion. A sensor detects the resulting pH change correlated with addition of each nucleotide base. (Bottom) For reversible dye terminator sequencing, the pooled, indexed libraries are hybridized to immobilized primers at millions of positions on a solid support (flow cell). Each molecule of DNA is then amplified in place by bridge PCR. The amplified templates are sequenced by synthesis with simultaneous addition of the four fluorescently color-coded nucleotides. Nucleotides complementary to each amplified template are added to the end of the growing chain. Nucleotides are blocked, preventing addition of more than one base with each round of synthesis. An image is made of the flow cell after each nucleotide addition. The blocking molecules and fluorescent signals from the nucleotides are then removed, followed by addition of the next round of nucleotides. The sequential images are converted to sequence information for each template.

Reversible Dye Terminator Sequencing

Reversible dye terminator technology is also called *sequencing by synthesis*. Sequencing templates are generated from the library in a final *bridge PCR* amplification reaction using primers immobilized at millions of locations on a glass support (flow cell) inside of the sequencing instrument. The immobilized primers are complementary to sequences added to the ends of the library fragments in the PCR steps of the library preparation. The result of the bridge PCR on the flow cell will be millions of clusters of immobilized amplicons. The amplicons are denatured to produce clusters of single-stranded sequencing templates.

Sequencing occurs on the immobilized templates by addition, detection, and removal of the four nucleotide labels **(Fig. 12–34B)**. Sequencing primers, DNA polymerase, and modified nucleotides are added to the sequencing reaction inside of the instrument. The nucleotides are modified by attaching fluorescent molecules to the nitrogen bases and a blocker on the ribose 3′ hydroxyl group. These bonds can be broken so that fluorescent labeling and 3′-OH blocking are reversible. The color (emission wavelength) of the fluorescent molecules is different for each nucleotide (A, C, T, or G).

Sequencing begins with primer hybridization to the complementary sites on each immobilized amplicon. DNA polymerase makes a single base extension of the primer with fluorescently labeled nucleotides complementary to the template. Further extension is temporarily blocked by the 3′-OH ribose modification. An image is made of the fluorescence emission from each cluster across the flow cell. Then, the fluorescent labels and blockers are removed, and the next bases (labeled and blocked) are added to each growing chain. This process is repeated 150 to 300 times to generate the sequence determined at each cluster location. This process, known as *massive parallel sequencing*, occurs simultaneously among all the clusters, allowing millions of sequences to be determined at one time.

Knowledge Check 12-10

What is the purpose of indexing in next-generation sequencing?

a. Production of template clusters
b. Identification of samples in pooled libraries
c. Selection of regions to be sequenced
d. Initiation of unbiased PCR amplification

Metagenomic Sequencing

Metagenomics is a microbiological application of NGS to detect multiple pathogens in a clinical sample. Metagenomic next-generation sequencing (mNGS) of plasma, bronchoalveolar lavage fluid, sputum, or tissue homogenates detects circulating cell-free DNA from pathogens. It is useful for rare, novel, and atypical clinical presentations of complicated infectious diseases. The advantage of mNGS in these cases is unbiased detection of a variety of organisms, which would otherwise require species-specific probes or primers. Samples are tested for all microbial nucleic acids that may be present. The resulting sequences can be compared with known genomic databases of bacterial, viral, fungal, and parasitic pathogens.

For metagenomic analysis, sample DNA is fragmented and subjected to library preparation and sequencing. There are targeted methods that make libraries of conserved 16s rRNA, 18s rRNA, or fungal internal transcribed spacer (ITS) regions; however, targeted analysis does not provide identification down to the species level. In contrast, "shotgun" mNGS libraries cover all sequences in the sample, including different parts of the genome of each organism present.

After sequencing, the genomes are assembled, and any genes present are analyzed to identify the organisms. By assessing particular gene structures, metabolic pathways, resistance factors, or other information may be determined. mNGS can be especially useful where standard testing fails to identify the pathogen in infected patients. Furthermore, it is not affected by prior antibiotic treatments, in contrast to culture methods. There are, however, some limitations to the method. Specificity can be low, so detection of sequences is compromised in immunosuppressed patients or in cases where mucosal barriers are damaged. In these conditions, multiple microbes may populate a sample, confounding identification of a target or causative microorganisms.

Knowledge Check 12-11

Which technology includes bridge PCR?

a. Reversible dye terminator sequencing
b. Sanger sequencing
c. Ion semiconductor sequencing
d. Pyrosequencing

Critical Thinking 12-2

The laboratory is investigating a failed NGS sequencing run. The reversible dye terminator sequencing began with long-range PCR performed on solid-phase–isolated DNA. The quantity of input DNA was confirmed to be adequate for sequencing by spectrophotometry, which also confirmed good purity. The products of the long-range PCR (5 to 6 kbp) were enzymatically fragmented, and common primer binding sites were added to the fragments. The 300 to 500 bp fragments were then used as templates for PCR with primers carrying adapter and barcode sequences on their 5′ end. The samples were analyzed for product size by electrophoresis and subsequently pooled. When the pool was subjected to reversible dye terminator sequencing, an error message of insufficient cluster intensity appeared on the sequencer, and no data were produced. Maintenance logs and instrument functional checks showed no instrument problems. What part of the protocol described might have affected the sequencing run? How might this step be corrected?

Sequence Data Analysis

The accuracy of sequencing data interpretation depends on the condition of the template, the efficiency of the sequencing reaction, and the quality of the sequence imaging. For all NGS methods, sequence data in the form of processed images or conductance scans are collected by instrument software. The quality of each base determination is assessed and then the sequence is called by a base caller algorithm. For clinical sequencing, a 1/1,000 probability of base calling error is recommended. The pertinent sequence data are then extracted and tabulated, after which indexing or other primer sequences may be trimmed from the sequence. The sorted sequences are then aligned with a reference sequence for variant calling. For typing or metagenomics, overlapping sequences are assembled into longer reads and matched to known reference sequences. Base calling, quality assessment, data extraction, trimming, assembly, alignment, variant calling, and matching are performed in software programs, which together compose a pipeline. There are a variety of programs for each of these tasks, depending on the sequencing application.

After a successful NGS run, areas of interest will have been sequenced from a few times to thousands of times. The number of times a region is sequenced is referred to as the *coverage*. Whole human genomes will have lower coverage (30 to 40×, 3 billion bp sequenced) than whole exome sequencing (sequencing of only protein coding regions; 50 to 100×, 30 to 50 million base pairs sequenced). Gene panels of a few hundred targeted genes are sequenced with higher coverage than genomes or exomes, depending on the number of genes included in the panel (e.g., 5,000× for the MHC locus). A 500× coverage is the minimal coverage required to call rare variants, such as might be present in mixed tissue samples (e.g., tumor tissue containing lymphocytes or other normal tissue). Cost is the limiting factor for the depth of coverage used. Not included in the sequencing cost are challenges of interpretation, reporting, and data storage.

A sequence variant (difference from the reference sequence) may be present in some or all the copies of the sequence covered. The percentage of sequences carrying the variant is the allele frequency in the sample. Somatic variants tend to have low allele frequencies, while germline (inherited) sequence changes will comprise 50% or 100% of the covered sequences.

Manufacturers have developed software programs to produce a finished report from targeted gene panels, with variants identified automatically along with quality, variant type, allele frequency (what percentage of the coverage contains the variant), and clinical significance. Nucleotide or protein sequence data may be stored as text files in the FASTA or FASTQ format (named after a DNA and protein sequence alignment software package first described in 1985). FASTA files are text of nucleotide sequence only. FASTQ files include a quality symbol for each base.

Regarding variant calling, NGS tends to be more error prone than Sanger sequencing, mostly due to the library preparation. Errors must be distinguished from true sequence variants in a sample. Variant frequency less than 2% may indicate sequence error. The error frequency will limit the sequencing method sensitivity, that is, only variants with frequencies greater than 2% will be called. Errors are minimized with adequate coverage, database information, and software algorithms.

Filters are designed to address accuracy issues before calling DNA alterations from a reference sequence. Filtering is the elimination or inclusion of sequence data based on parameters set by the user (variant frequency, coverage, quality scores).

Nucleic acid sequence data may be translated into the amino acid sequence using the genetic code. Intron or silent mutations that do not change protein sequence or conservative mutations that do not affect protein function or antigenicity are not likely to be biologically significant. Even variants that do change protein structure may not always be clinically significant. The medical significance of variants and the genes in which they are found is assessed by annotation. **Annotation** involves searching databases of variants and phenotypic associations to identify significant and reportable alterations. Different analysis systems may handle the sequence data differently such that reports may not be the same.

NGS has advanced the accuracy and extent of gene and allele identification, for example, in HLA typing. Once the sequencing is completed and samples identified from their bar codes, algorithms are used by designated software to determine genotypes. Analysis may include alignment and matching with known alleles from designated databases. Another type of algorithm performs sequence assembly from the short overlapping fragments without relying on a database to detect novel alleles. The increased informativity and throughput of NGS allow resolution of ambiguities that were not possible with previous molecular methods including Sanger sequencing.

Massive parallel sequencing has become a significant component of molecular testing in many areas of medicine. For example, whole exome sequencing is used to identify variants responsible for inherited disease conditions. Driver mutations that dysregulate cell growth factors are diagnostic and therapeutic targets in cancer. Genomic and metagenomic analysis not only includes known targets or target organisms but also reveals novel disease factors.

Knowledge Check 12-12

After sequence alterations are detected by next-generation sequence analysis, parameters such as coverage, allele frequency, and quality score are set to confirm sequence variants. What is this process called?

a. Annotation
b. Base calling
c. Coding
d. Filtering

Critical Thinking 12-3

Commercially available amplicon-based HLA typing kits use PCR to amplify specific HLA alleles for library preparation before sequencing. The accuracy of the sequencing technology is high; however, errors can occur, mostly from the library preparation. For example, specific amplification failure can occur if the amplification conditions are not optimal for a primer set in the multiplex reaction. Or, primer annealing may be compromised by template mutations or polymorphisms in the primer binding sites. How would failed amplification affect interpretation of the sequencing results at a heterozygous locus (i.e., presence of two different alleles for a particular trait)?

KEY CONCEPTS

Deoxyribonucleic Acid (DNA) and Ribonucleic Acid (RNA)

- The two main types of nucleic acids are DNA and RNA. They are polymers made up of chains of nucleotides.
- Nucleotides of DNA contain a deoxyribose sugar with one of the following bases: adenine (A), guanine (G), thymine (T), or cytosine (C).
- RNA is made up of nucleotides containing a ribose sugar bonded to one of four nitrogen bases: adenine, guanine, cytosine, or uracil (U; instead of thymine).
- DNA is double stranded and arranged in a double helix, whereas RNA is typically single stranded.
- In a DNA molecule, complementary base pairing occurs; adenine (A) pairs with thymine (T), and guanine (G) pairs with cytosine (C).
- When a DNA molecule replicates, the two daughter strands separate; each is a template for a newly synthesized complementary strand.
- The high specificity of detecting nucleic acid sequences through complementary base pairing is the basis of all nucleic acid diagnostic testing.
- The central dogma of molecular biology refers to the fact that DNA serves as the template for messenger RNA, which in turn codes for proteins.
- Mutations and polymorphisms are changes in nucleotide sequences that may affect specific protein structure and function.

Nucleic Acid Isolation

- There are two main approaches to isolation and purification of nucleic acids: extraction by precipitation from solution and collection by solid-phase binding.

Electrophoresis of Nucleic Acids

- Gel and capillary electrophoresis are used in many molecular methods. In these techniques, the negatively charged DNA fragments are separated by size under the force of an electric current in a semisolid gel or polymer solution.

Molecular Analysis

- Restriction fragment length polymorphisms (RFLPs) are changes in DNA that result in different sized pieces when cleaved by restriction enzymes.
- CRISPR-Cas9 is a gene-editing system that can be used to alter DNA at specific locations.
- Hybridization is the specific binding of two complementary DNA strands or a DNA strand and an RNA strand. Often a probe, which has a short known nucleic acid sequence, is used to detect an unknown nucleic acid sequence in a sample.
- Hybridization techniques include Southern blot analysis, microarray technology for simultaneous assessment of multiple genes, and fluorescent in situ hybridization (FISH) for analysis of specific genetic regions.
- Amplification involves making many copies of a specific nucleic acid sequence to obtain enough material for laboratory identification.
- Amplification methods include polymerase chain reaction (PCR), reverse transcriptase PCR (RT-PCR), quantitative PCR (qPCR), and digital PCR. All these methods amplify the target DNA.
- Relative amounts of target can be measured by qPCR with nonspecific DNA dyes or fluorescent-labeled target-specific probes. Absolute amounts can be measured by dPCR.
- In transcription-mediated amplification (TMA), the target is RNA instead of DNA. A cDNA copy is made of the original RNA and used to produce millions of RNA copies.
- Like TMA, loop-mediated amplification (LAMP) is an isothermal amplification method. High-temperature denaturation is replaced with the formation of single-stranded loops for annealing primers.

DNA Sequencing

- DNA sequencing involves determining the order of nucleotides in a DNA chain and is the most specific way of detecting polymorphisms and mutations.
- The Sanger chain termination sequencing method involves replicating a single DNA strand in the presence of fluorescent-labeled modified nucleotide bases called *dideoxynucleotide triphosphates*. DNA fragments of various sizes are generated from the original template, and the sequence is determined by detecting the fluorescent labels.
- Pyrosequencing is an alternate sequencing method that relies on the generation of light when nucleotides are added to a growing DNA chain.
- Next-generation sequencing (NGS) methods allow for rapid sequencing of many small DNA templates (library) at one time. The short sequences are then assembled into a complete sequence. NGS can be used to determine the sequence of specific genes using targeted gene panels, the sequence of only the coding regions within DNA (whole exome sequencing), or the sequence of an entire genome (whole genome sequencing) to identify mutations associated with a variety of diseases.
- Ion conductance sequencing and reversible dye terminator sequencing are the NGS technologies most frequently applied to clinical testing.
- After massive parallel sequencing, variants or mutations found in the sequence must be interpreted for technical quality and clinical significance. This includes how many times the variant region is sequenced (coverage), frequency and nucleotide characteristics of the variant (filtering), and previously reported disease associations (annotation).

Study Guide: Molecular Techniques and Their Applications

PROCESS	TECHNOLOGY	APPLICATIONS
Nucleic acid isolation	Solution extraction Solid-phase (filter/bead) systems	All nucleic acid testing
Electrophoresis	Agarose gel Polyacrylamide gel Capillary gel	Test result interpretation by presence and sizing of specific nucleic acids
DNA cleavage	RFLP CRISPR-Cas9	Microbe identification Epidemiology Human identification
Blotting/hybridization	Microarrays Bead arrays FISH	Virus panels Virtual karyotyping HLA typing Ancestry testing Genome-wide disease associations
Nucleic acid amplification	PCR, RT-PCR qPCR dPCR TMA LAMP	Cancer diagnosis/prognosis Infectious disease detection HLA typing Detection of genetic mutations Gene expression
Sequencing	Chain termination sequencing Pyrosequencing Next-generation sequencing	High-resolution HLA typing Cancer diagnosis, response to therapy Microbiome analysis

CRISPR-Cas9 = clustered regularly interspaced short palindromic repeats; dPCR = digital polymerase chain reaction; FISH = fluorescence in situ hybridization; HLA = human leukocyte antigen; LAMP = loop-mediated isothermal amplification; PCR = polymerase chain reaction; qPCR = quantitative polymerase chain reaction; RFLP = restriction fragment length polymorphism; RT-PCR = reverse transcriptase polymerase chain reaction; TMA = transcription-mediated amplification.

CASE STUDIES

1. A patient with a diagnosis of stage III lung cancer underwent surgery, and the tumor tissue was tested for the PD-L1 marker by immunohistochemistry (IHC). A section of tumor was placed in 10% buffered formalin for 24 hours, embedded in paraffin, and thin (4 micron) sections were cut from the fixed tissue in the paraffin block. The tissue sections were tested by IHC in an automated tissue stainer using rabbit IgG anti-human PD-L1 primary antibody that recognized PD-L1. Bound primary antibody was detected with an anti-rabbit isotype secondary antibody conjugated to an enzyme-labeled polymer to generate a color stain. Upon pathology review of the stained sections, it was determined that 60% of the tumor cells expressed PD-L1.

Questions

a. How would fixation adversely affect PD-L1 test results, and what procedure might counteract the adverse effects?

b. Describe positive and negative controls that would be used for detection of PD-L1.

2. A blood sample from a patient under treatment for HIV infection was submitted for virology testing. A laboratory test for the presence of HIV by qPCR was performed. The test can detect 50 to 1,000,000 viral copies per milliliter of plasma. Previous results over the course of treatment showed the virus present at sequential levels of 1,500; 600; 500; 220; and 100 copies per milliliter. The results of the qPCR test for the current specimen were negative; however, the internal amplification control for the qPCR test was also negative.

Questions

a. How would you interpret these results?
   i. The results are negative, consistent with the patient history.
   ii. The results are not interpretable because the amplification control is negative.

iii. The amplification control confirms that there is no contamination.
iv. The results are not correct based on the previous positive results.

b. The test was repeated, and this time, the target (HIV) amplification was negative while the amplification control was positive. How would you interpret these results?
i. The results show a true negative.
ii. The results are not interpretable because of contamination.
iii. The results are not correct based on the previous positive results.
iv. The amplification control confirms the presence of HIV.

c. Should 0 copies per milliliter be reported because nothing was detected by the qPCR test?

REVIEW QUESTIONS

1. In DNA and RNA, nitrogen bases are attached to which ribose carbon?
   a. C1
   b. C1′
   c. C3′
   d. C5′

2. What sequence is complementary to 5′GTACCAAA3′?
   a. 5′GTACCAAA3′
   b. 5′AAACCATG3′
   c. 5′TTTGGTAC3′
   d. 5′CATGGTTT3′

3. After elution from solid-phase columns, how might DNA concentration be increased?
   a. Phenol extraction
   b. Ethanol precipitation
   c. Mixing with detergent
   d. Denaturation with NaOH

4. To what does in situ hybridization refer?
   a. Probes react with intact cells within tissues.
   b. Probes are protected from degradation if hybridized.
   c. RNA polymerase copies messenger RNA.
   d. Hybridization takes place in solution.

5. The speed at which nucleic acids migrate in gel electrophoresis is determined by which property?
   a. Charge
   b. Fluorescence
   c. Absorption
   d. Size

6. What is the function of restriction endonucleases?
   a. They splice short DNA pieces together.
   b. They cleave DNA at specific sites.
   c. They make RNA copies of DNA.
   d. They make DNA copies from RNA.

7. Which of the following techniques uses RNA-guided enzymes?
   a. Microarray
   b. CRISPR
   c. Immunohistochemistry
   d. Restriction fragment mapping

8. Which best describes the principle of microarrays?
   a. Arrays contain multiple labeled probes on a solid support.
   b. An array contains multiple copies of only one unique probe.
   c. The sample is labeled with a fluorescent tag.
   d. Hybridization is detected by the presence of radioactivity.

9. Which best describes PCR?
   a. Probes are joined by a ligating enzyme.
   b. RNA copies of the original DNA are made.
   c. Labeled probes are used to select a target.
   d. Primers are used to make multiple DNA copies.

10. During PCR, what happens in the annealing step?
    a. The primers bind to the target DNA.
    b. Strands are separated by heating.
    c. An RNA copy is made.
    d. Protein is made from the DNA strands.

11. Which probe sequence will hybridize to 5′AGTCGATCGATGC3′?
    a. 5′TCAGCTAGCTACG3′
    b. 5′GCATCGATCGACT3′
    c. 5′AGTCGATCGATGC3′
    d. 5′CGTAGCTAGCTGA3′

12. Which is true of quantification using qPCR and dPCR?
    a. dPCR quantification is relative based on ΔCt.
    b. qPCR quantification is an endpoint measurement.

c. qPCR quantification range is much lower than that of dPCR.
d. dPCR quantification is absolute based on limiting dilution.

13. Which technique is an isothermal method based on RNA amplification?
a. PCR
b. TMA
c. dPCR
d. LAMP

14. Which is used in chain termination (Sanger) sequencing?
a. SYBR Green
b. ddNTP
c. PPi
d. Ethidium bromide

15. A pyrosequencer is this type of instrument.
a. Spectrophotometer
b. Fluorometer
c. Luminometer
d. Densitometer

16. What is an NGS sequencing library?
a. A database of clinically significant sequences
b. A collection of software programs used for sequence analysis
c. A collection of short templates to be sequenced simultaneously
d. A list of all variants found in a sequencing run

17. What type of signal is generated in reversible dye terminator sequencing?
a. Light
b. Fluorescence
c. Ionic conductance
d. Color

18. How are nucleotides distinguished in ion semiconductor sequencing?
a. Complementarity to template and release of H^+
b. Complementarity to template and release of PPi
c. Generation of specific fluorescent wavelength
d. Difference in visible light signal intensity

19. Metagenomics would be most useful in this scenario.
a. A child with strep throat
b. Prenatal testing
c. An elderly person with an unknown infection
d. Screening of a healthy person

20. In NGS, what is coverage?
a. The percentage of sequences carrying a variant
b. The number of genes sequenced
c. The number of times a region is sequenced
d. The percentage of the genome represented

Chapter 12 Answer Key

Answers to Knowledge Checks

12.1 c 12.2 d 12.3 a 12.4 b 12.5 d 12.6 b
12.7 d 12.8 d 12.9 b 12.10 b 12.11 a 12.12 d

Answers to Review Questions

1. b 2. c 3. b 4. a 5. d 6. b 7. b
8. c 9. d 10. a 11. b 12. d 13. b 14. b
15. c 16. c 17. b 18. a 19. c 20. c

13

Flow Cytometry and Laboratory Automation

Magenta Love, MS, MLS (ASCP), SCYM, and Audrey Grimaldi, DHSc, MS, MLS (ASCP)

LEARNING OUTCOMES

After finishing this chapter, you should be able to:

13.1 List and describe the functions of each of the major components of a flow cytometer.

13.2 Contrast intrinsic and extrinsic parameters in flow cytometry.

13.3 Explain the principles of hydrodynamic focusing and laminar flow and their importance within the flow cytometer.

13.4 Define the concept of fluorescence and how it is used in flow cytometry.

13.5 Explain the difference between forward light scatter (FSC) and side scatter (SSC) and the cellular properties they identify.

13.6 Interpret basic flow cytometry single-parameter histograms and dual-parameter dot plots.

13.7 Define immunophenotyping and describe the following steps of the procedure: sample preparation, incubation of the sample with antibodies, selection of the cells of interest, data acquisition, analysis, and reporting.

13.8 Apply knowledge of T- and B-cell surface antigens to identify various cell populations.

13.9 Given data, calculate the percentage and absolute numbers of a particular leukocyte population.

13.10 Discuss clinical applications of flow cytometry.

13.11 Discuss the advantages of automation in clinical immunology testing.

13.12 Discuss the factors considered by a laboratory in selecting an automated immunoassay instrument.

13.13 Explain the difference between a random-access analyzer and a batch analyzer.

13.14 Explain the methods by which sample carryover can be reduced in automated analyzers.

13.15 Define *accuracy*, *precision*, *reportable range*, *analytic sensitivity*, *analytic specificity*, and *reference interval*.

CHAPTER OUTLINE

You can go to **fadavis.com** keyword stevens for the laboratory exercises that accompany this text.

Instrumentation is an integral part of the modern clinical laboratory. Two types of instrumentation have played an essential role in the advancement of immunology testing: flow cytometry, which is needed to analyze cells of the immune system, and automated analyzers, which are used in immunoassays to evaluate serum proteins. In this chapter, we discuss the basic principles and clinical applications of these important technologies.

Flow Cytometry

Flow cytometry is a system that analyzes the intrinsic light-scattering characteristics of single cells (or beads) in a fluid suspension. The cells are simultaneously evaluated for their extrinsic properties (i.e., the presence of specific surface or cytoplasmic proteins) with fluorescent-labeled antibodies or probes. Flow cytometers, originally developed in the 1960s, did not make their way into the clinical laboratory until the early 1980s. At that time, physicians started seeing patients with a new mysterious disease characterized by a decrease in circulating helper T (T_H) cells, which was subsequently named AIDS. Since that time, flow cytometry has been used routinely for monitoring human immunodeficiency virus HIV infection status, and **immunophenotyping** cells by identifying their surface and cytoplasmic antigen expression. Over the years, applications of this field have grown tremendously, including characterization of leukemias and lymphomas, enumeration of hematopoietic stem cells, and detection of human leukocyte antigen (HLA) antibodies in transplantation, to give a few examples.

Flow cytometers can simultaneously measure multiple cellular or bead properties by using several different fluorochromes. A **fluorochrome,** or fluorescent molecule, absorbs light across a spectrum of wavelengths and emits light of lower energy across a spectrum of longer wavelengths. Each fluorochrome has a distinct spectral pattern of absorption (excitation) and emission. Using laser light facilitates the analysis and identification of different populations of cells or particles by their size, shape, and antigenic properties. A significant advantage of flow cytometry is that thousands of events can be analyzed in seconds because the flow rate of cells within the cytometer is so rapid, allowing for accurate detection of cells that are present in very small numbers.

We begin this section by describing the basic principles of conventional flow cytometry, then discuss some of its clinical applications, with a focus on immunophenotyping.

Instrumentation

A flow cytometer's major components include the fluidics system, the laser light source, and the optics and photodetectors. Computers perform data analysis and management.

Fluidics

For cellular parameters to be accurately measured in the flow cytometer, cells must pass through the laser light one cell at a time. To accomplish this, cells are processed into a suspension. The cytometer draws up the cell suspension and injects the sample inside a carrier stream of isotonic saline (sheath fluid) to form a smooth stream of fluid called a **laminar flow**, in which the cells move parallel to the sheath fluid and do not mix with it. The sample stream is constrained by the carrier stream and is thus **hydrodynamically focused** so that the cells pass single file through the intersection of the laser light source **(Fig. 13–1).** Each time a cell passes in front of a laser beam, light is scattered, and the interruption of the laser signal is recorded.

Laser Light Source

Solid-state diode lasers are typically used as light sources. The wavelength of monochromatic light emitted by a laser in turn dictates which fluorochromes can be used in an assay. Not all fluorochromes can be used with all lasers because each fluorochrome has distinct spectral characteristics. Newer instruments have up to five lasers—red, blue, violet, ultraviolet (UV), and yellow-green—each of which produces different colors when exciting a particular fluorochrome. This allows for as many as 20 fluorochromes, or colors, to be analyzed in a single tube at once.

Light Scatter

When a cell passes through the laser, light is scattered in many directions. The amount and type of light scatter (LS) can provide valuable information about a cell's physical properties. In the flow cytometer, scattered light is measured by photodiodes (semiconductors that produce an electrical current after absorbing particles called photons) located at two specific angles from the laser source:

- **Forward scatter (FSC),** which is measured in a forward direction at a slight angle from the axis of the laser beam (typically up to 20° from the light source).
- **Side scatter (SSC),** also called *right-angle* LS, because it is measured at 90° from the laser light.

FSC is proportional to the size of the cell because the incident light is diffracted along the cell's perimeter **(Fig. 13-2)**. The SSC signal is generated when the laser light is reflected off intracellular structures and correlates with the degree of granularity and complexity.

These two values can be used to characterize different cell types based on their inherent properties and are considered **intrinsic parameters.** Thus, in the blood, red blood cells (RBCs) have the smallest FSC and SSC, and granulocytes have the largest FSC and SSC. When the flow cytometer analyzes a sample of whole blood, the three major populations of white blood cells (WBCs)—lymphocytes, monocytes, and neutrophils—can be roughly differentiated from each other based solely on their intrinsic parameters (FSC and SSC) **(Fig. 13–3).**

Fluorescence

Unlike FSC and SSC, which represent light-scattering properties that are intrinsic to the cell, **extrinsic parameters** require addition of a fluorescent probe for their detection. Fluorescent-labeled antibodies bound to the cell can be detected with the laser. By using fluorescent molecules with different emission wavelengths, laboratorians can simultaneously evaluate an individual cell for several extrinsic properties. The clinical utility of such multicolor analysis is enhanced when the fluorescent data are analyzed in conjunction with FSC and SSC to enable more accurate subtyping. The combined data allow cells to be characterized according to size, granularity, antigens, total protein, surface receptors, and DNA content.

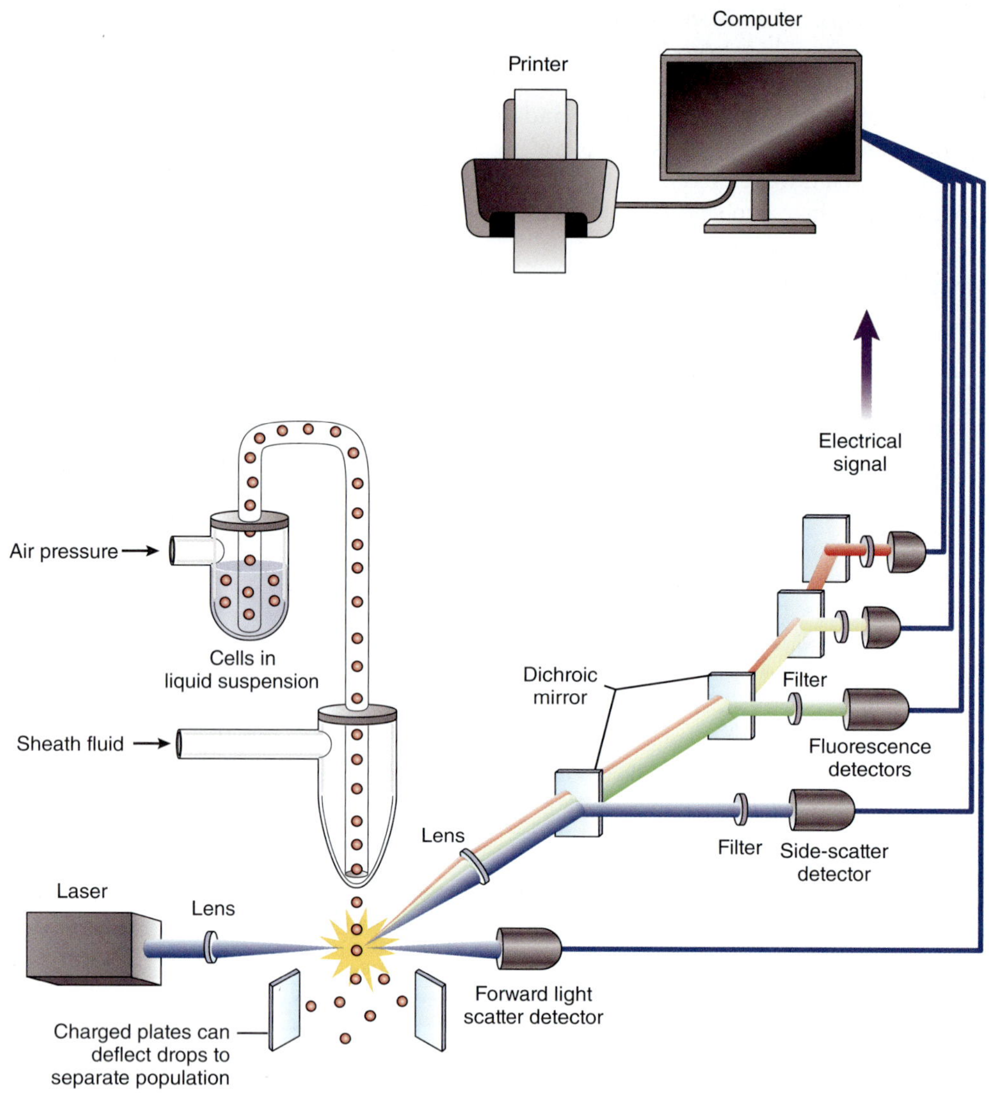

FIGURE 13-1 Flow cytometry. Components of a laser-based flow cytometer include the fluidics system for cell transportation, a laser for cell illumination, photodetectors for signal detection, and a computer-based data management system. Both forward and 90-degree light scatter are measured, indicating cell size and type.

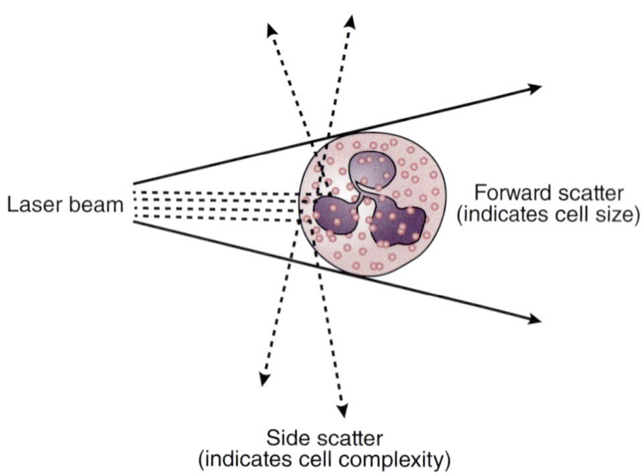

FIGURE 13-2 Light scatter properties. Forward scatter (FSC) is measured near the line of the laser beam and is proportional to cell size. Side scatter (SSC) is measured at a right angle from the laser source and correlates with the amount of granularity and complexity of a cell.

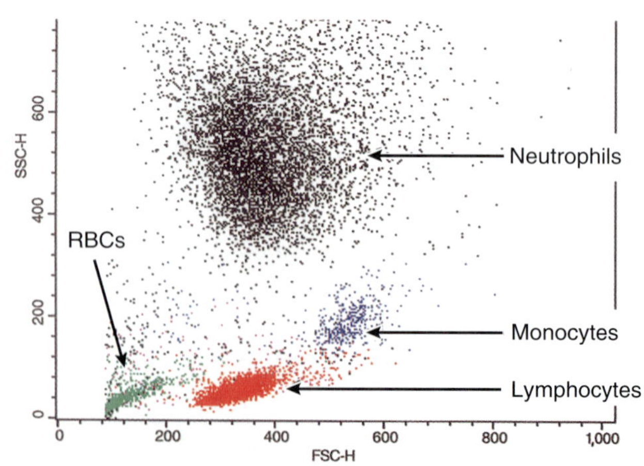

FIGURE 13-3 Peripheral blood leukocyte analysis by simultaneous evaluation of forward light scatter (FSC) and 90-degree LS (SSC). Based on the intrinsic characteristics of size (FSC) and complexity/granularity (SSC), the three main populations of WBCs (lymphocytes, monocytes, and neutrophils) can be differentiated into individual populations.

Antibodies labeled with fluorochromes are commercially made and can be purchased in multiple antigen-fluorochrome combinations. There is careful design when selecting reagents for flow cytometry experiments to optimize the number of antigens detected and the fluorochromes conjugated to the antibodies. **Table 13-1** presents the most commonly used fluorochromes. These fluorochromes emit strong signals at distinct wavelengths with minimal overlap with each other. Experimental design should also consider the dye's brightness. Bright dyes emit a high number of photons when excited by the laser. Brighter dyes should be paired with antigens that are in low amounts on the cell surface to increase visibility. Dim dyes do not emit as many photons and can be used for antigens that have a high density on the cell surface.

Knowledge Check 13-1

A heterogeneous mixture of cells can be differentiated by their intrinsic properties. Which two cell components are considered intrinsic parameters in flow cytometry?

a. Antigens and fluorochromes
b. Size and complexity
c. Maturity and lineage
d. DNA and RNA content

Optics and Photodetectors

The light scatter and fluorescence signals generated by the cells' interaction with the laser are detected by photodiodes for FSC and by photomultiplier tubes for fluorescence. The number of fluorochromes capable of being measured simultaneously depends on the number of photomultiplier tubes in the flow cytometer. The specificity of each photomultiplier tube for a given band length of wavelengths is achieved through the arrangement of a series of optical filters. The filters are designed to maximize collection of light derived from a specific fluorochrome while minimizing interference of light from other fluorochromes (Fig. 13-1). Specially placed mirrors or, in newer flow cytometers, fiber-optic cables direct the light to the detectors.

When fluorescence from labeled antibodies bound to cell surfaces reaches the photomultiplier tubes, it creates an electrical current that is converted into a voltage pulse. The voltage pulse is then converted into a digital signal using various methods, depending on the manufacturer. The digital signals are proportional to the intensity of light detected. The intensity of these converted signals is measured on a relative scale that is generally set into 1 to 256 channels, from the lowest energy level or pulse to the highest level.

Nontraditional Flow Cytometers

Advancements in technology have led to the development of flow cytometers that are based on alternative instrumentation. These include spectral flow cytometers, which capture the entire emission spectrum from each fluorochrome with solid-state multichannel detector arrays for each laser; flow cytometers that capture multicolor images of individual cells with cameras; and flow cytometers that use heavy metal isotope labels instead of fluorescent labels and perform time-of-flight measurements by mass spectroscopy. Instruments with such advanced technologies may allow clinical laboratorians to perform more precise analysis of cell populations in the future.

Immunophenotyping

The antigens on the surface of cells represent a range of different proteins, receptors, ligands, and cell components. The combined presence or absence of specific antigens determines a cell's **immunophenotype**. Historically, laboratories used individual naming systems to describe the antigens until a workshop in 1982 standardized the nomenclature by giving the antigens unique cluster of differentiation (CD) numbers that characterized their specific epitopes. **CD markers** are used to differentiate cells within a heterogenous population by identifying antigens specific for cell lineage, maturity, and activation. Some of the more commonly detected cell differentiation antigens are listed in **Table 13-2**.

Immunophenotyping involves four basic steps:

1. Sample preparation.
2. Incubation of the prepared sample with fluorescent-labeled reagent antibodies that bind to specific cell surface antigens.
3. Selection of a specific cell population for analysis by the flow cytometer on the basis of its light scatter and CD45 staining properties.
4. Data acquisition and analysis by the flow cytometer, followed by reporting of results.

Table 13-1 Commonly Used Fluorochromes

FLUOROCHROME	EXCITATION WAVELENGTH	EMISSION WAVELENGTH	BRIGHTNESS OF DYE
Fluorescein Isothiocyanate (FITC)	494 nm	518 nm	Moderate
Alexa Fluor 488	494 nm	517 nm	Moderate
Phycoerythrin (PE)	496 nm	576 nm	Very Bright
Phycoerythrin- Cyanine 5 (PECy5)	496 nm	670 nm	Very Bright
Peridinin-chlorophyll (PerCP)	481 nm	675 nm	Dim
Phycoerythrin- Cyanine 7 (PECy7)	496 nm	781 nm	Bright
Allophycocyanin (APC)	651 nm	660 nm	Very Bright

Table 13-2 Surface Markers on Leukocytes

ANTIGEN	CELL TYPE	FUNCTION
CD2	Thymocytes, T cells, NK cells	Involved in T-cell activation
CD3	Thymocytes, T cells	Associated with T-cell antigen receptor; role in TCR signal transduction
CD4	Helper T cells, monocytes, macrophages	Coreceptor for class II MHC; receptor for HIV
CD5	Mature T cells, thymocytes, subset of B cells (B1 cells)	Positive or negative modulation of T- and B-cell receptor signaling
CD7	T cells, thymocytes, NK cells, pre-B cells	Regulates cytokine production by T cells and NK cells
CD8	Thymocyte subsets, T_c cells	Coreceptor for class I MHC
CD10	Bone marrow stromal cells	Protease; marker for pre-B cells; CALLA
CD11b	Myeloid and NK cells	αM subunit of integrin CR3, binds complement component iC3b, myeloid cell adhesion
CD13	Myelomonocytic cells	Zinc metalloproteinase
CD14	Monocytic cells	Lipopolysaccharide receptor
CD15	Neutrophils, eosinophils, monocytes	Terminal trisaccharide expressed on glycolipids
CD16	Macrophages, NK cells, neutrophils	Low-affinity Fc receptor, mediates phagocytosis and ADCC
CD19	B cells, follicular dendritic cells	Part of B-cell coreceptor, signal transduction molecule that regulates B-cell development and activation
CD20	B cells, T-cell subsets	Binding activates signaling pathways, regulates B-cell activation
CD21	B cells, follicular dendritic cells, subset of immature thymocytes	Receptor for complement component C3d; part of B-cell coreceptor with CD19
CD22	B cells, B-ALL (surface and cytoplasmic), B-CLL, HCL, PLL	Involved in B-cell adhesion and B-cell signaling
CD23	B cells, monocytes, follicular dendritic cells	Regulation of IgE synthesis; triggers release of IL-1, IL-6, and GM-CSF from monocytes
CD25	Activated T cells, B cells, monocytes	Receptor for IL-2
CD33	Myeloid cells, monocytes, macrophages, granulocytes (weak), Pro-myeloid leukemia, AML, microglial cells	Cell adhesion and signaling; receptor that inhibits proliferation of myeloid cells
CD34	Hematopoietic progenitor cells, endothelial cells, immature leukemias	Cell adhesion, hematopoiesis
CD38	Plasma cells, thymocytes, NK cells, differentiated B lymphocytes, monocytes, multiple myeloma, ALL, AML	Regulates cell adhesion, activation, and proliferation
CD44	Most leukocytes	Adhesion molecule mediating homing to peripheral lymphoid organs
CD45	All hematopoietic cells	Tyrosine phosphatase, augments signaling
CD56	NK cells, subsets of T cells, neural tissue	Cell adhesion
CD57	NK-cell subsets, some T cell subsets, neuroectodermal cells	NK-cell maturation, T-cell differentiation
CD94	NK cells, subsets of T cells	Subunit of NKG2-A complex involved in inhibition of NK-cell cytotoxicity
CD103	Intraepithelial lymphocytes, HCL, adult T-cell leukemia	Ligand for E-cadherin, an adhesion molecule on epithelial cells

ANTIGEN	CELL TYPE	FUNCTION
CD138	Plasma cells, pre-B cells, epithelial cells, neural cells, breast cancer cells	Transmembrane proteoglycans that play a role in cell adhesion, migration, and proliferation
HLA-DR	B lymphocytes, activated T lymphocytes, monocytes; lack of expression is diagnostic of acute promyelocytic leukemia	T-cell activation
FCM7	B-cell subset, mantle lymphoma	In vitro response to antigens or mitogens
Kappa chains	B cells	Light chain part of antibody molecule on B cells
Lambda chains	B cells	Light chain part of antibody molecule on B cells

ADCC = antibody-dependent cellular cytotoxicity; ALL= acute lymphocytic leukemia; AML= acute myeloid leukemia; CALLA = common acute lymphoblastic leukemia antigen; CLL= chronic lymphocytic leukemia; Fc = fragment crystallizable; GM-CSF = granulocyte-macrophage colony-stimulating factor; HCL = hairy cell leukemia; IgE = immunoglobulin E; IL = interleukin; MHC = major histocompatibility class; NK = natural killer; PLL= prolymphocytic leukemia; TCR = CD3-αβ receptor complex.

We discuss each of these steps in the sections that follow.

Knowledge Check 13-2

Which lymphocyte population expresses CD4?
a. T helper cells
b. cytotoxic T (T_c) cells
c. All T cells
d. B cells

Sample Preparation

Samples commonly used for analysis include whole blood, bone marrow, and fluid aspirates. Whole blood should be collected into ethylenediaminetetraacetic acid (EDTA), the anticoagulant of choice for samples processed within 30 hours of collection. Heparin can also be used for whole blood and bone marrow and can provide improved stability in samples for up to 48 hours. Blood should be stored at room temperature (20°C to 25°C) before processing and should be well-mixed before being pipetted into staining tubes. Hemolyzed or clotted specimens should be rejected.

Whole blood contains about 1,000 times more RBCs than WBCs. Therefore, peripheral blood, bone marrow, and other samples with large numbers of RBCs require erythrocyte removal to allow for efficient analysis of the WBCs. Historically, density gradient centrifugation with Ficoll-Hypaque (Sigma, St. Louis, MO) was used to generate a cell suspension enriched for lymphocytes or lymphoblasts. However, this time-consuming method results in selective loss of some cell populations. Density-gradient centrifugation has been replaced by commercial and non-commercial erythrocyte lysis techniques. Samples are treated with lysing buffers to destroy the RBCs while leaving the WBCs intact.

Tissue specimens such as lymph nodes should be collected and transported in tissue culture medium (RPMI 1640) at either room temperature (if analysis is imminent) or 4°C (if analysis will be delayed). The specimen is then disaggregated to form a single cell suspension, either by mechanical dissociation or enzymatic digestion. Mechanical disaggregation, or "teasing," is preferred and is accomplished using a scalpel and forceps, a needle and syringe, or a wire mesh screen.

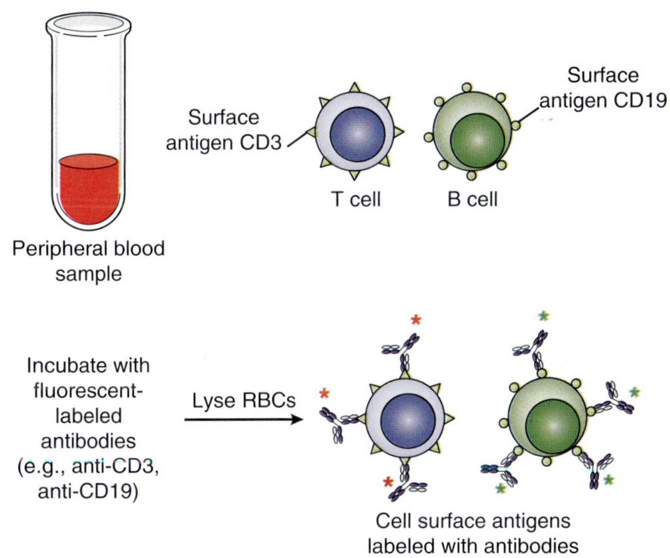

FIGURE 13-4 Immunophenotyping principle. Whole peripheral blood is incubated with a mixture of monoclonal antibodies, each specific for a different cell surface antigen and labeled with a different fluorochrome. The antibodies bind to their corresponding antigens. In this example, anti-CD3 is used to identify T cells, and anti-CD19 is used to identify B cells.

Antibodies are then added to the resulting cellular preparation, and the samples are processed for analysis. Monoclonal antibodies are preferable to polyclonal antibodies for immunophenotyping because the former are more specific. Each antibody binds to a different surface antigen and is labeled with a different fluorescent tag for differentiation (see **Figure 13-4**).

Data Acquisition and Analysis

Once the intrinsic and extrinsic properties of the cells have been collected, the data are digitized and ready for analysis. Typically, 10,000 to 20,000 "events" (i.e., the number of cells or particles that intersect the laser) are collected for each sample. Each parameter can be analyzed independently or in any combination. Graphics of the data can be represented in multiple ways.

The first level of representation is the **single-parameter histogram,** which plots a chosen parameter (generally fluorescence) on the *x*-axis vs the number of events on the *y*-axis; thus, only one parameter is analyzed using this type of graph **(Fig. 13–5).** The operator can then set a threshold value to differentiate cells that have low levels of fluorescence (negative) from cells that have high levels of fluorescence (positive) for a particular fluorochrome-labeled antibody. The computer will then calculate the percentage of "negative" and "positive" events from the total number of events collected.

The next level of representation is the bivariate histogram, or **dual-parameter dot plot,** where each dot represents an individual cell or event. Two parameters, one on each axis, are plotted against each other. The operator determines each parameter to be analyzed. Using dual-parameter dot plots, the operator can draw a **"gate"** around a population of interest and analyze various extrinsic and intrinsic parameters of the cells contained within the gated region **(Fig. 13–6).** The gate allows the operator to screen out debris and isolate subpopulations of cells of interest. Gates can be thought of as a set of filtering rules for analyzing a very large database. The operator

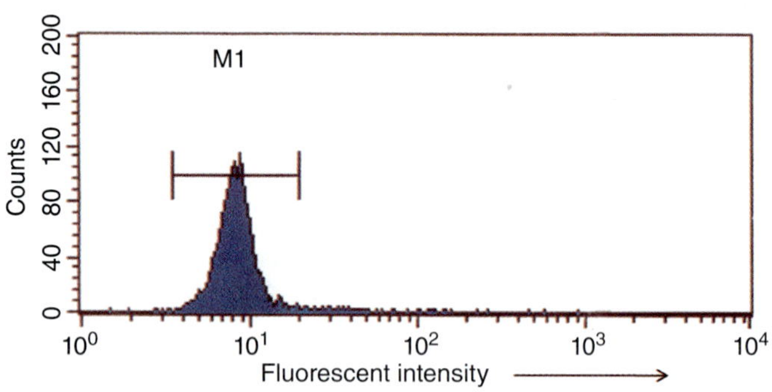

FIGURE 13–5 Example of a single-parameter flow histogram. The *y*-axis consists of the number of events. The *x*-axis is the parameter to be analyzed, which is chosen by the operator; it is usually an extrinsic parameter, such as a fluorescence. The operator can then set a marker to isolate the positive events. The computer will then calculate the percentage of positive events within the designated markers.

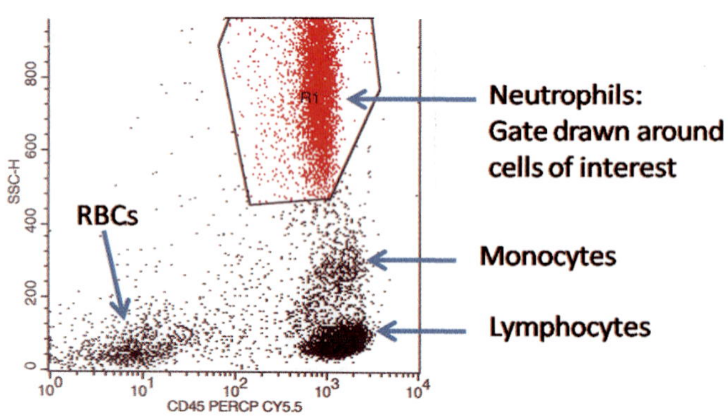

FIGURE 13–6 A dual-parameter dot plot. The operator chooses both parameters on the *x*- and *y*-axes. In this case, lysed whole blood is analyzed for CD45 (*x*-axis) and SSC (*y*-axis). The operator then draws a "gate" to isolate the population of interest (e.g., granulocytes) for further analysis.

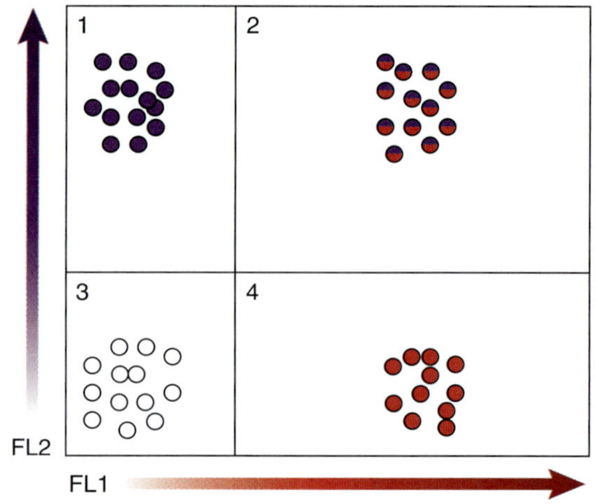

FIGURE 13–7 Quadrant analysis of a dual-parameter dot plot. The operator chooses which parameters to analyze on each axis. On each axis, there are fluorescent positive and fluorescent negative cells.

can filter the data in any way and set multiple or sequential filters (or gates).

When analyzing a population of cells using a dual-parameter dot plot, the operator chooses the parameters to examine on the *x*- and *y*-axes, divides the dot plot into four quadrants, and separates the positive events from the negative events in each axis **(Fig. 13–7):**

- Quadrant 1 consists of cells that are positive for fluorescence on the *y*-axis and negative for fluorescence on the *x*-axis.
- Quadrant 2 consists of cells that are positive for fluorescence on both the *x*- and *y*-axes.
- Quadrant 3 consists of cells that are negative for fluorescence on both the *x*- and *y*-axes.
- Quadrant 4 consists of cells that are positive for fluorescence on the *x*-axis and negative for fluorescence on the *y*-axis.

The computer and specialized software will calculate the percentage of cells in each quadrant based on the total number of events counted.

Analysis of Leukocyte Populations

To analyze leukocytes, the clinical sample—usually whole peripheral blood—is prepared and injected into the flow cytometer, which differentiates the various types of cells based on their staining with CD45 and light scatter properties (Fig. 13-6). CD45 is a pan-leukocyte marker present on all WBCs but with varying levels of expression based on the cell's maturity and lineage. Analysis of CD45 expression levels is useful in differentiating various populations of WBCs and, in combination with SSC, has replaced gating by FSC and SSC in many laboratories. However, it is always a good idea to examine the FSC and SSC plot to make sure a population is not being missed.

A gate is drawn around the cell population of interest, and the extrinsic characteristics of the gated population can then be analyzed. For example, **Figure 13-8** shows a dual-parameter dot plot in which a gated population of

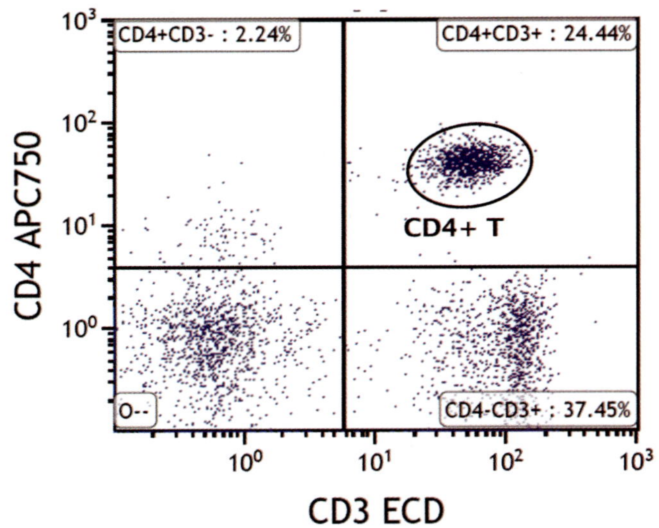

FIGURE 13–8 Example of a dual-parameter dot plot to identify CD4⁺ T cells: CD3 on the *x*-axis and CD4 on the *y*-axis. The cells in quadrant 2 that are positive for both CD3 and CD4 are true CD4⁺ T cells.

lymphocytes is analyzed for CD3 and CD4 expression to identify T_H cells.

Figure 13–9 illustrates the strategy used to analyze lymphocyte subsets with dual parameter plots. In this example, whole blood was incubated with fluorescent-labeled antibodies specific for CD3, CD4, CD8, and CD38. The sample was washed, treated with a lysis solution to remove RBCs, and analyzed on the flow cytometer. The sample was first plotted using FSC vs SSC, and a gate, or region, was drawn around the lymphocyte population (**Fig. 13-9A**). On the subsequent plots of fluorescent markers, only the gated lymphocyte population was analyzed. Each dot plot was divided into four quadrants to differentiate positive from negative populations. Then, the computer calculated the percentage of positive cells in each quadrant.

Three dual parameter plots were generated, each analyzing two different cell surface markers. In the dot plot on the left (**Fig. 13-9B**), quadrant 2 (upper right) identifies CD4⁺ CD3⁺ T-helper-cell lymphocytes. Quadrant 3 (lower left) includes B lymphocytes and natural killer (NK) cells. Quadrant 4 (lower right) identifies CD3⁺ CD4⁻ T-cell lymphocytes.

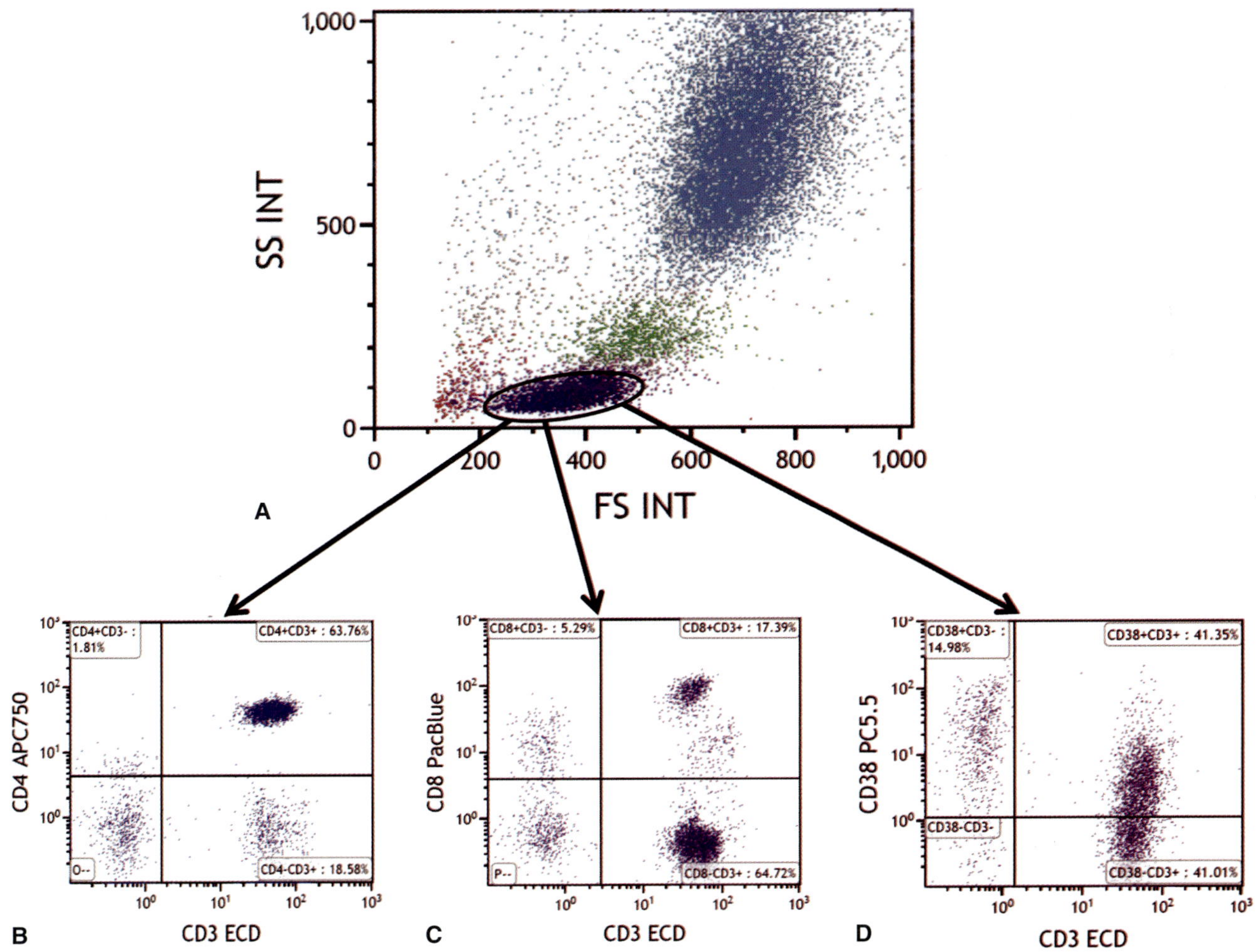

FIGURE 13–9 Gating strategy to analyze lymphocyte subsets in a sample of whole blood for CD3, CD4, CD8, and CD38 expression. (A) Selection of lymphocytes by gating based on forward scatter (FS) and side scatter (SS). On the subsequent plots of fluorescent markers, only the lymphocyte population is analyzed. (B) Analysis of CD3 and CD4 expression. (C) Analysis of CD3 and CD8 expression. (D) Analysis of CD3 and CD38 expression.

In the middle plot (**Fig. 13-9C**), quadrant 1 (upper left) identifies low-intensity $CD8^+$ $CD3^-$ NK cells. Quadrant 2 identifies $CD3^+$ $CD8^+$ T_c lymphocytes. Quadrant 3 contains lymphocytes that are $CD8^-$ $CD3^-$ (B-cell lymphocytes). Quadrant 4 contains $CD3^+$ $CD8^-$ T_H-cell lymphocytes.

In the plot on the right (**Fig. 13-9D**), quadrant 1 identifies $CD38^+$ $CD3^-$ B cells, quadrant 2 identifies $CD38^+$ $CD3^+$ activated T cells, quadrant 3 contains $CD38^-$ $CD3^-$ cells, and quadrant 4 identifies $CD3^+$ $CD38^-$ T cells, which are not activated.

Knowledge Check 13-3

What population in **Figure 13-10** is gated and labeled P1?
a. red blood cells
b. lymphocytes
c. granulocytes
d. monocytes

Result Reporting

Once the flow cytometer acquires the information, it analyzes the data from each cell population and expresses it in both percentages and absolute numbers. While these numbers are determined by the computer/software, an illustration of manual calculations follows to increase your understanding of how the results are obtained.

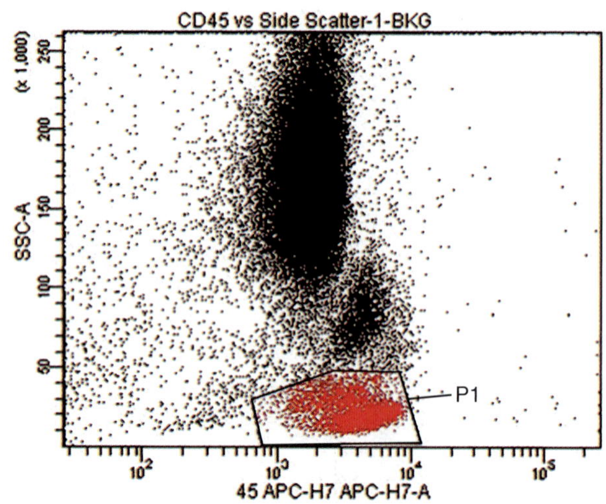

FIGURE 13-10 Flow cytometry image of whole peripheral blood analyzed for CD45 expression and side scatter. *(Courtesy of Upstate University Hospital Flow Cytometry laboratory, Syracuse NY).*

First, the percentage of fluorescent-positive cells is calculated as follows:

% Marker (+) Cells = (# Marker (+) cells counted ÷ Total # lymphocytes counted*) x 100

*Usually about 10,000

Example:

Suppose that out of 10,000 lymphocytes counted in a 1-mL blood sample by flow cytometry, 6,500 stained positive for the CD3 marker. What is the percentage of CD3-positive cells?

Solution:

% CD3 (+) cells = 6,500 ÷ 10,000 x 100 = 65%

The absolute count of a particular cell type—for instance, $CD3^+$ T lymphocytes—can then be obtained by multiplying the absolute cell count of the population of interest (e.g., lymphocytes; derived by the flow cytometer or a hematology analyzer) by the percentage of the fluorescent-positive cells in the sample (e.g., $CD3^+$ lymphocytes):

Absolute # Cells (e.g., CD3 T Cells) = WBC Count × % Lymphocytes × % Fluorescent -positive cells (e.g., CD3-FITC)

Example: Suppose the sample in the above example was found to have 4 x 10^3 WBC/µL. The differential showed that 30% of those cells were lymphocytes. What is the absolute number of T cells?

Solution:

Absolute # T cells = 4,000 x 0.30 x 0.65 = 780/µL

Finally, the patient's values are compared to reference ranges established by the testing laboratory. Typical ranges are shown in **Table 13-3**. You can see from the table that this patient would have a normal T-cell count.

This method is considered a dual-platform analysis. The disadvantage to this type of analysis is that it has a greater potential for added error associated with the use of two distinct methods to derive the absolute count. The single platform is now the method of choice to eliminate this type of error. Single platforms can be achieved by two types of methods: bead-based or volumetric. In the bead-based method,

Table 13-3 Reference Ranges for Lymphocyte Populations in Peripheral Blood[a]

MARKER	CELL POPULATION	% OF TOTAL LYMPHOCYTES	ABSOLUTE NUMBER OF LYMPHOCYTES (CELLS/µL)
CD19	B lymphocytes	6–23	91–610
CD3	Total T lymphocytes	62–87	570–2,400
CD4	Helper T cells[b]	32–64	430–1,800
CD8	Cytotoxic T cells[b]	15–46	210–1,200
CD16/CD56	NK cells	5–28	78–470

[a]*Reference values vary by age and testing laboratory. Values in table were obtained from ARUP Laboratories for individuals aged 16 to 64 years (http://ltd.aruplab.com/Tests/Pub/0095892; Accessed June 12, 2025).*

[b]*The ARUP reference range for the ratio of helper T to cytotoxic T cells (CD4:CD8) for persons 16 to 64 years is 0.80 to 3.90.*

commercially-available fluorescent microspheres of known concentration serve as an internal calibrator. A specific volume of the beads is added to an equal volume of the blood sample in each tube. The ratio of sample volume to microsphere volume is then used by the flow cytometer to calculate the absolute cell number directly from the individual flow cytometry tubes:

$$\# \text{ Cells}/\mu L = (\# \text{ Fluorescent } (+) \text{ cells} \div \# \text{ Fluorescent beads}) \times \text{Bead concentration (Beads}/\mu L)$$

In the volumetric method, the precise volume of the sample can be used to calculate the absolute number of events.

Clinical Applications

Routine applications of flow cytometry in the clinical laboratory can be divided into two categories: immunophenotyping of malignant leukocytes and immunophenotyping of nonmalignant cells. Malignant cell immunophenotyping refers to immunophenotypic characterization of leukemias, lymphomas, and other hematopoietic disorders. Nonmalignant cell immunophenotyping includes the characterization and enumeration of normal lymphocytes, such as $CD4^+$ T cells and $CD34^+$ stem cells.

Malignant Cell Immunophenotyping

Immunophenotyping by flow cytometry has become an important tool to initially evaluate patients with leukemias and lymphomas and subsequently monitor them after therapy has started. Immunophenotype characteristics have been incorporated into current leukemia and lymphoma classifications, beginning with the Revised European-American Lymphoma (REAL) classification in 1994 and, more recently, in the World Health Organization (WHO) classifications.

One of the most important components of flow cytometric analysis is the classification of hematopoietic malignancies by their lineage (i.e., B cell, T cell, or myeloid) and degree of differentiation (see Chapter 18). Detailed phenotypic analysis can determine the lineage, clonality, and degree of differentiation and activation of a specific cell population. This information is useful for differential diagnosis or clarification of closely related lymphoproliferative disorders. Immunophenotyping requires careful selection of combinations of individual markers based on a given cell lineage and maturation stage. Attempts to standardize individual marker panels, especially by European laboratory groups, are ongoing; however, the markers selected for inclusion in testing panels vary from institution to institution.

Knowing the unique characteristics of leukemias and lymphomas and pairing the specific markers that identify these characteristics can be useful in making a more reliable diagnosis. For example, in chronic lymphocytic leukemia (CLL), typically CD5 (a T-cell lymphocyte marker) is paired with CD20 (a B-cell lymphocyte marker) for analysis. The presence of a significant number of cells that are both $CD5^+$ and $CD20^+$ is an indication of CLL or mantle cell lymphoma.

Clonality of mature B cell malignancies can be determined by assessing kappa and lambda surface light chains. Healthy B cells express either kappa (κ) or lambda (λ) light chains on their cell surface; the normal range of κ-expressing B cells to λ-expressing B cells is between 3:1 and 0.3:1. In contrast, malignant B cells show an enlarged population of lymphocytes that all express either kappa or lambda. They are said to be monoclonal, and analysis provides an effective method to determine B-cell malignancy.

It is also useful to examine the expression of CD45, as this marker is present on all WBCs but in varying levels based on the cell's maturity and lineage. Immature WBCs known as blasts express lower levels of CD45 (low fluorescence) but show an increase of CD45 expression as the cell matures; therefore, mature WBCs have much brighter CD45 fluorescence compared with their earlier progenitor stages.

Immunophenotyping has also become an essential test in monitoring patients with leukemias and lymphomas. Patients who have been treated for a leukemia or lymphoma can be monitored for "minimal residual disease" (MRD) because small numbers of abnormal cells can be easily detected by flow cytometry.

Knowledge Check 13-4

Flow cytometry can be useful in the diagnosis and monitoring of leukemia patients by assessing which cell parameter(s)?

a. Maturity
b. Clonality
c. Lineage
d. All of the above

Critical Thinking 13-1

A laboratory would like to implement flow cytometry testing to identify immature B-cell malignancies. What antigens should be included in the experimental panel? What fluorochromes should be used for each antibody?

Immunophenotyping of Nonmalignant Cells

Immunophenotyping of leukocytes is also essential when an immunodeficiency in one or more WBC populations is suspected. Patient values are compared with reference ranges established by the clinical laboratory performing the testing. See Table 13–3 for typical ranges for B cells, T-cell subsets, and NK cells.

As we mentioned earlier, flow cytometry is essential in evaluating immunodeficiency caused by HIV, a virus that infects and destroys $CD4^+$ T cells, leading to AIDS in untreated individuals. Enumeration of peripheral blood $CD4^+$ T cells in patients infected with HIV by the flow cytometry laboratory is used to classify HIV disease stages and determine treatment options (see Chapter 24).

Flow cytometry is also the method of choice for the diagnosis of several inherited immunodeficiency diseases, including Bruton's tyrosine kinase deficiency (characterized by a lack of circulating mature B cells), DiGeorge syndrome (decreased T cells), and severe combined immunodeficiency disease (decreased T cells, with possible decreases in B cells and/or NK cells) (see Chapter 19). It is also used in chronic granulomatous disease (CGD), an X-linked or autosomal recessive disease in which neutrophils are defective in their oxidative burst. Unlike normal neutrophils, neutrophils from patients with CGD cannot oxidize the dye dihydrorhodamine 123 to form a fluorescent product which can be detected by flow cytometry.

Another example in which flow cytometry is used to evaluate nonmalignant WBCs is the enumeration of CD34 positive cells during hematopoietic stem cell (HSC) transplants. Donors for the transplants are stimulated to release more stem cells into their peripheral blood after receiving recombinant growth factors. Peripheral blood samples from such donors are sent to the flow cytometry laboratory, and a count of $CD34^+$ cells is performed to estimate the yield of stem cells collected. The CD34 count has also been found to be a good predictor of transplant success in the HSC recipients.

Other Clinical Applications

In addition to immunophenotyping, many other clinical applications have been developed for flow cytometry. Some examples of these are listed here:

- Diagnosis of paroxysmal nocturnal hemoglobinuria (PNH), an inherited disease characterized by a lack of the glycosylphosphatidylinositol (GPI) anchors, which some surface proteins need to attach to RBCs, neutrophils, monocytes, and other cells. Patients with PNH develop hemolytic anemia because their RBCs do not bind regulator proteins of the complement system and are susceptible to destruction (see Chapter 7). One flow cytometry test to detect PNH looks for the antigens that use the GPI anchor because these antigens will be missing or reduced in patients with PNH. Another test detects the GPI anchor itself by its ability to bind to fluorescent aerolysin (FLAER). Normal granulocytes and monocytes will be fluorescent because they possess the anchor, whereas the fluorescence in PNH cells missing the anchor will be reduced or absent.
- Determination of the DNA content or ploidy status (i.e., the number of chromosome sets) of tumor cells by incubating them with fluorescent DNA binding dyes (e.g., propridium iodide) and comparing the amount of fluorescence emitted by tumor cells to that of a normal cell population. This information can provide physicians with important prognostic information. Ploidy analysis is also useful in examining products of conception for molar pregnancies.
- HLA typing and crossmatching for solid-organ transplantation. Flow cytometry can perform this analysis much faster and more accurately than other serological methods (see Chapter 16).
- Detection of hemoglobin-F–positive cells in the case of a fetal-maternal hemorrhage; flow cytometry is much more sensitive than the traditional Kleihauer-Betke method.
- Cytometric bead arrays, which use beads of various sizes and different fluorescent levels to identify up to 100 analytes at the same time, such as anti-nuclear antibodies to different nuclear antigens, viral nucleic acids, and various genetic mutations (see Chapters 11, 12, and 15).

Critical Thinking 13-2

Explain why lymphocyte subset testing can aid in differentiating immunodeficiency disorders.

Immunoassay Automation

In addition to flow cytometry, automated technology has become more prevalent in clinical immunology testing with the advent of immunoassay analyzers. Reliable instrumentation for immunoassays using nonradioactive labels (e.g., enzyme, chemiluminescent, fluorescent) is available (see Chapter 11 for assay principles). Using a solid support to separate free and bound analytes, these instruments have made it possible to automate heterogeneous immunoassays even for low-level analytes such as peptide hormones. Currently, more than 60 different automated immunoassay analyzers capable of performing almost all common diagnostic immunoassays exist; they have largely replaced manual testing, especially in larger laboratories. As you will learn in the remaining chapters of this book, automation has a large impact on many areas of clinical immunology testing. Some of its major applications are listed in **Table 13–4**.

The driving motivation for the development of immunoassay analyzers has been the need to create an automated system capable of reducing or eliminating the many manual tasks required to perform analytical procedures and the demand to handle large volumes of samples. Eliminating manual steps decreases the likelihood of human error caused by fatigue or erroneous sampling. Laboratory professionals are also trying to streamline test performance to reduce test turnaround time and cost. Automation, in many cases, is more accurate and precise compared to manual methods; depending on the assay platform, it may be more sensitive as well. Other benefits of immunoassay automation include the ability to provide more services with less staff, save on controls, avoid duplicate and repeat testing, have a longer reagent shelf life and less disposal because of outdating, and better identification of samples with bar codes.

Because of the wide variety of available automated immunoassay analyzers, it can be difficult to determine the best instrument for any given laboratory. **Table 13–5** offers a partial list of the many factors to consider in determining what type of analyzer will fulfill a laboratory's needs. It is important for all those involved in the instrument's selection to prioritize the properties of any analyzer to meet the demands of the laboratory.

Characteristics of Automated Analyzers

The two main types of immunoassay analyzers currently available are batch analyzers and random-access analyzers.

Table 13-4 Applications of Automated Analyzers in Clinical Immunology Testing*

TESTING CATEGORY	COMMON CLINICAL APPLICATIONS	SELECT EXAMPLES
Allergy	Fluorometric enzyme-linked immunoassays for allergen-specific and total IgE	Allergen panels for peanuts, cow's milk, insect venom, wheat, sesame, egg, tree nuts, canine, feline
Autoimmune Diseases	ANA testing by IFA, ELISA, Fluorescent microbead immunoassay ANCA testing by IFA, ELISA Testing for other autoantibodies by ELISA or CLIA	Anti-double stranded DNA, anti-Sm, anti-RNP Anti-PR3 antigen, Anti-myeloperoxidase Anti-thyroglobulin and anti-TPO, Rheumatoid factor, Anti-mitochondrial antibodies
Immunodeficiency Diseases	Nephelometry and Immunoturbidimetry for Igs Immunophenotyping for CD markers by direct immunofluorescence and flow cytometry	Total serum IgG, IgA, and IgM Lymphocyte enumeration (e.g., B cells-$CD19^+$, T cells-$CD3^+$)
Immunoproliferative Diseases	IFE for detection of monoclonal antibodies Serum free light chain analysis by latex-enhanced immunoassays Immunophenotyping for CD markers by direct immunofluorescence and flow cytometry	Monoclonal IgG detection in multiple myeloma; Monoclonal IgM detection in Waldenström macroglobulinemia Quantitation of free monoclonal light chains in patients with immunoproliferative diseases Leukemia and Lymphoma classification
Infectious Disease Serology	Testing for IgM and IgG organism-specific antibodies or antigens by ELISA or CLIA to detect current and past infections and to assess immunity	ASO, CMV IgM/IgG, Rubella IgM/IgG, Rubeola IgM/IgG, *Toxoplasma gondii* IgM/IgG, anti-HBs, HBsAg
Transplantation Immunology	Detection of HLA antibodies in candidates and recipients of organ transplants by fluorescent microbead array	Elimination of organ donors with HLA antigens that could potentially react with a candidate's antibodies; Diagnosis and monitoring of antibody-mediated rejection in transplant recipients
Tumor Immunology	Testing for serum tumor markers by ELISA or CLIA to aid in cancer diagnosis, determine patient prognosis, monitor patient response to treatment, and identify tumor recurrence	AFP, CA-125, CEA, PSA

**AFP = α-fetoprotein; ANA = Antinuclear antibodies; ANCA = Anti-neutrophil cytoplasmic antibodies; ASO = Anti-streptolysin O; CA-125 = Cancer antigen 125; CEA = Carcinoembryonic antigen; CLIA = Chemiluminescence immunoassay; ELISA = Enzyme-linked immunosorbent assay; HBs = Hepatitis B surface antibody; HBsAg= Hepatitis B surface antigen; IFA = Indirect immunofluorescence assay; IFE = Immunofixation electrophoresis; Igs = Immunoglobulins; PSA = Prostate-specific antigen; RNP = Ribonuclear protein; Sm = Smith antigen; TPO = Thyroid peroxidase*

Batch analyzers examine multiple samples and provide access to the samples for the formation of subsequent reaction mixtures. However, they permit only one type of analysis at a time. In some cases, this may be considered a drawback; STAT samples cannot be loaded randomly, and multiple tests cannot be performed on any one sample. Partially for those reasons, the next generation of analyzers was designed in a modular system that could be configured to measure numerous analytes from multiple samples. These **random-access analyzers** can analyze many test samples and perform several different tests for any one sample.

Automation can occur in all three stages of laboratory testing: pre-examination (preanalytical), examination (analytical), and post-examination (post-analytical). For the purposes of this section, discussion is limited to automation within the examination stage of testing.

The tasks of the examination stage include introducing a sample, adding reagent, mixing the reagent and sample, incubating, detecting, calculating, and reporting the readout or results. All or some of these tasks may be automated on various immunoassay analyzers. **Automatic sampling** can be accomplished by several different methods; peristaltic pumps (older technology) and positive-liquid displacement pipettes (newer technology) are two examples. In most systems, samples are pipetted using thin, stainless-steel probes. Such probes have clot detectors that will automatically reject a sample if a clot is detected. They also have a liquid-level sensor that can detect the lack of sample in a tube, usually because of a short draw. Samples without the proper amount of liquid in them are also rejected.

A potential problem associated with reusable pipette probes is carryover or contamination of one sample with material from the previous samples. Various methods have been developed to reduce carryover, including using disposable pipette tips to initially transfer samples and flushing the internal and external surfaces of sample probes with diluent. *Continuous-flow analysis* refers to how the various liquids (analytes, reagents) are pumped through the analyzer. These liquids are pumped in a continuous stream at a constant rate. The term *continuous random access* refers to the analyzer's

Table 13-5 Factors for Consideration in Selecting an Automated Immunoassay Instrument

CATEGORY	FACTOR
Pre-Examination (Pre-Analytical)	Specimen type Specimen volume
Examination (Analytical)	Sensitivity Precision Accuracy and test standardization Linearity Interferences Carryover effects
Economic	Purchase cost Lease options Shipping and installation fees Maintenance costs Reagent costs Operator time and costs Costs for disposables Training for personnel Warranty
Instrument	Maintenance requirements Automation compatibility/LIMS compatibility Space requirements Utility requirements (electrical and HVAC) Reliability Clot error detection Hardware costs Non-warranty service
Manufacturer	Future product plans Speed of service response Reputation Technical support Menu expansion plans Purchase of a warranty/service contract
Operational	Test menu Throughput Reagent capacity Reagent stability Stat capability Reflex testing ability Reagent kit size/availability Training requirements Operating complexity Waste requirements Reagent storage requirements Reagent performance Downtime plans

HVAC = heating, ventilation, and air conditioning; LIMS = laboratory information management systems; STAT = from the Latin word statum, meaning "immediately"; in other words, testing should be done immediately; this is a commonly used abbreviation.

Adapted and Modified from Remaley AT, Hortin GL. Protein analysis for diagnostic applications. In: Detrick B, Hamilton RG, Folds JD, et al., eds. Manual of Molecular and Clinical Laboratory Immunology. 7th ed. Washington, DC: American Society for Microbiology; 2006:15; and Appold K. Checklist for buying a chemistry analyzer. Clin Lab Products. Nov. 2013:12–15.

capability for using one specimen to test for several analytes simultaneously. Other methods of analysis exist as well. For example, with ***discrete analysis***, each specimen is tested in a separate reaction chamber.

Reagent use in automated immunoassay analyzers requires consideration of the following factors: handling, preparing and storing, and dispensing. Some reagents come ready for use; if they do not, the analyzer must be able to properly dilute the reagents before they can be used. Most reagents come with bar codes the analyzer reads to reduce operator error; if the wrong reagent is loaded into the analyzer by mistake, the analyzer will detect the error and generate an error message. Reagents for many analyzers must be stored in laboratory refrigerators; however, in larger systems, there is a reagent storage compartment within the analyzer itself.

After reagents have been added to the samples, the next concern is proper mixing to obtain reliable results. Analyzers use different methods for mixing, including magnetic stirring, rotation paddles, forceful dispensing, and vigorous lateral shaking. Whichever method is used, it is imperative that no splashing between sample wells occurs to prevent erroneous results.

Timed incubation is then carried out at ambient temperatures. Some analyzers have built-in incubators for temperature-controlled incubation. Heated metal blocks are widely used to incubate reagent wells or cuvettes.

Detection of the final analyte depends on the chemistry involved in the immunoassay. In the past, colorimetric absorption spectroscopy was the principal means of measurement because of its ability to detect a wide variety of compounds. Newer methods of detection include fluorescence and chemiluminescence, both of which require fluorescence detectors. With the growing trend to offer flexibility in an automated analyzer, several companies have developed analyzers that can combine clinical chemistry and immunoassay testing on a single platform. Two examples are Beckman Coulter's UniCel DxC chemistry systems and Roche Diagnostics' Cobas analyzer series.

Instrumentation can reduce turnaround time for testing, remove the possibility of manual errors, and allow for greater sensitivity in determining the presence of low-level analytes. Batch analyzers may work best if only one type of test is performed on a large scale. Random-access analyzers allow for more flexibility and include rapid processing of STAT samples. In either case, any new instrument requires extensive validation before patient results can be reported with confidence.

Knowledge Check 13-5

A significant benefit of using an automated immunoassay analyzer is:

a. Reduction of quality control monitoring.
b. Elimination of reagent storage.
c. Reduction or elimination of manual steps required to perform analytical procedures.
d. Elimination of laboratory professional involvement.

Critical Thinking 13-3

Imagine that you are a medical laboratory professional working in a laboratory that performs serology testing. Your laboratory has a new automated immunoassay analyzer. Before using the analyzer to report patient results, you must perform assay validations. Two of the analytes you must evaluate are *Toxoplasma gondii* IgM and rubella virus IgG. Both can be performed on serum using noncompetitive indirect enzyme immunoassays (see Chapter 11). The analyzer's operational type is continuous random access.

Answer the following questions:

a. How many samples are required from each patient for analysis of each analyte (*T. gondii* IgM and rubella virus IgG)?
b. After the sensitivity validation is complete, what results (signal intensity/ colorimetric result) would you expect to see for specimens with high antibody concentrations and for specimens with low antibody concentrations?

Validation

Regardless of the instrumentation considered, the laboratory must always perform proper validation of new instrumentation or methodology. In performing the validation process, clinical laboratories must develop a protocol that complies with the Clinical Laboratory Improvement Amendments (CLIA) and their associated regulations for verifying the manufacturer's performance specifications. The CLIA, passed by the U.S. Congress in 1988 and modified several times thereafter, established quality standards to ensure accurate, reliable, and timely patient test results (see Chapter 8). The regulations apply to each nonwaived test or test system (categorized as moderate or high complexity) brought into the laboratory for the first time. In addition, laboratories must comply with their individual state's regulatory agency standards.

You can find detailed information on the CLIA and method validation from the organizations that administer the CLIA program (the Centers for Medicare and Medicaid Services [CMS], the U.S. Food and Drug Administration [FDA], and the Centers for Disease Control and Prevention [CDC]) and other agencies involved in the process from the following resources (websites accessed on June 12, 2025):

- CMS (https://www.cms.gov/medicare/quality/clinical-laboratory-improvement-amendments?redirect=/CLIA).
- CDC (https://www.cdc.gov/clia/php/about/)
- FDA (https://www.fda.gov/medical-devices/ivd-regulatory-assistance/clinical-laboratory-improvement-amendments-clia)
- The College of American Pathologists Laboratory Accreditation Program Inspection Checklist for Chemistry (https://www.cap.org/laboratory-improvement/accreditation/laboratory-accreditation-program)
- Clinical Laboratory Standards Institute Evaluation Standards (http://clsi.org)
- Westgard QC (https://westgard.com/clia-a-quality/clia-final-rule/247-cliafinalrule5.html) and (https://westgard.com/lessons/basic-method-validation/52-lesson24.html)

The laboratory must validate a new instrument or method before reporting patient results. As designated by CLIA, the required verifications to be determined for a new method are accuracy, precision, analytic sensitivity, and analytic specificity, including interfering substances, reportable range, and reference intervals:

- **Accuracy** refers to the test's ability to actually measure what it claims to measure (i.e., how close the test result is to the actual value). To determine accuracy, the assay may be tested using previously known positive or negative samples provided by proficiency testing or interlaboratory exchange. Parallel testing with an alternative method or technology can also be performed.
- **Precision** refers to the method's ability to consistently reproduce the same result on repeated testing of the same sample. See **Figure 13–11** for a pictorial representation of the difference between accuracy and precision. The CLIA specify that the standard deviation and coefficient of variation should be calculated from 10 to 20 day-to-day quality control data to estimate analytical errors. At least one normal control and one abnormal control (with known high or low analyte concentrations) should be included in the analysis.
- **Analytic sensitivity** in this context is defined as the lowest measurable amount of an analyte, also known as the *lower limit of detection*.
- **Analytic specificity** is the assay's ability to generate a negative result when the analyte is not present, while excluding other analytes.
- The **reportable range** is defined as the range of values that are reported by the laboratory as a positive result for the specimens assayed by the test procedure. Note that this may not include the entire dynamic range of the analytic instrument (i.e., from the minimum to the maximum detectable value) used to produce the result.
- The **reference interval** is the range of values found in healthy individuals, which is used as a guideline for clinical interpretation of positive and negative results.

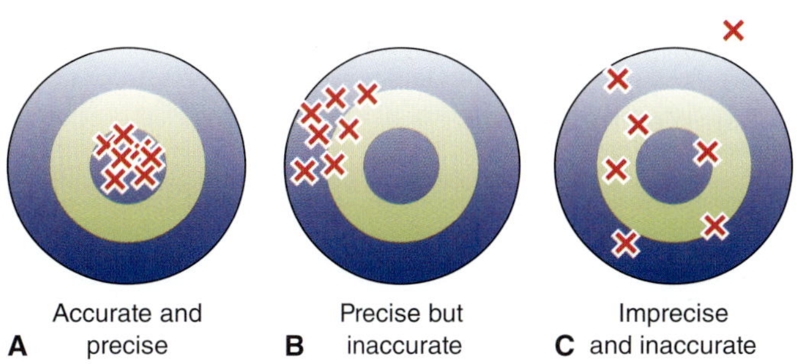

FIGURE 13–11 Pictorial representation of the difference between accuracy and precision. A. Accurate and precise—The darts consistently hit the target in the right place. B. Precise but inaccurate—The darts consistently hit the board, but in the wrong place, missing the target. C. Imprecise and inaccurate—The darts hit the board in various places, all incorrect.

Knowledge Check 13-6

According to CLIA 1988 regulations, when validating a new assay, the standard deviation and coefficient of variation should be calculated from:

a. 5 to 10 day-to-day quality control results.
b. 1 to 30 day-to-day quality control results.
c. 30 to 45 day-to-day quality control results.
d. 10 to 20 day-to-day quality control results.

KEY CONCEPTS

Flow Cytometry Instrumentation

- Flow cytometry is a powerful tool to identify and enumerate various cell populations. It was first used in clinical laboratories to perform $CD4^+$ T-cell counts in people with HIV.
- A flow cytometer measures multiple properties of cells suspended in a moving fluid medium.
- The flow cytometer has three major components: (1) the fluidics system, which carries cells or particles through the instrument in a single file; (2) the laser, which emits light to be scattered by the cells/particles and light excited by fluorochromes; and (3) the optics and photodetectors, which detect the amount of light scatter and fluorescence for each cell/particle.
- As each cell or particle passes single file through a laser light source, it produces a characteristic light pattern that is measured by multiple detectors for scattered light (forward and 90°) and fluorescent emissions if the cell is stained with a fluorochrome.
- Light scatter is an intrinsic parameter, as it measures properties inherent to a cell, whereas fluorescence is an extrinsic parameter because it requires addition of a fluorescent probe for detection.
- Scattered light in a forward direction is a measure of cell size, whereas the side scatter (at a right angle to the laser light) reflects a cell's internal complexity or granularity.

Immunophenotyping

- Immunophenotyping is a laboratory technique that uses fluorochrome-labeled antibodies to identify cells by their characteristic antigen expression.

Sample Preparation

- The most commonly used sample for flow cytometry is whole peripheral blood. The RBCs in the sample are destroyed with lysing buffers, and the WBCs are incubated with a mixture of monoclonal antibodies, each directed against a different surface antigen and labeled with a distinct fluorescent dye.

Data Acquisition and Analysis

- A gate is used to isolate a particular region of cells for further analysis, based on light scatter and fluorescent properties.
- Data can be analyzed using single- or dual-parameter plots. A single-parameter histogram plots a chosen parameter on the *x*-axis vs the number of events on the *y*-axis. A dual-parameter dot plot displays two parameters plotted against each other.
- The patient's results for each cell population analyzed are reported as both percentages and absolute numbers, and are compared to reference ranges established by the testing laboratory.

Clinical Applications

- The most common clinical applications of flow cytometry are immunophenotyping of malignant cells and nonmalignant cells.
- Quantification of an individual's lymphocyte populations is essential in diagnosing leukemias, lymphomas, inherited immunodeficiency diseases, and acquired immunodeficiencies such as AIDS.

Other Clinical Applications

- Other clinical applications of flow cytometry include diagnosis of PNH, DNA ploidy analysis of tumors, HLA typing and cross-matching, detection of hemoglobin F-positive cells, and cytometric bead arrays.

Immunoassay Automation

- Clinical laboratories have replaced many manual immunoassay procedures with a variety of automated immunoassay analyzers to allow for more accurate, precise, and sensitive testing of many analytes.
- Automation is incorporated in all stages of laboratory testing: pre-examination, examination, and post-examination.
- Automated analyzers are costly; however, they can reduce turnaround time and errors in the testing process.
- Many factors determine which analyzer will fill a particular laboratory's needs, including deciding whether a batch analyzer (which performs one test on multiple samples) or a random-access analyzer (which can run many different tests on multiple samples) can best serve testing needs.

Validation

- Once an analyzer has been purchased, a thorough validation of all assays to be performed must be done to ensure quality of testing. Validation should include a determination of accuracy, precision, analytic sensitivity, analytic specificity, reportable range, and reference interval.
- Accuracy refers to a test's ability to measure what it actually claims to measure.
- Precision is the ability to consistently reproduce the same result on a particular sample.
- Analytic sensitivity is the lowest measurable amount of an analyte, whereas analytic specificity is the assay's ability to give a negative result when the analyte is absent.
- The reportable range is the range of values that will generate a positive result for a test, whereas the reference interval is the range of values found in healthy individuals.

CASE STUDIES

1. A laboratory has just purchased a new immunoassay analyzer, and validation is being done before patient results can be reported. Twenty random patient samples are run by both the old and new methods. Three samples that were negative by the old instrument are positive by the new analyzer.

Questions

a. What sort of possible error—that is, sensitivity, specificity, accuracy, or precision—does this represent?

b. What steps should be taken to resolve this discrepancy?

2. A 3-year-old child is sent for immunologic testing because of recurring respiratory infections, including several bouts of pneumonia. The results show decreased immunoglobulin levels, especially of IgG. Although the patient's WBC count was within the normal range, the lymphocyte count was low. Flow cytometry was performed to determine if a particular subset of lymphocytes was low or missing. **Figure 13–12** shows the flow cytometry results obtained.

Questions

a. What do the flow cytometry patterns indicate about the population of lymphocytes affected?

b. How can this account for the child's recurring infections?

c. What further type of testing might be indicated?

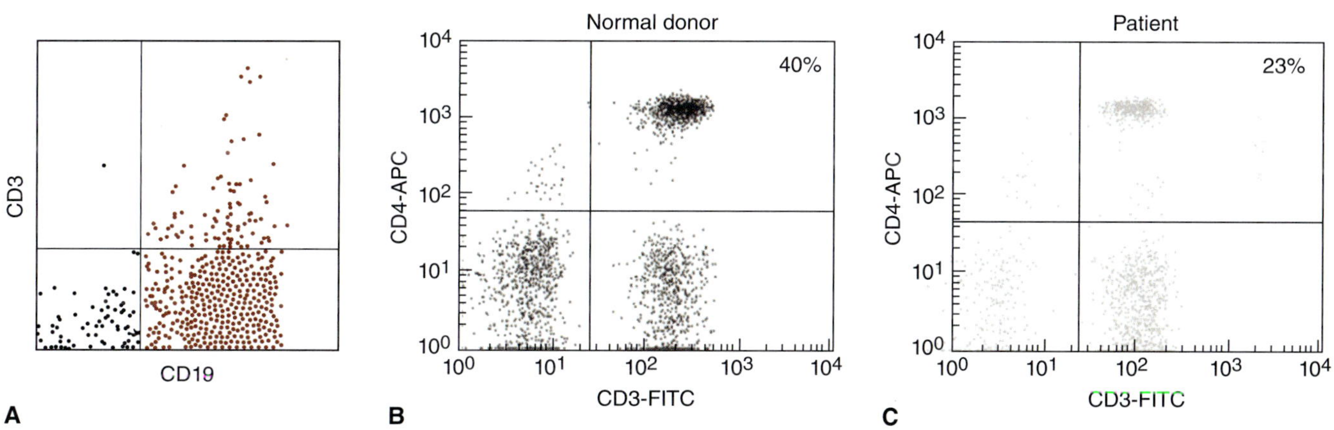

FIGURE 13–12 Flow cytometry patterns for the case study. (A) Patient plot of CD3 versus CD19. (B) and (C) Patient plots of CD3 versus CD4.

REVIEW QUESTIONS

1. Flow cytometers use different flow rates for diluent and sample injection to create
   a. Laminar flow
   b. Parallel flow
   c. Balanced flow
   d. Dynamic flow

2. Forward light scatter is an indicator of a cell's
   a. granularity.
   b. density.
   c. size.
   d. number.

3. For immunophenotyping, what reagent is added to the sample to detect cell surface antigens?
   a. Colorimetric dye
   b. Fluorochrome labeled antibodies
   c. Enzyme-linked antibodies
   d. Isotonic solution to burst red blood cells

4. Which statement represents the best explanation for a flow cytometer's ability to detect several cell surface markers at the same time?
   a. The forward scatter can separate out cells on the basis of complexity.
   b. One detector can be used to detect many different wavelengths.
   c. For each marker, a specific fluorochrome–antibody combination is used.
   d. Intrinsic parameters are separated out based on the amount of side scatter.

5. Which of the following cell surface markers would be present on a population of T helper (T_H) cells?
   a. CD3 and CD4
   b. CD3 and CD8
   c. CD3 only
   d. CD4 only

6. If an analyzer consistently indicates a positive test when the analyte in question is not present, this represents a problem with
   a. sensitivity.
   b. specificity.
   c. reportable range.
   d. precision.

7. All of the following are clinical applications for flow cytometry *except*
   a. fetal hemoglobin.
   b. immunophenotyping of lymphocyte subpopulations.
   c. HIV viral load analysis.
   d. enumeration of stem cells in a peripheral blood mononuclear cell product.

8. The fluorescent signals generated by cells intersecting with a flow cytometry laser are captured by
   a. bandwidth waves.
   b. wave channels.
   c. photomultiplier tubes.
   d. flow cells.

9. Data obtained by flow cytometric analysis of cells can be filtered by using a method of
   a. "gating" in a dot plot.
   b. banding of a histogram.
   c. single-parameter histogram monitoring.
   d. automatic sampling.

10. A flow cytometry technology that has the potential to detect 100 analytes from one sample of blood is called a/an
   a. RBC fragmentation assay.
   b. Dihydrorhodamine 123.
   c. sucrose test.
   d. cytometric bead array.

11. Which population of cells are lysed during the initial sample preparation steps for flow cytometry?
   a. Platelets
   b. White blood cells
   c. Epithelial cells
   d. Red blood cells

12. CD45 is a pan-leukocyte marker expressed on WBCs in varying levels or amounts of expression, based on the:
   a. size of a cell.
   b. granularity of a cell.
   c. maturity and lineage of a cell.
   d. malignancy of a cell.

13. Which of the following statements best describes a single-parameter histogram?
   a. Each event is represented by a dot.
   b. Data are distributed in four quadrants.
   c. Positive and negative events are plotted on the *x*- and *y*-axes.
   d. A chosen parameter is plotted versus the number of events.

14. What is the major function of the fluidics component of the flow cytometer?
   a. Regulates the temperature of the lasers
   b. Organizes scatter properties data for analysis
   c. Identifies positive fluorescent signals
   d. Suspends cells for transport past the laser

15. Which type of analyzer allows one to measure multiple analytes from numerous samples, loaded at any time?
   a. Batch analyzer
   b. Random-access analyzer
   c. Front-end-loaded analyzer
   d. Sequential access analyzer

16. Operational considerations when selecting automated analyzers for a laboratory include which of the following?
   a. Reagent stability
   b. Test menu
   c. STAT capability
   d. All of the above

17. Analyzers use different methods for mixing, including magnetic stirring, rotation paddles, and forceful dispensing. Whichever method is used, it is imperative that
   a. reagents should always be kept refrigerated.
   b. there is no splashing or carryover between samples.
   c. samples are kept at room temperature.
   d. multiple methods are not used simultaneously.

18. All of the following are benefits of automation *except*
   a. greater accuracy.
   b. reduced turnaround time.
   c. savings on reagents.
   d. No need for controls.

19. If an analyzer gets different results each time the same sample is tested, what type of problem does this represent?
   a. Sensitivity
   b. Specificity
   c. Accuracy
   d. Precision

20. If a research scientist wanted to study activated T cells after exposure to a virus, what CD markers could be used to identify the cells of interest in a whole blood sample?
a. CD10, CD19, CD34
b. CD16, CD56, CD45
c. CD2, CD5, CD25
d. CD15, CD14, CD13

21. Which quadrant would contain B cells if CD56 was plotted on the *x*-axis and CD19 on the *y*-axis?
a. Quadrant 1
b. Quadrant 2
c. Quadrant 3
d. Quadrant 4

22. A sample was sent from the hematology laboratory for flow cytometry testing. The patient was diagnosed with HIV, and the physician was interested in the CD4 absolute count. The following data was submitted from the CBC and differential:

WBC $9.5 \times 10^3/\mu L$
Differential:
Segmented neutrophils 56%
Band neutrophils 2%
Lymphocytes 20%
Monocytes 6%
Eosinophils 6%
After immunophenotyping the following populations were analyzed.

CD Marker	Percentage Positive (%)
$CD3^+$	65
$CD3^+/CD4^+$	17
$CD3^+/CD8^+$	48

What is the absolute lymphocyte count?
a. 190
b. 510
c. 1900
d. 4760

23. What is the absolute CD4 count in the example presented in Question 22?
a. 323
b. 1235
c. 32
d. 912

24. Calculate the absolute value of the $CD19^+$ positive cells based on the given data from the Hematology and Flow Cytometry laboratories.

CBC (complete blood count) and Differential from Hematology

Test	Result
WBC	$12.6 \times 10^3/\mu L$
Neutrophil	36%
Lymphocytes	22%
Monocytes	5%

Flow Cytometry Results from Immunology

Marker	Result
CD19	12%

The absolute count for the $CD19^+$ B cells in this sample is?
a. 49.9
b. 332.6
c. 1512
d. 33.2

Chapter 13 Answer Key

Answers to Knowledge Checks

13.1 b 13.2 a 13.3 b 13.4 d 13.5 c 13.6 d

Answers to Review Questions

1. a 2. c 3. b 4. c 5. a 6. b 7. c
8. c 9. a 10. d 11. d 12. c 13. d 14. d
15. b 16. d 17. b 18. d 19. d 20. c 21. a
22. c 23. a 24. b

Immune Disorders III

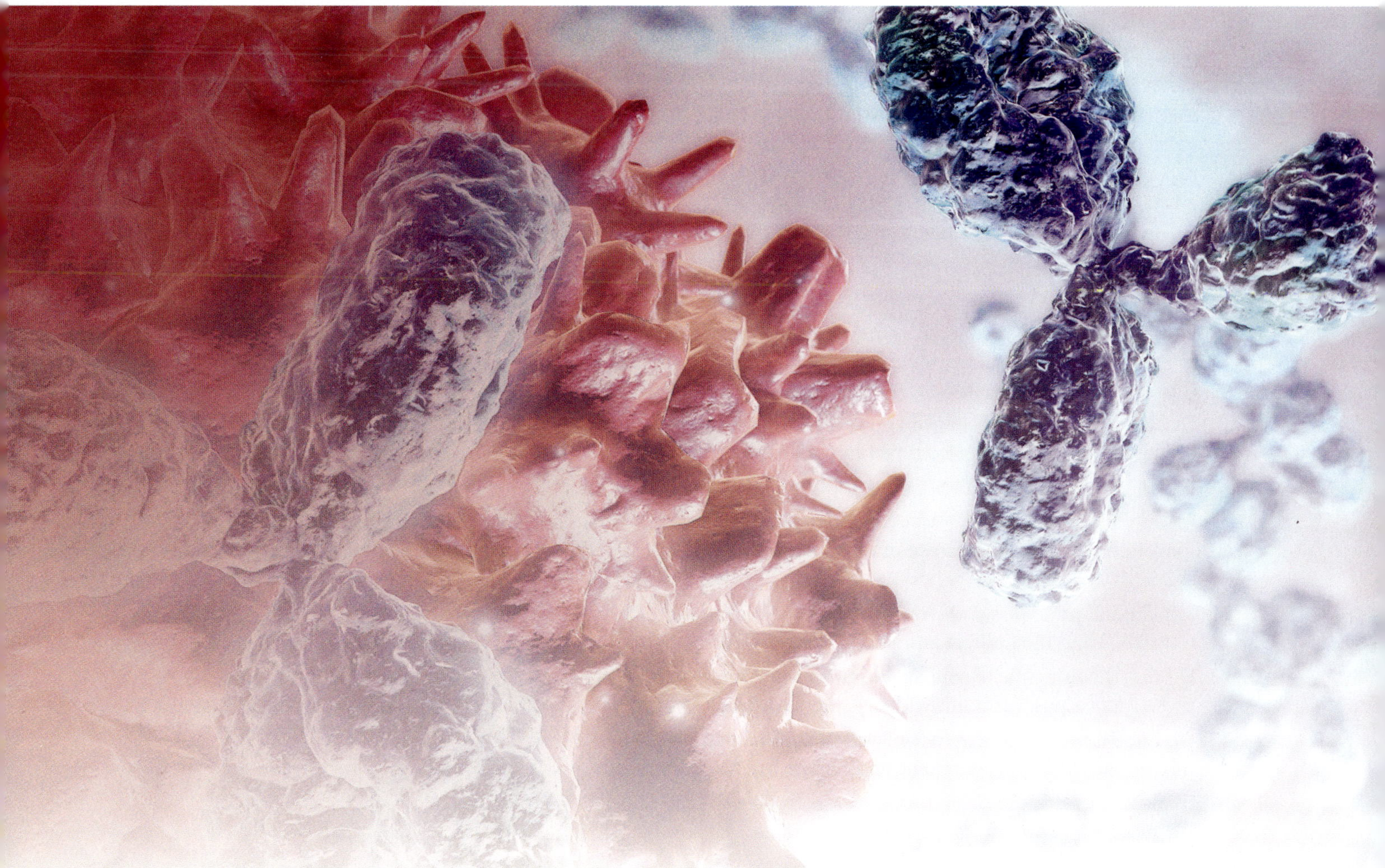

14 Hypersensitivity

Linda E. Miller, PhD, MB^{CM}(ASCP)SI

LEARNING OUTCOMES

After finishing this chapter, you should be able to:

14.1 Explain the concept of hypersensitivity.

14.2 Differentiate between the four types of hypersensitivity reactions in terms of antibody involvement, complement involvement, antigen triggers, and timing of the response.

14.3 Associate specific examples of clinical manifestations with each type of hypersensitivity.

14.4 Describe the immunologic mechanisms involved in each of the four types of hypersensitivity reactions.

14.5 Provide examples of preformed and newly synthesized mediators released from immunoglobulin E (IgE)-sensitized mast cells and basophils and discuss their effects.

14.6 Discuss the influence of genetic and environmental factors on susceptibility to type I hypersensitivity responses.

14.7 Explain the underlying mechanisms of pharmacological therapy, monoclonal antibody therapy, and allergy immunotherapy (AIT) in the treatment of allergies.

14.8 Discuss the procedure, clinical applications, advantages, and limitations of skin testing for type I hypersensitivity.

14.9 Describe the principles and clinical applications of allergen-specific and total IgE testing.

14.10 Explain how hemolytic disease of the fetus and newborn (HDFN) arises.

14.11 Explain the principles and clinical uses of the direct antiglobulin test (DAT) and the indirect antiglobulin test (IAT).

14.12 Discuss the principle of cold agglutinins testing and associate the presence of a positive result with specific disorders.

14.13 Describe how skin testing for delayed hypersensitivity is performed, its clinical applications, and how to interpret the results.

14.14 Explain the principle of interferon gamma release assays (IGRAs), their clinical utility, advantages, and limitations.

CHAPTER OUTLINE

You can go to **fadavis.com** keyword stevens for the laboratory exercises that accompany this text.

In previous chapters, we described immune responses as defense mechanisms that the body uses to rid itself of potentially harmful antigens. However, in some cases, the antigen can persist, and the immune response can cause damage to the host. This type of reaction, called **hypersensitivity,** is an exaggerated response to a typically harmless antigen that results in tissue injury, disease, or even death.

In the 1960s, British immunologists Philip Gell and Robin Coombs devised a classification system for hypersensitivity reactions based on their immunologic mechanisms. In this widely used system, these reactions are classified into four categories:

- **Type I hypersensitivity**—also known as *anaphylactic* hypersensitivity
- **Type II hypersensitivity**—also known as *antibody-mediated cytotoxic* hypersensitivity
- **Type III hypersensitivity**—also known as *complex-mediated* hypersensitivity
- **Type IV hypersensitivity**—also known as *cell-mediated* hypersensitivity

Hypersensitivity types I, II, and III are mediated by antibodies. Because symptoms associated with these types develop within a few minutes to a few hours after exposure to the inducing antigen, they are also known as **immediate hypersensitivity** reactions. In contrast, sensitized T cells, rather than antibodies, are responsible for type IV hypersensitivity. Clinical manifestations of type IV hypersensitivity typically do not appear until 24 to 48 hours after contact with antigen; therefore, this type is sometimes referred to as **delayed hypersensitivity.**

In this chapter, we review the nature of the immune reactants, clinical examples, and relevant testing for the four types of hypersensitivity. Knowledge about the underlying immunologic mechanisms of each type will help you understand how the tissue damage and resulting disease manifestations originate.

Type I Hypersensitivity

Type I hypersensitivity reactions are commonly thought of as *allergies.* A distinguishing feature of type I hypersensitivity is the short time span, usually minutes, between exposure to antigen and the onset of clinical symptoms. Some examples of these reactions are hay fever, allergic asthma, hives, and systemic anaphylaxis.

The antigens that trigger type I hypersensitivity are called **allergens.** Substances that can act as allergens are typically low-to-medium molecular weight proteins that are stable, highly glycosylated, and soluble in body fluids. Examples of common allergens include proteins in peanuts, eggs, pollen, and house dust mites. Some nonprotein substances, like the drug penicillin, can also stimulate type I hypersensitivity by acting as haptens that bind to self-proteins in the tissues.

In 1967, the serum factor responsible for type I hypersensitivity was identified as immunoglobulin E (IgE). Typically, patients who exhibit allergic hypersensitivity reactions produce a large amount of IgE antibody in response to a small concentration of allergen. IgE levels appear to depend on the interaction of both genetic and environmental factors. **Atopy,** a term derived from the Greek word *atopos* (meaning "out of place"), refers to an inherited tendency to develop classic allergic responses to naturally occurring inhaled or ingested allergens. The section that follows provides details about the immunologic mechanism that occurs in susceptible individuals to produce the symptoms of type I hypersensitivity reactions. While a similar reaction can occur in response to nonimmunologic stimuli, including exercise, cold temperatures, and some drugs, this chapter focuses on IgE-mediated hypersensitivity.

Immunologic Mechanism

Type I hypersensitivity is also known as *anaphylactic hypersensitivity,* based on its immunologic mechanism. The key components involved in this hypersensitivity type are IgE antibody, mast cells, basophils, and eosinophils. These components act together to produce an immediate type of reaction, which typically occurs within 30 to 60 minutes after antigen exposure. Type I hypersensitivity has two major phases: *sensitization* and *activation.* A *late-phase* reaction may also occur in some individuals.

Sensitization Phase

The steps of the sensitization phase are illustrated in **Figure 14–1.** The response begins when a susceptible individual is exposed to an allergen and produces specific IgE antibody. Langerhans and dendritic cells internalize and process the allergen, attach it to a major histocompatibility complex (MHC) class II molecule, and transport the complex to antigen-specific helper T (T_H) cells in the local lymphoid tissue. The T_H cells then produce cytokines that activate antigen-specific B

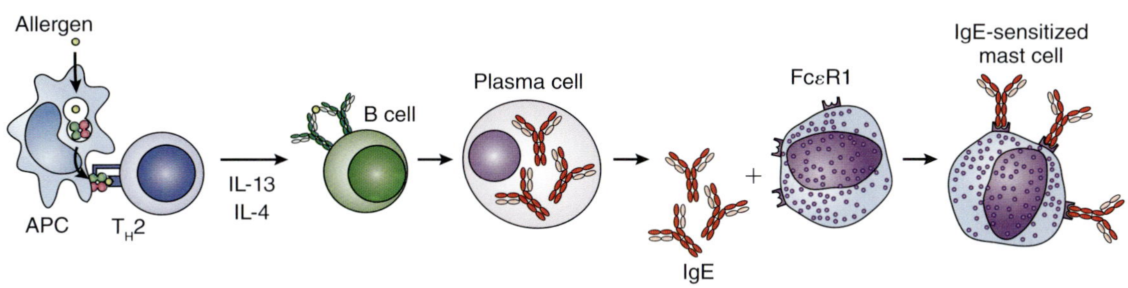

FIGURE 14–1 Type I hypersensitivity: Sensitization phase. Antigen-specific IgE is produced and attaches to Fc receptors on mast cells and basophils. APC = Antigen presenting cell.

cells to produce IgE antibody. IgE is mainly synthesized by B cells and plasma cells in the lymphoid tissue of the respiratory and gastrointestinal tracts and in the lymph nodes.

IgE production appears to be regulated by type 2 helper T cells (T_H2; see Chapters 5 and 6). In a normal immune response to microorganisms and other antigens, there is an appropriate balance between the activity of the T_H2 cells and the type 1 helper T cells (T_H1), which results in protective immunity that does not harm the host. However, in people with allergies, the immune response is shifted so that T_H2 cells predominate. This T_H2 type of response results in the production of several cytokines, including interleukin 4 (IL-4) and interleukin (IL-13). These cytokines are responsible for the final differentiation that occurs in B cells, initiating transcription of the gene that codes for the epsilon heavy chain of immunoglobulin molecules belonging to the IgE class. Additionally, IL-13 secreted by T_H2 cells stimulates increased mucus secretion by epithelial cells lining the airways and digestive tract.

In the sensitization phase, the IgE antibody produced attaches to high-affinity receptors called *FcεRI,* which bind the crystallizable fragment (Fc) region of the epsilon heavy chain. Large numbers of these receptors are found on mast cells and basophils, with a single cell having as many as 200,000 such receptors. Once bound to FcεRI, IgE functions as a receptor for the allergen.

Mast cells are the principal effector cells of immediate hypersensitivity. Found throughout the body and in most organs, they tend to be concentrated around the small blood vessels, lymphatics, nerves, and glandular tissue. Mast cells have abundant cytoplasmic granules that store numerous preformed inflammatory mediators. They are long-lived, residing for months in the tissues (see Chapter 1). Basophils are similar to, but distinct from, mast cells in their appearance and function. They are present in the peripheral blood, where they represent less than 1% of the total white blood cells (WBCs). They have fewer but larger granules than mast cells, and the concentrations of inflammatory substances in the basophil granules differ from those of mast cells. Basophils respond to chemotactic stimuli during inflammation and accumulate in the tissues, where they can persist for a few days.

Activation Phase

Upon repeated exposure to the allergen, the IgE-sensitized mast cells and basophils become activated and release chemicals that induce the symptoms of allergy. In the activation phase of the response, adjacent cell-bound IgE molecules are cross-linked by a bivalent or multivalent antigen, causing aggregation of the surface FcεRI receptors. This action, in turn, initiates complex intracellular signaling events involving multiple phosphorylation reactions, an influx of calcium, and the secretion of cytokines. The increase in intracellular calcium triggers rapid degranulation of the mast cells and basophils, which release chemical mediators that have been previously made and stored in the granules **(Fig. 14–2).** These preformed substances are referred to as *primary* mediators.

The most abundant preformed mediator is **histamine,** which makes up about 10% of the total weight of the granules in mast cells. Other primary mediators and their effects are listed in **Table 14–1.** Release of these substances is responsible for the early-phase symptoms seen in allergic reactions, which occur within 30 to 60 minutes after exposure to the allergen. The chemical mediators bind to receptors on target organs, most notably the skin, respiratory tract, and gastrointestinal tract, producing symptoms characteristic of an allergic response. The clinical manifestations depend on the target tissue and type of receptors activated. For example, in the skin, local swelling and redness, sometimes referred to as a ***wheal-and-flare*** reaction, can develop. Contraction of the smooth muscle in the bronchioles may result in airflow obstruction. Increased vascular permeability can cause hypotension or shock. Depending on the route by which an individual is exposed to the triggering allergen, one or more of these effects may be seen.

Late Phase

In addition to immediate release of preformed mediators, mast cells and basophils are triggered to synthesize other reactants from the breakdown of phospholipids in the cell membrane. These newly formed, or ***secondary,*** mediators include platelet-activating factor (PAF); prostaglandin (PG) D_2; **leukotrienes (LT)** B_4, C_4, D_4, and E_4; and cytokines (see Table 14–1). These products are more potent than the primary mediators and are responsible for a late-phase allergic reaction that can be seen in some individuals 6 to 8 hours after exposure to the antigen. In this phase of the reaction, numerous cells, including eosinophils, neutrophils, T_H2 cells, mast cells, basophils, and macrophages, exit the circulation and infiltrate the allergen-filled tissue. They release additional mediators that prolong hyperactivity and cause further tissue damage.

Eosinophils play an important role in the late-phase reaction. These cells are normally 1% to 3% of the circulating WBCs. During allergic reactions, T_H2 cells secrete IL-4, which stimulates recruitment of eosinophils to the tissues, and IL-5, which causes the bone marrow to increase eosinophil production. Thus, the number of eosinophils in the peripheral blood increases, creating a state called ***eosinophilia.*** The number of FcεRI receptors on eosinophils increases during the allergic response, enabling them to bind more IgE. The eosinophils release a variety of toxic molecules and inflammatory mediators from their granules, which contribute to the ongoing damage that occurs during chronic allergic conditions (Table 14–1).

In individuals with persistent inflammation resulting from the late-phase reaction, such as those with chronic asthma, tissue remodeling can result. This involves structural changes, such as thickening of smooth muscle, as well as changes in connective tissue, blood and lymphatic vessels, mucous glands, and nerves.

Knowledge Check 14-1

Type I hypersensitivity involves sensitization of mast cells by:

a. IgA
b. IgG
c. IgE
d. IL-4

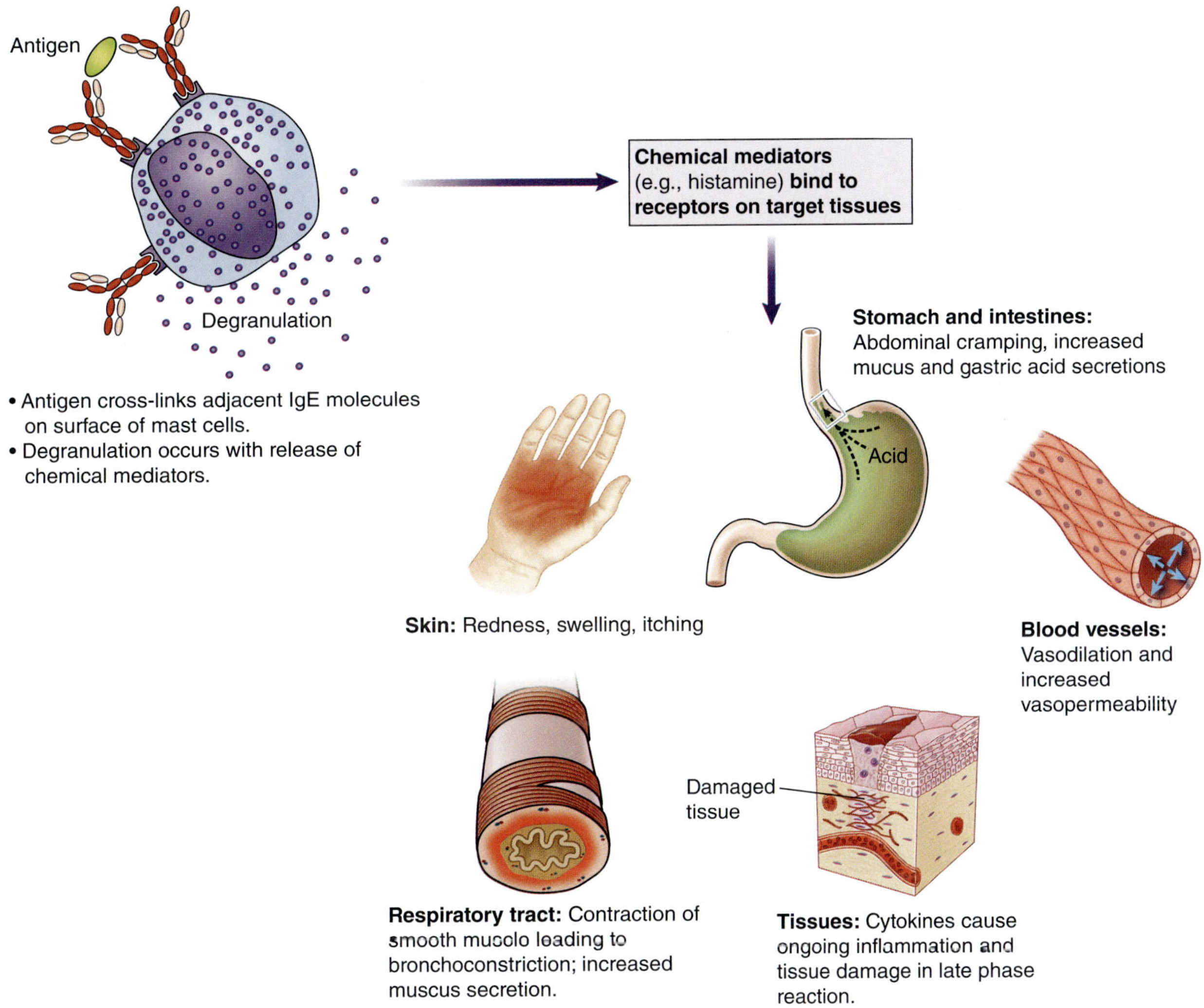

FIGURE 14–2 Type I hypersensitivity: Activation phase. Reexposure to the same antigen causes cross-linking of surface IgE, degranulation of mast cells and basophils, and release of chemical mediators that bind to target cells and cause allergy symptoms.

Genetic and Environmental Influences on Type I Hypersensitivity

The development of IgE responses and allergy appears to depend on complex interactions between genetic factors and environmental triggers. Several hundred genes associated with susceptibility to developing allergies have been identified. These genes affect different aspects of the immune response that contribute to the pathogenesis of type I hypersensitivity, including genes that affect the following:

- The structure of the body's protective skin and mucous membrane barriers and their ability to prevent penetration of microbes and potential allergens (e.g., gene for filaggrin)
- Recognition of the antigen by the innate immune system once the antigen has entered through the epithelial barriers (e.g., genes for CD14, and toll-like receptors TLR2 and TLR4)
- Cytokine production, the balance between T_H1 cells and T_H2 cells, and IgE production (e.g., genes for IL-4, IL-5, IL-13, IL-33, class II MHC)
- The process of tissue remodeling and repair (e.g., ADAM33)

Many environmental influences on the allergic response have also been identified. Exposure to infectious organisms appears to play a key role in the development of allergic disease. The increased prevalence of allergy in industrialized regions may be due, in part, to increased hygiene practices and use of antibiotics, with a consequent decrease in exposure to microbes. This, in turn, could have significant effects on the immune system by altering the microbial constituent of the gut and decreasing microbial diversity in the body. In utero or early life exposure to diverse microbes, such as those in a farming environment, appears to provide protection against allergies by inducing the development of regulatory T cells (Treg) and by directing the immune system toward beneficial T_H1 responses and away from T_H2 atopic reactions. Respiratory infections that damage pulmonary mucosal barriers, exposure to stress, variations in physical factors such as temperature, and contact with environmental pollutants such as cigarette smoke and diesel exhaust fumes can intensify clinical manifestations of allergy in susceptible individuals.

Table 14-1 Major Mediators of Type I Hypersensitivity

CATEGORY	EXAMPLES	EFFECTS
Preformed (primary) mediators produced by mast cells and basophils	Histamine	Smooth muscle contractions, vasodilation, increased vascular permeability
	Heparin	Stabilizes histamine, anticoagulation
	Enzymes: proteases (e.g., tryptases, chymase, cathepsin G, granzyme B), lysosomal enzymes	Activate complement proteins and cytokines, stimulate mucus production, tissue damage/ remodeling
	Cytokines (e.g., TNF-α, IL-4)	Recruit and activate inflammatory cells (e.g., neutrophils, eosinophils), induce IgE synthesis, induce apoptosis
Newly synthesized (secondary) mediators produced by mast cells and basophils	Prostaglandin PGD_2	Vasodilation, increased vascular permeability, bronchoconstriction, WBC chemotaxis
	Leukotrienes LTC_4, LTD_4, LTE_4	Increased vascular permeability, bronchoconstriction, mucus secretion
	PAF	Platelet aggregation, increased vasodilation and vasopermeability, WBC adhesion, chemotaxis
	Cytokines: IL-1, IL-3, IL-4, IL-5, IL-6, IL-8, IL-13, TNF-α, GM-CSF Chemokines (e.g., IL-8, CCL3)	Increase inflammatory cells in area; increase IgE production; increase myeloid cell production
Mediators produced by eosinophils	Enzymes (e.g., lysosomal hydrolases) Leukotrienes LTC_4, LTD_4, LTE_4 Cytokines and chemokines (e.g., IL-3, IL-5, GM-CSF, IL-8, IL-10, CCL3)	Tissue damage/remodeling Increased vascular permeability, bronchoconstriction, mucus secretion Increased production and activation of eosinophils WBC chemotaxis

GM-CSF = granulocyte-macrophage colony stimulating factor; IL = interleukin; PAF = platelet-activating factor; TNF = tumor necrosis factor; WBC = white blood cell.

Clinical Manifestations of Type I Hypersensitivity

Clinical manifestations of type I hypersensitivity are common. The prevalence of allergic diseases has been increasing worldwide for several decades, and a significant percentage of the world's population has allergic sensitization to common environmental antigens such as pollen or peanuts. In the United States alone, allergies have been reported as the sixth-leading cause of chronic illness, affecting nearly one in three adults and over one in four children.

The clinical manifestations of type I hypersensitivity are caused by the release of inflammatory mediators from mast cells and basophils and vary from a localized skin reaction to a severe systemic response known as **anaphylaxis.** Symptoms depend on variables such as the route of antigen exposure, allergen dose, and exposure frequency. If an allergen is inhaled, it is most likely to cause respiratory symptoms such as allergic rhinitis or allergic asthma. Ingestion of an allergen may result in gastrointestinal symptoms, whereas injection into the bloodstream can trigger a systemic response.

Allergic Rhinitis

Rhinitis is the most common form of atopy, or allergy. Symptoms include paroxysmal sneezing, rhinorrhea (runny nose), nasal congestion, and itching of the nose and eyes. Although the condition itself is merely annoying, complications such as sinusitis, otitis media (ear infection), eustachian tube dysfunction, and sleep disturbances may result. Pollen, mold spores, animal dander, and particulate matter from house dust mites are examples of airborne foreign particles that act directly on the mast cells in the conjunctiva and respiratory mucous membranes to trigger rhinitis. Seasonal allergic rhinitis, triggered by tree and grass pollens in the air during the spring in temperate climates, is called "hay fever."

Allergic Asthma

Asthma, derived from the Greek word for "panting" or "breathlessness," is caused by inhalation of small particles such as pollen, dust, or fumes that reach the lower respiratory tract. It can be defined clinically as recurrent airflow obstruction that leads to intermittent sneezing, breathlessness, and occasionally, a cough with sputum production. The airflow obstruction is caused by bronchial smooth muscle contraction, mucosal edema, and heavy mucus secretion. All these changes lead to an increase in airway resistance, making it difficult for inspired air to leave the lungs. The trapped air creates the sense of breathlessness.

Food and Drug Allergies

Food allergies are another example of type I immediate hypersensitivity reactions. Some of the most common food allergies are caused by cow's milk, eggs, nuts, soy, wheat, fish, and shellfish. Symptoms limited to the gastrointestinal tract include cramping, vomiting, and diarrhea, whereas spread of antigen through the bloodstream may cause urticaria (hives) and angioedema (swelling beneath the skin), asthma, rhinitis, or anaphylaxis (see the text that follows).

Drugs commonly implicated as triggers for type I hypersensitivity include penicillin and related antibiotics, sulfa drugs, anticonvulsants, NSAIDs (e.g., aspirin, ibuprofen), and chemotherapy drugs used to treat cancer. Symptoms can include skin rash, hives, itching, swelling, asthma, vomiting, dizziness, and anaphylaxis.

Skin Reactions

Local inflammation of the skin, or *dermatitis,* can also be caused by type I immediate hypersensitivity reactions. These reactions manifest as either acute urticaria or eczema. Urticaria appear within minutes after exposure to the allergen and are characterized by severe itching, erythema (redness) caused by local vasodilation, leakage of fluid into the surrounding area, and a spreading area of redness around the center of the lesion **(Fig. 14–3)**. Commonly called *wheal-and-flare,* this reaction is caused by the release of vasoactive mediators from mast cells in the skin following contact with allergens such as pet dander or insect venom. When these reactions occur deeper in the dermal tissues, they are known as *angioedema* **(Fig. 14–4)**. Urticaria can also appear because of other clinical manifestations, such as anaphylaxis and food allergies.

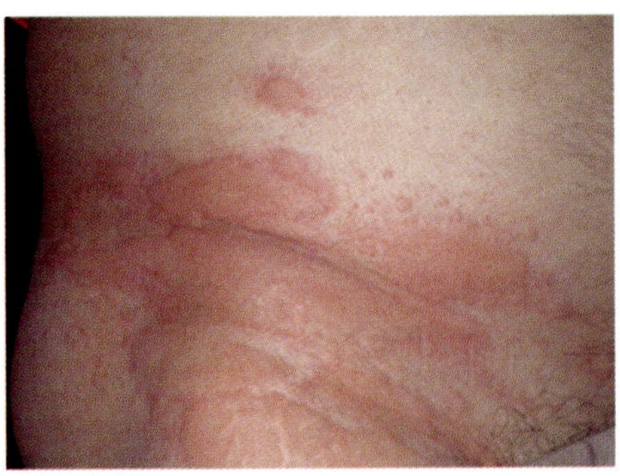

FIGURE 14–3 Urticaria (hives) caused by an immediate hypersensitivity reaction to a medication.

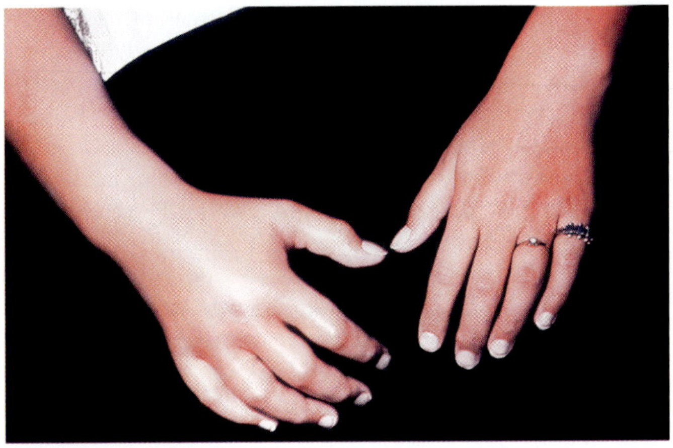

FIGURE 14–4 Angioedema caused by a yellow jacket sting on the right hand just above the middle finger. *(Courtesy of CDC/Margaret A. Parsons, Public Health Image Library.)*

Atopic eczema can take on various forms, from erythematous, oozing vesicles to thickened, scaly skin, depending on the stage of the reaction and the person's age. It is a chronic, itchy skin rash that usually develops during infancy, persists during childhood, and is strongly associated with allergic rhinitis and asthma.

Anaphylaxis

Anaphylaxis is the most severe type of allergic response because it is an acute reaction that simultaneously involves multiple organs. It may be fatal if not treated promptly. Anaphylactic reactions are typically triggered by glycoproteins or large polypeptides. Smaller molecules, such as penicillin, can also trigger anaphylaxis by acting as haptens that may become immunogenic by combining with host cell proteins. Typical agents that induce anaphylaxis include venom from bees, wasps, and hornets; drugs such as penicillin; and foods such as shellfish, peanuts, and dairy products.

Clinical signs of anaphylaxis begin within minutes after antigenic challenge and may include bronchospasm and laryngeal edema, vascular congestion, skin manifestations such as urticaria and angioedema, diarrhea or vomiting, and intractable shock because of the effect on blood vessels and smooth muscle of the circulatory system. The reaction's severity depends on the number of previous exposures to the antigen. This is because multiple exposures result in additional accumulation of IgE on the surface of the mast cells and basophils. Massive release of reactants from the granules, especially histamine, is responsible for the ensuing symptoms. Death may result from asphyxiation because of upper airway edema and congestion, irreversible shock, or a combination of these symptoms.

Latex Sensitivity

Natural rubber latex, an intracellular cytosol secreted from the rubber tree, *Hevea brasiliensis,* is used in the manufacture of many common items, including rubber gloves, balloons, condoms, and bandages. It contains many antigens that can trigger hypersensitivity. These reactions can be in the form of type I hypersensitivity or contact dermatitis caused by skin irritation or type IV hypersensitivity. Type I hypersensitivity reactions can manifest as urticaria, rhinoconjunctivitis (nasal congestion with runny nose and red eyes), asthma, angioedema, or anaphylaxis.

Latex sensitivity became a significant problem in the late 1980s after the implementation of Universal Precautions by the Centers for Disease Control and Prevention (CDC) and regulations by the Occupational Safety and Health Administration (OSHA) that required health care workers to wear gloves when performing laboratory procedures and working with patients. Sensitization to latex can occur because of direct skin contact or inhalation of airborne latex particles released when gloves are donned and removed. The risk of the latter occurring is increased when cornstarch powder is used in gloves because residual latex proteins can bind to the powder particles.

Groups at increased risk for latex allergy include health care workers, rubber industry workers, patients who have had multiple surgeries, and people who are allergic to certain foods that cross-react with latex allergens. The prevalence of latex sensitivity in the general population is estimated to be 4.3%, whereas it is thought to be more than 12% in health care workers and much higher in patients who have undergone multiple surgeries early in life. The incidence of latex sensitization has decreased in recent years in countries such as the United States where policies to avoid contact with latex have been implemented. These policies include the use of low-protein, powder-free gloves or gloves made from nonlatex materials, such as nitrile, neoprene, vinyl, or synthetic polyisoprene rubber.

Treatment of Type I Hypersensitivity

Allergen Avoidance

Avoidance of known allergens is the first line of defense. People can use environmental interventions such as encasing mattresses and pillows in allergen-proof covers and removing a harmful food from the diet. However, it is not always possible to eliminate contact with allergens. In these cases, pharmacological therapy is necessary to relieve acute symptoms, control chronic allergy manifestations, and in some cases, modulate the immune response to the allergen.

Drug Therapies

Drugs used to treat immediate hypersensitivity vary with the severity of the reaction. Localized allergic reactions, such as hay fever, hives, or rhinitis, can be treated with antihistamines and decongestants. Asthma is often treated with a combination of therapeutic drugs, including antihistamines and bronchodilators. In cases of persistent asthma, LT receptor antagonists and mast cell stabilizers are also used; in severe cases, corticosteroids can be added to block recruitment of inflammatory cells and their ability to cause tissue damage. Systemic anaphylaxis is a medical emergency that requires timely injection of epinephrine, a powerful vasoconstrictor, to quickly reverse symptoms that could potentially be fatal.

Monoclonal Antibodies

Another treatment approach is aimed at modulating the type I hypersensitivity response using monoclonal antibodies. Omalizumab, the first anti-IgE monoclonal antibody to be approved for clinical use, is a recombinant humanized antibody composed of human IgG framework genes recombined with complementarity-determining region genes from mouse anti-human IgE. This antibody binds to the Cε3 domain of human IgE, the site that IgE normally uses to bind to FcεRI receptors. Blocking this site prevents circulating IgE from binding to mast cells and basophils and sensitizing them. Treatment with omalizumab has also been shown to downregulate cellular expression of FcεRI receptors. Anti-IgE monoclonal antibodies have been used successfully to treat patients with moderate to severe asthma when added to conventional drug therapy.

Other monoclonal antibodies have been developed that target T_H2 cytokines involved in type I hypersensitivity. These include antibodies directed against IL-5 or its receptor, which reduce the number and activity of eosinophils, and an antibody directed against the alpha subunit of the IL-4 receptor, which blocks intracellular signaling by IL-4 and IL-13. These antibodies have been used to treat severe eosinophilic asthma and moderate to severe atopic dermatitis.

Recent advancements in antibody discovery technologies have led to development of IgG monoclonal antibodies that target specific allergens. These antibodies are thought to act by binding to epitopes on the surface of the allergens, preventing the allergens from cross-linking surface IgE antibodies and activating mast cells and basophils. Passive immunotherapy with such monoclonal antibodies offers a promising approach to treating allergies in the future.

Allergy Immunotherapy

If environmental control and drug therapy are not successful in managing the symptoms in an allergic person, **allergy immunotherapy (AIT)** may be considered. The goal of AIT, also known as ***allergen desensitization,*** is to induce immune tolerance to a specific allergen by administering gradually increasing doses of the allergen over time. AIT is believed to shift the patient's immune response to the allergen to a T_H1-type response and to induce the development of allergen-specific Tregs that release interleukin-10 (IL-10) and other immunosuppressive cytokines. These cytokines regulate T- and B-cell responses to the allergen and redirect the immune system to produce allergen-specific IgG4 or IgA "blocking" antibodies that combine with the antigen before it can attach to IgE-coated cells. Therefore, decreased activation of mast cells and basophils occurs, along with inhibition of eosinophil responses.

The standard practice for AIT has been to administer allergens subcutaneously (i.e., under the skin) over a period of 3 to 5 years. This practice has been shown to significantly reduce symptoms in patients with allergic rhinitis or asthma; however, it has the potential to induce anaphylaxis and must be administered in a physician's office. More recently, other routes of administration that pose a decreased risk of severe adverse reactions have been used, namely, oral and sublingual (placement of an allergen extract under the tongue). These delivery methods have been shown to reduce symptoms associated with allergic asthma and rhinitis and to significantly decrease or eliminate allergic reactions to certain food allergens, such as peanuts. Researchers are also investigating the use of purified, recombinant allergens and allergoids, which have been chemically altered to reduce reactivity with IgE. These approaches may further increase the effectiveness of AIT while decreasing the associated risk of severe reactions.

Testing for Type I Hypersensitivity

Evaluation of patients with an allergy begins with a medical history and physical examination to assess clinical symptoms. These assessments are followed by in vivo skin tests and in vitro tests for specific IgE antibodies to confirm the presence of an allergy and to determine the allergens to which a patient is sensitized. There are several types of in vitro IgE tests: allergen-specific IgE, allergen component IgE (also known as *molecular-based allergy diagnostics*), point-of-care rapid tests, and total IgE quantitation.

In Vivo Skin Tests

Testing for allergies typically begins with direct skin testing because this procedure is less expensive than serological testing and provides immediate results. Two types of skin tests are used in clinical practice: percutaneous tests (also known as *prick* or *puncture tests*) and intradermal tests.

Percutaneous tests can detect hypersensitivity to a wide variety of inhaled or food allergens. In these tests, the clinician uses a needle or pricking device to introduce a small drop of allergen extract into the upper layers of a person's skin on the inner forearm or the back. A panel of allergens is routinely used, with each applied to separate sites at least 2 cm apart. A negative control, consisting of the diluent used for the allergy extract, and a positive control of histamine are also included. After 15 to 20 minutes, the clinician examines the testing spots and records the reaction. In a positive test, a wheal-and-flare reaction will appear at the site where the allergen was applied **(Fig. 14–5)**. This reaction is mediated by IgE-sensitized mast cells in the skin. Scoring of the reaction is based on the presence or absence of erythema and the diameter of the wheal, with a diameter larger than 3 mm correlating best with the presence of allergy.

Intradermal tests are more sensitive than cutaneous tests and are more effective in detecting venom and drug allergies. They may also be performed if prick tests are negative and allergy is still suspected; however, they carry a larger risk (0.05%) for anaphylactic reaction than prick tests (0.03%). In intradermal testing, a 1-mL tuberculin syringe is used to administer 0.01 to 0.05 mL of test solution between layers of the skin. The test allergen is diluted 10 to 1,000 times more than the solution used for cutaneous testing. This test is performed on the inner forearm or upper arm so that if a systemic reaction occurs, a tourniquet can be applied to the arm to help stop the reaction. After 15 to 20 minutes, the site is inspected for erythema and wheal formation, and the wheal diameter is measured to determine a score.

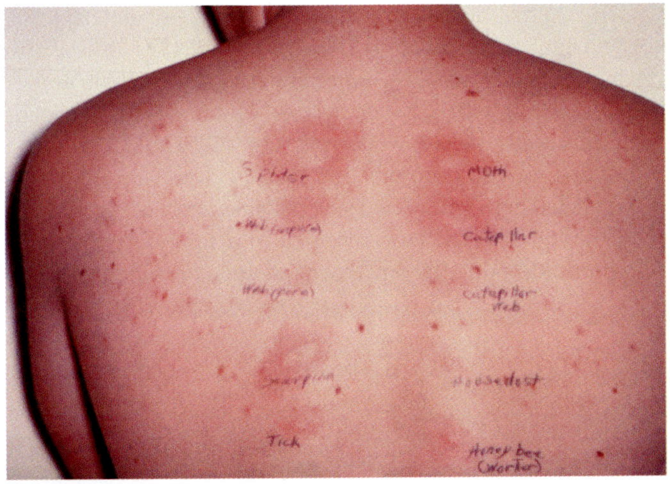

FIGURE 14–5 This individual is undergoing an allergen sensitivity test. The strongest positive reactions are to spider, moth, scorpion, caterpillar, and tick allergens, as indicated by the wheal-and-flare reactions at the sites of injection. *(Courtesy of the CDC/Dr. Frank Perlman and M.A. Parsons. Public Health Image Library.)*

Although skin testing is sensitive and relatively simple and inexpensive to perform, it has important limitations:

- There is slight risk that a systemic reaction can be triggered, so the test must be performed in the presence of an experienced medical professional.
- The test cannot be performed on patients who have severe skin conditions (e.g., urticaria, eczema, dermatographism [a condition in which scratching or pressure to the skin produces red swollen lines]) or tattoos on the arms that could interfere with interpretation of the results.
- Antihistamines and certain other medications must be discontinued a few days before testing because they can decrease or inhibit the skin reaction.
- False-negative results can be caused by absence of specific allergens in commercial extracts, improper technique, use of an inappropriate allergen dilution, or improperly stored allergen solutions.
- False-positive results can be caused by the patient's reaction to the diluent, preservative, or contaminants in the allergen extract or to physical trauma to the skin in patients with dermatographism.
- A positive skin test indicates sensitization to one or more allergens but does not necessarily mean clinical allergy; the diagnosis must be made through correlation of test results with clinical symptoms.

Allergen-Specific IgE Testing

Serological testing for allergen-specific IgE antibodies may be indicated when skin test results are not clear or do not correlate with the patient's clinical history. They may also be performed in cases where the risk of a harmful reaction is too large, skin disorders are present, or patients cannot discontinue medications before testing. These tests have excellent analytical sensitivity and are useful in detecting allergies to several common triggers, including ragweed, trees, grasses, molds, animal dander, foods, and insect venom.

The original commercial testing method for determining specific IgE, the ***radioallergosorbent test (RAST)***, was introduced in 1972. In this radioimmunoassay, patient serum was incubated with a paper disk to which various allergens were covalently linked. Following a washing step to remove unbound antibody, bound IgE was detected by adding a radiolabeled anti-IgE. After a second wash step, the amount of radioactivity detected was measured by a gamma counter and was proportional to the amount of allergen-specific IgE in the patient's sample.

Current immunoassays for serum IgE are also based on the classic sandwich technique but involve automated methods that use enzyme labels that react with substrates to produce fluorescence, chemiluminescence, or colorimetric reactions rather than radioactive labels. **Figure 14–6** illustrates the principle of these tests. The tests can be run with a single allergen or as a multiallergen screen using a panel of allergens in a single run. A commercial noncompetitive fluoroimmunoassay is considered by most allergy specialists to be the method of choice. In this assay, fluorescence is produced in proportion

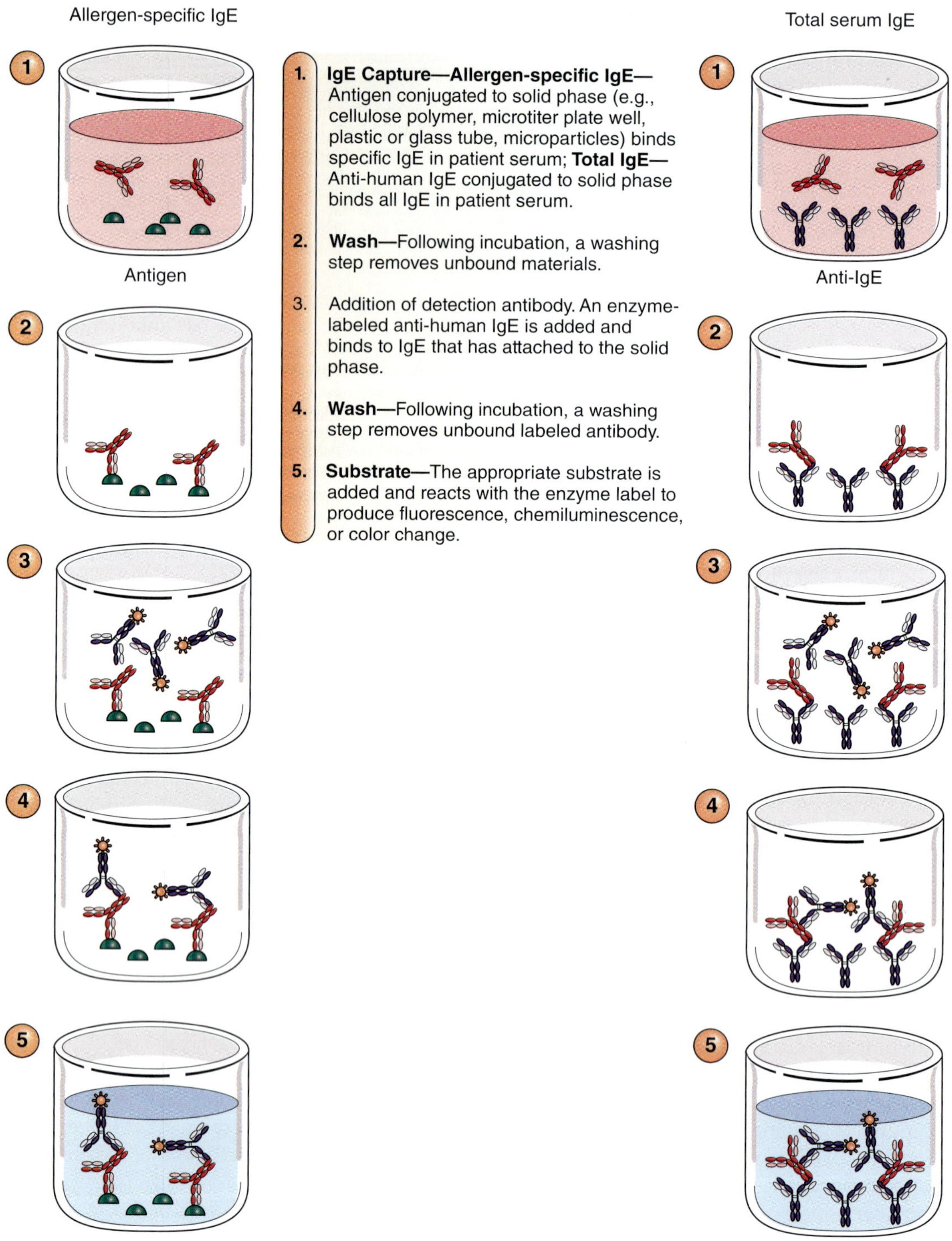

FIGURE 14–6 Comparison of noncompetitive immunoassays for allergen-specific IgE (formerly known as *RAST*) and total serum IgE (formerly known as *RIST*). IgE in the patient serum is shown in red for both tests.

to the amount of allergen-specific IgE in the sample. Patient results are derived from a standard calibration curve that is linked to the World Health Organization (WHO) IgE standard. Allergen-specific IgE values are reported in kilo international units (IU) of allergen-specific antibody per liter (kUA/L), where 1 unit is equal to 2.42 ng/mL of IgE. The method can detect IgE antibodies in the range of 0 to 100 kU/L, and 0.35 kU/L is commonly used as the cutoff for a positive test.

The results obtained by different immunoassays are not interchangeable because of differences in the composition of the allergen reagents. These reagents may consist of whole, natural extracts, or single allergen molecules derived by biochemical purification or recombinant DNA technology. The latter increase the diagnostic specificity of allergy testing but may miss reactions to antigens in their natural state.

Using advanced biochemical and molecular techniques, scientists have been able to characterize hundreds of allergens. This knowledge has led to the development of ***molecular-based allergy diagnostics*** that allow for parallel detection of IgE antibodies to more than 100 allergens using microarray formats. The principle of these assays is the same as singleplex testing except that patient serum is incubated with a polymer-coated glass slide or biochip containing miniature spots to which specific components derived from a wide variety of allergens have been applied (e.g., peanut proteins Ara h1, Ara3; grass pollen protein Phl p1; cat dander protein Fel d1). If specific IgE to a particular component is present, it will bind to the appropriate spots and be detected following addition of a labeled reporter anti-IgE reagent and substrate. Thus, molecular-based allergy diagnostics, also known as ***component IgE testing***, provides an extensive profile of sensitivities to many allergens. It is a highly specific type of testing that has been helpful in distinguishing between responses to true allergens and cross-reactivity, predicting the severity of clinical allergic responses based on the particular proteins to which individuals have been sensitized and providing guidance for selecting specific allergen immunotherapy and dietary restrictions. Using these tests has been especially helpful in the evaluation of peanut allergies.

Another development in IgE testing is a point-of-care lateral flow assay that can be used by primary care physicians to screen for reactivity to a few common allergens. In this assay, the allergen extracts are coated onto nitrocellulose strips encased in a cassette. A drop of blood from a finger prick is added to one well in the cassette, and a color-developing solution is added to a second well, driving the blood toward the antigen zone. In this semiquantitative test, the presence of allergen-specific IgE is indicated by a colored line in the corresponding allergen position. Patients with positive results can be referred to an allergist for further evaluation.

Regardless of the format of the specific IgE test used, the results should always be interpreted in light of the patient's medical history and clinical symptoms. This is because the presence of allergen-specific IgE antibody indicates sensitization to the allergen but not necessarily the presence of a clinical allergy.

Total IgE Testing

The first test for measuring total serum IgE was the competitive ***radioimmunosorbent test (RIST)***. The RIST used radiolabeled IgE to compete with patient IgE for binding sites on a solid phase coated with anti-IgE. Because of the expense and hazards of working with radioactivity, RIST has been replaced by noncompetitive solid-phase immunoassays or nephelometry assays with enhanced sensitivity (see Chapters 10 and 11). Figure 14–6 illustrates the principle of a commonly used fluorescent enzyme immunoassay.

Total IgE values are reported in kilo international units (kIU) per liter. One IU is equal to a concentration of 2.4 ng of protein per milliliter. IgE concentration varies with the person's age and exposure to allergens. The total IgE concentration is typically lower than 1 kU/L in cord blood, and serum IgE usually reaches adult levels at about 10 years of age. In adults, a cutoff value of 100 kU/L is considered the upper limit of normal. Levels above 100 kU/L are common in people with allergies. However, measurement of total serum IgE is not recommended for the routine clinical evaluation of patients with suspected allergies because values vary widely among patients and do not necessarily correlate with the presence of allergy. Patients with slightly elevated IgE levels may not have an allergy, and many patients with allergies have a total serum IgE concentration that falls within the reference range. Thus, allergen-specific IgE tests are considered to have more value in the diagnosis of allergies.

However, measurement of total serum IgE can be helpful in monitoring patients undergoing allergen immunotherapy or treatment with monoclonal anti-IgE antibody. Successful treatment results in significant reductions in total serum IgE levels and in the ratio of allergen-specific IgE to total IgE. Total serum IgE testing can also be used to evaluate patients with other conditions in which IgE levels may be elevated, such as helminth infections, and certain immunodeficiencies, such as Wiskott-Aldrich syndrome, DiGeorge syndrome, and hyper-IgE syndromes (see Chapter 19). Children living in areas where parasitic infections are endemic typically have serum IgE concentrations greater than 1,000 kU/L, whereas patients with hyper-IgE syndromes have extremely high IgE levels (2,000 to 50,000 kU/L).

Knowledge Check 14-2

Testing for type I hypersensitivity typically begins with:

a. A skin prick test
b. An immunoassay for total IgE
c. Allergen-specific IgE testing
d. Molecular-based allergy diagnostics

Critical Thinking 14-1

Suppose an adult patient had a total IgE level of 200 kU/L. What is the clinical significance of this value, and what other tests would be helpful in arriving at a diagnosis?

Type II Hypersensitivity

Type II hypersensitivity is also known as ***antibody-mediated*** or ***antibody-mediated cytotoxic*** hypersensitivity. It is an immediate form of hypersensitivity that typically occurs a few hours after exposure to antigen. The key components involved in these reactions are IgG and IgM antibodies, and complement.

Immunologic Mechanism

In type II hypersensitivity, IgG and IgM antibodies are produced against antigens found on cell surfaces or in the extracellular matrix. Because of the locations of these antigens, the clinical conditions produced by type II hypersensitivity are largely limited to a particular type of cell or organ. The antigens may be self-antigens, as in the case of autoimmune hemolytic anemia, or heteroantigens, such as red blood cell (RBC) antigens that stimulate transfusion reactions. Binding of the antibody to a cell can have one of three major effects, depending on the situation **(Fig. 14–7):**

1. The cell can be destroyed.
2. The function of the cell can be inhibited.
3. The function of the cell can be increased above normal.

Cell Damage

Cell damage can occur by several different mechanisms, some of which involve complement as well as antibodies:

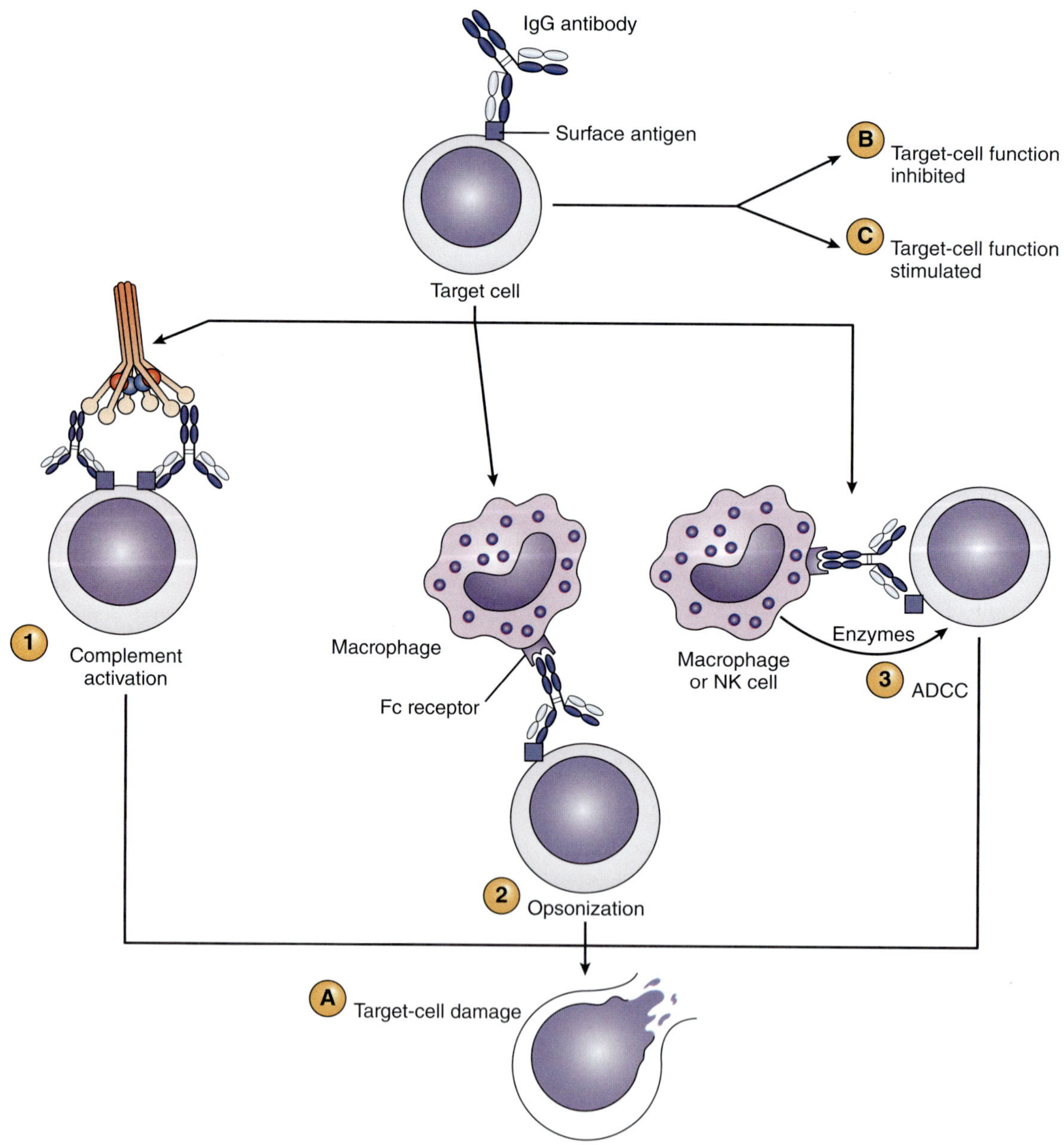

FIGURE 14–7 Type II hypersensitivity. In this reaction, IgG or immunoglobulin M (IgM) antibody binds to cell surface receptors, resulting in (A) cell damage from (1) complement activation, (2) opsonization, or (3) antibody-dependent cellular cytotoxicity (ADCC); (B) inhibition of cell function; or (C) stimulation of cell function.

1. Activation of the classical pathway of complement can lead to the formation of the membrane attack complex and cell lysis. Also, some of the complement proteins released after activation can opsonize cells or promote inflammation by recruiting neutrophils and macrophages.
2. Coating of the cell surface by antibodies can promote opsonization and subsequent phagocytosis of the cells. Opsonization can occur either through binding of IgG antibody to Fc receptors on macrophages and neutrophils or binding of cell surface C3b to complement receptors on phagocytic cells.
3. Cell damage can result from antibody-dependent cellular cytotoxicity (ADCC). ADCC is mediated through binding of IgG antibody to its corresponding antigen on the target cell and to Fc receptors on macrophages or natural killer (NK) cells. This binding stimulates the release of cytotoxic enzymes that destroy the cell.

Clinical examples that involve destruction of cells by type II hypersensitivity include blood transfusion reactions, hemolytic disease of the fetus and newborn, and autoimmune hemolytic anemia. We discuss these conditions in later sections.

Cell Inhibition

A second possible effect of type II hypersensitivity is that the cell surface antibody can inhibit the function of a cell. This can occur when antibody blocks the binding of a physiological ligand to its receptor, resulting in dysfunction of the cell. An example of this effect occurs in the autoimmune disease myasthenia gravis, which affects the neuromuscular junctions. Patients with this disease produce autoantibodies to receptors on muscle cells for the neurotransmitter acetylcholine (ACH). Normally, ACH is released from the nerve endings and binds to its corresponding receptors on muscle cells, stimulating contraction of the muscle fibers and muscle movement. However, in myasthenia gravis, attachment of the autoantibody to the ACH receptor blocks the binding of ACH, leading to muscle weakness (see Chapter 15).

Cell Stimulation

Sometimes, binding of an antibody to a self-antigen can have the opposite effect, stimulating the cell instead of inhibiting its function. This results in overproduction of the cell's product, such as a hormone. The classic example of this effect is an autoimmune disorder of the thyroid gland called Graves disease. Patients with Graves disease produce antibodies against the receptor for the thyroid-stimulating hormone (TSH) on thyroid cells. TSH, a hormone produced by the pituitary gland in the brain, binds to the TSH receptors and stimulates the thyroid cells to produce hormones that increase metabolism. Normally, this process is carefully regulated by a feedback loop that signals the pituitary gland to make less TSH in the presence of high levels of thyroid hormones. However, in Graves disease, the autoantibody binds to the TSH receptor, resulting in unregulated production of thyroid hormones. This leads to symptoms associated with increased metabolism, known as *hyperthyroidism* (see Chapter 15).

Knowledge Check 14-3

Type II hypersensitivity can result in:
a. Cell destruction
b. Decreased cell function
c. Increased cell function
d. All of the above

Clinical Examples of Type II Hypersensitivity

In the following sections, we discuss specific disorders associated with type II hypersensitivity and the mechanisms by which the antibodies produced cause pathology.

Transfusion Reactions

Transfusion reactions are examples of cell destruction that results from antibodies combining with heteroantigens. There are 36 different blood group systems with more than 380 different red blood cell (RBC) antigens. Some antigens are more likely to stimulate antibody production than others. Major groups involved in transfusion reactions include the ABO, Rh, Kell, Duffy, Kidd, MNS, and Diego blood group systems. Antibodies to some of these antigens are produced naturally with no prior exposure to RBCs, whereas other antibodies are produced only after contact with cells carrying that antigen.

The ABO blood group is of primary importance in considering transfusions. Anti-A and anti-B antibodies are naturally occurring antibodies, or **isohemagglutinins,** which are probably triggered by contact with similar antigenic determinants on microorganisms or environmental agents such as pollen. People do not make these antibodies to their own RBCs. Thus, a person who has type A blood has anti-B in their serum, and a person with type B blood has anti-A antibodies. An individual with type O blood has both anti-A and anti-B in the serum because O cells have neither of these two antigens. The antibody formed typically belongs to the IgM class, but IgG may also be made.

If a patient is given blood for which antibodies are already present, a transfusion reaction occurs. This reaction can range from acute massive intravascular hemolysis to an undetected decrease in RBC survival. The extent of the reaction depends on several factors, including the temperature at which the antibody is most active, the plasma concentration of the antibody, the immunoglobulin class involved, the extent of complement activation, the density of the antigen on the RBC, and the number of RBCs transfused. It is most important to detect antibodies that react at 37°C (i.e., normal body temperature). If a reaction occurs only below 30°C, it is not clinically significant because antigen-antibody complexes formed at colder temperatures tend to dissociate at 37°C.

Acute hemolytic transfusion reactions may occur within minutes or hours after receipt of incompatible blood. In this case, the person has been exposed to the antigen before the transfusion (e.g., through previous transfusion or pregnancy) and has preformed antibodies to it. Reactions that begin immediately are most often associated with ABO blood group incompatibilities, and the antibodies are of the IgM class. As soon as cells bearing the antigen are introduced into the patient, ***intravascular*** hemolysis *(inside the blood vessels)* occurs because of complement activation, resulting in the release of hemoglobin and vasoactive and procoagulant substances into the plasma. This may induce disseminated intravascular coagulation (DIC), vascular collapse, and renal failure. Symptoms in the patient may include fever, chills, nausea, lower back pain, tachycardia, shock, and hemoglobin in the urine.

Delayed hemolytic reactions occur days to weeks after a transfusion and are caused by an anamnestic (memory) response to the antigen to which the patient has previously been exposed. The type of antibody responsible is IgG, which was initially present in such low titer that it was not detectable with an antibody screen. Antigens most involved in delayed reactions include those in the Rh, Kell, Duffy, and Kidd blood groups. The Rh, Kell, and Duffy antigens may also be involved in immediate transfusion reactions. In a delayed reaction, antibody-coated RBCs are removed ***extravascularly*** by macrophages in the spleen or in the liver (i.e., destruction occurs ***outside of the blood vessels***). The patient may experience a mild fever, low hemoglobin, mild jaundice, and anemia. Intravascular hemolysis does not take place to any great extent because IgG is not as efficient as IgM in activating complement (see Chapters 3 and 7).

Hemolytic Disease of the Fetus and Newborn (HDFN)

Hemolytic disease of the fetus and newborn (HDFN) appears in infants whose mothers have been exposed to paternal blood group antigens on the baby's cells that differ from their own. The mother makes IgG antibodies in response to these antigens; these antibodies cross the placenta and destroy the fetal RBCs. When anemia becomes severe, erythropoiesis increases, and immature red blood cells are released from the bone marrow into the fetal circulation; thus, severe HDFN may be called ***erythroblastosis fetalis***. A major cause of severe reactions is the D antigen, a member of the Rh blood group. HDFN caused by ABO incompatibility is more common; however, the disease is milder, possibly because the A and B antigens on the fetus's RBCs are more poorly developed or reduced in number. Antibodies to more than 50 non-ABO blood group antigens have also been associated with HDFN, including anti-c, anti-C, anti-E, and anti-e and antibodies to the Kell, Duffy, MNS, and Kidd blood groups.

Sensitization of the mother to paternal blood group antigens may occur during pregnancy but occurs to a larger extent during the birth process, when fetal cells leak into the mother's circulation. Typically, the first child is unaffected because the first antibodies produced by the mother are IgM, which cannot cross the placenta; however, memory B cells

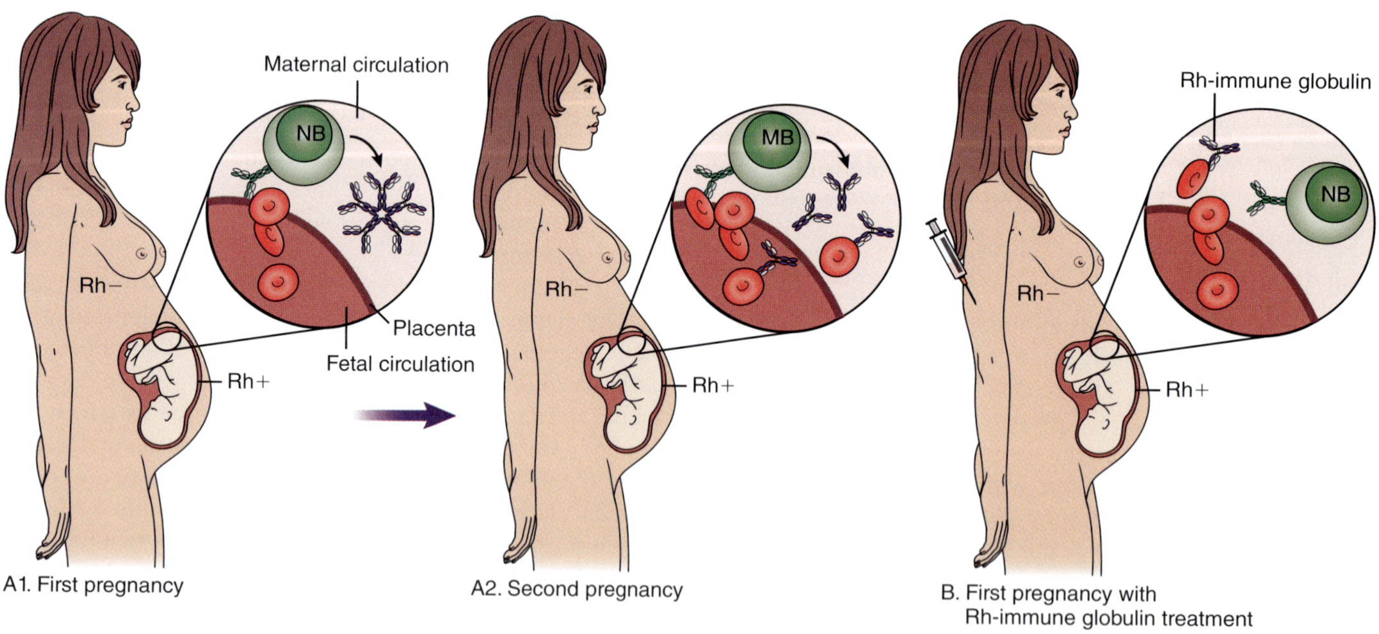

FIGURE 14–8 HDFN can develop in Rh-positive babies who are born to Rh-negative mothers if no treatment is administered. (A1) An Rh-negative mother may produce anti-Rh antibodies if a Rh-positive baby's RBCs enter her circulation late in gestation or during the birth process. In this primary immune response, naive B cells (NB) differentiate into plasma cells that secrete mainly anti-Rh IgM, which does not cross the placenta; therefore, a healthy baby is delivered. However, memory B cells (MB) are also produced, and (A2) if the mother becomes pregnant with another Rh-positive baby, these memory cells produce a strong secondary immune response and secrete mainly anti-Rh IgG, which crosses the placenta and destroys the baby's RBCs, resulting in HDFN. (B) Alternatively, passive immunization of the mother with anti-Rh immunotherapy during pregnancy and upon delivery prevents the mother from mounting an active immune response, allowing her future Rh-positive children to be born normally.

develop. These cells become activated upon reexposure to the same RBC antigen during a subsequent pregnancy, resulting in an anamnestic response and the production of IgG. This antibody can cross the placenta, attach to the fetal RBCs, and target them for hemolysis.

Depending on the degree of antibody production in the mother, the fetus may be aborted, stillborn, or born with evidence of hemolytic disease, as indicated by jaundice. As RBCs are lysed and free hemoglobin released, this is converted to bilirubin, which builds up in the plasma. There is too much of it to be conjugated in the liver, so it accumulates in the tissues. Excessive bilirubin may deposit in the brain and result in a severe neurological condition known as *kernicterus*. Treatment for severe HDFN involves an exchange transfusion to replace antibody-coated RBCs and phototherapy to break down the excess bilirubin into a water-soluble form. If serum antibody titrations during the pregnancy indicate a high level of circulating antibody, intrauterine transfusions can be performed.

To prevent the consequences of HDFN, all women should be screened at the onset of pregnancy. If they are Rh negative, they should be tested for the presence of anti-D antibodies monthly. To prevent development of HDFN, a commercially prepared product consisting of purified anti-D, called *Rh-immune globulin (RhIg)*, is administered prophylactically to at-risk Rh-negative pregnant women at 28 weeks of gestation and within 72 hours after delivery. The mechanism by which RhIg works is not completely known, but it is thought to facilitate clearance of fetal RBCs in the mother's circulation through opsonization and therefore suppress the production of maternal antibody **(Fig. 14–8).** This practice has dramatically reduced the incidence of HDFN cases caused by anti-D antibodies to less than 1%.

Autoimmune Hemolytic Anemia

People with **autoimmune hemolytic anemia** develop antibodies to antigens commonly found on their own RBCs, such as Rh proteins and the MNS blood group system. Warm autoimmune hemolytic anemia (AIHA) accounts for more than 70% of autoimmune anemias and is characterized by the formation of IgG antibody, which reacts most strongly at 37°C (normal body temperature). Some of these antibodies may be primary with no other disease association. Others may be secondary to another disease process such as viral or respiratory infections (e.g., infectious mononucleosis, cytomegalovirus, chronic active hepatitis), immunoproliferative disorders (e.g., chronic lymphocytic leukemia [CLL] and lymphomas), or autoimmune diseases (e.g., systemic lupus erythematosus). Often, the underlying cause of antibody production is unknown; this is referred to as *idiopathic autoimmune hemolytic anemia*.

Typical symptoms of warm AIHA include malaise, lightheadedness, weakness, unexplained fever, pallor, and possibly mild jaundice. These symptoms result from destruction of antibody-coated RBCs by macrophages in the liver and spleen. Hemolysis is primarily extravascular because IgG is not as efficient as IgM in activating complement; however, intravascular hemolysis can also occur if complement becomes activated. The severity of the hemolysis is affected by the subclass of IgG involved, with IgG3 and IgG1 being most destructive to the RBCs because they are best at binding complement.

Several types of drugs can also induce the production of antibodies that can cause hemolytic anemia, including antibiotics, NSAIDs, and anti-cancer drugs. These drugs can attach to the RBCs directly or form immune complexes that attach to the RBCs. Damage to the RBCs is believed to occur through several mechanisms. Some drugs, such as penicillins and cephalosporins, can act as haptens after binding to proteins on the RBC membrane. These drugs stimulate the production of anti-drug antibodies that destroy the RBCs, mainly through extravascular hemolysis. The cephalosporins are also thought to modify the RBC membrane by facilitating binding of immunoglobulins and complement. Other drugs, such as quinidine and phenacetin, can stimulate the production of anti-drug antibodies that bind to the drug to form soluble immune complexes. The complexes attach loosely to the surface of the RBCs, which are cleared by intravascular hemolysis after binding complement. Other drugs, such as methyldopa, can induce hemolytic anemia by stimulating production of autoantibodies against the RBC membrane.

Patients with warm AIHA are usually treated with corticosteroids to reduce antibody synthesis or, in more serious cases, with a splenectomy to decrease RBC clearance. Treatment with monoclonal anti-CD20 (rituximab) can be used for cases that cannot be managed effectively with corticosteroids. This antibody attaches to B cells and causes a decrease in antibody production. Symptoms of drug-induced AIHA resolve once the offending drug is discontinued.

Cold Agglutinin Antibodies

Cold agglutinins are a less frequent cause of immune hemolytic anemias. Cold agglutinins are autoantibodies that react with antigens on the RBC membrane at temperatures below 37°C. Most are specific for the I or i blood groups on RBCs. These cold-reacting antibodies belong to the IgM class and bind optimally to RBCs at temperatures between 4°C and 30°C. The reaction is reversible upon exposure to a warm temperature (37°C).

Cold agglutinins may be transient or chronic, depending on the cause. Polyclonal cold agglutinins can be produced secondary to certain infections, most notably *Mycoplasma pneumoniae* infection and infectious mononucleosis. In most cases, cold agglutinin production is transient and resolves in 2 to 3 weeks. Persistent, high-titer, monoclonal cold agglutinins have been associated with B-cell or plasma cell lymphoproliferative disorders, including B-cell CLL, B-cell lymphomas, Hodgkin disease, and Waldenström macroglobulinemia, and autoimmune diseases such as systemic lupus erythematosus (SLE). Chronic cold agglutinins can also be produced as a primary characteristic of a disease entity of unknown origin, known as *cold agglutinin disease* (CAD). CAD typically occurs in persons older than the age of 50 and is responsible for about 20% of autoimmune hemolytic anemia cases.

Cold agglutinins do not cause clinical symptoms unless the person is exposed to the cold, and they usually have their maximal effect when the temperature in the peripheral circulation falls below 30°C. Under these conditions, the antibodies can bind to the RBCs to form lattices, which can obstruct the small capillaries in the skin. The areas of the body most affected are those having the greatest exposure to the cold, most notably the fingers, toes, earlobes, and nose. These areas develop a blue coloration known as *acrocyanosis* and become numb, stiff, and slightly painful. The symptoms are quickly reversible when the patient returns to warm surroundings; however, in severe cases, peripheral necrosis may result.

Another consequence of cold agglutinins results from complement binding. Although complement activation cannot be completed in the cold, it can proceed once the cells recirculate and reach body temperature. If the RBCs become coated with C3b, opsonization can facilitate binding to macrophages and rapid clearance of the cells by the liver. Less commonly, the entire classical pathway is activated, and intravascular hemolysis occurs. Both processes lead to destruction of the RBCs and corresponding symptoms of autoimmune hemolytic anemia. Patients with this disease are usually treated by simply avoiding cold temperatures and keeping the extremities warm; drug therapy is only used if these measures are ineffective.

Immune Thrombocytopenic Purpura (ITP)

Immune thrombocytopenic purpura (ITP), previously known as *idiopathic thrombocytopenic purpura*, is a disorder in which antibodies develop against platelets, tiny cell fragments in the blood that form clots to stop bleeding. In children, acute ITP may develop after certain viral infections or immunizations and typically has a self-limited course, although a small percentage of cases may be more severe. In adults, ITP is a chronic condition caused by the formation of autoantibodies that recognize glycoproteins on the platelet membranes, including the (GP) IIb/IIIa complex, GP Ib/IIa, and GP VI. These antibodies bind to platelets and enhance their removal by macrophages in the spleen. Antibody production in chronic ITP may have no known underlying cause or may be secondary to a viral infection (e.g., HIV, cytomegalovirus) or autoimmune condition (e.g., antiphospholipid syndrome, SLE). Many drugs are also known to induce ITP by stimulating the production of anti-platelet antibodies on their own or by acting as haptens that bind to proteins on platelet membranes.

The normal number of platelets in the peripheral blood is generally considered to be between 150,000 to 450,000/μL. In ITP, destruction of the platelets results in a low platelet count, or *thrombocytopenia*, with small-vessel bleeding into the skin and mucous membranes. Depending on the amount of bleeding, the skin can develop small pinpoint hemorrhages, known as *petechiae*; round, midsize hemorrhages called *purpura;* or larger bruises known as *ecchymoses*. Symptoms in the mucous membranes can include nosebleeds, gum bleeding, heavy menstrual bleeding, and/or gastrointestinal bleeding; rarely, life-threatening bleeding from other areas of the body, including the central nervous system, can occur.

Symptoms of ITP usually vary with the degree of thrombocytopenia and determine the type of treatment administered. Mild cases of acute ITP usually do not require treatment and will resolve on their own, while patients with more significant symptoms can be treated with prednisone or other immunosuppressive drugs or with IV gamma globulin (IVIG), which blocks Fc receptors on phagocytic cells. Splenectomy may be required for patients with chronic ITP who do not respond to these treatments. Treatment of drug-induced thrombocytopenia involves discontinuing the offending drug; for severe cases, administering platelet transfusions and high-dose IVIG may be necessary.

Type II Reactions Involving Tissue Antigens

All the reactions we discussed thus far deal with individual cells that are destroyed when a specific antigen-antibody combination takes place. Some type II reactions involve destruction of tissues because of their combination with antibody. Organ-specific autoimmune diseases in which antibody is directed against a particular tissue are in this category. These include *Hashimoto disease,* in which antibodies to thyroid antigens destroy thyroid tissue; *myasthenia gravis,* in which antibodies to acetyl choline receptors block transmission of nerve impulses to the muscles; and *Graves disease,* in which antibodies bind to TSH receptors on thyroid cells and cause abnormally high thyroid function. We present the immunologic manifestations and detection of these and other autoimmune diseases that involve type II hypersensitivity in Chapter 15.

Testing for Type II Hypersensitivity

Laboratory testing for type II hypersensitivity varies with the clinical condition causing the reaction. Testing for autoantibodies associated with organ-specific autoimmune diseases is discussed in Chapter 15. Testing for ITP involves a complete blood cell count (CBC) to determine platelet number and additional testing to look for secondary causes of the condition. Serological testing for platelet antibodies is usually not performed, as the tests have low sensitivity.

Testing for hemolytic anemias typically begins by performing a CBC and peripheral blood smear. Expected results would show a low mature RBC count and hemoglobin concentration and an increase in immature RBCs called *reticulocytes*, as the bone marrow responds by producing new RBCs. Microspherocytes are typically seen on the peripheral blood smear due to membrane changes that occur as a result of immunoglobulins binding to the surface of the RBCs. Levels of free haptoglobin, which binds to hemoglobin released from dying RBCs, are typically low. Once these parameters support the presence of a hemolytic anemia, a direct antiglobulin test (DAT) must be performed to determine whether the cause of hemolysis is antibody mediated.

Direct Antiglobulin Test (DAT)

In 1945, Coombs, Mourant, and Race developed antiglobulin testing, which detects agglutination of RBCs after binding to reagent antibodies directed against specific antigens. The **direct antiglobulin test (DAT)**, sometimes referred to as the *direct Coombs test*, detects RBCs that have been sensitized with antibody or complement in vivo. The DAT is performed to detect transfusion reactions, HDFN, autoimmune hemolytic anemia, and drug-induced hemolytic anemia.

In this technique, illustrated in **Figure 14–9**, a suspension of patient RBCs is initially incubated with polyspecific anti-human globulin (AHG), a mixture of antibodies to IgG and the complement component C3d. The tube is centrifuged to enhance the reaction and is then observed for RBC agglutination. Positive agglutination indicates the presence of antibody or complement bound to the surface of the patient's RBCs in vivo. If agglutination occurs, the test is repeated using monospecific anti-IgG and anti-C3d to determine which of these is present. IgG with or without complement on the RBC surface is seen in warm AIHA or drug-induced AIHA. If the test is only positive for complement, the antibody attached to the RBCs is likely to be IgM, suggesting the presence of cold agglutinins. Negative agglutination results must be confirmed by adding commercially prepared antibody-coated check cells, which will agglutinate in the presence of the unused AHG.

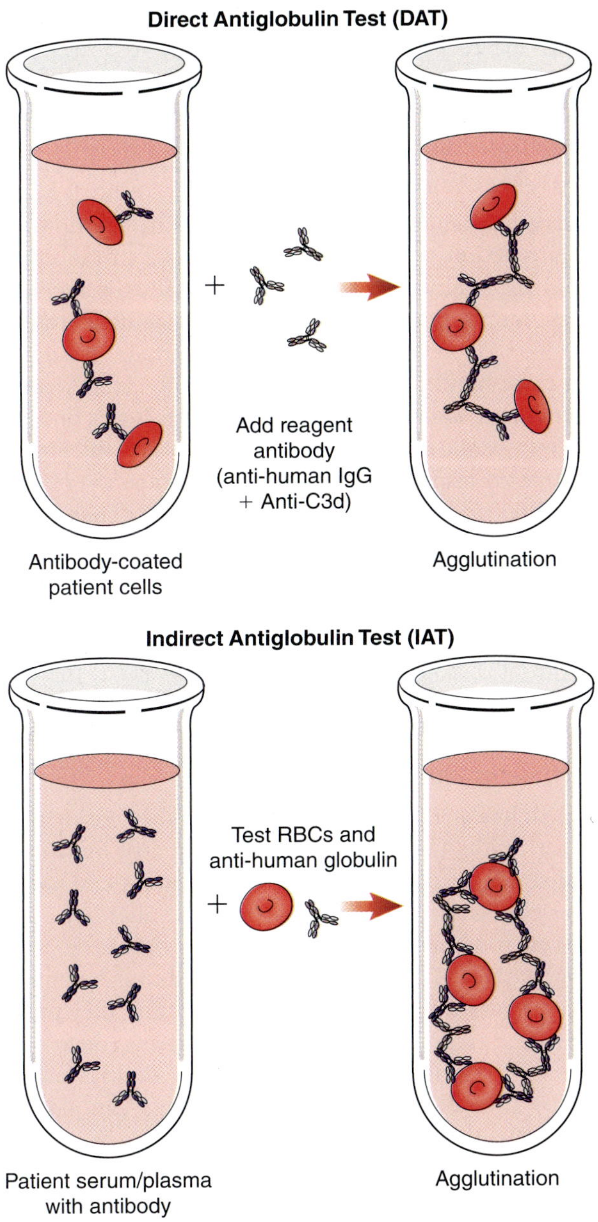

FIGURE 14–9 Principle of direct antiglobulin test (DAT) and indirect antiglobulin test (IAT). In the DAT, patient RBCs are combined with anti-human globulin to detect cell-bound antibodies or complement. In the IAT, RBC antibodies in patient serum are detected by incubation with test RBCs followed by addition of anti-human globulin. In either test, a positive result is indicated by RBC agglutination.

Indirect Antiglobulin Test (IAT)

The **indirect antiglobulin test (IAT)** has multiple applications. It is used (1) in the crossmatching of blood to prevent a transfusion reaction; (2) to determine the presence of a particular type of antibody in patient plasma, such as those in pregnant women that could cause HDFN; or (3) in typing patient RBCs. The method detects in vitro binding of patient antibody to reagent RBCs that have known blood group antigens. This method is a two-step process in which reagent RBCs and patient serum or plasma are allowed to combine at 37°C; the cells are then carefully washed to remove unbound antibody. AHG is added, and visible RBC agglutination occurs if antibody has been specifically bound (Fig. 14-9). Negative tests are confirmed by quality-control cells that are coated with antibody.

Cold Agglutinin Testing

To determine the titer of a cold agglutinin antibody, patient serum can be serially diluted and incubated overnight at 4°C with a dilute suspension of washed human type O RBCs. The tubes are then gently shaken and observed for agglutination. The last tube with agglutination represents the titer. Titers of 64 or higher are generally considered to be clinically significant. The agglutination should disappear after warming the tubes briefly in a 37°C water bath. Before testing, it is important to use prewarmed blood to separate the serum or plasma from the patient's RBCs. Failure to do so can result in binding of the cold agglutinins to the patient's own RBCs, producing false-negative results when the patient's serum is assayed for cold agglutinin reactivity against the reagent type O cells.

> **Critical Thinking 14-2**
>
> In the DAT and IAT tests, how can you be certain that the AHG reagent is working properly?

Type III Hypersensitivity

Type III hypersensitivity is also known as *complex-mediated* hypersensitivity. It is an immediate form of hypersensitivity that typically begins a few hours after exposure to antigen. Type III hypersensitivity reactions involve the formation of immune complexes containing IgG or IgM antibodies and complement.

Immunologic Mechanism

The mechanism underlying type III hypersensitivity involves three major steps.

Step 1: Development of Antibodies to Soluble Antigens in the Blood and Formation of Circulating Immune Complexes

This mechanism involves exposure to soluble antigens in the blood, such as foreign proteins derived from microbial pathogens or certain drugs, or in the case of some autoimmune disorders, self-antigens. The individual then produces specific IgM and IgG antibodies, which bind to the antigen to form complexes that circulate in the bloodstream.

Step 2: Deposition of the Complexes in the Tissues

You may recall from Chapter 10 that when soluble antigen combines with antibody, the size of the immune complexes formed is determined by the antigen:antibody ratio. If the concentrations of antigen and antibody are equivalent, large complexes are produced; in the body, such complexes are usually cleared by phagocytic cells. However, in the case of antigen excess, the complexes formed are smaller because there is a relative scarcity of antibodies with antigen-binding sites. Such small complexes, as well as complexes produced in high amounts, are not efficiently phagocytized and become deposited along the endothelial lining of the blood vessels. They can also migrate out of the blood and deposit in various tissues in the body. The basement membranes of the renal glomeruli and joints are particularly susceptible to immune complex deposition because at these sites, blood is filtered under high pressure to produce urine and synovial fluid, respectively.

Step 3: Activation of Complement and Production of an Inflammatory Reaction

Complement binds to the antigen-antibody complexes in the tissues, causing the formation of complement fragments that increase vasodilation and vasopermeability, attract macrophages and neutrophils, and enhance binding of phagocytic cells by opsonization (see Chapter 7). If the complexes are unable to be completely cleared by phagocytosis, the neutrophils will release enzymes from their lysosomal granules by a process known as *exocytosis*. This process results in damage to host tissue. Long-term changes include loss of tissue elements that cannot regenerate and accumulation of scar tissue. The mechanism of type III hypersensitivity is illustrated in **Figure 14–10**.

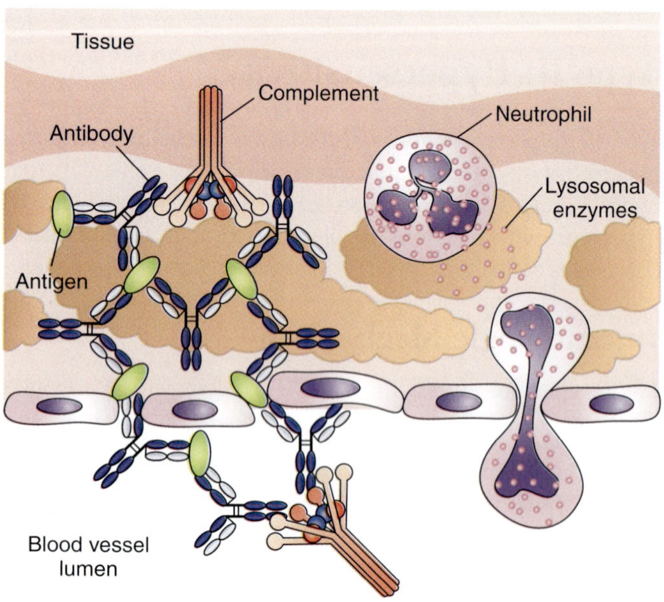

FIGURE 14–10 Type III hypersensitivity. Antigen and antibody combine to form immune complexes that deposit on the walls of blood vessels and tissues and activate complement. Complement fragments that are generated cause vasodilation, increased vascular permeability, and accumulation of neutrophils, which release their lysosomal enzymes and cause tissue damage.

Knowledge Check 14-4

Type III hypersensitivity differs from type II hypersensitivity in that:

a. Type III involves IgG antibodies, whereas type II involves IgM.
b. Type III involves soluble antigens, whereas type II involves cell surface antigens.
c. Type III is antibody mediated, whereas type II is cell mediated.
d. Complement is only involved in type III reactions.

Clinical Examples of Type III Hypersensitivity

Type III hypersensitivity reactions can be localized or systemic, depending on where the immune complexes deposit. In the following sections, we discuss examples of both types of reactions.

Arthus Reaction

The classic example of a localized type III reaction is the **Arthus reaction**, an inflammatory response in the skin discovered by Maurice Arthus in 1903. Arthus demonstrated this reaction in immunized rabbits with abundant circulating antibodies that were challenged with an intradermal injection of the corresponding antigen. The reaction, characterized by erythema and edema, peaks within 3 to 8 hours and is followed by a hemorrhagic necrotic lesion that may ulcerate. The inflammatory response is caused by a combination of antigen and antibody to form immune complexes that deposit in small blood vessels in the dermis and bind complement. Complement activation results in the recruitment of neutrophils, which release toxic products, such as oxygen-containing free radicals and proteolytic enzymes, and platelet aggregation to form thrombi; as a result, surrounding tissue in the skin is damaged. In humans, the Arthus reaction can rarely develop at the injection site after booster doses of some vaccines.

Serum Sickness

Serum sickness is a generalized type III hypersensitivity reaction that results from passive immunization of humans with animal serum. Before the advent of antibiotics and vaccines, serum sickness was observed more often because horse antiserums were used to treat infections such as diphtheria, tetanus, and pneumonia. These antisera were produced by immunizing horses with the corresponding antigen, and they provided immediate immunity to the people receiving them. Today, horse anti-venoms are still used to treat people who have been bitten by poisonous snakes. Serum sickness can also occur after treatment of patients with mouse monoclonal antibodies for diseases such as cancer or autoimmune disorders. Patients exposed to such animal sera can produce antibodies against the foreign animal proteins. These can combine with their corresponding antigen to form immune complexes that can deposit in the tissues and trigger the type III hypersensitivity response.

The classic symptoms of serum sickness are fever, skin rash, and joint pain; renal involvement can also occur. Symptoms appear 1 to 2 weeks after injection of the animal serum and usually resolve in a few weeks after the offending antigen is eliminated and the immune complexes are removed by phagocytic cells. However, previous exposure to animal serum can result in a more rapid reaction with increased severity.

Autoimmune Diseases and Other Causes of Type III Hypersensitivity

Type III hypersensitivity reactions can also be triggered by autologous antigens, as seen in several autoimmune diseases. SLE and rheumatoid arthritis (RA) are two such examples. Patients with these diseases commonly produce antibodies against nuclear constituents such as DNA and histones. They may also produce an antibody against IgG called *rheumatoid factor.* The autoantibodies combine with their corresponding antigen to produce immune complexes that trigger the type III hypersensitivity response. In SLE, immune complex deposition involves multiple organs; however, damage mainly occurs in the joints, skin, and kidneys. In RA, immune complexes primarily cause damage to the joints. Complement enhances tissue destruction in both diseases. See Chapter 15 for a detailed discussion of these two conditions.

Type III hypersensitivity can also be caused by several other factors. These include vaccine components, bee stings, treatment with certain drugs (e.g., penicillin and sulfonamides), and infections such as viral hepatitis and group A *Streptococcus*.

Testing for Type III Hypersensitivity

The laboratory methods associated with type III hypersensitivity are varied and depend on the condition being detected. For example, microbial cultures and serology tests for specific antibodies can be performed to detect infections that may cause immune complex development. In autoimmune diseases such as SLE and RA, the presence of antinuclear antibodies can be detected by various methods, including indirect immunofluorescence, enzyme-linked immunosorbent assay (ELISA), and fluorescent microbead multiplex immunoassays (see Chapter 15). Fluorescent staining of sections from tissue biopsies can be used to observe immune complex deposition in tissues such as the skin and kidneys. The staining pattern seen can help to identify the associated disease and determine its severity.

General methods to evaluate immune complex diseases include a CBC with a differential count, measurement of inflammatory markers such as C-reactive protein and the erythrocyte sedimentation rate (ESR), quantitative determination of serum immunoglobulins, and measurement of complement levels. During periods of high disease activity, complement levels in the serum may be decreased because some of the complement proteins are bound to antigen-antibody complexes. Reference laboratories may also perform specialized tests to detect circulating immune complexes. The results of these tests should be interpreted in conjunction with other laboratory and clinical findings to determine a specific diagnosis.

Type IV Hypersensitivity

Type IV hypersensitivity differs from the other three types of hypersensitivity in that sensitized T cells, rather than antibodies, play the major role in its manifestations. It is therefore known as *cell-mediated* hypersensitivity. Because symptoms begin more than 12 hours after exposure to antigen and peak between 48 and 72 hours, this reaction is also referred to as *delayed hypersensitivity.*

Immunologic Mechanism

Sensitization Phase

Although there are different mechanisms involved in type IV hypersensitivity, the classic type IV response involves CD4 T_H cells. An initial sensitization phase of 1 to 2 weeks takes place after the first contact with antigen. During this phase, Langerhans cells in the skin and macrophages in the tissues capture antigen and migrate to nearby lymph nodes, where they present the antigen to naive T_H cells. The antigen-presenting cells (APCs) also release cytokines that promote differentiation of the naive T cells into the T-cell subsets, T_H1 and T_H17, and stimulate their proliferation.

Effector Phase

The expanded T_H cells then migrate to the site where the antigen is located, and the effector phase of the response begins. At the site, activated T_H1 and T_H17 cells release several cytokines and chemokines that promote inflammation by recruiting macrophages and neutrophils to the area and inducing these cells to become activated. These include interleukin (IL-17), monocyte chemotactic protein (MCP-1/CCL2), interferon gamma (IFN-γ), and tumor necrosis factor (TNF); see Chapter 6 for further discussion of these proteins. The activated neutrophils release reactive oxygen species, nitric oxide, and lysosomal enzymes that damage surrounding tissues, while activated macrophages produce cytokines that stimulate further recruitment of WBCs and propagate the inflammatory response. The immunologic mechanism of type IV hypersensitivity is illustrated in **Figure 14–11.**

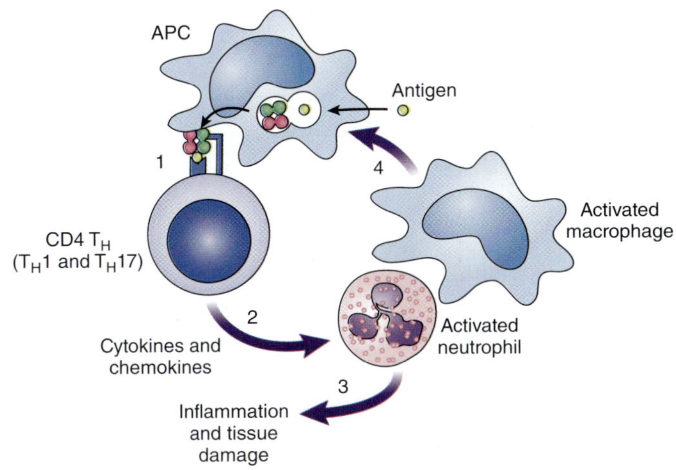

FIGURE 14–11 Type IV hypersensitivity. (1) APCs take up antigen and activate CD4 helper T (T_H) cells. (2) The T_H cells produce cytokines and chemokines that recruit and activate macrophages and neutrophils. (3) Neutrophils release lysosomal enzymes and other products that cause tissue damage. (4) Activated macrophages produce cytokines that prolong the inflammatory response and, in some cases, activate cytotoxic T cells to cause tissue damage (latter not shown).

Chronic Phase

Chronic persistence of antigen leads to the development of organized clusters of cells called **granulomas,** which consist of epithelioid-shaped and multinucleated fused macrophages with an infiltrate of lymphocytes or other WBCs. Many of these macrophages contain engulfed antigens, such as intracellular bacteria. Thus, the granuloma can function to wall off an infectious organism in a contained area, preventing its spread to other parts of the body. However, cells in the granuloma can release large amounts of lytic enzymes that can destroy surrounding tissue and promote fibrin deposition. Cytotoxic T cells are also recruited, and they bind with antigen-coated target cells to cause further tissue destruction.

Antigens That Induce Type IV Hypersensitivity

While the mechanism we described is an important immune defense, in certain situations, prolonged inflammation occurs that can result in harm to the individual. The antigens that can trigger type IV hypersensitivity are mainly intracellular pathogens or contact antigens. The intracellular pathogens can be bacteria, fungi, parasites, or viruses. Pathogens that commonly induce delayed hypersensitivity include *Mycobacterium tuberculosis, Mycobacterium leprae, Pneumocystis carinii, Leishmania* species, and herpes simplex virus. Contact antigens are those that come into direct contact with the skin. They include plants such as poison ivy and poison oak, metals such as nickel salts, and components of hair dyes and cosmetics. In the sections that follow, we discuss clinical manifestations of type IV hypersensitivity induced by these antigens. T-cell responses to self-antigens can also play a role in the pathogenesis of certain organ-specific autoimmune diseases, including RA and multiple sclerosis (see Chapter 15).

Knowledge Check 14-5

Type IV hypersensitivity differs from the other types of hypersensitivity in that it:

a. Involves IgE antibodies
b. Occurs within 30 minutes after antigen exposure
c. Does not cause tissue damage
d. Is mediated by T cells

Knowledge Check 14-6

Match each hypersensitivity type with its major characteristic:

a. Type I ____	1. Peaks at 48 hours after antigen exposure
b. Type II ____	2. Tissue deposition of antigen-antibody complexes
c. Type III ____	3. IgE binding to mast cells
d. Type IV ____	4. Antibodies produced against a cell surface receptor

Clinical Manifestations of Type IV Hypersensitivity

Type IV hypersensitivity reactions may involve the skin or internal organs. In the following sections, we discuss some clinical manifestations resulting from this mechanism.

Contact Dermatitis

Contact dermatitis is among the most prevalent skin disorders, affecting an estimated 15% to 20% of the general population. Reactions are usually caused by low molecular weight compounds that touch the skin. The most common causes include poison ivy, poison oak, and poison sumac, all of which release the chemical urushiol in the plant sap and on the leaves, causing allergic dermatitis on contact. Other common compounds that produce allergic skin manifestations include metals such as nickel; chemicals used in the manufacture of shoes and clothing; hair dyes; fabric finishes; cosmetics; fragrances; and topical medications, such as anesthetics, antiseptics, and antibiotics. Latex sensitization is also known to cause contact dermatitis.

Many of these substances function as haptens that bind to glycoproteins on skin cells. Langerhans cells in the skin process the hapten-protein complexes and migrate to the regional lymph nodes, where they present the antigen to T_H1 cells. Sensitization of the T_H cells takes several days; however, once it occurs, its effects can last for years because of immunologic memory. Cytokine production by the T_H1 cells causes macrophages to accumulate and release cytokines that promote proliferation of the T_H cells and a local inflammatory response.

Contact dermatitis typically begins with intense itching at the site of antigen contact. A skin eruption, characterized by erythema, swelling, and papule formation follows, appearing 24 hours to several days after the exposure **(Fig. 14–12)**. The papules may become vesicular, with blistering, peeling, and weeping. The dermatitis is first limited to skin sites exposed to the antigen, but then it expands to adjoining areas as the patient scratches the area and spreads the antigen. The reaction can last from several days to 3 weeks, depending on the degree of sensitization and the concentration of antigen absorbed. If the area is small and localized, a topical steroid may be used for treatment. For more severe cases, anti-histamine drugs or systemic corticosteroids may be administered. Patients need to avoid contact with the offending allergen in the future, as reactivity is usually lifelong.

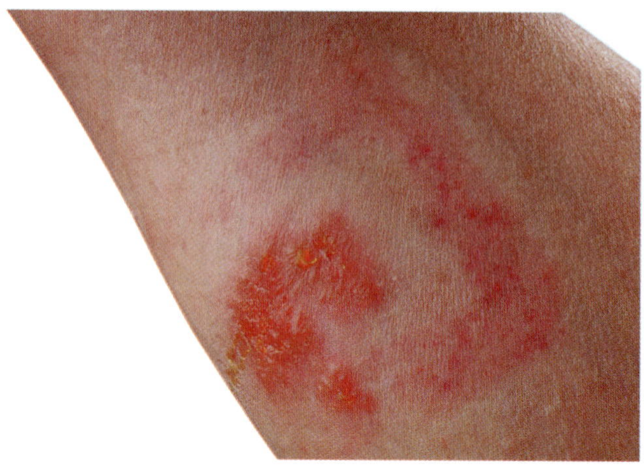

FIGURE 14–12 Contact hypersensitivity. Formation of papules occurs after exposure to poison ivy. *(Courtesy of Yong Choi/Thinkstock.)*

Hypersensitivity Pneumonitis

Hypersensitivity pneumonitis is mediated predominantly by sensitized T lymphocytes that respond to inhaled allergens. IgG and IgM antibodies are formed, but these are thought to play only a minor role in the pathogenesis of this disorder. Hypersensitivity pneumonitis is an allergic disease of the lung parenchyma characterized by inflammation of the alveoli and interstitial spaces. It is caused by chronic inhalation of a variety of antigens and is most often seen in people who are engaged in work or hobbies involving exposure to the implicated antigen.

Depending on the occupation and the particular antigen, the disease goes by several names: *farmer's lung, bird breeder's lung disease,* and *humidifier* or *air-conditioner lung disease.* The reaction is most likely caused by microorganisms, especially bacterial and fungal spores, to which individuals are exposed when working with moldy hay, pigeon droppings, compost, moldy tobacco, infested flour, and moldy cheese, to name a few examples. Symptoms of acute hypersensitivity pneumonitis include a dry cough, shortness of breath, fever, chills, and nausea, which may begin 4 to 8 hours after exposure of previously sensitized individuals to a high dose of the offending antigen. Long-term exposure to the antigen can lead to a chronic form of the disease characterized by difficulty breathing upon exertion, cough, fatigue, and weight loss caused by alveolar inflammation and interstitial fibrosis. Systemic corticosteroid therapy is used for treatment, and patients should take measures to avoid contact with the offending antigen.

Skin Testing for Delayed Hypersensitivity

Skin testing is used clinically to detect delayed hypersensitivity responses to a variety of antigens. The tests are based on a T-cell–mediated memory response. When antigen is injected intradermally or applied to the surface of the skin, previously sensitized individuals develop a reaction at the application site. This reaction results from infiltration of T lymphocytes and macrophages into the area. Blood vessels in the vicinity become lined with mononuclear cells, and the reaction reaches a peak by 72 hours after exposure. Skin testing has been used to determine antigen sensitivity in contact dermatitis, assess exposure to *M. tuberculosis,* and evaluate the competency of cell-mediated immune responses in patients with immunodeficiency diseases. We discuss each of these applications in the text that follows.

Skin Testing for Contact Dermatitis

The patch test is considered the gold standard in testing for contact dermatitis. This test must be done when the patient is free of symptoms or at least has a clear test site. A nonabsorbent adhesive patch containing the suspected contact antigen is applied on the patient's back, and the skin is checked for a reaction during the next 48 hours. Redness with papules or tiny blisters is considered a positive test. Final evaluation is conducted at 96 to 120 hours. All readings should be done by a skilled evaluator. False negatives can result from inadequate contact with the skin.

Skin Testing for Tuberculosis

Most people exposed to *M. tuberculosis* and related bacteria develop a latent infection that is asymptomatic; however, they have an increased risk (5% to 10%) of developing active tuberculosis (TB) disease with serious respiratory and other symptoms throughout the course of their lives (see Chapter 20). The tuberculin skin test (TST) has been used for more than 100 years to identify individuals infected with bacteria of the *M. tuberculosis* complex. Skin testing has been an important screening tool to detect exposure to TB in health care workers and other individuals at risk for the infection.

The TST is a classic example of a delayed hypersensitivity reaction, based on the principle that soluble antigens from *M. tuberculosis* induce a reaction in people who currently have TB or have been exposed to *M. tuberculosis* in the past. The test uses an *M. tuberculosis* antigen extract prepared from a purified filtrate of the organism's cell wall, called a ***purified protein derivative*** (PPD). The TST is routinely performed by the Mantoux method, in which 0.1 mL of 5 tuberculin units (TU) of PPD is injected intradermally into the inner surface of the forearm using a fine needle and syringe **(Fig. 14–13)**. The test site is examined between 48 and 72 hours for the presence of a hardened, raised area called ***induration***.

Interpretation of the reaction depends on the particular group in which the person is categorized. An induration reaction of 15 mm or more is considered a positive test in people with no risk factors, whereas a reaction of 10 mm or greater is considered positive in recent immigrants from high-prevalence countries, IV drug users, employees of health care and other high-risk facilities, persons with certain clinical conditions, and children younger than 5 years of age. An induration reaction of 5 mm or more is considered positive in persons who have HIV infection or other forms of immunosuppression, features on a chest x-ray consistent with TB, or recent contact with TB patients.

A positive TST indicates that the person has previously been exposed to *M. tuberculosis* or a related organism, but it does not necessarily mean that they have an active TB infection. Positive test results also occur in people who have previously received the bacille Calmette-Guérin (BCG) vaccine for TB. False-positive results can also occur in patients infected with nontuberculosis mycobacteria or if reactions are incorrectly measured or interpreted. False-negative results may occur in immunocompromised patients, those with very recent TB infection, people who have recently received certain vaccines, incorrect administration of the test, or incorrect test interpretation. A boosted reaction can also occur in some individuals who have decreased sensitivity to the PPD antigens due to receipt the BCG vaccine or infection with *M. tuberculosis* in the distant past; this is seen as an initial negative TST followed by a positive reaction in a subsequent TST caused by stimulation of a memory response to PPD. Two-step testing can reduce the chance that this result will be misinterpreted as a recent TB infection. This is performed by follow-up of a negative TST with a second TST 1 to 3 weeks later; if the second TST is positive, the person is considered to have a previous TB infection (as opposed to a recent infection) and should be treated for latent TB.

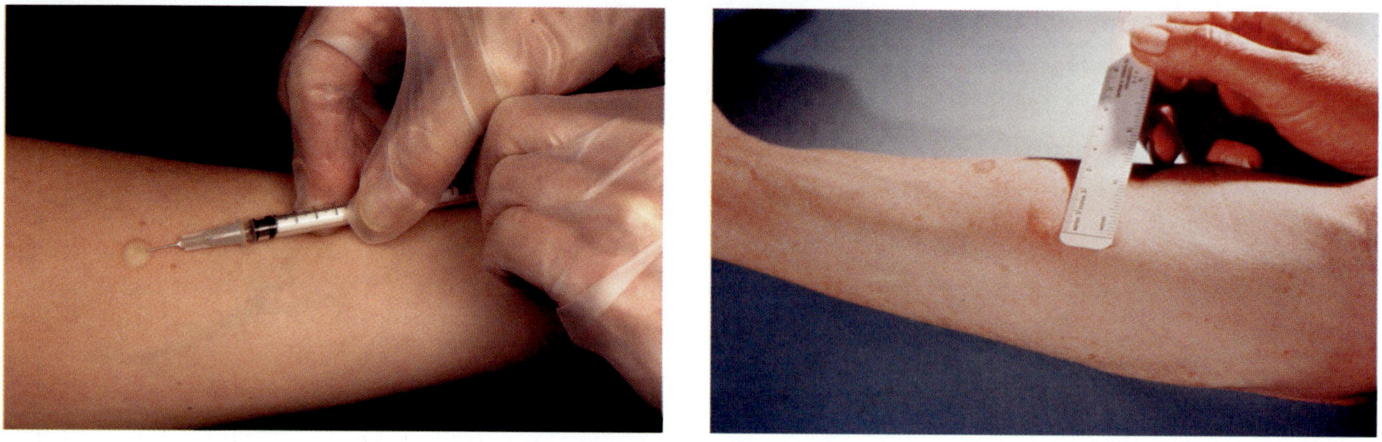

FIGURE 14–13 The Mantoux test. (A) PPD is injected into an individual's forearm, which causes a wheal (i.e., a raised area of the skin surface) to form at the injection site. (B) After 48 hours, the individual presented with an induration (hardened, raised area), indicating a positive reaction. *(A. Courtesy of the CDC/Gabrielle Benenson and Greg Knobloch, Public Health Image Library. B. Courtesy of the CDC/Donald Kopanoff, Public Health Image Library.)*

Skin Testing for Immunodeficiency

Skin testing can also be used to determine whether the cell-mediated arm of the immune system is functioning properly in individuals suspected of having immunodeficiency disorders. Antigens typically used for testing are from sources to which people have been commonly exposed, such as *Candida albicans,* tetanus toxoid, *Streptococcus* bacteria, and fungal antigens such as trichophyton and histoplasmin. The antigens are injected into separate sites in the skin by the Mantoux method; the injection sites are then examined at 48 hours for redness and induration. Healthy people should mount a memory response and develop a positive skin reaction to at least one of the antigens tested. Those with deficient cell-mediated immunity will display **anergy,** or the absence of positive reactions for all the common antigens used in the skin test. Negative results may also occur in individuals such as young children who have never been exposed to the antigens used in the test.

Interferon Gamma Release Assays (IGRAs)

Interferon gamma release assays (IGRAs) are in vitro methods that have been developed as an alternative to the TST to detect latent TB infection. The CDC recommends using IGRAs to detect latent TB in people who are at high risk of developing active disease, including those who were recently infected, health care workers, patients with HIV infection or certain medical conditions, and patients receiving immunosuppressive drugs. IGRA methods are more sensitive and specific than the TST, do not cause a boosting effect, and provide more objective results that are available sooner and are easier to interpret. IGRAs also produced fewer false positives in people who have received the BCG vaccine or have been infected with nontuberculous mycobacteria, and they require only a single visit to the clinic. However, none of the methods can differentiate between latent and active TB or predict which patients with latent infection will progress to develop active TB disease.

IGRAs detect a cell-mediated immune response by measuring the production of IFN-γ by patient T cells that have been stimulated with the *M. tuberculosis*–specific antigens, ESAT-6 and CFP-10. These antigens are not found in most strains of nontuberculous mycobacteria or in the bacteria used to make the BCG vaccine. Currently, there are two commercially available IGRAs that have been approved by the U.S. Food and Drug Administration (FDA): the QuantiFERON-TB Gold+ assay and the T-SPOT.TB test.

QuantiFERON-TB Gold+ Assay

In the QuantiFERON-TB Gold+ assay, patient blood is drawn into four special collection tubes:

1. A positive control that contains the T-cell mitogen, phytohemagglutinin (PHA)
2. A negative control (NIL) that does not contain TB antigens and adjusts for background
3. TB1, which contains peptides from the ESAT-6 and CFP-10 antigens, which stimulate CD4 T_H responses
4. TB2, which contains the ESAT-6 and CFP-10 peptides found in TB1 plus additional peptides from these antigens that stimulate CD8 cytotoxic T-cell responses

Patient blood is incubated in the tubes at 37°C for 16 to 24 hours. During the incubation, T cells from patients who have been infected with *M. tuberculosis* will respond to the TB antigens by producing the cytokine, IFN-γ. The tubes are then centrifuged to collect patient plasma, and the amount of IFN-γ in the plasma is measured by an ELISA. The test is considered positive if the amount of IFN-γ in either TB antigen tube is significantly higher than that in the negative control tube. Positive results suggest that the patient is likely infected with *M. tuberculosis* and should be followed with a clinical exam, chest x-ray, and microbiology tests to determine if active TB disease is present. False-positive results may occur in the presence of infection with some other types of mycobacteria. A low level of IFN-γ in the positive control tube indicates inability of the patient to make the cytokine because of immunosuppression and constitutes an indeterminate result.

T-SPOT.TB test

The T-SPOT.TB test is based on the enzyme-linked immunospot (ELISpot) technique. In this test, mononuclear cells are isolated from patient peripheral blood and placed into wells of a microtiter plate that have been precoated with antibody to IFN-γ. *M. tuberculosis*–specific antigens (ESAT-6 and CFP-10) are added to the wells, and the contents are incubated at 37°C for 16 to 20 hours in the presence of 5% CO_2. Positive and negative control wells are also included in the assay. During the incubation, T cells from patients exposed to *M. tuberculosis* release IFN-γ in their vicinity. After a wash step, an enzyme-labeled antibody to IFN-γ is added, and after another incubation and wash, substrate is added to the wells. Dark blue spots are produced where the IFN-γ–secreting cells were located in the wells, and the number of spots is counted under a magnifying glass or stereomicroscope (see Fig. 6–9).

Critical Thinking 14-3

Suppose the patient results that follow were obtained from an interferon gamma release assay. For the test to be valid, the NIL tube must give a value of <8.0 IU/mL, and the Mitogen tube minus NIL must give a value of >0.50 IU/mL.

Patient Results:

TB1 minus NIL – 0.10 IU/mL (Reference range = 0.00–0.35 IU/mL)

TB2 minus NIL – 0.40 IU/mL (Reference range = 0.00–0.35 IU/mL)

Mitogen minus NIL = 0.40 IU/mL

NIL = 0.02 IU/mL

What can you conclude about the clinical significance of these results?

KEY CONCEPTS

General Characteristics of Hypersensitivity

- Hypersensitivity is an exaggerated immune response to antigens that are usually not harmful. It results in cell destruction and tissue injury.
- Gell and Coombs devised a system for classifying hypersensitivity reactions into four types based on their immunologic mechanism and the nature of the triggering antigen.
- All four types of hypersensitivity represent defense mechanisms that stimulate an inflammatory response to an antigen that is seen as foreign. In many cases, the antigen is not harmful, but the response to it results in tissue damage.
- Hypersensitivity types I, II, and III are antibody mediated. Because they occur within minutes to hours after exposure to antigen, they are referred to as *immediate reactions*.
- Type IV hypersensitivity is a cell-mediated response involving T lymphocytes. Because the clinical manifestations do not appear until 24 to 72 hours after contact with the antigen, the type IV response is also referred to as *delayed hypersensitivity*.

Type I Hypersensitivity

- Type I hypersensitivity involves the production of IgE antibody to an allergen. In the sensitization phase of this response, the IgE binds to high-affinity FcεRI receptors on mast cells and basophils. In the activation phase, the receptors become cross-linked when the allergen binds to adjacent IgE molecules on the cell surface. Degranulation of the mast cells and basophils occurs, releasing preformed and newly synthesized chemical mediators that cause an inflammatory response. Cytokines produced during the response can cause a late-phase response of prolonged inflammation.
- Preformed mediators released from mast cells and basophils include histamine, heparin, and proteolytic enzymes such as tryptase. These factors cause contraction of smooth muscle in the bronchioles, blood vessels, and intestines; increased capillary permeability; chemotaxis of eosinophils and neutrophils; and decreased blood coagulability. Newly synthesized mediators such as prostaglandins, leukotrienes, and PAF potentiate the effects of histamine and other preformed mediators.
- Susceptibility to allergies is based on a combination of genetic factors that affect the immune response and environmental influences, such as exposure to infectious organisms.
- Clinical manifestations of type I hypersensitivity include localized wheal-and-flare skin reactions (i.e., urticaria or hives), rhinitis, allergic asthma, and a life-threatening condition called *systemic anaphylaxis*.
- Allergies can be treated with drugs such as antihistamines, decongestants, and corticosteroids. Monoclonal anti-IgE antibodies have been used to block the binding of IgE to mast cells and basophils in patients with moderate to severe asthma. Monoclonal antibodies to certain cytokines and their receptors have been used to reduce IgE synthesis and eosinophil recruitment.
- Allergen immunotherapy (AIT) can be administered to patients for whom drug therapy and environmental control measures are not successful. The goal of AIT is to induce immune tolerance by administering gradually increasing doses of the allergen through time.
- The preferred method of screening for allergies is an in vivo skin prick test, in which very small amounts of potential allergens are injected under the skin. A positive test produces a wheal-and-flare reaction within 20 minutes.
- In patients unable to tolerate skin testing, in vitro testing by noncompetitive solid-phase immunoassays for allergen-specific IgE can be performed. In these assays, patient serum is incubated with a solid phase to which a specific allergen has been attached.

Binding is detected with an enzyme-labeled anti-human IgE antibody and a colorimetric, fluorescent, or chemiluminescent substrate.

- Solid-phase immunoassays for total serum IgE can be used to monitor patients undergoing treatment with AIT or monoclonal anti-IgE and to detect patients with certain diseases characterized by elevated IgE levels. The principle of these tests is the same as that for allergen-specific IgE tests except that anti-IgE, rather than allergen, is attached to the solid phase.

Type II Hypersensitivity

- Type II hypersensitivity involves the production of IgG or IgM antibodies to antigens on the surface of host cells. These antibodies can destroy the cells through complement-mediated cytolysis, opsonization and phagocytosis, or antibody-dependent cellular cytotoxicity (ADCC). In other cases, binding of the antibody to the cell surface antigen can result in dysfunction or overstimulation of the cell.
- Examples of type II reactions that involve cell damage include autoimmune hemolytic anemia, transfusion reactions, hemolytic disease of the fetus and newborn (HDFN), and immune thrombocytopenic purpura (ITP). Myasthenia gravis is an example of a type II disorder in which the antibody blocks binding of a ligand to cell receptors, causing dysfunction of the cells. In contrast, antibodies in Graves disease stimulate cells after binding to their receptors.
- The direct antiglobulin test (DAT) is used to screen for transfusion reactions, autoimmune hemolytic anemia, and HDFN. In this test, washed patient RBCs are combined with anti-human globulin and observed for agglutination, indicating the presence of IgG or complement components on the cells.
- The indirect antiglobulin test (IAT) is used in antibody screening and identification and in crossmatching of blood to prevent transfusion reactions. It is also used to type patient RBCs for specific blood group antigens. The method detects in vitro binding of antibody to RBCs after addition of anti-human globulin to cause a visible agglutination reaction.
- Cold agglutinin antibodies bind to RBCs at temperatures below 30°C and cause micro-occlusions of small blood vessels or destruction of the RBCs, mainly through opsonization and extravascular clearance by macrophages in the liver. Production of cold agglutinins may be from unknown causes or may be associated with certain infections or B-cell/plasma cell lymphoproliferative disorders. Cold agglutinin titers can be determined by incubating patient serum with a dilute suspension of human type O RBCs overnight at 4°C and observing for agglutination.

Type III Hypersensitivity

- Type III hypersensitivity involves the formation of IgG or IgM antibody that reacts with soluble antigen under conditions of slight antigen excess to form small complexes that deposit in the blood vessels and tissues. These complexes activate complement, resulting in the migration of neutrophils to the site, with subsequent release of lysosomal enzymes and reactive oxygen species that damage the surrounding tissues.
- The Arthus reaction, characterized by deposition of antigen-antibody complexes in the blood vessels of the skin, is a classic example of a type III reaction. Other examples include serum sickness and autoimmune diseases such as SLE and RA.

Type IV Hypersensitivity

- Type IV hypersensitivity is a cell-mediated mechanism that involves the activation of CD4 T_H cells to release cytokines that recruit macrophages and other immune cells to the area. The resulting inflammatory reaction and, in some cases, cytotoxic T cells cause damage to the affected tissues.
- Contact dermatitis is an example of a type IV hypersensitivity reaction. It results from contact of the skin with chemicals released by plants such as poison ivy and poison oak, metals such as nickel, or components of hair dyes and cosmetics that act as haptens when bound to self-proteins. Hypersensitivity pneumonitis is a type IV hypersensitivity response that results mainly from occupational exposure to inhaled antigens.
- Skin testing is used to detect the type IV hypersensitivity responses in contact dermatitis and tuberculin (PPD) testing. It is also used to test for functional cell-mediated immunity to common antigens in patients suspected of having immunodeficiency diseases. Positive test results appear in 48 to 72 hours and indicate sensitization to the antigen(s) used in the test.
- Interferon gamma release assays (IGRAs) provide an alternative to tuberculin skin testing to detect latent *M. tuberculosis* infection. The IGRAs have several advantages compared with skin testing, including increased specificity, clearer result interpretation, and faster turnaround time to results.

Study Guide: Comparison of Hypersensitivity Reactions

	TYPE I	TYPE II	TYPE III	TYPE IV
Immune Mediators	IgE	IgG or IgM	IgG or IgM	T cells
Synonym	Anaphylactic	Antibody-mediated; or Antibody-mediated cytotoxic	Complex-mediated	Cell-mediated or delayed type
Timing	Immediate	Immediate	Immediate	Delayed
Antigen	Various heterologous allergens (e.g., certain drugs, proteins from foods, insect venom)	Cell surface: autologous or heterologous	Soluble: autologous or heterologous	Antigens that contact the skin, intracellular pathogens
Complement Involvement	No	Yes	Yes	No
Immune Mechanism	Release of mediators from IgE- sensitized mast cells and basophils	Cell destruction caused by antibody and complement, opsonization, or ADCC Cell function inhibited by antibody binding Cell function stimulated by antibody binding	Antigen–antibody complexes activate complement proteins. Neutrophils are recruited and release lysosomal enzymes that cause tissue damage.	Antigen-sensitized CD4 TH cells release cytokines that recruit macrophages and neutrophils and induce inflammation or activate cytotoxic T cells to cause direct cell damage.
Clinical Examples	Anaphylaxis, allergic rhinitis, allergic asthma, food allergies, urticaria	Transfusion reactions, hemolytic disease of the fetus and newborn, autoimmune hemolytic anemia, cold agglutinin disease, immune thrombocytopenic purpura, drug reactions, myasthenia gravis, Graves' disease	Arthus reaction, serum sickness, SLE, rheumatoid arthritis, drug reactions	Contact dermatitis, tuberculin and anergy skin tests, hypersensitivity pneumonitis

CASE STUDIES

1. A 13-year-old had numerous absences from school in the spring because of common cold symptoms that included head congestion and a cough. The adolescent had received antibiotic treatment twice but seemed to get one cold after another. A complete blood count (CBC) showed no overall increase in WBCs, but a mild eosinophilia was present. Because the patient had no fever or other signs of infection, the physician recommended allergy testing.

Questions

a. What would account for the eosinophilia noted?
b. What tests should be run for this patient?
c. If allergy immunotherapy was used, what test could be performed to monitor the patient's response over time?

2. A 55-year-old patient went to a physician complaining of feeling tired and run down. Two months previously, the patient had pneumonia and was concerned about an incomplete recovery. The patient's symptoms were only noticeable while going outside in the cold. A CBC count was performed, showing that the patient's WBC count was within normal limits; however, the RBC count was just below normal. A DAT performed on the patient's RBCs was weakly positive after incubating at room temperature for 5 minutes. When the DAT was repeated with monospecific reagents, the tube with anti-C3d was the only one that was positive.

Questions

a. What does a positive DAT indicate, and how do the DAT results relate to the patient's symptoms?
b. What is the most likely class of the antibody causing the reaction?
c. Why was the DAT positive only with anti-C3d when monospecific reagents were used?

REVIEW QUESTIONS

1. Which of the following is a general characteristic of hypersensitivity reactions?
   a. Immune responsiveness is depressed.
   b. Antibodies are involved in all reactions.
   c. An exaggerated immune response to an antigen occurs.
   d. The antigen triggering the reaction is a harmful one.

2. Which of the following is associated with an increase in IgE production?
   a. Transfusion reaction
   b. Allergic rhinitis
   c. Reaction to poison ivy
   d. Hemolytic disease of the fetus and newborn

3. Which of the following would cause a positive DAT test?
   a. Presence of IgG on RBCs
   b. Presence of C3d on RBCs
   c. A transfusion reaction caused by preformed antibody
   d. Any of the above

4. All of the following are associated with type I hypersensitivity *except:*
   a. Release of preformed mediators from mast cells
   b. Activation of complement
   c. Cell-bound antibody bridged by antigen
   d. An inherited tendency to respond to allergens

5. Which of the following is associated with anaphylaxis?
   a. Buildup of IgE on mast cells
   b. Activation of complement
   c. Increase in cytotoxic T cells
   d. Large amount of circulating IgG

6. To determine if a patient is allergic to ryegrass, the best test to perform is the:
   a. Total IgE test
   b. Skin prick test
   c. DAT
   d. Complement fixation

7. Which condition would result in hemolytic disease of the fetus and newborn?
   a. Buildup of IgE on mother's cells
   b. Sensitization of cytotoxic T cells
   c. Exposure to an antigen found both on mother's and baby's RBCs
   d. Prior exposure to a foreign RBC antigen

8. What is the immune mechanism involved in type III hypersensitivity reactions?
   a. Cellular antigens are involved.
   b. Deposition of immune complexes occurs in antigen excess.
   c. Only heterologous antigens are involved.
   d. Tissue damage results from complement-mediated lysis.

9. What is the immune phenomenon associated with the Arthus reaction?
   a. Tissue destruction by cytotoxic T cells
   b. Removal of antibody-coated RBCs
   c. Deposition of immune complexes in blood vessels
   d. Release of histamine from mast cells

10. Which of the following conclusions can be drawn about a patient whose total IgE level was determined to be 150 IU/mL?
    a. The patient definitely has allergic tendencies.
    b. The patient is subject to anaphylactic shock.
    c. Antigen-specific testing should be done.
    d. The patient will never have an allergic reaction.

11. Which of the following explains the difference between type II and type III hypersensitivity reactions?
    a. Type II involves cellular antigens.
    b. Type III involves IgE.
    c. IgG is involved only in type III reactions.
    d. Type II reactions involve no antibody.

12. Two days after administration of the tuberculin skin test, a health care worker developed an area of redness and induration 12 mm in size at the injection site. This result means that this individual has:
    a. An active case of TB
    b. Been exposed to *M. tuberculosis*
    c. Developed protective immunity against TB
    d. A result in the normal range for their risk group

13. A teenager developed red, itchy papules on the wrist 2 days after wearing a new bracelet. This reaction was caused by:
    a. IgE-sensitized mast cells in the skin
    b. Antigen-antibody complexes in the skin
    c. Damage to the skin cells by antibodies and complement
    d. An inflammatory response induced by cytokines released from T_H1 cells

14. Reactions to latex are caused by:
    a. Type I hypersensitivity
    b. Type IV hypersensitivity
    c. Skin irritation
    d. All of the above

15. To determine a cold agglutinin titer:
    a. Patient serum should be separated from whole blood at 4°C and tested at 4°C.
    b. Patient serum should be separated from whole blood at 4°C and tested at 37°C.
    c. Patient serum should be separated from whole blood at 37°C and tested at 4°C.
    d. Patient serum should be separated from whole blood at 37°C and tested at 37°C.

16. In vitro methods to detect a cell-mediated response to *M. tuberculosis* measure production of which of the following immunologic components?
    a. IgE antibody
    b. Interleukin-1
    c. Interleukin-2
    d. Interferon gamma

17. In type I hypersensitivity, histamine released from mast cells and basophils causes:
    a. Smooth muscle relaxation
    b. Increased vascular permeability
    c. Constriction of the blood vessels
    d. A late-phase reaction

18. In allergy immunotherapy (AIT), patients are given:
    a. Increasing doses of allergen
    b. Anti-histamine drugs
    c. Epinephrine
    d. Monoclonal antibodies to IgE

Chapter 14 Answer Key

Answers to Knowledge Checks

14.1 c 14.2 a 14.3 d 14.4 b 14.5 d
14.6 1-d; 2-c; 3-a; 4-b

Answers to Review Questions

1. c	2. b	3. d	4. b	5. a	6. b	7. d
8. b	9. c	10. c	11. a	12. b	13. d	14. d
15. c	16. d	17. b	18. a			

15 Autoimmune Diseases

Linda E. Miller, PhD, I, MB^{CM}(ASCP)SI

LEARNING OUTCOMES

After finishing this chapter, you should be able to:

15.1 Explain the mechanisms of central and peripheral tolerance that are essential in preventing the development of autoimmunity.

15.2 Discuss genetic and environmental factors thought to contribute to the development of autoimmunity.

15.3 Explain the relationship between microbial infections and the development of autoimmune disease.

15.4 Distinguish between organ-specific and systemic autoimmune diseases, providing examples of each and their associated target tissues.

15.5 Describe the immunopathology and clinical manifestations of each of the following diseases: systemic lupus erythematosus (SLE), rheumatoid arthritis (RA), granulomatosis with polyangiitis (Wegener granulomatosis), Graves disease, Hashimoto thyroiditis, type 1 diabetes mellitus, celiac disease, autoimmune hepatitis (AIH), primary biliary cirrhosis, multiple sclerosis (MS), myasthenia gravis (MG), and anti–glomerular basement membrane (anti-GBM) disease.

15.6 Associate each of the diseases listed in Learning Outcome 15.5 with its corresponding autoantibodies and laboratory findings.

15.7 Identify autoantibodies associated with Sjögren syndrome, systemic sclerosis (SSc), mixed connective tissue disease (MCTD), and the inflammatory myopathies.

15.8 Explain the principles of laboratory methods used to screen for and confirm the presence of anti-nuclear antibodies (ANAs).

15.9 Describe common immunofluorescence patterns seen in the indirect immunofluorescence (IIF) test for ANAs, along with their associated antibodies and clinical significance.

15.10 Describe the c-ANCA and p-ANCA patterns seen in the IIF test for ANCAs and their clinical significance.

15.11 Explain ways in which p-ANCA-associated antibodies can be differentiated from ANAs.

15.12 Discuss the composition and clinical significance of rheumatoid factor (RF) and anti-cyclic citrullinated peptide (anti-CCP).

CHAPTER OUTLINE

You can go to **fadavis.com** keyword stevens for the laboratory exercises that accompany this text.

In the early 1900s, Paul Ehrlich noted that the immune system could attack the very host it was intended to protect, a phenomenon he referred to as "horror autotoxicus," or "fear of self-poisoning." Such conditions later became known as *autoimmune diseases.* **Autoimmune diseases** are disorders in which immune responses are targeted toward self-antigens and result in damage to organs and tissues in the body. These harmful effects can be caused by T-cell–mediated immune responses or **autoantibodies** that are directed against host antigens. More than 100 autoimmune diseases have been discovered, and these can involve various organ systems. They are a leading cause of chronic illness and death, affecting about 4% of the world's population, including about 50 million people in the United States alone. We begin this chapter by discussing the factors that are thought to contribute to the development of autoimmunity so that you can gain a better understanding of the underlying pathology of autoimmune disease. We then discuss the clinical manifestations and immunopathology of specific autoimmune diseases and the laboratory tests used in their diagnosis.

Etiology of Autoimmune Disease

The underlying cause of autoimmune disease is unknown but is thought to involve interactions between an individual's genetic makeup and various environmental factors to which they are exposed. The result is a loss of immunologic tolerance to self-antigens. In the following sections, we discuss these concepts in more detail.

Self-Tolerance

As we discussed in Chapter 4, under normal circumstances, the immune system can differentiate between "self" and "nonself" or "foreign," so that self-antigens are not destroyed. Central to this phenomenon is **self-tolerance,** or the immune system's ability to accept autologous antigens and not initiate a response against them. Autoimmune disease is thought to result from a loss of self-tolerance.

Self-tolerance is a type of **immunologic tolerance**, or a state of immune unresponsiveness directed against a specific antigen, in this case, a self-antigen. For self-tolerance to develop, lymphocytes must be "educated" to distinguish between self-antigens and foreign antigens. This education occurs at two levels: central and peripheral.

Central tolerance occurs in the central or primary lymphoid organs, the thymus and the bone marrow. As T cells mature in the thymus, they encounter self-antigens that are normally present on the surface of thymic epithelial cells. In a process called *negative selection,* T cells that express T-cell receptors (TCRs) with a strong affinity for these self-antigens are deleted by apoptosis (see Chapter 5 and **Fig. 15–1**). **Apoptosis** is a normal process of cell death characterized by cell shrinkage, nuclear chromatin condensation, and formation of small structures that are phagocytized by macrophages; because apoptotic cells do not release their contents into the tissue environment, inflammation is not induced. Negative selection occurs with both the immature, double-positive $CD4^+/CD8^+$ T cells in the cortex and the more mature, single-positive $CD4^+$ or $CD8^+$ T cells in the medulla. During this process, some of the self-reactive $CD4^+$ T cells are not deleted but instead differentiate into regulatory T (Treg) cells that can specifically inhibit immune responses to self-antigens.

Similarly, as B cells mature in the bone marrow, those with receptors having a strong affinity for self-antigens are eliminated by apoptosis. Some self-reactive B cells are not deleted; rather, they are stimulated to rearrange their immunoglobulin genes so that their B-cell receptors are no longer antigen specific. This process is known as *receptor editing.* B cells with receptors that only weakly recognize self-antigens are induced to downregulate the expression of their receptors and develop a specific state of unresponsiveness to the antigens known as **anergy.**

Thus, central tolerance of T and B cells can be achieved in several ways. However, this process is not totally effective, and some self-reactive lymphocytes escape to the secondary lymphoid organs, such as the lymph nodes and spleen. Also, some self-antigens may not induce central tolerance because they are not expressed in high levels in the primary lymphoid organs. Therefore, a second level of protection is needed.

In this second level, known as **peripheral tolerance**, lymphocytes that recognize self-antigens in the secondary lymphoid organs are rendered incapable of reacting with those antigens. Peripheral tolerance of T cells can result from anergy caused by the absence or delay of a costimulatory signal from an antigen-presenting cell (APC) or binding of inhibitory receptors such as CTLA-4 (a molecule that prevents T-cell activation) to APCs. Peripheral T-cell tolerance can also result from inhibition of lymphocytes or APCs by Tregs or death by apoptosis. Self-reactive B cells in the periphery can be deleted by apoptosis, be rendered anergic after repeated stimulation with self-antigens, or receive inhibitory signals through receptors such as CD22.

In some individuals, self-tolerance can fail even after this second layer of protection; if this happens, autoimmunity can arise. The development of autoimmune disease is thought to be caused by complex interactions between genetic makeup, exposure to environmental factors, and defects in immune regulation. Next, we discuss some of the major factors thought to contribute to autoimmunity.

Knowledge Check 15-1

T cells that react strongly with self-antigens are normally eliminated in the thymus by:

a. Apoptosis
b. Receptor editing
c. Lack of costimulation
d. Inactivation of Tregs

Genetics

There is much evidence supporting a genetic basis for autoimmune disease. Autoimmune diseases are often more prevalent among family members than among unrelated individuals

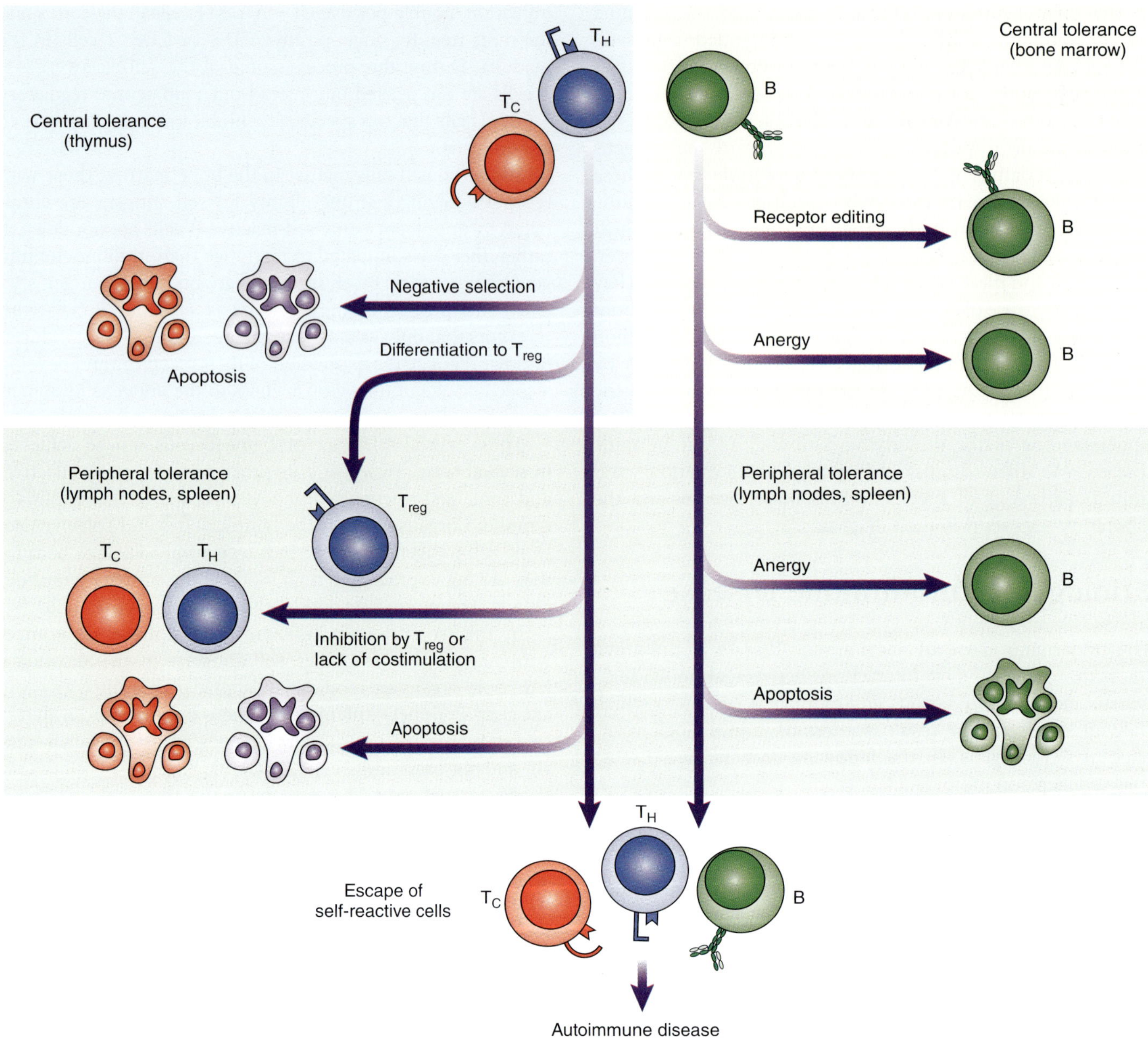

FIGURE 15–1 Mechanisms of central and peripheral tolerance. Central tolerance involves the elimination of immature T cells in the thymus and B-cell precursors in the bone marrow that have receptors for self-antigens. Peripheral tolerance occurs when mature, self-reacting T and B cells are inactivated in the secondary lymphoid organs such as the lymph nodes and spleen.

and are more prevalent among monozygotic (genetically identical) twins than dizygotic (nonidentical) twins or siblings. Researchers conducting molecular studies continue to identify specific genetic polymorphisms or mutations that are associated with autoimmune diseases.

Most of the research concerning humans has focused on genes in the major histocompatibility complex (MHC) (see Chapter 4). Investigators have found an association between the presence of certain human leukocyte antigen (HLA) types and the risk of developing a particular autoimmune disorder. The strongest link found is between the HLA-B27 allele and the development of ankylosing spondylitis, an autoinflammatory disease that affects the spine. People who possess HLA-B27 have over a 100 times greater chance of developing the disease than those who do not have that allele. We present other associations with specific MHC genes in Chapter 4 and in the sections on particular autoimmune diseases in this chapter. Differences in MHC genes are thought to influence the development of autoimmune disease because the specific structure of the MHC molecule can determine whether a self-antigen can attach to the peptide-binding cleft of the molecule and subsequently be processed and presented to T cells. Self-antigens may also be presented to T cells by class II MHC molecules that are abnormally expressed on cells where they are not typically found.

DNA sequencing and genome-wide association studies are revealing that the genetic basis of autoimmunity is complex, involving multiple genes, not only HLA genes but also several non-MHC genes. Some of these genes are associated with several autoimmune diseases, while others are linked to particular disorders. Variations in many of these genes influence the development of self-tolerance and regulation of immune responses, whereas others have more organ-specific effects. Examples of non-MHC genes associated with human autoimmune diseases and their functions include the following:

- Genes coding for signaling and transcription factors (e.g., *PTPN22*—T- and B-cell receptor signaling; *BLK*—B-cell activation; *IRF5*—production of type I interferons)
- Genes coding for cytokines and their receptors (e.g., *IL2RA*—T-cell activation and maintenance of Tregs; *IL23R*—differentiation of Th17 cells; *IL10*—inhibition of T_H1 cells)
- Genes involved in lymphocyte regulation (e.g., *CTLA4*—inhibition of T-cell activation; *AIRE* [autoimmune regulator] gene—promotes the development of T-cell tolerance in the thymus)
- Complement genes (e.g., *C1QA, C2, C4*—clearance of immune complexes)
- Genes involved in innate immunity (e.g., *NOD2*—receptor for bacterial peptidoglycans)

Although most autoimmune diseases involve multiple genes, single-gene mutations that can be inherited in a Mendelian fashion have been associated with rare autoimmune disorders.

Other Endogenous and Environmental Factors

Inheritance of specific genes may make an individual more susceptible to a particular autoimmune disease, but genetic makeup is not completely responsible because most people with a particular gene will not develop autoimmunity. Environmental and other factors are also thought to play a role in the development of autoimmune disease. In the sections that follow, we discuss some of the major factors thought to trigger autoimmune responses.

Hormonal Influence

Women are 2.7 times more likely to acquire an autoimmune disease than men; in fact, about 80% of patients with autoimmune diseases are female. Females also tend to develop autoimmunity at an earlier age and have a higher risk for acquiring more than one autoimmune disease as compared with men. They also have higher absolute $CD4^+$ T-cell counts and higher levels of circulating antibodies than men. These observations suggest there is a hormonal influence on the development of autoimmunity. Studies have shown that estrogens tend to direct the immune system in favor of a type 2 helper T cell (T_H2) response, resulting in more B-cell activation and antibody production, whereas androgens favor a type 1 helper T cell (T_H1) response with $CD8^+$ T-cell activation. Prolactin, a hormone that stimulates breast milk production in pregnant and nursing women, can stimulate both humoral and cell-mediated immune responses. The stimulatory effects of female hormones, and possibly defective X-chromosome inactivation, may place females at a greater risk for developing an autoimmune disease.

Tissue Trauma and Release of Cryptic Antigens

When immunologic tolerance to self-antigens occurs during the early development of lymphocytes in the thymus and bone marrow, some self-antigens may be *cryptic,* or hidden within the tissues of the host. Anatomical barriers shield the sequestered antigens from T and B lymphocytes, which are therefore not educated to develop tolerance to them.

Later in life, inflammation or tissue trauma could cause the cryptic antigens to be released and to suddenly be accessible to the uneducated lymphocytes, triggering an immune response. Tissue injury could be caused by factors such as infections, contact with environmental toxins, or physical injury from exposure to ultraviolet (UV) radiation. This concept has also been referred to as *immunologic ignorance* and may be responsible for the production of autoantibodies to the lens of the eye following an ocular injury, autoantibodies to sperm after a vasectomy, and autoantibodies to DNA after damage to skin cells caused by overexposure to UV rays from the sun.

As tissue damage progresses, more self-antigens may be altered and released, triggering further autoimmune reactions. This expansion of the immune response has been termed **epitope spreading.**

Microbial Infections

Scientists have been very interested in the association of microbial infections with the development of autoimmune disease because infections often precede the onset of autoimmunity. Bacteria, viruses, and other infectious pathogens may be able to trigger autoimmune responses in various ways:

- ***Similarities between microbial antigens and host antigens.*** This concept, known as **molecular mimicry,** refers to the fact that many bacteria or viruses have antigens that closely resemble the structure or amino acid sequence of self-antigens. Exposure to such foreign antigens may trigger immune responses that cross-react with similar self-antigens. Molecular mimicry has been postulated as a mechanism for several human autoimmune diseases. The best-known example is the association between the gram-positive bacterium *Streptococcus pyogenes* and rheumatic fever, an autoimmune disorder that mainly affects the joints and the heart. Some patients who have had scarlet fever or streptococcal pharyngitis develop rheumatic fever 2 to 4 weeks later if they are not treated adequately with antibiotics (see Chapter 20). Symptoms are thought to be caused by the production of antibodies to the M protein and *N*-acetylglucosamine components of the bacteria, which cross-react with cardiac myosin, causing damage to the heart.
- ***Innate immune signals.*** As we discussed in Chapter 2, upon exposure to microorganisms, receptors on innate immune cells bind to pathogen-associated molecular patterns, triggering a series of cellular signals that induce a local inflammatory response. As a result, leukocytes are recruited to the area, and APCs are stimulated to release cytokines that nonspecifically activate T and B cells. Some of the activated lymphocytes may have specificity for self-antigens.

- ***Stimulation of polyclonal lymphocyte responses.*** Some microbial proteins, called **superantigens**, can bind to both class II MHC molecules and T-cell receptors (TCRs), regardless of their antigen specificity. Examples are the staphylococcal enterotoxins that cause food poisoning and toxic shock syndrome. These superantigens act as potent T-cell mitogens by activating many T cells with different antigen specificities. If some of these T cells have specificity for a self-antigen, autoimmune responses might result. Likewise, some viruses, including the Epstein-Barr virus (EBV) and cytomegalovirus (CMV), can cause polyclonal activation of B cells.
- ***Influence of microbiota (normal flora).*** Recall from Chapter 2 that microbiota are commensal microorganisms that coexist with the host. Studies have shown that alterations in the microbial composition in various body sites (i.e., the microbiome) can disturb the normal homeostasis of the immune system. Expansion of certain types of endogenous microorganisms in the body has been associated with autoimmune diseases, possibly by disturbing the balance between helper T-cell (T_H) and regulatory T cell (Treg) activity, altering amino acid metabolism, and triggering autoantibody production.

Epigenetics and Modification of Self-Antigens

Recall from Chapter 12 that *epigenetics* refers to modifications in gene expression that are *not* caused by changes in the original DNA sequence. These changes are thought to be triggered by exposure to environmental toxins, ingestion of harmful foods or drugs, or the aging process. Such alterations include increasing or decreasing methylation of cytosine bases, modifying histones, and causing abnormal regulation by microRNAs. These modifications can result in changes in the level of gene expression by affecting transcription into mRNA, which is subsequently translated into proteins that influence an individual's phenotype. Over- or underexpression of certain genes in the immune system may result in homeostatic imbalances and a breakdown of self-tolerance, leading to autoimmunity.

Sometimes, exposure to environmental factors can lead to *post-translational (protein) modifications,* involving biochemical processes such as acetylation, lipidation, citrullination, and glycosylation. These modifications can alter the immunogenicity of an antigen, affecting its ability to be processed by APCs and presented to T cells. Such alterations of self-antigens can make them more immunogenic, leading to autoimmune responses. For example, citrullination of collagen might play a role in the pathogenesis of rheumatoid arthritis (RA), and glycosylation of myelin may be involved in the pathology of multiple sclerosis (see the "Rheumatoid Arthritis" and "Multiple Sclerosis" sections later).

Interactions Between Factors

Although the precise etiology of autoimmunity is unknown, much evidence suggests that this heterogeneous disease entity is caused by complex interactions between genetic and environmental factors **(Fig. 15–2).** Certain genes are thought to make individuals more susceptible to immune responses against self-antigens but are not sufficient by themselves to cause autoimmune disease. The individual's sex, tissue injury, and exposure to infectious microorganisms or other environmental agents are all believed to contribute to autoimmune responses in genetically susceptible individuals. As a result, immunologic tolerance is broken, autoreactive T cells recognize and proliferate in response to self-antigens, and B cells develop into plasma cells that secrete autoantibodies. Proinflammatory cytokines are released, and, together with dysfunctions in immunoregulatory cells, perpetuate the autoimmune responses. If these responses are not held in check, they can culminate in autoimmune disease. Tissue injury in these disorders results from hypersensitivity reactions involving autoantibodies to cell surface receptors, deposition of immune complexes containing self-antigens, and cell-mediated cytotoxicity (see Chapter 14). The immunopathological mechanisms vary with specific autoimmune diseases, as we discuss in the sections that follow.

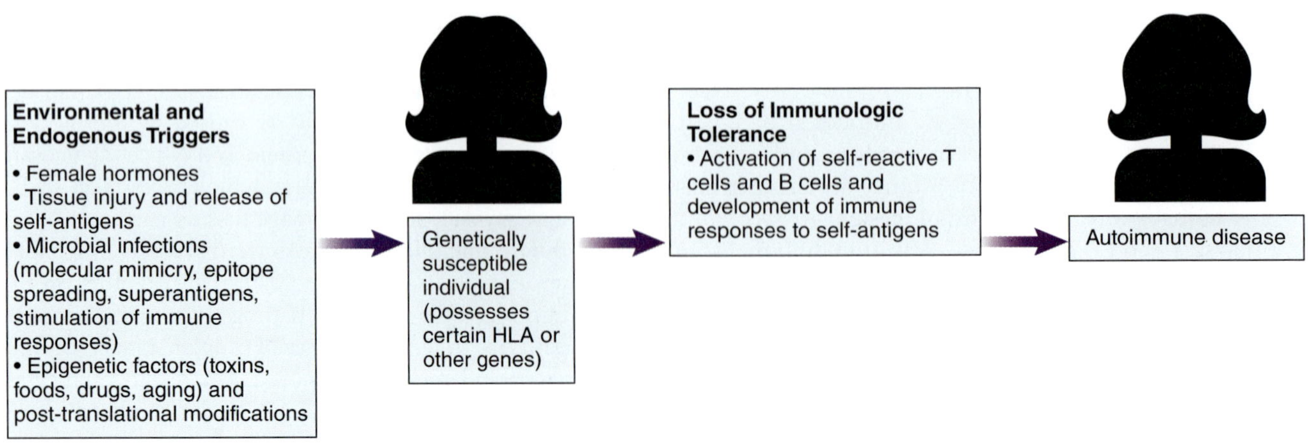

FIGURE 15–2 Interactions between genetic and environmental factors in the development of autoimmunity.

Knowledge Check 15-2

Microorganisms may play a role in autoimmunity by:
a. Inhibiting polyclonal lymphocyte responses
b. Suppressing innate immune signals
c. Stimulating immune responses against similar host antigens
d. Interfering with release of pro-inflammatory cytokines

Systemic Autoimmune Diseases

Autoimmune diseases are a diverse group of disorders that can be classified as systemic or organ specific, depending on the extent of pathology in the body. The systemic diseases affect multiple organs and tissues, whereas the organ-specific diseases mainly involve a single organ or gland. Two important groups of systemic diseases are the systemic autoimmune rheumatic diseases (SARDs), which involve inflammation of the joints and their associated structures, and the anti-neutrophil cytoplasmic antibodies (ANCA)-associated vasculitides, which are characterized by inflammation of the blood vessels. **Table 15–1** lists examples of systemic autoimmune diseases, along with their corresponding target tissues and associated autoantibodies. In the sections that follow, we discuss selected systemic autoimmune diseases and the laboratory tests that are essential to their diagnosis.

Systemic Lupus Erythematosus (SLE)

Systemic lupus erythematosus (SLE; lupus) is a chronic inflammatory disease that affects tissues and organs throughout the body. The estimated prevalence of the disease varies widely, depending on the population. The age of onset is usually between 15 and 45 years. Females are much more likely to be affected than males, by a ratio of about 9 to 1. SLE is also more common in African American, Asian American, and Hispanic people than in White people. With earlier diagnosis and improved treatments, the 5-year survival rate has increased from 50% in the 1950s to 95% today.

Etiology

The etiology of SLE is unknown, but it is thought to originate from complex interactions between environmental factors, genetic susceptibility, and immune system abnormalities. Environmental factors implicated in the pathogenesis of SLE include UV light, certain medications, prior infections (e.g., Epstein-Barr virus [EBV]), silica dust, pesticides, air pollutants, and cigarette smoking. Exposure to sunlight may alter DNA and is a well-known trigger of the photosensitive skin rashes seen in many patients with lupus. Certain drugs, such as procainamide (used to treat abnormal heart rhythms), hydralazine (used for high blood pressure), and the tuberculosis drug isoniazid, can induce a transient lupus-like syndrome that resolves once the drug is stopped. Hormones are also important, as indicated by the significantly higher incidence

Table 15-1 Examples of Systemic Autoimmune Diseases

DISEASE	TARGET CELLS AND TISSUES	ASSOCIATED AUTOANTIBODIES
Systemic Autoimmune Rheumatic Diseases (SARDs)		
Systemic lupus erythematosus (SLE)	Multiple cells and organs, including the skin, joints, kidneys, brain, heart, lungs	ANAs (e.g., anti-dsDNA, anti-Sm) Phospholipid antibodies Antibody to RBCs Antibody to platelets Antibody to lymphocytes Antibody to ribosomal components Antibody to endothelium RF
Rheumatoid arthritis (RA)	Joints, bone; other tissues in some cases	Anti-CCP RF ANAs
Sjögren syndrome	Eyes, mouth	ANAs, RF, anti-salivary duct antibodies, anti-lacrimal gland antibodies
Systemic sclerosis (SSc)	Connective tissue	ANAs: anti–Scl-70, anti-centromere antibody
Polymyositis/ dermatomyositis	Muscles, skin	ANAs (e.g., anti–Jo-1)
ANCA-Associated Vasculitides		
Granulomatosis with polyangiitis (Wegener granulomatosis)	Upper respiratory system, lungs, blood vessels	ANCA; c-ANCA pattern RF ANAs

ANAs = anti-nuclear antibodies; ANCA = anti-neutrophil cytoplasmic antibodies; CCP = cyclic citrullinated protein; RBC = red blood cells; RF = rheumatoid factor.

of SLE in females and an increased risk of developing lupus in females who have used estrogen-containing contraceptives or hormone replacement therapy. Hormones may help regulate the transcription of genes that are central to the expression of SLE.

Most people exposed to the environmental factors we mentioned do not develop lupus, and genetic makeup is believed to play an important role in susceptibility to SLE. Development of the disease is thought to be caused by interactions between environmental factors and multiple genes. Over 180 genetic loci that may play a role in human lupus have been discovered; of the HLA genes, certain HLA DR2 and HLA DR3 alleles appear to have the strongest association with a predisposition to SLE. Variations in other genes that may be involved in the pathogenesis of SLE include those that play a role in the clearance of immune complexes (e.g., genes for complement components C1q, C4, and C2), regulation of immune function, cytokine production (e.g., interferons), signaling of innate immune responses, and DNA repair. Specific genetic defects vary in individual patients but likely interact with environmental factors to alter self-molecules such as DNA, generate uncontrolled autoreactivity of T and B cells, and cause production of autoantibodies.

Immunopathology

The mechanisms by which SLE develops are not completely understood but are thought to begin with environmental factors such as infections that trigger innate immunity. Genetic defects in patients with SLE may result in abnormal clearance of nucleic acids and debris released from cells damaged during these responses and from neutrophil extracellular traps (see Chapter 2). Excessive amounts and altered forms of these self-antigens, along with the cytokines produced (e.g., type 1 interferons, TNF-α, IL-12), could potentially stimulate the adaptive immune system to make autoantibodies. The imbalance between Treg and helper T (T_H) cell activities in lupus drives further autoantibody production.

Over 100 autoantibodies associated with SLE have been discovered. The typical patient has several circulating autoantibodies, and autoantibody production can precede the onset of disease by several years. Antibodies produced in SLE include those with specificity for double-stranded DNA (dsDNA), histones and other nuclear components, lymphocytes, erythrocytes, platelets, phospholipids, ribosomal components, and endothelium. Antibodies to dsDNA are present in 70% of patients with lupus and are highly specific for the disease.

B cells and the autoantibodies they produce are believed to play a central role in the complicated pathogenesis of SLE. The antibodies combine with their respective antigens to form immune complexes, which cannot be cleared effectively by phagocytic cells. The complexes deposit in various body organs and activate complement, inducing the generation of chemotaxins such as C5a. As a result, neutrophils are recruited to the sites and release lysosomal enzymes and reactive oxygen species (ROS), causing injury to the surrounding tissues and promoting an inflammatory response. As you may recall from Chapter 14, this type of tissue damage is an example of type III hypersensitivity.

Autoantibodies can also cause cell destruction by other mechanisms. For example, antibodies to red blood cells (RBCs) can cause hemolytic anemia, and antibodies to platelets can cause thrombocytopenia by antibody-dependent cellular cytotoxicity (type II hypersensitivity). Antibodies to endothelial cells can cause inflammation and damage to the blood vessels, which may be responsible for the vasculitis and neuropsychiatric symptoms seen in some patients with SLE. Phospholipid antibodies are associated with increased miscarriage, stillbirth, and preterm delivery in pregnant women with lupus.

Neonatal lupus, which occurs in up to 8% of babies born to pregnant women with SLE, is associated with antibodies to the nuclear antigens, SS-A/Ro and SS-B/La. Symptoms are transient and resolve at 6 to 8 months of age when the maternal antibodies have been cleared from the infant's circulation. In utero heart block is a serious complication that occurs in 2% of fetuses whose mothers have anti–SS-A antibodies.

Clinical Signs and Symptoms

The clinical symptoms of SLE are extremely diverse, varying in terms of severity and the affected body areas. Nonspecific symptoms such as fatigue, weight loss, malaise, fever, and anorexia are often first to appear. The disease is marked by alternating relapses or flares and periods of remission. Most patients have polyarthralgias (pain in several joints) or arthritis, most commonly involving the hands, wrists, and knees. These symptoms usually do not lead to joint deformities.

Also common are skin manifestations, which can present in various forms. A photosensitive, erythematous rash may appear on any area of the body exposed to UV light. Less common but perhaps more dramatic is the classic butterfly rash across the nose and cheeks that appears in some patients with SLE **(Fig. 15–3).** This rash is responsible for the name *lupus*, derived from the

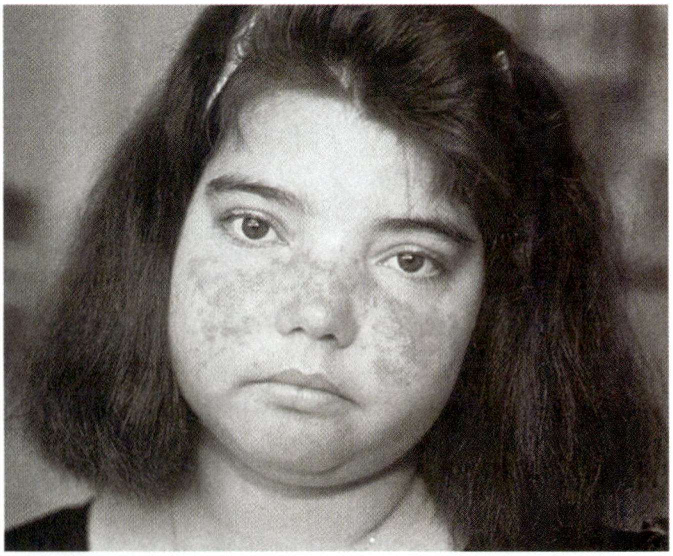

FIGURE 15–3 Butterfly rash in SLE. Characteristic rash over the cheekbones and forehead is diagnostic of SLE. The disease often begins in young adulthood and may eventually involve many organ systems. *(From Steinman L. Autoimmune disease.* Sci Am. *1993;269:107, with permission.)*

Latin term meaning "wolf-like." Discoid lupus is characterized by rough, raised skin lesions with central atrophy and scarring. Oral and nasal ulcers also develop frequently.

Renal involvement is present in about half of all patients with lupus, and nephritis (kidney inflammation) is a major cause of illness and death. There are several types of lesions, but the most dangerous is diffuse proliferative glomerulonephritis, characterized by cell proliferation in the glomeruli that can lead to end-stage renal disease. Other conditions involving the kidneys may include deposition of immune complexes in the subendothelial tissue and thickening of the basement membrane, both of which can lead to renal failure.

Other body areas that can be affected include the heart, lungs, central nervous system, gastrointestinal system, and eyes. Hematologic abnormalities such as anemia, leukopenia, thrombocytopenia, or lymphopenia can also be present because of antibodies to RBCs and white blood cells (WBCs).

Drug-induced lupus differs from the classic form of the disease, in that symptoms usually disappear once the drug is discontinued. Typically, this milder form of lupus usually manifests as fever, arthritis, or rashes; rarely are the kidneys involved. The most common drugs implicated are procainamide, hydralazine, chlorpromazine, isoniazid, quinidine, anticonvulsants such as methyldopa, and possibly oral contraceptives.

In 2019, the American College of Rheumatology (ACR) updated its previously published clinical and immunologic criteria to define SLE for the purposes of research and surveillance. The criteria, which were developed through collaboration of the ACR and the European League Against Rheumatism (now the European Alliance of Associations for Rheumatology [EULAR]), have a high level of sensitivity and specificity for the disease. These criteria begin with an absolute requirement that the patient has a current or previously positive ANA with a titer of at least 1:80 by indirect immunofluorescence (IIF) on HEp-2 cells (see section on "Anti-Nuclear Antibodies" that follows). Patients meeting this initial criterion are evaluated in seven clinical domains (constitutional, hematologic, neuropsychiatric, mucocutaneous, serosal, musculoskeletal, and renal) and three immunologic domains (anti-phospholipid antibodies, C3 and C4 complement protein levels, and SLE-specific antibodies—anti-dsDNA and anti-Sm). The domains are weighted, and patients are classified as having SLE if they meet at least one of the clinical criteria and have a total score of 10 or higher. The ACR will continue to update its criteria periodically. Although these criteria are not meant to be used for diagnosis, they reflect the major clinical and laboratory features of SLE and are useful in identifying patients who qualify for research studies and clinical trials.

Treatment and Prognosis

Various medications are used to treat SLE, including glucocorticoids, anti-malarial agents, nonsteroidal anti-inflammatory drugs (NSAIDs), immunosuppressive drugs, and monoclonal antibodies that target B cells. The drugs used depend on the body sites and severity of disease activity in individual patients. The anti-malarial drug hydroxychloroquine is recommended for all patients with SLE because it has immunomodulatory and anti-thrombotic effects. Systemic glucocorticoid and other immunosuppressive drugs are used to treat serious complications, such as acute fulminant (severe and sudden) lupus, lupus nephritis, or central nervous system (CNS) manifestations, due to their effectiveness in quickly suppressing the immune response. Patients must be monitored closely for side effects and drug doses tapered as clinical symptoms subside. The monoclonal antibodies, belimumab (directed against soluble B-lymphocyte stimulator [BlyS]) or rituximab (anti-CD20), inhibit B-cell proliferation and differentiation and may be used for patients who have not responded adequately to the previous treatments. New biological drugs continue to be evaluated.

The key to successful treatment is to control symptoms, prevent organ damage, and achieve remission. The most common causes of death are renal failure and infection, followed by heart disease. Treatments have come a long way in improving quality of life and long-term patient outcomes, as the 5-year survival rate has increased to about 95%, and 20-year survival to nearly 80%.

Laboratory Diagnosis of Systemic Lupus Erythematosus

General laboratory tests used in the initial evaluation of patients include a complete blood count (CBC), a platelet count, creatinine levels, and urinalysis to assess renal function. Some of the first laboratory findings in lupus patients are leukopenia and possible anemia and thrombocytopenia. Also, the erythrocyte sedimentation rate (ESR) may be elevated even though the C-reactive protein (CRP) level tends to be low or normal.

When SLE is suspected, the first test typically done is a screening test for **anti-nuclear antibodies (ANAs)** because these are present in most patients with the disease. When the screen is positive, further tests are done to differentiate the type of ANA. Antibodies to dsDNA and antibodies to the Sm nuclear antigen are highly specific for SLE. We discuss ANAs and the methods used to detect them in more detail in the section that follows. Phospholipid antibodies are present in some patients with lupus and are discussed in a later section.

After diagnosis, further tests are performed to monitor disease activity. Antibody to dsDNA can be measured in patients who are positive for this antibody, as titers often increase before a disease flare. Quantification of complement proteins such as C3 and C4 is also helpful for disease monitoring because serum complement levels decrease during disease flares as complement is bound by immune complexes (see Chapter 7). Additional laboratory tests are ordered based on the patient's clinical symptoms.

Knowledge Check 15-3

Which laboratory finding is characteristic of SLE?

a. Increased serum complement
b. Decreased C-reactive protein
c. Increased RBCs
d. Presence of anti-nuclear antibodies

Anti-Nuclear Antibodies (ANAs)

ANAs are autoantibodies directed against antigens in the nuclei of mammalian cells. ANAs are present in over 95% of patients with active lupus and are used as a major marker for the disease. However, ANAs are not specific for SLE because they can also be detected in a significant percentage of patients with other SARDs, including RA, mixed connective tissue disease (MCTD), Sjögren syndrome, scleroderma, and polymyositis-dermatomyositis. They are also found in some people with other conditions, including chronic infections, cancer, and pregnancy. Furthermore, up to 5% of healthy persons and up to 30% of older adults are ANA-positive.

Types of Anti-Nuclear Antibodies

ANAs are a heterogeneous group of antibodies with different antigen specificities. The nuclear antigens they are directed against include dsDNA and single-stranded DNA (ssDNA), histones, nucleosomes (DNA-histone complexes), centromere proteins, and extractable nuclear antigens (ENAs). Some of the more common ANAs and their associated features are discussed in the text that follows and listed in **Table 15–2.**

Double-stranded DNA (dsDNA) antibodies are the most specific for SLE because they are mainly seen in patients with lupus, and their levels correlate with disease activity. While only seen in 40% to 70% of patients, they are considered diagnostic for SLE, especially when found in combination with low levels of the complement component C3. Antibodies to dsDNA typically produce a homogeneous staining pattern on IIF. See the "Indirect Immunofluorescence (IIF)" section for further explanation.

Patients with lupus may also have **anti-histone antibodies.** Histones are nucleoproteins that are essential components

Table 15-2 Common Anti-Nuclear Antibodies

AUTOANTIBODY	ANTIGEN(S)	IMMUNOFLUORESCENT PATTERN	DISEASE ASSOCIATION
Anti-dsDNA	dsDNA	Homogeneous	SLE
Anti-ssDNA	ssDNA	Not detected on routine screen	SLE, many other diseases
Anti-histone	Different classes of histones	Homogeneous	Drug-induced lupus, other diseases
Anti-DNP	DNA-histone complex (nucleosomes)	Homogeneous	SLE, drug-induced lupus
Anti-Sm	Extractable nuclear antigen (uridine-rich RNA component)	Coarse speckled	Diagnostic for SLE
Anti-RNP	Proteins complexed with small nuclear RNA	Coarse speckled	SLE, mixed connective tissue disease
Anti–SS-A/Ro	Proteins complexed to RNA	Finely speckled	SLE, Sjögren syndrome, others
Anti–SS-B/La	Phosphoprotein complexed to RNA polymerase	Finely speckled	SLE, Sjögren syndrome, others
Anti-nucleolar	RNA polymerase, fibrillarin, PM-1	Prominent staining of nucleoli (can be smooth, clumpy, or speckled)	SLE, systemic sclerosis
Anti–Scl-70	DNA topoisomerase I	Compound pattern with speckling	Systemic sclerosis
Anti–Jo-1	Histidyl-tRNA synthetase	Fine cytoplasmic speckling	Polymyositis
Anti-centromere	CENP-A/B/C in the chromosome centromeres	Discrete speckled	Limited cutaneous systemic sclerosis (CREST syndrome)
DSF70/LEDGF	Lens epithelium-derived growth factor/transcription co-activator p75	Dense fine speckled	Usually indicates absence of SARDs

CREST = calcinosis cutis, Raynaud phenomenon, esophageal dysmotility, sclerodactyly, and telangiectasia; DNP = deoxyribonucleoprotein; dsDNA = double-stranded DNA; RNA = ribonucleic acid; RNP = ribonucleoprotein; SARDs = systemic autoimmune rheumatic diseases; SLE = systemic lupus erythematosus; ssDNA = single-stranded DNA.

Adapted from Ceribelli A, Tonutti A, Andrade LEC, Chan EKL. Standardization of fluorescent antinuclear antibody testing. In: Schmitz JL, Detrick B, O'Gorman MRG, eds. Manual of Molecular and Clinical Laboratory Immunology. *9th ed. Washington, DC: ASM Press; 2025:881–890; and ICAP International Consensus on ANA Patterns. https://www.anapatterns.org/. Accessed June 17, 2025.*

of chromatin. There are five major classes of histones: H1, H2A, H2B, H3, and H4. Antibodies to H2A and H2B can be detected in almost all patients with drug-induced lupus. The presence of anti-histone antibody alone or combined with antibody to ssDNA supports the diagnosis of drug-induced lupus. Although other patients with SLE have elevated levels of anti-histone antibodies, the titers are usually fairly low. High levels of anti-histone antibodies tend to be associated with more active and severe SLE. Anti-histone antibodies are also found in other SARDs, but the levels are usually lower. Anti-histone antibodies typically produce a homogeneous pattern in the IIF assay.

Nucleosome antibodies are stimulated by DNA-histone complexes known as *nucleosomes,* or deoxyribonucleoprotein (DNP). These antibodies are directed only against the complexes and not against DNA or the individual histones. Nucleosome antibodies are found in about 85% of patients with SLE, and their levels correlate with disease severity. They typically produce a homogeneous pattern in the IIF assay.

Extractable nuclear antigens (ENAs) are a group of nuclear antigens that were so named because they were isolated in saline extracts of mammalian tissues. They represent a family of small nuclear proteins associated with uridine-rich RNA and include ribonucleoproteins (RNPs), the Sm antigen, the SS-A/Ro and SS-B/La antigens, Scl-70, Jo-1, and PM-1.

Antibody to the **Sm antigen** is specific for lupus because it is not found in other autoimmune diseases. However, it is present in only 20% to 40% of patients with SLE, depending on the race of the population. Antibody to a preparation of this ENA was first described in a patient whose last name was Smith, hence the name *anti-Sm antibody.* The anti-Sm antibody produces a coarse speckled pattern of nuclear fluorescence on IIF.

Anti-RNP antibody is directed against RNP, which consists of several nonhistone proteins complexed to a small nuclear RNA called *U1-snRNP* (*U* for "uridine-rich"). RNP forms complexes with the Sm antigen in the nucleus, and antisera to these antigens produce a pattern of partial identity when they are reacted in the Ouchterlony double-immunodiffusion test (see discussion and Fig. 15–7 in the text that follows). In the IIF assay, anti-nRNP produces a coarse speckled pattern. Antibodies to RNP are detected in about one-fourth of patients with SLE but are also found at a high titer in individuals with MCTD and in lower levels in patients with other SARDs such as systemic sclerosis (SSc), Sjögren syndrome, and RA.

Patients with lupus can also produce antibodies to another family of ENAs called **SS-A/Ro** and **SS-B/La.** These antigens consist of small, uridine-rich RNAs complexed to cellular proteins and were given the prefix of SS- because a large percentage of patients with Sjögren syndrome have antibodies to the antigens. Anti–SS-A/Ro also appears in some patients with SLE and has been closely associated with the presence of nephritis, vasculitis, lymphadenopathy, photosensitivity, and hematologic manifestations such as leukopenia. Antibodies to SS-B/La are found in a small percentage of patients with SLE, all of whom have anti–SS-A/Ro. The SS-B/La antibody is most often found in patients with cutaneous SLE manifestations, especially photosensitivity dermatitis. Antibodies to both SS-A/Ro and SS-B/La can cross the placenta and have been associated with neonatal lupus. Newborns who have anti–SS-A/Ro are more likely to develop cardiac manifestations, whereas those who have anti–SS-B/La are more likely to have other symptoms, such as skin lesions. To detect the presence of these antibodies on IIF, it is necessary to use human tissue culture cells such as HEp-2 (human epithelial) because SS-A/Ro and SS-B/La antigens are not found in mouse or rat liver and kidneys. A finely speckled pattern is evident. Antibodies to the SS-A/Ro antigen are best detected on IIF using a special cell line, HEp-2000, which has been genetically transfected so that the cells hyperexpress the antigen.

The **nucleolus** is a prominent structure within the nucleus where transcription and processing of ribosomal RNA and assembly of the ribosomes take place. Staining of the nucleolus in IIF is mainly caused by antibodies to one of three nucleolar components: fibrillarin, RNA polymerase I, and PM-1. Antibody to fibrillarin is common in **systemic sclerosis** (**SSc** or *scleroderma*) and is indicated by clumpy nucleolar fluorescence in the IIF assay. SSc is an autoimmune disease that primarily involves the skin and blood vessels. Antibodies to RNA polymerase are also associated with SSc but produce a speckled nucleolar pattern in IIF. Homogeneous staining of the nucleolus is associated with antibodies to the PM-1 antigen (also known as *PM/Scl*) and is found in polymyositis and SSc.

Anti-centromere antibodies bind to proteins in the middle region of a chromosome where the sister chromatids are joined. They are directed against three centromere proteins called *CENP-A, CENP-B,* and *CENP-C.* They are found in over half of patients with limited cutaneous systemic sclerosis, or the **CREST syndrome,** a subset of scleroderma named after its five major features: *calcinosis* (deposition of calcium salts in the skin and subcutaneous tissues), *Raynaud phenomenon* (cold and numbness in the extremities due to decreased blood flow), *esophageal dysmotility* (problems swallowing due to dysfunctional movement of the smooth muscle in the esophagus), *sclerodactyly* (skin thickening and tightness), and *telangiectasia* (small red or purple clusters near the skin's surface due to capillary dilation). In the IIF assay, centromere antibodies produce discrete speckled staining in the nuclei of the cells.

Methods of ANA Detection

The various methods developed to detect ANAs in patient serum include IIF, enzyme-linked immunosorbent assay (ELISA), multiplex bead immunoassays, and immunodiffusion. We discuss these assays in the text that follows.

Indirect Immunofluorescence (IIF)

Fluorescent anti-nuclear antibody (FANA) testing is the most widely used and accepted test because it is highly sensitive, detects a wide range of antibodies, and is inexpensive and easy to perform. Also, the antigens are in their original form and location within the cells used in the test. IIF has three main applications: It has been used:

- As an initial test to determine the presence or absence of ANAs in patients who have symptoms of SARDs, aiding in their diagnosis
- To provide guidance in the selection of follow-up tests based on the immunofluorescence patterns obtained
- To determine an ANA titer because moderate to high titers have been better correlated with disease, whereas low titers are seen more often in the general population

The IIF test uses a commercially prepared microscope slide onto which nucleated cells have been fixed. The cell line, HEp-2 (derived from human larynx epidermal carcinoma), is the standard substrate for clinical laboratories worldwide. HEp-2 cells are used because they have large nuclei with high antigen expression, allowing for high sensitivity and facilitating visualization of results. HEp-2 cells at various stages of the cell cycle are used so that patterns in nondividing and dividing cells can be seen. Two variations of this cell line have also been developed: HEp-2000, an HEp-2 cell line genetically modified to increase expression of the SSA/Ro antigen, and HEp-20-10, which has an increased proportion of mitotic cells.

In the IIF method, patient serum is incubated with a microscope slide coated with HEp-2 cells, washed to remove unbound antibodies, and then allowed to react with an anti-human immunoglobulin (Ig) labeled with a fluorescent tag to detect bound IgG or total immunoglobulins from patient serum. Following a second incubation and wash, the slide is mounted and viewed under a fluorescent microscope using 400x magnification (40x objective and 10x eyepiece). Using a microscope with an LED light source can help to enhance the images. The principle of this assay is shown in **Figure 15–4**.

Most laboratories screen patient samples at a 1:80 or a 1:160 dilution, because the test has a high level of sensitivity. However, the 1:80 dilution has a low specificity for SARDs, because positive titers may be seen in some healthy persons or those with other medical conditions (e.g., hypertension, diabetes mellitus, gout, cancer). The screening dilution should be established by the testing laboratory with consideration for the population being tested. High ANA titers are generally considered to have a greater likelihood of clinical significance. Patient samples that are positive on the ANA screen are then serially diluted and retested to determine the antibody titer, specified as the highest dilution to show nuclear fluorescence. Inclusion of a 1+ endpoint control serum can help to standardize the readings by setting the minimum level of fluorescence that is considered positive.

In addition to the antibody titer, the pattern of fluorescence is also reported because it can provide clues about the autoantibody present and associated diseases. To standardize the interpretation of fluorescent patterns, an International Consensus on ANA Patterns (ICAP) was established by a committee of the International Union of Immunological Societies (IUIS) in 2014 in conjunction with the Centers for Disease Control and Prevention (CDC). ICAP conferences are held periodically, and updates on the international ANA classification system are

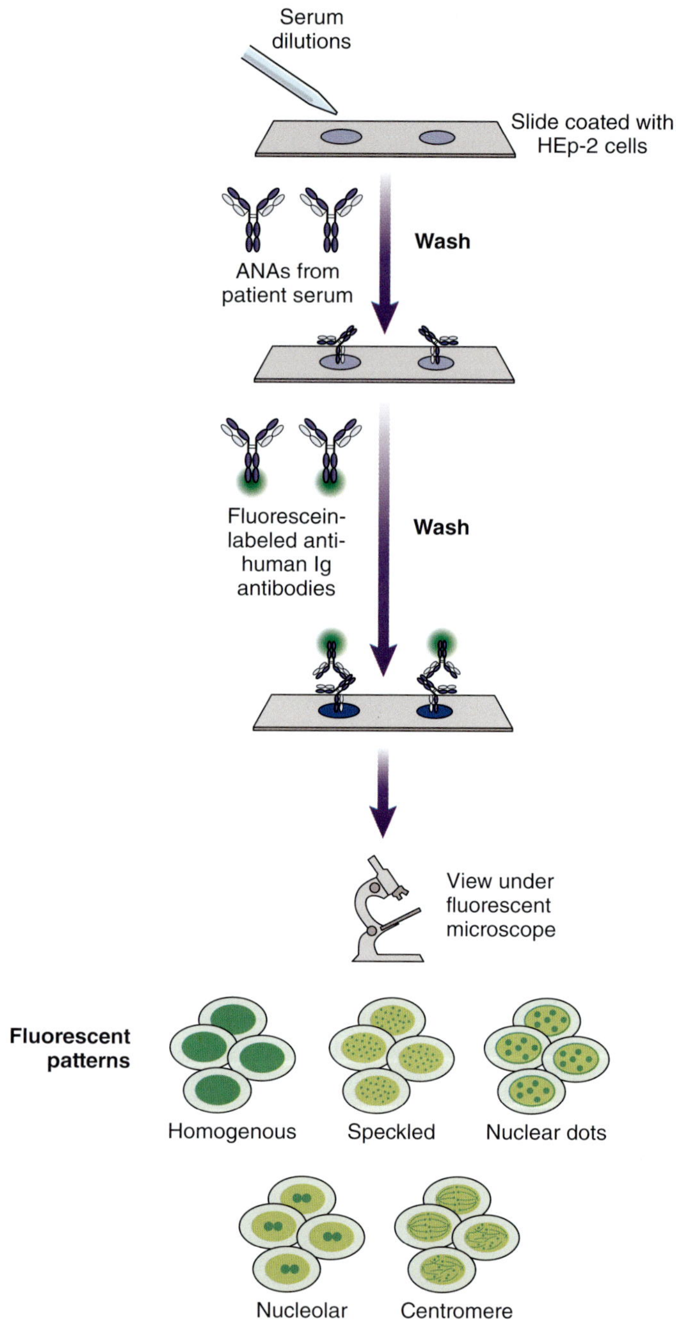

FIGURE 15–4 Fluorescent ANA test principle. Patient serum (containing anti-nuclear antibodies) is diluted and incubated on a microscope slide coated with HEp-2 cells. After washing, fluorescein-labeled anti-human Ig is added to detect bound autoantibodies. After a final wash, the slide is read under a fluorescent microscope. Five major patterns in nondividing cells are shown.

published on the website https://www.anapatterns.org/index.php. The system includes fluorescence patterns that may be detected not only within the nucleus but also in the cytoplasm or mitotic structures of the cell. Currently, 15 nuclear patterns, 9 cytoplasmic patterns, and 5 mitotic patterns have been identified and agreed on. The nuclear patterns have been classified into seven major groups and are further categorized into subgroups. Each pattern is assigned an AC (anti-cell) code ranging from AC-0 (negative) to AC-29, similar to the CD (cluster of differentiation) nomenclature used to identify WBC antigens. As new patterns are discovered, they are evaluated by the ICAP committee for inclusion in the classification system. Common nuclear groups are described in the list that follows and are depicted in **Figure 15–5.**

- **Homogeneous** (formerly called *diffuse*): This pattern is characterized by uniform staining of the entire nucleus in interphase (nondividing) cells and of the condensed chromosomal region in mitotic cells (dividing cells in metaphase, anaphase, and telophase). It is associated with antibodies to dsDNA, histones, and nucleosomes. The homogeneous pattern is found in patients with SLE, drug-induced lupus, chronic autoimmune hepatitis (AIH), and juvenile idiopathic arthritis.
- **Speckled:** The speckled group of patterns is characterized by discrete, fluorescent specks throughout the nuclei of interphase cells. It is divided into two subgroups depending on whether the specks are tiny/fine, or large/coarse. Staining is variable in the nucleolus and absent in the chromatin region of dividing cells. These patterns are associated with antibodies to ENAs and can be found in patients with SLE, Sjögren syndrome, SSc, and other SARDs.
- **Centromere:** Numerous discrete speckles are seen in the nuclei of interphase cells and the chromatin of dividing cells. Most cells have 46 speckles, representing the number of chromosomes. This pattern is caused by antibodies to proteins in the centromeres of the chromosomes and is found mainly in patients with the CREST syndrome subgroup, limited cutaneous SSc (see later discussion on "Other Systemic Autoimmune Rheumatic Diseases [SARDs]").
- **Nucleolar:** Prominent staining of the nucleoli within the nuclei of interphase cells is seen in this pattern. The size, shape, and number of the nucleoli per cell are variable, and staining can be smooth, clumpy, or speckled, depending on the type of antibody present. Staining may or may not be present in the dividing cells. The nucleolar patterns are primarily caused by antibodies to RNA and RNP and are seen mainly in patients with SSc but can also be present in patients with other SARDs.
- **Discrete Nuclear Dots:** This group is characterized by the presence of a few (1 to 6) or multiple (6 to 20) discrete nuclear dots per cell, depending on the subgroup. The multiple nuclear dot subgroup can be attributed to the presence of antibodies to the Sp-100, PML (promyelocytic leukemia) proteins, and MJ/NXP-2 antigens. This pattern has been associated with a broad spectrum of autoimmune diseases, including primary biliary cholangitis and dermatomyositis. The few nuclear dot subgroup pattern has not been strongly associated with any disease.
- **Dense Fine Speckled:** This pattern is associated with antibodies to the DFS70/LEDGF (lens epidermal-derived growth factor) antigen and is correlated with absence of a SARD on confirmatory testing.

Mixed patterns can also be observed; in some cases, one pattern may totally or partially obscure another (e.g., a homogeneous pattern might mask a speckled pattern). In these cases, titration of the patient serum can help to distinguish between the separate patterns, and an antibody titer would be reported for each one. If no clearly discernable fluorescent pattern is observed in the nuclei of the cells, the FANA test is considered negative. Up to 5% of patients with SLE test negative, so this test cannot be used to absolutely rule out SLE.

Although FANA has been considered the gold standard for ANA screening, it has some important limitations. The manual test is time consuming and requires significant expertise to correctly identify the fluorescent patterns. Discrepancy in results can be caused by subjective interpretation of the patterns; variations in the buffers, conjugate, and mounting medium supplied by different manufacturers of IIF assays; and the use of different fluorescent microscopes. Importantly, ANAs cannot be precisely identified only by the fluorescent patterns from the HEp-2 IIF test, so supplemental tests are needed to determine antibody specificity (see sections that follow).

Automated IIF ANA assays that provide computerized image acquisition (called *computer-aided diagnosis [CAD]*) help reduce subjectivity in result interpretation. Clinical laboratories are increasingly using these systems, and studies comparing them to the manual method show good overall agreement in discriminating between positive and negative results. CAD also provides a quantitative measure of fluorescence intensity, which can be used to estimate antibody titers. Although CAD systems can interpret a predefined set of patterns, they may have difficulty correctly interpreting samples with low titers and identifying rare nuclear patterns, cytoplasmic patterns, and mixed patterns. Thus, an experienced laboratorian must carefully interpret the results.

Solid-Phase Immunoassays

Clinical laboratories commonly use solid-phase assays (SPAs) for ANA detection, with ELISA and multiplex bead immunoassay formats. In these SPAs, the potential autoantigens are attached to polystyrene microtiter plate wells or synthetic beads. The antigens in commercial ANA kits are derived from tissue extracts or are produced by recombinant technology. Patient serum is incubated with the solid phase; then, following a wash step, bound autoantibodies are detected with anti-human Ig reagents to which an enzyme or fluorochrome has been attached (see Chapter 11).

ANA SPAs have two main uses in immunology testing. The first use is screening for the presence of ANAs as an alternative to the HEp-2 IIF method. Clinical laboratories have been increasingly using automated ELISAs for ANA screening because they fit well into the workflow and yield objective results. Screening assays use a mixture of antigens coated onto the solid phase to test for a broad range of ANAs. Because of the antigen preparations used, the sensitivity of ELISAs is generally less than the IIF, and false-negative results may occur. Differences can also be seen with kits from different manufacturers. For these reasons, clinical laboratories should specify the method they used when reporting results. Despite these

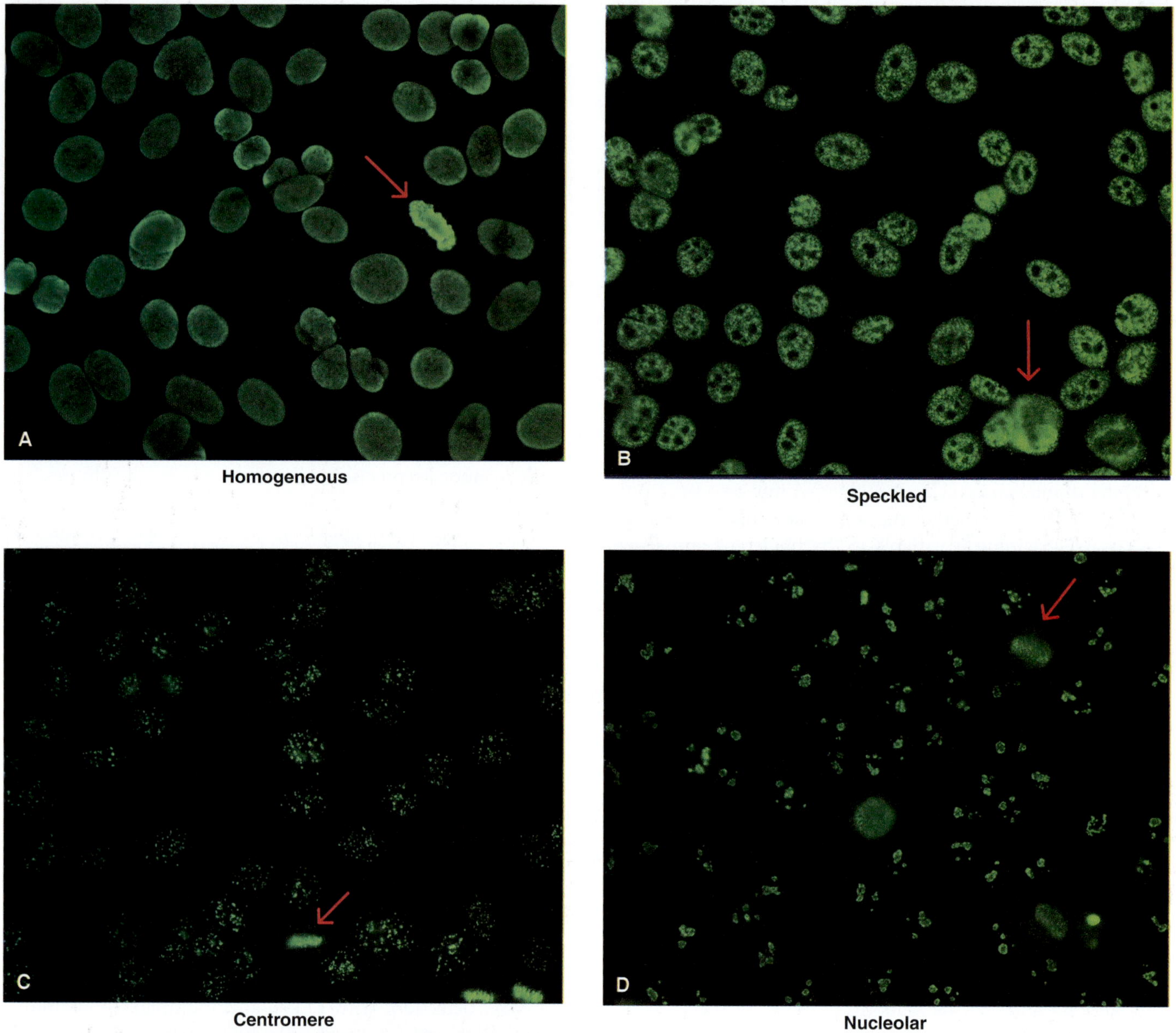

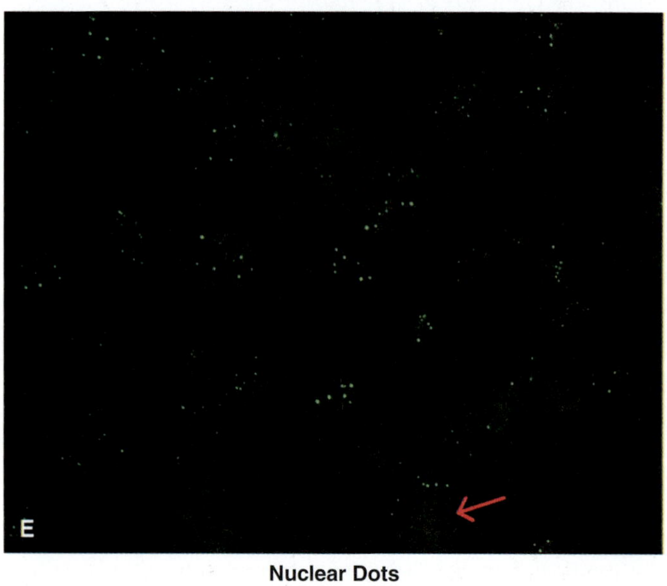

FIGURE 15–5 Photomicrographs of five common patterns of immunofluorescent staining for anti-nuclear antibodies: (A) homogeneous, (B) speckled, (C) centromere, (D) nucleolar, (E) nuclear dots. Arrows point to dividing cells. *(Courtesy of Upstate University Hospital Immunology/Core Laboratory, Syracuse, NY).*

limitations, studies have shown that ELISAs have a higher specificity than the HEp-2 IIF, and when both types of assays are used, the likelihood of obtaining clinically relevant results is increased.

The second use of SPAs is for confirmation of a positive ANA screen and further characterization of the ANA specificity. In these multiplex ELISAs or bead immunoassays, each microtiter well or bead is coated with a single antigen (e.g., dsDNA, Sm, RNP, SS-A/Ro, SS-B/La, Jo-1, Scl-70, PM/Scl, CENP-B, chromatin). Confirmatory testing may include a panel of these antigens or selected antigens based on the fluorescent pattern if HEp-2 IIF is used for screening.

Knowledge Check 15-4

Antibodies to extractable nuclear antigens (ENAs) such as Sm and RNP are associated with which pattern of fluorescence in the ANA IIF assay?

a. Homogeneous
b. Speckled
c. Centromere
d. Nucleolar

Immunofluorescence Using *Crithidia luciliae*

This assay is used to detect antibodies to dsDNA in patients who have symptoms suggestive of SLE and a positive ANA screen. This sensitive assay for dsDNA is an IIF test using a hemoflagellate organism called *Crithidia luciliae* as the substrate. The trypanosome has a circular organelle called a *kinetoplast* that is composed mainly of dsDNA **(Fig. 15–6).** In this test, patient serum is incubated on a microscope slide coated with *C. luciliae* organisms, and binding is detected with a fluorescent-labeled anti-Ig conjugate. Washing of the slide is performed after each step to remove unbound antibody. A positive test is indicated by a brightly stained kinetoplast. Dilutions of the patient serum can be used to determine antibody titer.

Ouchterlony Test

Immunodiffusion can detect some ANAs, particularly those associated with a speckled pattern in the HEp-2 IIF test. Ouchterlony double diffusion detects antibody to several of the small nuclear proteins, or ENAs, including Sm, RNP, SS-A/Ro, SS-B/La, Scl-70 (DNA topoisomerase I), and Jo-1 (see the previous descriptions and Table 15–2). In this method, a solution containing ENA antigens is placed in a central well of an agarose plate, and patient samples and controls are placed in the surrounding wells, as shown in **Figure 15–7.** A visible precipitate is formed between the ENA well and each surrounding well that contains antibodies to any of the ENAs present (e.g., anti-Sm, anti-RNP, or antibodies to other ENAs). If an outer well does not contain antibodies to any of the ENAs, no precipitate is formed between that well and the center well. Samples in the outer wells are identified as containing antibody to a particular ENA by comparing their reactivity patterns of identity, nonidentity, or partial identity to control sera containing specific ENA antibodies. A positive reaction is indicated by immunoprecipitation lines of serological identity. (Refer to Chapter 10 for a discussion of Ouchterlony test principles.) Although this type of testing is highly specific, it is not as sensitive and has a longer turnaround time to results (48 to 72 hours) as compared with the other techniques described.

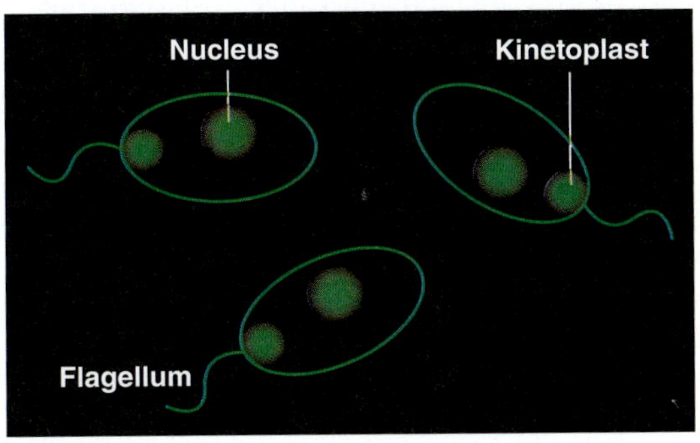

FIGURE 15–6 An illustration of *Crithidia luciliae* fixed to a microscope slide. A positive test for dsDNA will show green fluorescence in the nucleus and kinetoplast.

Anti-Phospholipid Antibodies

Anti-phospholipid antibodies are a heterogeneous group of antibodies that bind to phospholipids alone or phospholipids

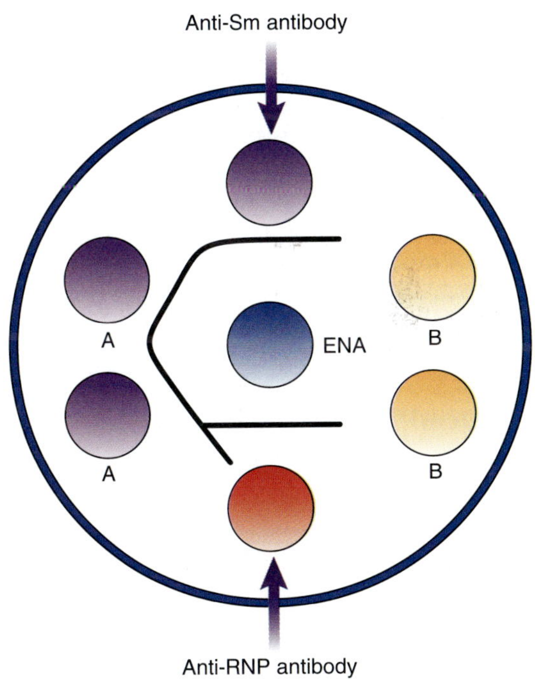

FIGURE 15–7 Extractable nuclear antibody immunodiffusion pattern. A mixture of ENAs, including RNP, Sm, and other soluble nuclear antigens, is placed in a central well in an agarose gel. Sm antibody and RNP antibody are run as positive controls, and patient samples A and B are placed between the controls. The pattern of precipitin lines formed indicates the antibodies present in patient serum. The arc of serological identity between the Sm control and serum from patient A indicates that serum A contains anti-Sm antibodies. The arc of partial identity formed between serum A and the RNP well occurs because RNP is always found complexed to Sm antigen. Thus, RNP antibodies are not present in serum A. Serum B contains neither Sm nor RNP antibody.

complexed with protein. They can affect every body organ, but they are especially associated with deep-vein and arterial thrombosis and with recurrent pregnancy loss. They are produced by patients with primary anti-phospholipid syndrome, and can be secondary to other autoimmune diseases (e.g., they have been found in up to 60% of patients with lupus). They can be identified by their ability to cause false-positive results in nontreponemal tests for syphilis (see Chapter 21), lupus anticoagulant tests, and immunoassays for antibodies to cardiolipin or other phospholipids.

The lupus anticoagulant (LA), one of several types of anti-phospholipid antibodies, was so named because it produces a prolonged activated partial thromboplastin time (APTT) and prothrombin time (PT). In patients with anti-phospholipid antibodies, the APTT may be prolonged, but it is not corrected by mixing with normal plasma. Ironically, patients with this antibody have an increased risk of clotting and spontaneous abortion. Platelet function may also be affected, and thrombocytopenia may be present.

The most commonly used screening test for the LA is the dilute Russell's viper venom time (dRVVT) assay, in which patient plasma is incubated with a snake venom, calcium, and other reagents to activate the common coagulation pathway, followed by measurement of the time to clot formation. Additionally, an APTT and a solid phase immunoassay to detect anti-phospholipid antibodies should be performed. If these antibodies are suspected, coagulation factor assays may also need to be performed to rule out any factor deficiencies or factor-specific inhibitors.

Critical Thinking 15-1

A patient with a slight fever, joint pain, and skin rash was tested for ANAs by an indirect immunofluorescence assay using HEp-2 cells. A bright homogeneous pattern was observed. What follow-up testing would you recommend?

Rheumatoid Arthritis (RA)

RA is another example of a systemic autoimmune disorder. It affects about 0.5% to 1% of the adult population worldwide, but prevalence varies with ethnicity and geographic location. Typically, it strikes people between the ages of 25 and 55. Females are three times as likely to be affected as males, and disease prevalence is highest in females who are over age 65. RA is mainly a chronic, symmetric, and erosive arthritis of the peripheral joints, but it can also affect multiple organs such as the heart and the lungs. Disease progress varies because there may be spontaneous remissions or an increasingly active disease in some people that rapidly progresses to joint deformity and disability. Over the last three decades, patients with RA have experienced less disability and a better quality of life because of advances in therapy and earlier treatment (see the "Treatment" section).

Etiology

Associations of RA with more than 100 genetic regions have been discovered. The strongest associations have been between certain HLA-DRB1 alleles (e.g., *0401), which may bind modified peptides more strongly, or *PTPN22* gene polymorphisms that affect T- and B-cell regulation. Epigenetic factors, such as altered DNA methylation affecting the transcription of critical genes, are also believed to play a role in the pathogenesis and severity of RA. The strongest environmental risk factor is believed to be cigarette smoking, which doubles the risk of developing the disease. Other factors have also been implicated, but their associations are weaker. Several infectious agents have been proposed as possible triggering antigens for RA, but a cause-effect relationship has not been proven.

Immunopathology

The pathology of RA is caused by an inflammatory process that results in the destruction of bone and cartilage. The joints in RA show an increase in cells lining the synovial membrane and formation of a *pannus,* a thick membrane of inflammatory granulation tissue that grows into the joint space and invades the cartilage and bone. Infiltration of the inflamed synovium with T and B lymphocytes, plasma cells, dendritic cells, mast cells, and granulocytes is evidence of immunologic activity within the joint.

Activated self-reactive T cells are thought to play an important role in the pathogenesis of RA by stimulating production of pro-inflammatory cytokines by macrophages and fibroblasts in the synovium, including interleukin (IL)-1, IL-6, IL-17, and tumor necrosis factor alpha (TNF-α) (see Chapter 6). TNF-α plays a key role in the inflammatory process by stimulating the production of other cytokines and facilitating migration of WBCs into the joint tissues. The pro-inflammatory cytokines also trigger fibroblasts and macrophages to release matrix metalloproteinases, enzymes that degrade important structural proteins in the cartilage.

Local bone erosion is another characteristic feature of RA. Multinucleated giant cells called *osteoclasts* are central to the structural damage seen in the bones. Osteoclasts absorb bone as part of the normal bone-remodeling process that occurs in the body in response to growth and repair of damaged bone. Normally, a good balance exists between bone production and destruction. However, in RA, osteoclasts become overly activated in the inflammatory environment of the joints. TNF-α, in conjunction with other cytokines and the molecule *RANKL* (receptor activator of nuclear factor kappa-B ligand), induces the differentiation of osteoclasts and inhibits bone formation. Local bone destruction and generalized osteoporosis throughout the body result.

Autoantibody synthesis is thought to be induced by cytokine overproduction. Two key antibodies found in the disease are *rheumatoid factor* and *anti-CCP.* **Rheumatoid factor (RF)** is an antibody that is most often of the IgM class and is directed against the Fc portion of IgG. Antibodies to cyclic citrullinated proteins **(anti-cyclic citrullinated peptide antibody [anti-CCP or ACPA])** are directed against an atypical amino acid called *citrulline,* which is generated when the enzyme peptidyl arginine deiminase (PAD) modifies the amino acid arginine by replacing an NH_2 group with a neutral oxygen. This enzyme is associated with granulocytes, monocytes, macrophages, and other types of cells. Death of granulocytes and macrophages triggers production of citrullinated proteins, and overexpression of these antigens may provoke an immune response in people with certain HLA-DRB1 alleles. These antibodies can react with citrulline-containing components of the matrix, including filaggrin, keratin, fibrinogen, and vimentin. ANAs are also present in some patients with RA (see the previous "Anti-Nuclear Antibodies" section).

The role of B cells and autoantibodies such as RF and anti-CCP in the pathology of RA is uncertain. The antibodies may combine with their specific antigens, forming immune complexes that deposit in the joints and bind complement. Complement proteins, in turn, can act as chemotactic factors for neutrophils and macrophages, resulting in type III hypersensitivity and amplifying the inflammatory response (see Chapter 14).

Clinical Signs and Symptoms

The initial symptoms of RA involve the joints, tendons, and bursae. Patients commonly experience nonspecific symptoms such as malaise, fatigue, fever, weight loss, and transient joint pain that begins in the small joints of the hands and feet. The joints are typically affected in a symmetric fashion. Joint stiffness and pain are usually present in the morning and improve with movement during the day. The disease can progress to the larger joints, often affecting the knees, hips, elbows, shoulders, and cervical spine. Joint pain can lead to muscle spasms and limit mobility. The ongoing inflammation, if left untreated, results in permanent joint dysfunction and deformity **(Fig. 15–8).** Osteoporosis (bone erosion) occurs in about 20% to 30% of patients with RA because of the inflammatory environment of the joints and activation of osteoclasts.

Many patients also develop clinical manifestations outside of the joints. These patients are most likely to have a history of smoking, have early disease onset, and test positive for anti-CCP or RF. Such manifestations include interstitial lung disease, pericarditis (inflammation of tissue surrounding the heart), and vasculitis. Some patients have small masses of tissue called *nodules* over the bones. Nodules can also be found in the myocardium, pericardium, heart valves, pleura, lungs, spleen, and larynx. About 10% of patients with RA develop secondary *Sjögren syndrome,* an autoimmune disorder characterized by dry eyes and a dry mouth in addition to connective tissue disease (see section on "Other Systemic Autoimmune Rheumatic Diseases [SARDs]"). A small percentage will develop *Felty syndrome,* a combination of chronic, nodular RA combined with neutropenia and splenomegaly. Patients with RA also have an increased risk of developing lymphoma. The most common cause of death in RA is cardiovascular disease, presumably because arteriosclerosis is accelerated by proinflammatory cytokines released during the disease process.

The ACR established diagnostic classification criteria for RA in 1987 to standardize identification of patients with RA for clinical trials. These criteria were revised in 2010 in collaboration with the EULAR to improve the identification of patients in the early stages of disease who could benefit from new treatments. The criteria are based on the number and types of joints involved, duration of symptoms, serology results for RF and anti-CCP, serum level of the acute-phase reactant, CRP, and the ESR. These important laboratory tests are discussed in more detail later.

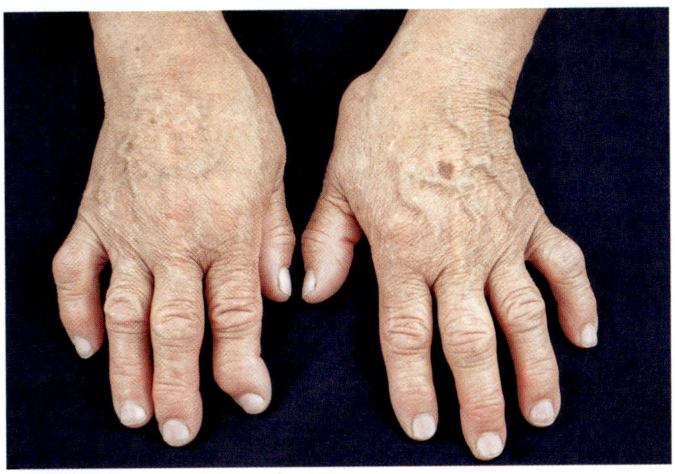

FIGURE 15–8 Hands of a patient with severe rheumatoid arthritis. *(GettyImages/Suze777)*

Treatment

In the past, therapy for RA was primarily based on NSAIDs such as salicylates (aspirin) and ibuprofen. Although these agents reduce local swelling and pain, they are no longer the dominant treatment for RA. The discovery that joint destruction occurs early in the disease has prompted more aggressive treatment and the development of new drugs to prevent disease progression. *Disease-modifying anti-rheumatic drugs (DMARDs),* most notably methotrexate, are now prescribed at the time of diagnosis. Methotrexate is thought to act by inhibiting adenosine metabolism and T-cell activation. If methotrexate alone does not work, it can be combined with other conventional DMARDs or with biological DMARDs. Short-term therapy with glucocorticoids such as prednisone can also be used in initial treatment or during acute disease flares.

Biological DMARDs have revolutionized how RA is treated because they target immune system components that are central to the disease pathogenesis. Several key RA therapies block the activity of the cytokine TNF-α. Agents that act against TNF-α are classified in two categories: (1) monoclonal antibodies to TNF-α (e.g., infliximab, adalimumab, certolizumab, golimumab) and (2) TNF-α receptors fused to an IgG molecule (etanercept; **Fig. 15–9**). Both types of agents specifically target and neutralize TNF-α and have demonstrated effectiveness in halting joint damage. Additional biological therapies for RA include monoclonal antibodies against the B-cell antigen CD20, T-cell costimulatory molecules on antigen-presenting cells, and the IL-6 receptor.

DMARDs have become the mainstay of RA treatment because they act on specific components of the inflammatory response and are effective in slowing the progression of joint erosion. These treatments have resulted in higher rates of disease-free periods (remission) and have dramatically improved the quality of life and prognosis of patients with RA. Although these agents are effective in treating RA, patients must be monitored closely because they are at greater risk for infection.

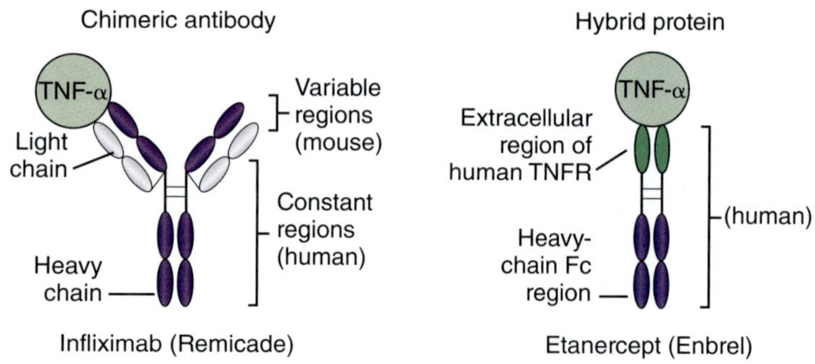

FIGURE 15-9 Biological agents that act against TNF-α. (A) Infliximab is a chimeric monoclonal antibody composed of human constant regions fused to mouse variable regions. The antibody binds to TNF-α, preventing it from interacting with the TNF receptor (TNFR). (B) Etanercept is a hybrid protein consisting of the extracellular (ligand binding) domains of the human TNFR (green), coupled with a human immunoglobulin constant region (blue). Etanercept acts as a decoy, sequestering bound TNF-α so it cannot interact with TNF receptors on target cells. *(Courtesy of Dr. Aaron Glass.)*

Laboratory Diagnosis of Rheumatoid Arthritis

Diagnosis of RA is based on a combination of clinical manifestations, joint imaging, and laboratory testing. RF is routinely tested for when making the initial diagnosis. The importance of testing for RF is also reflected in the fact that it is one of the classification criteria for RA. About 70% to 90% of patients with RA test positive for RF. Thus, a negative result does not rule out the presence of RA. Conversely, a positive test result is not specific for RA because RF is also present in about 5% of healthy people and in 10% to 25% of those over the age of 65. RF can also be found in patients with other SARDs, such as SLE, Sjögren syndrome, scleroderma, and MCTD, as well as in people with some chronic infections.

Manual agglutination tests using charcoal or latex particles coated with IgG were used for many years to detect RF. These tests, however, only detect the IgM isotype, found in about 75% of patients, and have largely been replaced by automated ELISA, CLIA, immunoturbimetric, and nephelometric methods, which have greater precision and sensitivity and can also detect other RF isotypes. Testing for IgG and IgA RFs increases test specificity. The presence of both IgM and IgA, or of all three isotypes, rarely occurs in other disease states, which may help in making a differential diagnosis. Testing for specific RF isotypes may also have prognostic value.

Laboratory testing for antibody to anti-CCP increases specificity for RA and is widely available. These assays are performed mainly by ELISA and use a circular synthetic form of citrullinated peptides to increase test sensitivity. Many RF-negative patients are positive for anti-CCP, and the presence of anti-CCP precedes the onset of RA by several years, making it a better marker for early disease. The presence of anti-CCP is also associated with an increased likelihood of developing clinically significant disease activity with a worse prognosis. Importantly, specificity of anti-CCP for RA is higher than RF, about 95%. Furthermore, the combination of anti-CCP and RF testing has a specificity of 98% to 100%, providing for a more accurate diagnosis of RA by allowing for better differentiation from other forms of arthritis.

Low ANA titers are present in about 40% of patients. The pattern most often identified is the speckled pattern directed against RNP. The significance of this group of autoantibodies remains unclear because they do not appear to be directly related to pathogenesis.

Once a diagnosis of RA is made, the most helpful tests for following the disease course are general indicators of inflammation, such as the ESR, CRP, and complement components. Typically, CRP and ESR are elevated during disease flares, and serum complement components are normal or increased because of increased acute-phase reactivity. CRP levels correlate well with disease activity because levels reflect the intensity of the inflammatory response.

Synovial fluid may also be analyzed to confirm an RA diagnosis and differentiate it from other forms of arthritis. Findings typically show an increase in WBCs (5,000 to 50,000 WBCs/mL), especially neutrophils, and absence of crystals or infection.

Knowledge Check 15-5

Which antibody is highly specific for RA?

a. RF
b. Anti-CENP-B
c. Anti-CCP
d. Anti-Sm

Other Systemic Autoimmune Rheumatic Diseases (SARDs)

Other SARDs include Sjögren syndrome, SSc, MCTD, and the inflammatory myopathies. **Sjögren syndrome** is characterized by chronic inflammation of the exocrine glands, most notably the ocular and salivary glands. This produces dry eyes and a dry mouth, also known as "sicca syndrome." The syndrome can be broadly classified into two groups, primary Sjögren syndrome, which occurs in the absence of other diseases, and secondary Sjögren syndrome, which occurs in patients who also have other diseases, most commonly SLE or RA. Most patients with the primary form of the disease test positive for RF and ANAs, exhibiting a fine speckled pattern of fluorescence associated with anti–SS-A/Ro and/or anti–SS-B/La. The presence of antibodies to SS-A/Ro is one component of the 2016 criteria established by the ACR and EULAR for the classification of primary Sjögren syndrome.

SSc, also known as *scleroderma,* is a rare SARD characterized by excessive fibrosis and vascular abnormalities that affect the skin and joints and progress over time to involve internal organs, most commonly the esophagus, lower gastrointestinal tract, lungs, heart, and kidneys. Symptoms include tightening and hardening of the skin, musculoskeletal pain, Raynaud phenomenon, and heartburn. Complications involving the internal organs often result in functional impairment, leading to death. Cases can be classified into one of two major groups, depending on the extent of skin involvement. In the first group, *diffuse cutaneous systemic sclerosis,* skin involvement extends from the fingers to the trunk; these patients are at risk of more rapid involvement of the internal organs. In the second group, *limited cutaneous systemic sclerosis* (i.e., *CREST syndrome*), skin involvement is restricted to the fingers, distal parts of the arms and legs, and face, and does not affect the trunk; progression to the internal organs is typically slower.

At least 13 different types of ANAs have been identified in patients with SSc. Three of these are included in the ACR/EULAR classification criteria for SSc and are useful in determining the diagnosis, subgroup, and prognosis of patients with the disease. Anti-centromere antibodies are found only in patients with limited cutaneous SSc and correlate with a better survival rate; antibodies to topoisomerase I (also known as Scl-70) are associated with diffuse cutaneous SSc and a poor prognosis; and antibodies to RNA polymerase III are associated with the diffuse form of the disease and rapid thickening of the skin but have a better prognosis than those with anti–Scl-70. Thus, these three ANAs are important biomarkers for SSc.

Mixed connective tissue disease (MCTD) is an overlap syndrome of limited cutaneous SSc combined with clinical features of SLE, polymyositis (inflammation of multiple muscles), and RA. MCTD is typically associated with high titers of autoantibodies to U1-RNP but absence of anti-centromere antibodies and generally has a better prognosis than limited cutaneous SSc.

The **inflammatory myopathies (IMs)** are a group of diseases characterized by chronic inflammation of the skeletal muscles ("myositis") and progressive muscle weakness. The muscles closest to the trunk of the body are generally affected first. Other organs, such as the skin, heart, lungs, gastrointestinal tract, and joints, are also frequently involved, and patients have an increased risk of malignancy. Two examples of IM are **polymyositis (PM)** and **dermatomyositis (DM).** DM differs from PM in that DM can present in children and adults and is characterized by the presence of a skin rash in addition to muscle involvement. Patients with DM and PM and other IMs can produce antibodies to various cellular antigens, some of which are myositis associated and found in other SARDs (e.g., SS-A/Ro, SS-B/La, PM-Scl, snRNPs) and others that are myositis specific, including antibodies to tRNA anti-synthetases, the most common being anti–Jo-1, which produces a fine speckled pattern in the cytoplasm of HEp-2 cells in the FANA test.

Granulomatosis With Polyangiitis (Wegener Granulomatosis)

Granulomatosis with polyangiitis (GPA), formerly known as **Wegener granulomatosis (WG),** is a rare autoimmune disease involving inflammation of the small- to medium-sized blood vessels, or *vasculitis.* The disease usually begins with local inflammation of the upper and lower respiratory tract. General symptoms include fever, malaise, arthralgias, anorexia, and weight loss. Most patients progress to develop a systemic form of the disease that can affect any organ system.

Almost all patients have symptoms that affect the upper respiratory system and lungs. Symptoms of the upper airway include severe or persistent rhinorrhea ("runny nose"), rhinitis, sinusitis, oral or nasal ulcers, and gingivitis. Damage to the nasal mucosa leads to drying of the nasal membranes, which become susceptible to infection and frequent bleeding. Chronic otitis media can cause perforation and scarring of the eardrums, causing hearing loss. Tissue damage can lead to perforation of the nasal septum or collapse of the bridge of the nose. Pulmonary infiltrates are commonly observed upon x-ray of the lungs. Although patients can experience coughing, shortness of breath, chest pain, or hemoptysis (coughing up blood), they may be asymptomatic.

As the disease progresses, other organ systems become involved. Most patients have renal involvement, ranging from mild glomerulonephritis with little functional impairment to severe glomerulonephritis that can rapidly lead to kidney failure. Most patients also experience pain and arthritis of the large joints, which is usually symmetric but not deforming. Patients may have skin lesions and many have eye involvement that can potentially lead to vision loss. Other areas of the body that can be affected include the nervous system, heart, and thyroid gland.

The etiology of GPA is unknown, but multiple genes are thought to be involved. The HLA-DPB1*0401 allele has a strong association with GPA in White patients, whereas the HLA-DRB1*0901 and HLA-DRB* 1501 alleles are associated with increased risk in Asian and African American populations, respectively. Although environmental factors have not been definitively identified, chronic nasal infection with *Staphylococcus aureus* bacteria has been associated with a greater rate of relapse in patients with GPA. *S. aureus* may induce molecular mimicry because it contains peptides that bear similarity to the proteinase 3 (PR3) autoantigen. Exposure to silica or to certain drugs, such as hydralazine and penicillamine, may also be risk factors.

Most patients with GPA have antibodies to neutrophil cytoplasmic antigens; in 80% of these, the antibody is directed against PR3, an enzyme in the azurophilic granules of neutrophils. Antibody to the PR3 antigen is thought to play a role in the pathophysiology of the systemic vasculitis seen in GPA. Events such as chronic infections can result in production of the pro-inflammatory cytokine TNF-α, which stimulates neutrophils and results in migration of the PR3 antigen from the granules to the neutrophil membrane. Binding of PR3 antibodies to the PR3 antigen and Fcγ-receptors on the cell surface results in activation of the neutrophils, which adhere to the endothelial cells lining the blood vessels. There, they release reactive oxygen species and proteolytic enzymes that damage the vascular endothelium. A T_H1 response follows, with release of cytokines that induce macrophage maturation and the formation of granulomatous lesions. Chronic activation of T cells within these lesions is thought to induce differentiation of autoreactive B cells into plasma cells that produce antibodies to PR3, thus perpetuating the response.

Therapy for GPA is directed toward suppression of this inflammatory response. Patients with severe forms of GPA should be treated initially with a combination of high-dose glucocorticoid drugs and the anti-CD20 monoclonal antibody rituximab or cyclophosphamide. Most patients attain remission with resolution of the inflammatory lesions after initial treatment and must then be maintained on a less potent immunosuppressive drug regimen. Immunosuppressive therapy has greatly improved patient outcomes, and 80% of patients survive at least 5 years.

Laboratory Diagnosis

General laboratory findings include a normochromic, normocytic anemia; leukocytosis; eosinophilia; and elevated ESR. There may also be a decreased concentration of albumin in the blood and mild to severe renal insufficiency. Urinalysis typically shows microscopic hematuria (blood in the urine), proteinuria (protein in the urine), and cellular casts.

Key to diagnosis is the presence of a positive anti-neutrophil cytoplasmic antibody (ANCA) test result, specifically antibody to PR3 (see the following section). Other serological findings include an elevated CRP; elevated immunoglobulin levels; and possibly other autoantibodies, such as RF and ANAs.

Anti-Neutrophil Cytoplasmic Antibodies (ANCAs)

Anti-neutrophil cytoplasmic antibodies (ANCAs) are autoantibodies against proteins that are present in the neutrophil granules. These antibodies are strongly associated with three syndromes involving vascular inflammation: GPA (WG), microscopic polyangiitis (MPA), and eosinophilic granulomatosis with polyangiitis (EGPA; formerly known as *Churg-Strauss syndrome*); these syndromes are collectively known as *ANCA-associated vasculitides (AAVs)*. In patients with GPA, ANCAs are mainly directed against the PR3 antigen, whereas in MPA and EGPA, they are usually specific for myeloperoxidase (MPO).

International consensus guidelines for ANCA screening were initially published in 1999 and updated in 2017 and 2020. The most recent guidelines recommend screening for ANCA with an automated immunoassay (ELISA, CLIA, or fluorescent microbead immunoassay) for antibodies to PR3 and MPO. ANCA testing should be performed on patients with clinical features of AAV or certain other disorders (anti-GBM disease; see later, idiopathic interstitial pneumonia and infective endocarditis associated with nephritis). If the test result is negative but small-vessel vasculitis is still suspected, a second immunoassay or an indirect immunofluorescence (IIF) can be performed to increase sensitivity.

IIF was also the method previously recommended for initial ANCA testing in the 1999 international consensus guidelines. In this method, patient serum is incubated with a microscope slide containing ethanol-fixed leukocytes. Ethanol treatment permeabilizes the granule membranes, allowing for migration of the contents out of the granules. After incubation, the slide is washed to remove unbound serum, and an anti-human IgG, fluorescein isothiocyanate (FITC)-labeled conjugate, is added. After a second incubation and wash step, the slide is viewed under a fluorescent microscope for staining of the neutrophils. Lymphocyte staining should not be present; if it is, it should be minimal.

Two patterns of fluorescence can be observed: *cytoplasmic*, or *c-ANCA*, and *perinuclear*, or *p-ANCA*. The c-ANCA pattern is mainly caused by PR3-ANCA and appears as diffuse, granular staining in the cytoplasm of the neutrophils **(Fig. 15–10A).** Staining is most intense in the center of the cell between the nuclear lobes and gradually fades at the outer edges of the cytoplasm. In the p-ANCA pattern, fluorescence surrounds the lobes of the nucleus, blending them together so that individual lobes cannot be distinguished **(Fig. 15–10B).** This is because the p-ANCA pattern is caused by antibodies against positively charged antigens such as MPO that are attracted toward the negatively charged nucleus. **Table 15–3** summarizes the main features of ANCAs.

It is important to distinguish the p-ANCA pattern from ANAs, which can also stain the nuclei of the neutrophils. With ANAs, the nuclear lobes may be more clearly separated, speckled staining may be present, and the nuclei of the lymphocytes will also be stained. If a true p-ANCA pattern is present, ANA testing using HEp-2 cells as the substrate in IIF should be negative. For more definitive differentiation, the test can be repeated using microscope slides with formalin-fixed leukocytes. Formalin is a cross-linking fixative that prevents the migration of antigens out of the granules. Therefore, in the presence of antibodies to MPO or other positively charged proteins, perinuclear staining will be prevented, and intense, granular staining of the cytoplasm that resembles c-ANCA will be seen.

Failure to detect ANCAs does not rule out the presence of AAV, and experts recommend performing biopsies of affected organs in ANCA-negative patients who are suspected of having an AAV. Also, ANCAs are not diagnostic for AAV and can be found in various other disorders, including other types of vasculitis; SARDs such as SLE and RA; autoimmune gastrointestinal and liver diseases; certain infections, including HIV and hepatitis C; cancer; and other diseases. Patients with these conditions often have ANCAs directed toward neutrophil antigens other than PR3 or MPO, which can also be detected by IIF. High ANCA titers correlate better with presence of disease and are useful in monitoring disease activity. Thus, a positive ANCA test must be combined with clinical manifestations and histological findings of biopsy tissue to make an accurate diagnosis. The clinical value of an ANCA test result is increased when the test is only performed on patients with specific clinical indications of AAV to reduce the probability of false-positive results.

Knowledge Check 15-6

The c-ANCA pattern of fluorescence is associated with which disease?

a. Sjögren syndrome
b. Eosinophilic granulomatosis with polyangiitis
c. Microscopic polyangiitis
d. Granulomatosis with polyangiitis (Wegener granulomatosis)

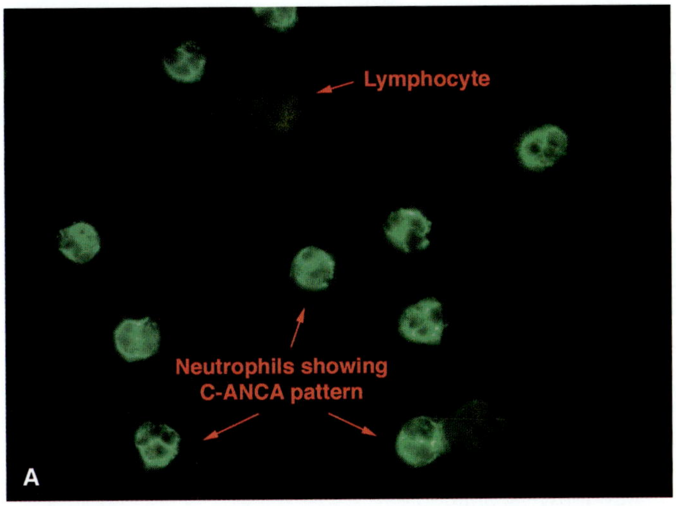

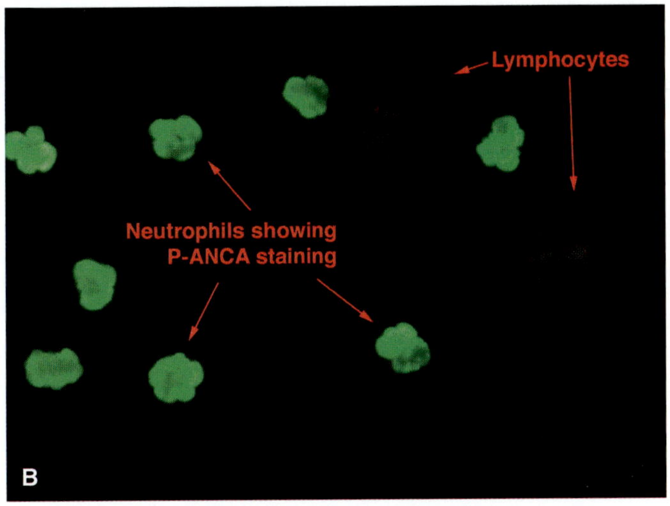

FIGURE 15–10 c-ANCA and p-ANCA fluorescent patterns. (A) c-ANCA (cytoplasmic pattern). Note the granular staining of the primary granules in the cytoplasm of the neutrophils and the more intense fluorescence between the lobes of each nucleus. The lymphocytes have negative staining. This pattern can be seen with either ethanol-fixed or formalin-fixed neutrophils. (B) p-ANCA (fluorescent pattern). This pattern is characterized by smooth or homogeneous staining of the multilobed nuclei in ethanol-fixed neutrophils as shown. (On formalin-fixed neutrophils, these antibodies would produce a granular cytoplasmic staining.) The lymphocytes are not stained. *(Reprinted with permission from Immuno Concepts.)*

Table 15-3 Anti-Neutrophil Cytoplasmic Antibodies (ANCAs)

PATTERN ON INDIRECT IMMUNOFLUORESCENCE WITH ETHANOL-FIXED LEUKOCYTES	APPEARANCE	AUTOANTIGENS	ASSOCIATED DISEASES
c-ANCA	Diffuse, granular staining in the cytoplasm of the neutrophils, fading toward the outer edges of the cells	PR3 antigen	Granulomatosis with polyangiitis (GPA; Wegener granulomatosis)
p-ANCA	Fluorescence surrounding the lobes of the neutrophil nuclei, blending them together	Positively charged antigens, including myeloperoxidase (MPO)	Microscopic polyangiitis (MPA) Eosinophilic granulomatosis with polyangiitis (EGPA; Churg-Strauss syndrome)

c-ANCA = cytoplasmic anti-neutrophil cytoplasmic antibody; p-ANCA = perinuclear anti-neutrophil cytoplasmic antibody.

Organ-Specific Autoimmune Diseases

In organ-specific autoimmune diseases, the immune response is directed against self-antigens that are mainly found in a single organ or gland. Although the clinical manifestations are largely related to the target area, systemic effects may sometimes also occur. Examples of organ-specific autoimmune diseases are listed in **Table 15–4**; we discuss several of these in more detail.

Autoimmune Thyroid Diseases (AITDs)

Autoimmune thyroid diseases (AITDs) include several different clinical conditions, most notably, Hashimoto thyroiditis and Graves disease. Although these conditions have different symptoms, both interfere with thyroid function, and they share some of the same antibodies. The thyroid gland is a bilobed, butterfly-shaped organ in the anterior region of the neck and is normally between 12 and 20 g in size. It is essential in regulating the body's metabolism, and controlling heart, muscle, and digestive functions; it also controls neurological development and helps maintain bone structure.

The thyroid gland is made up of spherical units called *follicles,* which consist of thyroid epithelial cells surrounding a protein-containing fluid (colloid). The primary constituent of the colloid is **thyroglobulin (Tg),** a large iodinated glycoprotein from which the active thyroid hormone *triiodothyronine*

Table 15-4 Organ-Specific Autoimmune Diseases

DISEASE	TARGET CELLS OR TISSUES	ASSOCIATED AUTOANTIBODIES
Addison disease	Adrenal glands	Antibody to adrenal cortical cells; antibody to 21-hydroxylase
Autoimmune hemolytic anemia	RBCs	Antibodies to RBCs
Autoimmune hepatitis (AIH)	Liver	AIH-1—smooth muscle antibodies; ANAs AIH-2—anti–liver-kidney microsomal antibody (anti-LKM-1); anti-liver cytosol type 1 antibody (anti-LC-1)
Autoimmune thrombocytopenic purpura	Platelets	Anti-platelet antibodies
Celiac disease	Small intestine and other organs	Anti-transglutaminase (tTG) Antibodies to deamidated gliadin peptides (DGPs) Endomysial antibodies
Anti–glomerular basement membrane disease (Goodpasture syndrome)	Kidneys, lungs	Antibody to type IV collagen in the renal and pulmonary basement membranes
Graves disease	Thyroid gland	Thyroid-stimulating hormone receptor antibodies (TRAbs) Anti-thyroglobulin Anti-thyroid peroxidase (TPO)
Hashimoto thyroiditis	Thyroid gland	Anti-thyroglobulin Anti-thyroid peroxidase (TPO)
Multiple sclerosis	Myelin sheath of nerves	Antibodies to myelin basic protein
Myasthenia gravis	Nerve-muscle synapses	Antibodies to acetylcholine receptors (AChR) Anti–muscle-specific kinase (MuSK) Antibody to the lipoprotein LRP4
Pernicious anemia	Stomach	Parietal cell antibody, intrinsic factor antibody
Poststreptococcal glomerulonephritis	Kidneys	Streptococcal antibodies that cross-react with kidney tissue
Primary biliary cholangitis	Intrahepatic bile ducts	Anti-mitochondrial antibodies (AMA)
Rheumatic fever	Heart	Streptococcal antibodies that cross-react with cardiac tissue
Type 1 diabetes mellitus	Pancreas	Anti-insulin Islet cell antibodies Anti–IA-2 and anti–IA-2βA Antibody to glutamic acid phosphatase (GAD) Anti-zinc transporter 8 (ZnT8)

(T3) and its precursor, *thyroxine (T4)*, are synthesized. The enzyme **thyroid peroxidase (TPO)** plays an important role in the synthesis of T3 and T4 by oxidizing iodine ions, which are then incorporated into the tyrosine residues of thyroglobulin, leading to production of the hormones.

Under normal conditions, T3 and T4 synthesis is tightly regulated by an endocrine feedback loop called the *hypothalamic-pituitary-thyroid axis* **(Fig. 15–11).** In this pathway, **thyrotropin-releasing hormone (TRH)** is secreted by the hypothalamus in the brain and stimulates the pituitary gland to release **thyroid-stimulating hormone** (**TSH;** also known as *thyrotropin*). TSH, in turn, binds to receptors on the cells of the thyroid gland, causing thyroglobulin to be broken down into T3 and T4, which are released into the blood; the released T4 can be converted into more T3 by the liver and kidneys.

If the concentrations of T3 and T4 in the blood are too low, TRH and TSH secretion increases, stimulating hormone production by the thyroid gland. In contrast, if the levels of T3 and T4 become too high, they feed back to the hypothalamus and pituitary to inhibit release of TRH and TSH, resulting in decreased production of the thyroid hormones. The presence of autoantibodies to components of the thyroid gland interferes with this process and causes under- or overactivity of the gland.

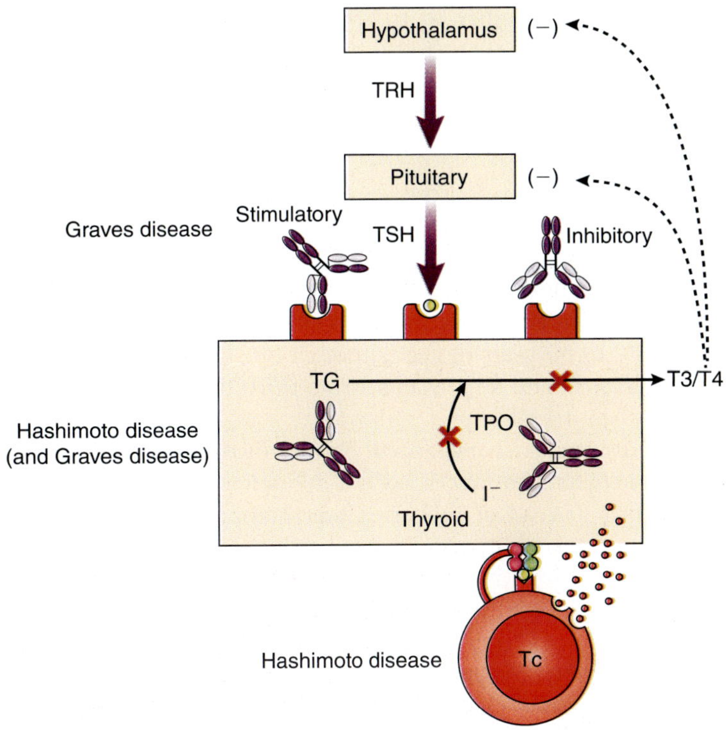

FIGURE 15–11 Autoimmune disorders in thyroid hormone synthesis and regulation. The actions of autoantibodies and cytotoxic T cells in the pathogenesis of Graves disease and Hashimoto disease are shown. Solid arrows = stimulation; dotted arrows = feedback inhibition.

Etiology

The genetic basis of AITDs is not completely understood but is thought to involve multiple genes related to immune regulation (e.g., HLA, *CTLA*-4, the costimulatory molecule CD40) or thyroid-specific antigens. For example, in White people, certain HLA-DR3 genes have been strongly associated with Graves disease, while polymorphisms in DR3, DR4, DR5, and DQ7 have been weakly associated with Hashimoto thyroiditis; however, these gene associations vary among different racial and ethnic populations. A unique feature of both Graves and Hashimoto disease is that HLA-DR antigens are expressed on the surface of thyroid epithelial cells, perhaps increasing the autoimmune response. Mutations in the thyroglobulin gene may allow for interaction of the protein with HLA-DR antigens, resulting in anti-thyroglobulin antibodies. These can be found in both Graves and Hashimoto disease. Also, in Graves disease, modifications in the TSH receptor gene may allow the immune system to recognize the receptor and produce antibodies against it.

Possible environmental triggers of AITDs include infections, certain medications, smoking, psychological stress, and pregnancy, but the strongest link is thought to be between high iodine intake and development of Hashimoto disease. Highly iodinated thyroglobulin is thought to be more immunogenic, possibly creating or exposing more epitopes and facilitating the antigen uptake and processing step of the adaptive immune response (see Chapter 5).

Clinical Signs and Immunopathology of Hashimoto Thyroiditis

Hashimoto thyroiditis, also known as *chronic lymphocytic thyroiditis,* was discovered in Japan in 1912 by Dr. Hakaru Hashimoto. It is a common autoimmune disease, affecting up to 4 out of every 1,000 individuals. Females are about four times more likely to develop the disease than males, and the disease prevalence increases with age. Patients develop an enlarged thyroid called a *goiter,* which is irregular and rubbery. Patients also produce thyroid-specific autoantibodies and cytotoxic T cells. Immune destruction of the thyroid gland occurs, resulting in a state of decreased thyroid function called *hypothyroidism*. Symptoms of hypothyroidism include dry skin, decreased sweating, puffy face with swollen eyelids, coarse skin with a yellow tinge, constipation, weight gain, fatigue, voice hoarseness, and brittle hair.

Several forms of Hashimoto disease have been described, each with distinct pathological features. In the classic form of the disease, the thyroid shows hyperplasia (increased number of cells), increased lymphocytes, activated T and B cells (with T cells predominating), macrophages, and plasma cells. Pathology to the thyroid gland is mediated mainly by $CD8^+$ cytotoxic T cells, which bind to the thyroid cells and destroy them by releasing enzymes that cause apoptosis or necrosis. Production of the cytokines TNF-α, IL-1, and interferon gamma (IFN-γ) is thought to promote inflammation and contribute to destruction of the thyroid cells. The immune response also results in the development of germinal centers that almost completely replace the normal glandular architecture of the thyroid and progressively destroy the gland. Many patients produce antibodies to Tg and TPO; these antibodies can bind complement, and this may result in an inflammatory response that perpetuates the tissue damage. A smaller percentage of patients produce antibodies against the TSH receptor that prevent binding of TSH. Injury to the thyroid gland and inhibition of its function result in the symptoms associated with hypothyroidism.

Clinical Signs and Immunopathology of Graves Disease

Graves disease, in contrast to Hashimoto thyroiditis, is characterized by *hyperthyroidism,* a state of excess thyroid function. Graves disease is one of the most frequently occurring autoimmune diseases and the most common cause of hyperthyroidism. The disease is typically diagnosed in people 20 to 50 years of age (although it can also occur in older persons), and its prevalence is 6 to 10 times higher in females than in males.

The disease is characterized by **thyrotoxicosis,** or an excess of thyroid hormones, with a diffusely enlarged goiter that is firm instead of rubbery. Clinical symptoms include nervousness, irritability, insomnia, weight loss, warm moist skin, sweating, rapid heartbeat, palpitations, breathlessness, fatigue, cardiac dysrhythmias, and menstrual abnormalities. Another sign, present in about one-third of patients, is *exophthalmos,* in which hypertrophy of the eye muscles (increased size) and increased connective tissue in the orbit cause the eyeball to bulge out so that the patient has a large-eyed, staring expression **(Fig. 15–12).** There is evidence that orbital fibroblasts express TSH receptor-like proteins that are affected by thyroid-stimulating immunoglobulin just as the thyroid is (see discussion that follows).

The thyroid shows uniform hyperplasia with a patchy lymphocytic infiltration. The follicles have little colloid but are filled with hyperplastic epithelium. Many of these cells express HLA-DR antigens on their surface in response to IFN-γ produced by infiltrating T cells. This allows presentation of self-antigens, such as the thyrotropin receptor, to activated T cells. B cells, in turn, are stimulated to produce antibodies.

The main antibodies involved in the pathogenesis of Graves disease are the **thyroid-stimulating hormone receptor antibodies (TRAbs).** There are three types of TRAbs. The type responsible for the hyperthyroidism seen in Graves disease is called **thyroid-stimulating immunoglobulin (TSI).** When TSIs bind to the TSH receptor, they mimic the action of TSH, resulting in uncontrolled receptor stimulation with excess release of thyroid hormones (see Fig. 15–11). Another type of TRAb, the *thyroid-blocking antibody (TBAb),* causes decreased thyroid function by preventing TSH from binding to its receptor. A third type of TRAb, designated as neutral, may induce apoptosis of thyroid cells. Patients with Graves disease may also produce anti-Tg and anti-TPO. Depending on the relative activities of stimulating and blocking autoantibodies, patient symptoms may vary from hyperthyroidism to euthyroidism (the state of normal thyroid function) to hypothyroidism, complicating patient diagnosis.

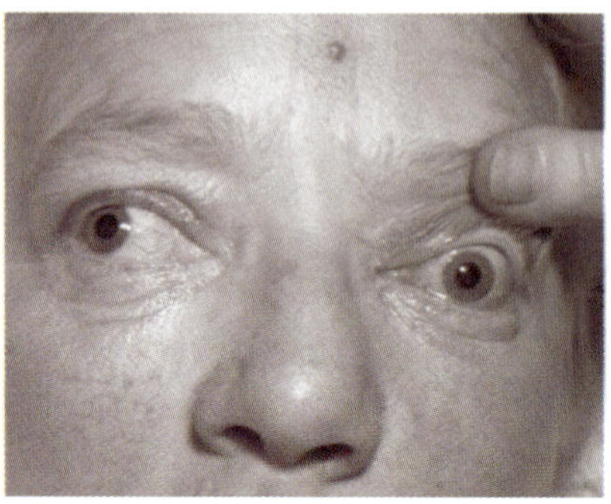

FIGURE 15–12 Exophthalmos indicative of Graves disease. *(Courtesy of CDC/Dr. Sellers/Emory University.)*

Treatment of Autoimmune Thyroid Diseases

Treatment for Hashimoto disease consists of daily oral thyroid hormone replacement therapy, with levothyroxine (T4) being the preferred drug. TSH levels should be monitored throughout treatment and are used to adjust the drug dose so that normal TSH levels are maintained.

Three types of treatment can be used for Graves disease: (1) radioactive iodine, which emits beta particles that cause local destruction of the thyroid cells; this is the preferred treatment in the United States; (2) anti-thyroid medications that inhibit the function of TPO and reduce production of thyroid antibodies; and (3) surgery to remove part of the thyroid (recommended for patients with a very large goiter, more severe disease, or resistance to other treatments). The choice of treatment(s) is individualized. Long-term remission is achieved in many people. Some patients, however, develop hypothyroidism; therefore, continued monitoring is essential.

Laboratory Diagnosis of Autoimmune Thyroid Diseases

Initial screening for AITDs involves measurement of circulating TSH levels. Recall that because of the hypothalamic-pituitary-thyroid axis, the TSH level is inversely related to the levels of T3 and T4. TSH is routinely measured with highly sensitive chemiluminescent immunoassays (CLIA) that can detect down to 0.01 mU/L. A normal TSH level indicates normal thyroid function, with rare exceptions. If the TSH level is abnormally high or low, laboratory tests for circulating thyroid hormone levels must be performed. Although immunoassays for total serum T3 and T4 are available, these hormones are mostly bound to carrier proteins (thyroid binding globulin, prealbumin, albumin), and alterations in these proteins can affect test results. Therefore, it is more useful to measure unbound thyroid hormone, usually free T4 (FT4). **Table 15–5** summarizes some of the main laboratory findings in Hashimoto disease and Graves disease.

Patients with Hashimoto thyroiditis have normal or high TSH levels and low FT4 levels. To differentiate the disease from other causes of hypothyroidism (e.g., certain medications or treatments), it is necessary to follow these findings by testing for thyroid antibodies. These antibodies are most commonly detected by sensitive ELISA, CLIA, or electrochemiluminescence immunoassays (ECLIAs; see Chapter 11). Antibodies to TPO are the best indicator of the disease because they are found in up to 95% of patients with Hashimoto disease but in

Table 15-5 Typical Laboratory Findings in Autoimmune Thyroid Diseases

DISEASE	TSH LEVEL	FREE T4 (FT4) LEVEL	AUTOANTIBODIES
Hashimoto thyroiditis	Normal or elevated	Decreased	Anti-thyroglobulin Anti-thyroid peroxidase (TPO)
Graves disease	Decreased or undetectable	Elevated	Thyroid-stimulating hormone receptor antibodies (TRAbs)[a] Anti-thyroglobulin Anti-thyroid peroxidase (TPO)

[a]*Diagnostic.*

only 10% to 15% of the general population. Antibodies to Tg are less sensitive and specific because they are detected in only 60% to 80% of patients with the disease and are found more frequently than TPO antibodies in healthy persons. Because anti-Tg antibodies are not found in all patients, a negative test result does not rule out Hashimoto disease.

In contrast, patients with Graves disease characteristically have low or undetectable levels of TSH and increased levels of FT4. Increased uptake of radioactive iodine also helps to confirm the diagnosis. Although antibodies to TPO and Tg are found in many patients, they are generally not useful in making the diagnosis. TRAbs, on the other hand, are highly indicative of Graves disease because they are present in 98% to 100% of patients; TRAbs are therefore included as one component of the diagnostic criteria for Graves disease.

Assays for TRAbs may be performed for diagnostic testing of patients with clinical symptoms and initial laboratory results suggestive of Graves disease, to evaluate patient response to therapy by monitoring TSI titers, clarify cases that are difficult to diagnose, or predict the risk of thyroid dysfunction in newborns born to mothers with Graves disease. There are two types of tests for TRAbs: binding assays and bioassays. In binding assays, such as automated ELISA, CLIA, or ECLIA, a labeled TRAb reagent competes with the patient antibody for TSH receptors bound to a solid phase. These assays measure serum levels of TRAbs and can be performed by routine clinical laboratories but they cannot determine the function of the antibodies. In contrast, bioassays can distinguish between TSI and TBAb. These assays require live cells and are performed by reference and research laboratories. Historically, they have been based on the ability of TSI to bind to TSH receptors on live cells and trigger cyclic adenosine monophosphate (cAMP)-dependent luciferase activity. Newer assays have been developed that are easier to perform and use biosensors to directly measure changes in cAMP levels in genetically modified cell lines that express human TSH receptors.

Critical Thinking 15-2

A patient with a goiter was experiencing restlessness, insomnia, rapid heartbeat, and weight loss. Laboratory testing revealed a decreased level of TSH and increased FT4. What disease do you suspect, and what additional testing would confirm the diagnosis?

Type 1 Diabetes Mellitus (T1D)

Diabetes mellitus is a group of common endocrine disorders characterized by *hyperglycemia* (a high level of glucose in the blood). The American Diabetes Association (ADA) has classified diabetes into four main categories based on the etiology of the disease: type 1 diabetes, type 2 diabetes, gestational diabetes, and diabetes because of other causes (e.g., neonatal diabetes, pancreatitis, drug induced). Most patients have type 2 diabetes, a non-autoimmune condition characterized by progressive loss of insulin secretion, insulin resistance, and metabolic syndrome; the prevalence of this form increases with age as a result of lifestyle factors (e.g., unhealthy diet, physical inactivity). Gestational diabetes develops in some women during the second or third trimesters of pregnancy.

About 5% to 10% of patients with diabetes mellitus are classified as having **type 1 diabetes mellitus (T1D)**, an autoimmune condition characterized by insulin deficiency due to destruction of pancreatic beta cells. Of these patients, 90% have an immune-mediated form of the disease, whereas the remaining 10% are idiopathic cases with no identifiable cause. In this section, we focus on the immune-mediated form of type 1 diabetes, which we refer to as *T1D*. T1D was previously known as *insulin-dependent diabetes* or *juvenile-onset diabetes* because it requires treatment with insulin and usually develops in children or young adults before the age of 30, although it can be seen at any age.

T1D is a chronic autoimmune disease involving selective destruction of the pancreatic beta cells. These cells are in clusters called the *islets of Langerhans* and are responsible for the production and secretion of the hormone insulin. Insulin plays a vital role in regulating the amount of glucose in the blood by promoting its absorption by skeletal muscles and fat tissue so that it can be converted into energy needed by our cells. The autoimmune destruction of beta cells in T1D results in insufficient insulin production, hyperglycemia, and harmful effects on the body. Early symptoms include increased hunger, thirst, and urination; unintentional weight loss; weakness and fatigue; and stomach pain. A life-treating diabetic coma can develop in patients with severely decreased insulin levels, as the body metabolizes fat as an energy source, releasing toxic ketones. Long-term effects include cardiovascular complications, renal disease, nerve damage, blindness, and infections of the lower extremities, which can lead to amputation.

Patients require lifelong insulin injections to control glucose levels and lower the risk of complications.

There is an inherited genetic susceptibility to T1D, likely attributable to multiple genes involved in immune function. Certain HLA-DR and HLA-DQ alleles are strongly associated with the disease. Patients with T1D are also susceptible to developing other organ-specific autoimmune diseases, most commonly, autoimmune thyroid diseases. Environmental factors have not been clearly defined, but possible influences include certain viral infections, proteins in cow's milk, and vitamin D deficiency.

Immunopathology

Progressive inflammation of the islets of Langerhans in the pancreas leads to fibrosis and destruction of most beta cells. The preclinical period may last for years. Hyperglycemia does not become evident until 80% or more of the beta cells are destroyed. Beta-cell death is mediated by cytotoxic T lymphocytes, pro-inflammatory cytokines (TNF-α, IFN-γ, and IL-1), and reactive oxygen species from phagocytic cells.

Autoantibody production precedes the development of clinically evident T1D by several years. Autoantibodies are produced against various components of the pancreatic islet cells and are present in newly diagnosed patients and in prediabetic individuals who are being monitored because they have a high risk of developing diabetes. Antibody production diminishes with time, however. Islet cell antibodies (ICAs) may be directed against insulin; the tyrosine phosphatase–like transmembrane proteins, *insulinoma antigen 2 (IA-2)* and *IA-2βA (phogrin)*; the enzyme *glutamic acid decarboxylase (GAD-65)*; *zinc transporter 8 (ZnT8)*; or various other islet cell proteins. Many of these antigens are components of the regulated pathway required for insulin secretion.

Treatment

The primary therapy for T1D involves multiple daily injections of insulin, with the goal of achieving normal blood glucose levels as much as possible. The insulin is prepared by recombinant DNA technology and consists of the amino acid sequence of human insulin or genetically modified variations with improved absorption and function. Clinical trials are investigating the use of immunosuppressive drugs and biological agents to inhibit the autoimmune responses that lead to beta-cell destruction and prevent disease progression in patients with T1D. In 2022, the U.S. Food and Drug Administration (FDA) approved the use of teplizumab, a monoclonal antibody directed against the T-cell antigen CD3, to delay progression of T1D in high-risk individuals. In 2023, the FDA approved Lantidra, an allogeneic cell therapy using pancreatic islet cells from deceased donors for treatment of T1D in adults who have had poor glucose control and repeated episodes of severe hypoglycemia (low blood sugar) despite other treatments. However, this treatment requires continual immunosuppressive therapy to prevent rejection, and the number of suitable donors is limited. Research on producing pancreatic islet cells from stem cells in vitro offers hope of curing T1D without the need for immunosuppression in the future.

Laboratory Diagnosis of Type 1 Diabetes Mellitus

According to the ADA, a person is considered to have diabetes if they meet one of four criteria: (1) a fasting glucose greater than 126 mg/dL on more than one occasion (normal value is lower than 100 mg/dL); (2) a random plasma glucose level of 200 mg/dL or more with classic symptoms of diabetes; (3) an oral glucose tolerance test of 200 mg/dL or more in a 2-hour sample with a 75-g glucose load; or (4) a hemoglobin A_{1c} value (Hb A_{1c}) greater than 6.5%. Hb A_{1c} is a glycated form of hemoglobin that is made when the RBC protein combines with glucose in the blood. The Hb A_{1c} plasma level is proportional to the life span of the circulating RBCs (up to 120 days) and reflects the average plasma glucose concentration over the previous 2 to 3 months.

Although T1D is usually diagnosed by demonstrating its main characteristic of hyperglycemia, it may be useful to perform serological tests for autoantibodies to distinguish T1D from type 2 diabetes. Most commonly, this involves testing for GAD antibody and at least one other antibody (IA-2, insulin, ZnT8). GAD antibodies are found in about 80% of patients with early-onset T1D but are also present in some patients with other autoimmune disorders; testing for more than one antibody increases specificity and sensitivity for the disease. Another use of serological testing is to predict the risk of developing T1D in children who have family members with the disease. The presence of two or more pertinent autoantibodies is associated with a high risk of developing T1D in these children.

ICAs have traditionally been detected by IIF using frozen sections of human pancreas. A competitive radiobinding assay is considered to be the gold standard in testing for ICAs but is labor intensive and involves radioactivity. Automated ELISA, radioimmunoassay (RIA), and electrochemiluminescence (ECLIA) assays are also available to measure individual ICAs. Multiplex ELISA, ECLIA, and agglutination-PCR (using antigen-DNA conjugates) that combine the tests for the four major ICAs into one assay have also been developed, making testing more efficient and having the potential to allow for earlier detection of T1D in the future.

Celiac Disease

Celiac disease is an autoimmune disease affecting the small intestine and other organs. It affects about 1% of the world's population, but this number is thought to be an underestimate because many cases go undiagnosed. Celiac disease is unique in that it is associated with a known environmental trigger—dietary gluten. Gluten is a protein complex found in wheat, barley, and rye that is poorly digested by the upper gastrointestinal system. It contains an alcohol-soluble component called *gliadin* that is rich in the amino acids glutamine and proline. Gliadin is resistant to digestive enzymes in the stomach, pancreas, and small intestine and therefore remains intact in the lumen, or space within the intestines, after ingestion. If there is an increase in the permeability of the intestinal walls, possibly because of an infection, undigested gliadin can pass through the epithelial barrier of the intestine and trigger an inappropriate immune response. The immunogenicity of gliadin is enhanced when it is acted on by **tissue transglutaminase (tTG),** an intestinal enzyme that converts the glutamine residues in gliadin to glutamic acid.

Almost all people with celiac disease have specific alleles that code for the haplotypes, HLA-DQ2 (HLA-DQ A1*05:01 or DQB1*02 or 01) or HLA-DQ8 (HLA-A1*03:02 or B1*03:02). The MHC II molecules coded for by these genes can strongly bind the immunogenic peptides generated from gliadin. The APCs from these individuals bind these peptides and present them to antigen-specific CD4 T cells, which produce cytokines that activate $CD8^+$ T cells and trigger an inflammatory response (see Chapter 5). As a result, injury to the intestinal villi occurs, and the architecture of the intestinal mucosa is damaged. Also, B cells are stimulated to produce antibodies to the deamidated gliadin peptides (DGPs), tTG, and endomysium (a layer of connective tissue surrounding the intestinal muscles).

However, most people with the previously mentioned genes do not develop celiac disease, so other factors must be involved. Environmental factors believed to play a role in the development of celiac disease include consuming large amounts of gluten at a young age, certain infections (e.g., rotavirus), and overgrowth of pathogenic bacteria in the gut. The disease is found more often in females than in males (ratio 2:1 to 3:1) and among those who have selective IgA deficiency, some chromosome abnormalities (Down syndrome, Turner syndrome, Williams syndrome), or certain autoimmune diseases (T1D, AITDs). Several non-HLA genes involved in immune function are also thought to contribute to the autoimmune response.

Clinical Symptoms and Treatment

Many of the clinical symptoms of celiac disease are related to malabsorption of nutrients by the small intestine, and the most common symptom is diarrhea. Infants typically present with diarrhea, abdominal distention, and failure to thrive but may also experience vomiting, irritability, anorexia, and constipation. Older children, teenagers, and adults may have the classic symptoms of diarrhea and abdominal pain or discomfort but often have other manifestations that make the condition difficult to diagnose. These include delayed puberty and short stature, arthritis or arthralgia, osteoporosis (due to malabsorption of calcium and vitamin D), neurological symptoms, iron-deficiency anemia, and dermatitis herpetiformis (a skin disorder with itchy blistering).

Treatment of celiac disease involves placing patients on a strict gluten-free diet. Elimination of gluten from the diet usually results in improvement of clinical symptoms within days or weeks and healing of intestinal damage in 6 months to 2 years. However, many patients do not adhere to a gluten-free diet because of expense, inconvenience, or social stigma; also, some patients have persistent symptoms despite adherence to the diet, and accidental ingestion of gluten from contaminated foods can occur. Alternative treatments are being investigated, including monoclonal antibodies or small molecule inhibitors of targeted points in the immune response.

Laboratory Diagnosis of Celiac Disease

Diagnosis of celiac disease is based on clinical symptoms, serological findings, duodenal biopsy, and typing for the disease-associated alleles. Serological testing is the initial approach to evaluate patients suspected of having celiac disease and helps differentiate these patients from those having conditions with similar symptoms, such as gluten sensitivity or wheat allergy. Patients should follow a regular diet before serological testing because false-negative antibody results can occur in people on a gluten-free diet.

Detection of IgA antibodies to tTG is the serological method of choice for initial testing because it is the most sensitive and specific marker for celiac disease. Testing for tTG is performed by automated immunoassays using recombinant tTG antigen (e.g., ELISA, particle-based multi-analyte technology [PMAT]). Serum IgA levels should be concurrently measured in people suspected of having celiac disease because some patients also have selective IgA deficiency and will therefore test negative in IgA-based assays. In patients who are IgA deficient, testing for IgG anti-tTG or for IgG antibodies to DGPs can be performed. Negative serology results do not exclude a celiac disease diagnosis, because antibody titers can decrease with time in patients following a gluten-free diet.

Despite their high specificity, false-positive results for anti-tTG can occur in patients with other autoimmune diseases and various other conditions. Therefore, positive anti-tTG results should be confirmed by another method. Guidelines published by the American College of Gastroenterology recommend that biopsy of the small intestine be performed to confirm the diagnosis. Initial biopsy results can also provide a baseline for comparing future samples for intestinal injury. Histological examination of biopsy tissue characteristically shows an increase in the number of intraepithelial lymphocytes, elongation of the intestinal crypts, and partial to total atrophy of the villi **(Fig. 15–13).** Determination of the T-lymphocyte count by CD3 staining and observation of IgA transglutaminase antibody deposits in the tissue can provide

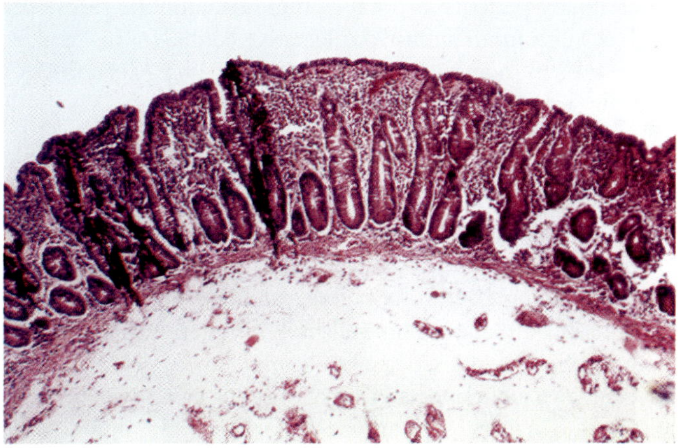

FIGURE 15–13 This photomicrograph depicts the cytoarchitecture exhibited by a section of intestinal epithelial mucosa that had been excised from an individual with gluten-induced enteropathy. Note the thickened, fused, and blunted morphology of the intestinal villi. *(Courtesy of CDC Public Health Image Library.)*

additional information to support the diagnosis. To minimize the occurrence of false-negative results, multiple biopsies should be obtained from different parts of the duodenum because mucosal injury may be patchy.

Detection of endomysial antibodies (EMAs), which are directed against the tissue that surrounds smooth muscle fibers, can be used to confirm the disease in children and adults who are unwilling to undergo biopsy. EMA tests are highly specific for celiac disease but are costly and labor intensive because they are based on IIF assays using monkey esophagus or human umbilical cord tissue as the substrate; therefore, they are not performed as commonly as anti-tTG.

HLA genotyping is not required for diagnosis but can be useful to differentiate celiac disease from other conditions, especially when antibody titers are weak or negative, or if there is a discrepancy between serological tests and biopsy results. Testing is commonly performed by PCR/sequence-specific oligonucleotide hybridization (see Chapter 16). The absence of HLA-DQ2 or HLA-DQ8-associated alleles virtually excludes a diagnosis of celiac disease because people who are negative for these haplotypes are highly unlikely to have the disease.

Following proper diagnosis and maintenance of patients with celiac disease on a gluten-free diet, clinical symptoms usually improve, antibody titers revert to negative, and histology can return to normal. However, about 5% of patients fail to improve, usually because of nonadherence to the diet (which can sometimes be unintentional) but sometimes due to refractory disease, incorrect diagnosis, disease complications, or simultaneous gastrointestinal disorders.

Autoimmune Liver Diseases

There are three major forms of **autoimmune liver disease: autoimmune hepatitis (AIH), primary biliary cholangitis (PBC),** and *primary sclerosing cholangitis (PSC)*. In AIH, the autoimmune process targets the hepatocytes; in PBC, it affects the small interlobular bile ducts; and in PSC, it affects the medium-sized intra- and extrahepatic bile ducts. There are also overlap syndromes that combine features of these diseases. Many patients also have other autoimmune disorders, such as Hashimoto disease or ulcerative colitis. In this section, we discuss in more detail two of these diseases, AIH and PBC, and the serological tests used in their diagnosis.

Autoimmune Hepatitis (AIH)

AIH, formerly known as *chronic active hepatitis,* is an immune-mediated liver disease that can lead to end-stage liver failure if untreated. The clinical features of AIH can be quite variable. About 25% of individuals are asymptomatic and are diagnosed only after abnormal liver function tests are found coincidentally when blood work is performed. Adults usually present with an unexpected onset of vague symptoms, including fatigue, nausea, weight loss, abdominal pain, itching, and maculopapular rashes. Less often, patients have symptoms of portal hypertension, such as gastrointestinal bleeding or hypersplenism. Jaundice may also be present. Rarely, the initial presentation is fulminant liver failure (severe disease with sudden onset) requiring liver transplantation.

Two types of AIH can be differentiated based on their autoantibody specificities: type 1 and type 2. Type 1 AIH accounts for two-thirds of all AIH cases, has a female:male ratio of 4:1, and mainly affects adults 40 years or older. Type 2 AIH has a female:male ratio of 10:1 and is seen mostly in children.

In White people, a higher risk of developing type 1 AIH is associated with the HLA-DRB1*03:01 and HLA-DRB1*04:01 alleles, whereas HLA-DQB1*02:01 has the strongest association with type 2 AIH; the susceptibility alleles vary in different ethnic populations. Low vitamin D levels, changes in microbiota, and exposure to certain drugs or viruses, most notably hepatitis C, may play a role in triggering AIH, the latter through molecular mimicry and cross-reactivity with liver antigens.

Common laboratory findings include elevated levels of the liver enzymes aspartate aminotransferase (AST) and alanine aminotransferase (ALT), with less prominent increases in serum bilirubin and alkaline phosphatase. Serum immunoglobulin levels, particularly IgG, are high; in adults, various autoantibodies may be present, including RF, ANAs, ANCAs, smooth muscle antibodies (SMAs), anti–liver-kidney microsomal antibody (anti-LKM-1), anti-liver cytosol type 1 antibody (anti-LC-1), and anti-mitochondrial antibodies (AMAs).

Autoantibody profiles can distinguish between type 1 and type 2 AIH. Type 1 patients are characteristically positive for SMAs and/or ANAs. Patients may also have an atypical p-ANCA. ANAs most commonly produce a homogeneous pattern on IIF but can sometimes produce a speckled pattern. The SMAs are directed against actin and other components of the cytoskeleton. They can be detected by ELISA, immunoblotting, multiplex bead immunoassays, or IIF on rodent kidney, stomach, or liver sections, where they produce fluorescent staining of the smooth muscle in the artery walls and other components, such as the glomeruli and tubules of the kidneys. Antibody titers are usually 1:80 or higher in adults but can be as low as 1:20 in children.

In contrast, patients with type 2 AIH characteristically produce antibodies against LKM-1, which are directed against cytochrome P450 2D6, or against LC-1. LKM antibodies can be detected by IIF, ELISA, or immunoblotting methods. On IIF using rodent tissue substrates, anti-LKM-1 stains the cytoplasm of the hepatocytes and the P3 portion of the kidney tubules. The resulting immunofluorescent pattern appears similar to that produced by mitochondrial antibodies but can be distinguished by experts when testing is performed on multiple tissue substrates, and the intensity of fluorescent staining of different components of the substrates is carefully examined. Clinically significant titers are 1:40 in adults and 1:10 in children; antibody titers correlate with disease activity. Antibodies to LC-1 are directed against a folate-metabolizing enzyme in the liver and stain the cytoplasm of liver cells in IIF. These antibodies can be masked by anti-LKM-1 if they are also present, and other methods, such as immunoblotting, may be required to detect them.

Liver biopsy is necessary to confirm the diagnosis of AIH and to assess the extent of liver damage. Inflammation at the portal-parenchymal boundary, known as *interface hepatitis,* is typical of AIH and is characterized by an infiltrate of lymphocytes, plasma cells, and histiocytes surrounding dying hepatocytes. Histological findings, along with detection of pertinent autoantibodies, elevated IgG, and exclusion of viral hepatitis, form a widely used simplified set of criteria recommended by the International Autoimmune Hepatitis Group for the diagnosis of AIH.

Laboratory findings are essential for early diagnosis, and treatment should be started promptly once the diagnosis is made. Most patients respond to the standard immunosuppressive treatment of prednisolone (with or without azathioprine) to induce remission, followed by azathioprine alone to maintain remission. However, patients must be monitored carefully because they are at increased risk of developing cirrhosis and possibly hepatocellular carcinoma. If untreated, AIH usually progresses to liver failure, at which point liver transplantation is required.

Primary Biliary Cholangitis (PBC)

PBC, formerly known as *primary biliary cirrhosis,* is the most common autoimmune liver disease, occurring about 10 times as often in females as in males. Many genes are thought to predispose individuals to PBC, with the strongest associations for HLA-DPB1*08 and HLA-DPB1*07 alleles. PBC is an autoimmune disease involving progressive destruction of the intrahepatic bile ducts. The destruction leads to chronic *cholestasis* (a condition in which the flow of bile is slowed or blocked), inflammation of the portal vein in the liver, and accumulation of scar tissue that can ultimately lead to cirrhosis and liver failure. Individual patients can be asymptomatic or have slowly or rapidly progressing disease. Symptoms include fatigue, pruritus (itchy skin), abdominal pain, and dry eyes and mouth; in the later stages, patients experience jaundice, ascites, and greasy stools. The standard initial therapy for PBC is ursodeoxycholic acid (UDCA), a bile acid that helps move bile through the liver. The use of UDCA has helped to slow disease progression and increase patient survival; other drugs may be used for patients who do not respond to UDCA. Liver transplantation is the only effective treatment for patients who have reached end-stage liver disease.

AMAs are found in most patients with PBC, and their presence is one of three diagnostic criteria for the disease established by the American Association for the Study of Liver Diseases. A diagnosis of PBC can be made if at least two out of three of these criteria are met. The first criterion is the presence of AMAs (titer of 1:40 or more), but a diagnosis of PBC cannot be based on AMAs alone because these antibodies have also been observed in patients with other conditions, such as SLE, RA, and graft-versus-host disease, and in a small percentage of healthy people.

The other two diagnostic criteria are a serum alkaline phosphatase level elevated at least 1.5 times the upper limit of normal for 6 months or more and liver biopsy showing destructive cholangitis (inflammation of the bile duct system) and interlobular bile duct injury. Patients commonly have elevated levels of aminotransferases and serum immunoglobulins, especially IgM, because of polyclonal B-cell activation. ANAs may also be positive and, depending on the antibodies present, can produce various patterns on FANA, including multiple nuclear dots (because of anti-Sp100), smooth nuclear envelope, or centromere.

Different methods have been developed to detect AMAs, including IIF, immunoblotting with mitochondrial preparations from mammalian tissue, ELISA, and fluorescent microbead immunoassay. Traditionally, AMAs have been detected by IIF with mitochondria-rich tissue substrates such as rodent liver, kidney, or stomach sections. These antibodies produce a bright, uniform granular cytoplasmic fluorescence in the distal renal tubules, gastric parietal cells, thyroid epithelial cells, and cardiac muscle. IIF uses antigens in their natural configuration and has fairly high levels of sensitivity and specificity; however, the method is manual, is time consuming, and requires a high level of expertise to correctly interpret the pattern. A small percentage of patients with PBC test negative for AMAs on IIF or may give atypical staining patterns that are difficult to interpret. ELISA testing for antibodies to the nuclear antigens GP210 or SP100 may be beneficial to the diagnosis of PBC in AMA-negative patients.

Since the development of IIF, the target antigens of AMAs have been identified as components of the 2-oxo-acid dehydrogenase complexes in mitochondrial energy-producing pathways. Identification of these antigens allowed for the development of automated solid-phase ELISA and fluorescence microbead immunoassays. These assays provide objective results, but their performance can vary because they do not include the full spectrum of antigenic epitopes available by IIF.

Multiple Sclerosis (MS)

Multiple sclerosis (MS) is an autoimmune disorder involving inflammation and destruction of the CNS. It affects almost 1 million Americans and over 1.8 million individuals worldwide. The disease most often begins between the ages of 20 and 40 and is twice as common in females as in males. Multiple genes are thought to contribute to the development of MS, but the disease is most closely associated with inheritance of the HLA allele, DRB1*1501. Environmental factors associated with MS include reduced exposure to sunlight, vitamin D deficiency, cigarette smoking, and infection with EBV after early childhood.

MS is characterized by the formation of lesions called *plaques* in the white matter of the brain and spinal cord, resulting in the progressive destruction of the myelin sheath of axons. T cells and macrophages predominate within the plaques, and activated CD8 cytotoxic T cells are found along the edges. Myelin-specific antibodies are produced and bind to the myelin membrane, where they may stimulate macrophages and specialized phagocytes called *microglial cells.* The T_H1 cytokines IL-2, TNF-α, and IFN-γ are believed to be central to the pathogenesis of the disease, promoting changes in the endothelial cells that facilitate adherence of activated T cells and their migration across the blood-brain barrier. T_H17 cells are also thought to play an important role in the inflammatory response of the CNS. The cascade of immunologic events results in acute inflammation, damage to the myelin sheath that surrounds the nerve fibers, and structural repair with recovery of some function, followed by post-inflammatory neurodegeneration.

Clinical Symptoms and Treatment

Damage to the CNS tissue can cause visual disturbances, weakness or diminished dexterity in one or more limbs, locomotor incoordination, dizziness, facial palsy, and sensory abnormalities, such as tingling or "pins and needles" that run down the spine or extremities, and flashes of light during eye movement. MS can be classified into three major subtypes based on the clinical course of the disease. About 90% of patients have relapsing-remitting MS, characterized by clearly defined episodes of neurological attacks with periods of full or partial recovery in between. Most patients with MS eventually develop progressive deterioration of the CNS and functional disability.

Treatment for MS is aimed at easing recovery from acute attacks and reducing the risk of future relapses. Acute exacerbations can be treated with glucocorticoids to reduce inflammation. Many disease-modifying therapies (DMTs), including monoclonal antibodies and sphingosine-1-phosphate (S1P) receptor modulators affecting various functions of the immune system, have been approved for long-term treatment of MS. These agents modulate the immune system through mechanisms that include sequestrating lymphocytes in the lymph nodes to prevent their entry into the CNS, interfering with lymphocyte proliferation by blocking DNA synthesis, depleting immune cells, and changing the cytokine pattern. Two examples of such therapies are the humanized monoclonal antibodies, ocrelizumab, which binds to CD20 and depletes mature B cells from the blood, and natalizumab, which is directed against an adhesion molecule of lymphocytes, preventing them from binding to endothelial cells and crossing the blood-brain barrier. S1P receptor modulators act by binding to their corresponding receptors on endothelial and other cells, causing internalization of the receptors and preventing lymphocyte migration. DMTs have had a large impact on reducing the severity of MS symptoms and improving long-term prognosis.

Laboratory Diagnosis of Multiple Sclerosis

The diagnosis of MS is based mainly on clinical symptoms, demonstration of disseminated lesions in the white matter of the brain and spinal cord by magnetic resonance imaging (MRI), and exclusion of other possible causes. A combination of laboratory tests can support the diagnosis, especially in cases in which the patient's symptoms or MRI findings do not meet the diagnostic criteria for MS:

- Immunoglobulins are increased in the cerebral spinal fluid (CSF) in most patients with MS, producing two or more distinct bands on protein electrophoresis that are not seen in the serum. These bands are referred to as *oligoclonal* and are identified by isoelectric focusing with immunoblotting **(Fig. 15–14)**.
- The IgG index, a calculated ratio of CSF IgG/albumin ÷ serum IgG/albumin, is typically elevated and may also be used in making a diagnosis, even though it is not specific for MS.

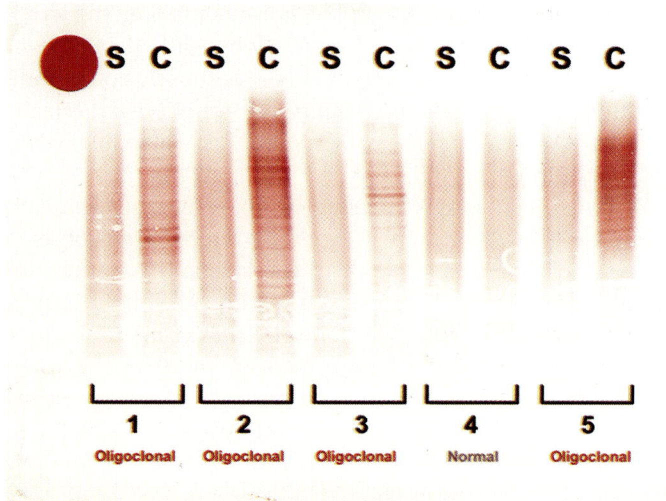

FIGURE 15–14 Isoelectric focusing and immunoblotting of serum (S) and CSF (C) samples from five patients. Patient 4 has normal results. Patients 1, 2, 3, and 5 have oligoclonal banding in the CSF that is not seen in the serum, a finding that supports a diagnosis of multiple sclerosis. *(Courtesy of Helena Laboratories.)*

- Although there is not one specific antibody that is diagnostic for MS, many patients produce antibody directed against a myelin basic protein peptide. Other antibodies, directed against components of oligodendrocytes and against myelin membranes, may also be produced.

Myasthenia Gravis (MG)

Myasthenia gravis (MG) is an autoimmune disease that affects the neuromuscular junction, the space in between the end of a motor neuron and a skeletal muscle. Patients with the disease experience weakness and fatigability of the skeletal muscles. The prevalence of MG ranges from 2 to 200 people per 1,000,000, depending on the population. The disease is heterogeneous in terms of its age of onset and sex. Early-onset MG (EOMG) occurs before the age of 50 and affects mainly females, whereas the late-onset form of the disease (LOMG) occurs after the age of 50 and is seen more often in males.

In MG, antibody-mediated damage to the acetylcholine receptors in skeletal muscle or to other proteins in the neuromuscular junction leads to progressive muscle weakness. Early signs are *ptosis* (drooping of the eyelids), *diplopia* (double vision), and the inability to retract the corners of the mouth, often resulting in a snarling appearance. Most patients progress to a generalized form of the disease involving more muscle groups, especially those in the upper limbs. Patients can also have difficulty speaking, chewing, and swallowing and may be unable to maintain support of the trunk, neck, or head. If respiratory muscle weakness occurs, it can be life threatening and require mechanical ventilation. Onset of symptoms can be acute, or they may develop and worsen over time.

Immunopathogenesis

About 85% of patients have antibodies to acetylcholine (ACh) receptors (AChRs), which appear to contribute to the disease pathogenesis by three mechanisms: blocking, binding, and modulating. Normally, ACh is released from nerve endings to generate an action potential that causes the muscle fiber to contract. When blocking antibodies combine with the receptor site, binding of ACh is thought to be prevented **(Fig. 15–15)**. Binding antibodies can activate complement and damage the postsynaptic muscle membrane, whereas modulating antibodies promote rapid endocytosis of the AChRs, resulting in reduced numbers on the muscle cell membranes.

Patients lacking anti-AChR may produce antibodies to other proteins involved in the neuromuscular junction. About 50% of patients have antibodies against muscle-specific kinase (MuSK), an enzyme that plays an important role in the development of the neuromuscular junction and in the clustering of AChRs on the muscle cell membrane, which enhances the transmission of the signals from the nerve cells. Consequently, there is fragmentation of the postsynaptic AChR clusters, resulting in muscle weakness and atrophy. Symptoms are usually severe, involving the facial, head, neck, and respiratory muscles. A smaller percentage of patients with generalized MG have antibodies against LRP4, a lipoprotein involved in the activation of MuSK. These patients are typically young females with a mild form of the disease. Antibodies to titin, a major protein in striated muscles, are found in up to 40% of patients with MG and are associated with LOMG.

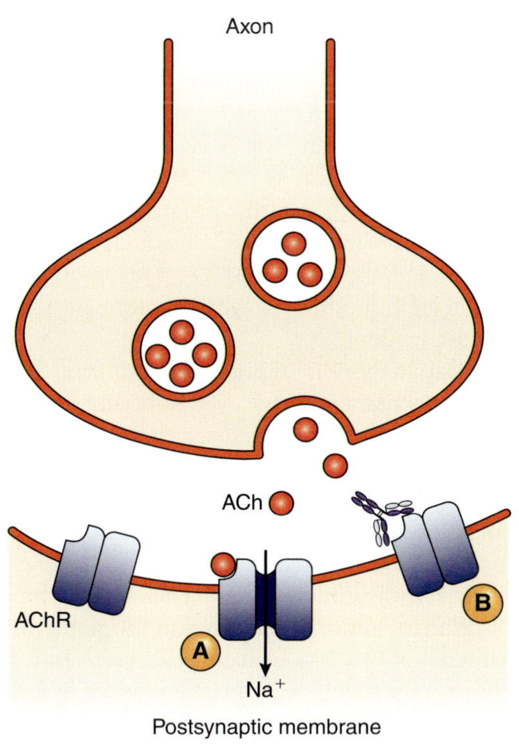

FIGURE 15–15 Blocking mechanism of immunologic injury in myasthenia gravis (MG). (A) Normal nerve impulse transmission: ACh is released from axon vesicles and binds to AChRs on the postsynaptic membrane, opening channels and allowing sodium ions to enter. (B) In MG, antibodies to the AchRs are formed, blocking transmission of nerve impulses.

The origin of MG is unknown, but the thymus appears to play a role in the autoimmune process of the disease. Thymic hyperplasia is common in patients with EOMG with AChR antibodies, and 10% to 15% of patients with LOMG have a *thymoma*, a tumor of the thymus. The follicles in the thymus expand and contain ectopic germinal centers with autoantibody-producing B cells. The autoimmune response may be triggered by myoid (muscle-like) cells in the thymus that express AChRs on their surface and may persist because of exposure to viruses such as EBV.

Genetic factors have been implicated in susceptibility to the disease. The HLA haplotype, A1, B8, DR3, has a strong association with EOMG, whereas the HLA antigens B7, DR2, and DR4 are more likely to appear in LOMG, and HLA-DR14-DQ5 may increase susceptibility to MuSK antibody production in MG.

Treatment

Most patients with MG can have a good quality of life with appropriate treatment. Anti-cholinesterase inhibitors to prevent destruction of the neurotransmitter ACh are used as the main therapy. Thymectomy can be performed on patients who have a thymoma but may also benefit those patients who do not. If these treatments are ineffective, immunosuppression is recommended. Treatment generally begins with high doses of glucocorticoid drugs followed by other immunosuppressive drugs, such as azathioprine or mycophenolate mofetil, to maintain the response. Plasmapheresis to remove the autoantibodies or IV immunoglobulin (whose mechanism of action is unknown) can be administered to patients in crisis. Biological agents such as monoclonal antibodies or fusion proteins targeted to specific components of the immune system involved in the pathogenesis of MG (e.g., the anti-CD20 agent, rituximab) may be given to patients with MG who are unresponsive to conventional therapies. These treatments have allowed patients with MG to maintain a quality of life that is nearly normal.

Laboratory Diagnosis of Myasthenia Gravis

Diagnosis of MG is based on clinical symptoms, electromyography (EMG), and laboratory testing for the disease-associated antibodies. EMG involves demonstration of decreased muscle response to repetitive stimulation of a motor nerve and increased muscle strength following inhibition of acetylcholinesterase, an enzyme that breaks down ACh.

The gold standard for detecting binding AChR antibodies is a quantitative radioimmunoprecipitation assay (RIPA) based on the reaction of patient serum with AChRs isolated from human muscle that are radiolabeled with α-bungarotoxin, a snake venom that binds with high affinity to a different site on the receptors. This highly sensitive assay can be used to determine antibody titers. Blocking and modulating AChR antibodies can be detected by RIPA or by a semiquantitative flow cytometry method in which patient serum is incubated with an AChR-expressing cell line, followed by addition of a fluorescent-labeled α-bungarotoxin. ELISAs for AChR antibodies have been developed but are not as sensitive as the other methods.

Patients who are negative for AChR antibodies should be tested for MuSK antibodies; this can be done by a quantitative RIPA. Testing for titin antibodies may also be useful in these patients and can be performed by a semiquantitative ELISA. IIF assays for LPR4 antibodies may also be performed but are not widely used. The use of additional markers, such as antibodies to agrin, a protein involved in the development and maintenance of the neuromuscular junction, is being studied.

Anti–Glomerular Basement Membrane Disease (Goodpasture Syndrome)

Anti–glomerular basement membrane (Anti-GBM) disease, also referred to as **Goodpasture syndrome**, is a small-vessel vasculitis characterized by the presence of an autoantibody to a basement membrane antigen in the glomeruli of the kidneys, alveoli of the lungs, or both. The basement membranes are composed of a thin, fibrous matrix that separates the epithelial cell layer within these organs from underlying connective tissue. Originally identified by Ernest Goodpasture in 1919, Goodpasture syndrome is a rare disorder that is found mainly in people of European ancestry. It mainly affects two age groups—males in their late 20s and males and females in their 60s and 70s.

The clinical presentation of patients varies, but most patients initially experience fatigue and malaise followed by clinical signs of kidney involvement, such as edema and hypertension, which can rapidly progress to acute renal failure if left untreated. Some patients develop chronic renal failure that requires lifetime hemodialysis or kidney transplantation. About 60% to 70% of patients with anti-GBM disease have pulmonary involvement with symptoms such as cough, shortness of breath, and hemoptysis (coughing up blood).

The standard treatment for anti-GBM disease involves administering high-dose corticosteroids to stop inflammation, followed by immunosuppressive drugs such as cyclophosphamide to inhibit further production of autoantibodies. Periodic plasmapheresis is performed to remove circulating autoantibodies from the blood. The monoclonal antibody rituximab (anti-CD20) has been used as a supplemental treatment in some patients. Prompt initiation of therapy is important because symptoms can be life threatening. If started early, therapy is successful in preventing acute renal failure in most patients. Long-term prognosis depends on the severity of symptoms at initial diagnosis and patient response to treatment.

Etiology and Immunopathology

Although little is known about the factors that trigger the autoimmune response in anti-GBM disease, there is a strong genetic association with HLA-DRB1*1501 and moderate association with HLA-DRB1*1502. Exposure to cigarette smoke and other pulmonary irritants, organic solvents, or infection has been implicated in disease pathogenesis by causing tissue injury that exposes critical antigenic epitopes. The autoantibodies produced in anti-GBM disease are specifically directed against the noncollagenous domain of the α-3 chain of type IV collagen. These autoantibodies react with collagen in the glomerular or alveolar basement membranes and bind complement. Complement proteins attract neutrophils, which mediate injury to the membranes by releasing chemically reactive oxygen-containing molecules and proteolytic enzymes. These reactants progressively destroy the renal tubular, glomerular, and pulmonary alveolar basement membranes. T-cell–mediated mechanisms are also thought to contribute to destruction of the basement membranes. Loss of membrane integrity causes blood and proteins to leak into the urine.

Laboratory Diagnosis

Laboratory evidence of renal involvement includes gross or microscopic hematuria, proteinuria, a decreased 24-hour creatinine clearance, and elevated blood urea and serum creatinine levels. Abnormally shaped RBCs and casts can be found in the urine sediment. In patients with pulmonary involvement, decreased total lung capacity and increased uptake of carbon monoxide are evident. An iron-deficiency anemia with decreased hemoglobin and hematocrit can develop if pulmonary hemorrhage is severe. The ESR and CRP level may be normal or increased.

Circulating antibodies to the GBM are found in most patients, and their detection plays an important role in disease diagnosis. GBM antibodies are detected by ELISA or fluorescent microbead immunoassays that use purified or recombinant α-3(IV) antigen substrates, or by an IIF assay that uses frozen kidney sections fixed to a microscope slide. The likelihood of detecting the GBM antibodies is increased when more than one assay is used. High-antibody titers are usually associated with rapidly progressing disease. Some patients are also positive for ANCAs, which are usually specific for MPO and show the p-ANCA pattern on IIF. ANCAs may be detected months to years before anti-GBM and symptoms are evident.

Histological analysis is important to confirm the diagnosis and to assess tissue damage. Tissue-bound anti-GBM can be detected by direct immunofluorescence on kidney or lung biopsy sections. In patients with renal disease, these antibodies are indicated by formation of a smooth, linear, ribbonlike pattern of fluorescence along the GBM. In contrast, glomerulonephritis caused by other autoimmune diseases shows a granular pattern of immunofluorescence caused by nonspecific deposition of immune complexes in the glomeruli. Examination of renal biopsy tissue also reveals crescent formations of inflammatory macrophages in the glomeruli. In patients with pulmonary involvement, linear IgG staining of the alveolar cell walls can be seen on direct immunofluorescence of lung biopsy tissue or bronchial washings. Laboratory testing plays a key role in differentiating anti-GBM disease from other diseases that can cause similar symptoms and in facilitating an early diagnosis that can lead to prompt treatment and better clinical outcomes.

Knowledge Check 15-7

Match each disease that follows with its characteristic autoantibody specificity:

a. Autoimmune hepatitis	____	1. Acetylcholine receptor
b. Celiac disease	____	2. TSH receptor
c. Diabetes mellitus (type 1)	____	3. TPO
d. Anti-GBM (Goodpasture) disease	____	4. Sm
e. GPA (Wegener granulomatosus)	____	5. CCP
f. Graves disease	____	6. Smooth muscle
g. Hashimoto thyroiditis	____	7. Neutrophil cytoplasmic antigens
h. Multiple sclerosis	____	8. Salivary glands
i. Myasthenia gravis	____	9. Islet cells
j. Primary biliary cholangitis	____	10. Tissue transglutaminase
k. Rheumatoid arthritis	____	11. Basement membranes
l. Sjögren syndrome	____	12. Myelin basic protein
m. Systemic lupus erythematosus	____	13. Mitochondria

KEY CONCEPTS

Etiology of Autoimmune Disease

- Autoimmune diseases result from a loss of self-tolerance, a delicate balance in the body that restricts the activity of T and B lymphocytes. Immunologic tolerance is achieved at two levels. Central tolerance affects potentially reactive B cells and T cells as they mature in the bone marrow and thymus, respectively, whereas peripheral tolerance occurs in the secondary lymphoid organs.
- Autoimmune disease is thought to result from complex interactions between the individual's genetic makeup, exposure to environmental factors, and defects in immune regulation. Associations between certain HLA types or polymorphisms in non-MHC genes involved in the immune response have been observed for several autoimmune diseases. Other factors, including sex hormones, tissue injury, and exposure to microbial infections, are thought to trigger the development of autoimmunity in genetically susceptible individuals.
- Infectious microorganisms are believed to trigger autoimmune responses in various ways, including molecular mimicry (a resemblance to self-antigens), epitope spreading (expansion of the immune response to additional self-antigens altered during autoimmune reactions), and the presence of superantigens that can bind to class II MHC molecules and TCRs with different antigen specificities.

Systemic Autoimmune Diseases

- Autoimmune diseases can be classified as organ specific or systemic, depending on whether tissue destruction is localized or affects multiple organs. SLE, RA, Sjögren syndrome, SSc, polymyositis, dermatomyositis, and GPA are examples of systemic diseases, whereas Hashimoto thyroiditis, Graves disease, type 1 diabetes mellitus, celiac disease, autoimmune hepatitis, primary biliary cholangitis, multiple sclerosis, myasthenia gravis, and anti-GBM disease are organ specific.
- Specific autoantibodies are strongly associated with the presence of certain autoimmune diseases and are useful in their diagnosis.

Systemic Lupus Erythematosus (SLE)

- SLE affects several organs in the body, most commonly the joints, skin, and kidneys. It most often begins in females of childbearing age.
- Patients with SLE make autoantibodies to various nuclear antigens, lymphocytes, erythrocytes, platelets, phospholipids, ribosomal components, and endothelium. Antibodies to double-stranded DNA are found in most patients with SLE and are specific for the disease.
- Autoantibodies are central to the pathology in SLE, forming immune complexes that deposit in the tissues and bind complement, causing tissue damage by type III hypersensitivity.

Anti-Nuclear Antibodies (ANAs)

- ANAs are found in most patients with SLE and in many patients with other systemic autoimmune rheumatic diseases. IIF using the human epithelial cell line HEp-2 as the substrate is considered the gold standard in ANA testing. Some of the main fluorescent patterns observed in IIF are homogeneous, speckled, nucleolar, centromere, and discrete nuclear dots. Each pattern is correlated with the presence of certain ANAs and should be followed up by confirmatory tests to more specifically characterize the antibodies.

- Other methods for ANA detection include ELISA, which can be used for ANA screening or ANA characterization, and multiplex bead immunoassays and immunodiffusion, which are used to identify specific ANAs.
- ENAs are ANAs that can be extracted from mammalian tissues with saline. Examples include Sm (specific for SLE), RNP, and SS-A and SS-B (commonly seen in Sjögren syndrome).

Anti-Phospholipid Antibodies

- Antibodies to phospholipids or phospholipid-protein complexes are made by many patients with SLE, and some patients with other diseases. These antibodies are associated with deep-vein and arterial thrombosis and recurrent pregnancy loss.
- Phospholipid antibodies can cause false-positive results in nontreponemal tests for syphilis, lupus anticoagulant assays, and cardiolipin antibody tests.

Rheumatoid Arthritis (RA)

- RA is a chronic inflammatory disease that mainly causes joint and bone damage but can also affect other organs.
- Two key antibodies made in the disease are rheumatoid factor (RF) and anti-cyclic citrullinated peptide (anti-CCP). RF, an autoantibody against the Fc portion of IgG molecules, is found in most patients with RA but is not specific for the disease. Anti-CCP, which is directed against a modified amino acid called citrulline, is found in many patients with RA and has high specificity for RA.

Other Systemic Autoimmune Rheumatic Diseases (SARDS)

- Other SARDS include Sjögren syndrome, characterized by dry eyes and a dry mouth; systemic sclerosis (SSc), a progressive disease in which excess fibrosis and vascular abnormalities affect the joints, skin, and internal organs; mixed connective tissue disease, an overlap syndrome of different SARDS; and the inflammatory myopathies, a group of chronic inflammatory diseases affecting the muscles (e.g., polymyositis, dermatomyositis).
- Antibodies to centromere proteins are specific for limited cutaneous SSc, also called the CREST syndrome, and produce the centromere pattern in the IIF test for ANAs.

Granulomatosus With Polyangiitis (GPA; Wegener Granulomatosus) and ANCAs

- GPA is a rare autoimmune disease involving blood vessel inflammation, or vasculitis. It mainly affects the upper respiratory system and lungs but can progress to other organs.
- Anti-neutrophil cytoplasmic antibodies (ANCAs) are strongly associated with autoimmune syndromes involving vasculitis, such as GPA.
- ANCAs can be detected by automated immunoassays (ELISA, CLIA, or fluorescent microbead immunoassay) or IIF. In IIF using ethanol-fixed leukocytes as the substrate, two patterns of fluorescence can result: c-ANCA, a diffuse, granular staining of the cytoplasm of the neutrophils, mainly caused by antibodies against PR3 and seen in most patients with GPA; and p-ANCA, characterized by fluorescence surrounding the nuclear lobes of the neutrophils, caused by antibodies to positively charged antigens such as myeloperoxidase (MPO). Fluorescence of the lymphocytes is absent.
- Three methods can distinguish a p-ANCA pattern from ANAs: An ANA IIF using HEp-2 cells should be negative; ANCA testing with formalin-fixed leukocytes will prevent perinuclear staining, producing cytoplasmic fluorescence; performance of automated ANCA immunoassays will reveal antigen specificity.

Organ-Specific Autoimmune Diseases

- In these diseases, the autoimmune response is mainly directed against a single organ or gland.
- In Hashimoto thyroiditis, immune destruction of the thyroid gland causes hypothyroidism; patients produce antibodies to thyroglobulin (Tg) and thyroid peroxidase (TPO). TSH levels are normal or high, and the thyroid hormones, FT4 and T3, are decreased.
- In Graves disease, disease-specific autoantibodies to the TSH receptor (TRAbs) bind to these receptors and stimulate the thyroid gland to produce excess FT4 and T3, resulting in hyperthyroidism. Patients have decreased or absent TSH due to feedback from the hypothalamic-pituitary-thyroid axis.
- Type 1 diabetes mellitus (T1D) is an autoimmune disorder characterized by destruction to the pancreatic beta cells, resulting in decreased insulin production and high blood glucose levels. Patients produce antibodies to insulin, insulinoma antigen 2 (IA-2) and IA-2βA (phogrin); glutamic acid decarboxylase (GAD-65); zinc transporter 8 (ZnT8); and pancreatic islet cells (ICAs). Laboratories perform glucose-related testing and testing for anti-GAD and one other autoantibody to confirm the diagnosis.
- Celiac disease affects the small intestine and other organs. It is caused by an autoimmune response to a component of gluten. Patients produce antibodies to gliadin, tissue transglutaminase (tTG), and endomysium. The initial laboratory test of choice is IgA-anti-tTG; IgA levels are concurrently tested to check for deficiency. Patients with negative results can be tested for IgG anti-tTG or IgG anti-deaminated gliadin peptides (DGPs). Endomysial antibodies can be detected by IIF for confirmation of positive results.

- In autoimmune hepatitis (AIH), the immune response targets the liver's hepatocytes. Patients with type 1 AIH produce smooth muscle antibodies (SMA), which can be detected by IIF on rodent kidney, stomach, or liver sections. Patients may also make ANAs or ANCAs. In type 2 AIH, patients make liver-kidney microsomal (LKM-1) and liver cytosol type 1 (LC-1) antibodies.
- Primary biliary cholangitis (PBC) is an autoimmune disease directed against the bile ducts. Antimitochondrial antibodies (AMAs) are found in most patients with PBC and are one of three diagnostic criteria for the disease.
- Multiple sclerosis (MS) involves inflammation and destruction of the CNS. Antibodies are made against a peptide in myelin basic protein, a component of the myelin sheath that surrounds nerve cells. Other characteristic findings are presence of oligoclonal bands upon isoelectric focusing and immunoblotting of CSF, and an elevated IgG index (the ratio of CSF IgG/albumin to serum IgG/albumin).
- Myasthenia gravis affects the neuromuscular junction and is characterized by muscle weakness. Most patients make antibodies to the acetylcholine receptors (AChR) on muscle cells, preventing muscle stimulation by acetylcholine released from nerve cells. Some patients make antibodies to muscle-specific kinase (MuSK) or the lipoprotein LRP4.
- Anti–glomerular basement membrane (anti-GBM) disease, or Goodpasture syndrome, is a small-vessel vasculitis in which patients make antibody to type IV collagen in the basement membranes of kidney glomeruli (GBM) and/or lung alveoli. Tissue-bound GBM antibodies can be detected in kidney biopsy samples by direct immunofluorescence and produce a smooth, linear pattern of fluorescence caused by immune complexes deposited along the GBM.

CASE STUDIES

1. A 25-year-old female consulted her physician because she had been experiencing symptoms of weight loss, joint pain in the hands, and extreme fatigue. The concentration of RF in the patient's serum was 50 IU/mL (reference range: 0 to 15 IU/mL); the ANA was positive by ELISA; the RBC count was 3.5×10^{12} per L (normal = 4.1 to 5.1×10^{12} per liter); the WBC count was 5.8×10^{9} per liter (normal = 4.5 to 11×10^{9} per liter).

   ### Questions

   a. What is a possible explanation for the RF and ANA results?
   b. What is the most likely cause of the decreased RBC count?
   c. Name two diseases that should be considered when making a diagnosis, and indicate what additional testing would help to distinguish between these.

2. A 40-year-old female went to her doctor because she was feeling tired all the time. She had gained about 10 pounds in the last few months and had some facial puffiness. Her thyroid gland was enlarged and rubbery. Laboratory results indicated a normal RBC and WBC count, but the TSH was increased, and the FT4 level was decreased.

   ### Questions

   a. What condition do these results likely indicate?
   b. What additional tests should be performed to support the diagnosis?
   c. How can this condition be differentiated from Graves disease?

REVIEW QUESTIONS

1. All of the following may contribute to autoimmunity *except:*
   a. Clonal deletion of self-reactive T cells
   b. Molecular mimicry
   c. Increased expression of class II MHC antigens
   d. Polyclonal activation of B cells

2. Which of the following is an organ-specific autoimmune disease?
   a. SLE
   b. RA
   c. GPA
   d. Hashimoto thyroiditis

3. SLE can be distinguished from RA based on which of the following?
   a. Joint pain
   b. Presence of anti-nuclear antibodies
   c. Immune complex formation with activation of complement
   d. Presence of anti-dsDNA antibodies

4. Which of the following supports a diagnosis of drug-induced lupus?
   a. Anti-histone antibodies
   b. Antibodies to Smith antigen
   c. Presence of RF
   d. Antibodies to SS-A and SS-B antigens

5. A speckled pattern of nuclear staining on IIF may be caused by which of the following antibodies?
   a. Anti-dsDNA
   b. Antibody to histones
   c. Centromere antibody
   d. Anti–SS-A/Ro antibody

6. Which of the following would be considered a significant finding in Graves disease?
   a. Increased TSH levels
   b. Antibody to TSH receptor
   c. Decreased T3 and T4
   d. Anti-thyroglobulin antibody

7. Destruction of the myelin sheath of axons caused by the presence of antibody is characteristic of which disease?
   a. Multiple sclerosis
   b. Myasthenia gravis
   c. Graves disease
   d. Anti–glomerular basement membrane disease

8. Blood was drawn from a 25-year-old patient with suspected SLE. A FANA screen was performed, and a speckled pattern resulted. Which action should be taken next?
   a. Report out as diagnostic for SLE.
   b. Report out as drug-induced lupus.
   c. Perform an assay for specific ANAs.
   d. Repeat the test.

9. Which of the following is a mechanism used to achieve peripheral tolerance?
   a. Negative selection of autoreactive T cells in the thymus
   b. Apoptosis of autoreactive B cells in the bone marrow
   c. Editing of B-cell receptors that weakly recognize self-antigens in the bone marrow
   d. Lack of a costimulatory signal to autoreactive T cells in the lymph nodes

10. Epitope spreading refers to:
    a. Post-translational modifications of self-antigens
    b. Changes in gene expression that are not caused by changes in DNA sequence
    c. Expansion of the immune response to additional self-antigens
    d. Cross-reaction of the immune response to a pathogen with a similar self-antigen

11. Anti-CCP (cyclic citrullinated proteins) is specifically associated with which autoimmune disease?
    a. Rheumatoid arthritis
    b. Myasthenia gravis
    c. Autoimmune hepatitis
    d. Systemic sclerosis

12. An IIF for ANCA showed diffuse granular cytoplasmic staining of the neutrophils that was not seen in the lymphocytes. This pattern of fluorescence is strongly associated with which disease?
    a. Systemic lupus erythematosus
    b. Granulomatosis with polyangiitis
    c. Microscopic polyangiitis
    d. Anti–glomerular basement membrane disease

13. A medical laboratory professional performs an IIF test for ANCAs and observes intense fluorescent staining of the nuclear lobes of the neutrophils. How can this type of staining be differentiated from an ANA?
    a. Perform the test on formalin-fixed leukocytes.
    b. Perform IIF with HEp-2 cells.
    c. Perform an ELISA for ANCAs.
    d. All of the above

14. A 20-year-old patient made an appointment to see a physician because of intermittent diarrhea. Laboratory testing revealed an iron-deficiency anemia. To determine if the patient has celiac disease, the doctor should order which of the following laboratory tests?
    a. Anti-tTG
    b. Anti-gliadin
    c. Anti-gluten
    d. All of the above

15. Anti-mitochondrial antibodies are strongly associated with which disease?
    a. Autoimmune hepatitis
    b. Celiac disease
    c. Primary biliary cholangitis
    d. Anti–glomerular basement membrane disease

16. Anti–SS-A/Ro are associated with which disease?
    a. Autoimmune hepatitis
    b. Sjögren syndrome
    c. Scleroderma
    d. Mixed connective tissue disease

Chapter 15 Answer Key

Answers to Knowledge Check

15.1 a **15.2** c **15.3** d **15.4** b **15.5** c **15.6** d
15.7 1-i; 2-f; 3-g; 4-m; 5-k; 6-a; 7-e; 8-l; 9-c; 10-b; 11-d; 12-h; 13-j

Answers to Review Questions

1. a **2.** d **3.** d **4.** a **5.** d **6.** b **7.** a
8. c **9.** d **10.** c **11.** a **12.** b **13.** d **14.** a
15. c **16.** b

16 Transplantation Immunology

John L. Schmitz, PhD, D(ABMLI), F(ACHI)

LEARNING OUTCOMES

After finishing this chapter, you should be able to:

16.1 Describe the histocompatibility systems relevant to clinical transplantation.

16.2 Discuss the polymorphic nature of the human leukocyte antigen (HLA) system and the roles of the class I and class II HLA proteins in the immune response.

16.3 Explain the inheritance of the HLA genes and its implications for transplantation.

16.4 Compare the mechanisms of direct and indirect alloantigen recognition.

16.5 Distinguish between an allograft, autograft, xenograft, and syngeneic graft (isograft).

16.6 Compare the immunologic mechanisms involved in hyperacute, acute, and chronic graft rejection.

16.7 Identify the types of grafts in which graft-vs-host disease (GVHD) could occur and discuss factors that impact the risk of developing GVHD.

16.8 List the major classes of immunosuppressive agents and their effects on the immune system.

16.9 Explain the principles of laboratory methods for HLA typing.

16.10 Describe laboratory methods for detecting and identifying HLA antibodies (i.e., antibody screening, identification, and crossmatching).

16.11 Deduce the suitability of a possible donor for a kidney-transplant recipient, based on results of ABO typing, HLA typing, and antibody identification.

16.12 Identify the preferred donor for a patient in need of a hematopoietic stem cell transplant.

16.13 Describe the nomenclature used for HLA antigens and alleles.

CHAPTER OUTLINE

You can go to **fadavis.com** keyword stevens for the laboratory exercises that accompany this text.

Transplantation is a lifesaving procedure for end-stage organ failure, cancers, autoimmune diseases, immune deficiencies, and various other diseases. Vascular composite allograft (VCA) transplantation (craniofacial, uterus, and limb) is also now a reality. In 2024, more than 48,000 organ and VCA transplants were performed in the United States. More than 50,000 hematopoietic cell transplants (HCTs; also termed bone marrow transplants) are performed worldwide each year for a variety of conditions, including cancer, autoimmune diseases, immunodeficiencies, and others. The number of transplants performed is a testament to the many developments during the past few decades in patient management before and after transplantation and in the technologies for organ or hematopoietic cell acquisition and sharing. Of critical importance has been the growing knowledge of the immunologic mechanisms of graft rejection and graft-vs-host disease (GVHD), including the role of the **human leukocyte antigen (HLA)** system. This information has led to the development of pharmacological agents that promote graft survival by interfering with various components of the immune system.

HLA molecules are the strongest immunologic barrier to successful allogeneic organ and HCT transplantation (see Chapter 4). These cell surface proteins play a central role in the thymic education of T lymphocytes, initiation of adaptive immune responses, and regulation of innate immune system components such as natural killer (NK) cells. Found on the surface of almost all nucleated cells, HLA proteins are antigenically very diverse, with tens of thousands of unique variants in the human population.

Most individuals have unique combinations of several different HLA proteins, and these proteins can elicit strong immune responses in people who have other HLA antigens. Because of the diversity and immunogenicity of the HLA proteins, transplanted cells or organs are recognized as foreign (non-self) by a recipient's immune system unless they happen to be HLA identical. Therefore, transplantation of a solid organ or hematopoietic stem cells (HSCs) into an allogeneic host is likely to result in graft rejection or GVHD without immunosuppressive therapy unless the donor and recipient are HLA identical.

Histocompatibility Systems

Humans have several antigen systems that influence the likelihood of graft rejection. These include the following:

- Major histocompatibility complex antigens (MHC antigens or HLA)
- Minor histocompatibility antigens (mHAs)
- MHC class I–related chain A (MICA) antigens
- ABO blood group antigens
- Non-HLA antigens

Major Histocompatibility Complex (MHC) Antigens

The classical (transplant) HLAs consist of the class I and class II MHC proteins. Class I proteins include HLA-A, HLA-B, and HLA-C; class II proteins consist of HLA-DRB1, HLA-DQB1, HLA-DQA1, HLA-DPB1, and HLA-DPA1. HLA proteins are encoded by a set of closely linked genes located on the short arm of chromosome 6 within the **major histocompatibility complex (MHC).** HLA genes are inherited as **haplotypes** from parental chromosomes **(Fig. 16–1).** A haplotype is a group of closely linked alleles on a single chromosome, for example, HLA-A1, HLA-Cw7, HLA-B8, HLA-DR3, and HLA-DQ2. Offspring receive one maternal and one paternal HLA haplotype. Based on Mendelian inheritance, there is a 25% chance that any two siblings will inherit the same two haplotypes (i.e., are HLA identical), a 50% chance of them being HLA haploidentical (i.e., sharing one of two HLA haplotypes), and a 25% chance of them being HLA nonidentical (i.e., sharing neither HLA haplotype).

HLA proteins are heterodimeric molecules consisting of two different polypeptide chains chemically bound to each other (see Chapter 4). Class I proteins are the product of the HLA-A, HLA-B, and HLA-C genes and are expressed on the cell surface covalently bound to β_2-microglobulin. Class I heterodimers are codominantly expressed on virtually all nucleated cells. Class II heterodimers are the products of the HLA-D region genes. Class II proteins are codominantly expressed, mainly on antigen-presenting cells (APCs; e.g., dendritic cells, monocytes, macrophages, B lymphocytes). For stable expression on the cell surface, both class I and II molecules also are complexed with a short peptide that can be derived from self-proteins or foreign proteins such as proteins from an infectious agent or other exogenous (non-self) protein.

As we discussed in Chapter 4, HLA proteins have critical roles in the development and functioning of the innate and adaptive immune systems. They serve as recognition elements for antigen receptors on T lymphocytes, thus initiating adaptive immune responses. They also serve as ligands

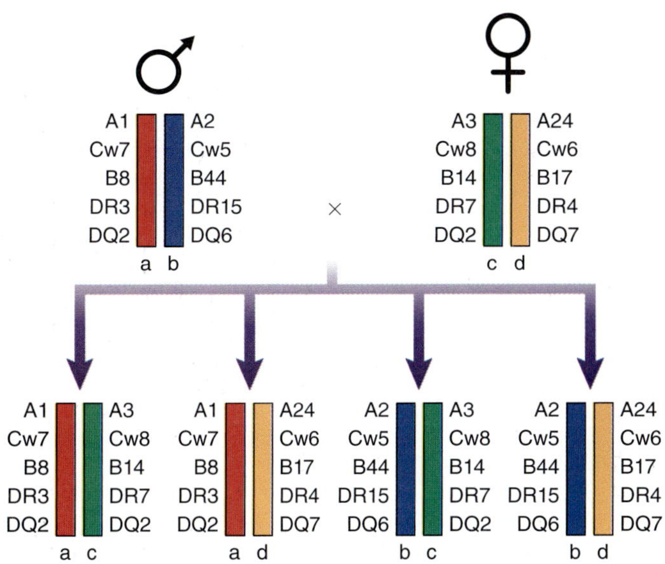

FIGURE 16–1 HLA genes are linked and inherited in Mendelian fashion as haplotypes. One paternal (a or b) and one maternal (c or d) haplotype is passed to each child. Four different combinations of haplotypes are possible in offspring. Elucidation of haplotype sharing between siblings is an important assessment in the search for a transplant donor. *(Figure courtesy of John Schmitz.)*

for regulatory receptors on NK cells in the innate immune response. The CD8 molecule on cytotoxic T lymphocytes (Tc) interacts with class I HLA proteins, whereas the CD4 molecule on helper T (T_H) cells interacts with class II HLA proteins.

A cardinal feature of the genes encoding HLA proteins is the extensive degree of allelic **polymorphism.** Polymorphism is the presence of two or more different genetic compositions among individuals in a population. The HLA system is the most polymorphic genetic system in humans; many HLA genes exist in the population, and numerous combinations of these genes are possible in individuals **(Tables 16–1** and **16–2).** The high degree of polymorphism is believed to have resulted from the benefit of initiating an immune response to a broad array of peptides of pathogenic microbes that populations encounter over time. In other words, the more antigens that can be presented to T cells by a diverse HLA repertoire, the more effectively the immune system can contain an infectious challenge. Although this has successfully enabled populations to survive infectious challenges, it severely restricts the ability to transplant tissues or cells between any two individuals because the HLA proteins are immunogenic and elicit robust allogeneic immune responses.

Knowledge Check 16-1

The biologic function of HLA proteins is to present foreign antigens to:
a. NK cells
b. T cells
c. Dendritic cells
d. B cells

Table 16-1 Approximate Number of HLA Antigens and Alleles Defined at the Classical Transplant Loci[a]

HLA LOCUS	NUMBER OF ANTIGENS	NUMBER OF ALLELES
A	28	8,640
B	62	10,446
C	10	8,743
DRB3	1	546
DRB4	1	292
DRB5	1	221
DQA1	—[b]	890
DQB1	9	2,858
DPA1	—[b]	779
DPB1	—[b]	2,859

[a]*Note: The number of HLA alleles identified has increased tremendously in recent years because of the availability of improved molecular techniques. The numbers in this table were current as of June 2025. To view the most up-to-date information about the HLA alleles discovered, access the websites https://www.ebi.ac.uk/ipd/imgt/hla/about/statistics/ and https://hla.alleles.org/pages/antigens/hla_antigens/*

[b]*HLA antigens encoded by genes in this locus were not previously phenotyped.*

Minor Histocompatibility Antigens (mHAs)

Researchers identified a second set of transplantation antigens based on studies in mice and humans that demonstrated tissue rejection in MHC-identical transplants and the development of GVHD in HLA-identical sibling HSC transplants. The scientists conducting these studies also noted that a "slower" rejection pace was mediated by these transplantation antigens, thus their name—**minor histocompatibility antigens (mHAs).**

The mHAs are non-HLA proteins that are polymorphic (demonstrate variation in the amino acid sequence between individuals). Both X-linked and autosomally encoded mHAs have been identified. Transplanting one individual's tissue or cells containing a polymorphic variant of one of these proteins into another individual possessing a different polymorphic variant can induce a recipient's immune response to the donor variant. CD4 and CD8 T cells recognize the variant protein in an MHC-restricted fashion and mediate the immune response. This response is analogous to the reaction to a microbial antigen. Several mHAs have been identified, including proteins encoded by the male Y chromosome, proteins for which the recipient has a homozygous gene deletion, proteins that are autosomally encoded, and proteins that are encoded by mitochondrial DNA.

MHC Class I–Related Chain A (MICA) Antigens

The MHC class I–related chain A (*MICA*) gene encodes a cell surface protein that is involved in gamma-delta T-cell, NK cell, and T_C cell responses. *MICA* is polymorphic, with more than 500 allelic variants encoding over 200 unique proteins. MICA proteins are expressed on endothelial cells, keratinocytes, fibroblasts, epithelial cells, dendritic cells, and monocytes, but they are not expressed on T or B lymphocytes. As such, MICA proteins could serve as targets for allograft immune responses. Antibodies to MICA antigens have been detected in as many as 11% of kidney-transplant patients and are associated with rejection episodes and decreased graft survival.

ABO Blood Group Antigens

The ABO system is the only blood group system that affects clinical transplantation. ABO blood group incompatibility is a barrier to solid-organ transplantation because antibodies can bind to their corresponding antigens that are expressed on the vascular endothelium. Binding activates the complement cascade, which can lead to very rapid rejection of the transplanted organ. This phenomenon, known as **hyperacute rejection,** occurs within minutes to hours after the vascular supply to the transplanted organ is established (see "Transplant Rejection"). Anti-A or anti-B antibodies develop in individuals lacking the corresponding blood group antigens. Thus, recipient-donor pairs must be ABO identical or compatible to avoid this adverse outcome. For example, a person of blood group A will possess anti-B antibodies and can thus receive an organ only from an ABO type A or type O donor. Likewise, a

Table 16-2 Listing of Individual HLA Antigens[a]

HLA-A		HLA-B			HLA-C	HLA-DR	HLA-DQ
1	68(28)	5	42	65(14)	w1	1	1
2	69(28)	7	44(12)	67	w2	103	2
203	74(19)	703	45(12)	70	w3	2	3
210	80	8	46	71(70)	w4	3	4
3		12	47	72(70)	w5	4	5(1)
9		13	48	73	w6	5	6(1)
10		14	49(21)	75(15)	w7	6	7(3)
11		15	50(21)	76(15)	w8	7	8(3)
19		16	51(5)	77(15)	w9(w3)	8	9(3)
23(9)		17	5102	78	w10(w3)	9	
24(9)		18	5103	81		10	
2403		21	52(5)	82		11(5)	
25(10)		22	53	Bw4		12(5)	
26(10)		27	54(22)	Bw6		13(6)	
28		2708	55(22)			14(6)	
29(19)		35	56(22)			1403	
30(19)		37	57(17)			1404	
31(19)		38(16)	58(17)			15(2)	
32(19)		39(16)	59			16(2)	
33(19)		3901	60(40)			17(3)	
34(10)		3902	61(40)			18(3)	
36		40	62(15)			51	
43		4005	63(15)			52	
66(10)		41	64(14)			53	

[a]Note: HLA antigen names begin with the prefix "HLA-" followed by the gene locus (A, B, C, or D) and the antigen number (e.g., HLA-A2). A "w" was originally placed after newly identified antigens at International Histocompatibility Workshops. The "w" has been retained for HLA-C antigen names to differentiate them from complement proteins (e.g., HLA-Cw1). The presence of a serological name that includes a second number in parentheses (e.g., A68[28] and A69[28]) identifies two serological specificities that were both originally classified as the "parent" (A28) antigen but were subsequently determined to be antigenically distinct (A68 and A69).

B-expressing individual has anti-A antibodies and can receive an organ only from an ABO type B or type O donor.

Some transplant centers perform ABO incompatible kidney transplants. This is a complex process involving plasmapheresis and IV immunoglobulin administration to reduce the anti-A/B titer and allow successful transplant.

Other Non-HLA Antigens

In addition to these well-described alloantigen systems, humoral immune responses to other non-HLA antigens in transplant recipients have been associated with poor transplant outcomes, although a direct causal relationship has yet to be firmly established. Among the several proteins to which antibodies have been described posttransplantation are angiotensin II type 1 receptor, vimentin, K-α_1-tubulin, collagen-V, and myosin.

Allorecognition

Transplantation of cells or tissues is classified by the genetic relatedness of the donor and the recipient.

- An **autograft** is the transfer of tissue from one area of the body to another in the same individual.
- A **syngeneic graft** (or **isograft**) is the transfer of cells or tissues between individuals of the same species who are genetically identical, for example, identical twins.
- An **allograft** is the transfer of cells or tissue between two genetically disparate individuals of the same species.
- Finally, a **xenograft** is the transfer of tissue between two individuals of different species.

Most transplants fall into the category of allografts. The HLA disparity between donor and recipient that occurs with allografts and xenografts will result in a vigorous cellular and humoral immune response to the mismatched (foreign) MHC antigens. This response is the main stimulus of graft rejection.

The recipient's immune system recognizes foreign HLA proteins via two distinct mechanisms: direct and indirect allorecognition **(Fig. 16–2).** In **direct allorecognition**, recipient T cells bind and respond directly to foreign (allo) HLA proteins on donor APCs. Direct allorecognition is characterized by a high frequency (up to 10%) of responding T cells compared with the responder frequency in a typical T-cell response to a foreign antigen. This may occur because T cells that recognize similar HLA antigens or viral antigens may also contribute to the response.

The **mixed lymphocyte reaction (MLR)** is an in vitro correlate of direct allorecognition. In this assay, lymphocytes from a person needing a transplant are incubated with lymphocytes from a potential donor that have been inactivated so they cannot proliferate. A disparity in the HLA-D antigens (class II antigens) found on the two populations of lymphocytes results in the proliferation of the recipient cells, which can be quantitated by incorporation of radiolabeled (^3H) thymidine into the DNA of the proliferating cells. The amount of radioactivity taken up by the cells increases in proportion to the amount of cell proliferation. Thus, a high level of radioactivity indicates that the recipient's T cells have divided in response to different HLA-D antigens on a potential donor's cells and that such a donor would be more likely to stimulate graft rejection.

Indirect allorecognition is the second pathway by which the immune system recognizes foreign (donor) HLA proteins. Indirect allorecognition involves the uptake, processing, and presentation of foreign HLA proteins by the recipient's APCs to the recipient's CD4 T cells (see Fig. 16–2). It is analogous to the normal mechanism of recognition of foreign antigens. Indirect allorecognition may play a predominant role in initiating alloantibody production and chronic rejection.

Transplant Rejection

The effector responses against transplanted allogeneic tissue include direct cytotoxicity, delayed-type hypersensitivity (DTH) responses, and antibody-mediated mechanisms. Antibodies can mediate antibody-dependent cellular cytotoxicity reactions and fix complement, resulting in cell death. Rejection episodes can be classified into three types according to the time of occurrence and the effector mechanism involved. In the sections that follow, we discuss these rejection types—hyperacute, acute, and chronic—in detail.

A third allorecognition pathway (semi-direct) has been suggested that involves the direct transfer of donor HLA proteins to recipient dendritic cells. It is expected that subsequent recognition by recipient T cells then occurs. The role of this pathway is being defined.

Hyperacute Rejection

As we previously discussed, hyperacute rejection occurs within minutes to hours after the vascular supply to the transplanted organ is established (in some cases, rejection may occur in an accelerated fashion several days after transplant and has been referred to as *accelerated vascular rejection*). This type of rejection is mediated by preformed antibody that reacts with donor vascular endothelium. ABO incompatibility or mismatched HLA antigens may be the antigenic target of

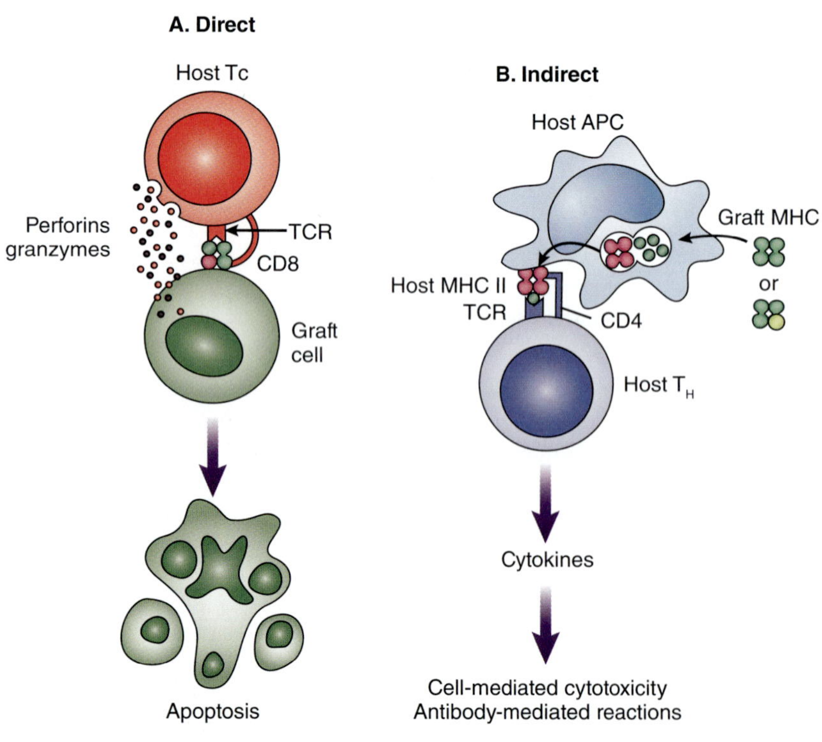

FIGURE 16–2 Direct vs indirect allorecognition. (A) In direct allorecognition, cytotoxic T cells from the host bind directly to foreign HLA (MHC I) proteins on graft cells. (B) In indirect allorecognition, APCs from the host present foreign MHC I or MHC II antigens to $CD4^+$ T_H cells, which produce cytokines that stimulate graft rejection.

hyperacute rejection. Antibodies to these antigens may be present because of blood transfusion, prior transplantation, or exposure of a pregnant woman to fetal antigens of paternal origin. Binding of preformed antibodies to the alloantigens activates the complement cascade and clotting mechanisms and leads to thrombus formation. The result is ischemia and necrosis of the transplanted tissue.

Hyperacute rejection is seldom encountered in clinical transplantation. Donor-recipient pairs are chosen to be ABO identical or compatible, and patients awaiting transplantation are regularly tested for the presence of preformed HLA antibodies. This facilitates donor matching that avoids organ offers from donors with mismatched HLA antigens for which the candidate has antibodies (e.g., donor = HLA-A2 positive, and recipient has anti-HLA-A2 antibodies). The absence of donor HLA-specific antibodies is also confirmed before transplant by the performance of a **crossmatch** test (see "HLA Antibody Screening, Identification, and Crossmatching"). These practices have virtually eliminated hyperacute rejection episodes.

Acute Rejection

Days to months after transplant, individuals may develop **acute rejection (AR).** AR can be mediated by an acute cellular (T-cell) response (ACR) or by donor-specific antibody (also known as *antibody-mediated rejection* [ABMR]). The pathological features of AR vary by organ, but several concepts are generalizable.

ACR is characterized by parenchymal and vascular injury. Interstitial cellular infiltrates contain a predominance of $CD8^+$ T cells, $CD4^+$ T cells, and macrophages. $CD8^+$ T cells likely mediate cytotoxic reactions to foreign MHC-expressing cells, whereas $CD4^+$ T cells likely produce cytokines and induce delayed-type hypersensitivity (DTH) reactions. Natural killer cells may also be involved in ACR. Antibody may be involved in acute graft rejection by binding to vessel walls and activating complement. The antibody induces necrosis and inflammation as opposed to the thrombosis typical of hyperacute rejection. Diagnostic criteria include characteristic histological findings, deposition of the complement protein C4d in the capillaries surrounding the renal tubules, and detection of donor-specific HLA antibody. The development and application of potent immunosuppressive drugs that target multiple pathways in the immune response to alloantigens have improved early graft survival of solid-organ transplants by reducing the incidence of AR and providing approaches for its effective treatment.

Chronic Rejection

Chronic rejection results from a process of graft arteriosclerosis characterized by progressive fibrosis and scarring with narrowing of the vessel lumen caused by proliferation of smooth muscle cells. Chronic rejection remains the most significant cause of graft loss after the first year of transplantation because it is not readily amenable to treatment. Several predisposing factors affect the development of chronic rejection, including prolonged cold ischemia, reperfusion injury, AR episodes, and toxicity from immunosuppressive drugs. Chronic rejection is also thought to have an immunologic component, presumably a DTH reaction to foreign HLA proteins. Studies support important roles for CD4 T cells, interferon gamma (IFN-γ), and B cells (HLA antibody) in this process. Cytokines and growth factors—secreted by endothelial cells, smooth muscle cells, and macrophages activated by interferon gamma—stimulate smooth muscle cell accumulation in the graft vasculature. Alloantibody production likely contributes to the development of chronic rejection as well.

Knowledge Check 16-2

Hyperacute rejection occurs:

a. Months after transplant due to preformed HLA antibody
b. Months after transplant due to donor-specific T cells
c. Hours after transplant due to preformed HLA antibody
d. Hours after transplant due to donor-specific T cells

Graft-vs-Host Disease (GVHD)

HCT transplants (and less commonly lung and liver transplants) are complicated by a unique allogeneic response—graft-vs-host disease (GVHD). In this condition, lymphoid cells in the graft mount an immune response against the host's histocompatibility antigens **(Fig. 16–3)**. Recipients of HCT transplants for hematologic malignancies typically have bone marrow ablated (depleted of cellular components) before transplantation to treat the malignancy and make room for incoming stem cells to repopulate the marrow. The individual receives an infusion of donor bone marrow or, more commonly, peripheral blood stem cells. The infused products often contain some mature T cells. These cells have several beneficial effects, including promotion of engraftment, reconstitution of immunity, and mediation of a graft-vs-leukemia (GVL) effect. The GVL effect is like the GVH response but targets the recipient's malignant cells instead of the recipient's healthy tissues, such as the skin and gastrointestinal tract. However, these mature T cells may also mediate GVHD.

Acute GVHD occurs during the first 100 days postinfusion and manifests in the skin, gastrointestinal tract, and liver. In mismatched allogeneic stem cell transplantation, the targets of GVHD are the mismatched HLA proteins, whereas in matched stem cell transplantation, mHAs are targeted. The infused T cells can mediate GVHD in several ways, including through a massive release of cytokines because of large-scale activation of the donor cells by MHC-mismatched proteins and by infiltration and destruction of tissue.

The incidence and severity of GVHD are related to the HLA match status of the donor and recipient and other factors. The recipient's medical team can take several approaches to reduce the incidence and severity of GVHD, including immunosuppressive therapy in the early posttransplant period and removal of T lymphocytes from the graft. T-cell reduction, achieved by purification of donor hematopoietic cells from the peripheral blood or bone marrow collection, is very effective in lowering the incidence of GVHD, but it can also reduce the GVL effect of the infused cells and increase the incidence of graft failure.

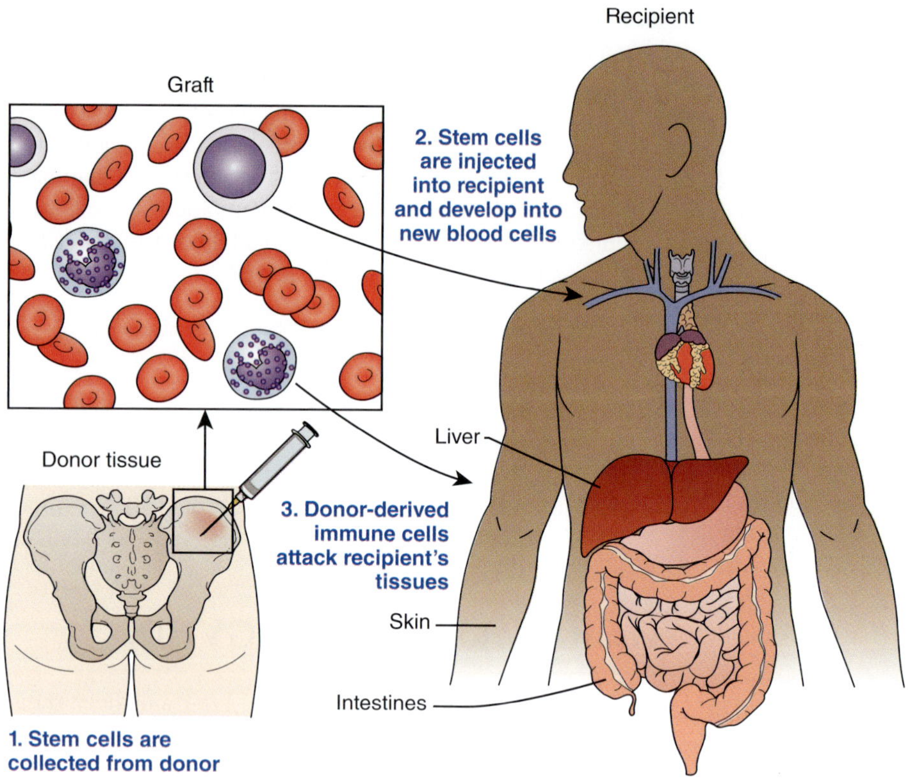

FIGURE 16–3 Graft-vs-host disease (GVHD). GVHD is caused by the reaction of T cells in the donor graft (e.g., bone marrow or peripheral blood stem cells) against mismatched HLA proteins in the recipient's tissues. This results in damage to the recipient's tissues, especially the skin, intestines, and liver.

Beyond 100 days' posttransplant, patients may experience chronic GVHD. This condition resembles autoimmune disease, with fibrosis affecting the skin, eyes, mouth, and other mucosal surfaces.

Critical Thinking 16-1

The following HLA typing results were obtained for a donor-recipient pair being worked up for a bone marrow (HCT) transplant. As you can see, there is an HLA mismatch at the HLA-A locus. Is this mismatch more likely to result in a graft-vs-host reaction or a host-vs-graft reaction?

	A	B	C	DRB1	DQB1
Patient	23:01	07:02	07:01	11:01	04:02
	23:01	42:01	17:01G	03:02	02:02
Donor	03:01	07:02	07:01G	11:01	04:02
	23:01	42:01	07:01G	03:02	02:02

Immunosuppressive Agents

The list of agents that suppress antigraft immune responses in solid-organ and HCT transplantation is growing. **Immunosuppressive agents** are used in several ways, including induction and maintenance of immune suppression and treatment of rejection. Combinations of different agents are frequently used to prevent graft rejection. However, the immunosuppressed state (and graft survival) induced by these agents comes at a price of increased susceptibility to infection, malignancies, and other associated toxic side effects. There are several classes of immunosuppressive agents:

- *Corticosteroids:* Corticosteroids are potent anti-inflammatory and immunosuppressive agents used for immunosuppression maintenance. At higher doses, they are used to treat AR episodes. Steroids act by blocking the production and secretion of cytokines, inflammatory mediators, chemoattractants, and adhesion molecules. These activities decrease macrophage function and alter leukocyte-trafficking patterns. However, long-term use is associated with several complications, including hypertension and diabetes mellitus.
- *Antimetabolites:* Antimetabolites interfere with the maturation of lymphocytes and kill proliferating cells. Azathioprine was the first such agent employed. It has been replaced in large part by mycophenolate mofetil, which has a more selective effect on lymphocytes compared with azathioprine and thus fewer side effects.
- *Calcineurin inhibitors:* Cyclosporine and tacrolimus are compounds that block signal transduction in T lymphocytes, resulting in impaired synthesis of cytokines such as interleukin (IL) 2, IL-3, IL-4, and IFN-γ. Inhibition of cytokine synthesis blocks the growth and differentiation of T cells, impairing the antigraft response. Rapamycin (sirolimus) is an agent that inhibits T-cell proliferation by binding to specific intracellular proteins, including mammalian target of rapamycin (mTOR). mTOR is an intracellular molecule involved in cellular functions such as proliferation and motility.
- *Monoclonal antibodies:* Several monoclonal antibodies that bind to cell surface molecules on lymphocytes are

used at the time of organ transplant and to treat severe rejection episodes after transplantation:

- Basiliximab binds CD25 (IL-2 receptor), interfering with IL-2–mediated T-cell activation. It may also deplete CD25-expressing cells.
- Alemtuzumab targets the CD52 receptor found on T and B lymphocytes and may be used for induction therapy at the time of transplantation.
- Rituximab, a chimeric antibody targeting the CD20 antigen on B cells, may be used for treatment of antibody-mediated rejection and as an induction agent (in highly sensitized candidates) to reduce the risk of antibody-mediated rejection.

A problem with some monoclonal antibody preparations is that patients can develop antibodies that may interfere with the effectiveness of these agents. The potential for this problem to occur is being reduced with increased use of humanized and fully human monoclonal antibodies (see Chapters 3 and 25):

- *Polyclonal antibodies:* Two polyclonal anti–T-cell antibody preparations have been used as induction agents or to treat severe rejection. Thymoglobulin is an antithymocyte antibody prepared in rabbits, and ATGAM is a polyclonal antiserum prepared from the immunization of horses. Both are potent immunosuppressive agents that deplete lymphocytes from the circulation. A drawback associated with the administration of polyclonal antibody preparations is the development of serum sickness because of antibody responses to the foreign immunoglobulins (see Chapter 14).

Clinical Histocompatibility Testing

Many studies have shown a significant improvement in graft survival when **HLA matching** is performed to maximize the HLA similarities between recipient and donor and when the recipient lacks antibodies to the donor's HLA antigens. Therefore, specialized testing to aid in the selection of the most appropriate donors for patients needing transplantation has been developed. Histocompatibility laboratories provide specialized testing for both solid-organ and HCT programs. Two main activities are carried out by these laboratories in support of transplantation: HLA typing and HLA antibody screening and identification.

HLA Typing

HLA typing is the identification of the HLA antigens (phenotype) or genes (genotype) in a transplant candidate or donor. For clinical HLA testing, phenotypes or genotypes of the classical transplant antigens or genes are determined (HLA-A, HLA-B, HLA-C, HLA-DR, HLA-DQ, HLA-DP). This information contributes to identification of the most immunologically suitable (lowest rejection risk) donor for a recipient in need of a solid organ transplant (SOT) or hematopoietic cell transplant (HCT). It must be stressed that other factors are also considered when choosing a particular donor for any given patient. For example, ABO compatibility and infectious disease status are important considerations in donor selection.

HLA Phenotyping

The classic procedure for determining the **HLA phenotype** is the **complement-dependent cytotoxicity (CDC)** test. Panels of antisera or monoclonal antibodies that bind to specific individual HLA antigens or groups of immunologically similar HLA antigens are incubated with lymphocytes from the person to be HLA typed in separate wells of a microtiter plate (Terasaki tray). Each well of the plate contains a different antibody preparation. It is important to note that multiple antisera are used for HLA typing. This requirement is based on the presence of both unique (private) epitopes on HLA molecules (those that identify a single specific HLA antigen) and public epitopes (epitopes that are present on more than one unique HLA protein). Because responses to public epitopes are common, multiple sera must be used to define a pattern of reactivity that correlates with a specific HLA antigen. T and B lymphocytes are used for HLA class I typing, whereas purified B lymphocytes are used for HLA class II typing because class II antigens are not found on most T cells.

Binding of antibody occurs only if the lymphocytes express the HLA antigen targeted by the antisera. After incubation with the antisera, reagent complement (from rabbit serum) is added. If the cells possess the HLA antigen recognized by the antibody in that well, complement is activated, and the cells are killed. A vital dye such as eosin red or trypan blue is added to distinguish live cells from dead cells, and the wells of the Terasaki tray are viewed microscopically. The dead cells, whose membranes have been made more permeable, can take up the dye and appear colored, whereas the live cells, whose membranes remain intact, cannot take up the dye and remain colorless. The proportion of dead cells is estimated by microscopic examination and scored according to the following scale, established by the American Society for Histocompatibility and Immunogenetics (ASHI):

- 1 = 0% to 10% cell death; negative
- 2 = 11% to 20% cell death; doubtful negative
- 4 = 21% to 50% cell death; weak positive
- 6 = 51% to 80% cell death; positive
- 8 = 81% to 100% cell death; strong positive
- 0 = unreadable

The principle of the CDC test is illustrated in **Figure 16–4.** Using this assay, an extensive array of HLA antigens can be defined (see Table 16–2).

The CDC method has several limitations for HLA typing. Viable lymphocytes must be used, which demands timely performance of the assay. Separation of T and B lymphocytes is required for differentiation of class I vs class II antigens. In addition, the source of antisera for HLA typing is not always consistent or reliable. Thus, reagents can vary in quality or quantity over time. Finally, the level of resolution (i.e., the ability to distinguish two closely related yet distinct HLA antigens) is limited. The limits of resolution do not significantly affect the role of this technology for matching solid-organ donors and recipients. However, for allogeneic stem cell transplantation, a higher level of resolution is required. DNA-based (molecular) HLA typing methods are now commonly used in histocompatibility laboratories because

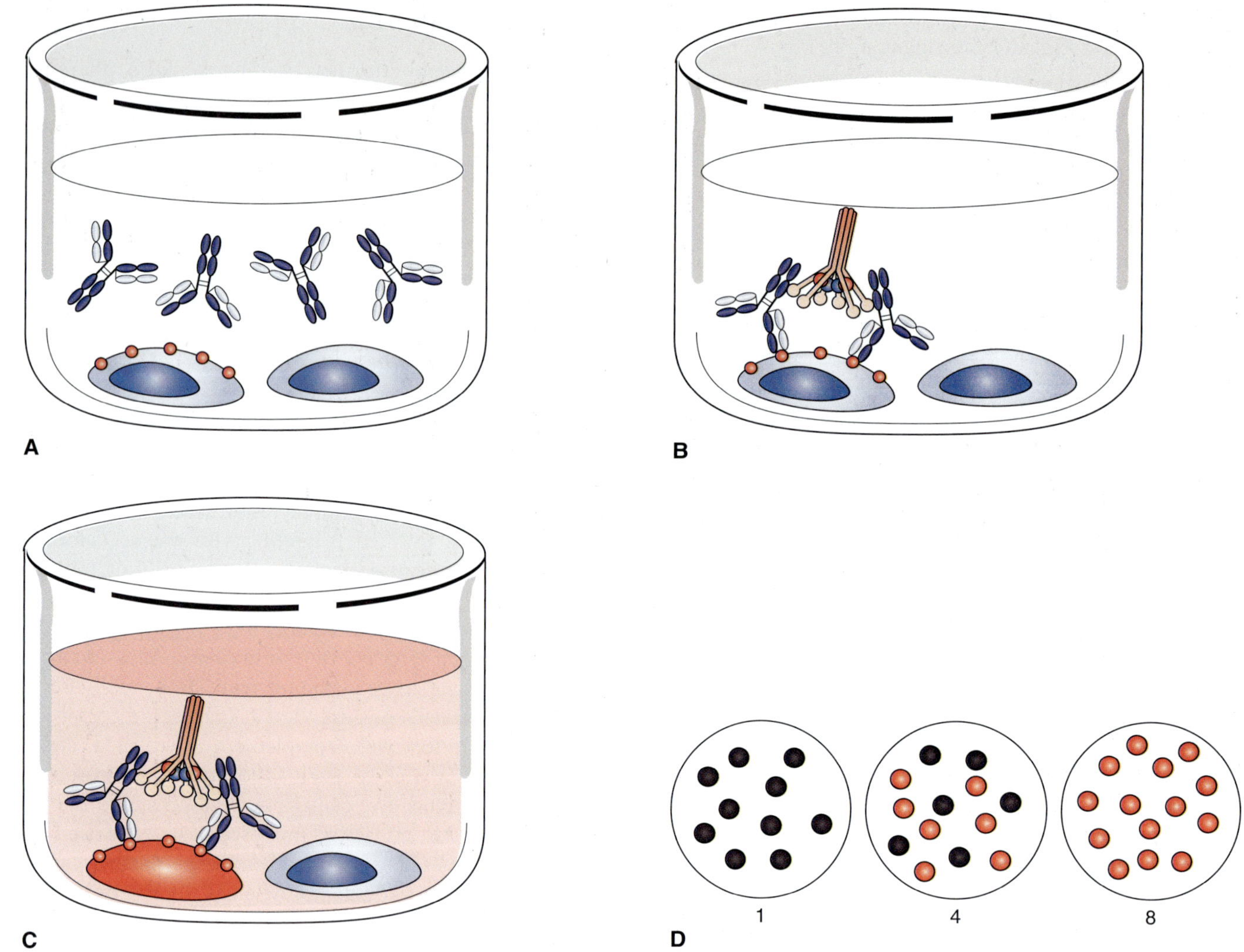

FIGURE 16–4 Principle of the complement-dependent cytotoxicity (CDC) test. (A) Addition of patient lymphocytes to wells containing specific HLA antisera. (B) Addition of reagent complement after binding of antisera to lymphocytes possessing the corresponding HLA antigen. (C) Addition of a vital dye. (D) Scoring of results.

their higher resolution, reagent quality and consistency, and amenability to higher throughput formats overcome the limitations of CDC-based methods. As such, relatively few laboratories continue to perform cytotoxicity-based HLA typing.

HLA Genotyping

Molecular HLA genotyping methods use polymerase chain reaction (PCR)-based amplification of HLA genes followed by analysis of the amplified DNA to identify the specific HLA allele or allele group (see Chapter 12). Three DNA-based HLA typing methods are in routine use: PCR with sequence-specific primers (PCR-SSP), PCR-sequence-specific oligonucleotide probe hybridization (PCR-SSOP), and sequence-based typing (SBT). The choice of methods is dictated in part by the level of typing resolution needed for the clinical application (i.e., SOT vs HCT).

One of the common approaches for analysis involves PCR amplification of HLA genes with panels of primer pairs, each of which amplifies specific alleles or related allele groups (PCR-SSP). Only those primer pairs that are perfectly base-pair matched to the target gene result in the generation of an amplification product **(Fig. 16–5).** Amplification is detected by agarose gel electrophoresis or a fluorescent label in a quantitative PCR (qPCR). The **HLA genotype** is then identified by determining the HLA alleles (allele group) that are amplified by the positive primer pairs (i.e., those demonstrating a specific band on the gel). A modification of the gel-based PCR-SSP replaces gel electrophoresis with DNA melt curve analysis after qPCR amplification (see Chapter 12). This method has the advantage of more rapid, automated analysis.

A second common approach for HLA genotyping is PCR-SSOP. This method involves a single PCR reaction that will amplify all HLA gene variants at a specific locus (referred to as a *generic amplification*). The amplified gene is then subjected to hybridization with a panel of DNA probes, each specific for a unique HLA allele or allele group. Only those probes that specifically hybridize to the amplified DNA will be detected. The HLA genotype is determined by assessing which probes are hybridized **(Fig. 16–6).**

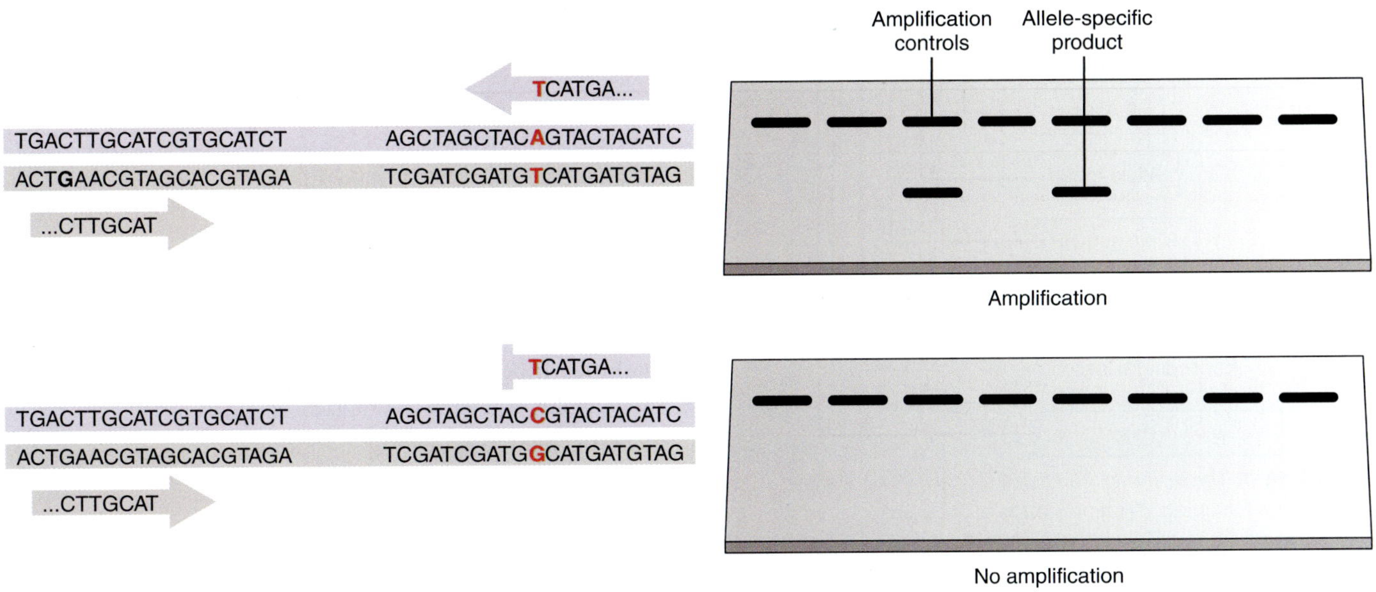

FIGURE 16–5 Principle of PCR-SSP. The sequence-specific primer ending in 3′ TCATGA . . . 5′ will be extended only from a template carrying the polymorphism shown in the top part of the figure.

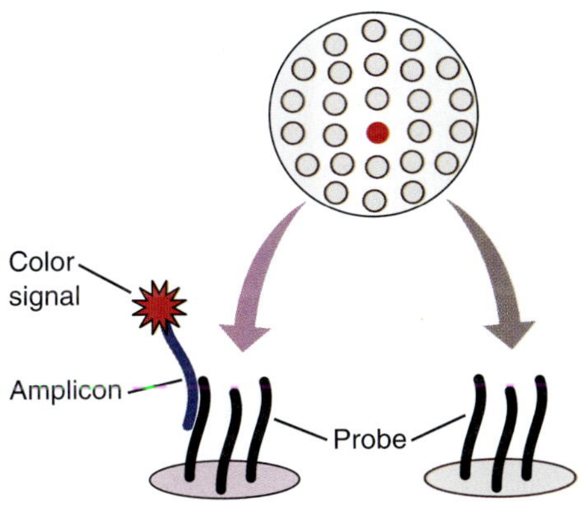

FIGURE 16–6 Principle of PCR-SSOP. Patient DNA is amplified using primers typically labeled with biotin at the 5′ end. The amplicons are then hybridized to panels of probes immobilized on a solid phase, most often a series of microbeads. If the sequence of the amplicon matches and hybridizes to that of the probe, a secondary reaction with fluorochrome conjugated streptavidin will generate a light signal when exposed to a laser (bottom left). If the sequence of the amplicon differs from that of the probe, no signal is generated (bottom right).

A third common method for HLA genotyping is SBT, which involves sequencing of PCR-amplified HLA genes. SBT can be carried out using Sanger dideoxy chain terminator sequencing (see Chapter 12). A generic amplification of the HLA gene of interest is conducted, followed by a sequencing reaction using dideoxy nucleotides. The dideoxy terminators are fluorescently labeled. Incorporation into the synthesized DNA molecule is detected using automated DNA sequencers with fluorescent detectors. The sequence of the target gene is compared with an HLA sequence database to determine the specific HLA allele for the patient.

SBT for HLA typing is considered the gold standard and can detect new allelic variants because it interrogates all nucleotides in the amplified target region as opposed to PCR-SSP and PCR-SSOP, which target small stretches of previously defined nucleotides. More recently, next-generation sequencing (NGS) technologies have been developed and used for HLA genotyping. This technology has the advantage over Sanger sequencing of providing unambiguous high-resolution/allele-level typing more consistently due to its ability to phase heterozygous base positions. NGS is rapidly becoming the most common HLA typing method, especially in laboratories that support HCT programs.

HLA genotyping overcomes the limitations of CDC-based HLA phenotyping. Cells do not need to be viable to obtain DNA for HLA genotyping. Typing reagents are chemically synthesized; thus, there is no reliance on human donors of antisera. HLA genotyping can provide varying levels of resolution that can be tailored to the specific clinical need. DNA-based typing can provide results at a level of resolution comparable with CDC-based typing (low-resolution antigen equivalent) or can provide results at the high-resolution or allele level, which are required for matching of unrelated hematopoietic (HSC) donors and recipients. Allele-level HLA typing has demonstrated the incredible extent of polymorphism within the HLA loci (see Table 16–1). The nomenclature used for HLA genotyping is explained in **Figure 16–7.**

Knowledge Check 16-3

In the allele HLA-B*07:02:01:37, what does the "02" represent?

a. The allele group
b. The specific allele number
c. A synonymous nucleotide variation
d. A polymorphism in an intron of the gene

HLA Antibody Screening, Identification, and Crossmatching

To prevent antibody-mediated graft rejection, the histocompatibility laboratory must test for the presence of HLA antibodies in a transplant recipient that could potentially react

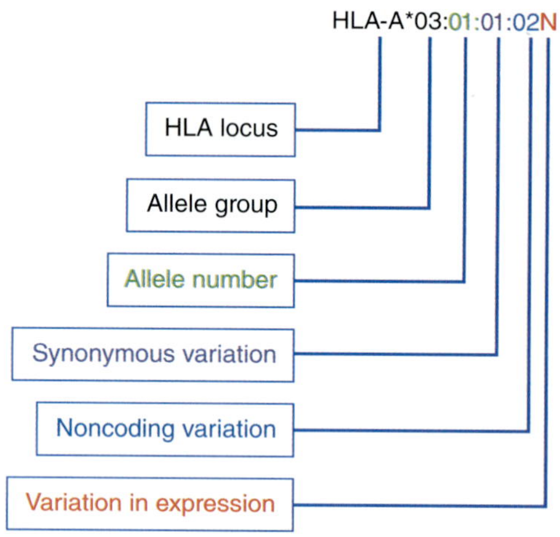

FIGURE 16–7 The nomenclature used for naming HLA alleles includes the following: (1) identification of the HLA locus, which is separated from the allele number by an asterisk (*). (2) The first two digits of the allele number, which typically correspond to the phenotypic group. (3) The next position after the ":" identifies the specific allele within the allele group. This position can accommodate up to three digits. (4) The next position identifies allelic variants resulting from synonymous nucleotide substitutions (i.e., they do not result in a change in the amino acid). (5) The next position identifies allelic variants resulting from polymorphisms in noncoding regions of the gene (i.e., introns). (6) Last, a letter may be added that indicates unique features of the allele, such as "N" indicating the allele is null (i.e., not expressed on the cell surface). *(Figure courtesy of John Schmitz.)*

with the donor graft. This process involves HLA antibody screening, identification, and crossmatching.

Antibody Screening and Identification

Antibodies to HLA antigens can be detected in candidates for and recipients of solid-organ transplants. These antibodies can develop in response to multiple blood transfusions or to prior HLA-mismatched transplants. They can also be produced by women who have had multiple pregnancies in response to paternally derived fetal antigens. Because of the potential adverse impact HLA donor-specific antibodies (HLA DSA) can have on graft survival, patients awaiting solid-organ transplantation are tested regularly for their presence with an **HLA antibody screen.** If detected, the HLA antigen specificity of the antibodies is then determined, typically by multiplex bead arrays, so that donors possessing those HLA antigens can be eliminated from consideration for donation to that patient. Antibody screening and identification are also performed after transplantation to aid in the diagnosis of antibody-mediated rejection or to assess the effectiveness of therapy for antibody-mediated rejection. Crossmatching is performed just before transplant to confirm the absence of donor-specific HLA antibody.

The methods used for antibody detection, identification, and crossmatching have changed significantly in recent years. The CDC method for HLA typing has also been used for HLA antibody detection and identification. In this case, panels of lymphocytes with defined HLA phenotypes are incubated with the patient's serum. If the serum contains HLA antibodies, they will bind to those lymphocytes in the panel that express the corresponding HLA antigen. Binding is detected by the addition of rabbit complement and a vital dye to assess cell death microscopically (see Fig. 16–4). Usually, 30 to 60 unique donor lymphocyte preparations are included in the panel; the proportion of these donor lymphocytes that are killed by antibody in the patient's serum is referred to as the *percent panel reactive antibody (%PRA)*. The specificity of the antibodies (i.e., what HLA antigens they bind to) may also be determined by evaluating the phenotype of the panel cells. Limitations of CDC antibody testing include the need for viable lymphocytes, manual nature of the testing, limited sensitivity, and poor ability to identify reactivity to specific HLA antigens if the patient has high levels of antibody (i.e., reacts to many different HLA antigens).

More recently, the determination of PRA for solid-organ allocation has been modified. Currently, a **calculated PRA (cPRA)** is determined for deceased donor kidney allocation. In this approach, the HLA antigens to which a candidate has HLA antibody are determined using solid-phase immunoassays. These antigens are then classified as unacceptable for that candidate. Accordingly, donors expressing those antigens are excluded from donation to that candidate. The proportion of potential donors in the population to which the transplant candidate belongs who possess one or more of the unacceptable antigens is determined and reported as the cPRA value. For example, a transplant candidate in the United States with an HLA-A2 antibody would have a cPRA value of 48% because 48% of people in the United States are projected to express HLA-A2, based on historic HLA typing data.

Solid-phase antibody detection and identification use flow cytometry or Luminex (multiplex bead array) technology. HLA-specific antibody in patient serum is captured on beads coated with purified HLA antigens, from a pool of donors, an individual donor, or a single purified or recombinant HLA protein. Beads coated with pooled HLA proteins are a sensitive qualitative screen for the presence of HLA antibody because they will detect antibodies to most common HLA antigens. Beads coated with purified or recombinant HLA proteins of a single HLA antigen type, called single-antigen beads, are then used to determine the specificity of the HLA antibodies in a patient's serum; this information is used to determine the cPRA. Patient serum is incubated with the beads, and bound antibody is detected by adding a fluorochrome-labeled anti-IgG reagent **(Fig. 16–8)**. A more recent version of flow cytometry–based antibody detection is the multiplex bead array (Luminex) system that can classify patient antibodies to up to 100 different HLA antigens in a single tube. Solid-phase single antigen bead arrays are the most sensitive technology for detecting HLA antibodies, and they provide the best determination of the specificity of HLA antibodies.

Crossmatching

Primarily for kidney transplantation, once a suitable donor has been identified for a particular patient, a donor-recipient crossmatch test is performed to confirm the absence of donor-specific antibody (DSA). To perform the crossmatch, donor T and B lymphocytes are incubated with recipient

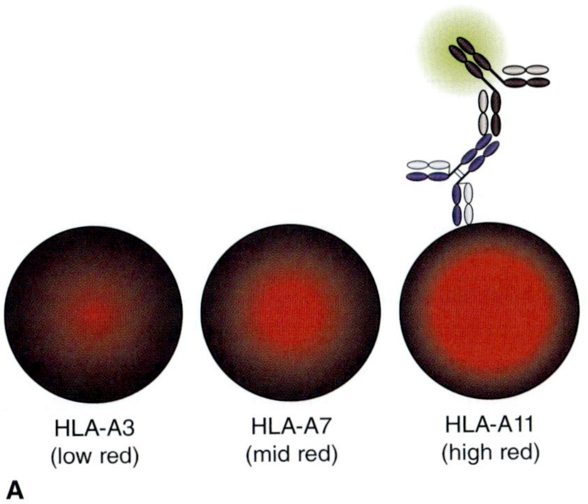

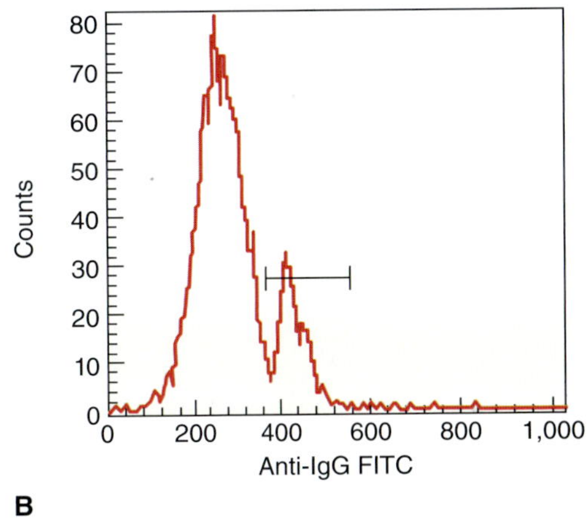

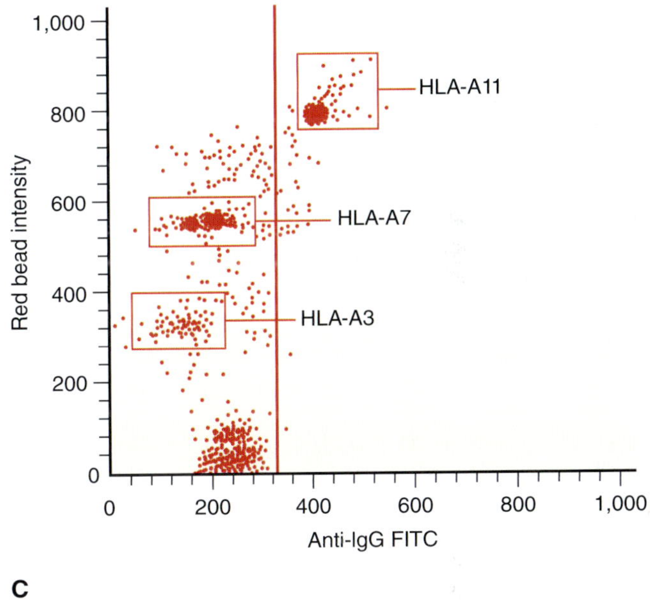

FIGURE 16–8 Flow cytometric detection and identification of antibodies. (A) Patient serum is incubated with a mixture of polystyrene beads coated with different HLA proteins (e.g., HLA-A3, HLA-A7, HLA-A11). The beads have been labeled with various amounts of a red dye for identification. Any HLA antibodies present in the serum will bind to the corresponding beads. After washing, patient antibodies bound to the beads are detected by the addition of a fluorescein isothiocyanate (FITC)-labeled anti-IgG reagent. After a second wash, the beads are analyzed for fluorescence on a flow cytometer. (B) Single-parameter histogram display of an HLA class I antibody screen using the three types of HLA-coated beads. The large peak represents beads with no bound antibody, whereas the smaller peak to the right indicates the presence of HLA antibody bound to approximately 29% of the HLA class I coated beads. This represents a positive HLA class I antibody screen. (C) The individual bead populations are identified in the dual-parameter dot plot. Note that the beads coated with HLA-A11 have shifted to the right relative to the other beads, indicating that the HLA antibodies in this patient's serum are specific for the A11 antigen.

serum in a CDC assay. Microscopic analysis is used to verify a lack of binding after the addition of complement and a vital dye to differentiate live cells from dead cells. Cell death is an indication of recipient antibody binding to donor HLA antigen(s), which signifies a positive crossmatch.

While CDC crossmatching is the classic method for identifying HLA antibodies, it has limited sensitivity. Alternatively, antibody binding can be detected by flow cytometry using a fluorochrome-labeled anti-IgG reagent to detect donor-specific antibody bound to donor T and/or B lymphocytes. As with antibody screening and identification, the flow cytometric crossmatch is the most sensitive method for detecting DSA. Although the flow cytometry crossmatch has been the "gatekeeper" for detecting the presence of DSA, it is being replaced, in certain situations, with a "virtual crossmatch." In this scenario, the recipient HLA antibody profile (i.e., the list of HLA antigens to which the patient has antibodies) is compared to the donor HLA type. If the recipient has antibodies targeting donor HLA antigens, a positive virtual crossmatch is defined. The lack of donor-specific HLA antibodies is considered a negative virtual crossmatch. Using this approach, some centers will proceed to transplant based on the virtual HLA DSA assessment alone.

Critical Thinking 16-2

Suppose you performed a flow cytometric crossmatch test for a patient donor pair in anticipation of a kidney transplant. The patient is known to have a high-level antibody to the class I antigen HLA-A2. The donor's HLA type includes the HLA-A2 antigen. When you perform the crossmatch and assess binding to T and B cells independently, what results (positive or negative) are expected for binding to the donor T cells and B cells?

Posttransplant Testing

Patients who received a SOT or HCT are intensely monitored after transplantation. Two types of histocompatibility tests are commonly performed after these transplants: HLA antibody testing in SOTs and chimerism after HCT.

SOT recipients are at risk of developing HLA antibodies to donor-specific antigens after transplantation. The development of DSAs after transplant has been associated with several outcomes. Some individuals have DSAs but no apparent clinical consequences. Others may experience antibody-mediated rejection or be at risk for acute cellular rejection. In the long term, posttransplant DSA development has been associated with lower graft survival compared with recipients who do not develop DSAs. The most common method to assess DSA involves the use of multiplex single-antigen bead arrays, as we already described.

The intent of HCT is to repopulate the recipient's immune system with donor-derived white blood cells and eliminate malignant cells in recipients with hematologic cancers. To monitor the patient for engraftment of donor cells, a blood sample can be assessed for the presence of donor-specific genetic markers. The relative quantity of donor cells vs recipient cells can be determined. Currently, the most common method to accomplish this is the use of short tandem repeat (STR) testing. STRs are short segments (two to six base pairs) of a specific, repeated DNA sequence. The number of repeats at a locus can vary from individual to individual; thus, determination of a repeat number can be used to distinguish donor from recipient DNA in the blood. To determine the relative STR length in a sample, PCR is used to amplify several different STR loci in the pretransplant recipient's DNA, the donor's DNA, and the recipient's posttransplant DNA. PCR amplicons are separated according to the size of the repeats by capillary electrophoresis (see Chapter 12). Posttransplant electropherograms are compared with individual donor and recipient electropherograms. The peak heights or areas are determined for donor and recipient loci and reflect the relative proportions in the posttransplant blood sample. In this fashion, donor engraftment, or lack thereof, can be determined.

Knowledge Check 16-4

The final check to confirm the absence of donor-specific HLA antibody before transplant is performed by:

a. Crossmatch
b. STR analysis
c. HLA genotyping of donor
d. HLA genotyping of recipient

The Histocompatibility Testing Process for Kidney Transplantation

Every year, thousands of people are waiting to be matched for a kidney transplant. When a patient with end-stage kidney disease is accepted by a transplant program for addition to the wait-list they will be HLA typed at the HLA-A, B, C, DRB1/3/4/5, DQB1, DQA1, DPB1, and DPA1 loci. This is considered the *pretransplant testing phase*. The patient will also be tested for the presence of HLA antibodies. If detected, the specific HLA antigens to which they bind are determined and referred to as *unacceptable antigens*. The list of these unacceptable antigens is used to determine the cPRA value for that patient. While patients are on the wait-list, they are tested periodically for any changes in their HLA antibody status during the pretransplant testing phase. The candidate's HLA typing and antibody results are part of the information used to allocate deceased donor kidneys.

In the *peri-transplant phase* of testing, when a deceased donor is identified, they will be HLA typed at the same loci as patients are typed. This information is a component of an extensive array of clinical and laboratory data that are used to allocate donor kidneys. When a potential recipient is identified and the kidney is offered, a crossmatch test is typically performed using donor lymphocytes and patient serum to confirm the absence of donor-specific antibody. If acceptable, that transplant may then take place.

As we previously discussed, the *posttransplant phase* of histocompatibility testing typically involves monitoring the recipient for development of donor-specific HLA antibodies using solid-phase testing methods. This information assists the clinician to manage immunosuppression and diagnose rejection.

The Histocompatibility Testing Process for Hematopoietic Stem Cell Transplantation

Patients in need of HCT are HLA typed using high-resolution molecular techniques. Likewise, donors are also typed at high resolution to allow identification of suitable donor-recipient combinations. For HCT, the primary loci assessed are HLA-A, B, C, and DRB1. The other loci are typically typed and considered for donor identification when multiple potential donors are identified. The preferred donor is an HLA-matched sibling donor. In the absence of such a donor, HLA-matched unrelated donors are identified by searching in bone marrow donor registries. If a matched unrelated donor is unavailable, mismatched donors are considered next. Each degree of mismatching (e.g., one-allele or two-allele mismatch) is associated with a reduction in the overall survival of patients getting an HCT. Another alternative donor is a *haploidentical* donor, which is one who shares one HLA haplotype with the patient. With advances in immunosuppressive therapies, haploidentical donors are in more common use.

HCT patients are also tested for HLA antibodies. If a patient has a donor-specific HLA antibody identified prior to transplant, an alternative donor is typically sought. This is due to the adverse impact of HLA antibodies on engraftment of stem cells from the infused bone marrow or peripheral blood stem cell collection.

KEY CONCEPTS

Histocompatibility Systems

- The immune system's ability to recognize and respond to the myriad of infectious agents that humans encounter has obvious benefits. However, the mechanisms that impart this ability make the transplantation of organs and cells between allogeneic individuals difficult.
- The targets of the response to transplanted tissues are HLA proteins and, to a lesser extent, minor histocompatibility antigens. HLA proteins play critical roles as antigen-presenting molecules for CD4 and CD8 T cells, resulting in the phenomenon of MHC restriction.
- Other non-HLA proteins that affect clinical transplantation include MICA, ABO blood groups, and others.

Allorecognition

- Although an individual's immune system develops to respond to the foreign proteins presented on its own MHC antigens, it responds intensely to foreign MHC proteins. Both the humoral and cellular branches of the immune system contribute to this allogeneic immune response and mediate graft rejection.
- The likelihood of developing an immune response to a graft depends on the genetic relatedness of the transplant donor and recipient. Autografts involve transfer of tissue from one area of the body to another in the same individual. Syngeneic grafts (isografts) involve the transfer of tissue between two genetically identical members of the same species. In allografts, tissue is transplanted between genetically nonidentical members of the same species, whereas in xenografts, tissue is transplanted between members of different species.

Transplant Rejection

- Because of the disparity in HLA antigens, allografts and xenografts have the potential to induce strong immune responses in transplant recipients.
- The recipient's immune system recognizes foreign HLA proteins by two mechanisms: direct and indirect allorecognition. In direct allorecognition, the recipient's T cells bind directly to foreign proteins on the donor's APCs. In indirect allorecognition, the foreign HLA proteins are taken up and processed by the recipient's APCs and presented to the recipient's T cells.
- Hyperacute rejection occurs within minutes to hours after transplantation and is mediated by preformed HLA antibodies that react with donor vascular epithelium, resulting in activation of the complement cascade and clotting mechanisms. Preformed antibodies can also cause accelerated rejection, which occurs during a span of several days.
- Acute rejection develops days to months after transplantation and is mediated by a cellular or humoral response to foreign HLA antigens, involving cytokine production by $CD4^+$ T cells, cytotoxic activity of $CD8^+$ T cells, and/or antibody-mediated effector mechanisms.
- Chronic rejection can occur after the first year of transplantation through cellular and humoral responses to foreign HLA proteins, resulting in graft arteriosclerosis, fibrosis, and scarring.

Graft-vs-Host Disease (GVHD)

- Graft-vs-host disease (GVHD) can occur in HLA-mismatched recipients of HSC transplants or, less commonly, via other transplants that contain lymphoid cells. In this condition, the donor's T lymphocytes destroy the recipient's cells, mainly in the skin, gastrointestinal tract, and liver.

Immunosuppressive Agents

- Despite intense immune responses, transplantation has become an effective treatment for many diseases because of the development of immunosuppressive agents that, in various ways, inhibit the immune system from responding to the allogeneic MHC proteins in the transplanted tissue.
- The classes of immunosuppressive agents include corticosteroids, antimetabolites, calcineurin inhibitors, monoclonal antibodies, and polyclonal antibodies. Unfortunately, these agents also interfere with immune responses to infectious organisms and tumors.

Clinical Histocompatibility Testing

- Identifying the MHC antigens of donors and recipients and monitoring the allospecific immune response are critical components of clinical transplantation. Greatly improved outcomes of transplantation are seen when donor and recipient are matched for HLA types as much as possible and when the recipient does not have preformed antibodies to the donor's HLA antigens.
- The classic method of HLA phenotyping is the complement-dependent cytotoxicity test (CDC), in which HLA antigens are typed by incubating the individual's lymphocytes with a panel of antisera and reagent complement. Positive cells are identified by their ability to bind specific antisera and complement, resulting in membrane permeabilization and uptake of vital stains.
- Molecular methods such as PCR-SSP, PCR-SSOP, and SBT provide greater resolution than HLA antigen typing by determining the HLA genotype at the allele level.
- Screening and identification of preformed HLA antibodies in transplant recipients can be performed by the CDC method through incubation of patient serum with panels of lymphocytes with known HLA antigens, flow cytometry, or Luminex technology.

- Crossmatching is performed by incubation of recipient serum with donor lymphocytes in a CDC assay to confirm the absence of donor-specific antibody.
- Engraftment of donor-derived white blood cells in an HCT recipient can be determined by testing for donor-specific genetic markers known as *STRs*.
- The histocompatibility testing process begins with a pretransplantation phase and continues through a peri-transplantation phase and a posttransplantation phase.

Study Guide: Classification of Grafts

TYPE OF GRAFT	DEFINITION	EXAMPLES
Autograft	Transfer of tissue within the same individual	Skin graft from a leg to the face of a burn patient Transfer of a saphenous vein from the leg of a cardiac bypass patient to their heart
Syngeneic (Iso) graft	Transfer of cells or tissues to a genetically identical individual	Transplant between identical human twins Grafts between genetically identical strains of mice
Allograft	Transfer of cells or tissues to a genetically nonidentical member of the same species	Human transplant from a deceased or living donor other than an identical twin Grafts between genetically nonidentical strains of mice
Xenograft	Transfer of cells or tissues to a member of a different species	Transplant of a pig valve into a human heart

Study Guide: Types of Graft Rejection

TYPE	TIMING (AFTER TRANSPLANT)	IMMUNOLOGIC MECHANISM
Hyperacute	Minutes to hours	Preformed antibodies to ABO, HLA, and certain endothelial antigens bind to donor vascular endothelium, activating complement and clotting factors. This leads to thrombus formation, ischemia, and necrosis of transplanted tissue.
Accelerated	Days	Same as for hyperacute rejection.
Acute	Days to months	Cell-mediated response to foreign MHC-expressing cells. CD4+ T cells produce cytokines and induce delayed-type hypersensitivity. CD8+ T cells mediate cytotoxic reactions. Antibodies produced against HLA antigens bind to vessel walls, activate complement, and induce transmural necrosis and inflammation.
Chronic	1 year or more	Delayed type hypersensitivity response, and possibly antibodies, to foreign HLA antigens on graft. Graft arteriosclerosis and smooth muscle proliferation occur, resulting in fibrosis, scarring, and narrowing of vessel lumen.
Graft-versus-host disease (GVHD)	100 days or more	T cells in HSC, lung, or liver transplants react against foreign HLA proteins in the recipient's cells, causing massive cytokine release, inflammation, and tissue destruction in various locations throughout the body.

Study Guide: Clinical Histocompatibility Testing

TYPE OF TEST	PURPOSE	METHODS
HLA Phenotyping	To identify the HLA antigens in a transplant candidate and potential donors.	Complement-dependent cytotoxicity (CDC)- Classic method for HLA typing. Donor and recipient lymphocytes are incubated separately with panels of reagent antibodies to HLA antigens. Reagent complement is added, followed by a vital stain to detect cell death, which if present in a specified percentage, indicates a positive result.
HLA Genotyping	Molecular methods are conducted to identify specific HLA alleles or allele groups in a transplant candidate and potential donors. Provides high-resolution typing required for HCT.	PCR-SSP- HLA genes are amplified using primers that bind to specific alleles; only those perfectly matched to the target gene will generate a product. PCR-SSOP- All HLA gene variants are amplified by PCR and incubated with a panel of labeled probes that are specific for a unique HLA allele or group. Only those probes that hybridize with the sample DNA will be detected. SBT- Sanger sequencing or NGS is conducted on DNA amplified by PCR to determine the nucleotide sequence of specific HLA alleles.
HLA Antibody Screening and Identification	Detects antibodies to HLA antigens in transplant candidates.	Patient serum is incubated with panels of lymphocytes with defined HLA phenotypes in a CDC method or solid phase immunoassay that uses microbeads coated with purified HLA antigens.
Crossmatching	To confirm the absence of antibodies in a transplant candidate or recipient to donor-specific HLA antigens.	Patient serum is incubated with donor T and B lymphocytes in a CDC method or solid phase immunoassay.

CASE STUDIES

1. An adult patient needs to have a second kidney transplant. The patient's first transplant was lost because of chronic rejection. The patient's HLA type, HLA antibodies, and ABO blood group status were determined. The patient was found to have antibodies to HLA-B35 by flow cytometric testing with HLA-B35–coated beads. The HLA type and blood group were also determined for two of the patient's siblings and two close friends who are interested in donating a kidney to the patient.

IDENTIFICATION	BLOOD GROUP	A	B	C	DR	DQ
Recipient	O	1,2	8,44	7,5	17,4	2,7
Sibling 1	O	1,11	8,35	7,4	17,1	2,5
Sibling 2	A	3,11	7,35	7,4	15,1	6,5
Friend 1	B	2,24	57,7	6,7	7,15	2,6
Friend 2	O	2,24	57,7	6,7	7,15	2,6

Question

a. From the available donors, who would likely be the most compatible with this patient?

2. A 59-year-old patient with leukemia needed an HCT to replenish hematopoietic cells destroyed by previous chemotherapy. Clinicians were hopeful that the patient's single sibling might be a suitable donor. However, the sibling was determined to be medically unsuitable for donation. As such, the transplant center conducted an unrelated donor search for this patient, and a potential donor was identified. The transplant registry provided the HLA type for the donor, which was determined using CDC-based testing (phenotyping). The patient's HLA type was determined at high resolution by SBT.

ID	HLA-A*	HLA- B*	HLA- C*	HLA-DRB1*	HLA-DQB1*
Patient	01:01	08:01	07:02	03:01	02:01
	02:01	44:02	02:01	15:01	06:02
Donor	1	8	7	3	2
	2	44	2	15	6

Questions

a. Is this donor-recipient pair HLA identical? Yes / No / Maybe

b. The transplant physician requested high-resolution HLA typing for the donor. Why?

REVIEW QUESTIONS

1. Which of the following responses is the type of allograft rejection associated with vascular and parenchymal injury with lymphocyte infiltrates?
   a. Hyperacute rejection
   b. Acute cellular rejection
   c. Acute humoral rejection
   d. Chronic rejection

2. Antigen receptors on T lymphocytes bind HLA class II + peptide complexes with the help of which accessory molecule?
   a. CD2
   b. CD3
   c. CD4
   d. CD8

3. Patients who received the following types of grafts are at risk for graft-vs-host disease (GVHD) *except* for recipients of:
   a. Bone marrow transplants
   b. Lung transplants
   c. Liver transplants
   d. Irradiated leukocytes

4. Which of the following properties is *not* exhibited by HLA molecules?
   a. They belong to the immunoglobulin superfamily.
   b. They are heterodimeric.
   c. They are integral cell membrane glycoproteins.
   d. They are monomorphic.

5. Kidney allograft loss from intravascular thrombosis without cellular infiltration 5 days posttransplant may indicate which primary rejection mechanism?
   a. Hyperacute rejection
   b. Accelerated humoral rejection
   c. Acute humoral rejection
   d. Acute cellular rejection

6. Which reagents would be used in a donor-recipient crossmatch test?
   a. Donor serum and recipient lymphocytes + rabbit serum complement
   b. Recipient serum and donor lymphocytes + rabbit serum complement
   c. Donor stimulator cells + recipient responder cells + complete culture medium
   d. Recipient stimulator cells + donor responder cells + complete culture medium

7. The indirect allorecognition pathway involves which one of the following mechanisms?
   a. Processed peptides from polymorphic donor proteins restricted by recipient HLA class II molecules
   b. Processed peptides from polymorphic recipient proteins restricted by donor HLA class I molecules
   c. Intact polymorphic donor protein molecules recognized by recipient HLA class I molecules
   d. Intact polymorphic donor protein molecules recognized by recipient HLA class II molecules

8. Which immunosuppressive agent selectively inhibits IL-2 receptor-mediated activation of T cells?
   a. Mycophenolate mofetil
   b. Cyclosporine
   c. Corticosteroids
   d. Basiliximab

9. Phenotyping for HLA class II antigens requires B lymphocytes because:
   a. B lymphocytes express HLA class II antigens.
   b. B lymphocytes do not express HLA class I antigens.
   c. B lymphocytes are exquisitely sensitive to complement-mediated lysis.
   d. B lymphocytes represent the majority of lymphocytes in the peripheral blood.

10. A renal transplant candidate was crossmatched with a donor who was mismatched for only the HLA-B35 antigen. The candidate was known to have an antibody specific for HLA-B35. Which of the following combinations of T- and B-cell flow cytometric crossmatch results would be expected?
    a. T-cell negative, B-cell negative
    b. T-cell positive, B-cell positive
    c. T-cell negative, B-cell positive
    d. T-cell positive, B-cell negative

11. Which of the following HLA alleles differs from A*02:01:02 by a synonymous nucleotide substitution?
    a. A*01:01:01:01
    b. A*02:01:03
    c. A*02:02
    d. A*02:03:01

12. Which of the following donors would be expected to elicit a positive mixed lymphocyte response in lymphocytes from a patient who has the HLA-DRB1*01:01, 01:03 alleles?
    a. DRB1*01:01, 01:03
    b. DRB1*01:01, 01:01
    c. DRB1*01:03, 01:03
    d. DRB1*01:01, 01:05

13. Which of the following donors would be the most appropriate, based on ABO compatibility, for a renal transplant candidate with the ABO type = O?
    a. O
    b. A
    c. B
    d. AB

14. Which of the following HLA antigens would be expected to elicit an HLA antibody response in a kidney-transplant recipient with the following HLA type: HLA-A*01,03; B*07,14; C*01,04N; DRB1*16,07?
    a. HLA-A*01
    b. HLA-B*14
    c. HLA-C*04
    d. HLA-DRB1*16

15. Suppose a 30-year-old person was found to be a suitable donor for a kidney transplant to a younger sibling. This transplant would be an example of a(an):
    a. Autograft
    b. Allograft
    c. Isograft
    d. Xenograft

16. What is the probability that two siblings are HLA identical?
    a. 0%
    b. 25%
    c. 50%
    d. 75%

17. An HCT from a parent (HLA-A1, 2; B8,35; DR17, 15) to a child (A1, 24; B8, 57; DR17, 4) is an example of:
    a. A haploidentical transplant
    b. An HLA-identical transplant
    c. An isograft
    d. A xenograft

18. The HLA allele HLA-A*03:01:01:02N is an example of a null allele. A null allele is:
    a. Overexpressed on the cell surface
    b. A secreted form of an HLA allele
    c. A novel, previously undescribed, allele
    d. An allele that is not expressed on the cell surface

19. Chronic allograft rejection is characterized by:
    a. Graft arteriosclerosis
    b. Occurrence a few days after transplant
    c. Recurrence of disease in the transplanted kidney
    d. An autoimmune response

20. The presence of donor-specific HLA antibodies in the potential recipient of an HCT is a risk factor for:
    a. A graft-vs-host reaction
    b. An acute rejection episode
    c. A chronic rejection episode
    d. Failure of engraftment

21. Of the four potential unrelated donors for a hematopoietic stem cell transplant (Unr 1, 2, 3, 4), which would have the lowest risk of inducing a GVHD response in the patient?

	HLA-A	HLA-B	HLA-C	HLA-DRB1
Patient	01:01	08:01	07:01	03:01
	11:01	55:01	03:03	04:03
Unr 1	01:01	08:01	07:01	03:01
	11:01	55:01	03:03	04:03
Unr 2	01:01	08:01	07:01	03:01
	11:01	55:01	03:03	07:01
Unr 3	01:01	08:01	07:01	03:02
	11:01	55:01	03:03	09:01
Unr 4	01:01	18:01	07:01	03:02
	11:01	55:01	03:03	09:01

Unr = unrelated donor.

    a. Unr 1
    b. Unr 2
    c. Unr 3
    d. Unr 4

Chapter 16 Answer Key

Answers to Knowledge Checks

16.1 b 16.2 c 16.3 b 16.4 a

Answers to Review Questions

1. b	2. c	3. d	4. d	5. b	6. b	7. a
8. d	9. a	10. b	11. b	12. c	13. a	14. c
15. b	16. b	17. a	18. d	19. a	20. d	21. a

17 Tumor Immunology

Linda E. Miller, PhD, I, MB^CM^(ASCP)SI

LEARNING OUTCOMES

After finishing this chapter, you should be able to:

17.1 Describe the process by which malignant cells are thought to develop and the characteristics that differentiate cancer cells from normal cells.

17.2 Differentiate between tumor-specific and tumor-associated antigens and recognize examples of each.

17.3 Discuss the uses of tumor markers in cancer screening, diagnosis, determining patient prognosis, predicting patient response to therapy, and monitoring patient responses to treatment.

17.4 Identify the characteristics that should be possessed by an ideal tumor marker and explain how nonideal features can affect the clinical utility of a marker.

17.5 Explain the principles of microscopic examination and immunohistochemistry and how they are used in oncology.

17.6 Distinguish the clinical applications of each of the following serum tumor markers: α-fetoprotein (AFP), cancer antigen 125 (CA 125), carcinoembryonic antigen (CEA), human chorionic gonadotropin (hCG), and prostate-specific antigen (PSA).

17.7 Discuss the advantages and limitations of immunoassays for serum tumor markers.

17.8 Discuss the uses of flow cytometry, cytogenetics, and molecular testing in oncology.

17.9 Recognize the clinical significance of specific cell surface and genetic markers for cancer.

17.10 Select the appropriate laboratory test to detect a specific type of tumor marker.

17.11 Describe the innate and adaptive immune responses that play a role in defense against tumors and how they contribute to immunosurveillance.

17.12 Discuss the process of immunoediting and mechanisms of tumor escape from the immune system.

17.13 Provide specific examples of active, passive, and adoptive cancer immunotherapy and describe how they work.

CHAPTER OUTLINE

You can go to **fadavis.com** keyword stevens for the laboratory exercises that accompany this text.

The field of tumor immunology focuses on the relationship between the immune system and cancer cells and encompasses several areas, including the following:

- The antigens associated with tumor cells
- The host's immune responses to tumors
- Mechanisms by which tumors are thought to escape these responses
- Therapeutic use of the immune system to destroy tumors

The field is of major interest to immunologists because cancer is a leading cause of morbidity and mortality, responsible for nearly 10 million deaths each year and accounting for one in every six deaths worldwide. Nearly 40% of people are estimated to develop cancer in their lifetime, and the number of new cancer cases is projected to double by 2045 due to population growth and increased prevalence of risk factors (e.g., tobacco use, obesity, physical inactivity, unhealthy diets, and air pollution).

Introduction to Tumor Biology

Tumor immunology is best understood with a background on the origin of cancer cells and their differences from normal cells. Normally, cell growth and division are carefully regulated processes that allow the body to rapidly produce new cells as needed. At the same time, cell division is inhibited when enough cells are present, and the life span of cells is limited through the normal physiological process of cell death, **apoptosis** (see Chapter 15). These activities allow the human body to perform functions necessary for life, such as generation of new skin cells to replace those that are dying, lymphocyte proliferation in immune responses, and regeneration of tissue during wound healing and repair. However, if these processes are allowed to continue unchecked, they can lead to excessive cell growth and division, resulting in development of an abnormal cell mass called a **tumor** (from the Latin, meaning "to swell") or **neoplasm** (from the Greek, meaning "new growth"). See **Figure 17–1.**

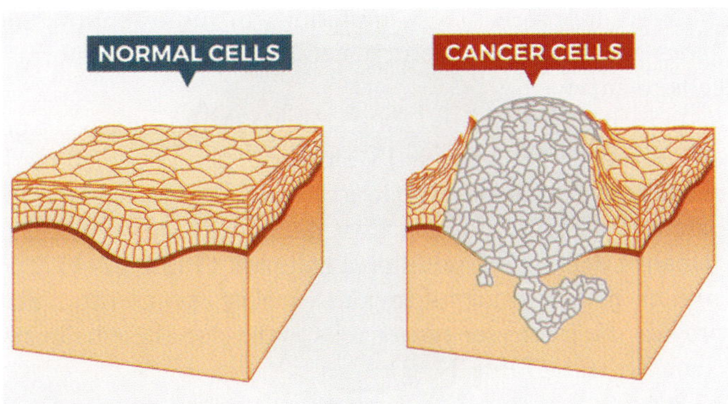

FIGURE 17–1 Cancer is a disease caused by cells dividing uncontrollably and spreading into surrounding tissues. *(Source: National Cancer Institute [NCI].)*

Tumors can be **benign** or **malignant.** Benign tumors are composed of slow-growing, well-differentiated cells with a similar organization to the normal tissue from which they originated. These tumors are surrounded by a capsule, which secures them in place and prevents them from circulating to other parts of the body. In contrast, malignant tumors, or cancer cells, are disorganized masses that are rarely encapsulated, allowing them to invade nearby organs and destroy their normal architecture. **Cancer,** named after the Latin word for "crab," derives its name from this property of invasiveness, which can resemble the legs of a crab when viewed in microscopic tissue sections. Also, malignant tumors commonly exhibit **metastasis,** or the ability of cells to break away from the original tumor mass and spread through the blood to nearby or distant sites in the body **(Fig. 17–2).** Malignant cells can vary in their degree of development, from completely differentiated, or mature, to undifferentiated cells that grow more aggressively and form tumors with a poorer prognosis.

Classification of Malignant Tumors

Malignant tumors are classified according to their tissue of origin. About 80% of cancers are **carcinomas,** derived from the skin or epithelial linings of internal organs or glands; about 9% are *leukemias* (circulating malignant white blood cells [WBCs] originating from bone marrow hematopoietic stem cells) or *lymphomas* (solid tumors arising from lymphoid organs; see Chapter 18); and about 1% are **sarcomas,** derived from bone or soft tissues such as fat, muscles, tendons, cartilage, nerves, and blood vessels. Other types of tumors include melanoma (malignant skin cells that make pigment), brain and spinal cord tumors, germ cell tumors (arising from cells involved in sperm and egg production), and neuroendocrine tumors (derived from cells that produce hormones after receiving signals from the nervous system).

To make a specific diagnosis and guide treatment decisions, physicians use staging systems based on the site and type of the primary tumor, tumor size, involvement of regional lymph nodes, presence or absence of metastasis, and degree of resemblance to normal tissue. The most widely used staging scheme for solid tumors is the TNM system of the American Joint Committee on Cancer (AJCC). For many types of cancer, the TNM criteria can be used to classify tumors into one of five stages: Stage 0—noninvasive (in situ) carcinoma; stage I—localized tumor; stage II—early, locally advanced cancer; stage III—late stage, locally advanced cancer; stage IV—cancer that has spread to distant body sites. In Chapter 18, we discuss the classification of hematologic malignancies.

The *cancer grade,* based on the microscopic appearance of the tumor cells, can also be used to determine patient prognosis and treatment. In general, lower-grade tumors, which have well-differentiated cells and relatively normal tissue structure, have a better prognosis than higher-grade tumors, with poorly differentiated cells and abnormal tissue structure.

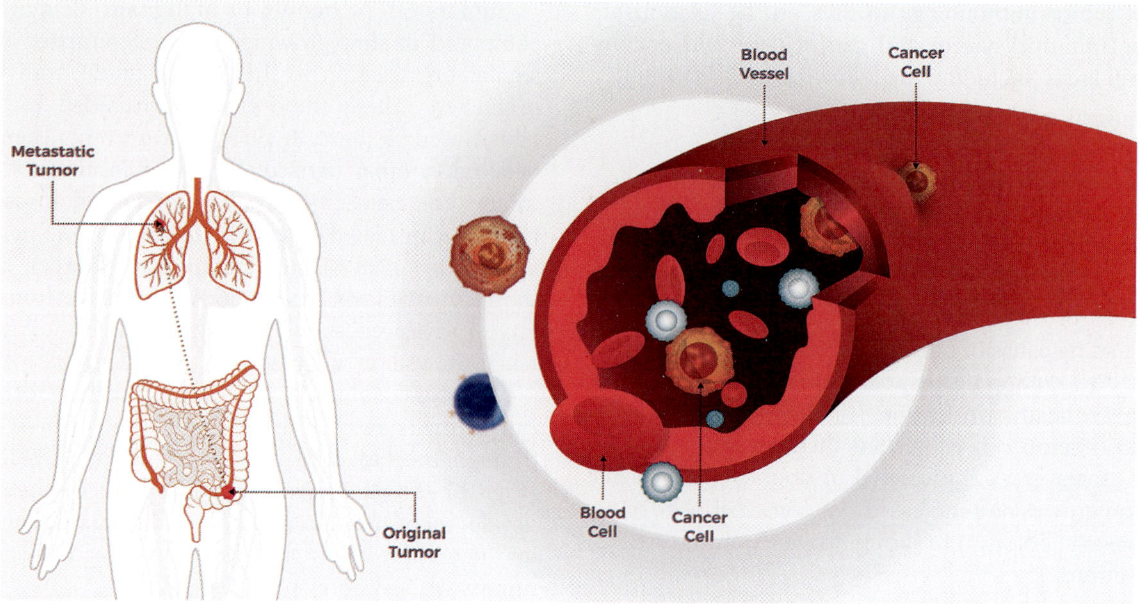

FIGURE 17–2 The process of metastasis. Cancer cells can break away from the original tumor and travel through the blood or lymphatic system to distant locations in the body, where they exit the vessels to form additional tumors. *(Source: National Cancer Institute [NCI].)*

Clinical Correlations

The TNM System

The system uses the letters TNM to describe the following:

T (Tumor): Describes the size of the primary tumor and the extent of its invasion into adjacent tissues, using a scale of T0 (noninvasive [in situ] tumor) and T1-T4 (showing progressive increase in size and invasiveness).

N (Nodes): Describes involvement of nearby lymph nodes, using a scale of N0 (no spread to regional lymph nodes) and N1 to N3 (showing progressive lymph node involvement).

M (Metastasis): Describes the extent to which the cancer has spread to other parts of the body, using a scale of M0 (no spread) to M1 (evidence of distant metastasis).

For example, breast cancer classified as T2N1M0 would involve a tumor between 2 to 5 cm in diameter that has spread to one to three regional lymph nodes but has not spread to distant sites.

Malignant Transformation

The transformation of a normal cell into a malignant tumor is thought to be a multistep process involving a series of genetic mutations that cause the cell's phenotype to change over time. This process, called **carcinogenesis,** is thought to be initiated by exposure of the host to environmental factors that induce genetic changes in the cell. These factors include chemical carcinogens (e.g., asbestos and cigarette smoke); radiation (ultraviolet rays from the sun and ionizing radiation from x-rays); and certain pathogenic viruses that have been linked to specific types of cancer (e.g., Epstein-Barr virus [EBV] and human papillomavirus [HPV]). These agents are believed to create genetic changes, or **mutations,** in our cells' DNA that affect the body's mechanisms that normally control cell growth.

Two major types of genes are involved in malignant transformation: proto-oncogenes and tumor suppressor genes. **Proto-oncogenes** are normal genes that stimulate cell proliferation and growth. Sometimes mutations in proto-oncogenes can convert them to oncogene-like genes, which have DNA sequences similar to those found in the *oncogenes* of transforming viruses. These genetic alterations—which include point mutations, chromosome translocations, and gene amplifications (see Chapter 12)—cause continual proto-oncogene activation, resulting in changes that allow cells to divide uncontrollably.

Excessive cell division is normally inhibited by the action of **tumor suppressor genes.** These genes control the entry of cells into the cell cycle and prevent cells from completing the cell cycle if they contain damaged DNA or other abnormalities. If a mutation causes the function of a tumor suppressor gene to be lost, normal growth-inhibitory signals are removed. Tumor suppressor genes also play an important role in recognizing damaged DNA in a cell and repairing it. If repair is not possible, the cell is induced to undergo apoptosis. Thus, mutations in tumor suppressor genes can result in genetic instability and allow abnormal cells to survive.

In their classic papers (2000 and 2011), the esteemed cancer researchers Hanahan and Weinberg defined eight hallmark characteristics that differentiate a cancer cell from a normal cell, based on scientific evidence from numerous reports. In 2022, Hanahan defined one additional hallmark **(Table 17–1).** The authors have also identified four *enabling characteristics* that provide the means for cancer cells to develop these hallmark characteristics **(Table 17–2).**

Research has shown that malignant tumors do not arise as a result of a single genetic mutation but rather from a series of mutations that accumulate in the same cell over a lifetime **(Fig. 17–3).**

Table 17-1 Hallmark Characteristics Differentiating Cancer Cells From Normal Cells

HALLMARK CHARACTERISTIC	DEFINITION
Sustaining proliferative signaling	Production of growth signals by the cancer cells themselves
Resisting cell death	Ability to escape apoptosis
Inducing or accessing vasculature	Ability to induce angiogenesis (development of new blood vessels) to provide oxygen and nutrients to the growing tumor
Enabling replicative immortality	Ability to divide indefinitely
Activating invasion and metastasis	Ability to spread to and grow in distant tissues
Evading growth suppressors	Ability to resist antiproliferative signals by escaping mechanisms that prevent progression through the cell cycle and by overexpressing growth-stimulating factors
Deregulating cellular metabolism	Using an aerobic glycolysis pathway to convert glucose into lactate to generate energy faster to support cell proliferation
Avoiding immune destruction	Escaping detection and elimination by the immune system
Unlocking phenotypic plasticity	Escaping progression to a state of terminal differentiation by reverting to a progenitor-like state, halting the differentiation process, or switching to a different differentiation pathway not associated with the cell of origin

Table 17-2 Characteristics That Enable Changes in Cancer Cells

ENABLING CHARACTERISTIC	DEFINITION
Genomic instability	Genetic mutations that promote excessive cell growth, alter cell function, and result in gains and losses of genes
Tumor-promoting inflammation	Infiltration of innate and adaptive immune cells into solid tumors, resulting in release of cytokines, reactive oxygen species (ROS), enzymes, and other bioactive molecules that promote inflammation, genetic changes, and tumor growth and survival
Nonmutational epigenetic reprogramming	Factors that promote tumor development by modifying chromosome structure to regulate the expression of key genes (see Chapter 12)
Polymorphic microbiomes	Changes in microbial populations that colonize the gut and other body sites and influence tumor growth

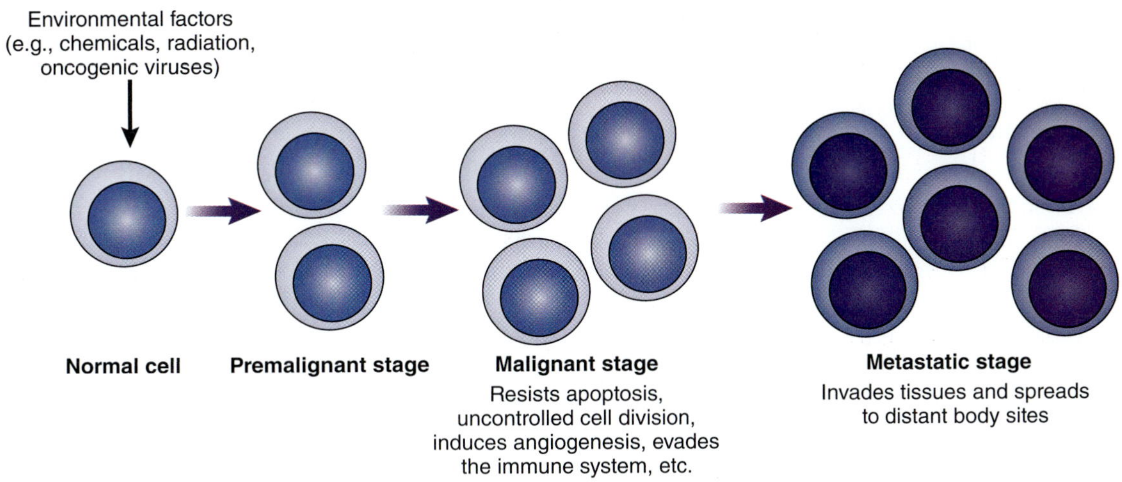

FIGURE 17–3 Genetic mutations in the evolution of cancer. As cells acquire an increasing number of mutations over time, they develop more of the characteristics that allow them to evolve into invasive cancer cells.

Cancer is not a single disease but rather a diverse group of more than 200 diseases that show variability in the characteristics we mentioned. In fact, heterogeneity is commonly found among different cancer cells in the same patient. The extent to which a tumor has these characteristics will determine its ability to survive, grow, and metastasize. This, in turn, influences disease aggressiveness, patient prognosis, and choice of therapy. The immune system has important effects on tumor growth. In this chapter, we discuss the interactions between tumors and the immune system in more detail and tumor antigens that can be used as markers for various cancer types.

Knowledge Check 17-1

Malignant tumors differ from benign tumors in that malignant tumors:

a. Are encapsulated
b. Involve cell proliferation
c. Undergo apoptosis
d. Can spread to distant tissues

Tumor Antigens

Tumor immunology is based on the premise that tumors possess antigens that the immune system recognizes as foreign. Some of these antigens, called **tumor-specific antigens (TSAs),** are unique to tumor cells, whereas others, the **tumor-associated antigens (TAAs),** are also found on normal cells. In this section, we describe different types of tumor antigens that fall into each of the two categories; **Table 17–3** summarizes their features.

Tumor-Specific Antigens (TSAs)

TSAs can be classified into several groups, depending on how they were derived. These include neoantigens, antigens of oncogenic viruses, and endogenous retroviral elements. In general, TSAs stimulate strong immune responses because they are not present on normal cells.

Neoantigens

Neoantigens, also known as *mutation-derived tumor antigens*, are created as a result of mutations in proto-oncogenes, tumor

Table 17-3 Types of Tumor Antigens

Tumor-Specific Antigens (TSAs)

ANTIGEN TYPE	DESCRIPTION	EXAMPLES[a]
Neoantigens (mutation derived)	Antigens created because of genetic mutations; these are unique to a tumor in a particular patient	p53, CASP-8
Fusion proteins	Antigens that result from the joining of two genes that are normally not adjacent to each other; they are unique to a particular type of tumor	*BCR/ABL* (CML, ALL, AML) *SYT-SSX1/SSX2* (synovial cell sarcoma) *TMPRSS2-ERG* (prostate cancer) *EML4-ALK* (non-small cell lung cancer)
Antigens of oncogenic viruses	Antigens expressed by cells infected with a cancer-causing virus	Epstein-Barr virus (EBV) antigens in EBV-associated B-cell lymphomas Human papillomavirus (HPV) antigens in cervical cancer, other genital cancers and anal cancer
Endogenous retroviral elements (ERVs)	Genomic DNA fragments created from integrated retroviral RNA	ERVH4, ERVH5, ERVH48-1

Tumor-Associated Antigens (TAAs)

ANTIGEN TYPE	DESCRIPTION	EXAMPLES[a]
Cancer/testis antigens	Expressed in gametes and in many tumors but not in somatic cells	MAGE (melanoma)
Differentiation antigens	Expressed on cells of a particular lineage but not in cells from other tissues	Tyrosinase (melanoma) MART-1 (melanoma) CEA (mainly in colorectal cancer) AFP (HCC) PSA (prostate cancer)
Overexpressed antigens	Found in higher levels on malignant cells than on normal cells	HER2 (mainly in some breast cancers)

AFP = α-fetoprotein; ALL = acute lymphoblastic leukemia; AML = acute myelogenous leukemia; CASP = caspase; CEA = carcinoembryonic antigen; CML = chronic myelogenous leukemia; HCC = hepatocellular carcinoma; HER2 = human epidermal growth factor 2; MAGE = melanoma antigen gene; MART = melanoma antigen recognized by T cells; PSA = prostate-specific antigen.

[a]Primary cancer associations are shown in parentheses.

suppressor genes, or unrelated genes. They have been discovered though advances in molecular methods, especially next-generation sequencing (NGS; see Chapter 12).

Most neoantigens originate from point mutations (i.e., genetic changes involving a single base pair), deletions in key genes that regulate cell proliferation, such as the tumor suppressor gene *p53*, and the gene coding for caspase 8, an enzyme important for apoptosis (both of which are associated with head and neck tumors and squamous cell carcinoma), or genes coding for DNA mismatch repair proteins (associated with some types of colorectal cancer). These antigens are patient-specific or restricted to very few patients and are highly immunogenic.

Neoantigens can also be produced by other types of mutations, including frameshifts, gene fusions, and splice variants. These mutations can result in the activation of genes that are involved in carcinogenesis. The proteins created are specific to a particular type or a few types of tumors.

Antigens of Oncogenic Viruses

Another group of TSAs consists of proteins encoded by cancer-causing viruses **(Table 17–4).** For example, antigens coded for by genes of the EBV can be found in cells from B-cell lymphomas associated with the virus. These antigens have been observed in the nucleus, cytoplasm, or plasma membrane of the associated tumor cells. The antigens are produced inside of the cells infected with an oncogenic virus and can be processed by class I MHC molecules and displayed on the tumor cell surface, where they are presented to cytotoxic T (T_c) cells.

Endogenous Retroviral Elements (ERVs)

Endogenous retroviral elements (ERVs) are DNA fragments that reside in the human genome as a result of infection with retroviruses. They make up about 8% of human DNA, but their expression is usually silenced in healthy cells. Research has shown that ERV gene products can be overexpressed in various cancer types, including bladder, colorectal, head and neck, lung squamous, ovarian, prostate, stomach, and uterine.

Table 17-4 Human Viruses Associated With Cancer

VIRUS	CANCER ASSOCIATIONS
Epstein-Barr virus (EBV)	Burkitt lymphoma Hodgkin lymphoma Leiomyosarcomas Posttransplant lymphoproliferative disease Nasopharyngeal carcinoma
Hepatitis B virus (HBV)	Hepatocellular carcinoma
Hepatitis C virus (HCV)	Hepatocellular carcinoma
Human herpesvirus 8 (HHV-8)	Kaposi sarcoma
Human papillomavirus (HPV)	Cervical cancer Other genital and anal cancers Oral cancers
Human T-lymphotropic virus I (HTLV-1)	Adult T-cell leukemia or lymphoma
Merkel cell polyomavirus	Merkel cell carcinoma (a type of skin cancer)

Tumor-Associated Antigens (TSAs)

Tumor-associated antigens (TSAs) are present in some types of normal cells but are overexpressed or abnormally expressed by cancer cells. These types include the cancer/testis antigens, differentiation antigens, and overexpressed antigens.

Cancer/Testis Antigens

Cancer/testis antigens are present in normal testicular germ cells (i.e., spermatogonia and spermatocytes), placental trophoblasts, and ovaries but not in normal somatic cells. They become tumor antigens when the transformation process causes them to be expressed on tumors originating from other cell types. These antigens have been identified on many tumors of epithelial or mesenchymal origin (cells that develop into connective tissue, blood vessels, and lymphatic tissue). Well-known examples of antigens in this category are the melanoma antigen gene (MAGE) proteins expressed by melanoma tumors.

Differentiation Antigens

Differentiation antigens are expressed in cells of a particular lineage but not in other tissues. Examples of antigens in this group are tyrosinase, an enzyme involved in melanin synthesis, and MART-1, a protein needed for melanosome function; both are present in normal melanocytes and malignant melanoma cells. This group of antigens also includes the **oncofetal antigens** that are normally expressed on developing cells of the fetus but not on cells in the adult. The genes coding for these antigens are silenced during embryonic development, but the process of malignant transformation allows them to be reexpressed. Examples of oncofetal antigens include carcinoembryonic protein (CEA), α-fetoprotein (AFP), and prostate-specific antigen (PSA). Many of these antigens are tumor markers that can be detected in the clinical laboratory (see "Clinically Relevant Tumor Markers").

Overexpressed Antigens

Overexpressed antigens are found in higher levels on some malignant cells than on normal cells. Genetic mutations occurring during transformation deregulate expression of these proteins, resulting in levels up to 100 times greater than normal. A well-known example of a tumor antigen in this category is the **human epidermal growth factor receptor 2 (HER2/neu)** protein, a transmembrane receptor that binds human epidermal growth factor. Amplification of the *HER2* gene in a certain type of breast cancer can result in increased production of this protein, which serves as a marker for detection and therapy (see "Immunotherapy" later).

An online database of tumor antigen peptides that have undergone comprehensive scientific study was initially developed by the Cancer Research Institute and is now maintained by the de Duve Institute. Researchers are continually discovering new tumor antigens by using molecular techniques. Some of these antigens can serve as targets for specifically directed therapies (see "Immunotherapy" later).

In addition to peptide TAAs, glycolipid and glycoprotein antigens may also be overexpressed in some tumors. Examples of these antigens include cancer antigen 125 (CA 125), associated with ovarian cancer, and cancer antigen 19-9 (CA 19-9), associated with pancreatic cancer. In the next section, we discuss clinical applications of some of these markers.

Clinically Relevant Tumor Markers

Tumor markers are biological substances in the blood, body fluids, bone marrow, or tissues that indicate the presence of a cancer or certain benign conditions. These substances can be produced by the tumor itself or by other body cells in response to the tumor or other conditions. Traditionally, clinical laboratories have measured tumor markers in the serum of patients who have been diagnosed with, or who are suspected of having, a specific type of cancer. These markers include proteins, carbohydrates, hormones, metabolites, and enzymes. Their concentration is related to the amount of tumor proliferation, the size of the tumor mass, the metabolic activities of the tumor, and release of the marker from dying tumor cells.

Receptors and other molecules on the surface of malignant cells can also be used as tumor markers. Increasingly, genetic alterations in tumor cells, including mutations, gene-expression patterns, and epigenetic changes, are being used as tumor markers.

Ideally, a tumor marker should have high sensitivity (i.e., it should easily detect most people who have a particular cancer) and high specificity (i.e., the marker should be absent in people without the malignant disease in question to minimize false-positive test results). These parameters are often not ideal, especially for serum markers, and should be kept in mind when considering the benefits and limitations of tumor marker testing.

We begin this section with a general discussion of the clinical uses of tumor markers before proceeding to specific examples of serum, cell surface, and genetic tumor markers and their clinical applications.

Clinical Uses of Tumor Markers

In general, tumor markers have five major applications in **oncology**, the medical field that specializes in cancer diagnosis and treatment:

1. **Screening:** Patient survival rates are usually higher when cancer is diagnosed in its earliest stages. Detecting cancer early, before it begins to invade normal tissues and is difficult to target, requires good screening methods. Ideally, tumor markers would be used to screen asymptomatic individuals in a population for the presence of cancer, but this is not usually performed because most markers are nonspecific and likely to produce false-positive results. Targeted screening of high-risk individuals (such as genetic testing of people with a family history of a specific type of cancer) is most effective.
2. **Diagnosis:** Tumor markers, combined with other laboratory tests and a patient's clinical symptoms, can be helpful in making an initial cancer diagnosis.
3. **Prognosis:** Tumor markers may provide information on patient prognosis, or the likely outcome of a cancer, to help guide treatment decisions. In general, an initial high concentration of a tumor marker or an increasing level of a tumor marker over time can indicate presence of a more aggressive cancer with possible metastasis, for which a rigorous treatment would be more effective.
4. **Predicting:** Some tumor markers can be used to predict whether a patient would likely benefit from a specific type of therapy that targets the marker. Testing for such markers is performed before therapy can begin.
5. **Monitoring:** One of the most important uses of tumor markers is to monitor known patients with cancer to determine whether their treatment is effective and to check for recurrence of the tumor. This can be done because the level of a serum tumor marker often correlates with the amount of tumor in the patient's body. The laboratory typically determines a baseline concentration of the marker before treatment begins, followed by serial measurements over time. A significant decrease in the concentration of a tumor marker after surgery, chemotherapy, or other treatment indicates that the therapy has been effective in reducing the tumor mass. In contrast, an increasing level of the marker after a return to normal indicates that the tumor has recurred and that more aggressive treatment may be needed. Elevation in a tumor marker can become evident several months before the cancer is detected by other methods.

The clinical significance of monitoring a tumor marker is illustrated in **Figure 17–4.** This figure shows tumor marker levels from the serum of a hypothetical patient with cancer who has been treated with surgery and two chemotherapy drugs. As expected, the level of the tumor marker declined after the initial tumor mass was removed by surgery. However, after a few months, the concentration of the tumor marker began to increase, indicating that the tumor had recurred. The tumor was unresponsive to chemotherapy 1, as reflected by the sustained elevation in the marker after treatment with that drug. This prompted a change in treatment to chemotherapy 2, which was successful in decreasing the amount of tumor present in the patient, as indicated by the decline in the tumor marker to an undetectable level.

Knowledge Check 17-2

All of the following are common clinical uses of tumor markers *except:*

a. Screening the general population for a particular type of cancer
b. Aiding in initial cancer diagnosis
c. Monitoring patient response to therapy
d. Predicting patient response to a targeted therapy

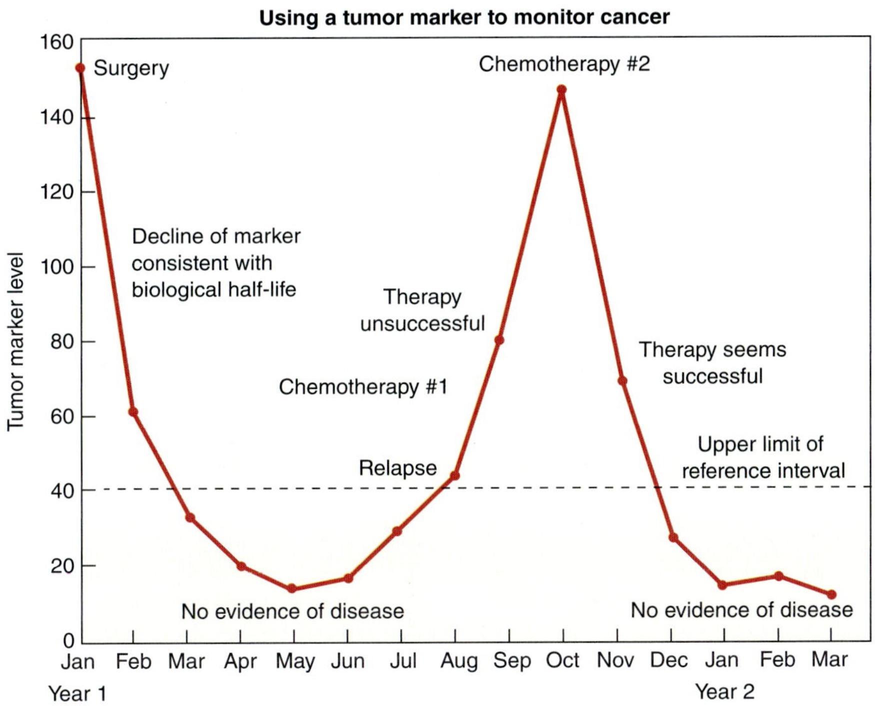

FIGURE 17–4 Tumor marker analysis. A curve showing a sample scenario monitoring a patient with cancer for tumor recurrence and for therapy effectiveness using levels of a circulating tumor antigen.

Serum Tumor Markers

Table 17–5 lists some of the more commonly used tumor markers that can be detected in patient serum and their clinical applications. We discuss some of these in more detail in the text that follows.

α-Fetoprotein (AFP)

α-Fetoprotein (AFP) is a 70,000-MW glycoprotein that is similar to albumin in its physical and chemical properties. It is classified as an oncofetal antigen because it is synthesized by the fetal liver and yolk sac and is abundant in fetal serum, but it declines to low levels (≤15 ng/mL, depending on laboratory method) by 12 months of age. AFP is frequently elevated in patients with primary hepatocellular carcinoma (HCC) and nonseminomatous testicular cancer but can also be elevated in other conditions, including pregnancy, ataxia telangiectasia, and nonmalignant liver diseases (e.g., viral hepatitis, cirrhosis).

AFP is a widely used tumor marker for HCC, serving as a tool in diagnosis, staging, prognosis, and monitoring patients undergoing therapy. The sensitivity of AFP for HCC is 41% to 65%, and its specificity ranges between 80% and 94%. Therefore, using AFP to screen for HCC has been most effective in populations with a high disease prevalence (e.g., China and Southeast Asia) and in patients with a high risk for HCC (e.g., patients with liver cirrhosis caused by hepatitis B or hepatitis C infection). The diagnostic utility of AFP may be improved by testing specifically for the isoform AFP-L3, which has a stronger correlation with HCC, and by combining AFP with other laboratory markers, such as des-γ-carboxy-prothrombin (DCP), the liver enzyme alanine aminotransferase (ALT), and a platelet count. High levels of AFP are associated with a poor prognosis in patients with HCC, whereas decreasing levels over time indicate a good response to therapy.

AFP is also an established tumor marker for nonseminomatous germ cell cancers of the testes (NSGCTs). This marker, along with other markers such as human chorionic gonadotropin (hCG; see section later in this chapter) and lactate dehydrogenase (LDH), plays an important role in patient diagnosis, tumor staging, therapeutic monitoring, and detection of relapse. AFP is elevated in 10% to 20% of patients with stage I NSGCT and in nearly all patients in later stages of the disease. As in HCC, increased concentrations are associated with a poor prognosis, whereas declining levels reflect responsiveness to therapy.

In addition to its applications as a tumor marker, AFP is widely used as a marker to detect fetal abnormalities. Increased AFP levels in the serum or amniotic fluid of pregnant women are seen with open neural tube defects such as spina bifida, whereas low levels of AFP are associated with Down syndrome.

Cancer Antigen 125 (CA 125)

A large, heavily glycosylated, mucin-like protein called **cancer antigen 125 (CA 125)** is the standard marker for ovarian cancer. It is not unique to ovarian tumors because it is also found in the normal ovary and other tissues, including the endocervix, endometrium, fallopian tubes, pleura, pericardium, and peritoneum, and the epithelial tissues of the colon, pancreas, lung, kidney, prostate, breast, stomach, and gallbladder. CA 125 can also increase during pregnancy or menstruation or because of benign gynecological conditions (e.g., endometriosis), nongynecological inflammatory conditions (e.g., hepatitis), and other malignancies.

CA 125 has multiple applications in ovarian cancer, ranging from screening and diagnosis to prognosis and monitoring response to therapy. Serum CA 125 levels greater than 38 U/L are typically considered to be above normal. Although 90% or more of women with ovarian cancer in stages II to IV have

Table 17-5 Common Serum Tumor Markers

MARKER	ASSOCIATED CANCER(S)	CLINICAL APPLICATIONS	NORMAL SOURCES	NONCANCEROUS CONDITIONS WITH ELEVATIONS
α-Fetoprotein (AFP)	Nonseminomatous testicular and other germ cell cancers Hepatocellular carcinoma (HCC)	Screening for HCC in high-risk populations Diagnosis and staging Prognosis Monitoring	Fetal liver and yolk sac, adult liver	Pregnancy, nonneoplastic liver diseases
β_2–Microglobulin	B-lymphocyte malignancies	Prognosis Monitoring	Part of class I MHC molecules	Inflammatory conditions and those with high cell turnover
Calcitonin and Ca^{++}	Medullary thyroid carcinoma	Diagnosis Monitoring	Thyroid	Hypercalcemia
Carcinoembryonic antigen (CEA)	Colorectal Thyroid Pancreatic Breast Lung Others	Prognosis Monitoring	Tissues of endodermal origin	Nonneoplastic liver and intestinal diseases, cigarette smoking
CA 125	Ovarian	Screening in women with a family history Diagnosis Prognosis Monitoring	Ovaries and various other tissues	Endometriosis, pelvic inflammatory disease, uterine fibroids, pregnancy, menstruation
CA 15-3	Breast cancer Can also be increased in pancreatic, lung, colorectal, ovarian, and liver cancers	Monitoring	Mammary tissue	Benign breast disease, nonneoplastic liver diseases
CA 19-9	Pancreatic Gallbladder Bile duct Gastric	Diagnosis Monitoring	Sialylated Lewis[a] blood group antigen	Benign hepatobiliary and pancreatic conditions
Human chorionic gonadotropin (hCG), intact and β-hcG forms	Nonseminomatous testicular cancer, ovarian germ cell, trophoblastic (hydatidiform mole, choriocarcinoma)	Diagnosis Prognosis (ovarian cancer) Monitoring	Placenta	Pregnancy
Monoclonal immunoglobulins (Ig) or free Ig light chains	Plasma cell, B lymphocytes	Diagnosis Monitoring Prognosis	Polyclonal immunoglobulins in the blood, few free light chains exist	Monoclonal gammopathy of undetermined significance (MGUS), amyloidosis, nonsecretory myeloma
Neuron-specific enolase (NSE)	Small cell lung cancer and neuroblastoma Pancreatic islet cell	Diagnosis Monitoring	Neuroendocrine tissues, RBCs	Creutzfeldt-Jakob disease (CSF)
Prostate-specific antigen (PSA)	Prostate	Diagnosis Monitoring	Prostate gland	Benign prostatic hyperplasia (BPH), prostatitis
Thyroglobulin	Thyroid	Monitoring	Thyroid gland	Hyperthyroidism

elevated CA 125, the marker is not recommended for screening of the general population because it lacks sensitivity and specificity. Elevated CA 125 levels are only seen in 50% to 60% of women with stage I ovarian cancer; therefore, generalized screening would miss about half of the women during the period when the disease is most treatable. However, annual CA 125 testing, together with a transvaginal ultrasound, is recommended for women with a family history of ovarian cancer because early detection and intervention are likely to be beneficial in this population. The sensitivity and specificity of testing are increased when CA 125 is combined with testing for human epididymis protein 4 (HE4), a glycosylated protein elevated in about 80% of patients with the epithelial subtype of ovarian cancer.

CA 125 also has other clinical applications. For example, an elevated CA 125 concentration combined with imaging is highly sensitive and specific for a differential diagnosis of ovarian cancer from benign pelvic masses, especially in postmenopausal women. Serial CA 125 testing is beneficial in monitoring patient responses to chemotherapy and is recommended before treatment is initiated, during treatment, and during patient follow-up. Rising concentrations of CA 125 over time can predict recurrence of the disease. Persistent elevations of CA 125 or an initial CA 125 value greater than 65 kU/L point to a poor prognosis.

Carcinoembryonic Antigen (CEA)

Carcinoembryonic antigen (CEA) is a glycoprotein with a molecular weight of 180,000 to 200,000, depending on the exact structure of its carbohydrate side chains. CEA was the first oncofetal antigen to be discovered. In 1965, Gold and Freedman described its presence in tissues from the fetal colon and colon adenocarcinoma, and its absence in colon tissues from healthy adults.

The serum CEA level is usually ≤3 ng/mL in healthy people. Increased CEA concentrations are associated with colorectal cancer, and CEA is the most widely used marker for that cancer. The main application of CEA is in monitoring patients undergoing therapy for colorectal cancer. A baseline CEA value should be obtained just before therapy, followed by regular CEA testing after treatment. Increasing CEA levels are a highly sensitive indicator of liver metastasis and can detect recurrent colorectal cancer by an average of 5 months before clinical symptoms appear. CEA measurement should be used in conjunction with clinical examination, radiological testing, and histological confirmation to maximize its sensitivity in detecting disease recurrence. CEA levels can also be used to determine the most appropriate treatment for patients with colorectal cancer because those with higher baseline levels before surgery tend to have a poorer prognosis.

However, CEA is not recommended for colon cancer screening because of its low sensitivity and specificity in this situation. CEA is not increased in all patients with colorectal cancer, and elevated CEA levels can occur in other conditions, including colitis, diverticulitis, irritable bowel syndrome, and nonmalignant liver disease. Cigarette smoking can cause an increase in CEA level to nearly twice that of nonsmokers. CEA levels can also be elevated in other cancers, notably those of the breast, thyroid, gastrointestinal tract, pancreas, and lung.

Human Chorionic Gonadotropin (hCG)

Human chorionic gonadotropin (hCG) is best known as the "pregnancy hormone" because it is made by trophoblasts, cells that contribute to development of the placenta and promote implantation of the embryo. It rises during the first few weeks of gestation, when it can be detected in the blood and urine of pregnant women. hCG can also be produced by certain malignant tumors; elevations are associated with germ cell tumors of the ovary and testes and choriocarcinoma, a rare type of cancer caused by malignant transformation of the trophoblast cells. In these tumors, testing for hCG is recommended as an aid in diagnosis, prognosis, monitoring response to therapy, and detection of recurrence.

hCG is a 45,000-MW glycoprotein composed of an α subunit, which is shared by luteinizing hormone (LH), follicle-stimulating hormone (FSH), and thyroid-stimulating hormone (TSH), and a β subunit that is unique to hCG. Most serological tests for hCG measure both intact hCG and the hCG β subunit to reduce the chance of obtaining false-negative results. Patients should be monitored using the same test because assays can vary in the hCG forms detected. Because hCG levels can also increase in men as the result of testes malfunction, it is important to observe rising values in sequential tests before making a diagnosis of testicular cancer. Elevations of hCG can also occur because of gonadal suppression caused by chemotherapy and do not necessarily indicate tumor recurrence.

Prostate-Specific Antigen (PSA)

Prostate-specific antigen (PSA), a 28,000-MW glycoprotein produced specifically by prostate gland epithelial cells, is the most widely used marker for prostate cancer. PSA was first discovered in semen, where it regulates seminal fluid viscosity and helps dissolve the cervical mucus cap to facilitate sperm cell mobility and entry through the cervix. Its presence was subsequently noted in serum, where it is commonly elevated in patients with prostate cancer.

The specificity of PSA for the prostate gland led to its routine use as a screening test for prostate cancer since 1994. Large clinical trials have found an increased detection rate of early-stage prostate cancer but only a modest reduction in patient mortality when PSA screening is performed in men aged 50 and older. Also, many prostate cancers are slow growing and unlikely to cause death during an older man's remaining life span. Therefore, using PSA to screen for prostate cancer has been a controversial issue because it may potentially lead to unnecessary testing and treatment.

There are several reasons for this concern. Although PSA is specific for prostate tissue, it is *not* specific for prostate cancer. PSA can also be elevated in other conditions affecting the prostate gland, such as *benign prostatic hyperplasia (BPH)*, an enlargement of the prostate gland that commonly occurs as men age, or prostatitis, an inflammation of the gland because of infection or irritation. Transient increases in PSA levels can also occur if samples are collected shortly after ejaculation, digital rectal examination (DRE), or prostate manipulation. As such, there is concern that general PSA screening can lead to the performance of unnecessary prostate biopsies and complications associated with overtreatment (e.g., urinary incontinence, erectile dysfunction, bowel dysfunction).

Many experts believe it may be better to carefully monitor the condition over time by active surveillance and observation ("watchful waiting") than to initiate treatment for early-stage prostate cancer that could decrease quality of life. Most professional organizations, including the American Cancer Society and the American Urological Association, recommend that the decision to receive PSA testing should be up to individual patients following a discussion with their physician about the benefits and harms of testing. Screening can be performed at regular intervals (e.g., 1 to 2 years) along with a digital rectal exam (DRE). The largest benefit is thought to be for men aged 55 to 69 and for men in high-risk groups (e.g., Black men or men with a first-degree relative with prostate cancer), in which screening should begin at age 40.

A total PSA value of 0 to 4 ng/mL is generally considered to be normal. If the PSA level is between 4 and 10 ng/mL, additional testing can be performed to assess the risk of developing prostate cancer and the need for a prostate biopsy:

- One test involves determination of the ratio of free PSA to total PSA (free PSA plus PSA complexed with α-1-anti-chymotrypsin); the smaller the ratio, the greater is the likelihood that prostate cancer is present, with a ratio of ≤0.1 indicating the highest probability.
- Another approach is to use risk calculators, such as the Prostate Health Index (PHI), based on a mathematical formula that incorporates free PSA, total PSA, and p2PSA, an isoform of free PSA that is more highly associated with prostate cancer; the higher the PHI value, the greater is the likelihood that cancer is present.
- The PSA velocity (PSAV) or the rate of increase in PSA values over time (concentration change/year) may also be calculated. PSA values will increase more rapidly if a growing tumor is present, and a PSAV value greater than 0.75 ng/mL/yr is more likely to be associated with the presence of prostate cancer.
- Molecular testing may also be performed to help determine the presence of prostate cancer or susceptibility to developing a hereditary form of prostate cancer.

A prostate biopsy is recommended for men with a total PSA value greater than 10 ng/mL. Regardless of the values of PSA and other tests, a biopsy and examination by a pathologist are required to make a definitive diagnosis.

PSA testing also plays an important role in the management of patients known to have prostate cancer. PSA values, in conjunction with histological observation of prostate biopsy tissue, can be used to define the prostate cancer stage and to guide physicians in determining optimal treatment. Also, a rapid rise in PSAV indicates more aggressive disease. A persistently high level of PSA after radical prostatectomy indicates that residual disease is present. When surgery is successful in removing the tumor, PSA will decrease to undetectable levels. Serial PSA measurements are used to monitor patients who have undergone surgery or other therapies for tumor recurrence: Rising PSA levels after treatment are a sign that the malignancy is recurring and can precede other indicators of disease recurrence by many years.

Cell Surface Markers

Many markers in clinical use are found on the surface of tumor cells. One group of commonly used markers are the CD antigens, which, as we discussed in previous chapters, are used to identify lymphocyte and myeloid populations. As you will see in Chapter 18, these markers are used to classify leukemias and lymphomas based on their cell lineage and maturation stage to aid in diagnosis and treatment decisions.

Another group of clinically useful markers are cell surface receptors that can bind to specific substances that cause a change in cell activity. For example, binding of estrogen and progesterone receptors (ER and PR) on the surface of normal breast cells to their respective hormones is important for breast development. ER and/or PR are overexpressed by some types of breast cancer cells, causing excess cell proliferation when their respective hormones are bound. Determining the receptor status of breast cancer cells is important because patients with cancers that are ER+ can be treated with drugs that inhibit estrogen synthesis or block attachment of estrogen to the receptors, whereas hormonal therapy is not beneficial in ER− cancers.

Some breast cancers also overexpress HER2, causing excess cell division in the presence of the growth factor. Determining the HER2 status of breast cancer is important because patients with HER2+ cancers can benefit from therapies that specifically target HER2 by preventing the growth factor from attaching to its receptor or by other mechanisms, whereas HER2− cancers will not respond to these therapies.

Likewise, some cancer cells have increased levels of the epidermal growth factor receptor (EGFR), a protein involved in the cell signaling that controls cell division. Overexpression of EGFR has been seen in various cancer types (non-small cell lung cancer, breast, ovarian, prostate, pancreatic, renal, head and neck, and colorectal cancer) and has been associated with a worse prognosis. Laboratory identification of EGFR overexpression has been instrumental in identifying patients who would benefit from treatment with EGFR inhibitors.

Genetic Markers

Some of the mutations seen in cancer cells can also serve as genetic markers that the laboratory can test for to characterize tumors and determine the most effective therapy for individual patients. One of the earliest genetic markers, discovered in 1960, is a chromosome translocation produced in certain types of leukemia cells but not in normal cells, producing what is commonly known as the *Philadelphia chromosome*. This mutation involves the *BCR* (breakage cluster region) gene on chromosome 9 and the c-*ABL* gene on chromosome 22. c-*ABL* is a cellular proto-oncogene that codes for tyrosine kinase, a key enzyme in cell-signaling pathways that promote cell division. During the translocation, the two chromosomes break and exchange parts so that the c-*ABL* gene is combined with part of the *BCR* to produce a hybrid gene that is constantly expressed, resulting in uncontrolled cell proliferation **(Fig. 17–5)**. The *BCR/ABL* gene rearrangements are found in most patients with chronic myelogenous leukemia (CML) and

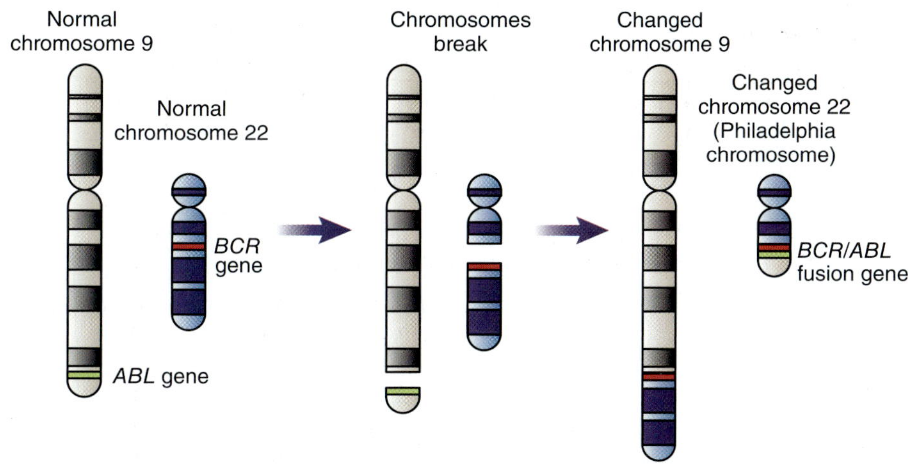

FIGURE 17–5 The *BCR/ABL* gene rearrangement characteristic of CML.

in some patients with acute lymphoblastic leukemia (ALL) or acute myelogenous leukemia (AML), and can be detected by fluorescence in situ hybridization (FISH) (see Chapter 18).

Scientific research has led to the discovery of thousands of genetic mutations and changes in gene expression that can serve as tumor markers. The Cancer Genome Atlas (TCGA) was established through a large-scale collaborative project funded by the National Cancer Institute and the National Human Genome Research Institute to catalog and characterize the genomic changes that occur in cancer. The project identified thousands of pertinent genomic alterations in several tumor types. This information has led to a better understanding of the molecular aspects of cancer and to the development of drugs targeted to specific genetic mutations associated with malignancy.

Increased knowledge of the human genome and advances in development of molecular techniques have revolutionized cancer diagnosis and treatment. Genetic markers play important roles in determining susceptibility of family members to hereditary forms of cancer, cancer diagnosis and prognosis, and identifying patients who would benefit from therapies that target a specific molecular abnormality. The field of genetic tumor markers is too extensive for discussion here, but a few examples of genetic markers and their clinical uses are presented in **Table 17–6.**

Table 17-6 Clinically Relevant Genetic Markers for Cancer

GENETIC MARKER	ASSOCIATED CANCER(S)	CLINICAL APPLICATIONS
BCR-ABL gene fusion	Chronic myeloid leukemia (CML), acute lymphoblastic leukemia (ALL), acute myeloid leukemia (AML)	Diagnosis, predicting response to targeted therapy, monitoring
BRAF V600 mutation	Melanoma, others	Predicting response to targeted therapy
BRCA1 and *BRCA2* mutations	Breast, ovarian, others	Screening high-risk individuals for hereditary cancer and defining options for preventative treatment
Chromosome p17 deletion	Chronic lymphocytic leukemia (CLL)	Diagnosis, prognosis, treatment options
HER2 gene amplification	Breast, ovarian, others	Predicting response to targeted therapy
Immunoglobulin gene rearrangements	B-cell malignancies	Diagnosis, monitoring
KRAS mutation	Colorectal cancer, non-small cell lung cancer, pancreatic cancer	Prognosis, predicting response to targeted therapy
Mutations in mismatch repair genes (e.g., *MSH2*)	Lynch syndrome (a hereditary disorder that predisposes people to developing a type of colorectal cancer and certain other cancers)	Screening family members for Lynch syndrome Prognosis Predicting response to targeted therapy
Messenger RNA for *PCA3*	Prostate	Diagnosis Monitoring to determine the need for repeat biopsy
T-cell receptor gene rearrangements	T-cell malignancies	Diagnosis, monitoring

Knowledge Check 17-3

Match each tumor with its primary cancer association:

a. *BCR-ABL*	____ 1. Colorectal
b. CA 19-9	____ 2. Testicular
c. CA 125	____ 3. Multiple myeloma
d. CEA	____ 4. CML
e. hCG	____ 5. Prostate
f. HER2	____ 6. Pancreatic
g. Monoclonal Ig	____ 7. Breast
h. *MSH2*	____ 8. Ovarian
i. PSA	____ 9. Lynch syndrome

Laboratory Testing in Oncology

Several types of laboratory methods are routinely used in oncology:

- Gross examination of the tumor sample
- Microscopic examination of tumor cell morphology and tissue characteristics
- Immunohistochemistry to detect tumor antigens in tissues
- Automated immunoassays for serum tumor markers
- Flow cytometry for identification of CD antigens in hematologic malignancies and determination of DNA ploidy
- Cytogenetic tests to detect chromosome abnormalities
- Molecular assays to identify genetic mutations in malignant cells

A combination of tests is routinely used to identify the specific type of cancer present and develop an effective treatment plan. Some of these tests are **companion diagnostics**, or tests that provide essential information for the safe and effective use of a particular therapy. In oncology, these tests identify patients who would most likely benefit from a therapy targeted toward a particular tumor marker. In the following sections, we discuss the types of laboratory tests commonly used in oncology and their applications.

Gross and Microscopic Examination of Tumor Tissues and Cells

Solid tumors or the tissue samples obtained from them (i.e., *biopsies*) by surgery or other procedures are sent to the pathology laboratory for *gross examination*. During this process, pathology professionals examine the specimen and record its size, color, consistency, and other characteristics. The samples are then processed for microscopic examination by the histology laboratory: They are placed in a container with a preservative such as formalin, put into small cassettes and embedded in paraffin wax to protect the tissue during storage, cut into very thin sections with a microtome, and adhered to microscope slides. The paraffin wax must be removed from the samples by a special process before the next step, staining of the microscope slides. Alternatively, samples that require rapid examination can be frozen prior to slicing with the microtome.

The microscope slides are then incubated with special dyes, commonly hematoxylin, a basic dye that binds to nucleic acids in cell nuclei, and eosin, an acidic dye that has an affinity for cytoplasmic components. Cytology samples from fine needle aspiration or body fluids can be concentrated, if needed, and smeared onto microscope slides prior to staining. Blood and bone marrow samples are smeared onto microscope slides and stained with Wright-Giemsa.

Pathologists then examine the slides for morphological characteristics that distinguish cancer cells from normal cells. These include a larger than normal nucleus with an irregular shape, prominent nucleoli, and chromatin changes; scant, intensely colored cytoplasm that frequently contains vacuoles; changes in organelles; appearance of atypical mitotic forms; and for solid tumors, changes in tissue architecture. These features can be used to determine the tumor grade. Evaluation of morphology and staining patterns can be subjective and requires considerable skill. Further laboratory testing is required to provide additional information and make an accurate diagnosis.

Immunohistochemistry

Immunohistochemistry (IHC) uses labeled antibodies to detect tumor antigens in formalin-fixed or frozen tissue sections of tumor biopsy material. Before testing, formalin-fixed sections must be treated to remove the paraffin and heated to make the antigen epitopes accessible. The indirect staining method is used because larger immune complexes are formed, providing more sensitive amplification of the signal than is achieved through direct staining (see Chapter 11). An unlabeled primary antibody specific for the antigen to be detected is applied to the tissue section on a slide. After an incubation and wash, a labeled secondary antibody directed against the Fc portion of the primary antibody is applied. The label can be an enzyme such as peroxidase, alkaline phosphatase, or glucose oxidase or a fluorescent dye such as fluorescein isothiocyanate (FITC), rhodamine, or Texas red. Immunofluorescence provides a greater dynamic range than immunochromatographic staining and is particularly useful for the identification and quantification of proteins located near each other. Binding is visualized by light microscopy after the addition of the appropriate chromogen in the case of enzyme labels and by fluorescent microscopy when fluorescent labels are used.

The use of positive and negative control tissues is essential for accurate results. Negative controls are necessary to ensure that the staining observed is because of antibody binding and not the background (i.e., nonspecific reactivity), whereas positive controls confirm that the antibody reagents are working properly. Normal tissue on the same slide can serve as an excellent internal control. Accuracy of the results is also increased when a broad panel of antibodies is used.

Immunohistochemistry is an effective technique for classifying tumors of uncertain origin because many tumors can have a similar appearance histologically. To be helpful in pathological diagnosis, the marker must be differentially expressed in the tumor of origin as compared with other tumors. The tumor can be broadly classified into one of three major lineages—*epithelial, mesenchymal,* or *hematopoietic*—by using stains for specific markers that are characteristic of each type of tissue. Routinely, *cytokeratins,* which are intermediate filaments found in all types of epithelial cells, are used as markers for tumors of epithelial lineage. There are 20 different cytokeratin subtypes, whose expression is often organ and tissue specific and depends on the stage of cell differentiation. *Vimentin,* an intermediate filament found in most mesenchymal cells, is used as a marker to indicate the presence of a sarcoma or melanoma, but its specificity is low because it is also expressed in some other tumor types. CD45, a WBC marker (see Chapter 13), can be used to identify hematopoietic malignancies.

Once the cell lineage is determined, antibodies for more specific markers can be used to precisely classify the neoplasm. For example, antibodies to numerous CD antigens can be used in IHC to identify the various lymphoid and myeloid cell types (see Chapter 18). Antibodies to estrogen receptors, progesterone receptors, and the HER2 antigen can be used in IHC as a companion diagnostic test to classify breast cancer and guide decisions about appropriate therapy **(Fig. 17–6).** Automated immunohistochemistry assays have been developed that allow for quantitation of the proteins expressed by different cell populations.

Immunoassays for Circulating Tumor Markers

Serum tumor markers are most commonly measured by labeled immunoassays using a sandwich format (see Chapter 11). These assays are automated, highly sensitive, and provide rapid results. Despite their advantages, as discussed in the following paragraphs, immunoassays can be affected by

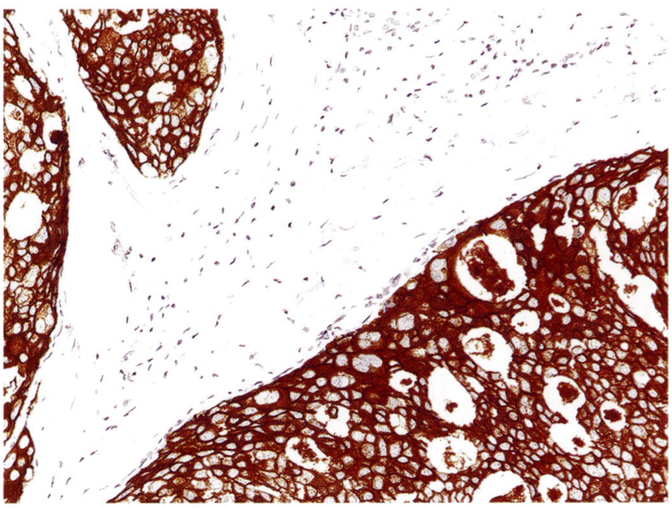

FIGURE 17–6 HER2 staining on breast cancer tissue by immunohistochemistry. Patients who are positive for the HER2 antigen are candidates for monoclonal anti-HER2 therapy. *(Photo by IHCantibody. Own work, CC BY 4.0, https://commons.wikimedia.org/w/index.php?curid=76076939.)*

several factors that need to be considered when the results are interpreted.

First, antibody reagents from different manufacturers can vary greatly in terms of what they detect, particularly if monoclonal antibodies are used. Thus, it is important to use the same method for monitoring patients over time because the results can be affected if patients change clinics or laboratories.

Second, false-positive or false-negative results can occur. Antibodies can cross-react with similar structures, potentially causing false-positive results. For example, the α subunit of hCG is virtually identical to the α subunit of LH, and the β subunits of the two hormones are 80% homologous. If the assay fails to measure the marker produced by the tumor, false-negative results can be produced. For example, methods that only detect intact hCG would miss tumors that produce free α and/or free β hCG chains.

A third factor that can affect immunoassay results is antigen excess. By virtue of their unchecked growth and aggressive metabolism, some neoplasms produce massive amounts of tumor marker molecules. When the measurements exceed the linear range of reportable results, a **high-dose hook effect** can be created, resulting in a falsely decreased measurement in the area of antigen excess (see Chapter 11, Fig. 11–8). In such cases, the sample must be diluted to determine its value within the reportable range. Criteria should be developed to identify situations in which the hook effect may be present so that specimens can be systematically diluted and accurate results obtained. A related problem of antigen excess in automated systems is sample carryover, so testing of the sample adjacent to the specimen with excessive antigen may also need to be repeated.

A fourth problem with immunoassays involves interference caused by heterophile, anti-animal, or autoantibodies in the patient sample. Significant interferences can result from human anti-mouse antibodies (HAMAs), high-affinity antibodies produced by some patients who have received passive immunotherapy with mouse monoclonal immunoglobulins (see Chapter 25). Because many immunoassays use mouse monoclonal antibodies as reagents, HAMAs in the patient sample can interfere profoundly with the reaction, causing either falsely elevated (most commonly) or falsely decreased test results. The principle of interference resulting in a false-positive result is illustrated in Figure 11–9.

To confirm the presence of interfering antibodies, the sample can be diluted and the linearity of the results analyzed. Specimens with interfering antibodies tend to exhibit nonlinear behavior. The laboratory can also test directly for the antibodies themselves. The likelihood of interference by endogenous antibodies can be reduced by pretreating the sample with commercial blocking reagents. These reagents are typically mouse or rabbit immunoglobulins that bind to the interfering antibodies and neutralize them. Interference with tumor marker tests can also be caused by factors that can affect other immunoassays, such as elevated bilirubin, lipemia, and hemolysis. In any case, patient results should not be reported until the interference issue is resolved.

Other recommendations should also be considered in the performance of tumor marker tests:

- Samples exhibiting lipemia or hemolysis should not be used, as these may create falsely decreased tumor marker concentrations.
- Cutoff values for screening tests are typically selected under the presumption that a relatively low number of people being screened actually have cancer and that it would be worse to miss a cancer than to do further testing on a healthy person to exclude cancer. Thus, a high number of false positives is expected because of low disease prevalence.
- Establishing a baseline level at initial diagnosis followed by serial testing over time can provide valuable information when a patient is being monitored for response to treatment or tumor recurrence. In this case, the upward or downward trend in the marker level is evaluated.
- When performing serial testing, each test should be performed by the same laboratory with the same test kit to minimize result variability.
- Testing for multiple markers, if possible, will increase sensitivity and specificity. The National Academy of Clinical Biochemistry (NACB) has published consensus guidelines for the clinical use of tumor markers.

Critical Thinking 17-1

A woman experiencing abdominal bloating and digestive problems was suspected of having ovarian cancer. Imaging and surgery confirmed the diagnosis; however, the patient's CA 125 level (32 U/mL) prior to surgery was within normal limits. Provide two explanations for this test result and explain how the laboratory can help differentiate between the two possibilities.

Flow Cytometry

As we discuss in detail in Chapter 18, flow cytometry plays an important role in the analysis of cancer cells in hematologic malignancies. To perform this analysis, peripheral blood and bone marrow cells from patients suspected of having leukemia or lymphoma are incubated with a panel of monoclonal antibodies directed against different CD antigens. These antibodies are labeled with different fluorochromes for identification and will attach to the cells that possess their corresponding markers in a direct immunofluorescence assay. The results are interpreted by flow cytometry and provide important information about the lineage of the malignant cell population (B cell, T cell, or myeloid) and its stage of differentiation (see Chapter 13). This information is used by physicians in patient diagnosis, monitoring, and selection of appropriate therapy.

Flow cytometry can also be used to determine the number of chromosome sets, or *ploidy,* in cancer cells by using fluorescent dyes that bind to DNA. Genetic changes in cancer cells over time can lead to a loss or gain of chromosomes, resulting in an abnormal chromosome number, or *aneuploidy.* This information can provide useful information about patient prognosis, as aneuploid cells tend to grow faster and may respond better to more aggressive therapy.

Cytogenetics Testing

Several types of tests are performed by the **cytogenetics** laboratory to study abnormalities in chromosome structure or numbers that may be associated with cancer: karyotype analysis, fluorescence in situ hybridization, and comparative genomic hybridization microarray. These tests provide information that is used in patient diagnosis, determining prognosis and treatment, and monitoring response to therapy.

Karyotype analysis involves visual interpretation of an image created by arranging a person's chromosomes according to their size, banding pattern, and centromere position **(Fig. 17–7).** In this method, chromosomes processed from the patient's tumor are stained and examined microscopically for various abnormalities. The number of abnormalities can increase as the disease advances. Structural abnormalities include *deletions* (loss of a chromosome segment), *duplications* (gain of a chromosome segment), *translocations* (transfer of a fragment from one chromosome onto a different chromosome), and *inversions* (reversal of the segment order in the same chromosome). In some cases, entire chromosomes can be gained or lost, resulting in *aneuploidy.*

Fluorescence in situ hybridization (FISH) detects chromosomal abnormalities more precisely at a molecular level. In FISH, interphase cells from the patient's tumor are incubated with fluorescent-labeled nucleic acid probes that are complementary to the sequence of interest. Cells containing the sequence will bind to the probes and are visualized with a fluorescent microscope. FISH is commonly used to detect very small deletions, chromosome translocations, such as the *BCR/ABL* rearrangement characteristic of chronic myeloid leukemia (CML; see Fig. 18–13), and gene amplifications, such as the *HER2* gene amplification seen in some cases of breast cancer, in which multiple copies of the fluorescent signal will be observed (see Fig. 12–20). Although FISH is a highly specific

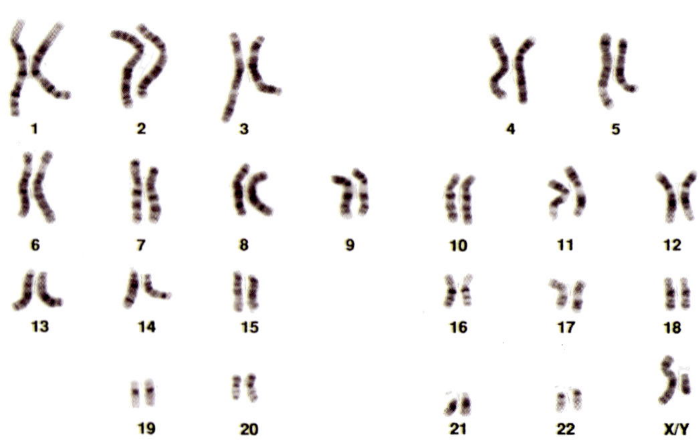

FIGURE 17–7 A normal male karyotype, containing 22 pairs of autosomal chromosomes and one pair of sex chromosomes. Karyotype analysis of tumor cells often reveals abnormalities in the number or structure of the chromosomes. *(Source: National Cancer Institute [NCI].)*

method, it can only detect gene sequences that are complementary to the probes used; as such, it may not detect less common abnormalities.

Comparative genomic hybridization (CGH) uses microarray technology to detect gains or losses of chromosomal material throughout the genome. In CGH, single-stranded DNA from the tumor is tagged with a fluorescent label and incubated with known nucleic acid sequences that have been spotted onto different areas of a membrane. The sample will hybridize to any complementary sequences on the tiny spots, allowing for simultaneous testing of the specimen for multiple genes. The microarray is interpreted with a fluorescent reader and analysis software, and the results are compared with a normal reference sample (see Fig. 12–17).

Molecular Tests

Advances in molecular testing have revolutionized cancer care. These tests identify precise changes in DNA or RNA that can be used as tumor markers to aid in cancer diagnosis and monitoring, detect predisposition to hereditary cancers, and identify patients for targeted therapies (i.e., treatments directed toward a particular genetic mutation). Commonly used methods in this category are next-generation sequencing (NGS), polymerase chain reaction (PCR), and microarrays.

NGS has become a standard method in the clinical management of patients with cancer. This technique, also known as *massively parallel sequencing,* simultaneously analyzes millions of DNA sequences in a sample of tumor tissue or blood from a patient with cancer (see Chapter 12). If the mutation is thought to be rare or unique, the entire genome or all the exons (the coding sequences in the genome) can be examined. Targeted NGS panels that examine selected genetic mutations commonly associated with a specific type or group of cancers have been developed by commercial manufacturers and can be used by laboratories as companion diagnostics to identify patients who could potentially benefit from targeted cancer therapy and patients who might be resistant to a particular therapy. For example, testing for certain *EGFR* mutations can identify patients with non-small cell lung cancer who would benefit from tyrosine kinase inhibitor therapies, whereas testing for *BRAF, KRAS,* and *NRAS* mutations in metastatic colorectal cancer can identify patients who would likely be resistant to treatment with anti-*EGFR* therapy. A list of approved companion diagnostic tests has been published by the U.S. Food and Drug Administration (FDA), and guidelines for their recommended uses have been developed by the National Comprehensive Cancer Network (NCCN), the American Society of Clinical Oncology (ASCO), and the College of American Pathologists (CAP).

NGS is also used to identify individuals with a high risk of developing a hereditary form of cancer. For example, people with a personal or family history of hereditary breast or ovarian cancer are routinely offered genetic testing for *BRCA1* and *BRCA2* mutations, which carry a 40% to 80% lifetime risk for developing breast cancer, and an 11% to 40% lifetime risk for ovarian cancer. Studies are also examining the use of NGS and other molecular methods to analyze cell-free DNA, or circulating tumor-derived DNA (ctDNA), shed from dying tumor cells into the bloodstream for mutations and other modifications (e.g., methylation) for early cancer detection, treatment selection, and monitoring of patients with cancer.

PCR methods and other amplification techniques have been used to detect genetic mutations known to be associated with cancer by using primers that bind specifically to the altered sequences and amplify them to detectable levels (see Chapter 12). Applications of PCR to oncology include detection of *BRAF V600E* for colon cancer, **microsatellite instability** in hereditary nonpolyposis colorectal cancer (HNPCC or *Lynch syndrome*), Ig gene rearrangements in B-cell malignancies, and T-cell receptor (TCR) gene rearrangements in T-cell malignancies. Microsatellite instability is caused by mutations in DNA mismatch repair (MMR) genes (e.g., *MSH1, MSH2, MSH6*) that can lead to replication errors that affect DNA sequences. Amplification of the MMR genes by PCR and detection by electrophoresis will show an increased number of bands (or peaks, if capillary electrophoresis is used) when the results of tumor tissue and normal tissue are compared **(Fig. 17–8).**

PCR detection of B- and T-cell malignancies is based on demonstration of clonality, as the malignant cells in a patient will produce an identical Ig or TCR. Normally, lymphocytes from an individual produce varying Ig and TCR gene rearrangements, which yield amplicons of different lengths that blend together to form a smear on electrophoresis, whereas patients with B- or T-cell malignancies will produce identical gene rearrangements that will be uniform in size and yield a predominant single band (see Fig. 18–14). Quantitative PCR can be used to determine patient response to treatment by estimating the tumor load over time.

In **gene-expression microarrays,** RNA from the tumor sample is tested in a microarray to analyze the expression of multiple genes and compare the results to a reference sample. This approach is uncovering molecular profiles that can characterize specific tumor types and subtypes to provide better information regarding patient diagnosis and prognosis. Gene-expression arrays, such as the MammaPrint, Oncotype

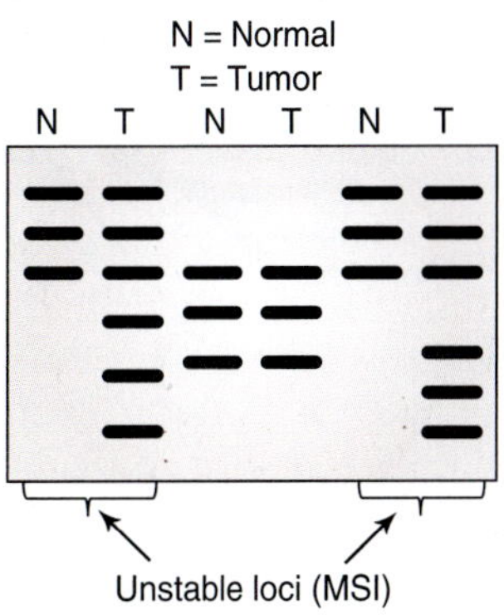

FIGURE 17–8 Microsatellite instability detected by PCR amplification of mismatch repair genes and gel electrophoresis. Note the increased number of alleles in the tumor samples as compared to the same alleles in normal cells.

DX, and BluePrint for breast cancer, can aid in predicting the likelihood of cancer recurrence and guiding treatment decisions for patients with cancer.

Interactions Between the Immune System and Tumors

In the 1950s, F. MacFarlane Burnet and Lewis Thomas independently proposed the theory of **immunosurveillance** to explain the role of the immune system in defense against cancer. This theory states that the immune system continually patrols the body for cancerous or precancerous cells and eliminates them before they become clinically evident. Burnet and Thomas based their hypotheses on early studies involving transplantation of tumor cells in genetically inbred mice. Cells of the immune system isolated from these mice or from humans have been shown to kill tumor cells in the laboratory. The protective role of the immune system against tumors has also been supported by clinical evidence in humans: a significantly higher incidence of cancer has been observed in transplant patients who received immunosuppressive therapy and patients with immunodeficiency diseases than in the general population. Also, the incidence of cancer rises significantly after the age of 60, when there is a decline in immune function. In this section, we discuss the types of immune defenses that are thought to protect the host against cancer. Ironically, some aspects of the immune response may actually promote tumor growth, and we discuss these in the section, "Immunoediting and Tumor Escape."

Immune Defenses Against Tumor Cells

Both innate and adaptive immune responses are thought to play a role in protecting the host from cancer. Protective mechanisms are believed to be mediated by CD8$^+$ cytotoxic T (T_C) cells, dendritic cells (DCs), CD4$^+$ helper T (TH1) cells, natural killer (NK) cells, and a subset of macrophages called M1. The role of antibodies is unclear. The mechanisms by which each of these components function are the same as those involved in the elimination of pathogenic organisms **(Fig. 17–9).**

Innate Immune Responses

NK cells are thought to be the key cells involved in innate immune responses to tumors, as people or laboratory animals with genetic defects in NK cells are more susceptible to developing tumors. As we discussed in Chapter 2, NK cells act in a manner that is similar to T_C cells (see the text that follows) but can kill tumor cells in a manner that is not antigen specific. They are activated to kill cells that lack class I MHC molecules, a property that is often seen in transformed cells (see "Immunoediting and Tumor Escape"). Activating receptors on NK cells bind to tumor antigens or substances released from dying

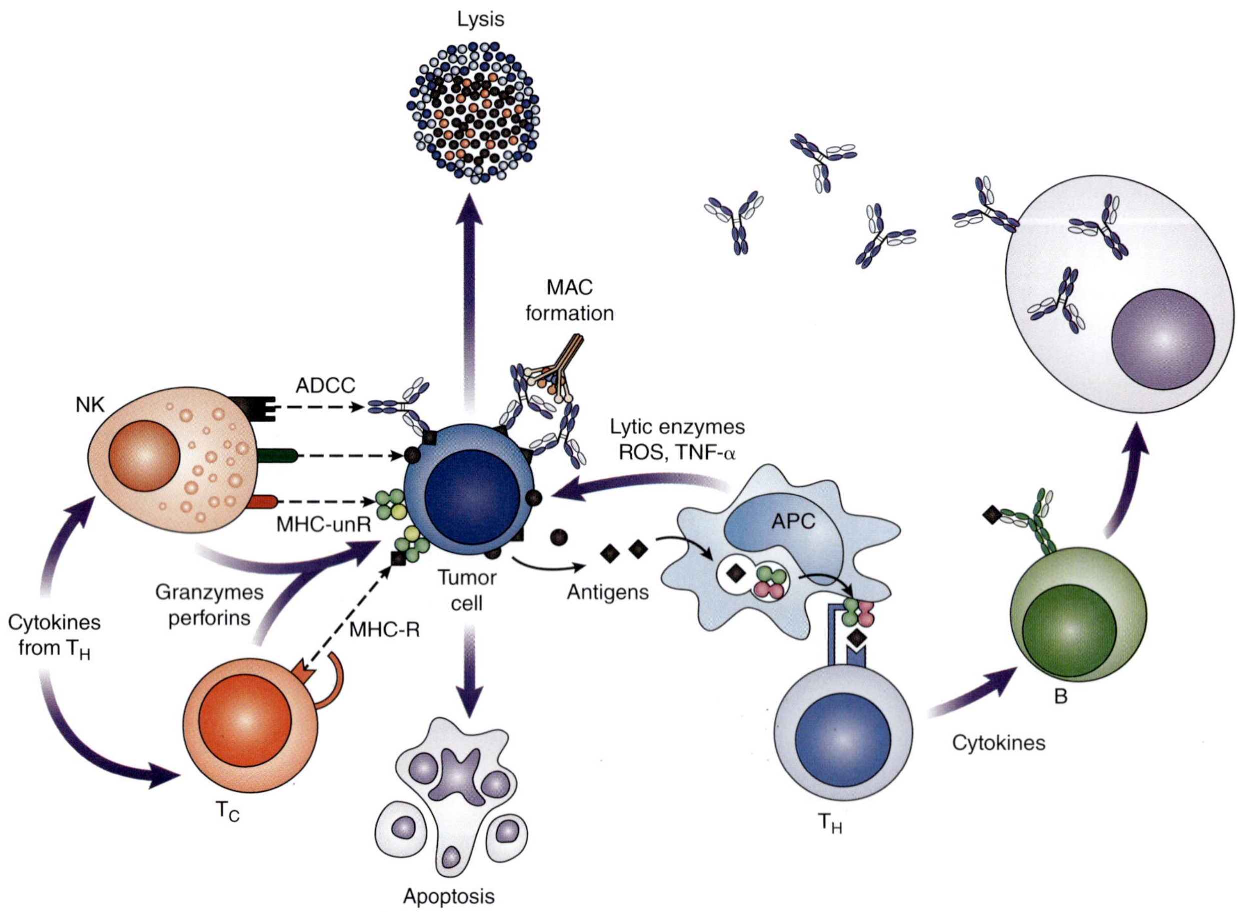

FIGURE 17–9 Immune defenses against tumor cells. MHC-R = MHC-restricted killing; MHC-unR = MHC unrestricted killing.

tumor cells, initiating intracellular signals that promote degranulation and the release of perforin and granzymes, which ultimately kill the cells by inducing apoptosis. NK-cell activity can be increased by interleukin (IL)-2. NK cells may also participate in antibody-dependent cellular cytotoxicity (ADCC) in the presence of tumor-specific antibodies (see the text that follows). NK cells are thought to be most effective against malignant cells circulating in the bloodstream during the early stages of tumor development. However, their effectiveness in eliminating well-established solid tumors is uncertain.

M1 macrophages may also play a role in innate immunity against tumors. M1 macrophages activated in vitro by interferon-gamma (IFN-γ) possess tumoricidal capabilities, killing tumor cells by the same mechanisms they use to kill infectious organisms, including release of lysosomal enzymes, reactive oxygen species, and nitric oxide. They also produce tumor necrosis factor alpha (TNF-α), a cytokine that can damage tumor cells by inducing local inflammation and thrombosis in the blood vessels within the cancerous mass. However, the significance of M1 macrophages in anti-tumor responses in the body is unclear.

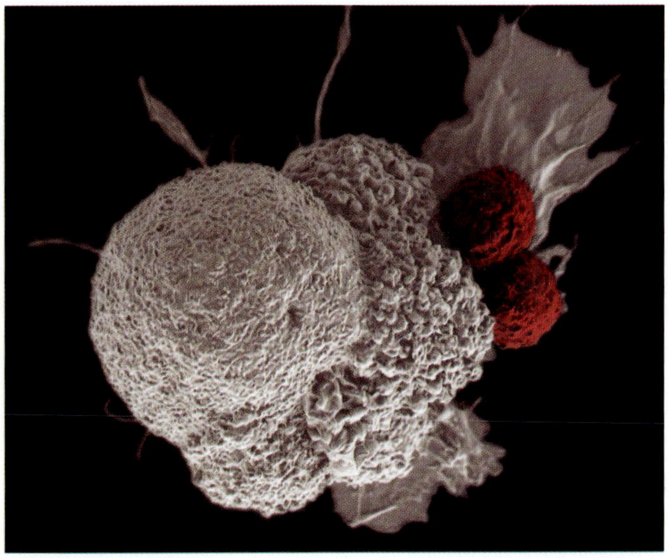

FIGURE 17–10 Tumor cell attack by cytotoxic T cells. Shown here is a pseudo-colored scanning electron micrograph of an oral squamous cancer cell (white) being attacked by two cytotoxic T cells (red). *(Source: National Cancer Institute [NCI].)*

Adaptive Immune Responses

The main mechanism of adaptive immunity against tumors is mediated by T_C cells. T_C-cell responses are initiated by DCs, which act as antigen-presenting cells (APCs) by processing tumor antigens and displaying the peptides derived from these antigens on their surface in combination with class I MHC molecules. This mechanism is known as *cross-presentation* because the exogenous tumor antigens are presented in context with class I MHC molecules rather than class II MHC molecules. The DCs present the tumor peptide-antigen complexes to specific TCRs on the surface of the T_C cells and provide costimulatory signals that promote T_C-cell maturation. The mature T_C cells use their antigen-specific TCRs to bind class I MHC-associated tumor antigens on the surface of the tumor cell. Within minutes, their granules migrate toward the plasma membrane and release cytotoxic proteins in the synapse formed between the T_C cell and the tumor cell. Among these proteins are perforin, which creates pores in the tumor cell membrane, and granzymes, which enter through the pores and cause apoptosis of the tumor target **(Fig. 17–10)**. A subpopulation of natural killer T (NKT) cells, which express properties of both NK cells and T cells, can destroy tumor cells in a mechanism that is similar to the T_C cells but is MHC independent.

DCs activate $CD4^+$ T_H1 cells through presentation of tumor antigens in combination with class II MHC molecules. The activated T_H1 cells may play a role in tumor immunity by secreting cytokines such as IL-2, which promote T_C-cell development and enhance NK-cell activity, and IFN-γ, which activates macrophages and increases class I MHC expression on the tumor cell surface.

Individuals with tumors can also produce antibodies against tumor antigens. In vitro studies have demonstrated that these antibodies can kill tumor cells by inducing complement-mediated lysis or ADCC. The latter mechanism occurs when the antibodies coat the tumor cells and bind to Fc receptors on the surface of macrophages, NK cells, or neutrophils, stimulating them to release enzymes that destroy the tumor targets. However, the relevance of these *antibodies* in vivo is unclear.

Knowledge Check 17-4

The most effective adaptive immune responses against tumors are mediated by:

a. Antibodies
b. Cytotoxic T cells
c. NK cells
d. M1 macrophages

Immunoediting and Tumor Escape

Despite the immune responses against tumors, cancer occurs at a high frequency in individuals who appear to be immunocompetent. Scientists have long been trying to find the answer to this intriguing puzzle. As the field of tumor immunology advances, they are recognizing that immunosurveillance is only part of a broader process that explains the complex relationship between the immune system and cancer. This process is thought to consist of three phases: *elimination, equilibrium,* and *escape*. It involves **immunoediting,** a process by which genetic and other changes in tumor cells allow them to escape the host's immune responses **(Fig. 17–11)**.

Elimination

The elimination phase of the immunoediting process is essentially the same as immunosurveillance. If the immunologic mechanisms involved in immunosurveillance are highly effective, they will likely result in complete elimination of the

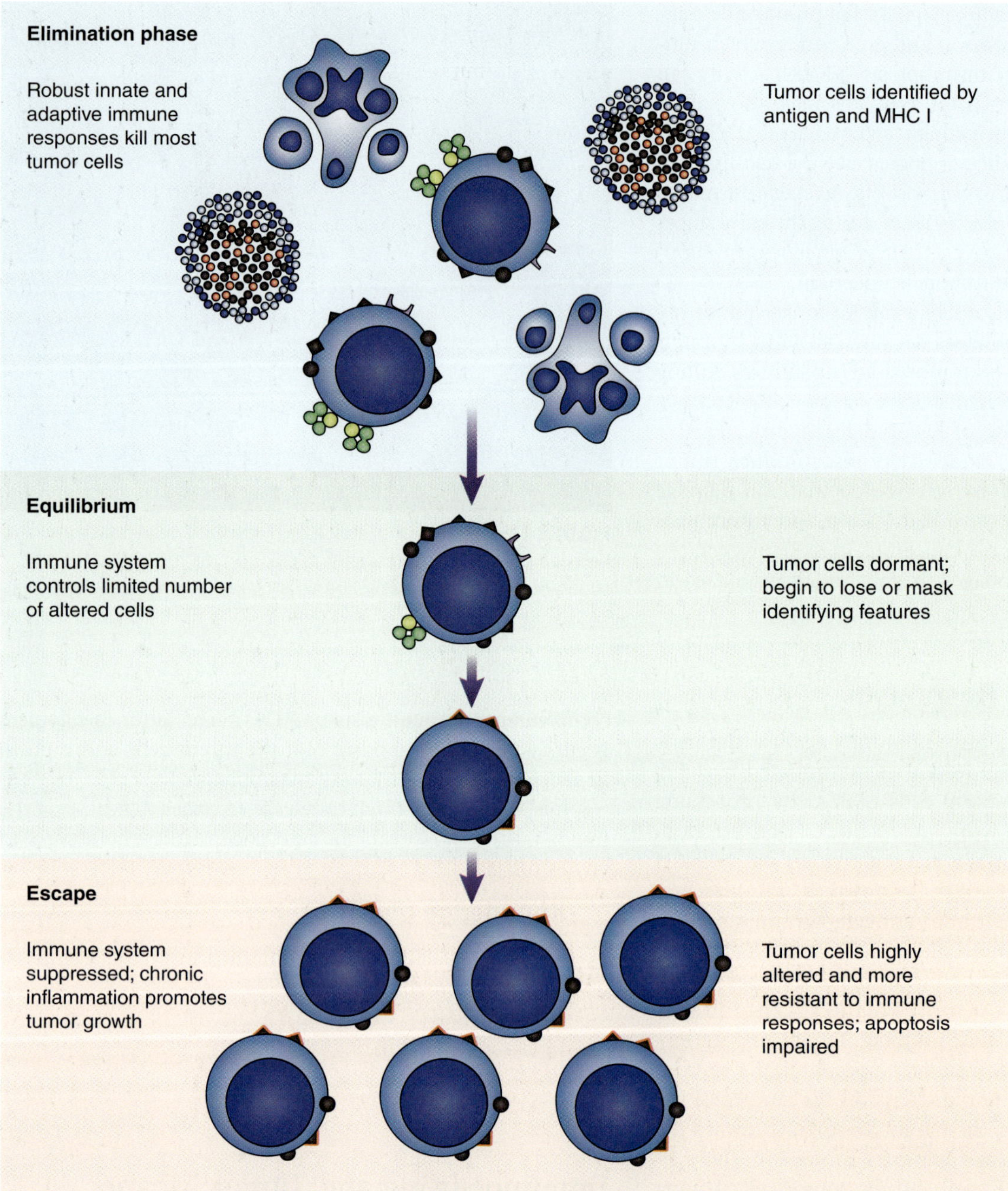

FIGURE 17–11 Relationship between the immune system and cancer: Immunoediting and mechanisms of tumor escape.

tumor. If the immune responses are not completely effective, some of the tumor cells will remain in the body. These cells are then thought to enter the equilibrium phase.

Equilibrium

In this phase, tumor cells are thought to enter a state of dynamic equilibrium with the immune system, which keeps the altered cells under control so that they are not clinically evident. During this period, tumor cells may remain dormant or evolve slowly over time. The dynamic interactions between the tumor and the immune system are thought to shape the phenotype of the tumor and its ultimate outcome, hence the term *immunoediting*. The tumor may eventually be eliminated by the body, establish permanent residence in the equilibrium phase, or evolve into a phenotype that can escape the immune system and cause disease.

During the equilibrium phase, mutations can occur in the genetically unstable transformed cells. Under selective pressure from immunologic forces of attack by cells in the **tumor microenvironment (Fig. 17–12)**, some of the tumor cells may develop into genetic variants that are resistant to immune defenses, similar to the development of antibiotic resistance by bacteria. These cells move past the equilibrium phase and enter the escape phase.

Escape

During this phase, the balance between immunologic control and tumor development is tipped in favor of the neoplasm, and tumor growth progresses, even in the presence of antitumor immune responses. Cancer is a heterogeneous disease, and tumors have developed a variety of strategies to evade the immune system (see Fig. 17–11). These mechanisms, which

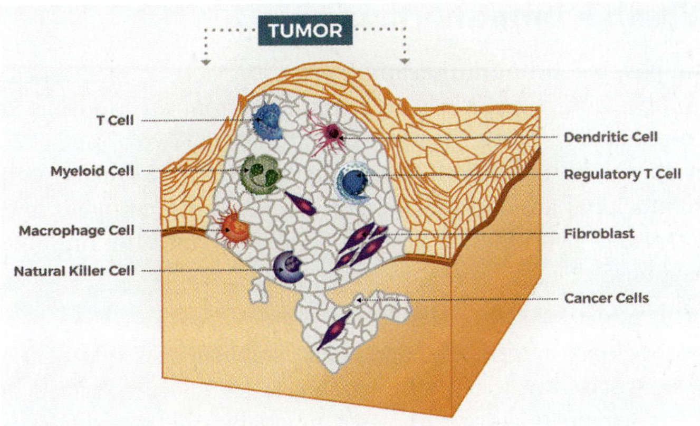

FIGURE 17–12 Within a tumor, cancer cells are surrounded by a variety of immune cells, fibroblasts, molecules, and blood vessels, known as the *tumor microenvironment*. Cancer cells can change the microenvironment, which in turn can affect how cancer grows and spreads. *(Source: National Cancer Institute [NCI].)*

mostly involve (1) loss of surface antigens or (2) inhibition of anti-tumor responses, are summarized here:

- Some tumors downregulate the expression of tumor antigens or MHC molecules on their cell surface, making them less likely to be recognized by T cells. Other modifications may involve defects in components of the antigen-processing machinery associated with class I MHC molecules.
- Tumors can suppress T-cell responses by engaging inhibitory receptors called *immune checkpoint molecules*. Normally, these molecules play a role in preventing autoimmunity and in regulating immune responses to microbes (see Chapter 15). Two well-studied molecules are cytotoxic T-lymphocyte antigen-4 (CTLA-4), which competes with CD28 for binding to CD80 (B7-1) and CD86 (B7-2) on APCs; and programmed death-1 (PD-1), which binds to programmed death-ligand 1 (PDL-1) on APCs.
- Many tumors secrete immunosuppressive substances, such as transforming growth factor-β (TGF-β; see Chapter 6).
- Regulatory T (Treg) cells and myeloid-derived suppressor cells that accumulate in the tumor, lymphoid tissues, and blood of individuals with cancer can inhibit protective immune responses.

Another factor that likely contributes to tumor progression is inflammation. Although acute inflammation may protect the host, chronic inflammation is believed to modify the cellular microenvironment in ways that promote tumor development. Pro-inflammatory cytokines and myeloid cells may contribute to tumorigenesis in several ways, including generation of free radicals that cause DNA damage, and production of factors that induce cell proliferation, increase tumor cell survival, enhance angiogenesis, modify the tissue to allow tissue invasion, and suppress adaptive immune responses.

The various defenses and escape mechanisms we discussed in the previous paragraphs are summarized in a study guide at the end of this chapter. A clear understanding of the evasion mechanisms used by tumors and of the immune responses they suppress is critical in developing rational approaches to targeted immunotherapy. In the section that follows, we present specific approaches taken to influence interactions between tumors and the immune system to promote tumor rejection.

Immunotherapy

Many different types of treatments are used for cancer. The therapy used for a particular patient depends on the type of tumor present and the disease stage. A combination of different treatments is typically used to maximize effectiveness. Conventional therapies include surgery to remove solid tumors, radiation and hormone therapies to reduce tumor size, and chemotherapy to destroy residual tumor cells and metastases. **Immunotherapy** (or *biological therapy*), based on the ability of the immune system to destroy tumor cells, has played an increasingly important role in cancer treatment in recent years. Increased knowledge of the genetic and protein changes that drive tumor growth have led to the development of **targeted therapies**, small molecule inhibitors and monoclonal antibodies that have revolutionized cancer treatment because they attack tumor cells more specifically, with fewer effects on normal cells. Small molecule inhibitors block the action of kinases or other molecules involved in cell signaling; an example is imatinib, which targets an abnormal kinase made in CML and certain other malignancies (see Chapter 18). Monoclonal antibodies are a type of passive immunotherapy that we discuss in more detail later.

Immunotherapeutic methods can be classified into three major types: active, passive, and adoptive. In active immunotherapy, the immune system is stimulated to mount a response against the tumor. Passive immunotherapy involves administration of tumor-specific antibodies or cytokines to attack the tumor. In adoptive immunotherapy, immune cells are provided to patients. Although it is well beyond the scope of this chapter to cover all the different protocols, in the following sections, we present the major types of immunotherapy and their applications to specific kinds of cancer.

Active Immunotherapy and Cancer Vaccines

The possibility of stimulating a patient's own immune system to respond to tumor antigens has long intrigued scientists. In 1891, the bone sarcoma surgeon William Coley began the first systematic study of immunotherapy. He noted that patients with cancer who developed an infection after surgery experienced tumor regression and had a better prognosis than patients who did not acquire an infection. Inspired by this knowledge, he developed a mixture of killed *Streptococcus pyogenes* and killed *Serratia marcescens* bacteria, which later became known as "Coley's toxins," to treat patients with inoperable bone and soft-tissue sarcomas. Although this treatment was successful in shrinking tumors in some patients, the results varied among physicians, and in 1962, the FDA no longer recognized the formulation as an effective cancer therapy. Despite criticism of Coley's work, the medical community later realized that his premise of stimulating the immune system to effectively treat cancer bore some merit. Today we acknowledge Coley as the "Father of Immunotherapy."

Coley's studies and numerous others that followed led to the development of **cancer vaccines,** formulations that stimulate the body's immune defenses against cancer. Cancer vaccines can be *prophylactic* or *therapeutic*. Prophylactic vaccines prevent infection with certain cancer-associated viruses. Two such vaccines in routine use are the HPV vaccine to prevent cervical and other HPV-associated cancers, and the hepatitis B vaccine to prevent HCC (see Chapter 25).

Therapeutic cancer vaccines are given to patients who have already developed cancer. These vaccines are designed to induce an immune response against tumor antigens, with the hope of eliminating existing tumor cells and producing long-lasting immunity. They can be made in several ways, including from bacteria, the patient's own tumor cells, TAAs associated with a particular type of cancer, antigens carried by the patient's DCs, mRNA coding for a tumor antigen, and oncolytic viruses (viruses that can infect, replicate in, and destroy cancer cells).

The most widely used therapeutic vaccine has been bacille Calmette-Guérin (BCG), a live but weakened strain of *Mycobacterium bovis* bacteria, used for noninvasive bladder cancer. Serial treatments in which BCG is directly delivered into the urinary bladder through a catheter are effective in reducing the progression of tumor growth and in delaying cancer recurrence in these patients. The exact mechanism by which BCG works is unknown, but it is believed to stimulate innate and T-cell–mediated immune anti-tumor responses and possibly destroy the tumor cells directly.

Other FDA-approved therapeutic cancer vaccines include the following:

- Sipuleucel-T (Provenge)—composed of patient DCs pre-incubated with the prostatic acid phosphatase (PAP) antigen and the cytokine granulocyte-macrophage colony-stimulating factor (GM-CSF), for men with metastatic prostate cancer
- Nadofaragene firadenovec (Adstiladrin)—a genetically modified, nonreplicating virus that contains a gene coding for IFN-α, for treatment of early-stage bladder cancer that has not responded to BCG therapy
- T-VEC (Imlygic)—an oncolytic herpes simplex type I virus that carries the gene for human GM-CSF, used to treat advanced melanoma

Many more cancer vaccines are in clinical trials. Development of effective therapeutic vaccines has been challenging because they are usually given to patients in advanced stages of disease who may have suboptimal immune responses, and they often target tumor antigens that are also shared by normal cells. Immunologists are hopeful that advances in DNA sequencing will help immunologists identify tumor-specific neoantigens that can be used to design more effective cancer vaccines in the future.

Passive Immunotherapy

In **passive immunotherapy,** as we previously mentioned, soluble components of the immune system are transferred to patients to boost their immune response. Two approaches used for patients with cancer involve (1) treatment with monoclonal antibodies to target specific tumor antigens and (2) use of cytokines to nonspecifically enhance the immune response.

Monoclonal Antibodies

Monoclonal antibodies have been established as one of the most successful therapeutic strategies for cancer because of their specificity. As we discussed in Chapter 3, these antibodies are derived from a single clone of cells that produce highly specific antibodies directed toward one epitope of an antigen. Monoclonal antibodies in cancer immunotherapy have been developed against different types of antigens, including CD antigens, glycoproteins, glycolipids, carbohydrates, vascular targets, stromal and extracellular antigens, growth factors, and immune checkpoint molecules. These antibodies have different mechanisms of action, depending on their targets. They can be used alone ("naked") or conjugated to a chemotherapy drug or radioactive particle. We discuss the major approaches to monoclonal antibody therapy in the text that follows (see **Table 17–7** for a summary).

Naked monoclonal antibodies, which are not attached to a toxic molecule, can exert their effects in different ways:

- Monoclonal antibodies directed against antigens on the tumor cell surface are thought to destroy the tumor through the same mechanisms used to attack infectious organisms—ADCC, opsonization, and complement-mediated cytotoxicity.
- Some monoclonal antibodies target surface receptors involved in intracellular pathways needed for cell growth and survival. These receptors are expressed at higher-than-normal levels on epithelial cancers of the colon, breast, lung, head, and neck. Therapeutic antibodies bind to these receptors and block signals needed to activate the molecular pathways.
- Monoclonal antibodies targeting antigens involved in angiogenesis block the formation of new blood vessels that provide oxygen and nutrients needed for tumor growth. Many of these antibodies are directed against the vascular endothelial growth factor (VEGF) family of proteins or their receptors.
- Some monoclonal antibodies, called **immune checkpoint inhibitors,** boost the immune response to the tumor by blocking inhibitory pathways that inactivate T cells. These antibodies bind to the inhibitory receptors CTLA-4 and PD-1 or its ligand PD-L1, which were discussed in a previous section. They are effective in treating several types of cancer. Their mechanism of action is illustrated in **Figure 17–13.**

Monoclonal antibodies against tumor antigens can also be linked to potent cytotoxic drugs or radioisotopes. These products, called **antibody-drug conjugates** or **immunotoxins,** deliver the toxic molecules directly to the tumor cells.

Table 17-7 Approaches to Cancer Immunotherapy Using Monoclonal Antibodies

ANTIBODY TARGETS	MECHANISM OF ACTION	EXAMPLES
Surface antigens on tumor cells	ADCC Opsonization Complement-mediated cytotoxicity	*Rituximab,* a MAb directed against the CD20 antigen on B cells; used to treat B-cell neoplasms *Alemtuzumab,* a MAb directed against the mature lymphocyte antigen, CD52; used to treat chronic lymphocytic leukemia
Cell surface receptors	Block signaling pathways involved in cell proliferation and survival	*Panitumumab,* a MAb directed against epidermal growth factor receptor (EGFR), used to treat colorectal cancer *Trastuzumab,* a MAb directed against HER2, used to treat breast and gastroesophageal tumors with overexpressed HER2
Antigens involved in angiogenesis	Inhibit formation of blood vessels needed to deliver oxygen and nutrients to the tumor	*Bevacizumab,* a MAb directed against vascular endothelial growth factor (VEGF); for treatment of colorectal, glioblastoma, lung, renal, cervical, and ovarian cancers
Immune checkpoint molecules—molecules on activated T cells or the tumor that block T-cell activation	Immune checkpoint inhibitors—enhance anti-tumor-specific T-cell responses by preventing T-cell inhibition	*Ipilimumab,* a MAb directed against cytotoxic T-lymphocyte antigen 4 (CTLA-4); for treatment of metastatic melanoma and renal cell carcinoma *Pembrolizumab* and *Nivolumab,* MAbs directed against programmed death-1 (PD-1); used to treat melanoma, colon cancer, and other tumors
Antibody-drug conjugates (immunotoxins) directed against tumor antigens	Deliver potent toxic molecules directly to tumor cells	*Brentuximab vedotin,* an immunotoxin directed against the CD30 antigen; used to treat Hodgkin lymphoma and anaplastic large-cell lymphoma *Trastuzumab emtansine,* an immunotoxin directed against the HER2 antigen; for treatment of HER2-positive metastatic breast cancer
Bi-specific T-cell engagers (BiTEs)—Bi-specific monoclonal antibodies with two different variable regions, one that binds to the tumor antigen and the other to a T-cell surface marker	Bring T cells close to tumor cells to facilitate direct contact and destruction of tumor cells	*Blinatumomab,* a MAb that binds to CD19 and CD3, approved for relapsed or refractory B-cell precursor ALL

ADCC = antibody-dependent cellular cytotoxicity; ALL = acute lymphoblastic leukemia; CD = clusters of differentiation; HER2 = human epidermal growth factor 2; MAb = monoclonal antibody.

Bi-specific T-cell engagers (BiTEs) are monoclonal antibodies produced by recombinant DNA technology that have two antigen-binding sites, one that attaches to the tumor antigen and the other that binds to a T-cell marker such as CD3. These antibodies are thought to bring T cells closer to the tumor cells of interest, so they can be more easily activated to attack the tumor cells.

Although monoclonal antibodies have had a large impact in cancer treatment, they have some limitations. Some patients develop hypersensitivity reactions to the antibody proteins. This problem has been substantially reduced as monoclonal antibody technology has evolved from making purely mouse antibody products to manufacturing fully human products (see Chapters 3 and 25). Monoclonal antibody treatment can also cause toxicity if the target antigen is expressed on normal cells. It may be ineffective if the antibodies are unable to permeate through tumor tissues or bind their target antigen molecules with high affinity. Finally, cancer cells can develop resistance to monoclonal antibodies, analogous to the way that bacteria develop resistance to antibiotics. Scientists are researching several new approaches to monoclonal antibody therapy that may overcome these limitations in the future.

Critical Thinking 17-2

A patient with metastatic non-small cell lung cancer received monoclonal anti-PD-L1 therapy and experienced a reduction in the size of their tumors. However, 1 year later, imaging studies revealed that the patient's tumors were increasing in size. Based on your knowledge of tumor biology, provide an explanation for these results.

Cytokines

As we discussed in Chapter 6, cytokines are small proteins that play an important role in regulating immune responses by serving as chemical messengers that affect cell interactions.

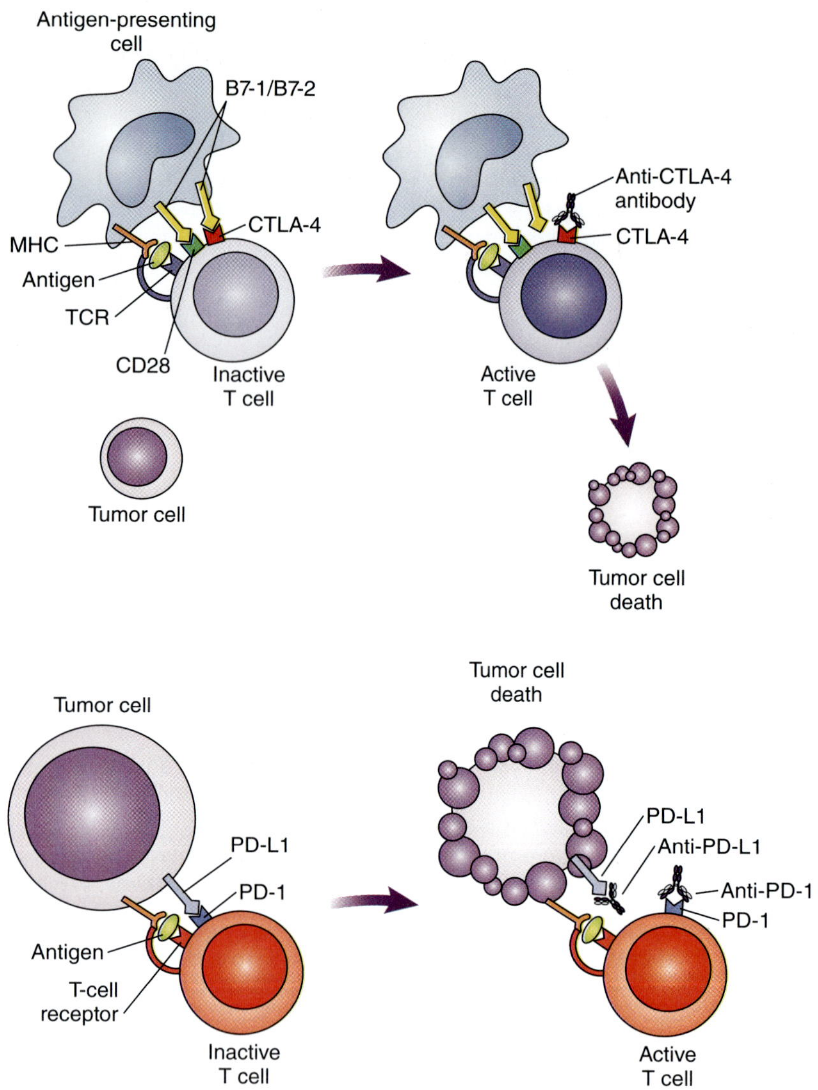

FIGURE 17–13 Immune checkpoint molecules and inhibitors. (A) CTLA-4. The CTLA-4/B7 binding inhibits T-cell activation. Blocking CTLA-4 enables the T cell to kill the tumor cell. (B) PD-1. The PD-L1 binds to PD-1 and inhibits the T cell from killing the tumor cell. Blocking PD-L1 or PD-1 enables the T cell to kill the tumor cell.

In cancer treatment, cytokines are used in two main ways, as hematopoietic growth factors and as therapeutic agents.

Because chemotherapy drugs inhibit cell division, they often adversely affect hematopoietic stem cell (HSC) development in the bone marrow, resulting in decreased production of WBCs, red blood cells (RBCs), and platelets. The **colony-stimulating factors (CSFs),** a type of **hematopoietic growth factor,** can be given to patients to help them recover from or prevent these toxicities. The main CSFs used to treat patients with cancer are granulocyte colony-stimulating factor (G-CSF), granulocyte-macrophage colony-stimulating factor (GM-CSF), erythropoietin, and IL-11 (see Chapter 6). G-CSF stimulates HSCs to develop into granulocytes, and GM-CSF stimulates HSCs to develop into granulocytes and monocytes, reducing the risk for severe infections. Erythropoietin stimulates RBC production from the bone marrow and can be used to treat patients with severe anemia. IL-11 stimulates megakaryocyte maturation, helping patients to recover from chemotherapy-induced thrombocytopenia.

The therapeutic application of cytokines is aimed at enhancing patients' immune responses to their tumors. Two cytokines that have been widely used are IFN-α and IL-2. IFN-α has been commonly used in cancer therapy to treat several types of cancer, including malignant melanoma, hairy cell leukemia, CML, and Kaposi sarcoma. It is thought to increase tumor immunogenicity, enhance DC responses to the tumor, enhance T_H1 responses and cell-mediated cytotoxicity, promote tumor apoptosis, and inhibit angiogenesis. Although high doses of IFN-α are associated with better clinical responses than low doses of the cytokine, they also generate strong adverse effects, including fever, asthenia (loss of muscle strength), neutropenia, and nausea and vomiting.

IL-2 induces T-cell proliferation and enhances T_c- and NK-cell function (see Chapter 6). However, systemic administration of IL-2 is limited because of its short half-life (less than 10 minutes) and serious adverse effects, including vascular leakage syndrome, marked fluid retention, and shock. Although this cytokine can be used to treat metastatic melanoma and advanced renal cancer, it is rapidly cleared from the body, and its most effective use may be to activate immunocompetent cells in vitro for adoptive immunotherapy (see "Adoptive Immunotherapy" later).

Although cytokines continue to be incorporated in immunotherapy, their use has been limited because of the serious and sometimes life-threatening side effects associated with high-dose systemic treatment. The cytokine network is very complicated, and administration of a cytokine can have multiple, and sometimes unwanted, effects. For example, in addition to its immunostimulatory effects, IL-2 is also necessary for the generation and maintenance of Treg cells, which can be involved in enhancing tumor growth. Studies using different approaches are under way to see if some of these obstacles can be overcome.

Adoptive Immunotherapy

Scientists have reasoned that because cell-mediated immunity is so important in defending against tumors, transferring T cells to patients with cancer may effectively assist them in eliminating tumor cells. This approach, known as **adoptive immunotherapy** or *T-cell transfer therapy*, uses T cells within the patient's tumor, called **tumor-infiltrating T cells (TILs)** or genetically modified T cells bearing chimeric antigen receptor T cells **(CAR T cells).** We discuss these therapies in the text that follows and also in Chapter 25.

TIL therapy is based on pioneering experiments conducted in humans in the late 1980s by Steven Rosenberg and his colleagues and earlier experiments conducted in mice, which demonstrated that TILs possessed potent cytolytic activity against genetically identical or autologous tumor cells. This therapy uses TILs isolated from a solid tumor that has been surgically removed from a patient. The T cells in the TIL population are activated by incubating them in vitro with dendritic cells from the patient that have been primed with neoantigens identified in the tumor **(Fig. 17–14).** The activated T cells are selected, expanded in culture with IL-2, and infused into the patient's bloodstream. The patient is given additional IL-2 to further stimulate the cells. Patients are treated with total body irradiation or high-dose chemotherapy before the adoptive cell transfer to remove cells that could suppress the anti-tumor responses and to create space for the infused cells to expand.

Adoptive therapy with autologous TILs has shown good clinical response rates in patients with malignant melanoma and has been approved by the FDA for patients with advanced melanoma who have not responded to other treatments. Clinical studies are being conducted to determine the effectiveness of TIL therapy for other solid tumors. Studies are also under way using T cells that have been genetically modified to express TCRs for tumor antigens commonly found on a particular type of tumor and displayed by a known HLA molecule.

In CAR T-cell therapy, a patient's peripheral blood WBCs are collected and enriched for T cells, which are then genetically modified to possess *chimeric antigen receptors (CARs)* and infused back into the patient. CARs are most often constructed by combining (1) the antigen-binding variable fragment of a monoclonal antibody directed against a specific tumor antigen with (2) intracellular domains of the TCR and (3) costimulatory molecules to provide activating signals to the T cells (see Chapter 25 for details). In this way, CAR T cells can target specific tumor antigens in an MHC-*independent* manner so the product can be universally used instead of being restricted for patients with a particular HLA type.

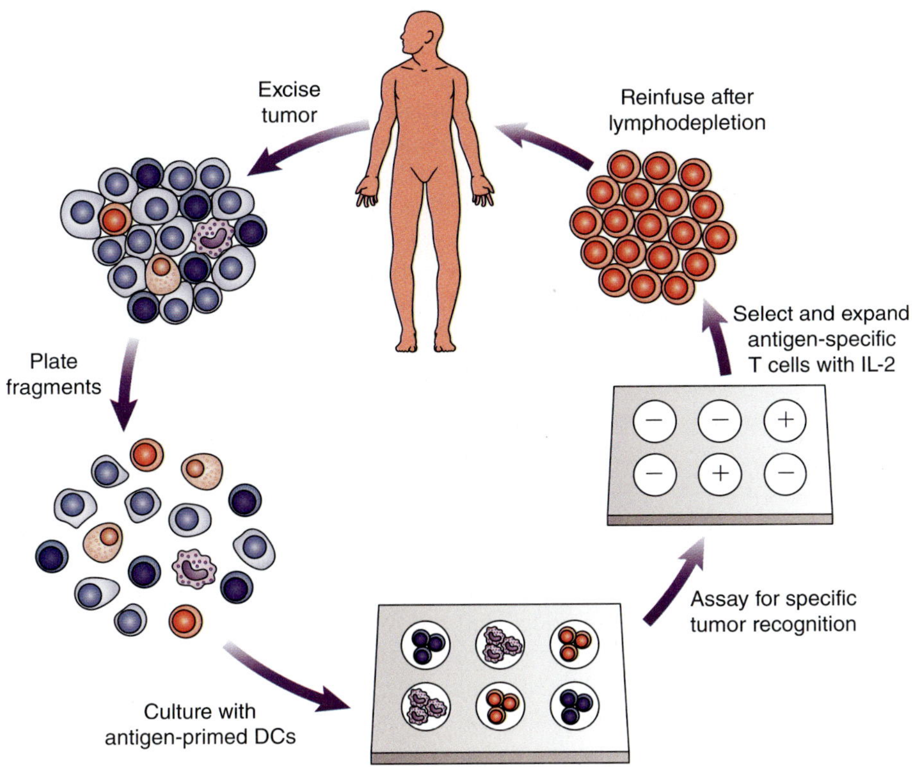

FIGURE 17–14 Adoptive immunotherapy with tumor-infiltrating lymphocytes (TILs). The patient's tumor is surgically removed and cut into fragments, which are cultured in vitro with antigen-primed dendritic cells (DCs). The cultures are screened for lymphocytes with potent anti-tumor activity. Positive cultures are expanded further in the presence of interleukin-2 (IL-2) and are infused into the patient. Before infusion, the patient is treated with high-dose chemotherapy or radiation to deplete immunosuppressive cells.

Several CAR T-cell therapies have been FDA approved for patients with hematologic malignancies for whom other treatments have not been effective; these include CAR T cells specific for the CD19 antigen, used for patients with certain B-cell malignancies, and CAR T cells specific for CD38 or BCMA (B-cell maturation antigen), for patients with advanced multiple myeloma. Studies are being conducted to determine if CAR T-cell therapy can also be used for other blood cancers or solid tumors. Research is also under way to see if genetically modified NK cells can be used in a similar manner.

Although adoptive immunotherapy holds much promise, it has some limitations. Toxicities have been reported; in CAR T-cell therapy, an intense inflammatory response resulting from excessive release of cytokines (see Chapter 6) or neurological complications can occur, and some patients with TIL therapy may experience capillary leak syndrome, causing dangerously low blood pressure and multiple organ failure. Resistance to the therapy may develop in some patients because the targeted antigen may be lost by tumor cells that have not been depleted by the treatment. Finally, adoptive cell-based therapies are expensive, personalized treatments that are available only in specialized laboratories and medical centers. Advances in technology and initiatives by the National Cancer Institute are making it possible to expand the production and uses of tumor-specific T cells.

Knowledge Check 17-5

Which of the following is an example of adoptive immunotherapy for cancer?

a. The BCG vaccine
b. The monoclonal antibody, Herceptin
c. Treatment with IL-2
d. CAR T-cell therapy

KEY CONCEPTS

Introduction to Tumor Biology

- A tumor is a cell mass resulting from excess cell growth and division. Benign tumors consist of slow-growing, well-differentiated cells that remain localized. Malignant tumors are disorganized masses that are not capsulated and can invade nearby organs; their cells can break away from the original mass and spread to distant sites, a process called metastasis.

Classification of Malignant Tumors

- Malignant tumors are classified by their tissue of origin: carcinomas derive from the skin or epithelial linings of the organs or glands; leukemias are malignant WBCs derived from bone marrow HSCs that circulate in the blood; lymphomas are solid tumors derived from lymphoid organs; sarcomas arise from bone or soft tissues; melanoma is derived from skin cells that make pigment; germ cell tumors arise from organs that make sperm and eggs; and neuroendocrine tumors come from hormone-producing cells.
- Cancer staging systems (e.g., TNM), which guide diagnosis and treatment, are based on the tumor's main site, type, and size; regional lymph node involvement; presence or absence of metastasis; and resemblance to normal tissue. The cancer grade, which is used to determine patient prognosis and treatment, is based on the microscopic appearance of the tumor cells.

Malignant Transformation

- Transformation of normal cells into malignant cells, or carcinogenesis, is a multistep process involving exposure to environmental factors (e.g., certain chemicals, radiation, and certain viruses) that induce a series of mutations, genetic changes in our cells' DNA.
- Two major groups of genes involved in malignant transformation are proto-oncogenes, which promote cell proliferation, and tumor suppressor genes, which regulate entry of cells into the cell cycle, maintain genetic stability, and repair damaged DNA.
- Malignant tumors contain immortal cells that resist apoptosis and proliferate in an unregulated manner. They can also induce angiogenesis, invade nearby tissues, spread to distant sites in the body, escape growth suppressor signals and immune destruction, deregulate metabolism, and escape progression to a terminal differentiation state. These characteristics are enabled by genetic mutations, genomic instability, inflammation, epigenetic changes, and changes in the microbiome.

Tumor Antigens

- The concept of tumor immunology is based on the premise that tumor cells possess antigens that can be recognized as foreign by the immune system. Some antigens are tumor specific (TSAs), or unique to a particular type of tumor cell, including neoantigens, and antigens induced by oncogenic viruses or endogenous retroviral elements. Others, called tumor-associated antigens (TAAs), are also expressed by normal cells and include the cancer/testis antigens, differentiation antigens, and overexpressed antigens.
- Neoantigens, created by mutations in proto-oncogenes, tumor suppressor genes, or other genes, are highly immunogenic proteins that are patient specific or restricted to few patients.
- Oncogenic viruses, such as EBV, are cancer-causing viruses whose genes code for antigens that are displayed on the tumor cell surface and recognized by T_c cells.
- Endogenous retroviral elements are DNA fragments derived from retroviruses that are found in the human genome. Their products are overexpressed in many cancer types.

- Cancer/testis antigens, such as the MAGE antigens on melanoma cells, are found in normal testicular germ cells, placental trophoblasts, and ovaries, and are overexpressed in some tumors.
- Differentiation antigens are expressed only in cells of a particular lineage. They include the oncofetal antigens (e.g., AFP, CEA, PSA) that are normally expressed on developing cells of the fetus but not on adult cells.
- Overexpressed antigens, such as HER2, are present in higher levels on some malignant cells than on normal cells.

Clinically Relevant Tumor Markers

- Tumor markers are biological substances that are increased in the blood, body fluids, or tissues of patients with a particular type of cancer. They include serum proteins, cell receptors, and genetic alterations.
- The ideal tumor marker should be highly sensitive, detecting most people with a particular type of cancer, and highly specific to minimize false-positive results. Many tumor markers do not have these characteristics, and this can affect laboratory results.
- Tumor markers have five main clinical applications: (1) providing targeted screening of high-risk individuals, (2) acting as an aid in cancer diagnosis, (3) providing information about patient prognosis, (4) predicting whether a patient is likely to benefit from a specific therapy, and (5) monitoring patients with cancer to check for treatment effectiveness and tumor recurrence.
- To monitor patient response to therapy, serial measurements are performed over time. If a therapy is effective, the amount of tumor marker will decrease. Ineffective therapy and tumor recurrence are indicated by an increase in the tumor marker level.
- Commonly used serum tumor markers and their primary cancer associations are presented in Table 17–5.
- Commonly used cell surface tumor markers are CD antigens for hematologic malignancies, HER2 and estrogen and progesterone receptors in breast cancer, and EGFR in various cancers.
- Genetic markers consist of gene mutations and changes in gene expression that are used in cancer diagnosis and prognosis, identification of patients who would benefit from targeted therapies, and identification of family members susceptible to hereditary cancers. Table 17–6 lists examples of clinically relevant genetic markers and their associated cancers.
- The Philadelphia chromosome is an example of a genetic marker. It arises from a chromosome translocation involving the *BCR* region on chromosome 9 and the c-*ABL* gene on chromosome 22. The abnormal gene codes for a tyrosine kinase that is overexpressed, resulting in excess cell proliferation. This chromosome abnormality is found in most patients with CML and in some patients with ALL or AML.

Laboratory Testing in Oncology

- Laboratory testing plays an essential role in cancer diagnosis and management. A combination of tests is routinely used. Some of these are companion diagnostics used to identify patients who would most likely benefit from a targeted therapy.
- Laboratory testing often begins with gross examination of solid tumors and microscopic examination of tumor cells for morphological characteristics that distinguish them from normal cells.
- Immunohistochemistry uses labeled antibodies to detect tumor antigens in formalin-fixed or frozen tissue sections from a tumor biopsy.
- Tests for circulating tumor markers are performed by highly sensitive, automated immunoassays. Their results can be affected by reagent variability among manufacturers, cross-reactivity with similar antigens, tumor antigen excess (producing a high-dose hook effect), or presence of heterophile, anti-animal, or autoantibodies in the patient sample.
- Detection of CD antigens for hematologic malignancies is performed by incubating peripheral blood or bone marrow cells with fluorescent-labeled antibodies and analyzing the results with flow cytometry. Flow cytometry can also be used to determine DNA ploidy in tumor cells.
- Cytogenetics testing detects abnormalities in chromosome structure and number by karyotyping, FISH, and CGH.
- Molecular testing most often uses NGS and PCR to identify cancer-associated gene mutations.

Interactions Between the Immune System and Tumors

- The hypothesis of immunosurveillance states that the immune system continually patrols the body for cancer cells and eliminates them before they become clinically evident.
- Innate and adaptive immune responses are activated against tumor cells. Innate responses are mediated by NK cells and possibly by M1 macrophages. Adaptive immune responses are mediated mainly by cytotoxic T cells and dendritic cells. Activated T_H cells and cytokines are also involved. The role of antibodies is unclear.
- Tumor cells are thought to escape these responses through the process of immunoediting, which allows some of the tumor cells to develop into genetic variants that are resistant to immune defenses.
- Mechanisms by which tumor cells can escape immune defenses include avoiding immune recognition by downregulating expression of surface

tumor antigens and class I MHC molecules and suppressing anti-tumor responses by T cells. Chronic inflammation is thought to promote tumor development by modifying the tumor microenvironment.

Immunotherapy

- Immunotherapy is based on the ability of the immune system to destroy tumor cells.
- Immunotherapeutic approaches include stimulating the immune system with cancer vaccines, passive therapy with monoclonal antibodies or cytokines, and adoptive immunotherapy with tumor-infiltrating lymphocytes (TILs) or genetically modified T cells bearing chimeric antigen receptors (CAR T cells).

Study Guide: Clinical Applications of Tumor Markers

CLINICAL APPLICATION	PURPOSE	BENEFITS	COMMENTS	EXAMPLE(S)
Screening	To identify cancer in high-risk asymptomatic individuals.	Detecting predisposition to hereditary cancers. Detecting cancer at an early stage.	False-positive results can lead to patient anxiety, unnecessary testing, and overtreatment. False-negative results can give misleading reassurance.	BRCA-1 and BRACA-2 for hereditary breast cancer. PSA for prostate cancer.
Diagnosis	To identify cancer in a particular patient.	Helps distinguish between conditions with similar clinical manifestations.	Presence of the marker or an elevation of the marker above normal levels suggests the presence of the cancer. Tests by themselves are not diagnostic and should be used in conjunction with other tests and clinical findings.	PSA
Prognosis	To predict the clinical outcome of a cancer patient and aid in therapeutic decision-making.	Used to identify the level (minimal to aggressive) and type of therapy that is best for a particular patient.	An initial high concentration or an increasing level of the tumor marker over time indicates a worse prognosis.	HER2
Predicting	To identify patients who would most likely respond to targeted cancer therapies.	Allows cancer therapy to be more precise.	Uses companion diagnostics, tests that must be performed in the identification process, so that targeted therapies are only given to patients with the targeted marker.	*BCR-ABL* gene fusion in CML.
Monitoring	To observe the response of a cancer patient to treatment.	Elevations can indicate tumor recurrence before other signs become evident.	The cancer must be positive for the marker before treatment begins. Effective treatment is indicated by decreasing levels of the marker over time. Increasing levels of the tumor marker indicate that the therapy is not effective.	CA 125

CA 125 = cancer antigen 125; CML = chronic myelogenous leukemia; HER2 = human epidermal growth factor 2; PSA = prostate-specific antigen.

Study Guide: Immune Defenses to Tumors and Escape Mechanisms

Defenses

INNATE DEFENSES	ADOPTIVE DEFENSES
NK Cells	**Cytotoxic T cells**
• Kill tumor cells that lack class I MHC • Release perforins and granzymes, which destroy tumor cells	• Most important adaptive defense against tumors • Bind specifically to surface tumor antigens complexed with class I MHC • Release perforins and granzymes, which destroy tumor cells
M1 Macrophages	**TH1 T helper cells**
• M1 macrophages may kill tumor cells through release of lysosomal enzymes, reactive oxygen species, nitric oxide, and the cytokine TNF-α	• May bind to tumor antigens in complex with class II MHC and release cytokines that activate cytotoxic T cells and enhance NK cell activity
	Antibodies
	• Role in tumor defense is unclear • May cause tumor cell destruction through complement-mediated lysis or ADCC
ESCAPE MECHANISMS	
Antigen Modulation	**Suppression/Alteration of Immune Response**
• Altered or downregulated expression of tumor antigens because of genetic mutations • Downregulated expression of class I MHC on tumor cell surface, making cells resistant to recognition and lysis by cytotoxic T cells	• Tumor cells produce immunosuppressive substances • Recruitment of Tregs and myeloid suppressor cells that suppress immune responses against the tumor • Upregulation of inhibitory receptors such as CTLA-4 or PD-1, which block protective T-cell responses • Chronic inflammation with release of proinflammatory cytokines may promote tumor growth

ADCC = antibody-dependent cellular cytotoxicity; APC = antigen-presenting cell; MHC = major histocompatibility complex; NK = natural killer; TNF = tumor necrosis factor; Treg = T regulatory.

CASE STUDIES

1. A 45-year-old woman went to her physician's office after noticing a lump during her breast self-examination. She had a strong family history of breast cancer. The lump, detected on mammography, was a 0.5-cm mass that adhered to her skin. Her CA 15-3 level was 60 IU/mL (reference range ≤38 IU/mL). After surgery, the CA 15-3 level dropped to 42 IU/mL. Analysis of breast biopsy tissue indicated abnormal morphology, increased HER2 expression, and negative estrogen and progesterone receptor expression.

Questions

a. Is a residual tumor likely? If so, why?
b. In addition to chemotherapy, what other therapy would be recommended? Why?
c. What type of therapy is unlikely to be successful? Why?

2. A 66-year-old male went to his urologist complaining of frequent urination with small volumes of urine, creating great urgency. During the digital rectal exam, the urologist felt an enlarged prostate with no distinct nodules or abnormal areas. The patient's PSA level was determined and compared with the level from the previous year. The physician also asked that the free-to-total PSA ratio be determined. The test results are shown in the data that follow.

Laboratory Results

Test	Patient Results	Reference Interval
Current PSA	4.2 ng/mL	0–4 ng/mL
PSA 1 year ago	3.9 ng/mL	0–4 ng/mL
PSA velocity	0.30/ng/mL/yr	<0.35 ng/mL/yr
Free PSA/total PSA	0.26	N/A[a]

PSA = prostate-specific antigen.
[a]Values less than 0.1 are associated with the highest probability of finding prostate cancer on prostate biopsy.

Questions

a. What is the source of PSA?
b. Do the findings in this case indicate the need for a prostate biopsy, and is it likely that the patient has prostate cancer? Explain your answer.

REVIEW QUESTIONS

1. How can normal cells become malignant?
   a. Overexpression of proto-oncogenes
   b. Mutations in tumor suppressor genes
   c. Viral infection
   d. All of the above

2. Which statement best summarizes the concept of tumor development through immunoediting?
   a. Tumor cells produce cytokines that are toxic to T cells.
   b. Tumor cells that can escape the immune system have a growth advantage over tumor cells that are destroyed during immunosurveillance.
   c. T-cell activity causes increased MHC expression on tumor cells, allowing them to escape the immune response.
   d. Secreted tumor antigens saturate T-cell receptors, making T cells incapable of binding to tumor cells.

3. Which of the following is a tumor-specific marker?
   a. *BCR/ABL* fusion protein
   b. CEA
   c. CA 125
   d. PSA

4. Most tumor markers are not used to screen the general population because they:
   a. Cannot be inexpensively measured
   b. Do not rise to high enough levels in the presence of cancer
   c. Can also be elevated in conditions other than the cancer
   d. Vary too much between patients belonging to different ethnic populations

5. Both AFP and hCG exhibit serum elevations in:
   a. Pregnancy
   b. Ovarian germ cell carcinoma
   c. Nonseminomatous testicular cancer
   d. All of the above

6. Suppose a patient with ovarian cancer had a serum CA 125 level of 50 kU/L at initial diagnosis. After surgical removal of the tumor, the CA 125 level declined to 25 kU/L. The patient received chemotherapy drug 1; after 1 year, the CA 125 level was 40 kU/L. She was then given chemotherapy drug 2, and the CA 125 level rose to 60 kU/L. These results indicate that:
   a. Surgery was effective in removing the patient's tumor.
   b. Chemotherapy drug 1 was more effective than chemotherapy drug 2.
   c. Both chemotherapy drug 1 and chemotherapy drug 2 were effective.
   d. Neither chemotherapy drug 1 nor chemotherapy drug 2 was effective.

7. The hook effect that can occur in immunoassays for circulating tumor antigens is caused by which of the following in the patient sample?
   a. An excess of tumor antigen
   b. A very low concentration of tumor antigen
   c. Heterophile antibodies
   d. Autoantibodies

8. Which laboratory method is used to identify CD antigens in hematologic malignancies?
   a. Microscopic examination
   b. Karyotyping
   c. Flow cytometry
   d. PCR

9. Expression of the HER2 antigen in breast tissue is routinely detected by:
   a. FISH
   b. NGS
   c. Sandwich immunoassays
   d. Flow cytometry

10. Which marker(s) could be elevated in nonmalignant liver disease?
    a. AFP
    b. CEA
    c. CA 15-3
    d. All of the above

11. Each of the following markers is correctly paired with a disease in which it can be used for patient monitoring *except:*
    a. CEA/choriocarcinoma
    b. CA 15-3/breast adenocarcinoma
    c. CA 125/ovarian adenocarcinoma
    d. CA 19-9/pancreatic adenocarcinoma

12. Which marker is used in immunohistochemical staining to identify tumors of epithelial origin?
    a. Cytokeratin
    b. Vimentin
    c. CD45
    d. CD10

13. Which assay would you recommend to test for chromosome rearrangements such as the *BCR/ABL* translocation seen in CML?
    a. PCR
    b. FISH
    c. Microarray
    d. NGS

14. Innate immune responses thought to be involved in defense against tumors include:
    a. NK-cell–mediated apoptosis
    b. MHC-I–restricted T-cell–mediated destruction
    c. ADCC
    d. All of the above

15. A woman with breast cancer is treated with a monoclonal antibody to HER2. This is an example of:
    a. A cancer vaccine
    b. An immunotoxin
    c. Passive immunotherapy
    d. Active immunotherapy

16. Mutations in which gene are associated with the microsatellite instability seen in Lynch syndrome?
    a. *BRAF*
    b. *MSH2*
    c. *KRAS*
    d. *PCA3*

Chapter 17 Answer Key

Answers to Knowledge Checks

17.1 d 17.2 a 17.3 1-d; 2-e; 3-g; 4-a; 5-i; 6-b; 7-f; 8-c; 9-h 17.4 b 17.5 d

Answers to Review Questions

1. d 2. b 3. a 4. c 5. d 6. d 7. a
8. c 9. a 10. d 11. a 12. a 13. b 14. a
15. c 16. b

18 Immunoproliferative Diseases

Linda E. Miller, PhD, I, MB^{CM}(ASCP)SI, and Stephen M. Wiesner, PhD, MT(ASCP), FACSc

LEARNING OUTCOMES

After finishing this chapter, you should be able to:

18.1 Differentiate between leukemias, lymphomas, and plasma cell dyscrasias, and provide examples of each type of malignancy.

18.2 Describe some of the cellular and genetic changes that occur during malignant transformation of hematologic cells.

18.3 Explain the criteria on which the current classification schemes for identification of the hematopoietic neoplasms are based.

18.4 Describe cell surface markers and cytogenetic abnormalities commonly associated with acute lymphoblastic leukemia, chronic lymphocytic leukemia, and hairy cell leukemia.

18.5 Describe the relationship between monoclonal B-cell lymphocytosis and hematologic malignancies.

18.6 Differentiate between Hodgkin lymphomas and various types of non-Hodgkin lymphomas in terms of their cellular characteristics and surface markers.

18.7 Correlate selected cluster of differentiation (CD) markers with their associated cell type.

18.8 Describe the relationship between monoclonal gammopathy of undetermined significance (MGUS), smoldering multiple myeloma (SMM), and multiple myeloma, and the laboratory and clinical criteria that differentiate these conditions.

18.9 Define *Bence Jones proteins.*

18.10 Correlate clinical manifestations and laboratory results with multiple myeloma, Waldenström macroglobulinemia, primary cold agglutinin disease, and heavy chain diseases.

18.11 Recommend laboratory tests that can be used to diagnose and follow the progression of immunoproliferative disorders.

18.12 Recognize laboratory results that indicate the presence of a malignant clone of hematologic cells.

18.13 Explain the underlying principles of serum and urine protein electrophoresis (SPE and UPE), immunofixation electrophoresis (IFE), immunosubtraction (immunotyping), and serum free light chain (sFLC) analysis.

CHAPTER OUTLINE

You can go to **fadavis.com** keyword stevens for the laboratory exercises that accompany this text.

18.14 Interpret SPE and IFE results of samples from patients with monoclonal gammopathies.

18.15 Discuss the types of genetic abnormalities frequently seen in hematologic malignancies and the laboratory methods used to detect them.

The immunoproliferative diseases refer to a diverse group of hematologic malignancies that arise from hematopoietic cells of a lymphoid or myeloid lineage. Our focus in this chapter is on the lymphoid malignancies, which can be broadly classified as leukemias, lymphomas, and plasma cell dyscrasias. **Leukemias** are malignancies that originate from hematopoietic cells in the bone marrow, which migrate to the peripheral blood. In contrast, **lymphomas** are solid tumors whose cells usually arise in the lymph nodes and other lymphoid tissues, such as the tonsils and spleen, where they proliferate. There can be an overlap between the sites affected by leukemias and lymphomas, as leukemic cells can also be found in the lymphoid tissues and other organs in the body, and lymphoma cells may also be seen in the peripheral blood, especially when the malignancy is far advanced. However, it is generally most useful to classify the malignancy according to the site where it first arose, rather than the sites it can ultimately involve.

The **plasma cell dyscrasias,** also known as *plasma cell disorders* or *monoclonal gammopathies*, are malignancies of the plasma cells and associated premalignant conditions. These commonly involve the bone marrow, lymphoid organs, and other nonlymphoid sites. They are considered biologically distinct from the leukemias and lymphomas.

In this chapter, we introduce some of the lymphoid malignancies that are commonly evaluated by the clinical laboratory. (We do not intend to provide a comprehensive discussion of hematologic malignancies.) We also describe key principles and applications of some of the laboratory tests that are essential to the diagnosis and monitoring of patients with lymphoid malignancies.

Malignant Transformation of Hematologic Cells

Hematologic malignancies are characterized by excessive accumulation of cells in the blood, bone marrow, or other lymphoid organs. The increased cell number may occur because of rapid proliferation and excess cell production or failure of the cells to undergo apoptosis, a normal physiological process of cell death, or both. Malignancy may reflect the result of an initially normal process in which regulatory steps to control the level of cell proliferation have failed. Mutations can also result in arrested maturation of a cell. Thus, some malignant hematopoietic cells may not develop into properly functioning mature cells but may remain at an earlier stage of differentiation and continue to replicate.

Cells of the immune system are at great risk for malignant transformation because the features that characterize the development of malignancy are also a normal part of the immune response. For example, as we discussed in Chapter 5, proliferation of T and B lymphocytes is an integral part of the immune response to an antigenic stimulus. Also, gene rearrangements are a normal part of lymphocyte maturation, and somatic hypermutations occur in the immunoglobulin (Ig) genes of the B cells during Ig class-switching and the generation of high-affinity antigen receptors (see Chapter 3).

The immune system is naturally diverse and heterogeneous in its response against a wide range of potential pathogens. Normal immune responses are **polyclonal,** meaning that cells with different antigen specificities all proliferate in response to an immune stimulus. In contrast, hematologic malignancies are **monoclonal,** arising from excessive proliferation of a single mutant parent cell to form a clonal population of genetically identical cells that are similar in their appearance and surface markers. Elevated numbers of a specific population of lymphocytic cells in the bloodstream, bone marrow, or lymphoid tissues raise the suspicion of a hematologic malignancy.

Cell Properties

Despite being affected by abnormal regulation, malignant lymphoid cells generally retain some or all the morphological and functional characteristics of their normal counterpart (e.g., their characteristic cell surface antigens or immunoglobulin secretion). These characteristics are often used to classify lymphoid malignancies. Malignant and premalignant proliferation of cells can occur at any stage in the differentiation of the lymphoid lineages, and determining the stage of differentiation aids in patient diagnosis, treatment, and prognosis.

Immune System Modulation

As in many malignancies, leukemias and lymphomas modulate the immune system. Patients with chronic inflammatory conditions exhibit an overall suppressive cytokine environment. The inflammatory environment produced by leukemia and lymphoma suppresses hematopoiesis and modulates the immune system to be less responsive to the presence of malignant cells. This allows the tumor to establish itself and proliferate. The overall suppression of hematopoiesis and the immune system also make the patient more susceptible to infections. Infectious complications are a significant cause of illness and death in patients with cancer, and particularly so in patients with immune system neoplasms. Patients are at increased risk of infection and are more susceptible to infection by a broader spectrum of opportunistic organisms that would usually be considered normal flora.

Genetic Changes

As we discussed in Chapter 17, malignant transformation is thought to be a multistep process, sometimes involving exposure to environmental agents such as chemical carcinogens and radiation, which induce a series of genetic mutations. Recall that the key genes involved are the **proto-oncogenes,** which promote cell growth, division, resistance to apoptosis, and growth factor independence; and the **tumor suppressor genes,** which control cell division by regulating progression of cells through the cell cycle. The latter also maintain the genetic stability of the cells by repairing damaged DNA. Changes in these genes can result in uncontrolled cell proliferation or prolonged life span of the malignant cells as a result of resistance to apoptosis.

The genetic alterations in malignant cells of hematopoietic origin include point mutations involving a change in a single nucleotide base, duplications or deletions of specific genes or portions of genes, and chromosomal abnormalities, including inversions or translocations in which chromosomes break apart and rearrange their genetic material (see Chapter 12). Additions or deletions of whole chromosomes may also occur, resulting in abnormal chromosome numbers, a condition referred to as *aneuploidy.* Although aneuploidy is thought to be caused by common secondary events that are not specific to a particular hematologic malignancy, its presence can provide valuable prognostic information.

The detection of translocations is of particular value in the diagnosis of several hematologic malignancies. Many translocations in immunoproliferative diseases involve an exchange between the immunoglobulin (Ig) or T-cell receptor (TCR) loci and various partner chromosomes, leading to abnormal proto-oncogene expression. For example, some of the hematologic malignancies are characterized by translocations involving the proto-oncogene *MYC,* which stimulates the transcription of several other genes involved in cell proliferation. Overexpression of the *MYC* gene can occur because of a rearrangement in which *MYC* is placed under the control of a different gene promoter sequence. For example, a translocation involving the *MYC* gene on chromosome 8 and the immunoglobulin μ gene on chromosome 14, denoted as t(8;14), is implicated in the pathogenesis of Burkitt lymphoma (BL), a B-cell malignancy. Because of persistent *MYC* expression, several genes involved in cell proliferation are activated beyond normal levels. The resulting high levels of MYC protein drive the affected cells to continually proliferate and, along with other genetic changes, result in a malignant phenotype.

Other hematologic malignancies are associated with genes that affect apoptosis. For example, most cases of follicular lymphoma have a t(14;18) gene translocation, in which portions of chromosome 14 (which contains the Ig heavy chain genes) and chromosome 18 (which contains an anti-apoptotic gene called *BCL-2*) are exchanged, resulting in the rearrangement and constitutive overexpression of *BCL-2.* The *BCL-2* gene induces the production of an inner mitochondrial membrane protein that blocks apoptosis. Therefore, the cells affected by this translocation do not die normally. Even though the altered cells do not proliferate at an increased rate, an excessive number of cells accumulates because their survival is prolonged compared with normal cells.

Other characteristic translocations result in the production of novel fusion proteins. For example, chronic myeloid leukemia is characterized by a translocation between the *BCR* (Breakpoint Cluster Region) on chromosome 9 and the *ABL1* proto-oncogene on chromosome 22 (see Fig. 17–5). This results in a BCR/ABL fusion protein, which codes for a continuously activated tyrosine kinase enzyme, causing unregulated cell division. The *BCR* and *ABL1* genes are fused in a slightly different arrangement in some lymphoid leukemias. Scientists have developed anti-cancer drugs such as imatinib mesylate, marketed under the brand name Gleevec, to specifically target the abnormal protein produced by this gene translocation. These drugs slow cell growth by inhibiting the activity of the altered kinase.

Classification of Hematologic Malignancies

The classification of hematologic malignancies has undergone many changes over the years with the development of new laboratory techniques and acquisition of knowledge about these diseases. In the 1950s and 1960s, classification and diagnosis were based primarily on abnormalities in the morphological features of the malignant cells, which were viewed on peripheral blood or bone marrow samples fixed onto microscope slides and treated with stains such as Wright-Giemsa. Advances in understanding basic lymphocyte biology led to a major rethinking of the use of classification schemes based solely on cell morphology. The discovery of surface markers on T and B lymphocytes in the 1970s and 1980s allowed this information to be incorporated into the diagnosis of hematologic malignancies. The 1990s and 2000s witnessed a tremendous expansion of knowledge about the genetic changes of the tumors. Therefore, investigators and clinicians today are using a combination of morphological, immunologic, cytogenetic, and molecular techniques to assist in the classification of hematologic malignancies.

Several classification schemes have been used over the years. In 1976, the French-American-British (FAB) Cooperative Group consensus criteria for leukemias and myelodysplastic syndromes, based on cell morphology alone, was introduced, and they remain relevant today. The Revised European American Lymphoma (REAL) classification for leukemias and lymphomas scheme, adopted in 2001 and updated in 2008, 2016, and 2022 by the World Health Organization (WHO), became the basis for classifying all types of hematologic malignancies. This widely accepted system is considered by many to be the "gold standard" in the classification of tumors for diagnosis and determination of appropriate therapy.

The WHO system classifies hematologic malignancies into several major groups and numerous subgroups. The groupings are based on cell lineage, and specific cancers are further defined by their immunologic markers and genetic features, in addition to their morphological and cytochemical staining properties. The major groupings for the tumors of lymphoid origin are as follows:

- The precursor lymphoid neoplasms
- The mature B-cell neoplasms
- The mature T- and natural killer (NK)-cell neoplasms
- Hodgkin lymphomas
- Immunodeficiency-associated lymphoproliferative disorders

In addition to the WHO classification, the International Consensus Classification (ICC) was proposed in 2022. The ICC and the WHO classification are similar in many respects. The differences are mainly in the classification of some of the disease states rather than diagnostic criteria, with a notable expansion of subcategories of multiple myeloma/plasma cell myeloma in the ICC as compared to the WHO classification. The expansion of subcategories in the ICC is based on recurring molecular and cytogenetic changes found in myeloma.

In this chapter, we discuss some of the recognized types of lymphomas, leukemias, and plasma cell dyscrasias in more detail. The classification schemes continue to evolve as new knowledge is gained about the characteristics that typify the various disease entities.

Knowledge Check 18-1

Which classification scheme relies solely on the morphological appearance of cells on a Wright-Giemsa–stained smear?

a. WHO
b. REAL
c. FAB
d. ICC

Leukemias

Leukemias can be broadly divided into two groups based on the cell type from which they originated: myeloid and lymphoid. The myeloid leukemias are derived from the common myeloid progenitor and encompass the granulocytic, monocytic, megakaryocytic, and erythrocytic leukemias. We do not cover the myeloid leukemias in detail but briefly present a classic genetic change associated with chronic myeloid leukemia (CML) and how it is identified in the clinical laboratory. The focus of this section is the lymphoid leukemias, which originate from mature lymphocytes or their progenitors.

The lymphoid and myeloid leukemias can be further divided into *acute* and *chronic* types. In acute leukemias, the malignant cells multiply rapidly in the bone marrow and crowd out normal hematopoietic precursors, resulting in a decrease in red blood cells (RBCs; anemia) and fatigue; decreased neutrophils with subsequent infections and fever; and decreased platelets (thrombocytopenia), causing bleeding abnormalities. The acute lymphoid leukemias involve immature/precursor cells called *lymphoblasts* (or *blasts*) that multiply rapidly in the bone marrow and are present in the peripheral blood. They are small to medium-sized cells that contain little cytoplasm, dense nuclear chromatin, and indistinct nucleoli **(Fig. 18–1)**. The acute lymphoid leukemias progress rapidly and can become fatal in weeks or months if left untreated; however, they have a high response rate to therapy, so prompt diagnosis is important.

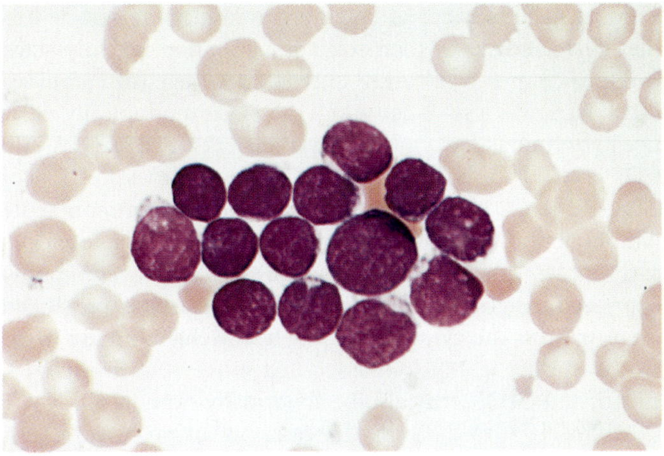

FIGURE 18–1 Lymphoblasts in the peripheral blood.

In contrast, chronic leukemias generally involve mature cells. They usually present with variable nonspecific symptoms and progress more slowly. In this section, we discuss examples of acute and chronic lymphoid leukemias.

Critical Thinking 18-1

Compare the lymphoblasts in Figure 18–1 to the normal lymphocyte shown in Figure 1–8. Why do you think laboratory testing in addition to observation of morphological features is needed to make an accurate diagnosis of a hematologic malignancy?

Acute Lymphoblastic Leukemias (ALLs)

Acute lymphoblastic leukemia (ALL) (also known as *acute lymphocytic leukemia*) is characterized by the presence of poorly differentiated precursor cells (blasts) in the bone marrow and peripheral blood. These cells can also infiltrate soft tissues, leading to organ dysfunction. ALL is usually seen in children between 2 and 5 years of age and is the most common form of leukemia in this age group. ALL is a treatable disease with a high rate of remission and a 5-year survival of about 90% in children, of whom 20% will relapse. Remission and cure rates are lower in adults with ALL. The main type of treatment is chemotherapy, though, in some cases, chemotherapeutic regimens have been combined with targeted molecular drugs or chimeric antigen receptor T-cell (CAR T-cell) therapy, which involves the administration of genetically modified T cells (see Chapter 25).

Most ALL cases are of B-cell origin, and these can be further characterized by their stage of maturation, as early-stage (pre-pro or pro) B-cell ALL, intermediate-stage (or common) B-cell ALL, and pre–B-cell ALL. The blasts are typically positive for terminal deoxynucleotidyl transferase (TdT), HLA-DR, CD79a, CD19, and CD22 and show variable expression of CD34. The CD10 marker, originally named "common acute lymphoblastic leukemia antigen" or "CALLA," is found in early stages of B-cell differentiation and is also commonly expressed. Slightly more mature B cells, at the pre–B-cell stage, express the cytoplasmic μ Ig heavy chain but are negative for surface Ig. Myeloid-associated antigens, such as CD13, CD15, and CD33, may also be abnormally expressed.

About 10% to 20% of ALL cases are of precursor T-cell origin and occur most commonly in teenage males as a lymphoma or as a combined leukemia/lymphoma. T-cell precursor ALL is characterized by the presence of TdT, and the T-cell markers, CD7 and CD3. CD4 and CD8 are usually positive, and CD2 and CD5 have variable expression. Knowledge of the antigen expression pattern at the time of diagnosis is very important in monitoring patients for possible recurrence of the tumor (i.e., minimal residual disease, measurable residual disease) after treatment.

The WHO and the ICC classify ALL into several subtypes based on the genetic abnormalities associated with the cells, to precisely determine diagnosis. Molecular and cytogenetic analysis also provide information that aids in the prognosis of patients with ALL. For example, *hyperdiploidy,* in which the malignant cells contain more than 46 chromosomes, is associated with a good prognosis, whereas *hypodiploidy* (less than 46 chromosomes) is associated with a poorer prognosis. The most common translocation in ALL of B-cell origin, t(12:21)(p13;q22), also known as *ETV6/RUNX1* (or *TEL-AML-1*), is associated with an excellent prognosis in children. This translocation is difficult to detect and is identified by fluorescence in situ hybridization (FISH) rather than traditional cytogenetic karyotyping.

Knowledge Check 18-2

A common CD marker found on B-lymphoblastic leukemias is:

a. CD3
b. CD4
c. CD8
d. CD10

Monoclonal B-Cell Lymphocytosis

Monoclonal B-cell lymphocytosis (MBL) is a premalignant state that includes three entities: low-count MBL, CLL/SLL type MBL, and non-CLL/SLL. In low-count MBL, there is a clonal expansion of lymphocytes (less than 0.5×10^9 clonal cells/L) without any other features of a B-cell lymphoproliferative disorder. In CLL/SLL (chronic lymphocytic leukemia/small lymphocytic lymphoma) type (high count) MBL, there is a clonal expansion of greater than 0.5×10^9 clonal cells/L and a total B-cell count less than 5×10^9 cells/L without any other features of a B-cell lymphoproliferative disorder. Non-CLL/SLL is characterized as any monoclonal non-CLL/SLL phenotype expansion without any other features of a B-cell lymphoproliferative disorder. Low-count MBL is an indolent disease, and there is a lower but nonetheless significant risk of progression. Conversely, CLL/SSL-type MBL precedes virtually all cases of CLL/SLL.

Chronic Lymphocytic Leukemia (CLL)/ Small Lymphocytic Lymphoma (SLL)

The mature lymphoid neoplasms may involve B cells, T cells, or NK cells. They include chronic lymphocytic leukemia (CLL) and small lymphocytic lymphoma (SLL). CLL and SLL are considered a single disease with different clinical presentations. CLL is the most common leukemia in adults living in Western countries of the world. It mainly occurs in patients over 50 years of age and has a two-to-one male-to-female predominance.

The malignant clone in CLL/SLL is derived from small mature B lymphocytes. The cells appear to be cytologically normal but are dysfunctional and accumulate in the bone marrow, blood, spleen, lymph nodes, and other organs. Patients usually present with an increase in the peripheral blood lymphocyte count, which may be an incidental finding on a routine physical examination. Lymph node enlargement is prominent early in the disease. Anemia and thrombocytopenia are usually absent at the time of diagnosis. However, as the malignant lymphocytes continue to increase in number, replacement of normal elements in the bone marrow leads to decreased numbers of RBCs and platelets. Treatment includes chemotherapy, monoclonal antibodies directed against the CD20 antigen, and targeted agents directed against various proteins involved in biological pathways that control cell proliferation, including Bruton tyrosine kinase (the *BTK* gene product) and B-cell leukemia 2 (the *BCL2* gene product). CLL is compatible with a long survival, greater than 10 years, as treatments can help control or reduce symptoms; however, they are not curative. Autoimmune hemolytic anemia is a common complication in CLL, and some patients progress to more aggressive disease, referred to as *Richter transformation,* in which prolymphocytes predominate. Hence, an increased prolymphocyte number in the peripheral blood smear is of significant concern with respect to prognosis.

The malignant cells in CLL/SLL express the B-cell markers CD19, CD20 (weaker expression), CD23, and CD200, and are negative for CD10. Typically, the cells are dimly positive for surface Ig. They abnormally express the T-cell marker CD5. CD23 status is particularly important because it distinguishes CLL from mantle cell lymphoma, which has a much less favorable prognosis. Cytogenetic analysis shows that patients whose malignant B cells have undergone somatic hypermutations in the variable Ig heavy chain genes (see Chapter 3) have a better prognosis than those whose cells have not undergone such mutations. Another abnormality associated with an adverse patient outcome is a deletion in chromosome 17 that involves the *TP53* tumor suppressor gene (del[17q][TP53]).

Knowledge Check 18-3

Which of the following is true?

a. CLL is defined as a T-cell neoplasm because CD5 is typically expressed.
b. CLL is more common in males than females.
c. CD20 is usually overexpressed in CLL.
d. CLL cells are negative for surface Ig.

Hairy Cell Leukemia

Hairy cell leukemia is a rare, slowly progressive disease characterized by infiltration of the bone marrow and spleen by leukemic cells without involvement of the lymph nodes. It has a male predominance and is most often seen in individuals over 50 years of age. The clinical presentation can resemble several other B-cell neoplasms, including CLL/SLL and splenic marginal-zone lymphoma. Patients usually present with bone marrow disease and pancytopenia (a condition in which there are low numbers of RBCs, WBCs, and platelets in the blood) because of bone marrow infiltration; however, the blood lymphocyte count is usually not very high. A monocytopenia (low absolute monocyte count in the blood) occurs in most patients at presentation. Splenomegaly (enlarged spleen) is striking, whereas lymphadenopathy (enlarged lymph nodes) is generally absent. A so-called dry tap, or failure to obtain a bone marrow aspirate, is more common in hairy cell leukemia than in some other lymphoproliferative diseases, and efforts must be made to obtain evaluable material for microscopic examination by other means, such as a touch preparation of a core biopsy specimen.

The malignant lymphocytes are medium-sized cells with round- to oval-shaped nuclei that occupy a large percentage of the cell volume. The cells often have irregular, "hairy" cytoplasmic projections from their surfaces **(Fig. 18–2)**. They can be seen in the peripheral blood or bone marrow but are typically present in low numbers and may be difficult to find.

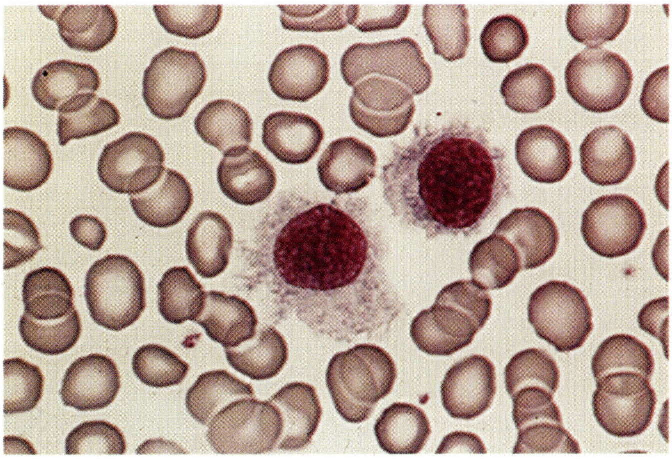

FIGURE 18–2 Hairy cell leukemia.

The malignant cells express the B-cell markers CD19, CD20, and CD22, and the interleukin (IL)-2 receptor CD25, which are not specific for the disease. The classic type of hairy cell leukemia is also positive for CD103 and CD123, and these markers are particularly helpful in making a specific diagnosis when used in combination with the other markers.

Immunohistochemistry staining of bone marrow biopsy tissue with anti-CD20 can help identify the malignant B cells, and staining with antibody to annexin A1 can help differentiate them from other mature B-cell neoplasms. An accurate diagnosis is made in most cases because of the cytomorphological and immunophenotypic characteristics. Polymerase chain reaction (PCR) for the detection of the mutated gene *BRAF-V600E* has been shown to be a sensitive and reliable test to aid in the diagnosis of hairy cell leukemia. The mutation codes for an overly active kinase that enhances cell proliferation and is the target for a small molecule inhibitor that can be given to patients who do not respond to other therapies.

Knowledge Check 18-4

Which CD marker, in combination with other markers, contributes most to the diagnosis of hairy cell leukemia?

a. CD19
b. CD20
c. CD103
d. CD22

Lymphomas

The lymphomas have commonly been referred to as **Hodgkin lymphoma (HL)** and the **non-Hodgkin**, or **lymphocytic, lymphomas (NHLs).** We discuss each of these entities in more detail in the text that follows.

Hodgkin Lymphomas (HLs)

The HLs were first described by Thomas Hodgkin in 1832. The disease entity is common, with a yearly incidence of about 80,000 cases worldwide. Studies suggest that HL has an infectious etiology, having possible association with the Epstein-Barr virus (EBV), which is known to preferentially infect B cells and immortalize them.

HL can occur in both young and older adults and has a slight male predominance. The peripheral lymph nodes are primarily involved, although many organs, such as the liver, lung, and bone marrow, can be affected. Advances in chemotherapy and radiation therapy have made it possible to cure HL in most cases. The WHO classification recognizes two major types of HL: *classic HL*, which comprises the majority of cases, and *nodular lymphocytic-predominant HL (NLPHL)*. In the ICC, NLPHL is classified as *nodular lymphocyte predominant B-cell lymphoma (NLPBL)*. In both classifications, classic

HL is further divided into four subtypes: *nodular sclerosis, mixed cellularity, lymphocyte-rich,* and *lymphocyte-depleted HL,* based on the types of cells that make up the background in which the tumor exists.

Classic HL is characterized by the presence of Reed-Sternberg (RS) cells in affected lymph nodes and lymphoid organs. RS cells are typically large, with one, two, or multiple nuclei containing a prominent nucleolus **(Fig. 18–3).** These abnormal cells are not usually found in the peripheral bloodstream. RS cells are typically surrounded by an inflammatory, mixed population of lymphocytes, histiocytes, eosinophils, and plasma cells, which presumably have been attracted to the tumor in its immunoproliferative environment. The nontumor cells often account for most of the cells in the tumor biopsy.

Molecular studies have shown that the malignant RS cells are primarily of B-cell lineage, despite their lack of typical B-cell markers. RS cells in all subtypes of classic HL have a similar antigenic profile, being positive for CD30 and often for CD15. CD20 expression is typically weak or absent.

The malignant cells of NLPHL/NLPBL have a different morphology from those found in classic HL and are referred to as *lymphocytic and histiocytic (L&H) cells.* L&H cells are large, with a moderate amount of cytoplasm and a single, folded nucleus that resembles popcorn; thus, they are often referred to as "popcorn cells." These cells rarely express CD30 but instead express the mature B-cell antigens CD20 and CD22, as well as CD45. They are often surrounded by small lymphocytes.

Non-Hodgkin Lymphomas (NHLs)

NHLs include a wide range of neoplasms, and these may involve the B cells, T cells, or NK cells. B-cell lymphomas represent about 85% to 90% of all NHL cases, and the NK-cell malignancies are the most infrequent. Over two-thirds of the patients are older than 60 years of age, and the incidence is greater in men than in women. Immunosuppression seems to be the greatest risk factor for NHL; in fact, an increase in cases corresponded to the emergence of HIV. Other conditions associated with increased risk for NHL include certain

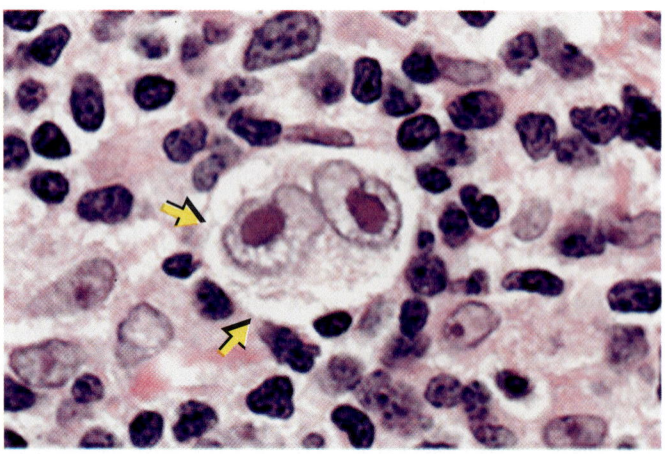

FIGURE 18–3 Hodgkin Reed-Sternberg cell with two nuclei, each containing prominent nucleoli, giving the cell an "owl's-eyes" appearance (arrows).

autoimmune diseases, congenital immunodeficiency disorders, organ transplantation, and exposure to certain infectious agents.

Non-Hodgkin B-Cell Lymphomas

B-cell lymphomas generally begin in the germinal centers of lymph nodes. Although these lymphomas can begin in any tissue, the gastrointestinal tract is the most common site for NHL outside of the lymph nodes. Three characteristics usually identify lymphomas as having a B-cell origin: (1) surface Ig, which is found on no other cell type; (2) other cell surface proteins, such as CD19 and CD20, that are sensitive and specific for B cells; and (3) rearranged Ig genes. In almost all cases, both the surface Ig and the rearranged Ig genes have features of clonality such as light chain restriction (kappa or lambda) or specific V-D-J gene segment utilization.

B-cell malignancies include *diffuse large B-cell lymphoma (DLBCL), follicular lymphoma, mantle cell lymphoma,* and *Burkitt lymphoma.* The most common NHL is DLBCL, which accounts for 30% to 40% of NHL. DLBCL is a heterogeneous group of diseases characterized by diffuse growth of large atypical cells. The malignant cells display a mature B-cell phenotype, with surface Ig and B-cell markers such as CD19, CD20, and CD22. The cells are rapidly growing, but prompt, aggressive treatment with chemotherapy and monoclonal antibody to CD20 results in a high cure rate. CAR T-cell therapy, involving the administration of genetically modified T cells directed toward the CD19 antigen, is approved for patients who do not respond to other treatments (see Chapters 17 and 25). The 5-year survival rate for DLBCL is about 65%. The median age at diagnosis is 66 years, and like many hematologic malignancies, there is a slight male predominance.

The next most common type of B-cell lymphoma is follicular lymphoma, which originates in the germinal centers within the follicles of the lymphoid organs. The cells have a mature B-cell phenotype and are positive for surface Ig, CD19, CD20, and CD22. The disease is associated with the chromosomal translocation t(14;18)(q32;q21), in which the Ig heavy chain gene on chromosome 14 has been placed next to the *BCL-2* gene on chromosome 18. This results in overexpression of the BCL-2 protein, which allows the malignant cells to survive by inhibiting apoptosis. Patients with the disease are typically asymptomatic at the time of diagnosis, except for painless lymphadenopathy. However, the disease has usually disseminated to the spleen, liver, and bone marrow, and though 5-year survival rates are as high as 90%, the disease has a poor long-term prognosis.

Mantle cell lymphoma was so named because the malignant cells resemble lymphocytes in the mantle zone surrounding the germinal centers in terms of their morphology and immunophenotype. The classic form of this cancer is characterized by a diffuse infiltration of the lymph nodes with intermediate-sized cells that have irregular, cleaved nuclei. Small-cell and blastoid-cell variants (the latter which has blast morphology) also occur. The cells express B-cell antigens, such as CD19, CD20, CD22, CD79a$^+$, and surface Ig as well as the T-cell marker CD5. Importantly, MCL cells lack CD23, distinguishing this disease from CLL. The cells strongly express the anti-apoptotic protein BCL-2 and are identified by their characteristic chromosome translocation, t(11;14)(q13;q32), between the Ig heavy chain gene and the cyclin D1 gene. Most patients have an aggressive clinical course that is unresponsive to therapy, but some may have a slower disease progression that does not require therapy for several years.

Burkitt lymphoma (BL) is a malignancy of the mature B cells that can occur in three forms: endemic, sporadic, and immunodeficiency associated. The endemic form, discovered by Denis Burkitt, represents the prototype of the disease. It is the most common childhood tumor in equatorial Africa and other areas of the world where malaria is endemic. The tumor typically grows in the jaw or maxilla **(Fig. 18–4)** and is associated with EBV infection at an early age. The immunodeficiency-associated form is associated with EBV infection in patients with HIV/AIDS or other conditions involving profound immunosuppression. In contrast, the sporadic form is not associated with EBV infection and typically involves the abdomen. The malignant cells in BL have a characteristic morphology. They are medium-sized cells with finely clumped chromatin, numerous nucleoli, and a deeply basophilic cytoplasm containing several distinct vacuoles. Bone marrow and lymph node tissue may have a "starry sky" appearance, resulting from a mixture of the cells from the tumor with macrophages that have phagocytized apoptotic cells. The cells are typically positive for the B-cell antigens CD19, CD22, CD20, CD79a, and often CD10, as well as surface Ig. Most cases display the characteristic chromosome translocation, t(8;14)(q24;q32), involving the *MYC* oncogene on chromosome 8 and the *IGH* gene (Ig heavy chain gene) on chromosome 14. This translocation causes *MYC* to be expressed under the control of the Ig heavy chain gene promoter, resulting in uncontrolled cell proliferation. Laboratory testing plays a critical role in diagnosis, as BL is a fast-growing tumor that is rapidly fatal if untreated but has a high cure rate if recognized early and treated with chemotherapy.

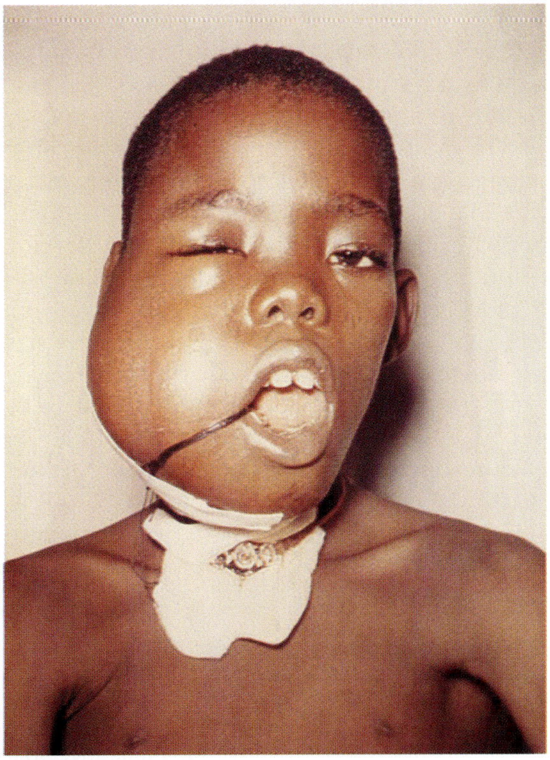

FIGURE 18–4 Child from Nigeria with a large facial tumor, caused by Burkitt lymphoma, a form of non-Hodgkin lymphoma. The solid tumor is composed predominantly of abnormal B cells. *(Courtesy of the CDC Public Health Image Library/Robert S. Craig.)*

Non-Hodgkin T-Cell Lymphomas

T-cell lymphomas are a diverse group of more rare disorders that include *mycosis fungoides (MF), Sézary syndrome (SS),* and *adult T-cell leukemia/lymphoma (ATLL).* MF and SS are cutaneous T-cell lymphomas that involve the skin. Patients develop dermatitis lesions that form plaques, which develop into ulcerative tumors over time. Although MF is a slowly progressive disease that is mostly confined to the skin, it can disseminate to the lymph nodes, liver, spleen, and other organs in the later stages. SS is a systemic disorder in which the malignant cells are present in the peripheral blood; it has a worse prognosis than MF. The malignant cells in both MF and SS are mature $CD4^+$ T cells that display TCR gene rearrangements. They appear abnormal, having irregular-shaped, folded (cerebriform) nuclei. Treatment in the early stages involves topical application of steroid creams or phototherapy. In the later stages, patients are treated with various chemotherapy agents and monoclonal antibodies in an attempt to improve the clinical outcome.

Critical Thinking 18-2

Think about mechanisms that are involved in lymphocyte maturation and activation (discussed in Chapter 5). How might our understanding of diseases in which these mechanisms are not functional lead to new approaches in the treatment of lymphoproliferative disorders?

ATLL is a T-cell malignancy that is endemic in Japan, the Caribbean, and certain other areas of the world. It is associated with infection with the retrovirus HTLV-I, which is transmitted through the placenta or breast milk, IV drug use, blood transfusion, or sexual contact (see Chapter 24). The malignancy develops in a small percentage of infected persons after a long latency period. The disease's acute form has an aggressive clinical course in which there is extensive involvement of the lymph nodes, blood, skin, and bones. The malignant cells are moderately large blasts with convoluted or clover-leaf–shaped nuclei and condensed chromatin, called "flower cells" because of their appearance. The cells have the phenotype of mature helper T cells, being positive for CD3 and CD4 and TCR gene rearrangements. The acute form of the disease does not respond well to chemotherapy and has a low survival rate, but allogeneic stem cell transplant and targeted therapies show promise for the future.

Clinical Correlations

Advancements in Treatments for Leukemias and Lymphomas

Treatment for leukemias and lymphomas is evolving. Traditional treatments include standard chemotherapeutic regimens, many of which use DNA damaging agents to induce tumor cell death. These compounds preferentially target rapidly dividing cells to reduce tumor growth. However, these approaches are not selective, and other dividing cells in the body are equally affected, including normal hematopoietic cells and epithelium. Since the introduction of imatinib mesylate (Gleevec), the drug that targets the BCR-ABL oncoprotein in CML, and anti-CD20 antibodies such as rituximab (Rituxan), the drug that targets B cells in lymphoid neoplasms, there has been an expansion of targeted molecular therapies. Some examples are as follows:

- *Bruton tyrosine kinase inhibitors (BTKi):* These drugs target the BTK protein that is essential for B-cell development.
- *Venetoclax:* This drug binds to and blocks BCL2, a protein that initiates apoptosis and promotes tumor cell survival.
- *Nutlins:* These are small molecules that interfere with degradation of p53, a tumor suppressor protein that halts cell cycle progression in the event of DNA damage (see Chapter 17). Importantly, nutlins are only effective if the TP53 gene is unmutated or is not absent due to a chromosomal deletion. Therefore, laboratory evaluation of TP53 status is crucial to determine the potential efficacy of nutlin therapy.

Many of the targeted therapeutics have significantly fewer long-term side effects when compared to standard chemotherapy. Many are more easily tolerated by patients, especially patients who are not good candidates for aggressive chemotherapy. As the library of targeted molecular therapeutics expands, laboratory testing will become increasingly important in assessing the status of cellular pathways for which targeted therapies are available to determine which may be most effective for a particular patient.

Plasma Cell Dyscrasias

The plasma cell dyscrasias are plasma cell disorders that include several related syndromes: multiple myeloma, Waldenström macroglobulinemia, primary cold agglutinin disease, heavy chain diseases, and the premalignant conditions **monoclonal gammopathy of undetermined significance (MGUS)** and smoldering multiple myeloma (SMM). These conditions are characterized by overproduction of a single immunoglobulin component called a *myeloma protein* **(M protein)**, or **paraprotein** (i.e., abnormal protein), by a clone of identical plasma cells. Therefore, these disorders are also known as **monoclonal gammopathies.** Although monoclonal immunoglobulins may also be produced in other lymphoproliferative disorders of B-cell origin, laboratory detection and characterization of M proteins play an important role in the diagnosis, differentiation, and monitoring of the plasma cell dyscrasias.

Monoclonal Gammopathy of Undetermined Significance (MGUS) and Smoldering Multiple Myeloma (SMM)

As with other types of cancer, multiple myeloma is thought to arise from a multistep process in which plasma cells in the bone marrow undergo genetic changes that lead to their malignant transformation. As this process progresses, the cells are thought to evolve into the premalignant condition, MGUS, followed by an intermediate state, SMM, before they eventually develop into cancer.

MGUS is a common condition that is present in about 3.5% of people aged 50 or older. People with MGUS produce a monoclonal immunoglobulin but do not have symptoms of organ damage or other laboratory findings associated with multiple myeloma or the other plasma cell dyscrasias. MGUS is usually diagnosed incidentally when patients with various nonspecific symptoms undergo laboratory testing such as serum protein electrophoresis (SPE). The International Myeloma Working Group (IMWG) has identified three criteria that define the presence of MGUS:

1. A serum monoclonal protein (IgG or IgA) concentration less than 3 g/dL
2. A plasma cell count of lower than 10% of the total cells in the bone marrow
3. The absence of signs or symptoms associated with multiple myeloma

Studies have found that people with MGUS have an average lifetime risk of developing multiple myeloma or other related disorders of about 1% per year. Patients with MGUS who produce a monoclonal IgG or IgA typically progress to multiple myeloma, patients who produce a monoclonal IgM can develop Waldenström macroglobulinemia or other lymphoproliferative disorders, and patients with monoclonal light chains can develop light chain multiple myeloma, amyloidosis (buildup of misfolded monoclonal light chain fibers in organs and tissues), or light chain deposition diseases. Greater risk of disease progression is associated with the production of an M protein that is not IgG, a monoclonal Ig concentration of 1.5 g/dL or greater, and an abnormal free light chain (kappa:gamma) ratio (see section on "Serum Free Light Chain [sFLC] Analysis").

SMM is an intermediate stage in the malignant transformation process and has a higher risk of progression than MGUS:

Clinical Correlations

CRAB Features

The clinical findings associated with multiple myeloma are commonly referred to as "CRAB," with each letter in the acronym standing for one of the features: increased serum calcium, renal failure, anemia, and lytic bone lesions.

About 10% of people with SMM have been observed to progress to malignant disease within 5 years after diagnosis. The IMWG has identified the following criteria for SMM:

1. A serum monoclonal IgG or IgA concentration of greater than or equal to 3 g/dL or a urine monoclonal protein greater than or equal to 500 mg in a 24-hour collection
2. A plasma cell count between 10% and 60% of the total cells in the bone marrow
3. The absence of signs or symptoms associated with multiple myeloma

SMM has a higher risk for rapid progression to malignancy if any of the following are present: the serum monoclonal protein levels are more than 30 g/L, the monoclonal antibody is IgA; there is a progressive increase in the monoclonal Ig concentration over 6 months; there is an abnormal free light chain ratio (greater than 8); there are high numbers of bone marrow plasma cells (~50% to 60%); the plasma cell phenotype is abnormal; or certain cytogenetic abnormalities are present.

Currently, no standardized treatments to prevent or delay the progression of MGUS or SMM exist. Lifelong follow-up of patients with medical examinations and pertinent laboratory testing (e.g., SPE, complete blood count [CBC], kidney function tests, serum calcium levels) is recommended to identify the development of malignancy before serious complications occur. SMM patients with high-risk factors can be offered clinical trials to receive treatment options with the hope that disease progression can be prevented.

Multiple Myeloma

Multiple myeloma, sometimes called *plasma cell myeloma,* is a malignancy of mature plasma cells that accounts for about 10% of all hematologic cancers and nearly 2% of all cancers diagnosed. It is the most serious and common of the plasma cell dyscrasias. Multiple myeloma occurs most often after the age of 60, and men are more likely than women to develop it. The National Cancer Institute estimates that more than 35,000 newly diagnosed cases and more than 12,000 myeloma-related deaths occur annually in the United States.

Patients with multiple myeloma typically have excess plasma cells in the bone marrow, a monoclonal immunoglobulin component in the plasma and/or urine, and lytic bone lesions. Plasma cells infiltrating the bone marrow may be morphologically normal or may show atypical or bizarre cytological features. The malignant plasma cells phenotypically express CD38, CD56, and CD138. About 20% of myeloma cells express CD20. Unlike normal plasma cells, myeloma cells can slowly divide.

The immunoglobulin produced by the malignant clone can be of any type, with IgG being the most common (50% of cases), followed by IgA and light chains only. Very often, production of heavy and light chains by the malignant plasma cells is not well synchronized, and an excess of kappa or lambda light chains may be produced. In about 10% of cases, the myeloma cells produce light chains exclusively. These monoclonal light chains can be found in the blood at low levels, but about 60% to 70% of myeloma patients rapidly excrete them in the urine, where they are known as **Bence Jones proteins.** Rarely do myelomas produce IgM, IgD, IgE, or heavy chains only. Also rarely, two or more distinct M proteins are produced or a myeloma might not produce a detectable secretory product. The serum and urine M proteins are routinely detected and characterized by protein electrophoresis, immunofixation, and free light chain assays (see sections that follow). The levels of normal immunoglobulins are often decreased in proportion to the amount of monoclonal immunoglobulin in the serum because of the large number of myeloma cells.

The clinical manifestations of multiple myeloma are primarily skeletal, hematologic, and immunologic. Hematologic problems are often related to the failure of the bone marrow to produce a normal number of hematopoietic cells because myeloma cells progressively replace them **(Fig. 18–5).** The low number of hematopoietic precursors in the bone marrow leads to anemia, thrombocytopenia, and neutropenia. High levels of M protein can interfere with coagulation factors, leading to abnormal platelet aggregation and abnormal platelet function. These abnormalities, coupled with thrombocytopenia, make hemorrhaging, bruising, and purpura common complications of multiple myeloma.

Multiple myeloma preferentially involves bone, producing multiple lytic lesions that often lead to bone pain and pathological fractures **(Fig. 18–6).** Bone loss is caused by a complex interaction between the myeloma cells and normal cells in the bone. The myeloma cells trigger increased activity of the osteoclasts, whose function is to resorb bone tissue during the normal bone-remodeling process, and decreased activity of the osteoblasts, which help to replace the degraded bone with new bone tissue. Therefore, bone tissue is degraded faster than it can be replaced, and bone disease is a major contributing factor to disease morbidity. Bone pain, usually involving the spine or chest, is the most common presenting symptom of multiple myeloma. Hypercalcemia is very common because calcium is released as the bones degrade. In advanced disease, the hypercalcemia itself can reach life-threatening levels. Despite the dependence of multiple myeloma cells on the

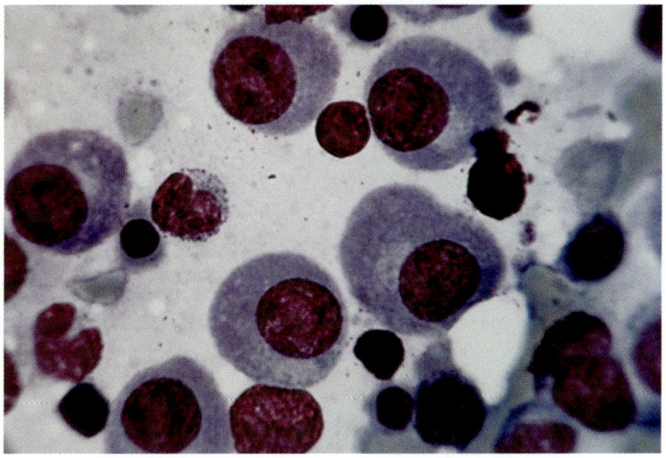

FIGURE 18–5 Bone marrow biopsy sample from a patient with multiple myeloma, showing replacement of marrow by plasma cells.

bone marrow, tumors may occasionally be found in the spleen and liver. These tumors are typically more aggressive.

When immunoglobulin levels in the blood are sufficiently high, they may cause the formation of rouleaux, stack-like formations of RBCs that can be seen on examination of a peripheral blood smear. Excess production of the abnormal immunoglobulin is accompanied by a progressive decrease in the normal immunoglobulins, leading to a deficiency of normal antibody responses and a higher incidence of infections.

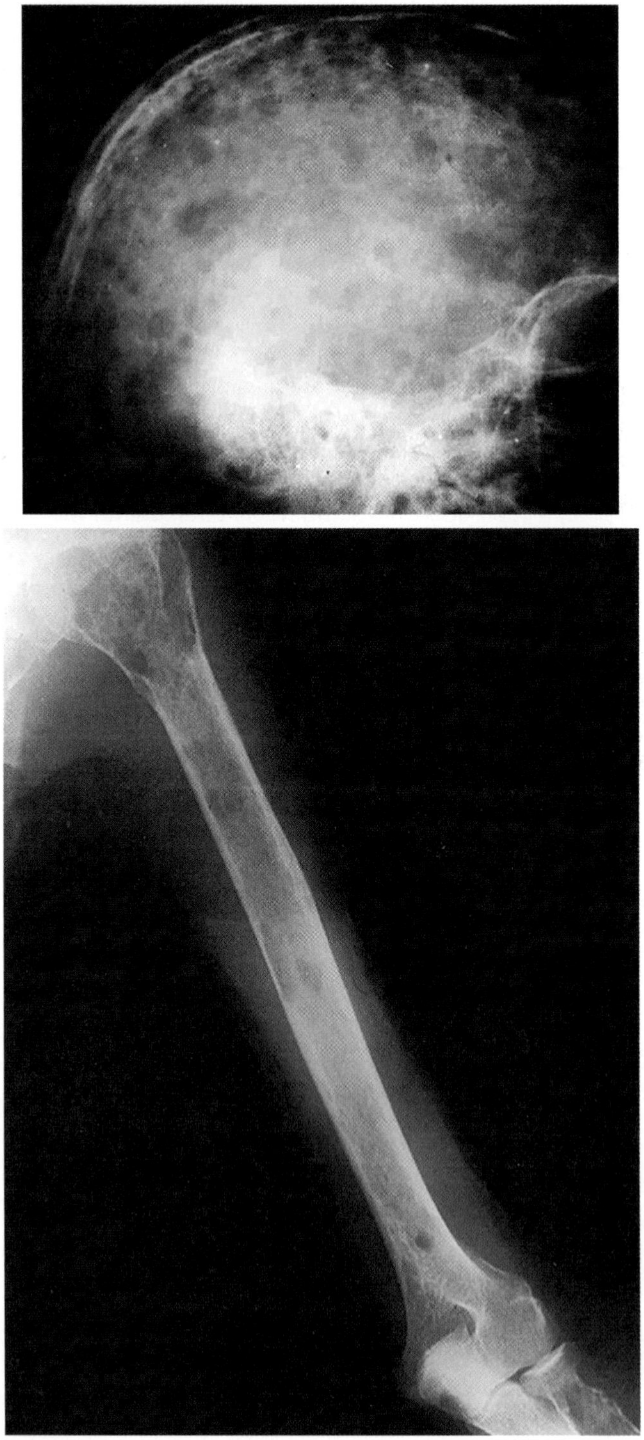

FIGURE 18–6 Bone lesions seen in a patient with multiple myeloma. (A) Lytic skull lesions. (B) Left humerus.

Hyperviscosity can develop when the level of M protein in the plasma is high. Because viscosity depends on the concentration and size of the molecule in solution and IgM is the largest of the immunoglobulins, hyperviscosity is most often seen with IgM-producing tumors. Hyperviscosity syndrome is also sometimes seen with an IgG3-producing myeloma because IgG3 is the largest of the IgG subclasses.

Up to 15% of patients with multiple myeloma develop light chain deposition disease or amyloidosis. These are two related disorders in which free light chains or immunoglobulin fragments are deposited in the tissues. Amyloid fibers stain with the dye Congo red and show apple-green birefringence when viewed with a polarizing microscope. Light chains can be identified in tissue sections by immunofluorescence or immunohistochemical staining with specific antibodies. The deposition of antibody-derived material results in organ dysfunction. The kidneys are most often affected, but every tissue in the body can develop amyloid deposits. Cardiomyopathy (disease of the heart muscle), peripheral neuropathy (peripheral nerve pain, numbness, or weakness), hepatosplenomegaly, and ecchymoses (areas of skin discoloration caused by blood in the tissues) are the most common manifestations.

Patients with multiple myeloma can develop either acute or chronic renal failure. As many as two-thirds of patients with multiple myeloma exhibit some degree of renal insufficiency. Patients with myelomas that produce light chains or IgD are much more likely to develop renal failure than those with other types. Renal insufficiency caused by Bence Jones proteins is seen in about 50% of patients. After infection, this is the second-leading cause of death. Bence Jones proteins are thought to be directly toxic to tubular epithelial cells and can damage the kidneys by precipitating in the tubules, causing intrarenal obstruction.

The IMWG identified the following criteria for the diagnosis of multiple myeloma:

1. Clonal bone marrow plasma cells present at greater than or equal to 10% or plasmacytoma observed in a biopsy within or outside of the bone marrow
2. One or more of the following:
   a. Presence of end-organ damage (CRAB features)
   b. Clonal bone marrow plasma cell percentage greater than or equal to 60% in the absence of end-organ damage
   c. Serum free light chain (sFLC) ratio greater than or equal to 100, with the monoclonal free light chain concentration greater than or equal to 100 mg/L (see section on "Serum Free Light Chain [sFLC] Analysis")
   d. More than one focal lesion of at least 5 mm in size on magnetic resonance imaging (MRI) studies

The overall 5-year survival rate for patients with multiple myeloma is about 60%. Patients with localized disease tend to survive longer than those diagnosed with disease that has metastasized. The prognosis is generally worse in patients who are diagnosed in the later stages of disease or who show evidence of renal damage. Cytogenetics analysis of chromosomal abnormalities provides valuable information regarding patient prognosis. For example, the presence of trisomies (three copies of a single chromosome) or the translocations (t[11;14] or t[6;14]) are considered a standard risk for disease progression, whereas a deletion in the short arm of chromosome 17 or the translocations (t[14;16] or t[14;20]) indicate a high risk for more aggressive disease. These and other molecular and cytogenetic changes are the basis for the ICC subclassification of myeloma of mature lymphoid neoplasms.

Different treatment options are available for multiple myeloma and are directed by the level of risk for disease progression. Various combinations of drugs are often used, along with supportive treatments, such as bone-strengthening and pain medications to manage patient symptoms. Therapies include immunomodulating agents such as thalidomide and lenalidomide; proteasome inhibitors such as bortezomib that stop enzyme complexes from degrading proteins that control cell division; and monoclonal antibodies, such as daratumumab, which is directed against the plasma cell marker CD38, as well as chemotherapy and autologous stem cell transplantation. Measurements of M proteins are conducted along with other laboratory tests to monitor patients and determine treatment effectiveness. Successful treatment will result in a decrease in the M protein concentration, sometimes to undetectable levels. Although multiple myeloma is an incurable disease, increased treatment options have improved the mortality rate.

Waldenström Macroglobulinemia

Waldenström macroglobulinemia, also known as a *lymphoplasmacytic lymphoma,* is a malignant proliferation of IgM-producing lymphocytes. It is a rare condition; only about 1,500 cases are reported annually in the United States. More cases occur in males than in females, and the median age at onset is about 70 years. Most patients (greater than 90%) have a genetic mutation in the *MYD88* gene, and about 30% of cases exhibit a mutation in the *CXCR4* gene. Both genes code for proteins that are involved in cell signaling pathways that regulate cell division and apoptosis; overexpression of these proteins results in increased cell proliferation and survival. The presence of MGUS increases the risk of Waldenström macroglobulinemia 200-fold over the general population.

The malignant cells in Waldenström macroglobulinemia possess the B-cell markers CD19, CD20, CD22, and CD79a and stain brightly for cytoplasmic IgM. They are also positive for CD38 and do not express CD3, CD5, CD10, and CD103. The tumor cells can have various presentations, described as small lymphocytes, plasmacytoid lymphocytes, and cells resembling mature plasma cells. Typically, one morphotype will predominate. The cells always infiltrate the bone marrow and are sometimes found in the spleen and lymph nodes. In bone marrow aspirates, the lymphocyte count can be within the reference range or severely elevated.

The clinical signs and symptoms of Waldenström macroglobulinemia are variable and are caused by infiltration of the malignant cells into the bone marrow, spleen, liver, and lymph nodes as well as the overproduction of monoclonal IgM. Accumulation of the cells in these organs can produce splenomegaly, hepatomegaly (enlargement of the liver), and lymphadenopathy. Signs and symptoms often include weakness, fatigue, anemia, bleeding, and occasionally plasma hyperviscosity. Anemia is attributed to overgrowth of tumor cells in the bone marrow, displacing erythropoiesis. Thrombocytopenia and leukopenia are less commonly seen. Bleeding can be caused by a combination of thrombocytopenia and interference of platelet function by monoclonal IgM.

The monoclonal IgM can accumulate in any tissue, forming deposits that lead to inflammation and tissue damage. Because early diagnosis is possible, hyperviscosity is uncommon. Lytic bone lesions, hypercalcemia, and renal tubular abnormalities are rare, differentiating this disease from multiple myeloma. About 20% of the patients have peripheral neuropathy. It appears that the monoclonal IgM in these cases is directed against glycoproteins or glycolipids of the peripheral nerves, causing symptoms of neuropathology.

All individuals with Waldenström macroglobulinemia have an elevated serum monoclonal IgM that migrates in the gamma region during SPE. However, the concentration varies widely and does not differentiate this disease from other B-cell lymphoproliferative disorders. IgM levels do not affect survival rate or correlate with symptoms; patients with serum IgM concentrations over 5,000 mg/dL can be asymptomatic, whereas patients with levels of 500 mg/dL can have significant bone marrow infiltration and pancytopenia. The presence of IgM paraprotein is not specific for Waldenström macroglobulinemia. SPE should be used to evaluate the amount of monoclonal protein, and the presence of IgM should be confirmed by immunofixation electrophoresis (IFE; see the section on IFE in the text). In 70% to 80% of patients, the light chain is kappa. Bence Jones proteinuria is present in about 10% of cases. Serum β_2-microglobulin levels are generally above 3 mg/dL, the upper limit of the reference range.

In 10% to 20% of patients, the IgM paraproteins behave as **cryoglobulins.** Cryoglobulins precipitate at cold temperatures and can occlude small vessels in the extremities in cold weather. Occlusion of small vessels can lead to hypoxia and the development of skin sores or even necrosis of portions of the fingers or toes. Cryoglobulins can also contribute to plasma hyperviscosity. Cryoglobulins can be detected when a blood or plasma sample is refrigerated in the clinical laboratory. The precipitate forms at cold temperatures and dissolves upon warming.

Some of the clinical symptoms are caused by autoantibody activity of the monoclonal IgM antibody. The antibodies can bind to RBCs, producing an autoimmune hemolytic anemia. Coating of the RBCs can produce rouleaux, which can be demonstrated on peripheral blood smears. Some IgM paraproteins, called *cold agglutinins,* have specificity for the *i* or *I* antigens and will agglutinate RBCs in the cold. A thrombocytopenic purpura-like syndrome can develop from binding of the paraprotein to thrombocytes. In addition, IgM can be demonstrated against polyclonal IgG. This results in immune complex disease characterized by vasculitis, affecting small vessels of the skin, kidneys, liver, and peripheral nerves.

Asymptomatic patients do not require treatment, but they should be monitored. Treatment includes chemotherapy, targeted therapies such as immunomodulating agents and proteosome inhibitors (see discussion on multiple myeloma), monoclonal antibodies directed against CD20, and plasmapheresis to reduce blood viscosity. With these treatments, the 5-year survival rate of patients with the disease is close to 80%.

Primary Cold Agglutinin Disease

Primary cold agglutinin disease (CAD) is recognized as a lymphoproliferative neoplasm that presents as an autoimmune hemolytic anemia usually caused by IgM antibodies directed against the I antigen on RBCs (see Chapter 14). Rarely, IgG or IgA forms of the disease occur. Binding of IgM to the surface of RBCs activates the classical complement cascade causing RBC lysis. Patients are often asymptomatic unless they are exposed to cold temperatures causing IgM binding in the extremities or other exposed areas of the body. The disease is caused by a clonal population of mature B cells, most of which use the heavy chain variable gene *VH4-34* and the kappa light chain variable genes *IGKV3-20* or *IGKV3-15*. The *VH4-34* region carries the sequences for binding the I antigen. Specific genetic mutations in these and other genes have been associated with primary cold agglutinin disease. Notably, a mutation of *MYD88*, found in Waldenström's macroglobulinemia, excludes a diagnosis of CAD. Cold agglutinins often occur in the context of other disorders, including other mature B-cell neoplasms. Other diseases must be ruled out to confer the diagnosis of primary CAD.

Heavy Chain Diseases

The **heavy chain diseases** are rare B-cell lymphomas characterized by production of a monoclonal Ig heavy chain. Genetic mutations in the affected B cells result in the production of abnormal heavy chains that have lost part of their CH1 or variable domain, so they are incapable of binding to Ig light chains. These diseases are classified according to the type of heavy chain produced, which can be alpha (α), gamma (γ), or mu (μ).

Alpha heavy chain disease, the most common type, is seen most often in young adults in their 20s or 30s with heritage from the Mediterranean region, including northern Africa and the Middle East. It has been associated with chronic bacterial and parasitic infections arising from inadequate sanitation. The disease is a lymphoma that involves the mucosal-associated lymphoid tissue (MALT) and can occur as one of three forms: gastrointestinal, respiratory, or lymphomatous. Most patients have the gastrointestinal form, characterized by intestinal malabsorption with diarrhea, abdominal pain, and weight loss. The monoclonal α chains can be identified in patient serum through reaction with anti-IgA in IFE (see the section on IFE). Because of their abnormal structure and tendency to polymerize, they may not be evident by SPE, which can appear normal or demonstrate a broad band that migrates to the α-2 or β region. Histological testing of biopsy tissue obtained from the small intestine or other affected areas demonstrates an infiltration of plasma cells and mature B cells. Early diagnosis is important because treatment with antibiotics in the early stage of the disease can improve prognosis. Patients unresponsive to antibiotics or those who have progressed to later stages of the disease are treated with chemotherapy.

Critical Thinking 18-3

Aside from the immunosuppressive effects of leukemias and lymphomas, what other factors may contribute to the susceptibility of patients with these diseases to infection?

Gamma chain disease is a rare disorder that has been found in people worldwide, usually appearing between the ages of 60 and 70. One-fourth of the patients also have an autoimmune disease such as rheumatoid arthritis (RA). The disease is heterogeneous and can present in one of three forms: disseminated lymphoma with lymphadenopathy and generalized symptoms such as fever and weight loss; localized disease with lymphoma limited to the bone marrow; or localized disease involving areas outside of the lymph nodes, such as the skin. The abnormal gamma chains tend to migrate to the β region on SPE, where they may be masked by other proteins. Serum IgG is elevated, and the abnormal protein can be seen by IFE, which demonstrates a monoclonal γ band in the absence of monoclonal light chains. Immunohistochemistry studies reveal the presence of malignant B cells and plasma cells in the bone marrow, spleen, lymph nodes, or other involved areas such as the skin. Patients are treated with chemotherapy, and the prognosis is highly variable, ranging from 1 month to many years.

Mu heavy chain disease is an extremely rare disorder that has been diagnosed in a very small number of people globally, mainly White males aged 50 to 60 years. Most patients also have a lymphoid malignancy that resembles CLL or SLL. Patients have symptoms related to the associated lymphoma, such as splenomegaly, hepatomegaly, and anemia. More than half of patients have a normal SPE pattern, but IFE typically reveals μ polymers of various sizes that are not associated with kappa or gamma light chains. The urine does not usually contain μ heavy chains but demonstrates the presence of free monoclonal light chains (Bence Jones proteins) in more than half of patients. Bone marrow aspirates reveal a mixture of plasma cells containing prominent cytoplasmic vacuoles and small round lymphocytes resembling those of CLL. Patients are treated with chemotherapy, and overall survival is variable, ranging from under 1 month to many years.

Role of the Laboratory in Evaluating Immunoproliferative Diseases

The diagnosis of a hematologic malignancy is usually suggested by a patient's medical history and clinical symptoms and confirmed by laboratory testing. Laboratory evaluation of a patient suspected of having an immunoproliferative disorder begins with a CBC and differential and examination of the cell populations on a peripheral blood smear. Blood samples from some patients with hematologic malignancies may show a decrease in RBCs (anemia) or platelets (thrombocytopenia) because of crowding out of normal hematopoietic precursors by the malignant cell population. A decrease in normal white blood cells (WBCs) may also be evident and can result in increased susceptibility to infections. Microscopic examination of cell morphology in the peripheral blood smear can provide important clues about the lineage of the malignant cell population. Cells of monocytic or granulocytic origin can be differentiated from those of lymphoid origin with various cytochemical stains, such as peroxidase and Sudan Black B. Once abnormalities are detected in the CBC and differential, a bone marrow aspirate and biopsy are obtained to confirm the diagnosis. Although microscopic examination of the bone marrow cells can confirm the presence of a malignant population, specialized tests are required to more precisely identify the cells of interest.

In this section, we discuss three types of specialized tests used to diagnose and monitor patients with lymphoproliferative disorders: immunophenotyping by flow cytometry, evaluation of immunoglobulins, and genetic testing. The laboratory can assess the immunophenotype of hematopoietic cells in the blood, bone marrow, or lymphoid tissues by flow cytometry. This is done by detecting cell surface antigens that are characteristic of a specific lineage and stage of differentiation. This technology serves as a complement to microscope-based traditional diagnostic methods and adds distinctive discriminatory capabilities that are unmatched by any other diagnostic technique. By performing immunophenotyping, the laboratory can determine whether the malignant cell population consists of B cells, T cells, NK cells, plasma cells, or cells of myeloid origin.

A second role of the laboratory is to evaluate the amounts and characteristics of the immunoglobulins produced by malignant B cells or plasma cells. Because the B-cell lineage develops into plasma cells that produce antibodies, B-cell malignancies are sometimes associated with excess or abnormal antibody production. Thus, the concentrations and characteristics of the immunoglobulins in the patient's serum or urine can be used to diagnose and evaluate the plasma cell dyscrasias.

Third, the laboratory is involved in assessing genetic and chromosomal abnormalities in hematologic malignancies. Genetic techniques play an important role in routine clinical practice. Cytogenetic analyses are used to detect chromosomal abnormalities such as translocations. Molecular techniques such as microarray and PCR can be used to detect mutant sequences within genes that have been linked to particular diseases.

Immunophenotyping by Flow Cytometry

Immunophenotyping, or the analysis of cell surface marker expression, is commonly used in the diagnosis and classification of leukemias and lymphomas. Because the malignant cells express markers that often correspond to those of their normal precursors, insight into their lineage of origin and stage of maturation can often be determined by this technique (see Chapter 13).

Cluster of differentiation (CD) antigens on the surface of hematopoietic cells are routinely detected by flow cytometry. **Table 18–1** lists some of the clinically relevant markers. In immunophenotyping, clinical samples containing cells that are potentially neoplastic are incubated with panels of antibodies that are specific for the relevant antigens. The laboratory must use a panel of carefully selected antibodies because no single surface marker specific for a particular hematologic malignancy exists. The clinical laboratory determines the specific antibodies used for testing based on the suspected disease, the type of sample, and the amount of sample available. Each antibody in a single reaction tube is labeled with a different fluorescent dye. Thus, cells that express a specific antigen bind to the corresponding antibody and emit fluorescence of a particular color. Fluorescence, cell size, and other cell characteristics are analyzed by flow cytometry (see Chapter 13), determining the antigenic profile, or immunophenotype, of the cell population. **Table 18–2** lists the CD markers typically found on selected hematologic malignancies of lymphoid origin. **Figure 18–7** shows flow cytometry results from a patient with B-cell ALL.

B cells that express immunoglobulins in their cytoplasm or on their surface are subject to heavy and light chain restriction. As we discussed in Chapter 3, each B cell can only express one type of heavy chain and one type of light chain. The ratio of kappa light chains to lambda light chains in a normal population of B cells is usually about 2:1 because the kappa light chain undergoes somatic recombination first, and the lambda

Table 18–1 Markers Commonly Detected by Flow Cytometry in the Analysis of Hematologic Malignancies[a]

CELL TYPE	COMMONLY ASSOCIATED MARKERS
T cells	CD1, CD2, CD3, CD4, CD5, CD7, CD8, TCR alpha-beta, TCR gamma-delta
B cells	CD10, CD19, CD20, CD22, CD23, CD79a, CD103, HLA-DR, kappa (surface and cytoplasmic), lambda (surface and cytoplasmic)
Myeloid cells and monocytes	CD11b, CD13, CD14, CD15, CD33, CD64, CD117, HLA-DR, myeloperoxidase
Miscellaneous	CD11c, CD16, CD25, CD26, CD30, CD34, CD38, CD41, CD42b, CD45, CD56, CD57, CD61, glycophorin, TdT, CD103, CD123, CD138, CD200

[a]Modified from ARUP Laboratories. Laboratory Test Directory. Leukemia/Lymphoma Phenotyping by Flow Cytometry. https://ltd.aruplab.com/Tests/Pub/3001780. Accessed November 26, 2024. TCR = T-cell receptor; TdT = terminal deoxynucleotidyl transferase.

Table 18–2 Surface Markers Characteristic of Selected Leukemias and Lymphomas

HEMATOLOGIC MALIGNANCY	CHARACTERISTIC SURFACE MARKERS[a]
Classic Hodgkin lymphoma	$CD15^+$ (most), $CD30^+$, $CD3^{+/-}$, $CD20^-$ or weak, $CD45^-$
Nodular lymphocytic-predominant Hodgkin lymphoma (NLPHL)	$CD20^+$, $CD22^+$, $CD45^+$, $CD15^-$, $CD30^-$
B-cell acute lymphocytic leukemia (B-ALL)	$CD10^+$, $CD19^+$, $CD22^+$, $CD34^{+/-}$, $CD79a^+$, TdT^+, $HLA\text{-}DR^+$
T-cell acute lymphocytic leukemia (T-ALL)	$CD2^{+/-}$, $CD3^+$ (surface or cytoplasmic), CD4 (usually +), $CD5^{+/-}$, $CD7^+$, CD8 (usually +), TdT^+
Chronic lymphocytic leukemia (CLL)	$CD5^+$, $CD19^+$, CD20 (weak +), $CD23^+$, $CD200^+$
Mantle cell lymphoma (MCL)	$CD5^+$, $CD19^+$, $CD20^+$, $CD79a^+$, $CD23^-$
Hairy cell leukemia	$CD19^+$, $CD20^+$, $CD22^+$, $CD25^+$, $CD103^+$, $CD123^+$
Multiple myeloma	$CD38^+$, $CD56^+$, $CD138^+$, ~20% are $CD20^+$
Waldenström macroglobulinemia	$CD19^+$, $CD20^+$, $CD22^+$, $CD38^+$, $CD79a^+$, $CD3^-$, $CD5^-$, $CD10^-$, $CD103^-$

[a]*CD = cluster of differentiation; + = positive; – = negative; TdT = terminal deoxynucleotidyl transferase.*

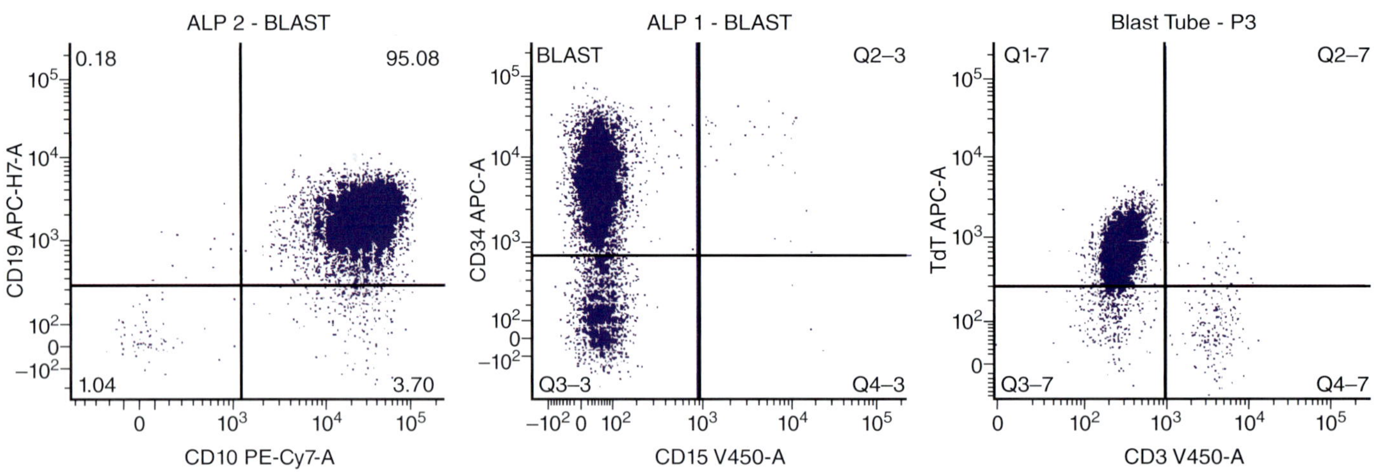

FIGURE 18–7 Flow cytometry histograms from a peripheral blood sample of a patient with B-cell ALL. Note that the malignant cells are positive for CD19, CD10, CD34, and TdT (terminal deoxynucleotidyl transferase).

light chain is only used when kappa light chain recombination fails. When examining a population of B cells in which a proliferative disorder is suspected, both anti-kappa and anti-lambda light chain antibodies are included. A kappa:lambda ratio of greater than 10:1 or less than 0.1:1 is strong evidence of a clonal immunoproliferative disease. Further characterization by additional CD markers helps to narrow the diagnosis.

Similarly, T cells that express the T-cell receptor can use one of two beta chain constant regions during somatic recombination. An antibody against the T-cell beta constant 1 (TRBC1) chain is used to detect T-cell clonality.

Flow cytometry is ideal for fluids such as blood, in which cells are naturally suspended, but it is also useful for lymphoid tissues, from which single-cell suspensions can be easily made. The advantages of flow cytometry are largely based on its ability to very rapidly and simultaneously analyze multiple cell properties, including size, granularity, and surface and intracellular antigens, even in small samples. The quantitative nature of the data produced, with regard to expression of individual cell antigens and distribution of cell populations, offers objective criteria to interpret results.

However, laboratorians and clinicians must recognize that malignant cells can differ from their normal counterparts (e.g., B-cell ALL versus normal B cells) in terms of the antigens that they characteristically express. This difference can occur in any of the following ways:

1. There may be a gain of antigens not usually expressed by the normal cell type or lineage.
2. There may be abnormally increased or decreased levels of the antigens expressed by the malignant cells or, in some cases, a complete loss of normal antigens.
3. The malignant cells may express antigens at inappropriate times during the maturation process.
4. There may be a homogeneous expression of antigens that are typically heterogeneously expressed by the normal counterpart.

Knowledge Check 18-5

Helper T cells in the peripheral blood commonly express all of the following *except:*

a. CD3
b. CD4
c. CD5
d. CD7
e. CD10

Evaluation of Immunoglobulins

As we discussed in Chapter 3, the basic immunoglobulin unit consists of two identical heavy chains and two identical light chains, covalently linked by disulfide bonds. The five antibody classes (and Ig subclasses) are defined by the structure of their heavy chain (e.g., gamma heavy chain in IgG, μ heavy chain in IgM, etc.). The two types of light chains (κ and λ) can each occur in combination with any of the heavy chain types (e.g., IgG_κ or IgG_λ). Recall that the heavy chains and light chains each contain constant and variable regions. The constant region contains the part of the immunoglobulin that binds to cell receptors and the part involved in complement fixation. The variable regions contain the *idiotypes,* which are responsible for the antigen specificity of the antibody. Normally, the pool of immunoglobulins in plasma is heterogeneous because it contains several classes of antibodies and immunoglobulins with different idiotypes that recognize a variety of antigens. This variability means that the immunoglobulins also vary in their physical characteristics, such as molecular weight and charge.

As we discussed in Chapter 5, B cells differentiate into antibody-producing plasma cells by maturation through several stages. Each B cell recognizes only a single antigenic site or epitope. An early B-cell precursor is stimulated to proliferate and mature when it encounters the epitope that it recognizes. When a foreign molecule enters the body, the many different epitopes on it each stimulate a B-cell response, leading to the production of an array of different antibodies. However, in monoclonal gammopathies such as multiple myeloma, the proliferation of one clone of transformed plasma cells leads to the overproduction of an immunoglobulin of a single class and antigen specificity. These M proteins are found mainly in the gamma region of an SPE analysis. All the antibody proteins produced by the clone of plasma cells are identical in terms of their heavy chains, light chains, and idiotype.

The initial tests used to screen for the presence of a monoclonal gammopathy are serum immunoglobulin levels and SPE (see the section that follows). Quantitative measurement of immunoglobulin levels in the serum is routinely performed by automated nephelometric or immunoturbidimetric methods (see Chapter 10). Because each plasma cell produces only one type of immunoglobulin, the persistent presence of an elevated amount of a single immunoglobulin class suggests malignancy. In contrast, an increase in the amount of total immunoglobulin, without an increase in any one specific class, is characteristic of nonmalignant conditions such as infections or autoimmune diseases.

Serum Protein Electrophoresis (SPE)

SPE separates serum proteins based on their size and electrical charge, as we discussed in Chapter 3. SPE results in five regions: albumin, plus the α_1, α_2, beta, and gamma globulins. IgG, IgM, IgD, and IgE migrate in the gamma globulin region, whereas IgA migrates as a broad band in the beta and gamma regions. **Figure 18–8,** panel A, shows a stylized drawing of the protein distribution in normal serum. As you can see by looking at the gamma region, immunoglobulins normally show a range of mobilities because they are derived from many clones of plasma cells (i.e., they are polyclonal) and have different variable-region sequences. Panel B shows the SPE pattern for a polyclonal increase in serum immunoglobulins. Note the broad mobility and increased height of the gamma globulin peak. Polyclonal increases in serum immunoglobulins are seen in a variety of disorders, including infections, autoimmune diseases, liver diseases, and some immunodeficiency states (e.g., hyper-IgM syndromes). Panel C depicts a monoclonal immunoglobulin, which is increased in concentration and has a narrow range of mobility because an identical clone of plasma cells produces it. This is illustrated by the tall, narrow peak in the gamma region.

Immunofixation Electrophoresis (IFE)

Additional evaluation of serum immunoglobulins by IFE is performed if the SPE shows a monoclonal component, if there is a significant quantitative abnormality of serum

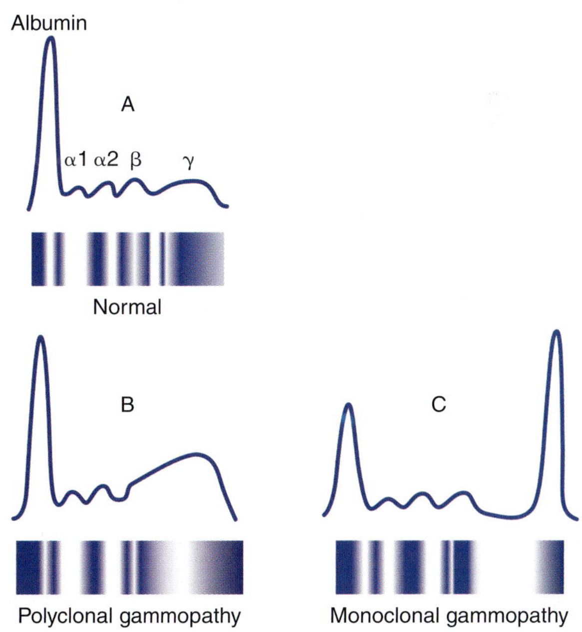

FIGURE 18–8 Serum protein electrophoresis of normal and abnormal samples. The lower portion of each panel is a representation of a stained agarose electrophoresis gel. The staining intensity corresponds to the amount of protein in each region of the gel. In the upper portion of each panel is a densitometer tracing of a gel similar to the one beneath it. In the upper panel showing a normal serum sample, the largest peak is albumin. The globulin regions are as indicated.

immunoglobulins, or if the clinical picture strongly suggests a plasma cell dyscrasia. Myeloma cases in which only light chains are produced may not be detected on SPE because the light chains are rapidly cleared in the urine. Therefore, additional studies on a random or 24-hour urine sample may be indicated even in the presence of a normal SPE.

Serum Immunofixation Electrophoresis (IFE)

IFE is a highly sensitive and specific assay that is used to identify the type of monoclonal protein present in a sample. It can be performed manually or by automated capillary electrophoresis systems. In IFE, serum samples are electrophoresed in six separate lanes on an agarose gel, and specific anti-sera are applied directly to the lanes. The antisera used are selected to detect the most common M proteins and are directed against the following:

- Whole human serum (lane 1)
- Anti-γ (to detect IgG) (lane 2)
- Anti-α (to detect IgA) (lane 3)
- Anti-μ (to detect IgM) (lane 4)
- Anti-κ (to detect kappa light chains) (lane 5)
- Anti-λ (to detect lambda light chains) (lane 6)

The antibodies combine with the immunoglobulin proteins in the sample to form complexes that are visualized by staining. **Figure 18–9** illustrates the principle of IFE. Areas of diffuse staining indicate polyclonal immunoglobulins, whereas monoclonal bands produce narrow, intensely stained bands **(Fig. 18–10).**

Interpretation of IFE results requires a high level of expertise. When the monoclonal protein is in high concentration and the amount of polyclonal immunoglobulin of the same class is low, the bands produced in IFE gels are usually clear and easy to identify, as shown in Figure 18–10. However, the presence of higher levels of normal immunoglobulins can make it difficult to distinguish a minor monoclonal band against a background of normal proteins. These M proteins can sometimes be identified by a technique called *immunosubtraction* (see section that follows). Poorly resolved bands can also be caused by poor technique during the electrophoresis or antisera application steps. Other situations can also affect the quality of the results. For example, plasma is not recommended because fibrinogen can adhere to the β region of the gel and cause monoclonal proteins to stick nonspecifically, resulting in distinct bands in all the antisera tracks. Samples with large amounts of rheumatoid factor or immune complexes can also produce unusual results, such as precipitin bands at the position of sample application. An extreme excess of monoclonal immunoglobulin can cause a *postzone* effect that produces a clear zone in the center of the band **(Fig. 18–11).**

Immunosubtraction

A variation of immunofixation, called **immunosubtraction** or **immunotyping,** is a sensitive procedure that uses capillary electrophoresis to identify monoclonal immunoglobulin components. In this technique, antibodies to each heavy or light chain isotype are added to separate capillary runs of the patient's specimen. Binding of the antibody to its heavy or light chain antigenic target changes the electrophoretic mobility of the patient's immunoglobulin molecule. Thus, monoclonal peaks "disappear" in the presence of antibodies to their components, allowing typing to occur by subtraction of peaks. **Figure 18–12** shows an example of a monoclonal IgG κ protein detected by immunotyping.

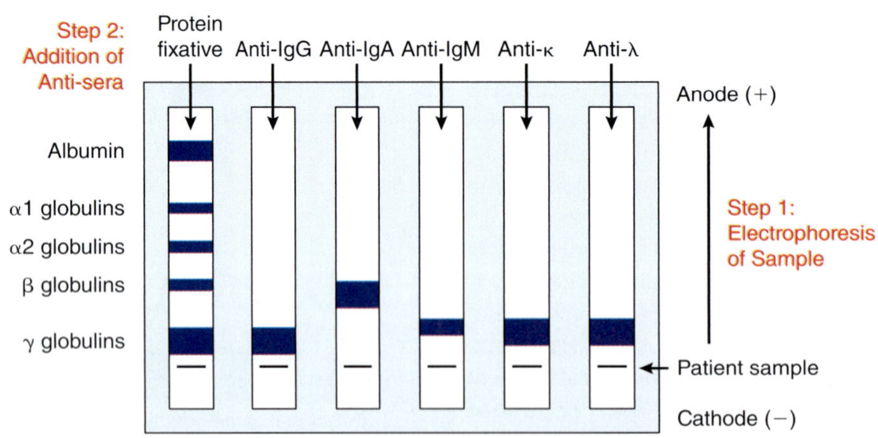

FIGURE 18–9 Principle of immunofixation electrophoresis (IFE). IFE involves two major steps. In step 1, proteins in the clinical sample (serum, urine, or cerebrospinal fluid) are applied to an agarose gel and separated according to their surface charge under the influence of an externally applied electrical field. At a pH of 8.6, the proteins acquire a negative charge and move toward the positively charged anode. Five major protein fractions result: gamma globulins, beta globulins, α_1-globulins, α_2-globulins, and albumin. Immunoglobulins are located mainly in the gamma globulin fraction but can also migrate into the beta globulin fraction. In step 2, specific antisera are added to each one of the lanes and react with their corresponding protein to produce a precipitin band. A protein fixative is added to lane 1, which binds to all the major protein fractions. The precipitin bands can be visualized after staining the gel with a protein stain and destaining with acetic acid to remove background color. *(Courtesy of Dr. Linda Miller.)*

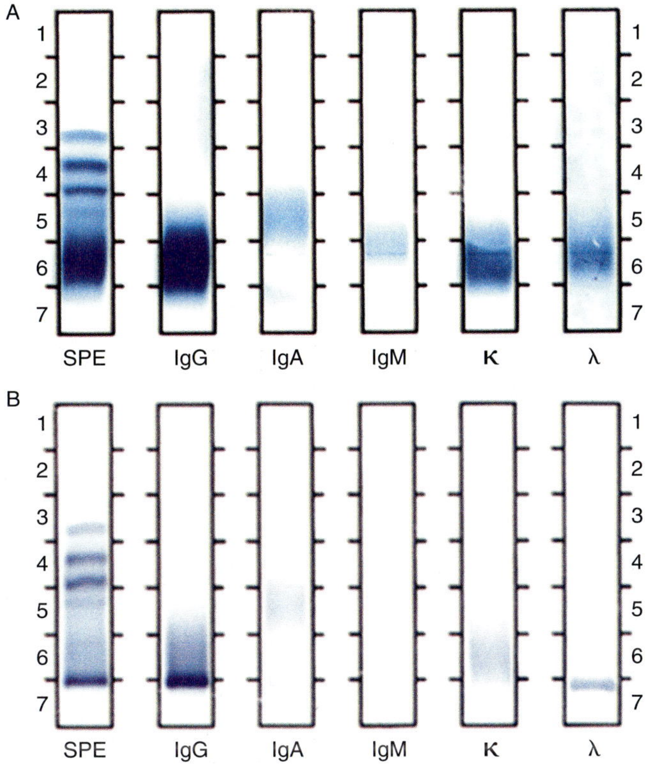

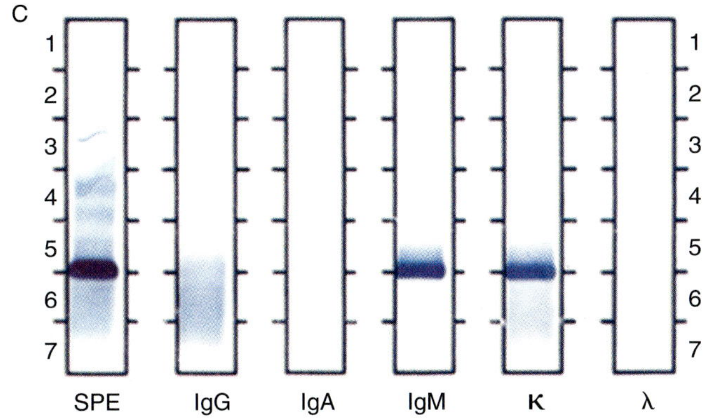

FIGURE 18–10 Sample IFEs from normal serum and sera from patients with monoclonal gammopathies. (A) Normal serum. Note the broad, diffuse bands in all the immunoglobulin lanes. These represent polyclonal antibodies that are heterogeneous in terms of their antigen specificity and structure and therefore migrate to slightly different positions on the gel. (B) Serum from a patient with a monoclonal IgG, λ antibody. Note the discrete, narrow bands in the IgG and λ lanes. The monoclonal antibody molecules produced by the patient are all identical and migrate to the same position on the gel. (C) Serum from a patient with monoclonal IgM, κ antibody. Note the discrete, narrow bands in the IgM and κ lanes. *(Courtesy of Dr. Linda Miller.)*

Clinical Correlations

Postzone Effect in IFE

Recall from Chapter 10 that equivalent amounts of antigen and antibody are required for optimal formation of immune complexes and precipitation. Extreme antigen excess results in the formation of small immune complexes that cannot be visualized. This is called a *postzone* effect. When a sample with a very large concentration of an M protein is reacted with antisera on an IFE gel, precipitation will be visible on the outer edges of the band, where the reaction is in equivalence, but will not appear in the center of the band, where the reaction is in the postzone area. The problem can be corrected by diluting the sample and repeating the IFE procedure.

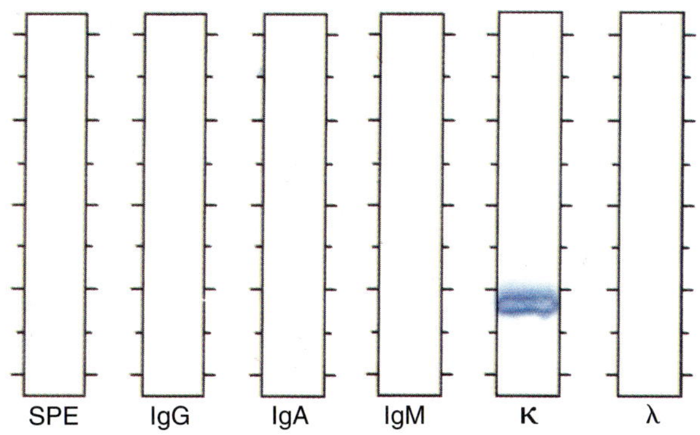

FIGURE 18–11 Postzone effect in immunofixation electrophoresis (IFE). IFE was performed on a 24-hour urine sample that was concentrated 50× by manual ultrafiltration (original protein concentration = 22 mg/dL). Note the clear area in the center of the κ band on the gel, reflecting decreased immunoprecipitation caused by an excess of κ chains relative to the amount of anti-κ reagent used in the κ lane. *(Courtesy of Dr. Linda Miller.)*

Urine Immunofixation Electrophoresis

Urine protein electrophoresis (UPE) and urine IFE also play important roles in the diagnosis of multiple myeloma and other plasma cell dyscrasias. As we previously discussed, some patients with these disorders produce an excessive amount of free monoclonal Ig light chains (i.e., Bence Jones proteins). Because these proteins are rapidly cleared from the circulation, they may be undetectable on serum IFE. However, the excess light chains are excreted into the urine and can be identified using UPE and urine IFE. The free light chains are believed to contribute to renal disease by depositing in the glomeruli and tubules of the kidneys and by their involvement in the development of renal casts. Therefore, UPE and urine IFE can be used to monitor patients with plasma cell dyscrasias. These tests can also be used to assess the effect of therapy on the production of free monoclonal light chains and can indicate more extensive renal damage when large proteins such as intact immunoglobulins, which are normally retained in the blood, are demonstrated in the urine.

Urine samples for UPE and IFE are typically collected over a 24-hour period. The total protein concentration is determined, and the sample is treated by filtration or centrifugation to remove any sediment that could interfere with performance of the tests. The samples must also be concentrated so that enough protein is present to produce visible bands on the gel. Concentration can be accomplished by one

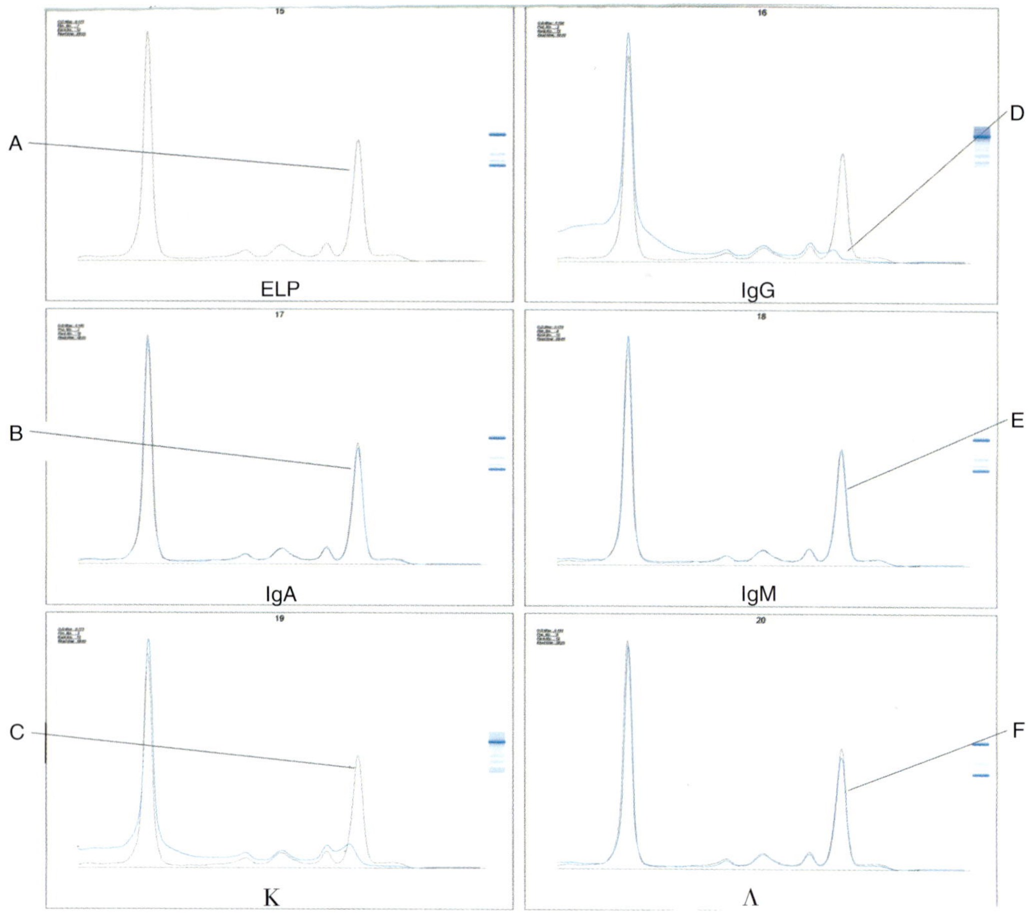

FIGURE 18–12 Immunotyping of a monoclonal IgG, κ protein. Panel A: Serum protein electrophoresis (SPE). The arrow points to the M-spike in the gamma region. Panel B: Electrophoresis with anti-alpha heavy chain. This pattern is overlaid with the original SPE. The patterns are identical. Panel C: Electrophoresis with anti-kappa light chain. The M-spike has disappeared, indicating the peak contains a kappa light chain (see arrow). Panel D: Electrophoresis with anti-gamma heavy chain. The M-spike has disappeared, indicating the peak contains IgG (see arrow). Panel E: Electrophoresis with anti-mu heavy chain. This pattern is overlaid with the original SPE. The patterns are identical. Panel F: Electrophoresis with anti-lambda light chain. This pattern is overlaid with the original SPE. The patterns are identical. *(Courtesy of Dr. Thomas Alexander.)*

of two ways. The first way involves the use of urine concentrators with ultrafiltration membranes that can retain large proteins (usually 10,000 daltons or more) but allow water, salts, and other small molecules to pass through, thus reducing the sample volume. In the process, the sample flows through a chamber containing the absorbent membranes and is collected when it reaches the desired volume and concentration. The second way involves centrifugal concentrators that concentrate the sample by high-speed filtration. Centrifugal concentrators are faster than ultrafiltration membranes and can produce higher concentration factors. They are recommended for the preparation of urine samples in capillary electrophoresis systems.

In both techniques, the desired concentration factor is based on the amount of protein in the urine sample and is determined by dividing the starting sample volume by the final volume. The concentrated sample is then applied to the electrophoresis gel, and the tests are completed as previously described for SPE and serum IFE.

Serum Free Light Chain (sFLC) Analysis

Although UPE and urine IFE are sensitive methods for detecting free monoclonal light chains, they have some limitations. For example, the requirement for a 24-hour urine collection can delay results. Also, interpretation of the results is subjective and can be difficult when a low level of free light chains is present with a high level of proteinuria, creating a high degree of background staining. Automated tests for sFLC offer advantages over the traditional methods for urine testing.

The sFLC assays are latex-enhanced immunoassays that measure free kappa and lambda light chains in the serum. The assays use polyclonal antibody reagents that recognize a diverse range of FLC epitopes that are normally hidden when the light chains are bound to heavy chains in intact immunoglobulins. This allows for quantitative measurement of free kappa and free lambda chain concentrations, and calculation of a κ/λ ratio, which is normally between 0.26 and 1.65. An abnormal κ/λ ratio outside of the reference range, along with an increase of either κ or λ, is a sensitive indicator for the presence of a malignant plasma cell clone.

The sFLC assays are highly sensitive, being capable of detecting concentrations lower than 1 mg/L. This sensitivity allows them to detect monoclonal FLCs in patients previously thought to be negative for monoclonal Ig production by serum or urine IFE. Based on the quantitative nature and high level of sensitivity of sFLC testing and clinical studies, the IMWG developed consensus guidelines that recommend the use of a sFLC assay along with SPE and serum IFE to screen for multiple myeloma and related disorders. The group also stated that the sFLC can replace the 24-hour urine IFE to screen for most plasma dyscrasias (except for light chain amyloidosis). The experts also concluded that sFLC measurements are valuable in monitoring patients with plasma cell disorders and in helping to determine patient prognosis.

However, sFLC assays have some drawbacks and require caution when interpretating the results. sFLC assays have been shown to have a %CV as high as 30%, depending on the assay used. Clinicians must be informed of the degree of variability in the assay used to avoid overinterpreting small changes in results. Also, some assays are susceptible to false-negative results and nonlinearity due to antigen excess.

Knowledge Check 18-6

Which of the following techniques is used to characterize the heavy chain component of an M protein?

a. Serum protein electrophoresis (SPE)
b. Immunofixation electrophoresis (IFE)
c. Urine protein electrophoresis (UPE)
d. Serum free light chain (sFLC)

Evaluation of Genetic and Chromosomal Abnormalities

As we previously discussed, researchers have identified the specific mutations associated with malignant transformation for many of the hematologic malignancies. These genetic alterations are an integral part of the diagnosis, as outlined in the WHO and ICC criteria. The detection of chromosome translocations is of particular value in diagnosing hematologic malignancies. **Table 18–3** lists chromosome translocations that are characteristic of selected leukemias and lymphomas.

Often, these translocations can be detected by cytogenetic techniques. Malignant lymphoid cells can be stimulated to proliferate in vitro, and their metaphase chromosomes can be examined for grossly visible abnormalities that correspond to characteristic translocations. Traditional cytogenetic evaluation by karyotyping has been supplemented by **fluorescence in situ hybridization** (**FISH;** see Chapter 12). FISH is used to directly identify a specific region of DNA in a cell. It involves the preparation of short sequences of single-stranded DNA, called *probes,* which are complementary to the DNA sequences of interest. The probes bind to the complementary chromosomal DNA in the patient sample and, because they contain a fluorescent label, allow the location of those DNA sequences in the chromosomes to be visualized with a fluorescent microscope. **Figure 18–13** shows an example of a FISH result obtained from a patient with a hematologic malignancy. Probes can be used on chromosomes, interphase nuclei, or tissue biopsies. FISH on interphase chromosomes is quite sensitive and rapid because it does not require cell culture. However, it only provides information about the specific DNA sequence being detected by the probe used in the test.

Lymphoid malignancies can also be evaluated by molecular techniques to identify abnormalities that are too subtle or diverse to be detected by karyotyping or FISH. Laboratorians use molecular methods to find microdeletions or clonal rearrangements of the immunoglobulin genes in B-cell malignancies or of the TCR genes in T-cell malignancies. PCR is a widely used technique to detect these gene rearrangements.

To detect B-cell clonality, for example, the PCR amplifies the Ig heavy chain gene sequence containing the variable and joining genes. Recall from Chapter 3 that rearrangements in the Ig heavy and light chain genes occur during B-cell maturation. The rearrangements occur randomly so that each B cell has a unique sequence of variable-heavy (V), diversity (D), and joining (J) gene segments. This unique sequence is retained as the B cell proliferates. Thus, the sequence can be used as a marker for the B-cell clonality characteristic of B-cell malignancies. It appears as a band of distinct size when it is amplified by PCR and run on gel electrophoresis. **Figure 18–14** illustrates the presence of a malignant B-cell clone in the samples run in lanes 3, 6, 9, and 10, which show a sharp band that migrates to a specific position on the gel, representing a unique V-D-J Ig heavy chain (IgH) gene rearrangement. In contrast, normal polyclonal B cells produce a diverse array

Table 18–3 Cytogenetics Characteristics of Selected Leukemias and Lymphomas

HEMATOLOGIC MALIGNANCY	CHARACTERISTIC CYTOGENETICS[a]
Burkitt lymphoma	Most commonly t(8;14) *[IGH/MYC]*; also t(2;8) and t(8;22)
Follicular lymphoma	t(14;18) *[IGH/BCL2]*
Mantle cell lymphoma	t(11;14) [*IGH*/cyclin D1]
B-cell acute lymphoblastic leukemia (B-ALL)	t(12;21) *[ETV6/RUNX1]*
Chronic myelogenous leukemia (CML)	t(9;22) *[BCR/ABL]*

[a]IGH = immunoglobulin heavy chain gene; t = translocation.

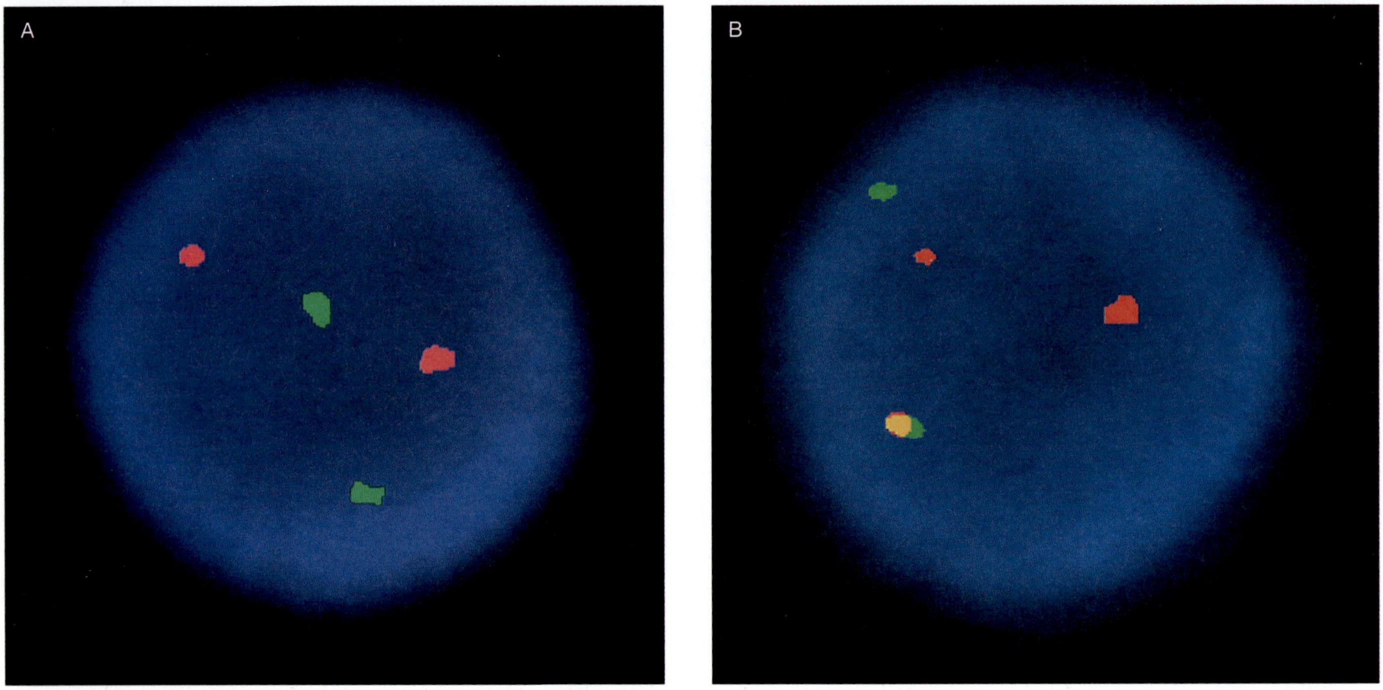

FIGURE 18–13 Fluorescence in situ hybridization (FISH) demonstrating a chromosomal translocation. In this assay, interphase cells were hybridized with molecular probes complementary to specific regions on chromosomes 9 and 22. The green signal represents the *BCR* (breakpoint cluster region) on chromosome 22, and the red signal represents the *ABL1* proto-oncogene on chromosome 9. A yellow signal represents the *BCR/ABL1* fusion caused by a 9;22 chromosome rearrangement. (A) A normal test result, showing two green signals representing two copies of chromosome 22 and two red signals representing two copies of chromosome 9. (B) Result from a patient with a translocation between chromosomes 9 and 22 (t[9;22][q34.1;q11.2]). The yellow signal indicates the fusion between the *BCR* and *ABL1* loci on the rearranged chromosome 22, also known as the *Philadelphia chromosome*. The smaller red signal detects the residual *ABL1* sequences present on the rearranged chromosome 9. This translocation is found in patients with chronic myelogenous leukemia (CML) as well as some individuals with acute myeloid leukemia (AML) and acute lymphoblastic leukemia (ALL). *(Courtesy of the Cytogenetics Laboratory, SUNY Upstate Medical University.)*

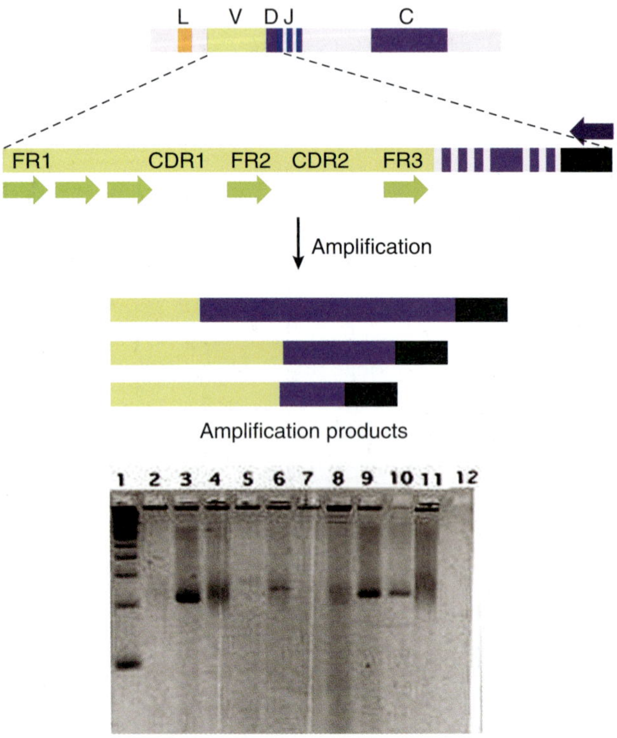

FIGURE 18–14 Immunoglobulin heavy chain gene rearrangement by PCR with amplification from the variable region. Forward primers complementary to the variable region and reverse primers complementary to the joining region are used to amplify the diversity region (top). In a polyclonal specimen, amplification products in a range of sizes will result. These products produce a dispersed band pattern on an ethidium bromide–stained agarose gel (lanes 4, 8, 11). If at least 1% of the sample represents a monoclonal gene rearrangement, that product will be amplified preferentially and revealed as a sharp band by gel electrophoresis (lanes 3, 6, 9, and 10).

of V-D-J IgH gene rearrangements, which migrate to different positions on the gel, producing a smear (Fig. 18–14, lanes 4, 8, and 11). Similarly, unique rearrangements in the TCR genes can be amplified by PCR to detect a malignant T-cell clone.

Although PCR and FISH are used to detect abnormalities in targeted genes, other molecular techniques can assay larger areas of the genome. In particular, microarrays and next-generation sequencing (NGS) provide a more comprehensive analysis of the neoplastic genome, resulting in better patient diagnosis and more precise, targeted therapies for the hematologic malignancies.

DNA microarray technology enables efficient analysis of thousands of genes in the human genome in a single hybridization experiment. Genomic DNA is isolated from a clinical sample, labeled with a fluorescent dye, and incubated with a microarray membrane or slide to which unique molecular probes have been attached at different locations (see Chapter 12). The probes are complementary to portions of specific genes or chromosome regions so that fluorescent spots will be visible in the locations where the sample DNA has bound. This technique is being used clinically to detect small genetic changes called *single nucleotide polymorphisms* (SNPs), and larger chromosome deletions or additions that result in *copy number variations* (CNVs) that may occur in hematologic malignancies.

NGS of tumor cells is also making its way into routine clinical practice. This technique is being used to analyze the nucleotide sequence of all the genes (i.e., whole genome sequencing), the coding regions of the genome (referred to as *exome sequencing*), or the transcriptome (i.e., messenger RNA) in samples from patients with cancer, including those with hematologic malignancies. The tremendous amount of data resulting from these analyses is allowing clinicians to identify genetic profiles associated with specific hematologic malignancies and is revealing new genetic changes associated with the pathobiology of lymphoid neoplasms.

KEY CONCEPTS

Introduction

- The immunoproliferative diseases are a diverse group of malignancies that arise from hematopoietic cells of a lymphoid or myeloid lineage.
- Leukemias originate from hematopoietic cells in the bone marrow that migrate to the peripheral blood, whereas lymphomas are solid tumors that usually arise in the lymph nodes and affect other lymphoid tissues. However, there is often overlap in the sites affected by these malignancies.

Malignant Transformation of Hematologic Cells

- Malignant transformation of hematologic cells results from genetic changes that promote cell proliferation or failure to undergo apoptosis.
- Lymphocytes are at high risk for malignant transformation because they undergo genetic changes as they mature and are stimulated to proliferate during immune responses.
- Malignant lymphoid cells may retain some or all the morphological characteristics of their normal counterparts but may have been arrested at an earlier stage of maturation.

Classification of Hematologic Malignancies

- The WHO and the ICC classifications of hematologic malignancies are based on their morphological features, cytochemical staining, immunophenotype as determined by flow cytometry, and genetics.

Leukemias

- The acute lymphocytic leukemias (ALLs) are characterized by the presence of poorly differentiated precursor cells called "blasts" that migrate rapidly in the bone marrow and are found in large numbers in the peripheral blood. They usually originate from immature precursors belonging to the B-cell lineage.
- Monoclonal B-cell lymphocytosis (MBL) includes three entities: low-count MBL (lymphocytes less than 0.5×10^9 clonal cells/mL), high-count MBL (CLL/SLL; lymphocytes greater than 0.5×10^9 clonal cells/mL), and non-CLL/SLL.
- Chronic lymphocytic leukemia (CLL)/small lymphocytic lymphoma (SLL) is a slowly progressive malignancy derived from mature B lymphocytes.
- Hairy cell leukemia is a rare, slowly progressive disease that mainly affects the bone marrow and spleen. The malignant cells express mature B-cell markers and have irregular hairy cytoplasmic projections from their surface.

Lymphomas

- Classic Hodgkin lymphoma is characterized by the presence of abnormal lymphocytes of B-cell origin called *Reed-Sternberg (RS) cells* in the lymph nodes and other lymphoid organs. It can be divided into four subtypes based on the population of cells that surround the RS cells in the affected tissues.
- Nodular lymphocytic-predominant Hodgkin lymphoma (NLPHL) is characterized by the presence of large, lymphocytic and histiocytic (L&H) cells that express mature B-cell antigens and are surrounded by small lymphocytes. L&H cells have a single, folded nucleus that resembles popcorn and are often referred to as "popcorn cells."
- Non-Hodgkin lymphomas include a wide range of neoplasms involving the B cells, T cells, or NK cells. They are most commonly found in immunosuppressed patients and include the B-cell malignancies, diffuse large B-cell lymphoma, follicular lymphoma, mantle cell lymphoma, and Burkitt lymphoma; and the T-cell malignancies, adult T-cell leukemia/lymphoma, mycosis fungoides, and Sézary syndrome.

Plasma Cell Dyscrasias

- The plasma cell dyscrasias, also known as *monoclonal gammopathies,* are plasma cell malignancies or premalignant conditions of the plasma cells characterized by production of a monoclonal immunoglobulin (M protein or paraprotein).
- Two premalignant conditions, monoclonal gammopathy of undetermined significance (MGUS) and smoldering multiple myeloma (SMM), are plasma cell dyscrasias that are associated with an increased risk of progressing to multiple myeloma. They are defined by a specific concentration of monoclonal immunoglobulin and percentage of plasma cells in

the bone marrow in the absence of clinical features associated with multiple myeloma.

- Multiple myeloma is a plasma cell malignancy characterized by an increased number of plasma cells in the bone marrow that crowd out normal hematopoietic precursors. The cells produce an M protein, usually IgG, IgA, or free light chains. The clinical features of multiple myeloma are known as "CRAB" (increased serum **c**alcium, **r**enal failure, **a**nemia, and lytic **b**one lesions).
- Waldenström macroglobulinemia is a malignancy of plasmacytoid lymphocytes that produce an IgM paraprotein.
- The heavy chain diseases are rare B-cell lymphomas that produce a monoclonal immunoglobulin heavy chain (alpha, gamma, or mu), which is incapable of binding to a light chain.
- Some patients with plasma cell dyscrasias produce free monoclonal light chains (kappa or lambda) and excrete the excess chains in the urine, where they are known as *Bence Jones proteins*.

Role of the Laboratory in Evaluating Immunoproliferative Diseases

- The cellular origin of a lymphoid malignancy is determined in the laboratory by flow cytometry. Fluorescent-labeled antibodies are used to identify CD markers on the surface of the malignant cells to determine their lineage, stage of maturation, and presence of abnormal antigen expression. This procedure is called *immunophenotyping*.
- Identification and quantification of a paraprotein are central to the diagnosis and monitoring of patients with monoclonal gammopathies. Serum protein electrophoresis (SPE) is used to detect the presence of an M protein, which is then characterized by immunofixation electrophoresis (IFE). In IFE, the presence of a monoclonal immunoglobulin is indicated by a discrete, narrow band that migrates to a restricted position on the gel, whereas polyclonal immunoglobulins are diverse and produce broad, diffuse bands.
- Immunosubtraction, or immunotyping, is a procedure in which antibodies to heavy and light chain isotypes are added during capillary electrophoresis of the sample. Existence of an M protein is indicated by the disappearance of a monoclonal peak in the presence of its corresponding antibody.
- Analysis of urine by UPE and IFE is important in the detection of Bence Jones proteins, which can contribute to renal damage. Before testing, the urine must be concentrated by manual filtration or high-speed centrifugal filtration to yield enough protein to produce visible banding on the gel.
- Serum free light chain (sFLC) assays are latex-enhanced automated immunoassays that measure free kappa and lambda light chains in patient serum. These sensitive assays can rapidly detect low levels of free light chains. An increase in κ or λ, along with an abnormal κ:λ ratio, indicate the presence of a malignant plasma cell clone.
- Genetic and chromosomal abnormalities can be detected by cytogenetic and molecular techniques, including FISH, PCR, microarray, and NGS. These methods allow for the detection of chromosome translocations, nucleotide deletions, and unique V-D-J gene rearrangements that are characteristic of specific hematologic malignancies.

CASE STUDIES

1. A 73-year-old patient visits a primary care physician complaining of fatigue and shortness of breath, upper back pain, and a cough that has become productive over the last 2 days. The patient was febrile and appeared acutely ill. A chest x-ray revealed pneumonia, and the following significant laboratory results were found:

   RBC count of 4.1×10^{12}/L (reference range 4.6 to 6×10^{12}/L), hemoglobin 13 g/dL (reference range 14 to 18 g/dL), WBC count of 4.8×10^9/L (reference range 4.5 to 11×10^9/L), and an erythrocyte sedimentation rate of 12 mm/hr (reference range 0 to 9 mm/hr).

   Based on the patient's clinical picture and lab results, the physician then ordered serum immunoglobulin levels. The following results were reported: IgG = 3,250 mg dL (reference range 600 to 1,500 mg/dL), IgM = 48 mg/dL (reference range 75 to 150 mg/dL), and IgA = 102 mg/dL (reference range 150 to 250 mg/dL).

   #### Questions

   a. What disease should you suspect? Why?

   b. What additional tests could help confirm the diagnosis, and what results would you expect to find?

2. A 47-year-old patient presented with fever, pneumonia, and an enlarged spleen. The hemoglobin was 11.5 g/dL (reference range 14 to 18 g/dL), the WBC count was 2.7×10^9/L (reference range 4.5 to 11×10^9/L), and the platelet count was 70×10^9/L ($150–450 \times 10^9$/L). A bone marrow biopsy revealed, among the normal bone marrow cells, numerous diffuse cells 10 to 14 µm

CASE STUDIES CONTINUED

in diameter with abundant, clear to lightly basophilic or eosinophilic cytoplasm. Delicate broad projections were seen on the surface of the cells. The nuclei were oval and indented with variable chromatin and no prominent nucleoli. Immunohistochemical analysis revealed that the leukemic cells were positive for CD20, DBA44 (a B-cell marker), CD68, and annexin A1. Expression of CD20, CD11c, CD25, and CD103 was demonstrated by flow cytometry.

Questions

a. Based on the laboratory results, what disease is most likely in this patient?

b. What is the significance of the immunophenotyping results?

REVIEW QUESTIONS

1. Bence Jones proteins consist of:
   a. Monoclonal IgG
   b. IgG-IgM complexes
   c. Free kappa or lambda light chains
   d. Free μ heavy chains

2. Which of the following is the best indicator of a malignant clone of cells?
   a. Overall increase in antibody production
   b. Increase in IgG and IgM only
   c. Unique V-D-J IgH gene rearrangement by PCR
   d. Decrease in overall antibody production

3. Which of the following laboratory techniques is routinely used to identify chromosome translocations associated with specific hematologic malignancies?
   a. FISH
   b. IFE
   c. Immunosubtraction
   d. PCR

4. All of the following features are commonly used to classify lymphoid neoplasms *except:*
   a. Cell of origin
   b. Presence of gene translocations
   c. Exposure of the patient to carcinogens
   d. Morphology or cytology of the malignant cells

5. Hodgkin lymphoma is characterized by:
   a. Proliferation of T cells
   b. Excess immunoglobulin production
   c. An incurable, rapidly progressive course
   d. Presence of Reed-Sternberg cells in the lymph nodes

6. Chronic lymphocytic leukemia (CLL) is characterized as:
   a. Usually being of B-cell origin
   b. Being curable with chemotherapy
   c. Usually occurring in children
   d. Following a rapidly progressive course

7. Which of the following is characteristic of heavy chain diseases?
   a. Usually of B-cell origin
   b. Rare lymphomas
   c. Production of abnormal Ig heavy chains
   d. All of the above

8. Flow cytometry results for a patient reveal a decreased number of peripheral blood cells with CD2 and CD3. These results indicate a reduced number of what type of cells?
   a. B cells
   b. T cells
   c. Monocytes
   d. Natural killer cells

9. Which of the following is true of Waldenström macroglobulinemia?
   a. Monoclonal IgM production may be associated with hyperviscosity syndrome.
   b. Multiple Ig-producing clones are found.
   c. The malignant cells produce monoclonal free heavy chains.
   d. Bence Jones proteins are never produced.

10. The presence of anemia, bone pain, thrombocytopenia, and lytic bone lesions is suggestive of:
    a. Hodgkin lymphoma
    b. Hairy cell leukemia
    c. Chronic lymphocytic leukemia
    d. Multiple myeloma

11. The presence of an M protein on immunofixation electrophoresis (IFE) is indicated by:
    a. Broad, diffuse banding
    b. A narrow, discrete band
    c. A few well-defined bands in the IgG lane
    d. A single band at the point of application in all of the lanes

12. Surface immunoglobulin on a leukemic cell indicates presence of a:
    a. B cell
    b. T cell
    c. Macrophage
    d. Plasma cell

13. Which of the following is *not* a requirement for urine testing by IFE?
    a. Collection of a 24-hour sample
    b. Concentration of the sample
    c. Dilution of the sample
    d. Removal of sediment

14. Multiple myeloma is characteristically preceded by:
    a. Chronic hypogammaglobulinemia
    b. EBV infection
    c. Non-Hodgkin lymphoma
    d. Monoclonal gammopathy of undetermined significance

15. Which serum free light chain (sFLC) assay result indicates the presence of a malignant plasma cell clone?
    a. An abnormal κ:λ ratio
    b. A decrease in κ and λ concentrations
    c. A decrease in IgG, IgA, and IgM concentrations
    d. An increase in immunoglobulin concentrations over a 24-hour period

16. Which of the following is best characterized as a plasma cell dyscrasia?
    a. Chronic lymphocytic leukemia/small cell lymphoma
    b. Waldenström macroglobulinemia
    c. Follicular lymphoma
    d. Diffuse large B-cell lymphoma

17. A patient presents with a lymphocyte clonal expansion of 0.9×10^9/L and a B-cell count of 4.3×10^9/L. The cells appear as small lymphocytes with a high nuclear/cytoplasmic ratio, clumped chromatin, and clear, blue cytoplasm. All other parameters are within normal limits. These findings suggest which of the following?
    a. Hodgkin lymphoma
    b. Hairy cell leukemia
    c. Multiple myeloma (plasma cell myeloma)
    d. CLL/SSL type MBL

18. Chromosomal translocations that occur in Burkitt lymphoma, mantle cell lymphoma, and follicular lymphoma often involve chromosome 14. How do these translocations drive the development of neoplasms?
    a. The gene involved at the breakpoint region of chromosome 14 gets activated.
    b. The gene on the reciprocal chromosome is placed under the control of a different promoter and causes overexpression of the gene.
    c. There is a tumor suppressor gene on chromosome 14 that becomes inactivated, causing resistance to apoptosis.
    d. The translocation causes the deletion of a regulatory element in the genome that controls cellular maturation.

Chapter 18 Answer Key

Answers to Knowledge Checks

18.1 c 18.2 d 18.3 b 18.4 c 18.5 e 18.6 b

Answers to Review Questions

1. c	2. c	3. a	4. c	5. d	6. a	7. d
8. b	9. a	10. d	11. b	12. a	13. c	14. d
15. a	16. b	17. d	18. b			

19 Immunodeficiency Diseases and Inborn Errors of Immunity

Linda E. Miller, PhD, I,MB[CM](ASCP)SI

LEARNING OUTCOMES

After finishing this chapter, you should be able to:

19.1 Differentiate between primary and secondary immunodeficiencies.

19.2 Define inborn errors of immunity (IEIs) and describe the International Union of Immunological Societies (IUIS) classification system for the IEIs.

19.3 Describe the modes of inheritance, immunologic defects, clinical manifestations, and appropriate therapies associated with selected IEIs.

19.4 Indicate the types of infections, and in some cases, malignancies, typically associated with defects in B cells, T cells, neutrophils, or complement.

19.5 Select appropriate laboratory tests to determine numbers and functions of B cells, T-cell populations, and phagocytic cells.

19.6 Correlate laboratory results with the presence of different types of IEIs.

CHAPTER OUTLINE

You can go to **fadavis.com** keyword stevens for the laboratory exercises that accompany this text.

Immunodeficiencies are disorders in which a part of the body's immune system is missing or dysfunctional. People with these conditions have a decreased ability to defend themselves against infectious organisms and are more susceptible to developing certain types of cancer. The clinical symptoms associated with immunodeficiencies vary; depending on the disease and the individual patient, they may be absent or very mild, chronic with recurrent infections, or severe, with life-threatening infections and failure to thrive.

Immunodeficiencies can be inherited or acquired after exposure to certain environmental factors. The acquired disorders, or **secondary immunodeficiencies,** have various causes, including certain infections, malignancies, nutrient deficits, burns that compromise the skin barrier, and immunosuppressive therapies (e.g., steroids, chemotherapy, monoclonal antibodies, or small molecule inhibitors that target immune components). In Chapter 24, we discuss a notable example of a secondary immunodeficiency, AIDS, caused by HIV.

In this chapter, we focus on the inherited immunodeficiencies, or **primary immunodeficiency diseases (PIDs).** Several PIDs show X-linked inheritance (caused by an abnormal gene on the X chromosome) and, therefore, mainly affect males, who have only one X chromosome. Others are autosomal recessive (caused by defective genes on a chromosome other than X or Y, inherited from both father and mother) or autosomal dominant (having only one defective gene on a non-sex chromosome inherited from a parent), and affect both sexes equally. Gene expression is also affected by other factors, such as epigenetics (see Chapter 12), mosaicism (existence of normal and abnormal versions of the gene in different body cells), and exposure to environmental factors.

The PIDs can affect innate immunity, adaptive immunity, or immune regulation and are associated with distinct clinical features, depending on the component(s) involved. Because these components interact extensively in various immune responses, a defect in one branch of the system may also affect other aspects of immune function. A deficiency in one component may also be accompanied by hyperactivity of other components. This may occur because persistent infections continuously stimulate the available immune cells or because a compensatory mechanism has been activated to correct for the deficient immune function.

Figure 19–1 illustrates points in the development of the immune system at which several PIDs exert their main effects.

Inborn Errors of Immunity (IEIs)

The PIDs, also known as **inborn errors of immunity (IEIs),** are a diverse group of inherited conditions caused by abnormalities in single genes that affect immune function, resulting in immunodeficiency, and possibly exaggerated or dysfunctional immune responses as well. These disorders may also affect other organs, notably those of the central nervous, digestive, renal, or pulmonary systems. While most IEIs are rare diseases, studies are revealing that when considered collectively, they are quite common; an estimated 1 in every 1,200 to 2,000 people are thought to have some form of IEI. With increased use of next-generation sequencing (NGS) and other genetic technologies in recent years, discovery of these disorders has been rising at an extraordinary rate; at the time of this writing, more than 550 different IEIs have been identified.

The International Union of Immunological Societies (IUIS) has grouped the IEIs into categories based on their immunologic defects. Some diseases are listed in more than one category because they have overlapping features. Included in the classification system are tables listing the IEIs along with their genetic defects, mode of inheritance, laboratory results, and other associated features, to aid in patient diagnosis. The classification system is updated every 2 years. The 10 categories of the 2024 IUIS classification are as follows:

- Category 1: Combined Immunodeficiencies
- Category 2: Combined Immunodeficiencies With Syndromic Features
- Category 3: Predominantly Antibody Deficiencies
- Category 4: Diseases of Immune Dysregulation
- Category 5: Congenital Defects of Phagocytes
- Category 6: Defects in Intrinsic and Innate Immunity

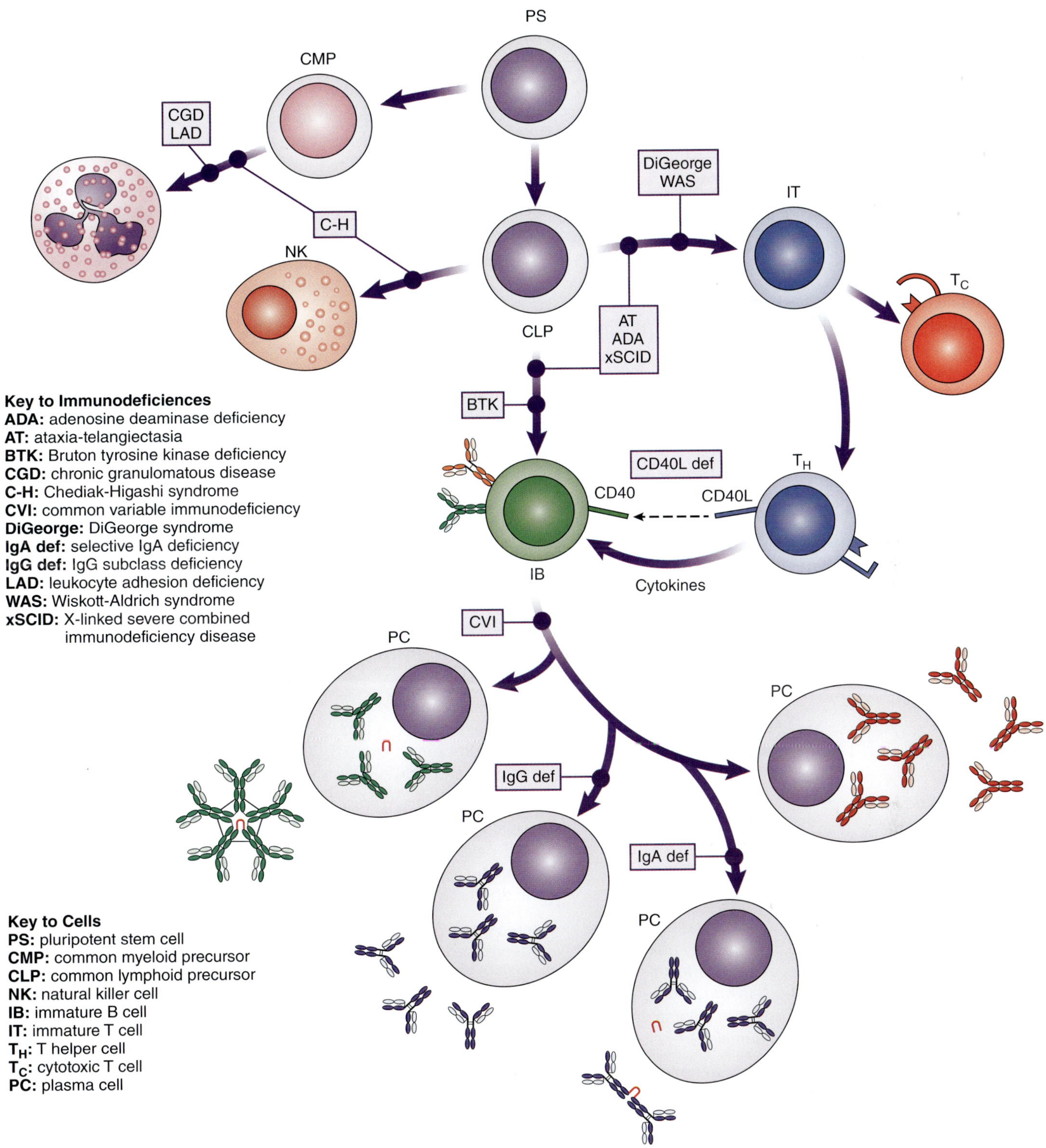

FIGURE 19–1 Examples of primary immunodeficiency diseases and their effects on the immune system.

- Category 7: Autoinflammatory Diseases
- Category 8: Complement Deficiencies
- Category 9: Bone Marrow Failure
- Category 10: Phenocopies of Inborn Errors of Immunity

Clinical diagnosis of the IEIs can be challenging but important because early detection and treatment can help prevent serious, long-term tissue damage and overwhelming infections. Early diagnosis may also provide opportunities for appropriate genetic counseling, carrier detection, and prenatal diagnosis for other family members. While the types of infection and symptoms displayed by a patient can give important clues about the specific IEI present, the clinical laboratory plays an essential role in identifying these important diseases. In this chapter, we discuss some of the better-known IEIs and the laboratory methods used to detect these disorders.

Knowledge Check 19-1

All of the following are characteristic of inborn errors of immunity (IEIs) *except:*

a. Are inherited disorders of immunodeficiency
b. Are caused by a defect in a single gene
c. May be acquired as a result of a viral infection
d. May affect adaptive or innate immunity

B-Cell/Antibody Deficiencies

B-cell deficiencies are classified by the IUIS as Category 3: Predominantly Antibody Deficiencies. As we discussed in earlier chapters (Chapters 1, 3, and 5), B cells play a central role in humoral immunity and are responsible for antibody production. Thus, the diseases in this group are characterized by decreased or undetectable levels of serum immunoglobulins. Because immunoglobulins migrate to the "gamma region" after serum protein electrophoresis (see Chapter 3), immunoglobulin (Ig) deficiencies have also been termed **agammaglobulinemias.**

Genetic defects that affect B-cell maturation, differentiation, or interactions with T cells cause agammaglobulinemias. In some cases, only a single Ig class is deficient, whereas all the other classes are normal. In general, defects in humoral immunity result in pyogenic (i.e., pus-forming) bacterial infections, often with encapsulated bacteria. Upper and lower respiratory tract infections are common, including recurrent sinusitis, otitis media (i.e., ear infections), and pneumonia; some infections may be severe and require hospitalization. Infections typically begin after 6 months of age, when the level of maternal antibodies begins to wane, although they may appear in adulthood in some conditions. Other complications include abnormal lymphocyte activation or proliferation, leading to autoimmunity, lymphoproliferative disorders, or malignancy.

Critical Thinking 19-1

Recurrent bacterial infections in B-cell deficiencies are not seen at birth but develop after a few months of age. Explain why this occurs.

A wide range of Ig deficiency states have been reported. In this section, we describe the more common, well-characterized syndromes and summarize their main characteristics in **Table 19–1.**

Table 19–1 Characteristics of Selected B-Cell/Antibody Deficiencies

DISEASE	DEFECT	LABORATORY FINDINGS	CLINICAL PRESENTATION
Transient hypogammaglobulinemia of infancy	Unknown genetic abnormality Delayed development of helper T-cell function in some patients	Decreased IgG and, in some cases, decreased IgA and IgM Normal numbers of circulating B and T cells	Recurrent respiratory infections and food allergies appearing at 5 to 24 months; resolves by 2 to 6 years
Bruton tyrosine kinase (Btk) deficiency (X-linked agammaglobulinemia)	X-linked inheritance of defective *BTK* gene Blocks differentiation of B-cell progenitors	Lack of mature $CD19^+$ B cells; normal number of T cells Decreased levels of all antibody classes	Recurrent bacterial infections beginning around 6 months of age
Common variable immunodeficiency	Group of diverse disorders with mostly unknown genetic defects B-cell failure to differentiate into plasma cells or insufficient T-cell help	Decreased IgG, along with decreased IgA and/or IgM in some cases Normal numbers of $CD19^+$ B cells and T cells	Variable—most patients have recurrent bacterial infections; some have lymphoproliferative or autoimmune disorders Usually diagnosed at 20 to 30 years of age
Selective IgA deficiency	Unknown genetic defect Ig class switching; IgA and B-cell differentiation	IgA decreased; some patients also have reduced IgG2 Patients may develop IgE–anti-IgA antibodies if exposed to blood products containing IgA	Often asymptomatic, but some patients have respiratory and gastrointestinal tract infections and are more likely to develop autoimmune diseases or allergies
Isolated IgG subclass deficiency	Unknown genetic defects Defective Ig class differentiation	Reduced IgG1, IgG2, IgG3, or IgG4	Variable—most patients are asymptomatic Patients with IgG1 or IgG3 deficiencies may not respond sufficiently to bacterial or viral proteins Those with IgG2 deficiency may be susceptible to bacteria with polysaccharide-containing capsules

Transient Hypogammaglobulinemia of Infancy With Normal Numbers of B Cells

All infants have low Ig levels from about 3 to 6 months of age as maternal IgG declines. However, some babies, especially those born prematurely, do not begin synthesizing Ig promptly, and the low levels persist for a longer time. These children, said to have **transient hypogammaglobulinemia of infancy (THI)**, have reduced levels of IgG, and in some cases, IgA and IgM, resulting in recurrent infections, especially of the respiratory tract; food allergies may also be seen. Ig levels usually normalize spontaneously by 2 to 6 years of age. This observation and the elimination of other antibody deficiencies are essential for diagnosis of THI. Treatment typically includes antibiotics; IV Ig therapy (intravenous or subcutaneous Ig preparations; see Chapter 25) may be given for more severe infections.

The mechanism of THI is unknown. Although more common in males, it does not appear to be X-linked, and a genetic association has not been identified. Patients have normal numbers of circulating B and T cells, but there may be a delay in the development of helper T (T_H) cell function or synthesis of cytokines that are important for antibody production.

X-Linked Bruton Tyrosine Kinase (Btk) Deficiency

Bruton tyrosine kinase (Btk) deficiency, also known as **X-linked agammaglobulinemia,** was first described in 1952 by Ogden Bruton. The defective gene is on the X chromosome, so this syndrome affects males almost exclusively. About half of the patients have a family history of the disease. Patients lack circulating mature $CD19^+$ B cells and have undetectable or low levels of all Ig classes. They have no plasma cells in their lymphoid tissues but have pre-B cells in their bone marrow. Because of the lack of B cells, the tonsils and adenoids are small or entirely absent, and lymph nodes lack normal germinal centers. T cells are normal in number and function.

Patients develop recurrent bacterial infections beginning in infancy as maternal antibody is cleared. Respiratory infections caused by encapsulated organisms such as streptococci, pneumococci, and *Haemophilus influenzae* are common. Patients may also develop infections of the skin or gastrointestinal (GI) tract, with diarrhea. In some cases, infections may become severe, spreading through the blood and affecting other organs. Patients may also be susceptible to certain types of viral infections and should not receive live virus vaccines. The syndrome can be effectively treated with Ig replacement therapy and vigorous administration of antibiotics to treat and prevent infections.

Btk deficiency results from arrested differentiation at the pre–B-cell stage, leading to a complete absence of mature B cells and plasma cells. Mutations in the *BTK* gene result in a deficiency of the Btk enzyme in B-cell progenitor cells, causing a failure of Ig variable heavy chain (V_H) gene rearrangement (see Chapter 3). Btk deficiency can be differentiated from THI by its absence of $CD19^+$ B cells in the peripheral blood, abnormal lymphoid tissue histology, and persistence beyond 2 years of age. About 15% of patients with agammaglobulinemia caused by a lack of B cells have defects in other genes involved in B-cell maturation, which are inherited in an autosomal recessive manner. These patients have symptoms and laboratory findings similar to Btk deficiency.

Common Variable Immunodeficiency (CVI)

Common variable immunodeficiency (CVI) is a diverse group of disorders with a prevalence of about 1 in 25,000. Although this is a low incidence, CVI is the most common PID with a severe clinical syndrome. Patients usually begin to have symptoms in their 20s and 30s, but children and older adults can also develop the disease. The disorder is sporadic in most cases, but up to 25% of patients may have a family history. It occurs with equal frequency in males and females. While the genetic cause is unknown in most patients, defects in single genes associated with immune function have been identified in about 10% of cases.

CVI is characterized by **hypogammaglobulinemia** (low Ig levels in the blood) that leads to recurrent bacterial infections, particularly sinusitis and pneumonia. Patients are usually deficient in IgG and IgA but may have low levels of only IgG, or of IgG, IgA, and IgM, depending on the individual. Intestinal malabsorption and diarrhea are often present. CVI is also associated with an increased risk of lymphoproliferative disorders, gastric carcinomas, and autoimmune disorders. The most common autoimmune manifestations of CVI are immune thrombocytopenia and autoimmune hemolytic anemia. Other symptoms may include lymphadenopathy, splenomegaly, and intestinal hyperplasia.

CVI is often a diagnosis of exclusion, after other PIDs have been ruled out. Patients have a low serum IgG level and recurrent bacterial infections. The blood group **isohemagglutinins** (naturally occurring IgM antibodies to ABO blood group antigens) are typically absent or low. In contrast to Btk deficiency, most patients with CVI have normal numbers of mature B cells. However, the B cells do not differentiate normally into Ig-producing plasma cells. Multiple types of cellular defects have been found in patients with CVI. Intrinsic B-cell defects may be responsible for some cases, while in others, T_H cells may fail to provide adequate support for the differentiation of B cells into plasma cells and memory cells.

CVI can usually be effectively treated with Ig replacement therapy. However, because secretory IgA levels are low, patients are still susceptible to respiratory and GI infections, which should be treated vigorously with antibiotics.

Selective IgA Deficiency

Selective IgA deficiency is the most common PID in North America and Europe, occurring in about 1 in 500 persons of European descent. These individuals have decreased IgA concentrations but usually have normal levels of IgG and IgM. Most patients are asymptomatic and may be unaware of their condition. Those with symptoms usually have respiratory and GI tract infections and are more likely to develop autoimmune diseases such as systemic lupus erythematosus (SLE), rheumatoid arthritis (RA), celiac disease, and thyroiditis. Allergies and malignancy are also more common.

About 20% of patients who are IgA deficient and develop infections also have an IgG2 subclass deficiency. If the serum IgA is lower than 5 mg/dL, the deficiency is considered severe. If the IgA level is two standard deviations (SDs) below the age-adjusted mean but greater than 50 mg/dL, the deficiency is partial. Although the genetic defect has not been established, experts have hypothesized that the lack of IgA is caused by impaired Ig heavy chain gene switching and development of IgA-producing plasma cells.

IgE antibodies specifically directed against IgA are produced by 30% to 40% of patients with severe IgA deficiency, who respond to IgA as a foreign protein if they are exposed. These antibodies can cause life-threatening anaphylactic reactions when blood products containing IgA are transfused (see Chapter 14). Because many patients with severe IgA deficiency have no other symptoms, the IgA deficiency may not be detected until the patient experiences a transfusion reaction, resulting in anti-IgA production. Products for transfusion to known IgA-deficient patients should be collected from IgA-deficient donors, and cellular products should be washed to remove as much donor plasma as possible.

Most gamma globulin preparations contain significant amounts of IgA. However, replacement IgA therapy may not be beneficial because the half-life of IgA is short (around 7 days), and intravenously administered IgA is not transported to its normal site of secretion at mucosal surfaces. Because IgA-containing products may provoke anaphylaxis, subcutaneous administration of Ig replacement therapy is preferred for patients with severe infections. Broad-spectrum antibiotics can also be provided.

Isolated IgG Subclass Deficiency

IgG subclass deficiencies are conditions in which the levels of one or more of the four IgG subclasses are more than two SDs below the age-adjusted mean level. The genetic abnormalities involved in these conditions are largely unknown. Normally, about 66% of the total IgG is IgG1, 23% IgG2, 7% IgG3, and 4% IgG4. Therefore, a single subclass deficiency may not result in a total IgG level below the normal range, and most individuals are asymptomatic. In patients with recurrent infections, IgG subclass levels should be measured if the total IgG level is normal but the clinical picture suggests Ig deficiency.

Most IgG antibodies directed against protein antigens are of the IgG1 and IgG3 subclasses, whereas most IgG antibodies against carbohydrate antigens are IgG2 or IgG4. Thus, deficiencies involving IgG1 or IgG3 lead to a reduced ability to respond to bacterial toxins and viral infections, whereas selective IgG2 deficiency can result in recurrent infections with polysaccharide-encapsulated bacteria such as *Streptococcus pneumoniae* and *H. influenzae*. Patients can be treated with antibiotics to clear the infections and, possibly, with Ig replacement therapy if infections persist.

Knowledge Check 19-2

B-cell immunodeficiencies are characterized by:
a. Decreased or absent immunoglobulins
b. Increased number of $CD19^+$ cells
c. Increased B-cell activation
d. Persistent infections with intracellular organisms

T-Cell Defects and Combined Immunodeficiencies

As we discussed in earlier chapters, T cells are classified into different subpopulations and have many important roles in the immune response. Therefore, low T-cell numbers or defects in T-cell function affect multiple aspects of the immune system, including cell-mediated immunity and regulation of immune responses through their cytokine secretion. Because T_H cells provide helper functions that are necessary for normal B-cell development and differentiation, antibody production is also affected. Thus, T-cell deficiencies are considered to be combined defects; some of these diseases also involve nonimmunologic body components. The IUIS classifies these disorders in categories 1 and 2.

In general, congenital defects in T-cell–mediated immunity result in recurrent infections with intracellular viral, fungal, bacterial, and parasitic organisms. Patients almost always develop mucocutaneous candidiasis, a yeast infection that involves the skin, nails, and mucous membranes. They are also prone to disseminated viral infections, especially with latent viruses such as herpes simplex, Epstein-Barr virus (EBV), varicella zoster, and cytomegalovirus (see Chapter 23). Vaccines consisting of live, weakened viruses, such as those for measles, chickenpox, and rotavirus, should not be administered to these patients because they can cause severe infections. Because T cells also play an important role in tumor immunity, patients with these conditions are more susceptible to developing certain types of cancer, especially those of lymphoid origin.

Primary T-cell immunodeficiencies are more difficult to treat than defects in humoral immunity, and differentiation from HIV-induced immunodeficiency is essential for proper treatment. While Ig replacement therapy is often very effective in treating antibody deficiency, treatment for deficiencies in cell-mediated immunity must include transplantation of immunologically intact cells to reconstitute immune function. These therapies most often involve infusions of hematopoietic stem cells (HSCs) from bone marrow or peripheral blood, preferably from a human leukocyte antigen (HLA)-compatible donor.

A potential risk of HSC transplants from incompatible HLA donors is graft-vs-host disease (GVHD). As we discussed in Chapter 16, GVHD results from an immune response of donor T lymphocytes in the HSC transplant to dissimilar HLA antigens on the recipient's cells. A severe T-cell defect in the patient allows the donor T lymphocytes to survive, proliferate, and attack the tissues of the recipient as foreign. Severe damage to the patient's tissues, such as the skin, GI tract, and liver, can result, leading to serious, lifelong complications and possibly death. The closer the match between the genetic constitution of the patient and the graft donor, the less severe the GVHD is likely to be. Irradiation of cell-containing blood products (platelet concentrates, packed red blood cells [RBCs], and whole blood) before transfusion destroys the ability of the donor lymphocytes to proliferate and prevents the development of GVHD in immunodeficient recipients.

In the sections that follow, we discuss selected immunodeficiencies from IUIS categories 1 and 2; their main characteristics are summarized in **Table 19–2.**

Severe Combined Immunodeficiency (SCID)

Severe combined immunodeficiency (SCID) refers to a group of life-threatening diseases caused by a lack of mature T cells. Scientists have discovered at least 20 different genetic mutations that can cause SCID by affecting different steps in T-cell development (see Chapter 5). A lack of B cells and/or natural killer (NK) cells can also be present in different forms of SCID. These are referred to by a shorthand notation of $T^{+/-}B^{+/-}NK^{+/-}$, with the $^{+}$ superscript denoting a normal number of the cell type and the $^{-}$ sign indicating a very low number. About half of SCID cases are inherited by an X-linked recessive mode (seen only in males), while the other types are autosomal recessive (seen in both males and females). Characteristics of five of the more common types of SCID, listed in order of their frequency, are summarized in **Table 19–3.** Other defects include those involving the CD3 chains, CD45, and the Artemis gene, which codes for genes needed for DNA repair.

Patients with SCID present early in infancy with infections by nearly any type of organism. Oral *Candida* yeast infections, pneumonia, and diarrhea are the most common manifestations. The latter can lead to malnutrition, weight loss, and failure to thrive. Without prompt diagnosis and treatment, patients with SCID typically die before they are 2 years old.

HSC transplantation is the standard treatment for SCID, producing greater than 90% long-term survival if administered during the first few months of life, prior to development of serious infections. Patients must be pretreated with chemotherapy or monoclonal antibodies to destroy any lymphocytes that might cause GVHD and to make room in the bone marrow for the transplanted HSCs to engraft. Enzyme replacement therapy can be used as a temporary treatment for patients with ADA deficiency prior to HSC transplantation. Extreme measures must also be taken to prevent infections, such as maintaining a high level of environmental and personal hygiene and avoiding contact with sick individuals. Gene therapy has been developed for treatment of ADA deficiency, X-linked SCID, and a few other types of SCID. This type of therapy is performed by transfecting the normal version of the disease-causing gene into the patients' T cells or HSCs and reinfusing the gene-corrected cells into the patient. It has resulted in sustained immune reconstitution and fewer infections in several patients but may be associated with significant side effects and is only available through enrollment in clinical trials.

> **Clinical Correlations**
>
> **The Story of David Vetter**
>
> David Vetter was a young boy who captured the public's attention after being born with SCID in 1971. Because he had a brother who died in infancy from SCID the year before, David was placed in germ-free chambers (which the public referred to as "bubbles") immediately after birth and for most of his life following confirmation of his diagnosis. In October 1983, after advances in transplantation had been made, David received a bone marrow transplant from his younger sister, in the hope that it would help restore his immune system. Unfortunately, David died from complications of the transplant in February 1984, and it was later discovered that his sister's bone marrow had transferred EBV, which caused a lymphoma to develop in David's body. Research on David's tissue samples led to discovery 9 years later of the gene that causes X-linked SCID. A combination of scientific research and public influence over the years has resulted in newborn screening and successful HSC transplantation for this otherwise lethal disease.

CD40 Ligand (CD154) Deficiency

Several of the combined immunodeficiencies have less profound effects than SCID. One example of these is CD40 ligand (CD40L or CD154) deficiency. This disease is one of the *hyper-IgM syndromes (HIGM)*, rare disorders characterized by decreased IgG, IgA, and IgE levels and normal or increased IgM. CD40L deficiency is inherited as an X-linked recessive form involving a mutation of the gene that codes for CD40L. Recall from Chapter 5 that CD40L is a surface T-cell molecule that is required for B-cell activation in the T-dependent antibody response. Thus, B cells from patients with this form of the disease are unable to undergo Ig class switching or produce high-affinity antibodies. These patients also have defective T-cell activation in cell-mediated immune responses. Less commonly, HIGM are inherited as autosomal recessive forms involving other genes involved in Ig class switching and affinity maturation (e.g., genes that code for CD40 on B cells, activation–induced deaminase [AID], or uracil *N*-glycosylase [UNG]). Some patients also develop neutropenia (decreased neutrophils in the blood), for unknown reasons.

Recurrent infections, especially of the respiratory and GI tracts, are common in patients with HIGM. Patients may develop severe opportunistic infections with organisms such as *Pneumocystis jiroveci*, a fungus that causes pneumonia, or *Cryptosporidium*, a parasite that causes GI problems and

Table 19–2 Characteristics of Selected Immunodeficiencies in IUIS Categories 1 and 2

DISEASE	DEFECT	LABORATORY FINDINGS	CLINICAL PRESENTATION
Category 1: Combined Immunodeficiencies			
Severe combined immunodeficiency (SCID)	Defects in various genes (see Table 19–3) X-linked (most common) and autosomal recessive forms exist	Severe decrease in T cells, and possibly B cells and/or NK cells	Severe, recurrent infections early in infancy Without HSC transplantation or gene therapy, patients usually die by 2 years of age
CD40 ligand (CD154) deficiency	X-linked inheritance of CD40L gene *(CD40LG)*	T-cell numbers are normal to low Memory B cells are absent Impaired T- and B-cell activation Defective isotype switching with increased or normal IgM but decreased concentrations of other Ig classes	Recurrent respiratory and GI tract infections; opportunistic infections; increased risk of autoimmunity and cancer
Category 2: Combined Immunodeficiencies With Syndromic Features			
Ataxia-telangiectasia (AT)	Autosomal inheritance of mutated *ATM* gene, resulting in defective DNA repair	Reduced IgG2, IgA, IgE, and increased IgM Progressive decrease in T-cell numbers Increased α-fetoprotein	Recurrent lung and sinus infections Poor muscle control Capillary swelling in eyes and face Progressive neurological deterioration Chromosome instability Increased risk of cancer
DiGeorge syndrome	Chromosome 22 deletion (region 22q11.2), affecting embryonic development of the thymus, parathyroid glands, and face	T cells decreased or normal B cells normal Immunoglobulins normal or decreased	Varies: Hypocalcemia, cardiac defects, abnormal facial features, and cognitive delay may be seen Patients with complete absence of the thymus (less than 1% of cases) develop life-threatening infections
Hyper-IgE syndromes (HIES)/ Job syndrome	Autosomal dominant inheritance of *STAT3* mutation; other HIES involve autosomal recessive inheritance of other genetic mutations	Very high IgE levels Decreased memory B cells and specific antibody responses Decreased T_H17 and T_{FH} cells Defective neutrophil chemotaxis	Recurrent eczema, skin abscesses, and lung infections; distinct facial features, bone fractures, dental abnormalities
Wiskott-Aldrich Syndrome (WAS)	X-linked inheritance; mutations in the Xp 11.22-23 locus	Progressive decrease in T-cell number and function Normal B-cell number Decreased IgM; IgA and IgE often elevated Decreased antigen-specific antibody responses and isohemagglutinins Increased serum alpha-fetoprotein Prolonged bleeding time Decreased NK-cell cytotoxicity Decreased neutrophil chemotaxis	Recurrent infections, thrombocytopenia and small platelet size, eczema Increased risk of developing autoimmunity and lymphomas

Table 19-3 Characteristics of Selected Forms of SCID

SCID TYPE	GENE DEFECT(S)	PHENOTYPE	OTHER COMMENTS
X-linked SCID	Interleukin-2 receptor gamma (*IL2RG*)	$T^-B^+NK^-$	Most common form of SCID *IL2RG* codes for the γ chain common to receptors for several interleukins, causing impaired lymphocyte maturation. B cells are normal or high in number, but their function is impaired, leading to reduced Ig production.
Adenosine deaminase (ADA) deficiency	*ADA*	$T^-B^-NK^-$	Deficiency of ADA enzyme leads to impaired metabolism of purines and accumulation of toxic metabolites that kill lymphocytes.
RAG deficiency	*RAG-1* or *RAG-2*	$T^-B^-NK^+$	Deficiency in recombinase activating enzymes is needed for TCR or Ig gene rearrangements during T- and B-cell maturation.
IL7R deficiency	*IL7R*	$T^-B^+NK^+$	Defect in receptor for IL-7, impairs signaling needed for T-cell development.
JAK3 deficiency	*JAK3*	$T^-B^+NK^-$	JAK3 codes for the enzyme Janus kinase 3, needed to transmit intracellular signals from IL-2 to induce lymphocyte proliferation and differentiation. Dysfunctional B cells lead to reduced Ig levels.

liver disease. They also have an increased risk of developing an autoimmune disease and cancer. Treatment involves Ig replacement therapy and antibiotics; HSC transplantation has been successful in restoring lymphocyte function in severe cases.

Ataxia-Telangiectasia (AT)

Ataxia-telangiectasia (AT) is a complex, autosomal recessive syndrome that affects the nervous system and the immune system. It is characterized by ataxia (poor muscle control) and telangiectasias (capillary swelling, resulting in red skin blotches). Blood vessels in the whites of the eyes may be dilated, and there may also be a reddish butterfly-shaped area on the face and ears. Progressive deterioration of the nervous system occurs, causing difficulties in speaking, swallowing, coughing, walking, and fine motor control.

Most patients have increased levels of serum α-fetoprotein. Patients have a combined defect of humoral and cellular immunity that results in increased susceptibility to infections, especially those of the lungs and sinuses. Antibody response to antigens, especially polysaccharides, is blunted. IgG2, IgA, and IgE levels are often low or absent, and IgM is increased, although the pattern can be quite variable. Patients also show a decrease in the number of circulating T cells over time.

Although the disease incidence is rare, as much as 1% of the population is heterozygous for the genetic mutation associated with the condition. Mutations in the *ATM* gene (chromosome 11, region q22) produce a defective kinase, an enzyme involved in DNA repair and in cell cycle control. Errors that occur during gene rearrangements may not be repaired properly, and the lymphocytes often have chromosomal breaks and other abnormalities involving the TCR genes in T cells and the Ig genes in B cells.

AT is also associated with a significant risk of lymphoid malignancy, presumably because the failure to repair damaged DNA leads to the accumulation of mutations. Ig replacement therapy may be given to patients with low Ig levels, but there is no cure for AT. Death usually occurs in early adult life from either pulmonary disease or malignancy, but treatments aimed at managing the symptoms are allowing some patients to live longer.

DiGeorge Syndrome (DGS)

DiGeorge syndrome (DGS), named after Angelo DiGeorge, who reported the condition in 1965, is a congenital disorder caused by abnormal development of the thymus and other tissues during embryonic development. DGS is estimated to occur in 1:4,000 to 1:6,000 live births. Ninety percent of the cases result from a sporadic microdeletion in chromosome 22, region q11.2, which codes for over 90 genes. The deletion can be detected by fluorescence in situ hybridization (FISH), comparative genomic hybridization (CGH) microarray, or other molecular techniques (see Chapter 12). The syndrome has also been known by several other names, including **22q11.2 deletion syndrome**, velocardiofacial syndrome, Shprintzen syndrome, and conotruncal anomaly face syndrome because of variations in the clinical features that may be seen.

The clinical features of DGS vary widely but most often involve the thymus, heart, parathyroid glands, and face. The cardiac defects often require surgical correction, and the parathyroid deficiency can be managed by calcium and vitamin D supplementation. Facial abnormalities include cleft palate, increased distance between the eyes and downward-slanting eyelids, small low-set ears and hearing loss, underdevelopment of the upper jawbones, and a short philtrum (groove between the nose and upper lip). Developmental delays in cognitive and motor function and behavioral problems may be seen, and patients are at increased risk of developing psychiatric disorders later in life.

Most patients have a smaller than normal thymus, resulting in low T-cell numbers; however, the T cells that are present are functionally normal. In less than 1% of patients, the thymus is completely absent. These patients are susceptible to developing life-threatening infections and require isolation precautions, antibiotics, Ig replacement, and human thymus tissue or HSC transplants; however, transplantation may be associated with complications, such as development of autoimmunity or GVHD. Although many patients with DGS live into adulthood, the prognosis varies, depending on the severity of the clinical abnormalities present.

Hyper-IgE Syndromes (HIES)

The hyper-IgE syndromes (HIES) are rare PIDs characterized by elevated serum IgE, increased eosinophils, eczema, recurrent skin abscesses caused by *Staphylococcus aureus*, and frequent lung infections. Mucocutaneous candidiasis is also common (see Chapter 22). The most common HIES is an autosomal dominant condition commonly known as **Job syndrome,** as its features resemble those of the biblical figure Job. Job syndrome is caused by genetic mutations in the *STAT3* gene, which codes for a key protein involved in the JAK-STAT pathway of signal transduction induced by several cytokines, hormones, and growth factors. Several autosomal recessive forms of HIES caused by mutations in other genes and having similar features have also been identified.

Job syndrome also involves connective tissue and skeletal abnormalities, causing characteristic facial features (a prominent chin and forehead, deep-set eyes, broad nose, thick skin, and high-arched palate), joint hyperextensibility, bone fractures, and retention of the primary teeth. In addition to high IgE levels, there is a decrease in antigen-specific antibody responses (e.g., to vaccine antigens), normal B-cell numbers but reduced memory B cells, decreased T_H17 and follicular helper T (Tfh) cells, and defective neutrophil chemotaxis. Treatment involves long-term use of antimicrobial drugs to prevent and promptly treat infections, incision and drainage of abscesses, skin care including topical steroid and moisturizing creams, and clinical management of bone and dental problems. With these measures, patients typically survive 50 years or longer.

Wiskott-Aldrich Syndrome (WAS)

Wiskott-Aldrich syndrome (WAS), described by Alfred Wiskott in 1937, is a rare X-linked recessive syndrome with an estimated incidence of 1:100,000 live male births. Over 300 mutations have been described in the *WAS* gene (Xp 11.22-23 locus) that codes for the WASp protein in blood cells other than RBCs. Defects in the protein result in abnormalities in the actin filaments of the cytoskeleton in WBCs and platelets, disrupting cell movement and intercellular cell signaling.

The classic, most severe form of WAS is defined by three main clinical features:

- Immunodeficiency, causing recurrent bacterial, viral, and fungal infections and failure to thrive
- Thrombocytopenia (decreased number of platelets) and small platelet size, causing increased bleeding tendency, especially bloody diarrhea
- Extensive eczema, an itchy skin rash

Patients also have an increased tendency to develop autoimmune disorders and lymphomas. Two milder variants have also been described: X-linked thrombocytopenia and X-linked neutropenia.

The laboratory features of WAS include a decreased platelet number and size, prolonged bleeding time, and a normal or increased number of megakaryocytes (platelet precursors) in the bone marrow. Abnormal immunologic findings include decreased T-cell numbers and function, defective antibody responses, especially to polysaccharide antigens, impaired NK-cell cytotoxicity, and reduced chemotaxis of phagocytic cells. In patients with classic WAS, B-cell numbers are usually normal, but there is a progressive decrease in T cells with time. Serum IgG is usually normal, but IgM is decreased, and IgA and IgE are often elevated. Patients have a severe deficiency of isohemagglutinins. Patients also have persistently increased levels of serum α-fetoprotein, which can be a useful diagnostic feature.

Treatment includes antimicrobial drugs, Ig replacement therapy, platelet transfusions and sometimes splenectomy to manage the thrombocytopenia and prevent bleeding, and topical steroids to relieve eczema. In the past, patients with classic WAS usually died in childhood because of infection, hemorrhage, or malignancy. More recently, treatment advances have improved quality of life and patient survival. HSC transplants, especially from an HLA-matched sibling in patients younger than 5 years old, have been successful in restoring lymphocyte and platelet function. Gene therapy using the patient's own bone marrow cells genetically modified to carry the *WAS* gene offers hope for a cure in the future.

Knowledge Check 19-3

Which statement about T-cell immunodeficiencies is true?

a. They only affect cell-mediated immune responses.
b. There is an increased number of $CD3^+$ cells.
c. They are caused by increased T_H cell activation.
d. They may involve nonimmunologic body systems.

Diseases of Immune Dysregulation

Recall from earlier chapters that the immune system must achieve an appropriate balance between activation and suppression so that it can destroy foreign invaders but not harm the body. Deficiencies in regulation of the immune response can result in not only recurrent infections but also a loss of immunologic tolerance (see Chapter 15), autoimmunity, excessive inflammation, high levels of lymphocyte proliferation, malignancy, and allergy. These disorders are classified in IUIS category 4; a few examples are listed here:

- The *autoimmune lymphoproliferative syndrome (ALPS)* is caused by mutations in genes involved in lymphocyte apoptosis (i.e., those coding for the cell surface molecule FAS, FAS-ligand, caspase 8, or caspase 10). These defects lead to production of autoantibodies against RBCs, platelets, and neutrophils and decreased numbers of those cells, and enlargement of the lymph nodes and spleen due to proliferation of autoreactive double-negative T cells.

- The *CD25 deficiency,* an autosomal recessive disorder caused by genetic mutations in the *IL2RA gene,* is characterized by a lack of Treg cells and impaired cytotoxic T (T_c) cell proliferation, leading to lymphoproliferation and autoimmunity.
- *Chédiak-Higashi syndrome* is a rare autosomal recessive PID caused by mutations in the *LYST* (CHS1/lysosomal trafficking regulator) gene, leading to defective transport of lysosomes in cells. Patients have enlarged lysosomal granules in all granule-containing cells, including granulocytes (as seen in a peripheral blood smear), platelets (causing bleeding problems), and melanocytes, causing hypopigmentation (loss of skin color). Decreased neutrophil number and chemotaxis, and NK-cell and T_c activity are seen. Some patients develop progressive neurological symptoms and/or hemophagocytic lymphohistiocytosis (HLH), a life-threatening condition caused by overactivation of lymphocytes and macrophages, excessive inflammation and cytokine production, and multiorgan failure.
- *IPEX syndrome,* named after its characteristics (immune dysregulation, polyendocrinopathy, enteropathy X-linked), is caused by X-linked recessive inheritance of a defective *FOXP3* gene. This gene codes for the forkhead box P3 (FOXP3) protein, a transcription factor needed for proper development and function of Treg cells. Patients have decreased Treg numbers and/or function and are susceptible to developing severe autoimmune conditions at a young age, especially type 1 diabetes, autoimmune enteropathy (of the intestinal linings), thyroiditis, hemolytic anemia, thrombocytopenia, and eczema. IgE and IgA are elevated.
- Several IEIs are caused by genetic mutations that trigger abnormal immune responses to EBV infections, including the *X-linked lymphoproliferative syndromes* (XLP1 [SAP deficiency] and XLP-2 [XIAP deficiency]). The most notable characteristic of these syndromes is uncontrolled lymphocyte proliferation in various organs that can lead to fulminant infectious mononucleosis, B-cell lymphomas, or HLH.

Treatment varies, depending on the disease, but may involve immunosuppressive biologic drugs or HSC transplantation along with symptom management.

Deficiencies in Innate Immunity

Deficiencies in innate immunity may involve phagocytic cells, NK cells, inflammatory cytokines, pattern recognition receptors (PRRs) such as the toll-like receptors (TLRs), or complement proteins. In general, phagocytic cell defects are associated with susceptibility to bacterial and fungal infections and immune dysregulation; PRR defects disrupt cell signaling, leading to viral, bacterial, or fungal infections; abnormal inflammatory cytokine production can result in autoinflammatory syndromes; and complement deficiencies can cause bacterial infections and autoimmunity. In this section, we discuss examples of diseases involving phagocytic cells, innate cytokines, and PRRs. The characteristics of some of these diseases are summarized in **Table 19–4.** For a discussion of complement deficiencies, see Chapter 7.

Table 19–4 Characteristics of Selected Deficiencies in Innate Immunity

DISEASE	DEFECT	LABORATORY FINDINGS	CLINICAL PRESENTATION
Chronic granulomatous disease (IUIS category 5)	X-linked recessive inheritance of an abnormal *CYBB* gene that codes for a component of the NADPH oxidase enzyme complex (NOX) accounts for 70% of cases; the rest involve autosomal recessive inheritance of other NOX components	Decreased generation of ROS (H_2O_2 and O_2^-) in neutrophils and monocytes, causing a decreased DHR test result	Recurrent infections, especially with catalase-positive bacteria; inflammatory bowel disease; granuloma development
Leukocyte deficiency syndrome I (LADI; IUIS category 5)	Autosomal recessive inheritance of the *ITGB2* gene, which codes for CD18, an adhesion molecule subunit of CD11a, CD11b, and CD11c	Decreased CD18 and CD11 on WBCs by flow cytometry	Delayed umbilical cord separation; delayed wound healing; chronic skin, intestinal, and respiratory tract infections; periodontitis
Chronic mucocutaneous candidiasis (IUIS category 6)	Autosomal recessive or dominant inheritance of variations in genes coding for IL-17 and its receptors or other genes that code for molecules needed for development of T_H17 cells or cell responses to IL-17	Selective inability of T cells to respond to *Candida* antigens in vitro or by delayed-type hypersensitivity skin testing	Persistent *Candida* infections of the mucous membranes (e.g., oral thrush), skin, scalp, and nails; increased susceptibility to autoimmune endocrine disorders

DHR = dihydrorhodamine; H_2O_2 = hydrogen peroxide; NADPH = nicotinamide adenine dinucleotide phosphate; O_2^- = superoxide anion; ROS = reactive oxygen species.

Phagocytic Cell Deficiencies

Phagocytic cell deficiencies can result from decreased phagocyte numbers, function, or both, and are classified in IUIS category 5. Neutrophils are the most affected, as they constitute the majority of the phagocytes. To destroy invading organisms, neutrophils must adhere to vascular endothelial cells in the blood vessels, migrate through the capillary wall to a site of infection, and ingest and kill the microbes (see Chapter 2); deficiency disorders may affect any of these steps. In general, patients experience bacterial and fungal infections of the skin, respiratory tract, and lymph nodes early in life; the infections can range from mild to life threatening (e.g., bacterial sepsis). In this section, we describe two conditions of phagocyte dysfunction.

Chronic Granulomatous Disease (CGD)

Chronic granulomatous disease (CGD) is a group of disorders in which the neutrophils are incapable of generating an oxidative burst, the process by which neutrophils make reactive oxygen species (ROS) such as hydrogen peroxide (H_2O_2) and superoxide anion (O_2^-), which have microbiocidal effects (see Chapter 2). This occurs because of a defect in nicotinamide adenine dinucleotide phosphate (NADPH) oxidase (NOX), an enzyme complex central to ROS generation. Scientists have discovered mutations in six different genes that code for NOX subunits. About 70% of CGD cases are due to a mutation in the gene that codes for the β subunit of the cytochrome b gene (*CYBB*) and are inherited by an X-linked recessive mode. The remaining cases, which are autosomal recessive, are caused by mutations in genes that code for other NOX components.

Infections in CGD usually begin in the first year of life, initially involving the skin, lungs, GI tract, and lymph nodes that drain those organs; they may then spread to other organs such as the liver, spleen, kidneys, bones, and brain. Patients are especially susceptible to catalase-positive bacteria such as *Staphylococcus aureus, Burkholderia cepacia, Chromobacterium violaceum,* and *Serratia marcescens,* and to fungi such as *Aspergillus* and *Nocardia,* which are also catalase positive. Catalase is an enzyme that inactivates H_2O_2, allowing the organisms to survive in the presence of H_2O_2 possibly made by CGD patients (albeit in reduced amounts) or by the microbes themselves. Some patients develop chronic inflammatory bowel disease and perianal disease and form granulomas that can obstruct the respiratory, GI, or genitourinary tracts. While the clinical presentation of CGD varies, the X-linked form tends to be more severe.

CGD was historically diagnosed by measuring the ability of a patient's neutrophils to reduce the yellow dye nitroblue tetrazolium (NBT) to a deep blue product called formazan, which could be detected microscopically in a peripheral blood smear. Today, a more objective, quantitative flow cytometric assay is more commonly used. In this assay, neutrophils are labeled with dihydrorhodamine (DHR), a dye that fluoresces when it is reduced. The neutrophils are then activated using phorbol myristate acetate (PMA), which is mitogenic for neutrophils. The resultant oxidative burst reduces the DHR, producing fluorescence that can be quantitated by flow cytometry. Neutrophils from patients with CGD are unable to undergo the oxidative burst and thus show less fluorescence than normal neutrophils.

Patients with CGD are given antibiotics and antifungal drugs to treat and prevent infections. Administration of cytokines, such as interferon gamma, may increase the oxidative burst activity in some patients. HSC transplantation may result in a permanent cure, and success rates are highest in young, disease-free patients. These treatments, along with prompt detection and infection management, are allowing patients to live well into adulthood (40 years and more). Clinical trials using gene therapy offer added hope for the future.

Leukocyte Adhesion Deficiency (LAD) Syndromes

The leukocyte adhesion deficiency (LAD) syndromes are rare PIDs characterized by a deficiency in WBC adhesion proteins that enable the WBCs to adhere to the endothelial lining of the blood vessels during an inflammatory response. As a result, the WBCs fail to leave the vasculature and migrate to a site of emerging infection, and peripheral blood WBC and neutrophil numbers are increased.

The LAD syndromes have been classified into three types based on their genetics and clinical symptoms. LADI is caused by mutations in the integrin beta-2 gene (*ITGB2*) that codes for CD18, a subunit of the adhesion molecules CD11a, CD11b, and CD11c on neutrophils, monocytes, and lymphocytes. LAD II is characterized by a deficiency in carbohydrate molecules involved in adhesive interactions (e.g., sialyl-Lewis X [CD15a] and H [Bombay] antigen caused by mutations in the *SLC35C1* gene, which affects transport of the sugar fucose to the Golgi apparatus). In LAD III, genetic mutations in the *FERMT3* gene result in defective activation of the β-integrins on WBCs.

LADI, the most common of the LADs, is transmitted through autosomal recessive inheritance and has variable severity, depending on the amount of CD18 expression. Its clinical manifestations begin shortly after birth and include delayed umbilical cord separation, absent pus formation and delayed wound healing, chronic skin infections, intestinal and respiratory tract infections, and periodontitis. Diagnosis is confirmed by genetic testing and demonstration of decreased CD11/18 antigen on patient WBCs by flow cytometry. Antibiotic administration is essential in treating and preventing infections in these patients. HSC transplantation is the only corrective therapy for severe cases of LADI; if it is not performed, such patients usually die in infancy.

Other Defects of Innate Immunity

The IUIS has classified deficiencies in components of innate immunity other than phagocytes and complement in category 6. These diseases include defects in cytokines and their receptors, signaling molecules, and TLR molecules, and they are subdivided according to the types of infections they are most likely to predispose patients to. For example, mutations in genes coding for IL-12 and the IL-23 receptor predispose patients to mycobacterial disease; genetic mutations causing defects in the signaling molecules STAT1, STAT2, and IRF7 lead to decreased interferon production and predispose patients to severe viral infections; and genetic abnormalities associated with TLR molecules (e.g., TLR3 deficiency) or TLR signaling pathways (e.g., MyD88, IRAK1, and TLR7) result in increased susceptibility to bacterial infections. Diagnosing these entities is based on clinical presentation, which leads to molecular analyses to identify specific genetic mutations.

Another condition in this category, **chronic mucocutaneous candidiasis (CMC),** has been associated with different genetic mutations, including those affecting IL-17 and its receptors, and STAT1, a signaling molecule important to the development of IL-17–producing T cells. In CMC, immune responses to *Candida* and related fungi are impaired (as can be demonstrated by a selective inability of T cells to respond to *Candida* antigens by proliferation in vitro or in delayed-type hypersensitivity skin testing), but other immune responses are normal. As a result, patients have persistent *Candida* infections involving the mucous membranes, skin, scalp, and nails. Oral thrush is common and presents soon after birth. Autoimmune conditions, mostly involving the endocrine glands, may also develop. Life expectancy is usually normal, but lifelong treatment with antifungal drugs is required to manage the infections.

Knowledge Check 19-4

DHR reduction is a specialized laboratory test that measures:

a. Phagocytosis
b. NADPH oxidase activity
c. Chemotaxis
d. Leukocyte adhesion

Autoinflammatory Disorders

Autoinflammatory disorders, classified by the IUIS in category 7, develop as a result of inappropriate activation of antigen-independent inflammatory responses. Patients with these conditions present with recurrent fevers and systemic inflammation involving multiple organs, including the skin, joints, serosal membranes lining the abdominal and chest cavities, GI tract, and central nervous system (CNS). Specific symptoms, treatment, and prognosis vary with the disease. The disorders are grouped according to whether they have abnormalities in interferon production and signaling, involve the inflammasome, or have other defects not involving the inflammasome.

Type I interferonopathies are a diverse group of disorders involving mutations in various genes that cause excessive production of type I interferons (IFN-α and IFN-β). The resulting inflammatory symptoms often mimic those of autoimmune diseases like SLE. Inflammatory markers such as C-reactive protein (CRP) are often elevated, and autoantibodies are commonly produced; thus, gene sequencing is important in making an accurate diagnosis.

Inflammasomes are complexes that contain caspase enzymes and other proteins involved in inflammation and cell death. They are found in many innate cell types (e.g., macrophages, dendritic cells, neutrophils, and epithelial cells). Once inflammasomes are activated by microbial substances or cellular stress, they stimulate the production of the proinflammatory cytokines IL-1 and IL-18. Genetic defects involving the inflammasome include the following:

- *Familial Mediterranean fever*, an autosomal recessive or autosomal dominant disorder caused by mutations in the *MEFV* gene, which result in abnormal activation of the pyrin inflammasome
- *Muckle-Wells syndrome*, an autosomal dominant disorder caused by mutations in the *NLRP3* gene, resulting in abnormal activation of the cryopyrin inflammasome

Examples of autoinflammatory disorders that do not involve the inflammasome include the following:

- *Tumor necrosis factor (TNF) receptor-associated periodic syndrome (TRAPS),* an autosomal dominant or sporadic disorder caused by mutations in the *TNFRSF1A* gene that codes for a TNF receptor, resulting in decreased binding of the cytokine, TNF-α
- *ADAM17* deficiency, an autosomal recessive disorder caused by mutations in the *ADAM17* gene, resulting in decreased TNF-α production

Primary Immunodeficiencies Involving Bone Marrow Failure

Deficiencies resulting from failure of the bone marrow to generate hematopoietic stem cells can either be inherited or acquired as a result of various factors, including exposure to chemotherapy or radiation for cancer treatment, toxic chemicals, and autoimmune responses; the acquired disorders may also have no known cause. Inherited immunodeficiencies of bone marrow failure (IUIS category 9) are a group of rare disorders involving genetic mutations that affect hematopoietic lineage pathways. As a result, there is a decrease in RBCs (anemia), platelets (thrombocytopenia), and WBCs (leukopenia). Thus, common symptoms are fatigue and pallor, bleeding, and susceptibility to infections and malignancies. Features characteristic of each syndrome but unrelated to the bone marrow are often also seen.

The most common of the inherited bone marrow deficiencies is *Fanconi anemia,* a group of rare disorders caused by genetic mutations in one of 22 genes (*FANCA* to *FANCW*) involved in repair of damaged DNA; most cases are autosomal recessive. The genetic instability leads to dysregulation of the cell cycle and cell death. Patients have various physical abnormalities, progressive bone marrow failure, and increased risk for certain cancers, including acute myeloid leukemia and squamous cell carcinomas of the head and neck, GI tract, or gynecologic organs. Diagnosis is based on clinical evaluation, hematologic findings, cytogenetic analysis, and NGS for the specific gene mutations. Supportive treatments for patient symptoms are provided, and HSC transplant can provide a cure. However, complications related to transplantation and other features of Fanconi anemia arise, and many children with the disease die before the age of 10.

Knowledge Check 19-5

Match each disease listed with its major characteristic:

a. Bruton tyrosine kinase deficiency	___	1. Delayed development of antibody production
b. Common variable immunodeficiency	___	2. Defective HSC generation from bone marrow
c. Transient hypogammaglobulinemia of infancy	___	3. Giant lysosomal granules
d. Severe combined immunodeficiency	___	4. Selective defect in T-cell responses to *Candida* antigens
e. Ataxia-telangiectasia	___	5. Abnormal inflammasome activation
f. DiGeorge syndrome	___	6. X-linked disorder caused by lack of mature B cells
g. Wiskott-Aldrich syndrome	___	7. Lack of mature T cells and possibly NK and/or B cells
h. Chédiak-Higashi syndrome	___	8. Defective development of thymus, parathyroid glands, heart, and facial features
i. Autoimmune lymphoproliferative syndrome	___	9. Defect in neutrophil NADPH oxidase
j. Chronic granulomatous disease	___	10. Recurrent infections, thrombocytopenia, eczema
k. Chronic mucocutaneous candidiasis	___	11. Defect in lymphocyte apoptosis
l. Familial Mediterranean fever	___	12. Decreased antibody production usually appearing in adulthood
m. Fanconi anemia	___	13. Progressive decrease in T-cell function, neurological deterioration, capillary swelling

Phenocopies of Primary Immunodeficiencies

Phenocopies of primary immunodeficiencies (IUIS category 10), unlike PIDs, are not caused by caused by germline mutations; rather, they are the result of somatic mutations (genetic alterations that occur in body cells after fertilization) or autoantibodies directed against cytokines. These abnormalities cause clinical manifestations that are similar to diseases in other IUIS categories. Two examples, which we previously mentioned, are *autoimmune lymphoproliferative syndrome* (ALPS; also included in category 4), which, in some patients, is caused by somatic mutations in the *TNFRSF6I* gene, and *chronic mucocutaneous candidiasis* (CMC; also included in category 6), which can also be caused by autoantibodies to IL-17 and/or IL-22. Other examples, which were discussed in Chapter 7, are *acquired angioedema,* caused by autoantibodies to the C1 inhibitor of complement, and *atypical hemolytic uremic syndrome,* caused by autoantibodies to factor H; both conditions are also included in IUIS category 8.

Knowledge Check 19-6

Phenocopies of primary immunodeficiencies differ from the other IEIs in that they are:

a. Not hereditary
b. Caused by a mutation in a single gene
c. Caused by increased activation of Tregs
d. Defects in nonimmunologic body systems

Laboratory Evaluation of Immune Dysfunction

The evaluation of possible immunodeficiency starts with a patient history to assess clinical manifestations, followed by a complete blood count (CBC) with a WBC differential, and a complete metabolic panel. If reduced numbers of hematopoietic cells are seen in the CBC, additional tests are performed to determine the numbers and functional capabilities of the individual cell populations. In the sections that follow, we discuss various laboratory tests used in the diagnosis of immunodeficiencies. **Table 19–5** lists laboratory tests commonly used to evaluate different components of the immune response. When performing some of these tests, it is important for laboratorians to compare the patient results with age-matched reference ranges, as the values can change with age. In some cases, evaluation of hematopoietic cells in a bone marrow biopsy may also be performed.

Laboratory Tests for Evaluation of B-Cell Function and Numbers

Assessment of B-cell function begins with measurement of serum IgG, IgM, IgA, and IgG subclass levels by automated nephelometric or immunoturbidometric methods to screen for defects in antibody production; it may also be performed by radial immunodiffusion (RID; see Chapter 10). Decreased Ig levels are also evident in serum protein electrophoresis (SPE; γ and/or β regions) and immunofixation electrophoresis (IFE). A lack of bands indicates a deficiency in one or more Ig classes (see Case Study 2 later). SPE can also be quantitative if the total serum protein is determined, and the results are read using a densitometer.

When interpreting quantitative Ig results, it is important to remember that Ig levels vary with age. The serum

Table 19–5 Laboratory Tests for Immunodeficiencies

COMPONENT ASSESSED	LABORATORY TESTS
All WBCs	CBC count, WBC differential
B cells	Serum IgG, IgA, IgM levels; IgG subclass levels Isohemagglutinin titers (IgM) IgG antibody response to protein and polysaccharide antigens Flow cytometry for B-cell markers (e.g., CD19, CD20, CD21)
T cells	Flow cytometry for T-cell markers (e.g., CD3, CD4, CD8) TREC newborn screening Lymphocyte activation assays (mitogen; interferon gamma release) Delayed hypersensitivity skin tests (e.g., *Candida*, diphtheria, tetanus)
NK cells	Flow cytometry for NK-cell markers (e.g., CD56, CD16) NK-cell cytotoxicity assays
Neutrophils	Peripheral blood smear Flow cytometry for neutrophil markers (e.g., CD15, CD18) DHR reduction test
Complement	Assays of complement function (e.g., CH50 for the classical pathway) Serum complement protein levels (e.g., C3, C4)

CBC = complete blood cell; DHR = dihydrorhodamine; Ig = immunoglobulin; NK = natural killer; TREC = T-cell receptor excision circles; WBC = white blood cell.

level of IgG at birth is about the same as the adult level, reflecting transfer of maternal IgG across the placenta; it then declines during the first 6 months of life, as maternal antibody is catabolized. IgA and IgM levels are very low at birth. All Ig concentrations gradually rise when the infant begins to produce antibodies at a few months of age in response to environmental antigens. IgM reaches normal adult levels first, around 1 year of age, followed by IgG at about 5 to 6 years of age. In some children, IgA levels do not reach normal adult values until adolescence. Therefore, it is important to compare a child's Ig levels to age-matched reference ranges.

If Ig levels are low but detectable, additional tests can be performed to determine if antibody responses to specific antigens are functional. Testing for isohemagglutinins can be performed by the transfusion service. By the age of 2, a child should have naturally occurring IgM antibodies against ABO blood group antigens. Absence of these antibodies suggests an abnormal IgM response. Antibody responses to vaccine or other antigens to which the population is commonly exposed can also be measured. This can be done by measuring specific antibody titers to routine childhood vaccines. In unimmunized children, the development of tetanus or diphtheria antibodies can be determined 2 weeks after immunization. In a previously immunized patient, the response to a booster injection can be evaluated at 4 to 8 weeks postvaccination. Antibody responses to other protein and polysaccharide antigens can also be determined to evaluate a possible IgG subclass deficiency. Recall that IgG1 and IgG3 respond best to protein antigens, whereas IgG2 responds best to polysaccharide antigens.

Direct immunofluorescence assays involving incubation of the patient's peripheral blood cells with monoclonal antibodies to B-cell antigens and analysis by flow cytometry are performed to enumerate the B cells as part of an immunophenotyping panel (see Chapter 13). Recall that CD19, CD20, and CD21 are found on mature B cells, CD38 is found mainly on plasma cells, and various marker combinations can be used to determine the numbers of B cells in different developmental stages. Patient results must be compared with age-matched reference ranges. An absence of $CD19^+$ B cells suggests a Btk deficiency. However, secondary immunodeficiencies are more common than PIDs. For example, a common cause of absent B cells in adults is treatment with rituximab, a monoclonal anti-CD20 antibody used to treat patients with certain autoimmune diseases (see Chapter 15). The antibody destroys B cells, resulting in no detectable $CD19^+$ or $CD20^+$ cells, as seen in **Figure 19–2**, a flow cytometry histogram from a patient treated with rituximab.

Clinical Correlations

Isohemagglutinins

Isohemagglutinins are antibodies, mainly of the IgM class, produced by individuals against antigens of the ABO system that they do not possess. People who are blood type A lack the B antigen on their RBCs and normally have anti-B antibodies in their serum. Likewise, type B individuals lack the A antigen and normally have anti-A in their serum. Type O persons lack both the A and B antigens and therefore produce both anti-A and anti-B. Isohemagglutinins are present in the serum of newborns and are commonly tested for when looking for a humoral immunodeficiency. Their origin is unclear, but they may be produced spontaneously by a subset of B lymphocytes (thus, they have been called natural antibodies) and/or by adaptive immune responses to cross-reacting bacterial or food antigens.

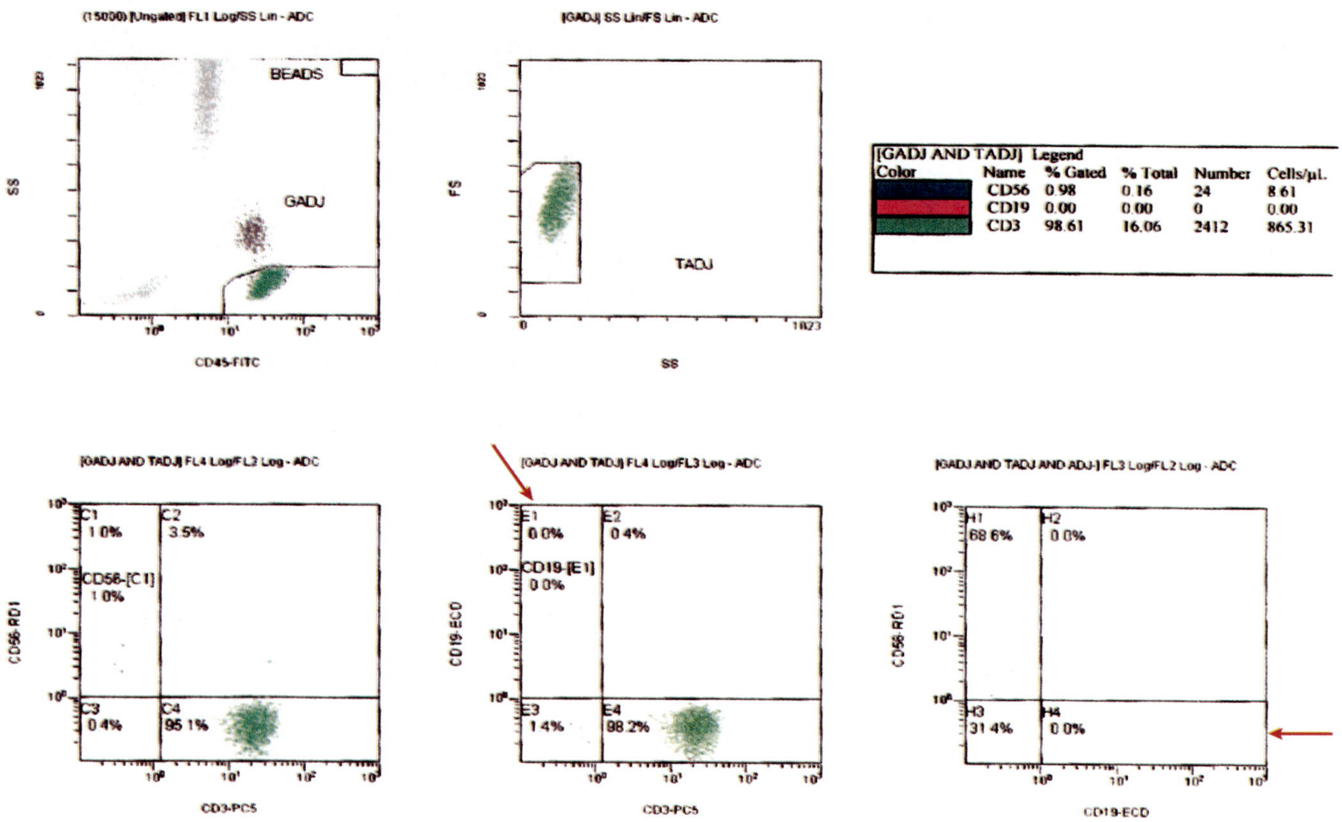

FIGURE 19–2 Flow cytometry histogram of peripheral blood stained with antibodies to CD3, CD19, and CD56. No $CD19^+$ cells are detected in this patient sample, as indicated by the red arrows. *(Courtesy of Dr. Thomas Alexander.)*

Tests for Evaluation of T-Cell Numbers and Function

Direct immunofluorescence and flow cytometry are routinely used to determine the total T-cell number by detecting CD3 and T-cell subsets ($CD3^+CD4^+$ T_H cells and $CD3^+CD8^+$ T_c cells). Patient values are compared to age-matched reference ranges.

Also, all states in the United States determine T-cell numbers by another method as part of their newborn screening programs. In this system, **T-cell receptor (TCR) excision circles (TRECs)** are detected in newborn blood by quantitative polymerase chain reaction (PCR) (**Fig. 19–3**; see also Chapter 12). Recall from Chapter 5 that the TCR for antigen contains an α chain and a β chain. During T-cell maturation, rearrangement of specific V and J genes coding for the variable region of the α chain and specific V, D, and J genes coding for the variable region of the β chain occur to produce a TCR that is antigen specific. In the process, the intervening sequences are removed and joined at their ends to form circular by-products called *TRECs*. The absence or a severely low number of TRECs indicates a lack of functional T cells, allowing early identification of T-cell–related deficiencies, most notably, SCID.

Specialized tests may also be performed to assess T-cell function. For example, proliferation of peripheral blood T cells from a patient after stimulation with an antigen or T-cell mitogens can be measured in culture. A **mitogen** is a substance that stimulates mitosis in all T cells or all B cells, regardless of antigen specificity. Examples of commonly used T-cell mitogens are phytohemagglutinin (PHA) and concanavalin A (Con A). Following incubation with the mitogen, the T-cell response is measured by quantitating the uptake of radioactive thymidine, a nucleoside incorporated into DNA. Increased thymidine uptake suggests cell division and activation; decreased thymidine uptake is seen in patients with functional T-cell defects, as compared to thymidine uptake by normal control cells tested simultaneously. This assay requires experienced technologists, a radioactive materials license, and laboratory-determined reference ranges.

Another test, the Cylex ImmuKnow assay, measures intracellular adenosine triphosphate (ATP) production in patient CD4 T cells stimulated by PHA. This test is most often used to monitor organ transplant patients receiving immunosuppressive therapy. An individual's response to *Mycobacterium tuberculosis* antigens can be measured by the QuantiFERON-TB Gold Plus assay or the T-SPOT assay (see Chapter 14).

Finally, as we also discussed in Chapter 14, delayed-type hypersensitivity skin testing can be performed by clinicians to assess the cell-mediated immune response to common environmental or vaccine antigens, such as *Candida*, mumps, or tetanus toxoid. Failure to develop a reaction of redness and

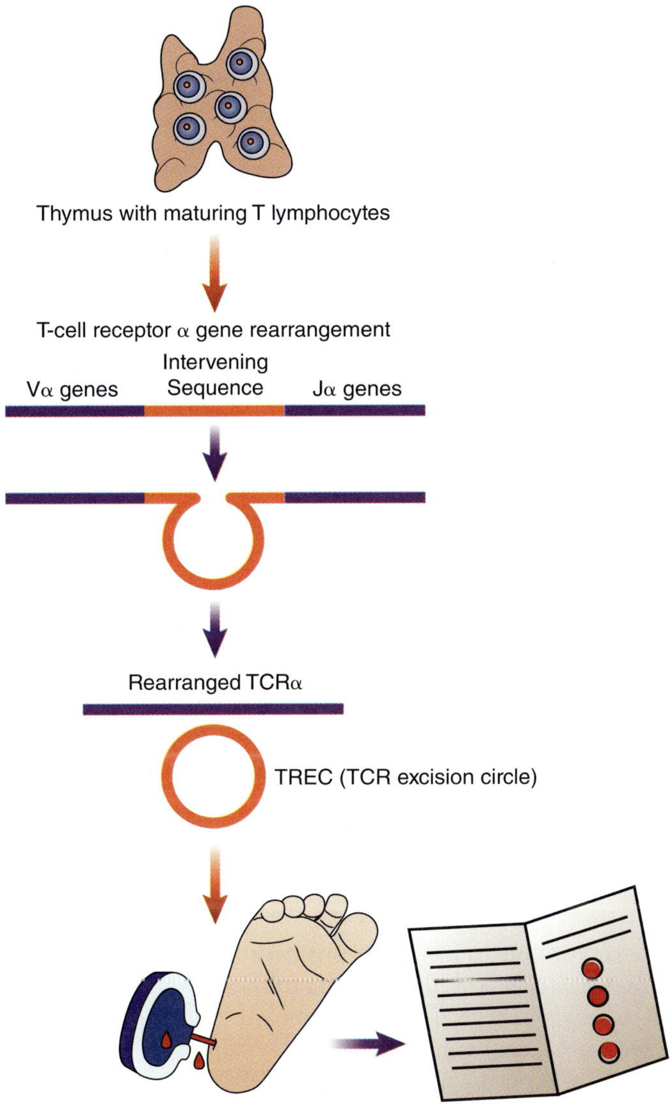

FIGURE 19–3 Newborn testing for T-cell receptor excision circles (TRECs) formed by normal T-cell receptor gene rearrangements.

induration at the injection sites within 48 to 72 hours suggests a T-cell deficiency. Importantly, skin testing should not be performed in infants or very young children, as lack of previous exposure to these antigens can also result in a negative reaction.

Laboratory Assessment of Innate Immunity

Laboratory tests to evaluate the various components of innate immunity include those for complement, phagocytic cells, NK cells, and TLRs. As we discussed in Chapter 7, screening for complement deficiencies usually begins with assays that detect functional abnormalities in the complement pathways (e.g., CH50). Low functional activity may indicate a deficiency in a specific component of the classical (and possibly an alternative) pathway of complement and can be followed by automated nephelometric or immunoturbidimetric assays to measure individual complement proteins. The laboratorian should be aware, however, that low CH50 levels may be caused by complement consumption and do not, by themselves, indicate a hereditary complement deficiency. If phenocopies of IEI involving complement are suspected, tests for complement autoantibodies may also be performed.

Various tests can be done to evaluate phagocytic cell number and functions. To determine absolute neutrophil and monocyte numbers in peripheral blood, a CBC and differential can be performed; neutrophils are considered to be decreased if their absolute number is less than 1 to 1.5 × 10^9/L, and severe neutropenia is present if the number is less than 0.5 × 10^9/L. A peripheral blood smear can be used to detect abnormal cell morphology, such as the giant lysosomal granules characteristic of the Chédiak-Higashi syndrome. In CGD, defects in neutrophil oxidative burst activity may be detected by the DHR test. Flow cytometry can be used to confirm a diagnosis of LADI, characterized by decreased WBC expression of CD18 and CD11, and LADII, in which CD15 is absent. Although difficult to perform, in some cases, specialized tests for chemotaxis may be done to evaluate neutrophil defects such as LAD, Chédiak-Higashi syndrome, and WAS.

NK-cell numbers can be determined by flow cytometry; mature NK cells have dim CD56 expression and are positive for CD16, whereas immature NK cells are brightly positive for CD56. Specialized assays that measure NK-cell cytotoxicity may also be performed. TLR defects can be assessed by stimulating peripheral blood mononuclear cells with TLR-specific ligands (see Chapter 2) in vitro and then measuring the cytokines released by enzyme-linked immunosorbent assay (ELISA) or microbead immunoassays, although these tests are not available for routine laboratory testing.

Knowledge Check 19-7

Which laboratory test is used to enumerate B cells?

a. Nephelometry
b. CBC and differential
c. Flow cytometry analysis of $CD19^+$ cells
d. Immunofixation electrophoresis

Family History and Genetic Testing

It is very important to obtain a complete family history as part of the IEI diagnosis process. The mode of inheritance, if known, can rule in or rule out many of the IEIs. Genetic testing provides the ultimate confirmation of an IEI diagnosis and helps to determine the appropriate therapy for individual patients. Testing typically begins with panel-based NGS to examine a set of preselected genes that may be associated with the suspected condition. If large deletions or duplications are observed, copy number variation (CNV) assays, commonly comparative genomic hybridization (CGH) or single nucleotide polymorphism (SNP) microarrays, can be performed to confirm the results (see Chapter 12). While panel-based NGS is cost effective, it fails to detect genetic variants not included in the test. In these cases, more expensive whole exome sequencing (sequencing of the coding regions of all the human genes) or whole genome sequencing (sequencing of all coding and noncoding regions in the human genome) may be required to detect the mutation.

Genetic testing of family members of affected patients can help identify individuals who may be at risk of developing the disease or passing it on to their offspring. Thus, a team approach among the family, clinicians, medical geneticists, and laboratory is required to make an accurate diagnosis.

Critical Thinking 19-2

A patient with *Candida* infections of the skin and mouth was given antifungal treatments, but the infections kept returning. Genetic testing for hereditary immunodeficiency was negative. What are possible reasons for this result?

KEY CONCEPTS

- Immunodeficiencies are disorders in which part of the body's immune system is missing or dysfunctional. There are two types of immunodeficiencies: primary (i.e., inherited) and secondary (acquired because of other factors, such as infections, malignancies, or immunosuppressive drugs).
- Immune system deficiencies can affect the humoral and/or cell-mediated branches of the adaptive immune system, or various components of the innate defense system (e.g., phagocytic cells, complement).

Inborn Errors of Immunity

- The International Union of Immunological Societies (IUIS) has classified the primary immunodeficiencies into 10 categories based on their clinical features, immunologic defects, and genetic abnormalities.

B-Cell/Antibody Deficiencies

- B-cell deficiencies (IUIS category 3), or agammaglobulinemias, are characterized by decreased or undetectable Ig levels. Decreases may occur in all Ig classes or in a single Ig class or subclass.
- Reduced Ig typically leads to recurrent infections with pyogenic bacteria, particularly of the respiratory and intestinal tracts, usually beginning at about 6 months of age when maternal antibodies have waned.
- Patients are typically treated with antibiotics and Ig replacement therapy.
- Transient hypogammaglobulinemia of infancy, Bruton tyrosine kinase (Btk) deficiency, common variable immunodeficiency, selective IgA deficiency, and isolated IgG subclass deficiencies are examples of diseases in which there is mainly a B-cell defect and decreased antibody production.

T-Cell Defects and Combined Immunodeficiencies

- Deficiencies in T-cell number or function also affect other aspects of immunity, notably antibody and cytokine production; thus, they are referred to as combined immunodeficiencies. Some of these diseases also involve parts of the body that are not part of the immune system.
- Defects in T-cell–mediated immunity generally lead to recurrent infections with intracellular pathogens, such as viruses, fungi, and intracellular bacteria.
- Treatment of T-cell/combined immunodeficiencies often involves HSC transplantation, preferably from an HLA-matched donor to prevent GVHD.
- The combined immunodeficiencies (IUIS category 1) include several forms of severe combined immunodeficiency disease (SCID) and CD40L deficiency.
- The combined immunodeficiencies with syndromic features (IUIS category 2) include ataxia-telangiectasia, DiGeorge syndrome, hyper-IgE syndromes, and Wiskott-Aldrich syndrome.

Diseases of Immune Dysregulation

- Diseases of immune dysregulation (IUIS category 4) are caused by defects in Treg cells or other regulatory components and result in autoimmunity, excessive inflammation, high levels of lymphocyte proliferation, and increased risk of malignancy and allergy.
- Diseases in this category include ALPS, CD25 deficiency, IPEX syndrome, Chédiak-Higashi syndrome, and X-linked lymphoproliferative syndromes.
- Treatment may involve immunosuppressive drugs or HSC transplantation.

Deficiencies in Innate Immunity

- Deficiencies in innate immunity may involve phagocytic cells, NK cells, inflammatory cytokines, TLRs, or complement proteins.
- Defects in phagocyte numbers and/or function (IUIS category 5) generally lead to pyogenic bacterial infections, often of the skin. Immunodeficiency states range from mild to lethal and include chronic granulomatous disease (CGD) and leukocyte adhesion deficiency (LAD) syndromes.
- Complement deficiencies (IUIS category 8) result from mutations in genes coding for individual complement proteins (including regulatory proteins). These deficiencies typically result in recurrent bacterial infections or autoimmunity.
- Other defects in innate immunity (IUIS category 6) include defects in cytokines or their receptors (e.g., chronic mucocutaneous candidiasis), signaling molecules, and TLRs.

Autoinflammatory Disorders

- Autoinflammatory disorders (IUIS category 7) are caused by inappropriate activation of innate immunity, resulting in recurrent fevers and systemic inflammation.
- Diseases in this category include the type I interferonopathies, inflammasome-mediated diseases (e.g., familial Mediterranean fever, Muckle-Wells syndrome), TRAPS, and ADAM17 deficiency.

Primary Immunodeficiencies Involving Bone Marrow Failure

- Bone marrow defects result in failure to generate sufficient HSCs, producing anemia, thrombocytopenia, and leukopenia.
- They can be inherited (IUIS category 9; e.g., Fanconi anemia) or acquired after exposure to chemotherapy, radiation, toxic chemicals, or other factors.

Phenocopies of Primary Immunodeficiencies

- Phenocopies of primary immunodeficiencies (IUIS category 10) are caused by somatic mutations or autoantibodies, rather than hereditary mutations.
- Diseases in this category include ALPS, chronic mucocutaneous candidiasis, acquired angioedema, and atypical hemolytic uremic syndrome.

Laboratory Evaluation of Immune Dysfunction

- Evaluation of immunodeficiencies begins with a patient history, CBC and WBC differential, and complete metabolic panel.
- B-cell numbers are determined by flow cytometry for B-cell markers (e.g., CD19). B-cell function is assessed by serum Ig levels, isohemagglutinin titers, and antibody responses to specific antigens.
- T-cell numbers are determined by flow cytometry for T-cell markers (e.g., CD3, CD4, CD8). Tests for T-cell function include T-cell mitogen assays (e.g., PHA), interferon gamma release assays, and delayed-type hypersensitivity skin tests.
- Newborn screening for deficiencies in T-cell number (e.g., SCID) involves detection of TRECs, T-cell receptor excision circles that have been removed during normal TCR gene rearrangements that occur during T-cell development.
- NK-cell numbers are determined by flow cytometry for NK-cell markers (e.g., CD16, CD56). NK-cell function can be assessed using cytotoxicity assays.
- Neutrophils are assessed on a peripheral blood smear, by flow cytometry for neutrophil markers (e.g., CD15, CD18), and functional assays such as the DHR reduction test, which evaluates NADPH oxidase activity.
- Evaluation of complement involves assays for complement function (e.g., CH50) and quantitation of individual serum complement proteins by automated nephelometry or immunoturbidimetry.

Study Guide: Inborn Errors of Immunity

IUIS CATEGORY	DESCRIPTION	DISEASE EXAMPLES
1. Combined Immunodeficiencies	Low to absent humoral and cell-mediated immunity due to T cell deficiencies	SCID (common gamma chain deficiency, *JAK3* deficiency, ADA deficiency) CD40L deficiency
2. Combined immunodeficiencies with syndromic features	T cell defects with low to absent humoral and cell-mediated immunity and additional, non-immunologic abnormalities	Ataxia-telangiectasia, DiGeorge syndrome, Hyper IgE syndromes, Wiskott-Aldrich syndrome
3. Predominantly antibody deficiencies	One or more immunoglobulin classes are decreased	Bruton's thymidine kinase (Btk) deficiency, transient hypogammaglobulinemia of infancy, common variable immunodeficiency, selective IgA deficiency, IgG subclass deficiencies
4. Diseases of immune dysregulation	Loss of T regulatory or other immune controlling mechanisms	Chediak-Higashi syndrome, autoimmune lymphoproliferative syndrome (ALPS), CD25 deficiency, IPEX Syndrome
5. Congenital defects of phagocytes	Reduction in phagocytic function, number, or both	Chronic granulomatous disease, leukocyte adhesion deficiency (LAD)
6. Defects in intrinsic and innate immunity	Interruption in signaling pathways of innate immune cells	Chronic mucocutaneous candidiasis, TLR3 deficiency, IRAK1 deficiency
7. Autoinflammatory disorders	Diseases usually associated with recurrent fevers and systemic inflammation	Type I interferonopathies, familial mediterranean fever, TNF-receptor–associated periodic syndrome (TRAPS)
8. Complement deficiencies	Defective production of individual complement components	C2 deficiency, C3 deficiency, C6 deficiency, hereditary angioedema

9. Bone Marrow Failure	Failure to produce bone marrow HSC cells, resulting in anemia, thrombocytopenia, and leukopenia	Fanconi anemia
10. Phenocopies of IEIs	IEI associated with an acquired mutation or autoantibody	ALPS, chronic mucocutaneous candidiasis associated with autoantibodies

ADA = adenosine deaminase; IEI = inborn error of immunity; IPEX = Immune dysregulation, polyendocrinopathy, enteropathy X-linked; IUIS = International Union of Immunological Societies; SCID = severe combined immunodeficiency.

CASE STUDIES

1. A 7-month-old male child was diagnosed with bacterial meningitis. Previously he had been hospitalized with bacterial pneumonia. Laboratory results were as follows: RBC count: normal; WBC count: 22 × 10^9/L (normal is 5 to 24 × 10^9/L); differential: 70% neutrophils, 15% monocytes, 5% eosinophils, and 10% lymphocytes; SPE: no gamma band present.

Questions

a. What is the most likely condition, based on the patient's clinical presentation, history, and laboratory results?
b. What further testing do you recommend to confirm the patient's diagnosis?
c. What treatment should be provided for the patient?

2. A 37-year-old adult presents with a long history of recurrent upper respiratory infections and occasional diarrhea, beginning in childhood. The patient has received countless antibiotic regimens through the years. The physician orders an SPE and Ig levels. A low gamma level and no monoclonal proteins are seen in the SPE. IgG, IgM, and IgA concentrations are below the reference ranges. The physician then orders an immunofixation assay (IFE).

Question

a. **Figure 19–4** shows the results of four IFE gels. Region 1 is the normal control serum. Which of the remaining regions best represents the expected pattern for this patient?
b. Explain why you chose this answer.

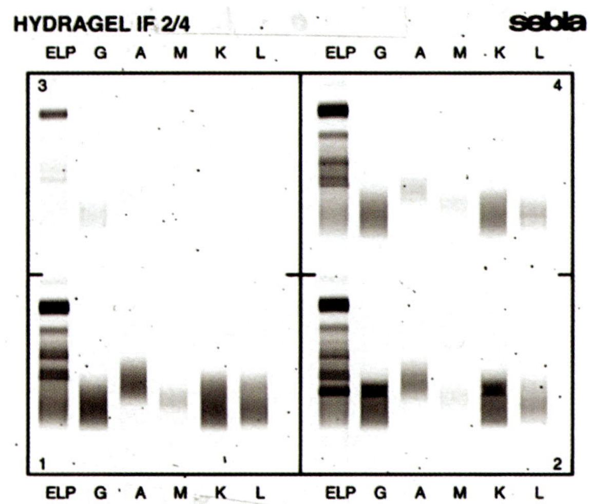

FIGURE 19–4 Case Study 2: Four different immunofixation patterns.

REVIEW QUESTIONS

1. Inborn errors of immunity refer to what type of disease?
   a. Autoimmune
   b. Allergic
   c. Immunodeficiency
   d. Immunoproliferative

2. T-cell subset enumeration by flow cytometry would be most useful in making the diagnosis of which disorder?
   a. Bruton tyrosine kinase (Btk) deficiency
   b. Selective IgA deficiency
   c. Severe combined immunodeficiency (SCID)
   d. Chronic granulomatous disease (CGD)

3. Which of the following would be seen in a patient with NADPH oxidase deficiency?
   a. Defective T-cell function
   b. Inability to produce IgG
   c. Defective NK-cell function
   d. Defective neutrophil function

4. Defects in which branch of the immune system are most commonly associated with severe illness after the administration of live virus vaccines?
   a. Cell-mediated immunity
   b. Humoral immunity
   c. Complement
   d. Phagocytic cells

5. Which of the following statements applies to Bruton tyrosine kinase (Btk) deficiency?
   a. It typically appears in females.
   b. There is a lack of circulating $CD19^+$ B cells.
   c. T cells are abnormal.
   d. There is a lack of pre-B cells in the bone marrow.

6. The DiGeorge syndrome is characterized by all of the following *except:*
   a. Autosomal recessive inheritance
   b. Cardiac abnormalities
   c. Decreased parathyroid gland function
   d. Decreased number of mature T cells

7. A 3-year-old boy is hospitalized because of recurrent bouts of pneumonia. Laboratory tests are run, and the following findings are noted: prolonged bleeding time, decreased platelet count, increased level of serum α-fetoprotein, and a deficiency of naturally occurring isohemagglutinins. Based on these results, which is the most likely diagnosis?
   a. Common variable deficiency
   b. Selective IgA deficiency
   c. Severe combined immunodeficiency (SCID)
   d. Wiskott-Aldrich syndrome

8. Which of the following is associated with ataxia-telangiectasia?
   a. Autosomal recessive inheritance
   b. Defect in both cellular and humoral immunity
   c. Chromosomal breaks in lymphocytes
   d. All of the above

9. A 4-year-old boy presents with recurrent skin and respiratory infections with catalase-positive organisms. Which of the following assays should be considered for diagnosing his presumed immunodeficiency?
   a. DHR reduction
   b. CD4 quantitation
   c. CD19 quantitation
   d. CD56 quantitation

10. Which of the following is an example of a secondary immunodeficiency?
    a. DiGeorge syndrome
    b. Acquired immunodeficiency syndrome (AIDS)
    c. Common variable immunodeficiency
    d. Chronic granulomatous disease

11. Phenocopies of inborn errors of immunity are caused by:
    a. Autoantibodies
    b. Somatic mutations
    c. Inheritance of a single mutation
    d. a and b

12. The PHA mitogen assay is useful in determining the functional capabilities of which cell type?
    a. T cells
    b. B cells
    c. NK cells
    d. Neutrophils

13. Which disorder involves abnormal activation of inflammasomes?
    a. Leukocyte adhesion deficiency (LAD)
    b. Type I interferonopathy
    c. Familial Mediterranean fever
    d. Tumor necrosis factor receptor-associated periodic syndrome (TRAPS)

14. Chédiak-Higashi syndrome is an IEI that involves:
    a. Autoantibodies
    b. Decreased antibody production
    c. Decreased production of reactive oxygen species
    d. Defective lysosome transport

15. TREC screening for SCID is used to determine the number of which type of cell?
    a. B cells
    b. T cells
    c. NK cells
    d. Neutrophils

Chapter 19 Answer Key

19.1 c **19.2** a **19.3** d **19.4** b **19.5** 1-c 2-m 3-h 4-k 5-l 6-a 7-d 8-f 9-j 10-g 11-i 12-b 13-e **19.6** a **19.7** c

Answers to Review Questions

1. c **2.** c **3.** d **4.** a **5.** b **6.** a **7.** d **8.** d **9.** a **10.** b **11.** d **12.** a **13.** c **14.** d **15.** b

IV

Laboratory Diagnosis of Infectious Disease

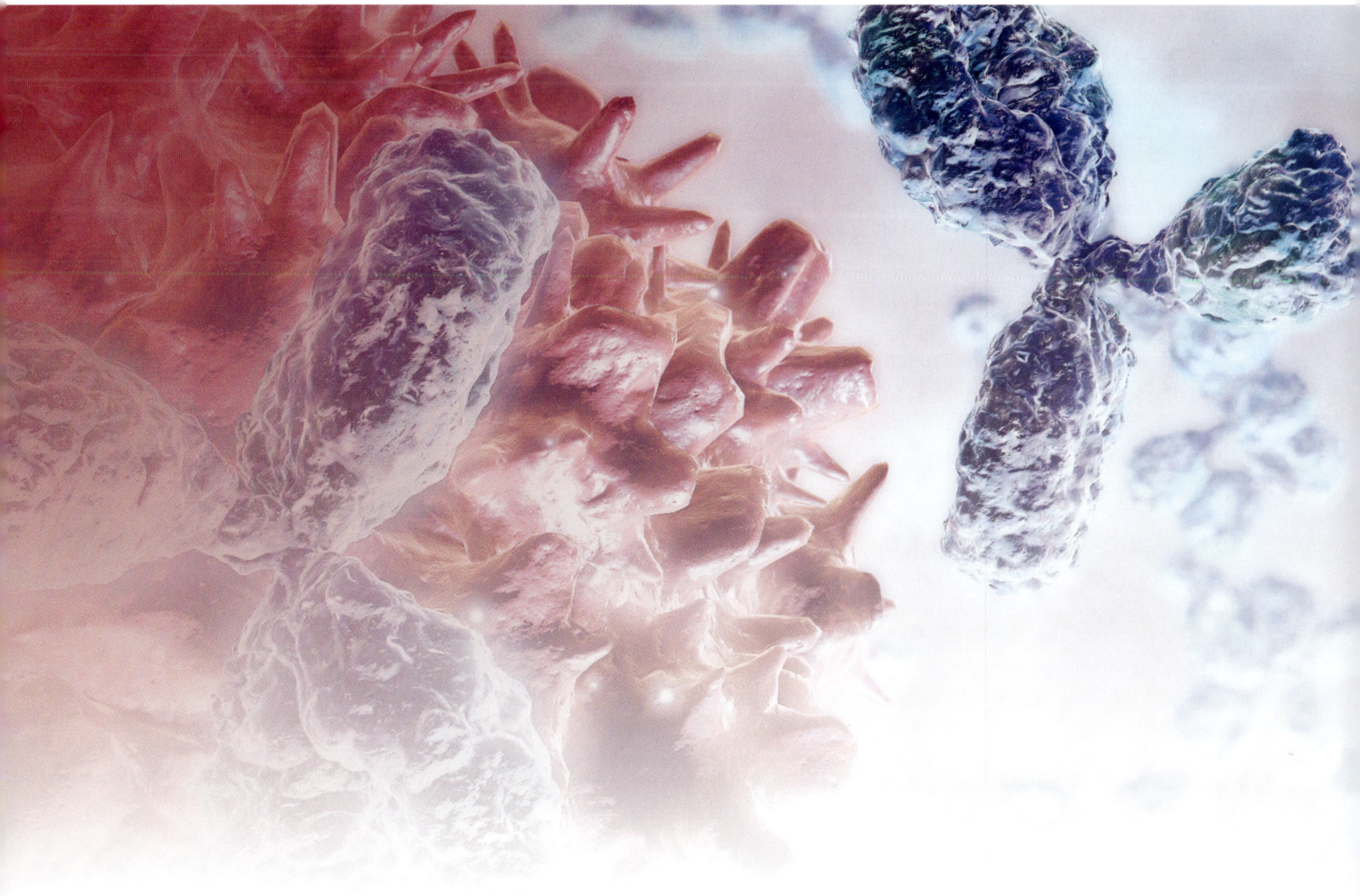

20 Laboratory Detection of Bacterial Infections

James L. Vossler, MS, MLS[CM](ASCP) SM[CM]

LEARNING OUTCOMES

After finishing this chapter, you should be able to:

20.1 Differentiate between commensalistic, mutualistic, and parasitic relationships.

20.2 Differentiate between pathogenicity, virulence, and infectivity.

20.3 Define the term *opportunistic pathogen.*

20.4 Cite structural features of bacteria that contribute to increased virulence.

20.5 Describe host defenses against bacteria and the means by which bacteria can evade the immune system.

20.6 Compare and contrast endotoxins and exotoxins with respect to biological activity, immunogenicity, and genetic encoding for the production of the two toxin categories.

20.7 Cite the five general laboratory means of detecting the causative agent of a bacterial infection.

20.8 List the exotoxins produced by group A streptococci and the roles they play in contributing to the virulence of *Streptococcus pyogenes.*

20.9 Describe the symptoms and pathogenesis of acute rheumatic fever and poststreptococcal glomerulonephritis.

20.10 Explain the principle, interpretation, and clinical significance of the anti-streptolysin O (ASO) and anti-deoxyribonuclease B (anti-DNase B) tests.

20.11 Describe the respiratory and dermatologic manifestations of *Mycoplasma pneumoniae* infections.

20.12 Discuss the use of serology for the diagnosis of *M. pneumoniae* infections, including the clinical value of detecting cold agglutinins.

20.13 Describe the epidemiology of Rocky Mountain spotted fever (RMSF) with respect to its etiologic agent, transmission, and pathogenesis.

20.14 Discuss the clinical use and principles of serological and molecular techniques to diagnose Rocky Mountain spotted fever.

20.15 Compare the general characteristics of mycobacteria to those of other groups of bacteria.

20.16 Describe the pathogenesis of tuberculosis (TB).

CHAPTER OUTLINE

You can go to **fadavis.com** keyword stevens for the laboratory exercises that accompany this text.

20.17 Differentiate between TB disease, latent tuberculosis infection (LTBI), and reactivation tuberculosis.

20.18 Differentiate between multi-drug resistant (MDR) and extensively drug-resistant (XDR) tuberculosis.

20.19 Discuss the laboratory methods and testing available for the detection of mycobacteria.

The collection of microorganisms that exists on the body—bacteria, viruses, and single-celled prokaryotic organisms (e.g., yeast and fungi)—is referred to as the human **microbiome.** The bacteria comprising the human microbiome keep us healthy in many ways. They protect us against disease-causing bacteria, aid in food digestion, produce certain vitamins, and stimulate both the innate and adaptive immune systems. The establishment of an organism that leads to host injury is referred to as an "infection." When a microbe causes damage to host cells or alters physiology that results in clinical signs and symptoms of disease, the phrase "infectious disease" applies.

Determining the cause of a bacterial infection has traditionally relied largely on growing the organisms in culture, biochemical testing, and using stains to view them under the microscope. These infections can also be identified by immunoassays that detect bacterial antigens or antibodies and by molecular or proteomic techniques that detect nucleic acid or proteins from the organisms, respectively. We begin this chapter with an introduction to the human-microbe relationship and factors that influence the interactions between bacteria and the immune system. We then discuss laboratory methods that are commonly used to detect bacterial infections in the context of selected pathogenic bacteria.

Human-Microbe Relationships

When an individual is born, a dynamic relationship begins between the human host and the bacteria in the environment. Very quickly, various bacteria establish themselves on the surfaces of an individual, including the gastrointestinal tract, creating a **symbiotic** relationship. The bacteria and the host "live together," often maintaining a long-term interaction. Symbiotic bacteria that reside on and colonize these surfaces are referred to as the **indigenous microbiota** (also known as "normal flora"). The bacterial populations that exist on the body are not homogenous; they vary in composition and numbers, depending on the area of the body.

The microbial populations outnumber human cells by 10 to 1. Collectively, they may account for 2 to 6 pounds of an individual's body weight. Although it was previously thought that a relatively limited number of bacteria make up the human microbiome, we now know that the microbial community is actually very diverse. Furthermore, more than 90% of the bacteria that comprise the human microbiome cannot be cultured in vitro, most likely because their growth depends on specific conditions or substances that have not been duplicated in the laboratory.

Our relationship with our indigenous microbiota exists through coevolution, coadaptation, and codependency between the bacteria and the host. For a microorganism to survive, the organism needs to colonize the host and acquire nutrients. Importantly, it must not stimulate the host's immune response (in the case of the indigenous microbiota) or it must avoid or circumvent the immune responses. Once established, it must be able to replicate and disseminate to a preferred body site for survival and eventually be transmitted to a new susceptible host.

Three types of symbiotic relationships exist between humans and bacteria. In **commensalistic** relationships, there is no apparent benefit or harm to either organism. The indigenous microbiota are often referred to as "commensals" or the "commensalistic bacteria," describing bacteria that are recovered in culture that do not represent a pathogen. An example of a commensalistic organism is *Staphylococcus epidermidis,* which colonizes and inhabits the human skin. In a **mutualistic** relationship, both humans and the bacteria benefit. One example is the *Lactobacillus* species that colonizes the epithelial surfaces of the vaginal canal. The human host provides conditions such as appropriate temperature, atmosphere, and nutrients that allow the bacteria to grow and multiply. In exchange, the bacteria produce lactic acid, which prevents colonization of bacteria and yeast that may cause disease. Another example is the gram-negative rod *Escherichia coli* that resides in the gastrointestinal tract. *E. coli* relies on intestinal contents for nutrients, and humans derive certain vitamins from *E. coli,* particularly vitamin K, which is required for the formation of blood clotting factors. Although most of the interactions between the host and members of the microbiome are harmless, the encounter with specific organisms or viruses occasionally results in harm to the host. In this case, a **parasitic** relationship exists between the other organisms and the host.

As we previously mentioned, the establishment of an organism that leads to host injury is referred to as an *infection.* Although there is harm to the host, not all infections are symptomatic. Often, the infection may be *subclinical;* in other words, there are no signs or symptoms. An example is infection with *Chlamydia trachomatis,* a sexually transmitted organism. Only about 10% of infected males and up to 30% of infected females will show symptoms when infected with *C. trachomatis.* The organism may then be transmitted to other people or may result in complications such as pelvic inflammatory disease in women.

Several terms are used to describe the interaction between the infecting organisms and the host. *Infectivity, pathogenicity,* and *virulence* are often used interchangeably; however, each term has different meanings when discussing an organism's ability to cause an infection. **Infectivity** refers to an organism's ability to establish an infection. More specifically, infectivity describes the proportion of individuals exposed to a pathogen through horizontal transmission (i.e., person-to-person spread) who will become infected. Another term with similar meaning is *contagious.* For example, the measles virus is extremely contagious, having a high degree of infectivity.

Pathogenicity refers to the inherent capacity of an organism to cause disease. This is a qualitative trait of the organism determined by its genetic makeup. Some organisms, such as HIV, are primary or true pathogens that can cause harm to most people who have intact immune systems. Although an organism may be pathogenic in nature, it may not always cause disease. The outcome of the host-pathogen interaction is determined by several factors, including the host's immunologic status. Some microorganisms, known as "opportunistic pathogens," may only cause disease or infection in individuals who have compromised immune systems because of factors such as chemotherapy, radiation therapy, or various chronic diseases.

Virulence is a quantitative trait that refers to the extent of damage, or pathology, caused by the organism. For example, *Yersinia pestis,* the causative agent of bubonic and pneumonic plague, is considered extremely virulent and is likely to cause severe illness and death upon infection unless antibiotics are administered. If the bacterial strain is not capable of causing disease, the organism is said to be "avirulent." Not all members of a bacterial species may be capable of causing disease. For example, *E. coli* resides as commensal bacteria in the gastrointestinal tract, but only some strains of *E. coli* can cause diarrheal disease.

The degree of damage is mediated by specific virulence factors. **Virulence factors** may increase an organism's pathogenicity by contributing to the organism's ability to establish itself on or in the host, invade or damage host tissue, or evade the host immune response.

Knowledge Check 20-1

What is the term used to describe the relationship that bacteria that colonize the skin (e.g., *Staphylococcus epidermidis*) have with the human host?

a. Commensalistic
b. Mutualistic
c. Parasitisitic
d. Symbiotic

Bacterial Virulence Factors

Factors that increase a bacterium's virulence may be classified as either structural components or as extracellular substances produced by the bacteria. Various types of bacterial virulence factors are discussed in the sections that follow and summarized in the Study Guide at the end of the chapter.

For an organism to be pathogenic, it must possess genetic determinants that allow it to produce either the structural components or the extracellular products that contribute to its virulence. Genetic determinants located on the bacterial chromosome are generally responsible for the production of structural or surface molecules, which help the organism to attach to and colonize the host. The genetic information needed to produce these extracellular virulence factors is most often located on independent genetic elements called *plasmids.*

Plasmids are self-replicating extrachromosomal DNA molecules that are located in the bacteria's cytoplasm and contain a limited number of genes. Plasmids are mobile genetic elements that can also be transferred between bacteria through various mechanisms. Acquiring exogenous DNA that codes for the production of virulence factors can convert an avirulent strain into a virulent strain.

Structural Virulence Features

Bacterial cells are classified as prokaryotic cells, whereas human cells are classified as eukaryotic cells. Although prokaryotic bacterial cells are relatively simple, they have a well-developed cell structure and contain several structural and genetic features not found in eukaryotic cells. One significant difference is that the bacterial chromosome is not enclosed inside a membrane-bound nucleus but instead resides inside the bacterial cytoplasm. Also housed in the cytoplasm are internal cellular structures, such as ribosomes, mesosomes, other cytoplasmic inclusion bodies, and potentially plasmids. Bacterial cells do not contain membrane-bound organelles such as the mitochondria found in eukaryotic cells **(Fig. 20–1)**.

Other significant differences between eukaryotic and prokaryotic cells are features of the cell membrane and the presence of a cell wall in bacteria. Like the plasma membrane in eukaryotic cells, the bacterial plasma membrane plays a regulatory role in transporting molecules in and out of the cell. The cell membrane in bacteria also contains various enzyme systems responsible for energy generation. In eukaryotic cells (except for plants and fungi), the plasma membrane is the outer surface of the cell. In contrast, bacteria have a cell wall as their outermost feature. The bacterial cell wall prevents osmotic lysis and confers shape and rigidity to the bacteria. Peptidoglycan is the primary component providing shape and rigidity. Most antibiotics used to treat bacterial infections target the production of peptidoglycan in the cell wall.

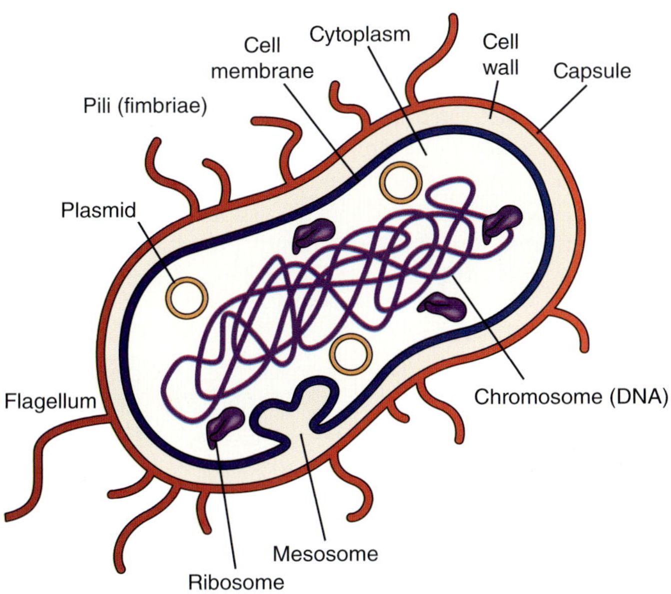

FIGURE 20–1 Cross section of a bacterial cell.

The bacterial cell wall structure has two different variations, classified as either gram positive or gram negative, depending on their staining characteristics with the Gram stain. Gram-negative cell walls have features that increase an organism's virulence, as we discuss later. One of the features found in the cell wall of gram-negative bacteria is the lipopolysaccharide (LPS) layer. The three components that make up LPS are an outer core polysaccharide, an inner core polysaccharide, and lipid A. When released from dead or dying cells, a portion of LPS called lipid A is exposed. Lipid A, also referred to as **endotoxin**, is a powerful stimulator of cytokine production that leads to various systemic manifestations and potentially fatal endotoxic (gram-negative) shock (discussed later in this section).

To successfully establish an infection, bacteria must first adhere to and colonize the host tissue. To persist in the host, they must also be capable of evading the immune system. Structural features are generally involved in the adherence of bacteria or the evasion of the immune system. Whiplike structures called *flagella* can facilitate adherence and movement of the bacteria toward a host cell.

Bacteria have surface structures or molecules that can bind specifically to complementary receptors on specific cells of host tissues. The most common surface structures involved in attachment are fimbriae, which are composed of protein. The fimbriae involved in specific attachment to prokaryotic surface ligands are referred to as the *common pili*. Other pili used to exchange genetic information, called the *F* or *sex pili*, are fewer in number than common pili. The sex pili may also help attach bacteria to host cells.

In addition to allowing the organism to attach to and colonize tissues, pili play a role in resisting phagocytosis by white blood cells (WBCs) and may undergo antigenic variation to evade the adaptive immune response. For example, the pili of *Neisseria gonorrhoeae* specifically adhere to human mucosal epithelial cells. *N. gonorrhoeae* can evade the immune response and resist phagocytosis by rearranging portions of its genome, which change the pili's antigen makeup. Most strains of *E. coli* that colonize the gastrointestinal tract do not adhere to epithelial cells of the small intestine. The ability of certain strains of *E. coli* to cause gastrointestinal disease is associated with expression of specific pili that allow for adherence to the epithelial cells of the small intestine. For example, enterotoxigenic *E. coli* (ETEC) strains have factor antigen I (CFA) pili that adhere to the cells in the small intestine; the organism then produces the toxins that cause diarrhea.

Attachment may also occur via adhesions or surface molecules on the bacterial cell, referred to as *afimbrial* (non–pili dependent) *attachment*. Host-cell receptors recognized by bacterial surface molecules include proteoglycans, laminins, collagens, elastin, and hyaluronan. Glycoproteins such as fibrinogen, fibronectin, and vitronectin are also potential receptors for bacteria. The ability of ***Streptococcus pyogenes*** pili to attach to host cells is caused by the production of

F protein, which attaches to fibronectin. In addition to aiding in attachment, surface M protein, the major virulence factor of *S. pyogenes,* allows the organism to resist phagocytosis.

A major structural feature that increases an organism's virulence is the presence of a capsule, which is usually polysaccharide in nature. Capsules contribute to the organism's ability to resist innate and adaptive immune responses through a variety of means. They can block the attachment of antibodies, inhibit complement activation, or act as a decoy when capsular material is released into the surrounding host environment. One of the most important features of a capsule is its role in blocking phagocytosis by WBCs. For example, the primary determinant of the virulence of *Streptococcus pneumoniae* is a polysaccharide capsule that prevents the ingestion of pneumococci by alveolar macrophages. Also, extracellular capsular antigens are released and bind to immunoglobulins, reducing the effective immune response against the organism itself. Bacterial strains that do not possess a capsule are, in most cases, avirulent and not able to produce disease.

Clinical Correlations

Capsular Antigens and Vaccine Development

Most capsules evoke a strong humoral immune response and are used in the development of vaccines. For example, the vaccines for *Haemophilus influenzae* type b, *S. pneumoniae,* and certain types of *Neisseria meningitidis* consist of antigens derived from bacterial capsules (see Chapter 25).

Extracellular Virulence Factors

Extracellular substances produced by bacteria also contribute to an organism's virulence by breaking down the body's primary or secondary defenses, damaging the host tissues and cells, or facilitating the growth and spread of the organism. Substances that perform the latter function are called *invasins.* Hyaluronidase, collagenase, phospholipases, lecithinases, coagulase, and various kinases are examples of invasins.

Endotoxin and Exotoxins

Bacteria may also produce two types of toxins—endotoxin and exotoxins. Endotoxin (lipid A) is found in the LPS layer of the cell walls of all gram-negative bacteria. When the cell dies, the LPS layer is removed from the cell, releasing endotoxin in the host. The effects of endotoxin are complex. Endotoxin induces a variety of host responses, including the production of cytokines such as interleukin (IL)-1, IL-6, IL-8, tumor necrosis factor (TNF), and platelet-activating factor, which stimulate the production of prostaglandins and leukotrienes. This results in inflammation, increased heart rate, increased body temperature (fever), and decreased blood pressure. Endotoxin also activates the complement cascade, resulting in formation of the anaphylatoxins C3a and C5a, which cause vasodilation and increase vascular permeability. The alternative coagulation cascade is also activated, producing coagulation, thrombosis, and acute disseminated intravascular coagulation (DIC), leading to hemorrhage and shock. A potential consequence of endotoxin release is septic shock, a life-threatening illness usually resulting from a gram-negative *bacteremia,* or presence of bacteria in the blood. With septic shock, there is a large-scale release of inflammatory mediators that results in massive vasodilation and hypotension, sometimes referred to as a "cytokine storm" (see Chapter 6). If the condition worsens, there is widespread organ damage, including renal failure, liver dysfunction, heart damage, and eventual death. Endotoxin is immunogenic but does not elicit a protective immune response, so no vaccine is available against this bacterial component.

Unlike endotoxin, which has multiple effects on the body, **exotoxins** have a specific and targeted activity. They are proteins released from living bacteria (mostly gram positive bacteria) and are some of the most potent molecules known to harm living organisms. Exotoxins may be classified as neurotoxins, cytotoxins, or enterotoxins, according to their effect on cells. Exotoxins bind to specific receptors on host cells. Most exotoxins have several subunits that bind to these receptors (i.e., the B subunits) and a subunit that is actually responsible for the specific activity of the toxin (the A subunit). An example of a cytotoxin is the diphtheria toxin, produced by *Corynebacterium diphtheriae* (a gram-positive rod), which interferes with protein synthesis in epithelial cells. Neurotoxins include the tetanus toxin, produced by *Clostridium botulinum* (a gram-positive rod), which prevents the release of inhibitory transmitters from the presynaptic membrane of neuromuscular cells, leading to continuous excitement of muscle cells and spasms. Botulism toxin, produced by *Clostridium tetani,* a gram-positive rod, works in a reverse manner—the toxin prevents the release of acetylcholine (ACh) from nerve cells, resulting in paralysis of the motor system. Examples of enterotoxins are toxins A and B produced by *Clostridioides difficile* (previously *Clostridium difficile*), which cause fluid secretion (diarrhea), mucosal injury, and inflammation **(Fig. 20–2).** Exotoxins are extremely immunogenic and induce the production of protective antibodies. Inactivated exotoxins called "toxoids" are used for some vaccines. For example, the toxin of *Corynebacterium diphtheriae* is used in the vaccine to prevent diphtheria.

Some exotoxins may act as "superantigens." Unlike other antigens, superantigens are not processed by antigen-presenting cells (APCs). Instead, they bind directly to class II major histocompatibility molecules (MHC II) on APCs outside of the normal antigen-binding groove. The MHC II molecule binds to the T-cell receptor (TCR) with the whole antigen (toxin) attached. Normally, only 0.0001% of T cells are activated in an immune response. However, a superantigen induces activation of up to 20% of T cells, resulting in a massive release of cytokines. The systemic events brought on by the release of large amounts of cytokines lead to what is referred to as "toxic shock syndrome." Examples include the TSST-1 toxin produced by *Staphylococcus aureus* and the superantigens produced by *Streptococcus pyogenes,* the cause of streptococcal toxic shock syndrome (STSS).

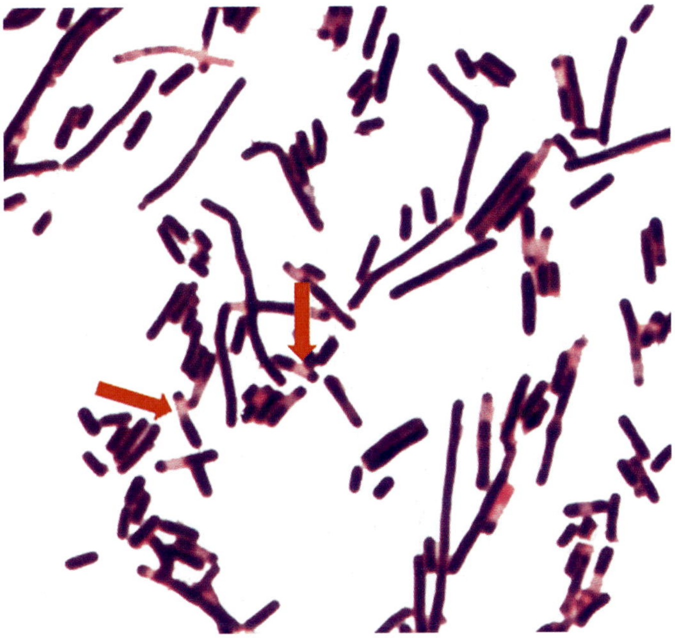

FIGURE 20–2 Gram stain of *Clostridioides difficile* (a gram-positive rod). Arrows point to the clear areas in the cell, which represent a spore. Spores are resistant to disinfectants and contribute to the spread of the organism from person to person. *(Courtesy of James Vossler.)*

Immune Defenses Against Bacterial Infections and Mechanisms of Evasion

Immune Defense Mechanisms

Although bacteria may possess various features that increase their virulence, they must be able to circumvent or overcome the host's defense mechanisms. As we discussed in previous chapters, both innate and adaptive responses may occur after an encounter with potential pathogens.

Innate Defenses

The first line of defense involves intact skin and mucosal surfaces that serve as structural barriers. In addition, the epithelial surface may have enzymes and nonspecific anti-microbial peptides (AMPs), such as defensins, and other proteins that have anti-microbial activity. One example of an enzyme with specific anti-microbial activity is lysozyme, which is found in many secretions, including tears and saliva. Lysozyme destroys the peptidoglycan in the cell wall of bacteria, especially gram-positive bacteria. Other enzymes such as ribonucleases, which destroy RNA, have anti-microbial and anti-viral activities.

The body excretes a wide variety of AMPs and proteins that play a role in innate defenses. Some of these substances are only secreted by specific tissues or cells. For example, one group of soluble peptides, called *defensins,* is produced continuously by different cells in the body. There are three main classes of defensins: alpha, beta, and theta. α-Defensins are produced by neutrophils, certain macrophage populations, and Paneth cells of the small intestine. This class of defensins is believed to disrupt the microbial membrane. β-Defensins are produced by neutrophils and the epithelial cells lining various organs, including the bronchial tree and genitourinary system. They are believed to increase resistance of epithelial cells to colonization. θ-Defensins are not found in humans.

Many anti-microbial proteins contribute to the innate immune response. For example, complement proteins can promote chemotaxis. Interleukins help regulate immune responses and inflammatory reactions. Prostaglandins induce dilation or constriction of blood vessels and modulate inflammation. Leukotrienes are involved in inflammation and fever.

Acute phase reactants also play important roles. For example, C-reactive protein (CRP) activates the complement system and promotes phagocytosis by macrophages. Haptoglobin binds free plasma hemoglobin, which deprives the bacteria of iron. Ceruloplasmin is a glycoprotein that binds copper and has bactericidal activities.

Bacteria, fungi, and viruses possess pathogen-associated molecular patterns (PAMPs), which are structures consisting of carbohydrates, nucleic acids, or bacterial peptides. PAMPs are recognized by pattern recognition receptors (PRRs) expressed on the cells of the innate immune system (e.g., the toll-like receptors [TLRs]; see Chapter 2). Engagement of a PRR with the appropriate PAMP triggers the release of immune mediators such as cytokines and chemokines, boosts production of various defensins and proteins, and initiates phagocytosis. The phagocytic process is enhanced by activation of the alternative complement cascade, which is triggered by microbial cell walls or other products of microbial metabolism.

Adaptive Immune Responses

Adaptive immune responses include the production of antibodies directed against bacterial surface antigens or extracellular products produced by bacteria such as exotoxins. Antibody formation is the main defense against extracellular bacteria. The mechanisms by which antibodies can attack invading bacteria are discussed in Chapter 3.

Cell-mediated immunity (CMI), the other branch of the adaptive immune response, is helpful in attacking intracellular bacteria, such as *Mycobacterium tuberculosis, Legionella pneumophila, Listeria monocytogenes,* and *Rickettsia* species. Through the mechanism of delayed-type hypersensitivity, CD4 T cells produce cytokines, which activate macrophages to release enzymes that destroy the bacteria (see Chapter 14). Recruitment of inflammatory cells results in the formation of granulomas that surround the bacteria-infected cells to help prevent the spread of infection. Cytotoxic T cells are also recruited to the site of infection and mount an antigen-specific attack on the cells containing intracellular bacteria.

Bacterial Evasion Mechanisms

Bacteria have developed several ways to inhibit the immune system or make it more difficult for immune responses to occur. Three main mechanisms used by bacteria are avoiding

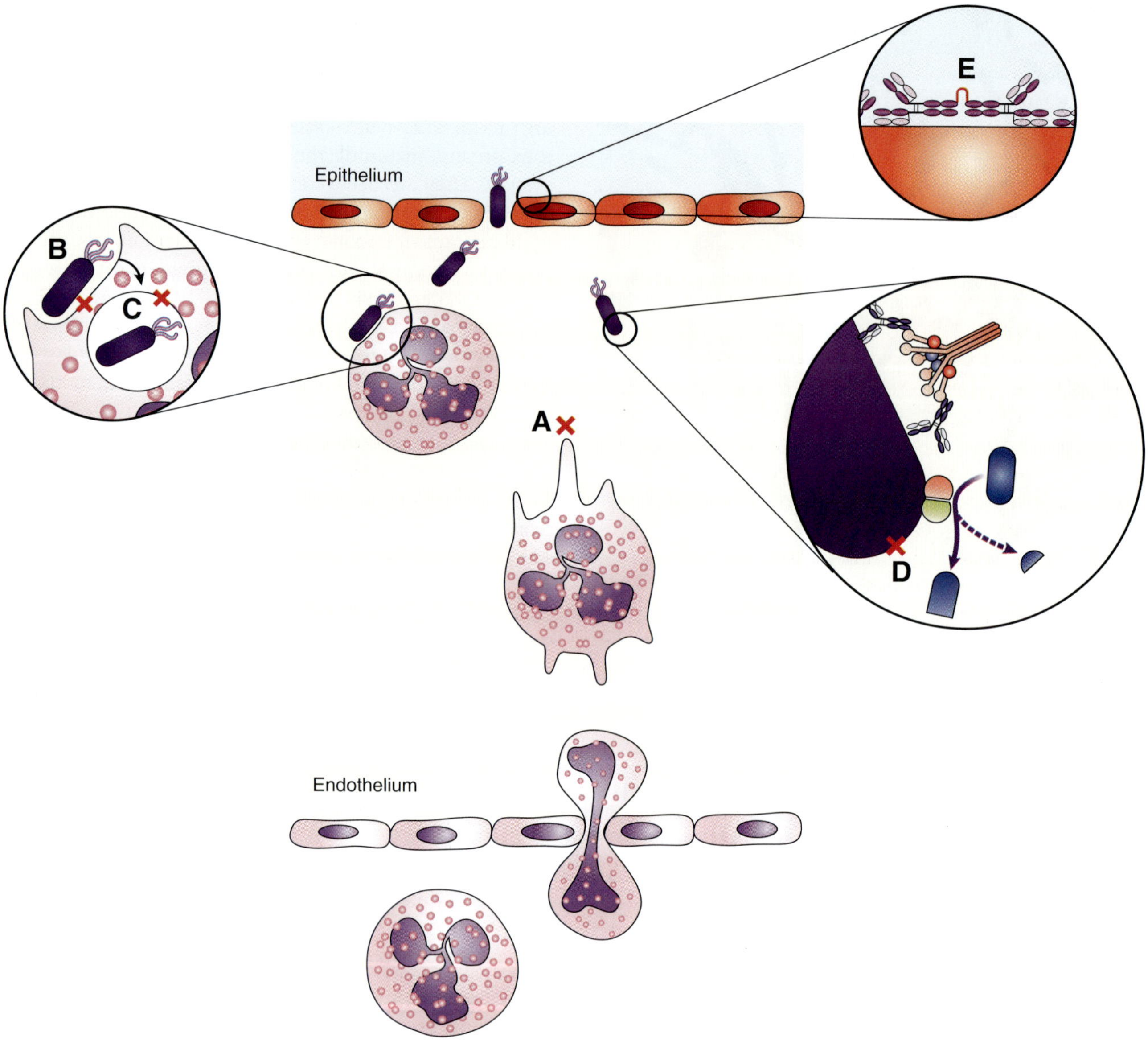

FIGURE 20–3 The strategies bacteria use to evade host defenses. (A) Inhibiting chemotaxis. (B) Blocking adherence of phagocytes to the bacterial cells. (C) Blocking digestion. (D) Inhibiting complement C3b binding. (E) Cleaving immunoglobulin A (IgA).

antibodies, blocking phagocytosis, and inactivating the complement cascade **(Fig. 20–3)**. Bacteria can evade antibodies by altering their bacterial antigens, a process called *antigenic variation*. Some bacteria can also coat themselves with host proteins such as fibrin or immunoglobulins (e.g., *S. aureus*) or fibronectin (e.g., *Treponema pallidum*) or hide their surface molecules through antigenic disguise (e.g., the hyaluronic acid capsule of *S. pyogenes*). Bacteria can also evade the specific immune response by decreasing expression of MHC molecules on host cells and producing proteases that degrade IgA. *N. gonorrhoeae, H. influenzae,* and *Streptococcus sanguinis* are examples of bacteria that can cleave IgA.

Most evasion mechanisms target the process of phagocytosis. Bacteria can mount a defense at several stages in the phagocytic process, including chemotaxis, adhesion, and digestion. Some pathogens such as *N. gonorrhoeae* inhibit the release of chemotactic factors that would bring phagocytic cells to the area. The cell walls of *S. pyogenes* produce an M protein that interferes with adhesion to the phagocytic cell. The presence of a polysaccharide capsule found in such organisms as *N. meningitidis, S. pneumoniae, Yersinia pestis,* and *H. influenzae* inhibits the binding of neutrophils and macrophages needed to initiate phagocytosis.

Microorganisms use several different mechanisms to resist digestion. Some bacteria can block fusion of lysosomal granules with phagosomes after being engulfed by the phagocyte. *Salmonella* species, *Mycobacterium tuberculosis* and *Mycobacterium leprae* (the causative agent of leprosy), can all do this. In *M. tuberculosis* and *M. leprae* infections, each bacillus is contained in a membrane-enclosed fluid compartment called a *pristiophorus vacuole* (PV), which does not fuse with lysosomes because of the complexity of the cell wall. Mycobacteria have a thick cell wall primarily composed of fatty molecules known as mycolic acids. The presence of the mycolic acids in the cell wall allows the bacterium to grow inside macrophages, effectively hiding it from the host immune system. The mycolic acids also allow mycobacteria to resist decolorization by acids used in staining the organisms; hence, they are referred to as "acid-fast bacilli" (AFB).

Another mechanism of resisting digestion involves the production of extracellular products after the bacteria are phagocytized. Their main effect is the release of lysosomal contents into the cytoplasm of the phagocytic cells, subsequently killing the WBC. Examples include leukocidin, produced by *S. aureus;* listeriolysin O, produced by *L. monocytogenes;* and streptolysin, produced by *S. pyogenes.*

Another major defense some bacteria use is to block the action of complement. Organisms that produce a capsule do not bind the complement component C3b, which is important in enhancing phagocytosis. These organisms cannot easily be phagocytized unless coated by other opsonins (e.g., IgG). Also, some organisms express molecules that disrupt one or more of the complement pathways. For example, protein H, produced by *S. pyogenes,* binds to C1 but does not allow the complement cascade to proceed further. Another example is *Streptococcus agalactiae,* also known as *group B streptococcus (GBS).* GBS has a capsule that is rich in sialic acid (a common component of host-cell glycoproteins), causing degradation of C3b and making the organism resistant to complement-mediated phagocytosis.

Laboratory Detection and Diagnosis of Bacterial Infections

The clinical laboratory provides health care professionals with information from patient samples about the causative agent(s) responsible for an infection. This information allows doctors to better manage patient therapy to control infections because specific pathogenic microorganisms and viruses are detected.

Traditional ways to detect the agents responsible for an infection include (1) culture or growth of the causative agent, (2) microscopy, (3) biochemical testing, (4) detection of bacterial antigens in the clinical sample, and (5) serology to detect antibodies produced in response to the infection. The COVID-19 pandemic has highlighted the need for readily available, accurate, and fast diagnostic testing methods to detect and characterize infectious agents. More recently, methods that allow for more rapid detection and increased sensitivity have been developed. These include molecular techniques that detect bacterial and viral DNA or RNA and proteomics to detect bacterial proteins from clinical samples. In this chapter, we review both traditional and newer methods for determining the causative agent of an infection.

Bacterial Culture

Traditional means of determining the cause of a bacterial infection rely largely on growing the organism in culture and biochemical testing (e.g., detecting specific enzyme activity, carbohydrate utilization, oxidation/reduction). Various broth and solid media may be used to recover the organism. Some media may contain substances that enhance the growth of certain organisms and are referred to as *enriched media. Selective media* contain substances or antibiotics that suppress the growth of commensalistic bacteria and support the growth of other bacteria. *Differential media* contain substrates that allow for the differentiation of bacteria based on their ability to use the substrate. For example, MacConkey agar selects for gram-negative bacteria and differentiates between lactose-fermenting and non–lactose-fermenting bacteria. Some organisms, such as *Bordetella pertussis,* the causative agent of whooping cough, have specific growth requirements for which specialized media must be used.

Although culture is the primary laboratory means of diagnosing bacterial infections, culturing of bacterial pathogens has limitations. There are several bacterial pathogens for which clinically useful culture systems are not available. For other organisms, recovery in culture may take too long to be clinically useful. For example, although *Mycoplasma pneumoniae,* a leading cause of community-acquired pneumonia, can be cultured, culturing is a challenge. The organism is extremely fastidious (difficult to grow) and may take weeks to recover in the laboratory. Other organisms present a danger to the laboratorian if they are not grown and handled using the most rigorous safety precautions. An example is *Yersinia pestis,* the causative agent of pneumonic plague, infamous for causing a pandemic in the 1300s that killed millions of people in Europe and North Africa (the "black death").

Microscopic Visualization

Visualization of the causative agents with microscopic techniques is most often done using differential or fluorescent stains. A common example is the Gram stain for differentiating gram-positive bacteria, which stain purple with crystal violet from gram-negative bacteria, which stain pink with safranin **(Fig. 20–4)**. Other examples are the acid-fast stain for detecting *M. tuberculosis* **(Fig. 20–5),** and the Giemsa stain for detecting the causative agents of malaria. Direct fluorescent antibody (DFA) assays involve the use of antibody conjugated with a fluorescent label to detect specific bacteria in a sample. Many DFAs are being replaced by molecular tests because they lack sensitivity or because the reagents are not widely available. Although the various staining methods are not difficult to perform, a trained microscopist is necessary for proper interpretation. Another limitation of microscopy is that not all organisms may be visualized through microscopic means.

Biochemical Testing

Biochemical testing is an essential component of bacterial identification. It involves analyzing metabolic activities that are characteristic of certain bacterial species because of the enzymes they possess. For such tests, a positive or negative biochemical reaction in the presence of a particular substrate is used to identify the organism. Some examples of commonly used biochemical tests are those for:

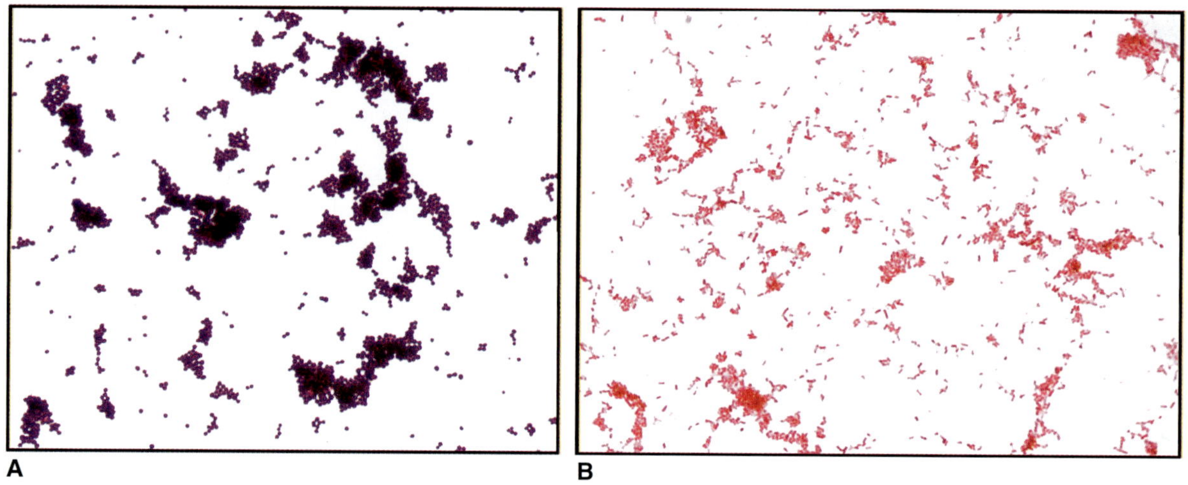

FIGURE 20–4 (A) Gram stain of *Staphylococcus aureus* showing gram-positive cocci in clusters. (B) Gram stain of *Escherichia coli* showing gram-negative rods. *(Courtesy of James Vossler.)*

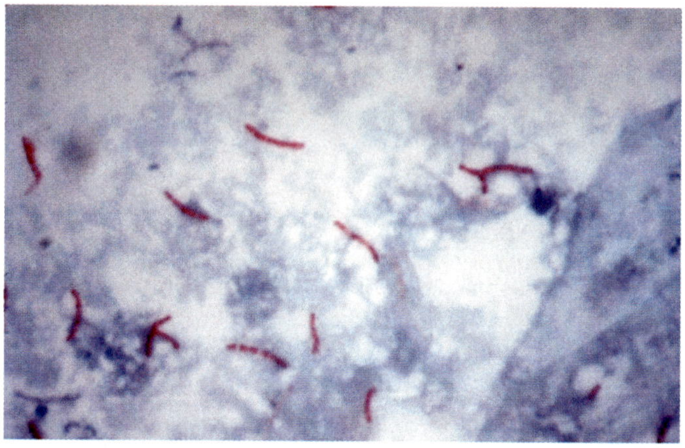

FIGURE 20–5 Photomicrograph of *Mycobacterium tuberculosis* bacteria using acid-fast Ziehl-Neelsen stain; magnified 1,000×. The acid-fast stains depend on the ability of mycobacteria to retain the dye when treated with mineral acid or an acid-alcohol solution. *(Courtesy of the CDC/Dr. George P. Kubica, Public Health Image Library.)*

- Amylase: Checks for starch hydrolysis.
- Bile Esculin Agar: Detects hydrolysis of esculin in the presence of bile.
- Catalase: Based on the ability to break down hydrogen peroxide.
- Indole: Detects indole production from tryptophan.
- Lactose fermentation: Based on the ability to break down lactose into simpler sugars.
- Oxidase: Detects cytochrome oxidase, which is involved in electron transport.
- Urease: Based on hydrolysis of urea to produce ammonia.

Antigen Detection

Antigen detection assays are available for a wide variety of bacteria, viruses, parasites, and fungi in clinical samples. Testing methods include latex agglutination (LA), enzyme-linked immunosorbent assay (ELISA), and lateral flow immunochromatographic assays (LFAs) that detect the presence of an analyte (e.g., bacterial antigen) in a sample. Advantages of the LA assay and LFA are the relative ease by which they can be performed, their low cost, and the rapid turnaround time. Many of the LA assays and LFAs are classified as "CLIA waived" tests. Under the Clinical Laboratory Improvement Amendments (CLIA), simple, low-risk tests can be "waived" (i.e., laboratories performing the testing are not subject to routine inspection) and may be performed in physicians' offices and various other locations (see Chapter 8). Bacteria for which antigen detection is widely used include *S. pyogenes* (strep throat) and *L. pneumophila* (Legionnaires' disease). Antigen detection assays are highly specific, and because of advances in technology, the sensitivities of the assays have improved dramatically. In many cases, antigen detection assays, particularly LFAs, have replaced other methods used to detect bacterial, fungal, and viral infections.

Molecular Detection

Developments in the field of molecular diagnostics have allowed for increased availability and use of nucleic-acid–based assays in the clinical laboratory to detect bacteria, viruses, and parasitic agents responsible for human infections. Compact hybridization and gene amplification assays that are easy to perform have made their way into physicians' office laboratories. A common molecular technology is the polymerase chain reaction (PCR), in which specific genetic sequences are amplified and detected. With quantitative PCR (qPCR), results can be obtained in a few hours. For some bacteria, such as *Neisseria gonorrhoeae* and *Chlamydia trachomatis,* nucleic-acid–based assays are widely available and are more sensitive than traditional culture methods. Molecular assays are now the method of choice for the detection of *Clostridioides (Clostridium) difficile.*

In recent years, the U.S. Food and Drug Administration (FDA) approved an increasing number of molecular-based assays, allowing for rapid detection and identification of bacterial infections. Molecular assays are also available to detect genes that are responsible for anti-microbial resistance (e.g., methicillin-resistant *Staphylococcus aureus* [MRSA] and vancomycin-resistant enterococci [VRE]) directly from clinical specimens.

Although nucleic-acid–based assays are more sensitive than other methods, there are limitations associated with nucleic-acid–based testing. These include the high cost of reagents and equipment; the need for highly skilled personnel; false-negative results due to a small number of organisms, improper sample collection or storage, or reaction inhibitors; and false-positive results due to contamination. Test results may also remain positive after live organisms have been eliminated from the body, as their nucleic acid can persist.

Serological Diagnosis

Serology has historically been used to detect and confirm infections from organisms that are difficult to culture or for which other laboratory methods of diagnosing the infection are not available. Serology may also be useful in determining the causative agent when clinical symptoms are not specific enough to identify the cause of the infection. For certain organisms (e.g., *Anaplasma, Ehrlichia, Chlamydophila pneumoniae, Chlamydophila psittaci, Coxiella burnetii, Leptospira, Ricksettia* spp., and *T. pallidum*), serological testing remains useful and, in some cases, is the best means of detecting exposure to, or infection with, an organism. Detection of IgM and IgG antibodies may help distinguish between recent or previous exposure to an organism, and antibody titers may be used to assess reactivation or reexposure to an infectious agent (see Chapter 3).

The main disadvantage of using serology in diagnosis is that there is usually a delay between the start of the infection and the production of antibodies to the infecting microorganism. Although IgM antibodies may appear relatively early (7 to 10 days after exposure), some infections have a rapid course, and therapy may need to be initiated before IgM antibodies can be detected. In some cases, demonstration of a high IgG antibody titer in the initial stage of infection is diagnostic; however, the high titer may be caused by a past infection, and the patient's symptoms may have an entirely different cause. When testing for the presence of IgG antibodies, it is ideal to collect serum samples during both the acute and convalescent phases of an illness so that a rising titer to the suspected pathogen can be observed. Another limitation of serology is that immunosuppressed patients may be unable to mount an antibody response.

Proteomics

The **proteome** is the total complement, or set of proteins expressed by an organism or cell. **Proteomics** is the analysis and study of the proteins expressed by an organism's genome. Proteomics can be used to detect biomarkers—biological molecules in blood, other body fluids, or tissues that are a sign of a normal or abnormal process or of a condition or disease.

The use of proteomic analysis for clinical samples is relatively new in the laboratory diagnosis of infectious diseases. Proteomics has the potential to be used to detect agents causing an infectious disease, monitor the effectiveness of treatment, or identify changes in a disease caused by a microorganism or virus. Advances in proteomic analysis are attributable largely to the introduction of mass spectrometry (MS) platforms capable of screening complex biological fluids for individual protein and peptide biomarkers. Research on the use of proteomics to detect biomarkers for the detection of bacterial, viral, parasitic, or fungal infections is ongoing. Specific protein biomarkers may also reveal the biological state of a particular organism (e.g., reproducing or dormant) or pathological changes within an infected host.

Proteomics platforms used in clinical settings include matrix-associated laser desorption ionization time-of-flight mass spectrometry (MALDI-TOF MS) and surface-enhanced laser desorption ionization time-of-flight MS (SELDI-TOF MS). The most important application of **MALDI-TOF** is the identification of bacterial and fungal isolates growing from a culture.

To perform MALDI-TOF MS, the sample is placed on a solid surface matrix. The matrix is then placed in an instrument, where pulses of laser light vaporize the specimen, generating high molecular weight ions that absorb energy from the proteins and carbohydrates in the sample in a process known as *desorption*. The ions are then accelerated by an electrical field and a vacuum. Because the ions have the same energy, yet a different mass, they reach the detector at different times. The smaller ions reach the detector first because of their greater velocity, whereas the larger ions take longer due to their larger mass. Hence, the analyzer is called "TOF" because the mass is determined from the ions' "time of flight" from being ionized to reaching the detector **(Fig. 20–6).** Identification of a microorganism in the sample is based on the generation of a characteristic "protein fingerprint" called a *profile* **(Fig. 20–7).**

A variant of MALDI-TOF, SELDI-TOF, has a higher sensitivity for low molecular weight proteins. Research has shown that MALDI-TOF and SELDI-TOF can be used to detect certain parasitic and fungal infections in patients. The use of MALDI-TOF and SELDI-TOF to detect biomarkers associated with bacterial, viral, fungal, and parasitic agents shows promise for the diagnosis of infections caused by these agents.

In the remainder of this chapter, we review the infections caused by specific bacteria and the clinical laboratory tests used to detect these infections.

Knowledge Check 20-2

What is the primary purpose of culturing a sample from the blood or tissue of a patient suspected of having a bacterial infection?

a. Identifying the species of bacteria in the sample
b. Recovering the organism causing the infection
c. Determining whether an organism is virulent or avirulent
d. Determining the number of organisms present in a sample

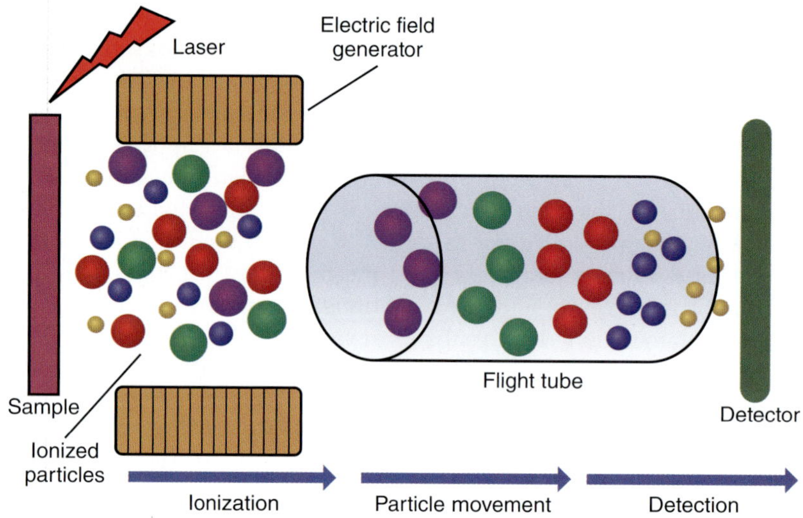

FIGURE 20–6 MALDI-TOF. The sample is ionized with a laser beam, breaking it into various-sized particles. The particles are accelerated in a tube with a magnetic field. Particles move through the tube via a vacuum. Smaller particles move faster through the tube (time of flight). The number of particles of each size is measured, creating a pattern unique to each organism and allowing for identification of the organism. *(Courtesy of James Vossler.)*

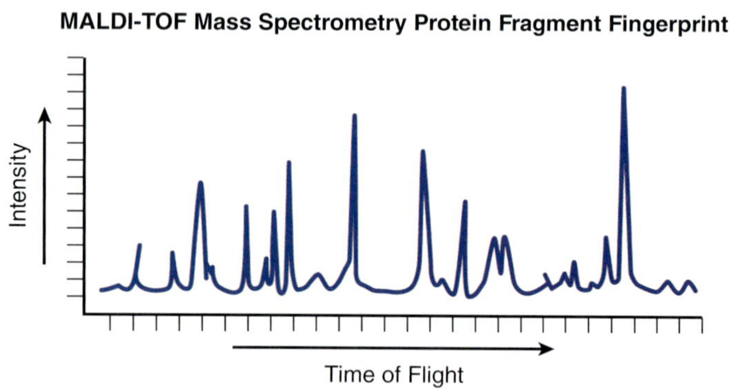

FIGURE 20–7 An example of a profile or pattern generated with MALDI-TOF. The pattern is compared with a database of known profiles, allowing for microorganism identification. *(Courtesy of James Vossler.)*

Knowledge Check 20-3

Which type of laboratory test should be used to determine if a patient has had a previous bacterial infection?
a. Molecular test for bacterial DNA
b. Rapid antigen test
c. Serology test for antibodies
d. Proteomics testing

Group A Streptococci (*Streptococcus pyogenes*)

Classification and Structure

Streptococci are gram-positive cocci; these spherical, ovoid, or lancet-shaped organisms are often arranged in pairs or chains when observed on a Gram stain **(Fig. 20–8)**. The streptococci are initially differentiated by their effect on sheep red blood cells (RBCs) when grown in culture. Those that completely lyse or hemolyze the blood cells are classified as being β-hemolytic. If the organisms only partially hemolyze the cells, causing them to appear green, they are classified as α-hemolytic. If the organisms exhibit no effect on the cells, they are referred to as γ-hemolytic. The β-hemolytic streptococci are further classified according to a group-specific carbohydrate composition that divides the bacteria into 20 groups designated A through H and K through V. These are known as the **Lancefield groups,** based on the pioneering work of Dr. Rebecca Lancefield.

A member of the β-hemolytic streptococci is *S. pyogenes*, a major cause of bacterial pharyngitis (a throat infection) and childhood impetigo (a skin infection). Because *S. pyogenes* has a group A carbohydrate, the organism is also referred to as **group A streptococcus (GAS).** Other cell wall components, the M and T proteins, allow for further classification and differentiation **(Fig. 20–9).** The M protein is a filamentous molecule consisting of two α-helical chains twisted into a ropelike structure that extends out from the cell surface. Some strains have a hyaluronic acid capsule outside the cell wall that contributes to the bacterium's antiphagocytic properties.

Serotyping and molecular techniques can be used to identify a particular strain of GAS. Serotyping involves identifying the M protein antigens by precipitation with type-specific antisera. More than 100 different serotypes have been identified by this method. However, serotyping has limitations, including limited availability of typing sera, new M protein types that do not react with the antisera, and difficulty in interpreting the results. Genotyping techniques involving PCR amplification of a portion of the *emm* gene, which codes for the M protein, followed by sequence analysis circumvents these problems. Pulsed-field gel electrophoresis (PFGE) has also been used for epidemiological studies. In PFGE, DNA from GAS is separated by using an alternating current to obtain a unique pattern or "fingerprint." The patterns from multiple sources may be compared when there is a group A streptococcal outbreak.

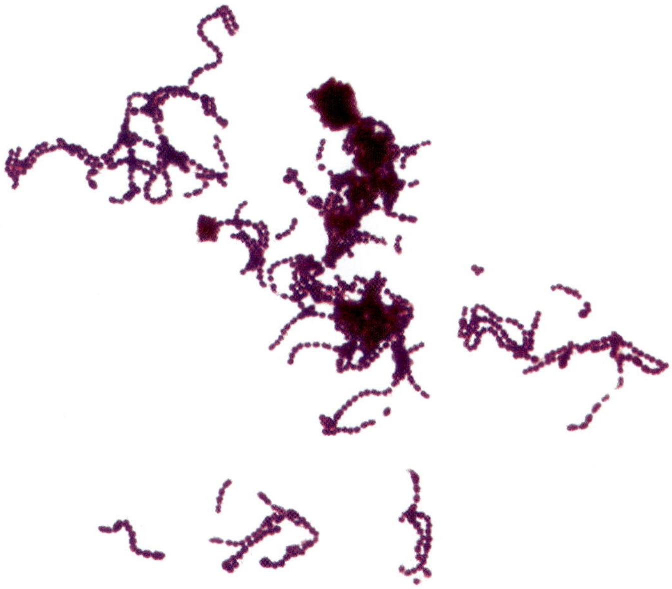

FIGURE 20–8 Gram stain of *Streptococcus pyogenes,* also known as group A streptococci, which are gram-positive cocci that grow in pairs and chains. *(Courtesy of James Vossler.)*

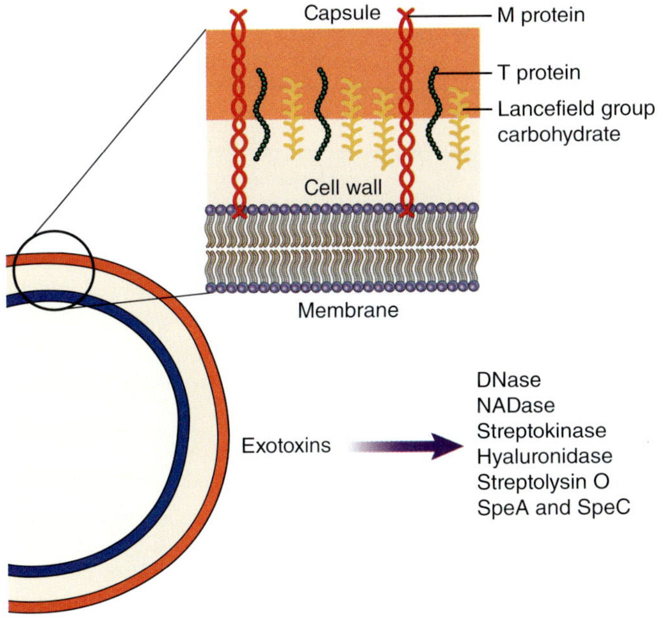

FIGURE 20–9 Diagram of antigenic components of *Streptococcus pyogenes.*

Virulence Factors

GAS is one of the most common and ubiquitous pathogenic bacteria and causes a variety of infections. The M protein is the major virulence factor of GAS and has a net-negative charge at the amino-terminal end that helps to inhibit phagocytosis. The M protein also limits deposition of C3 on the bacterial surface, thereby diminishing complement activation. The M protein, along with lipoteichoic acid and protein F, help GAS attach to host cells. Immunity to GAS appears to be associated with antibodies to the M protein. There are more than 100 serotypes of this protein, and immunity is serotype specific. Therefore, infections with one strain will not provide protection against another strain.

Additional virulence factors include various exotoxins that may be produced during the course of an infection. *S. pyogenes* produces several pyrogenic (fever-inducing) exotoxins called Spe A, B, and C. SpeA and SpeC are superantigens that induce inflammation by nonspecifically activating T cells and stimulating production of inflammatory cytokines. SpeB is believed to contribute to the invasion of GAS into tissues, cellular apoptosis, and recurrent infection with GAS. Other extracellular substances include the enzymes **streptolysin O,** deoxyribonuclease B (DNase B), hyaluronidase, nicotinamide adenine dinucleotide (NAD), and streptokinase. Antibodies produced against these substances are useful in the diagnosis of infection and complications or sequelae associated with GAS infection (discussed later in the chapter).

Clinical Manifestations of Group A Streptococcal Infection

S. pyogenes is responsible for infections ranging from pharyngitis (inflammation of the pharynx resulting in a sore throat) to life-threatening illnesses such as necrotizing fasciitis and streptococcal toxic shock syndrome. The two major sites of infections in humans are the upper respiratory tract and the skin, with pharyngitis ("strep throat") and streptococcal pyoderma (a skin infection) being the most common clinical manifestations. Symptoms of pharyngitis include fever, chills, severe sore throat, headache, tonsillar exudates, petechial rash on the soft palate, and anterior cervical lymphadenopathy **(Fig. 20–10).** The most common skin infection is *streptococcal pyoderma* (also known as **impetigo**), characterized by vesicular lesions on the extremities that become pustular and crusted **(Fig. 20–11).** These infections tend to occur in young children. Other complications include otitis

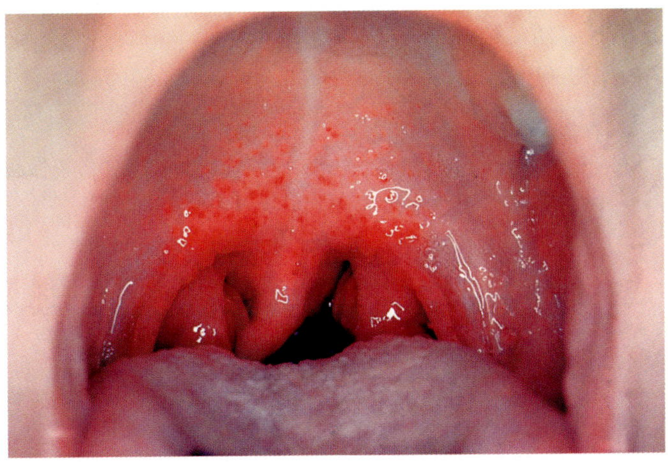

FIGURE 20–10 Pharyngitis, or sore throat, is characterized by swelling and reddening of the pharynx. Note the inflammation of the oropharynx and petechiae, or small red spots on the soft palate caused by *Streptococcal pharyngitis. (Courtesy of the CDC/Henry F. Eichenwald, Public Health Image Library.)*

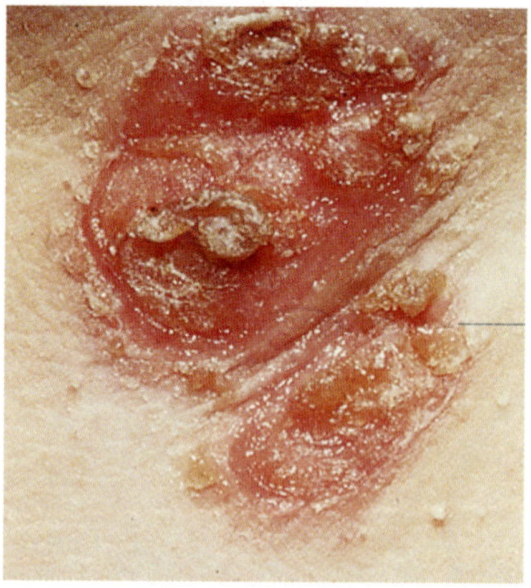

FIGURE 20–11 Impetigo is a dermatologic streptococcal infection that is characterized by thick, golden-yellow discharge that dries, crusts, and sticks to the skin. It is also caused by the *S. aureus* bacteria. *(Courtesy of the CDC/Dr. Herman Miranda, Public Health Image Library.)*

media (inflammation of the ear), erysipelas (superficial skin infection), cellulitis (infection of the deeper layers of the skin), puerperal sepsis (genital tract infection that can occur after delivery of a child), and sinusitis (inflammation of the tissues in the sinuses). Septic arthritis, acute bacterial endocarditis, and meningitis also can result from a pharyngeal infection. Humans are the primary reservoir for GAS, and transmission of GAS is from person to person.

A small percentage of individuals develop **scarlet fever.** Although usually associated with pharyngeal infections, scarlet fever may occur with streptococcal infections at other sites. Symptoms include a fever of higher than 101°F, nausea, vomiting, headache, and abdominal pain. A distinct scarlet rash initially appears on the neck and chest and then spreads all over the body. Scarlet fever results from infection with a GAS that elaborates streptococcal pyrogenic exotoxins (erythrogenic toxins). Two of those toxins, SpeA and SpeC, can act as superantigens that may induce toxic shock syndrome. Toxic shock syndrome is a life-threatening multisystem disease that often begins as a skin or soft tissue infection and may proceed to shock and renal failure because of cytokine overproduction.

Necrotizing fasciitis may occur when a GAS skin infection invades the muscles in the extremities or the trunk. The onset is acute and is a medical emergency. Exotoxins produced by *S. pyogenes* cause a rapidly spreading infection deep in the fascia, resulting in ischemia, tissue necrosis, and septicemia if not treated promptly. The disease may be associated with predisposing conditions such as chronic illness in older adults or varicella (chickenpox) in children, but healthy persons can be affected as well. Reporting of necrotizing fasciitis and toxic shock syndrome is part of a surveillance program conducted by the Centers for Disease Control and Prevention (CDC). Although the incidence of this syndrome has declined in the United States, a significant number of cases are still reported each year.

Group A Streptococcal Sequelae

GAS has the potential to develop into two serious sequelae: **acute rheumatic fever** and **poststreptococcal glomerulonephritis (PSGN).** *Sequelae* are conditions that are the consequence of a previous disease or injury. The sequelae result from the host's immune response to infection. Serological testing plays a major role in the diagnosis of these two diseases because the organism itself may no longer be present by the time symptoms appear.

Acute rheumatic fever can develop if strep throat, scarlet fever, and GAS skin infections (impetigo) are not treated properly. Acute rheumatic fever develops as a sequela to pharyngitis or tonsillitis in 2% to 3% of infected people. It is associated with the M antigen serotypes 1, 4, 12, and 25. The latency period is typically 1 to 3 weeks after onset of the sore throat. Characteristic features of acute rheumatic fever include fever, pain caused by inflammation in the joints, and inflammation of the heart. If it is not treated promptly, rheumatic heart disease may develop. Rheumatic heart disease weakens the heart valves, and if severe enough, may require surgery or in advanced cases result in death.

Acute rheumatic fever is most likely caused by antibodies or cell-mediated immune responses originally produced against streptococcal antigens that cross-react with antigens in human heart tissue. Chief among the antibodies thought to be involved are those directed toward the M proteins, which have at least three epitopes that resemble antigens in heart tissue, permitting cross-reactivity to occur. Titers of some antibodies may remain high for several years following infection.

The second potential sequelae following a streptococcal infection is PSGN, a condition that affects the kidneys. PSGN is thought to be caused by a type III hypersensitivity reaction that is triggered by production of SpeB and nephritis-associated plasmin receptor (NAPlr). PSGN is associated with the nephrogenic strains of *S. pyogenes* with the M antigen serotypes 2, 42, 49, 56, 57, and 60. PSGN may range from being asymptomatic to a full-blown acute nephritic syndrome. Symptoms of glomerulonephritis may include hematuria, proteinuria, edema, and hypertension. Patients may also experience malaise, backache, and abdominal discomfort. Renal function is usually impaired because the glomerular filtration rate is reduced, but renal failure is not typical.

The most widely accepted theory for the pathogenesis of poststreptococcal glomerulonephritis is that it results from deposition of immune complexes containing streptococcal antigens in the glomeruli. These immune complexes stimulate an inflammatory response involving release of lysosomal contents from WBCs and complement activation, resulting in kidney damage and impaired function.

Laboratory Diagnosis

Culture

Diagnosis of acute streptococcal infections typically is made by culturing the organism from the infected site. The specimen is plated on sheep blood agar and incubated. If GAS is present, small translucent colonies surrounded by a clear zone of β-hemolysis will be visible **(Fig. 20–12).** Identification is based on susceptibility to bacitracin, testing for L-pyrrolidonyl-β-naphthylamide (PYR) activity, or Lancefield typing.

Detection of Group A Streptococcal Antigens

As an alternative to culture, rapid assays have been commercially developed to detect group A streptococcal antigens directly from throat swabs. The group A antigens are extracted by enzymatic or chemical means, and the process takes anywhere from 2 to 30 minutes.

Lateral flow immunochromatographic assays (LFAs) are increasingly being used to detect bacterial, viral, fungal, and parasitic antigens in clinical samples (see Chapter 11), and have largely replaced enzyme immunoassay (EIA) and LA assays. LFAs are widely used in outpatient clinics, physician offices, and urgent care facilities for rapid diagnosis of streptococcal pharyngitis.

The assays are technically easy to perform, allow for single-sample testing because of the incorporation of an internal control, and in many cases, are more sensitive than traditional laboratory methods and other antigen detection methods (see Fig. 11–16). An example of an LFA used for the detection of GAS from a throat swab is shown in **Figure 20–13.**

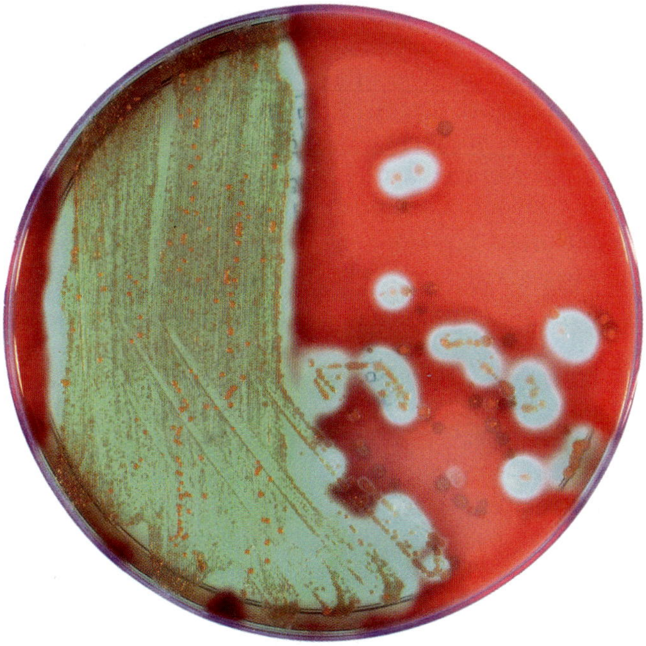

FIGURE 20–12 Throat culture plate showing a positive result for β-hemolytic group A streptococci *(S. pyogenes).* Bacterial colonies not producing β-hemolysis represent indigenous microbiota of the oropharynx. *(Courtesy of James Vossler.)*

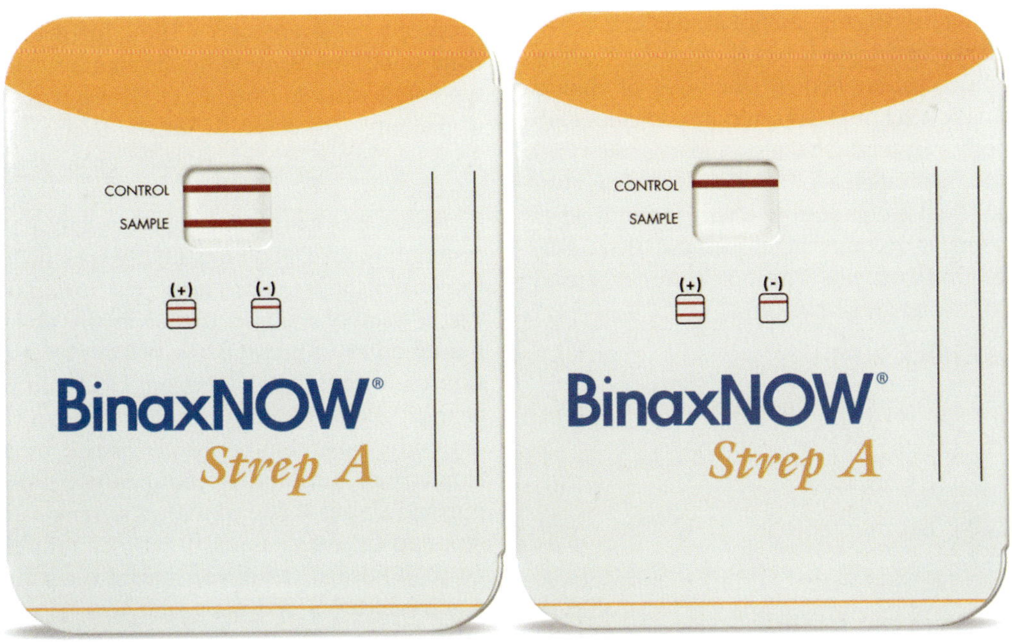

FIGURE 20–13 BinaxNOW lateral flow assay. The BinaxNOW Strep A rapid immunochromatographic assay for the qualitative detection of *Streptococcus pyogenes* group A antigen from throat swab specimens. To perform the test, a throat swab is inserted into the test card. Extraction reagents are added from dropper bottles. The test card is closed to bring the extracted sample in contact with the test strip. Strep A antigen captured by immobilized anti-strep A binds conjugated antibody in the test area. Immobilized species antibody captures the second visualizing conjugate in the control zone. The test is interpreted by the presence or absence of visually detectable pink-to-purple colored lines. A positive result is indicated by production of both a sample line and a control line (shown on left), whereas a negative assay will produce only the control line (shown on right). *(BinaxNOW is a trademark of Abbott, Inc. Used with permission.)*

Many of the assays require no more than 2 to 5 minutes of hands-on time. The specificity and sensitivity of the assays in many instances are higher than other methods. Although the assays have high sensitivity, cultures should be performed when rapid test results are negative. Molecular methods, including hybridization of specific rRNA sequences and qPCR, have also been developed to rapidly detect GAS in clinical specimens.

Detection of Streptococcal Antibodies

Culture or rapid screening methods are very useful for diagnosis of acute pharyngitis. However, serological assays must be used to identify acute rheumatic fever and PSGN because the organism is unlikely to be present in the pharynx or on the skin at the time symptoms appear. Group A streptococci elaborate more than 20 exotoxins, and the antibody response to one or more of these is used as documentation of nonsuppurative (non-pus forming) disease. Some of the exotoxin products include streptolysins O and S; deoxyribonucleases A, B, C, and D; streptokinase; NADase; hyaluronidase; diphosphopyridine nucleotidase; and pyrogenic exotoxins.

The antibody response to these streptococcal products is variable because of several factors, such as age of onset, site of infection, and timeliness of antibiotic treatment. The most diagnostically important antibodies are anti-streptolysin O (ASO) and anti-DNase B. After a pharyngeal infection, the ASO and anti-DNase B titers are commonly elevated. Only the anti-DNase B titer is typically increased after a skin infection. During group A streptococcal infections, other antibodies are made to cellular antigens, such as the group A carbohydrate and the M protein, but these antibodies are not detected routinely because commercial reagents are not available.

Serological evidence of disease is based on an elevated or rising titer of streptococcal antibodies. The onset of clinical symptoms of rheumatic fever or PSGN typically coincides with the peak of antibody response. If acute- and convalescent-phase sera are tested in parallel, a fourfold rise in titer is considered significant. The use of at least two tests for antibodies to different exotoxins is recommended because detectable ASO is not produced in all patients. The most commonly used tests are those for ASO and anti-DNase B.

Knowledge Check 20-4

Serological testing for group A streptococcal antibodies is useful for the diagnosis of which condition?

a. Pharyngitis
b. Impetigo
c. Acute rheumatic fever
d. Scarlet fever

Anti-Streptolysin O (ASO) Testing

ASO tests detect antibodies to the streptolysin O enzyme produced by GAS. This enzyme is able to lyse RBCs. The presence of antibodies to streptolysin O indicates recent streptococcal infection in patients suspected of having acute rheumatic fever or PSGN following a throat infection. ASO titers typically increase within 1 to 2 weeks after infection and peak between 3 to 6 weeks after the initial symptoms (e.g., sore throat). However, an antibody response occurs in only about 85% of patients with acute rheumatic fever within this period. ASO titers usually do not increase in people with skin infections, possibly because free cholesterol in the skin binds to streptolysin O and decreases its immunogenicity.

The first test developed to determine the **ASO titer** was a manual test based on the ability of antibodies in dilutions of the patient's serum to neutralize the hemolytic activity of streptolysin O on reagent RBCs. Because of the labor-intensive nature of this test and because the streptolysin O reagent and the RBCs used were not stable, today ASO testing is most commonly performed by nephelometry or immunoturbidimetry (see Chapter 10). These methods are automated procedures that provide rapid, quantitative measurement of ASO titers. The antigen used in this technique, purified recombinant streptolysin, is attached to polystyrene particles. When antibody-positive patient serum combines with the antigen reagent, immune complexes are formed, resulting in an increase in light scatter or a reduction in light transmission. Results are reported in international units per milliliter (IU/mL) based on the World Health Organization international standard.

ASO titers tend to be highest in school-age children and young adults. The range of expected normal values varies, depending on the patient's age and geographic location. Thus, individual laboratories must establish their own upper limits of normal for specific populations.

Anti-Deoxyribonuclease B (Anti-DNase B) Testing

Testing for **anti-DNase B** is usually performed in conjunction with ASO testing. Detection of anti-DNase B is clinically useful in patients suspected of having glomerulonephritis preceded by streptococcal skin infections because, as we mentioned, ASO antibodies often are not stimulated by this type of disease. Antibodies to DNase B may also be detected in patients with acute rheumatic fever who have a negative ASO test result. Titers typically peak at 6 to 8 weeks after infection.

DNase B is mainly produced by group A streptococci, so testing for anti-DNase B is highly specific for group A streptococcal sequelae. The classic test for anti-DNase B activity was a manual method based on the ability of anti-DNase B antibodies to neutralize a reagent DNase B enzyme, preventing it from depolymerizing DNA and producing a color change. As with ASO testing, testing for anti-DNase B is currently most commonly performed by automated nephelometry or turbidimetry by incubating patient serum with purified DNase B bound to polystyrene particles. Results are reported in international units per milliliter (IU/mL). The range of normal values varies with the patient's age and geographic location and must therefore be established by individual testing laboratories.

Critical Thinking 20-1

Suppose an anti-DNase B test performed on a serum sample from a patient suspected of having a recent group A streptococcal infection is positive, but an ASO titer done on the same sample is negative. What are possible causes of these discrepant results?

Mycoplasma pneumoniae

Mycoplasma is a member of a unique group of organisms that belong to the class *Mollicutes*. Mycoplasmas represent the smallest known free-living life forms (150 to 250 nm) and have a small genome. Various members colonize plants, animals, and insects in addition to being human pathogens. These extracellular parasites attach to and exist on the surface of host cells using attachment organelles and adhesion molecules specific for their host cells. They absorb their nutrients from the host cells to which they are attached. The organisms lack cell walls (thus lacking peptidoglycan), have sterols in their cell membrane, and have complex growth requirements, making culture difficult and time consuming.

Mycoplasma pneumoniae Pathogenesis

The best-known *Mycoplasma* is *M. pneumoniae,* which is a leading cause of respiratory infections worldwide. *M. pneumoniae* infections are found in all age groups, with a majority involving the upper respiratory tract. *M. pneumoniae* is spread from one person to another by respiratory droplets. Relatively close association with an infected individual appears to be necessary for transmission of the organism. The incubation period is 1 to 3 weeks. The infection has an insidious onset, which differs from the acute onset observed with respiratory viruses such as influenza and adenovirus. Typically, an individual develops a fever, headache, malaise, and cough—the clinical hallmark of a *M. pneumoniae* infection. Depending on the age, about 5% to 10% of individuals progress to tracheobronchitis or pneumonia.

Originally, pneumonia caused by *M. pneumoniae* was referred to as "atypical pneumonia" because the infection could not be treated with penicillin. This is because the organism lacks the cell wall to which penicillin is directed against. In many cases, the pneumonia is mild, often appearing as a common cold, and symptoms are generally mild enough that bedrest or hospitalization is not required. The infection has been referred to as "walking pneumonia" because individuals often do not stay home from work or school and still participate in their daily activities. Although many infections are mild, *M. pneumoniae* accounts for 20% of all hospitalizations for pneumonia in the United States. *M. pneumoniae* may remain in the respiratory tract for several months after resolution of the infection, causing chronic inflammation and a lingering cough. *M. pneumoniae* may also initiate or exacerbate asthma.

Dermatologic Manifestations

Up to 7% of individuals with *M. pneumoniae* develop Stevens-Johnson syndrome, or erythema multiforme major, a condition in which the top layer of the skin dies and sheds. The syndrome is considered a medical emergency that usually requires hospitalization. The conjunctivae as well as the joints and various organs in the genitourinary and gastrointestinal tract may also be involved. The basis of Stevens-Johnson syndrome is not clearly known, but it may be caused by the immune response of the host or by augmented sensitivity to antibiotics while being treated for *M. pneumoniae*.

Another manifestation of *M. pneumoniae* infection is Raynaud syndrome, a transient vasospasm of the digits in which the fingers turn white when exposed to the cold. Although the exact cause is unclear, it may be related to the development and action of cold agglutinins in the body (see Chapter 14). Other extrapulmonary manifestations of Raynaud syndrome include arthritis, meningoencephalitis, pericarditis, and peripheral neuropathy.

Immunology of *Mycoplasma pneumoniae* Infection

In addition to stimulating the production of many proinflammatory and anti-inflammatory cytokines and chemokines, several classes of antibodies are produced in the course of an *M. pneumoniae* infection. As with any infection in which there is a humoral response, the body produces antibodies that neutralize the microorganism. *M. pneumoniae* also induces the production of autoantibodies, including agglutinins directed against the lungs, brain, cardiolipins, and smooth muscle.

The cold agglutinins observed with *M. pneumoniae* infection are oligoclonal IgM antibodies directed against the altered I antigens found on the surface of human RBCs. These antibodies can agglutinate the RBCs at temperatures below 37°C (see Chapter 14). Development of the antibodies is thought to result from cross-reaction of antibodies formed against *M. pneumoniae* and the I antigen on human RBCs, or from alteration of the RBC antigen by the organism.

Laboratory Diagnosis of *Mycoplasma pneumoniae* Infection

Laboratory means of detecting *Mycoplasma* infection may involve culturing the organism, detecting *M. pneumoniae*–specific antibodies in serum, and identifying *M. pneumoniae* nucleotide sequences directly in patient specimens.

Detection of *Mycoplasma pneumoniae* by Culture

Although culturing has been considered the gold standard for diagnosis, culturing for the organism is rarely carried out in the clinical laboratory because of the fastidious nature of *M. pneumoniae*. Collection and transport of the specimen differ from traditional methods used for other microorganisms. The transport media may be trypticase soy broth with 0.5% albumin, SP4 medium, or a viral transport medium. If the sample cannot be plated immediately, it should be frozen at –70°C. Culturing requires the use of specialized media designed for the recovery of *Mycoplasma*. The organism takes several weeks to grow in most cases. If the culture is successfully performed, the growth produces a "mulberry" colony with a typical "fried egg" appearance. Because of the difficulty in culturing for the organism and the time required for the organism to grow, culturing for the organism is rarely used for human clinical samples but is widely used in veterinary diagnostic laboratories.

Detection of Antibodies to *Mycoplasma pneumoniae*

M. pneumoniae–specific antibodies can be detected about 1 week after infection, peak at 3 to 6 weeks, and then decline gradually. Several methods have been developed to detect these antibodies. The most widely used are qualitative EIAs for point-of-care testing and ELISA for measurement of IgM and IgG antibodies. *M. pneumoniae*–specific IgM likely indicates a recent infection, but paired acute and convalescent-phase serum testing is considered the best serological approach for confirming recent infection. Although IgM is the primary immunoglobulin response to infection, testing for IgG antibodies is also necessary; the reason is that adults may only elicit an IgG response because of reinfection with the organism.

For many years, before the development of antigen-specific serological tests, laboratory diagnosis of *M. pneumoniae* involved testing for cold agglutinins. Cold agglutinins develop in about 50% of patients with *M. pneumoniae* infection. These antibodies are produced early in the disease (7 to 10 days) and can typically be detected at the time the patient seeks medical attention. The titer peaks at 2 to 3 weeks, and antibodies are present for 2 to 3 months after infection. A titer of 1:64 or greater, along with the clinical presentation of the patient, suggest infection with *M. pneumoniae*. Although once considered the primary means of diagnosing *Mycoplasma* infection, testing for cold agglutinins is no longer recommended because the test is not very sensitive or specific; these antibodies are also associated with other conditions, including some viral infections (e.g., infectious mononucleosis and cytomegalovirus) and collagen vascular diseases.

Molecular Diagnosis of Mycoplasma Infections

Since 2012, the number of FDA-approved molecular tests for the detection of *M. pneumoniae* genes has increased. One widely used method is the BioFire FilmArray Respiratory Panel, developed by BioFire Diagnostics, Inc., now part of bioMérieux SA. Using nested multiplex PCR, the assay can detect 20 respiratory viruses and bacteria, including *B. pertussis*, *C. pneumoniae*, and *M. pneumoniae*. Another popular method is the Illumigene Mycoplasma Direct by Meridian Bioscience, which uses loop-mediated isothermal amplification (LAMP) technology to detect *M. pneumoniae* in throat swab specimens (see Chapter 12). As additional assays are developed and receive FDA approval, molecular testing will become more widespread and will likely become the primary means of diagnosing *M. pneumoniae* infections.

Knowledge Check 20-5

What is the best laboratory method for diagnosing a current *M. pneumoniae* infection?

a. IgM-specific *M. pneumoniae* antibodies by rapid EIA
b. IgG-specific *M. pneumoniae* antibodies by ELISA
c. Cold agglutinin titers
d. Molecular testing for *M. pneumoniae* DNA

Rickettsial Infections

Members of the *Rickettsiaceae* family cause a variety of infections in humans and animals. Because of advances in molecular technology, various members originally belonging to the genus ***Rickettsiae*** have been reclassified. These obligate intracellular, gram-negative bacteria now include the genera *Rickettsia* (rickettsiosis) and *Orientia* (*Orientia tsutsugamushi* causing scrub typhus). Additional members are the *Ehrlichia* group including *Ehrlichia* (ehrlichiosis), *Anaplasma* (anaplasmosis), *Neorickettsia* (associated with helminths), and *Neoehrlichia*.

Agents of *Rickettsia*-Related Disease

Two distinct groups compose the genus *Rickettsia:* the spotted fever group (SFG) and the **typhus** group (TG). Each is responsible for a different set of diseases **(Table 20–1).** In the United States, the main rickettsial disease is **Rocky Mountain spotted fever (RMSF),** caused by *R. rickettsia* (SFG). Epidemic typhus, caused by *Rickettsia prowazekii* (TG), is the most prevalent member of the TG globally. Typhus fever (also known as *epidemic typhus*) occurs in conditions of poor hygiene and overcrowding, such as in prisons and refugee camps. Epidemic typhus was responsible for more than 3 million deaths in World War I. Once prevalent throughout the globe in the first half of the 20th century, epidemic typhus exists mainly in developing countries of the world today. People traveling to areas with large homeless populations and regions that have recently experienced war or natural disasters leading to poor hygiene and crowded conditions (such as refugee camps) are at risk of acquiring typhus fever.

Each of the species responsible for the various rickettsial diseases has a variety of animal reservoirs. The vectors responsible for the transmission are arthropods (ticks, mites, lice, or fleas) that transmit the organism through their bite after feeding on an infected animal **(Fig. 20–14).** The one exception is typhus fever (epidemic louse-borne typhus), which is transmitted when an infected human body louse excretes *R. prowazekii* onto the skin while feeding, and the individual becomes infected by rubbing louse fecal matter or crushed

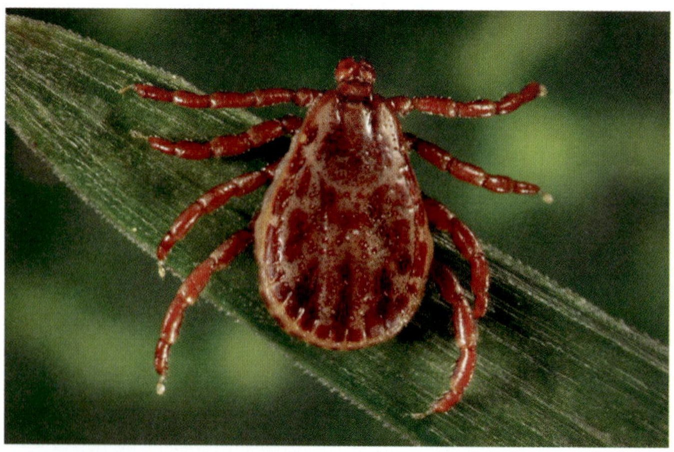

FIGURE 20–14 The Rocky Mountain wood tick, *Dermacentor andersoni*, is a known North American vector of *Rickettsia rickettsii*. *(Courtesy of the CDC/Dr. Christopher Paddock and James Gathany, Public Health Image Library.)*

lice into the bite wound. Except for *R. prowazekii* (epidemic typhus), humans are accidental hosts for *Rickettsia* and *Rickettsia*-related organisms. *Rickettsia* and *Rickettsia*-related organisms have worldwide distribution; however, certain members have a specific geographic distribution. For example, *Rickettsia japonica* is found only in Japan, whereas *R. rickettsii* is found in the Western hemisphere. Some species, such as *Rickettsia typhi*, are found worldwide.

The members of the *Rickettsia* genus and *Anaplasma* and *Ehrlichia* cause several clinical diseases. Because of the prevalence of RMSF in North and South America, this chapter focuses on RMSF.

Table 20-1 Classification of Selected *Rickettsiae* Known to Cause Disease in Humans

ANTIGENIC GROUP	DISEASE	SPECIES	VECTOR	ANIMAL RESERVOIR(S)	GEOGRAPHIC DISTRIBUTION
Anaplasma	Human anaplasmosis	*Anaplasma phagocytophilum*	Ticks	Small mammals, rodents, and deer	Worldwide, primarily United States
Ehrlichia	Human monocytic ehrlichiosis	*Ehrlichia chaffeensis*	Ticks	Deer, wild and domestic dogs, domestic ruminants, and rodents	United States, possibly elsewhere worldwide
Neoehrlichia	Human neoehrlichiosis	*Neoehrlichia mikurensis*	Ticks	Rodents	Europe, Asia
Neorickettsia	Sennetsu fever	*Neorickettsia sennetsu*	Trematodes	Fish	Japan, Malaysia, possibly other parts of Asia
Scrub typhus	Scrub typhus	*Orientia tsutsugamushi, Orientia chuto*	Trombiculid mites and chiggers (mite larvae)	Rodents	Asia-Pacific region (north Australia, China, Indonesia, maritime Russia); Middle East (Afghanistan); possibly several countries in sub-Saharan Africa; United Arab Emirates (UAE)
Spotted fever	Rocky Mountain spotted fever	*Rickettsia rickettsii*	Ticks	Rodents	North, Central, and South America
	Rickettsiosis	*Rickettsia aeschlimannii*	Ticks	Unknown	Africa (South Africa); North and South America; Asia (Korea); southern and eastern Europe (Balkans, Turkey, Ukraine, and former Soviet Union)
	Queensland tick typhus	*Rickettsia australis*	Ticks	Rodents	Australia, Tasmania
	Mediterranean spotted fever (Boutonneuse fever)	*Rickettsia conorii*	Ticks	Dogs, rodents	Africa; southern Europe; southern and western Asia (India)
Typhus	Epidemic typhus, sylvatic typhus	*Rickettsia prowazekii*	*Human body louse, flying squirrel ectoparasites*	Humans, flying squirrels	Central Africa; North, Central and South America; Asia
	Murine typhus	*Rickettsia typhi*	Fleas	Rodents	Temperate, tropical, and subtropical areas worldwide

Adapted from Centers for Disease Control and Prevention. *2024 Yellow Book for Rickettsia*. Online version at https://wwwnc.cdc.gov/travel/yellowbook/2024/infections-diseases/rickettsial-diseases. Accessed December 2, 2024.

Rocky Mountain Spotted Fever

Epidemiology

Rocky Mountain spotted fever (RMSF) is caused by *R. rickettsii*, which is transmitted to the human host by a tick bite. In the United States, the organism is transmitted by the American dog tick *(Dermacentor variabilis)*, the Rocky Mountain wood tick *(Dermacentor andersoni)*, and the brown dog tick *(Rhipicephalus sanguineus)*. Although called *Rocky Mountain* spotted fever, five states—North Carolina, Oklahoma, Arkansas, Tennessee, and Missouri—account for more than 60% of RMSF cases in the continental United States. The occurrence of the disease has seasonal variation corresponding to tick activity, being most prevalent between May and September. The organism is transmitted transstadially in the tick (i.e., it remains present in the tick as the tick progresses from the nymph state to the adult) and is transmitted transovarially (from generation to generation through the eggs of the tick), allowing for maintenance of the organism in the tick population. Transmission occurs when the tick bites the host for a blood meal. When the tick has fed after 6 to 10 hours, the organism is injected into the host from the salivary glands.

Pathogenesis

Once introduced into the skin, the organisms spread via the lymphatic and circulatory systems, where they attach to and invade their target cells, the vascular endothelium, by means of the OmpA and OmpB ligands. The organisms multiply by binary fission inside the endothelial cells, are released, and infect adjacent cells. This leads to hundreds of contiguous infected cells, producing the lesions and skin rash associated with the infection. The main pathophysiological event caused by the infection is endothelial cell damage, which leads to increased vascular permeability, resulting in edema, hypovolemia (low extracellular fluid volume), hypotension (low blood pressure), and hypoalbuminemia (decreased level of blood albumin).

Clinical Manifestations

The symptoms observed with RMSF occur approximately 2 to 14 days (median 7 days) after a tick bite. Before the development of the hallmark rash, a large percentage of patients will experience a severe headache, nausea, vomiting, abdominal pain, diarrhea, and abdominal tenderness. The fever usually begins within the first 3 to 5 days after the onset of symptoms, and the rash usually appears 3 to 5 days after the onset of the fever. The rash typically starts on the hands and soles of the feet and proceeds to the trunk, although it may start on the trunk in some people **(Fig. 20–15)**. With the classic form of RMSF, death occurs 7 to 15 days after the onset of symptoms if appropriate therapy is not provided. With the fulminant (i.e., severe and sudden onset) form of RMSF, death occurs within the first 5 days. The resolution or fatal outcome of the disease is largely related to the timeliness of initiating appropriate therapy. Immediate treatment with doxycycline reduces the severity of the infection.

Diagnosis of RMSF

Initial diagnosis is often made clinically after ruling out various other conditions, including typhoid fever, measles, rubella, enteroviral infection, and respiratory tract infection.

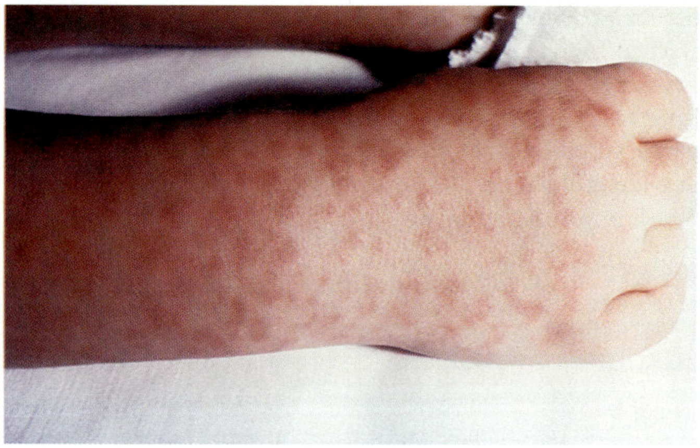

FIGURE 20–15 The characteristic spotted rash of Rocky Mountain spotted fever, the most severe and most frequently reported rickettsial illness in the United States. The disease is caused by *Rickettsia rickettsii. (Courtesy of the CDC, Public Health Image Library.)*

The overlapping symptoms, or clinical presentation, during the initial stages of the disease can make the diagnosis of RMSF extremely difficult. The diagnosis of fulminant RMSF is even more difficult because of its rapid course. The rash develops shortly before death, if at all; therefore, antibodies to *R. rickettsii* do not have time to develop.

Serological and Molecular Diagnosis

The organism infects the endothelial cells and does not circulate until the disease has severely progressed. Therefore, culturing for the organism is not of any value in the diagnosis of RMSF. If the patient has a rash, immunohistochemistry (IHC) assays can be performed on skin biopsies of a rash lesion. IHC assays for the detection of *R. rickettsii* are only available at specialized laboratories. Serology is the usual method for confirming the diagnosis of RMSF, but this is a retrospective diagnosis. Antibodies to *R. rickettsia* develop 7 to 10 days after the onset of symptoms, and most patients do not have detectable antibodies during the first week of illness. For a successful outcome, therapy needs to be initiated before that time.

The gold standard for the serological diagnosis of RMSF is the indirect immunofluorescence assay (IFA) with *R. rickettsii* antigen, performed on paired acute and convalescent serum samples collected 2 to 4 weeks apart to demonstrate a fourfold rise in antibody titers. The test is specific for *R. rickettsii* IgM and IgG antibodies and is widely available in the United States. In this test, patient serum is incubated with a microscope slide to which *R. rickettsii* antigen has been bound. Following a wash step, a fluorescein-labeled anti-human immunoglobulin is added; after a second incubation and wash, the slide is examined with a fluorescence microscope. For many years, antibodies produced in patients with rickettsial infections were detected by an agglutination test known as the Weil-Felix test, which was based on cross-reactivity of the patient's antibodies with polysaccharide antigens present on the OX-19 and OX-2 strains of *Proteus vulgaris* and the OX-K strain of *Proteus mirabilis*. This test has largely been replaced with new serological methods, although it continues to be used in countries where more advanced methods are unavailable. In late 2023, the FDA approved a qPCR assay that was developed by the National Center for Emerging and Zoonotic Infectious Diseases (NCEZID) to identify rickettsial DNA in blood samples in the early stages of the infection. This test provides more rapid results than serological testing for antibodies, enabling earlier diagnosis of the infection.

Knowledge Check 20-6

The indirect immunofluorescence assay (IFA) is commonly used in RMSF diagnosis. What does it detect?
a. *Rickettsia rickettsii* antigens in the skin
b. Antibodies against *Rickettsia rickettsii*
c. *Rickettsia rickettsii* antigens in the blood
d. DNA fragments of *Rickettsia rickettsii* in the blood

Mycobacteria

Mycobacteria are a group of organisms that have very complex cell walls, as compared to other bacteria. They are classified as gram positive, with a thick peptidoglycan layer, but their cell walls also have an outer layer composed mainly of mycolic acids. The mycolic acids are waxlike, giving the mycobacteria several unique characteristics. For example, they are able to resist decolorization with acid alcohol during staining. Because of this property, the mycobacteria are referred to as **acid-fast bacilli** (AFB). The Ziehl-Neelsen stain and the Kinyoun stain are the most commonly used stains to detect *Mycobacterium* species in clinical specimens. The stains dye the acid-fast bacilli bright red, which makes them distinct against a blue or green background (refer to Fig. 20–5). The mycolic acid layer also contributes to the pathogenicity of mycobacteria, allowing them to resist destruction by phagocytic cells and survive inside macrophages, where they can hide from the immune system. The mycolic acids also make the bacteria less susceptible to antibiotics.

Mycobacterium tuberculosis Complex (MTB Complex)

Within the genus *Mycobacterium,* there are over 200 recognized species, and these can be classified as part of the *Mycobacterium tuberculosis* complex or the *nontuberculosis mycobacteria.* The ***Mycobacterium tuberculosis* complex (MTB complex)** has 11 different species, with the most recognized being *Mycobacterium tuberculosis,* a primary cause of tuberculosis (TB) in humans. *Mycobacterium bovis,* another member of the MTB complex, is the main cause of TB in cattle, deer, and other mammals. The organism can also be responsible for TB in humans. The other significant pathogen is *M. leprae,* the cause of leprosy.

Nontuberculosis Mycobacteria (NTM)

The other *Mycobacterium* species are collectively referred to as the **nontuberculosis mycobacteria (NTM).** NTM are free-living organisms found everywhere in the environment. About 200 NTM species have been identified. NTM can be responsible for four clinical syndromes in humans:

1. Pulmonary disease mainly observed in patients with cystic fibrosis and older adults with or without underlying lung disease. Infections are primarily caused by *Mycobacterium avium* complex (MAC; a group of bacteria containing *Mycobacterium avium* and *Mycobacterium intracellulare*), *Mycobacterium abscessus,* and *Mycobacterium kansasii.*
2. Lymphadenitis (especially cervical) in children, caused mostly by MAC, *Mycobacterium scrofulaceum,* and in Northern Europe, *M. malmoense* and *M. haemophilum.*
3. Disseminated disease in patients who are severely immunocompromised, mostly caused by MAC and less commonly by the rapidly growing mycobacteria (RGM), *M. abscessus, M. fortuitum,* and *M. chelonae.*
4. Skin and soft tissue infections, usually from direct inoculation and caused primarily by *M. marinum* and *M. ulcerans,* and the RGM.

Pathogenesis of Tuberculosis (TB)

TB infection begins with the inhalation of *M. tuberculosis* from aerosol droplets. Only one to 10 bacilli are necessary for transmission. Following deposition in the lungs, the bacilli are phagocytized by alveolar macrophages, where they are usually destroyed or inhibited. If they are not destroyed, infected macrophages may be carried by the lymphatic system to other areas of the body, including the lymph nodes, kidneys, and epiphyses of the long bones. Within 3 to 8 weeks, the body's immune system usually halts multiplication, preventing further spread. Hypersensitivity develops during this period, indicating the development of cell-mediated immunity. At this point, although the infection is present throughout the body, people do not have symptoms or signs other than a positive TB skin test and are said to have **latent TB infection (LTBI).** If the immune system fails to keep the organism in check, it can multiply and cause symptomatic, active tuberculosis. Of those exposed to a person with active disease, the likelihood of developing a latent infection is thought to be 90% to 95% and that of developing active TB disease, 5% to 10%.

Latent Tuberculosis Infection, TB Disease, and Reactivation Tuberculosis

Once *M. tuberculosis* bacilli are inhaled, there are four possible outcomes:

1. Clearance of the organism
2. Development of a latent infection; LTBI, a clinical state that is asymptomatic
3. Development of active disease, also known as primary tuberculosis
4. **Reactivation tuberculosis,** or development of active disease many years after a period of latent infection

Latent TB Infection (LTBI)

About one-quarter of the global population and up to 13 million people in the United States are thought to have LTBI. The duration of latency varies, and healthy people can harbor MTB bacilli for a lifetime. Previously contained latent infection with *M. tuberculosis* can provide up to 80% protection against TB disease from a subsequent exposure. People with LTBI are not infectious and cannot transmit the organisms to others. However, about 5% to 10% of individuals with LTBI will develop active disease later in life. Thus, people with LTBI are a major reservoir for new active TB cases in the United States.

Tuberculosis (TB) Disease

Tuberculosis (TB) is the leading cause of death from a bacterial infection worldwide, causing 1.25 million deaths and an estimated 10.8 million illnesses in 2023. In the United States, over 10,300 cases of TB were reported to the CDC in 2024, and more than 80% of these cases resulted from long-standing, untreated latent TB infection.

When pulmonary TB occurs, clinical manifestations of TB most often appear 1 month to 2 years after infection. Symptoms include fatigue, fever, loss of appetite, weight loss, cough with sputum production that may be bloody, night sweats, and chills. If the body does not clear the organism, a cell-mediated immune response develops, but antibodies to *M. tuberculosis* are not produced.

Reactivation Tuberculosis

Reactivation occurs when a subclinical latent infection progresses to active TB disease. People with LTBI and no underlying medical problems have about a 5% risk of developing active TB in the first 2 to 5 years after infection and another 5% risk of developing active TB over their remaining lifetime. Persons with LTBI who have an impaired immune system caused by conditions such as HIV infection, cancer, and immunosuppressive therapy have an increased risk of developing reactivation tuberculosis.

Multi-Drug Resistant (MDR) and Extensively Drug-Resistant (XDR) Tuberculosis

Treatment of tuberculosis involves the simultaneous use of several drugs. Most commonly, isoniazid (INH) combined with three other drugs—rifampin (RIF), pyrazinamide (PZA), and ethambutol (ETH)—are used to treat active TB. These drugs are considered first-line treatment for TB. Prophylaxis with isoniazid (INH) reduces the risk of developing TB in people exposed to infection or with latent infection. Second-line drugs for TB are given if first-line treatment is unsuccessful in eliminating the organism; however, these treatments are more costly and have more adverse effects.

Drug resistance in bacteria may develop through random mutations or natural selection of bacteria that become resistant during or after treatment. With increased drug usage over the years, TB strains that are resistant to one or more drugs have appeared. Several factors have led to increased drug resistance, including patients failing to complete their treatment for tuberculosis, and dissemination of the resistant strains because of increased global travel and crowded conditions in large metropolitan areas. **Multi-drug resistant TB (MDR-TB)** is defined as disease due to *M. tuberculosis* that is resistant to INH and RIF. MDR-TB occurs worldwide, with China, India, and the countries of the former Soviet Union and Russia having the highest number of MDR-TB cases. **Extensively drug-resistant tuberculosis (XDR-TB)** is defined as disease caused by strains that are resistant to INH, RIF, pyrazinamide, and ethambutol. MDR-TB and XDR-TB take much longer to treat than drug-susceptible TB and require the use of second-line anti-TB drugs. Some strains have also emerged that are resistant to one or more of the second-line agents.

Critical Thinking 20-2

A patient who recently traveled to India was diagnosed with tuberculosis. The patient started a standard anti-TB drug regimen but failed to show improvement after 2 months of treatment. Explain why treatment likely failed and what can be done next to treat this patient. What are the disadvantages to second-line treatment?

Tuberculosis Vaccines

Currently only one approved vaccine to prevent tuberculosis exists: the **Bacille Calmette-Guérin (BCG) vaccine,** first used on humans in 1921. The vaccine consists of attenuated (weakened) strains of *Mycobacterium bovis,* a bacillus that is related to *M. tuberculosis* and mostly causes tuberculosis in cattle (although strains that are not weakened may sometimes cause TB in humans). BCG vaccination is not recommended in the United States due to the low incidence of TB, but it is often given to infants and small children in other countries where TB is common and is usually part of the routine newborn immunization schedule. The vaccine has a low degree of effectiveness, likely caused by genetic changes in the strains of bacteria used to produce the vaccine over time. Research is ongoing to develop a vaccine with increased efficacy.

Laboratory Detection of Mycobacteria

Culture is the gold standard for detecting mycobacteria in clinical specimens. The CDC recommends that three sputum samples collected at least 12 hours apart be submitted to the laboratory for culture. Sputum or tissue samples must first be decontaminated and liquefied to remove fast-growing nonmycobacterial organisms. Samples submitted for culture are also treated with an AFB stain. It should be noted that the stain sensitivity for *M. tuberculosis* is only about 45% to 75%, depending on the number of bacteria shed in the respiratory tract.

The most commonly used media for culture of mycobacteria are Löwenstein-Jensen, a solid agar-based media, and Middlebrook 7H12, a liquid broth media. The media are made selective for mycobacteria by adding antibiotics. Mycobacteria are slow-growing organisms that multiply every 24 to 48 hours; therefore, detecting their growth in the laboratory takes a few days. Liquid broth cultures require about 10 days of incubation for AFB-positive, and 20 days for AFB-negative, specimens for detection of organisms, as compared with solid media, which require 3 to 8 weeks. Cultures for mycobacteria are examined up to 8 weeks before being determined to have no growth. Identification of the bacteria from cultures is traditionally based on biochemical testing, but that has been replaced with molecular methods, mainly DNA sequencing.

Faster detection of MTB from clinical specimens can be performed by PCR or a target-amplified nucleic acid probe test. For example, the GeneXpert MTB/RIF assay (Cepheid, Sunnyvale, CA), only takes about 2 hours to obtain results. The test uses qPCR to amplify an *M. tuberculosis* gene and also detects the gene for rifampin resistance, an indicator of MDR-TB. As compared with culture, the GeneXpert MTB/RIF assay had an overall sensitivity of 89% and specificity of 99% for detection of *M. tuberculosis* in sputum samples. MTB isolates are also routinely tested for susceptibility to first-line drugs—INH, RIF, pyrazinamide (PZA), and ethambutol (EMB)—to detect drug-resistant strains.

Testing for *M. tuberculosis* Infection

There are two types of tests that can be used to determine if a person has been exposed to *M. tuberculosis:* skin testing and blood testing for interferon gamma (IFN-γ) production. Both types evaluate the individual's cell-mediated immune response to the organism. Skin tests are referred to as the *Mantoux test*, *TB skin test*, *tuberculin skin test (TST)*, and *PPD (purified protein derivative) test.* Mantoux refers to the technique for administering the test, which involves injecting a small amount of PPD solution just beneath the surface of the skin, usually on the forearm. The solution contains an inactivated protein extract from *M. tuberculosis* cultures. Most people infected with *M. tuberculosis* develop a red, swollen skin reaction at the injection site over 2 to 3 days (see Chapter 14). Some people who were exposed to TB in the distant past may have a false-negative skin test because the immune response to TB has weakened over time. If a first skin test is negative, a second skin test may be done 1 to 2 weeks later. In this two-step skin testing method, the first PPD test may "boost" the response if it has faded over time, allowing reactivity to occur on the repeat test in people who have been previously exposed to TB. People who have received the BCG vaccine or have been infected with cross-reacting NTM may also test positive with the PPD test. HIV infection or other causes of immunosuppression can cause false negative results.

Per the CDC guidelines, annual TB testing of health care personnel is not recommended unless there is a known exposure or ongoing transmission at a health care facility. Health care personnel with untreated latent TB infection should receive an annual TB symptom screen. Health care workers with a previously negative TB test who have been exposed to an individual with active TB should be tested immediately and retested 8 to 10 weeks after the last known exposure. If the TST is used to test health care personnel upon hire, two-step testing should be used. If an interferon-γ release assay (see later) is used upon hire, only one test is needed.

The other type of tests that may be used to determine TB exposure are interferon-γ release assays (IGRAs). IGRAs are in vitro methods that measure a type IV cell-mediated immune response to antigenic peptides derived from *M. tuberculosis.* The QuantiFERON-TB Gold Plus test (QFT-Gold-Plus) test and the T-SPOT.TB test (T-Spot) tests are both FDA-approved IGRAs. The two tests differ in their methodologies (see **Fig. 20–16** and Chapter 14). Both tests can be positive when there is active disease or latent disease. Individuals will test positive with the QFT test 2 to 8 weeks after exposure, as compared to 4 to 10 weeks with the PPD test. The T-SPOT.TB has comparable sensitivity and specificity to the QFT test. An advantage of the two tests is that they will not be positive in people who have received the BCG vaccine and will be less likely to test positive in people previously infected with NTM.

Critical Thinking 20-3

A health care worker develops a persistent cough and fever. Sputum AFB stains are negative, but the chest x-ray reveals suspicious lesions. Cultures remained negative after 3 weeks of incubation. Do the test results rule out tuberculosis? What additional laboratory tests would help to determine whether the worker has TB?

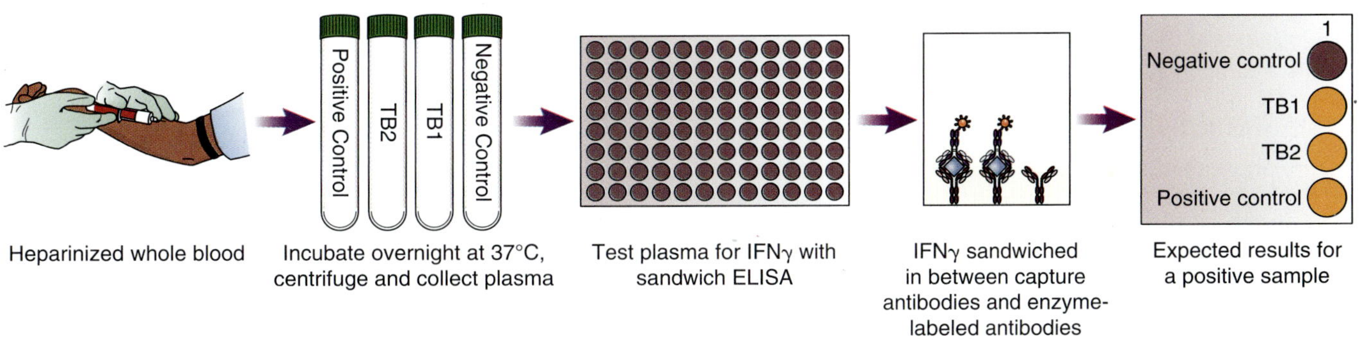

FIGURE 20–16 QuantiFERON-TB Gold Plus test principle. Peripheral blood from the patient is drawn into four specialized tubes: Negative Control; TB1 (contains TB antigens that stimulate CD4 T cells); TB2 (contains TB antigens that stimulate CD4 and CD8 T cells); and Positive Control (contains a T-cell mitogen). Following overnight incubation, the tubes are centrifuged to collect plasma, which is then tested for IFN-γ by a sandwich ELISA. A positive test is reported if TB1 and/or TB2 have an elevated IFN-γ result, and the control tubes work as expected.

KEY CONCEPTS

Human-Microbe Relationships

- The indigenous microbiota vary at different sites in the body.
- The symbiotic relationship that exists between bacteria and humans is beneficial in protecting against infection, stimulating the immune system, aiding in digestion of food, and producing various vitamins.
- Humans exist in a commensalistic relationship with the bacteria that make up the human microbiome. Encounters with some microbial organisms result in a parasitic relationship in which there is harm to the host that may result in an infection.

Bacterial Virulence Factors

- *Pathogenicity* refers to the ability of an organism to cause disease, *virulence* refers to the extent that a pathogen causes damage to the host, and *infectivity* refers to the ability of an organism to spread from one host to another.
- To be virulent, an organism must possess structural features or produce extracellular substances that allow it to invade or cause damage to the host. These are referred to as *virulence factors.*
- Live bacteria may produce exotoxins that are generally specific to a particular organism and have specific modes of action on the host. Exotoxins are highly immunogenic, and antibodies formed against them are protective.
- Endotoxin, or lipid A, is part of the gram-negative bacterial cell wall that is released from dead bacteria. Endotoxin has a broad range of systemic effects on the body because it induces the release of cytokines that can lead to septic shock. Endotoxin, although immunogenic, does not result in the production of protective antibodies.

Immune Defenses Against Bacterial Infections and Mechanisms of Evasion

- Innate immune defenses (phagocytosis, production of anti-microbial defense peptides, various proteins) contribute greatly to the body's ability to overcome a bacterial infection.
- Adaptive immunity plays a major role in defense against bacteria when the innate defenses are not sufficient in preventing infection.
- Antibodies attack bacteria by several mechanisms, including complement-mediated lysis, opsonization, and neutralization of bacterial toxins.
- Cell-mediated immunity plays an important role in attacking intracellular bacteria.
- Bacteria have developed several ways to escape immune responses, including avoiding antibodies, blocking phagocytosis, and inactivating complement.

Laboratory Detection and Diagnosis of Bacterial Infections

- Laboratory detection of the causative agent of a bacterial infection includes culturing the organism, microscopic visualization of the bacteria in clinical specimens, testing for bacterial antigens in the clinical specimen, detecting the pathogen's DNA or RNA, proteomics, and serological tests for antibodies formed against the agent.
- Highly sensitive, rapid lateral flow immunochromatographic assays (LFAs) are commonly used to detect bacterial, viral, fungal, and parasitic antigens.

Group A Streptococcus (*Streptococcus pyogenes*)

- *Streptococcus pyogenes* (group A streptococcus [GAS]) is the primary cause of bacterial pharyngitis. It is also a primary cause of a skin infection called *impetigo.* Untreated GAS infections may result in sequelae known as *acute rheumatic fever* and *poststreptococcal glomerulonephritis.*
- The production of exotoxins contributes to the infections caused by GAS. Streptolysin O, hyaluronidase, deoxyribonuclease B (DNase B), and streptokinase play a role in the infections associated with GAS.
- Scarlet fever occurs in a small percentage of people infected with GAS and is caused by the production of erythrogenic exotoxins that may also result in toxic shock syndrome.
- The laboratory diagnosis of GAS infection includes culture and antigen detection for acute infection, and anti-streptolysin O and anti-DNase B antibody detection for GAS sequelae.

Mycoplasma pneumoniae

- *Mycoplasma pneumoniae* is a leading cause of community-acquired pneumonia. Infection with *M. pneumoniae* may not require bedrest or hospitalization and is often referred to as "walking pneumonia."
- Infection with *M. pneumoniae* may result in dermatologic manifestations causing Stevens-Johnson syndrome. Raynaud syndrome, another manifestation that may be observed with *M. pneumoniae,* is a reversible variable vasospasm of the digits in which the fingers turn white when exposed to the cold.
- Detection of *M. pneumoniae*–specific IgM immunoglobulin is the most useful diagnostic assay because it likely indicates a recent infection.
- Production of cold agglutinins is observed in 50% of people with *M. pneumoniae.* Demonstration of cold agglutinins is neither specific nor sensitive when detecting infection by the organism.
- Molecular methods for the detection of *M. pneumoniae* in clinical samples are becoming more widely available for routine use for the diagnosis of *Mycoplasma* pneumonia.

Rickettsial Infections

- Rocky Mountain spotted fever (RMSF) is caused by *Rickettsia rickettsii* and is transmitted to the human host by a tick bite.
- The main pathophysiological event caused by RMSF is endothelial cell damage leading to increased vascular permeability, which then results in edema, hypovolemia, and hypotension. Various cytokines are released, and damage to the host may have a fatal outcome if therapy is not initiated in a timely fashion.
- The gold standard for the serological diagnosis of RMSF is the indirect immunofluorescence assay (IFA) for *R. rickettsii* antibody performed on two paired serum samples to demonstrate a significant (fourfold) rise in antibody titers.

Mycobacteria

- Mycobacteria have complex cell walls that resist decolorization with acid alcohol in the Gram stain. Therefore, they are referred to as "acid-fast bacilli" and must be stained with special dyes in the laboratory.
- The genus, *Mycobacterium,* contains the *Mycobacterium tuberculosis* (MTB) complex and the nontuberculosis mycobacteria (NTM). *Mycobacterium tuberculosis,* the major cause of tuberculosis in humans, is the most widely recognized organism in the MTB complex.
- *M. tuberculosis* is transmitted by inhaling the organism in aerosols from an infected individual. Its primary infection is in the lungs, but it can spread to other organs, including the kidneys and bones. The main immune defense against the organism is cell-mediated immunity, which can keep the organism in check.
- *M. tuberculosis* can result in latent tuberculosis infection (LTBI, which is asymptomatic and non-transmissible), active tuberculosis disease (in which patients exhibit symptoms of TB such as fever, cough, and bloody sputum), or reactivation tuberculosis (development of active TB disease in a person who had LTBI due to immune system suppression).
- The most common treatment of TB is isoniazid combined with three other drugs. Multi-drug resistant TB (MDR-TB) can develop if *M. tuberculosis* becomes resistant to isoniazid and another first-line drug, rifampin. Extensively drug-resistant TB (XDR-TB) can develop if the organism becomes resistant to all four first-line drugs; in that case, second-line drugs must be used.
- Bacille Calmette-Guérin (BCG) is a weakened strain of mycobacteria that is used as a tuberculosis vaccine in some parts of the world.
- Laboratory detection of mycobacteria involves culturing the organisms (which are slow-growing) in special media, staining with an acid-fast dye, and using molecular methods for faster identification of the organisms in clinical samples.
- TB infection (both latent or active) can be determined by two methods: (1) a skin test to detect a cell-mediated immune response to injected purified proteins (PPD) from *M. tuberculosis* or (2) a blood test to detect interferon-γ release from T lymphocytes that have been activated in vitro with antigens from the organism. A positive skin test is indicated by redness and induration at the site of injection in 2 to 3 days. The blood test (QuantiFERON-TB Gold) provides more rapid results than skin testing and also, unlike the skin test, is negative in people who have received the BCG vaccine.

Study Guide: Immune Defenses Against Bacterial Infection

INNATE DEFENSES	ADAPTIVE IMMUNE RESPONSES
Skin and mucosal surfaces	Antibodies produced against bacterial antigens promote opsonization and complement binding.
Antimicrobial defense peptides and proteins on epithelial surfaces (e.g., lysozyme, defensins)	Antibodies produced against bacterial exotoxins have neutralizing activity.
Other proteins (e.g., complement proteins, interleukins, prostaglandins, leukotrienes)	T-cell–mediated immune responses attack intracellular bacteria.
Acute-phase reactants (e.g., CRP, haptoglobin)	
Pattern recognition receptors (e.g., TLRs on macrophages and dendritic cells)	
Phagocytosis by neutrophils and macrophages	

Study Guide: Bacterial Virulence Factors

VIRULENCE FACTOR	DESCRIPTION	MECHANISM OF PATHOGENESIS	EXAMPLE(S)
Pili	Hair-like structures on the surface of bacteria	Adherence to and colonization of host tissue Resistance to phagocytosis Transfer of genetic material	Enterotoxigenic *E. coli* pili adhere to cells in small intestine.
Adhesion molecules	Molecules on surface of bacteria	Attach to a variety of host cell receptors, such as proteoglycans, collagen, fibrinogen	Fibronectin binding proteins of *S. pyogenes* facilitate attachment to host cells.
Capsule	A polysaccharide layer surrounding the cell wall of some bacteria	Blocks phagocytosis Blocks attachment of antibodies for opsonization Inhibits complement activation Acts as a decoy when released	Capsule of *S. pneumoniae* bacteria prevents phagocytosis by alveolar macrophages.
Endotoxin	Lipid A component of lipopolysaccharide on cell walls of gram negative bacteria; released when bacteria die	Powerful stimulator of cytokine production	Gram-negative bacterial infection involving bacteremia can cause septic shock.
Exotoxins	Neurotoxins, cytotoxins, and enterotoxins released from live bacteria	Bind to specific receptors on host cells Some can act as superantigens that activate numerous T cells	Tetanus neurotoxin prevents transmitter release from neuromuscular cells, resulting in continuous muscle spasms. Exotoxins from *S. pyogenes* can cause toxic shock syndrome.

CASE STUDIES

1. A 6-year-old child was brought to the pediatric clinic. The mother indicated that the child had been ill for several days with fever and general lethargy. The morning of the visit, the child experienced back pain and had what appeared to be blood in the urine. History and physical examination indicated an unremarkable health history other than a severe sore throat with fever 3 weeks prior that was medicated with aspirin and throat lozenges. The child's temperature was 101.5°F, and the physician noted edema in the child's hands and feet. Blood and urine specimens were collected for a complete blood cell count (CBC), urinalysis, rapid GAS antigen test, ASO titer, and anti-DNase B titer. Laboratory test results were as follows:

CBC Results

RBC count: normal
Platelet count: normal
WBC count: 12.7×10^9/L (normal = $4.8 - 10.8 \times 10^9$/L)

Urinalysis

Color: red (normal = straw)
Clarity: cloudy (normal = clear)
Protein: 2+ (normal = negative/trace)
Blood: large (normal = none)

Rapid GAS Antigen Test

Negative

ASO Titer

1:200 IU/mL (reference range less than 250 IU/mL)

Anti-DNase B Titer

1:1,400 IU/mL (reference range less than 300 IU/mL)

Questions

a. What disorder is indicated by the child's history, physical examination, and laboratory test results?
b. What was the most likely causative agent of the sore throat preceding the current symptoms?
c. Discuss the most widely accepted theory explaining the physiological basis for this disease. Why didn't the physician order a throat culture?
d. What is the significance of the urinalysis results?
e. What is the significance of the ASO and anti-DNaseB test results?

2. A 36-year-old adult was seen by a physician because of flu-like symptoms along with a sore throat and chills for the past 3 days. The patient also had difficulty breathing along with a temperature of 100.2°F and was producing a moderate amount of sputum. The physician decided that the probable diagnosis was some type of pneumonia and ordered the following laboratory tests: CBC, sputum culture, tests for influenza virus, and *M. pneumoniae* and cold agglutinin titers. The results were as follows:

CBC Results

RBC: normal
WBC: 11.7×10^9/L (normal = $4.8 - 10.8 \times 10^9$/L)

Sputum Culture

Negative

Mycoplasma Titers

IgM: none detected
IgG: 1:16

Cold Agglutinin Titer

Positive 1:128

Questions

a. What is the most probable cause of the pneumonia?
b. What is the significance of the *Mycoplasma* titer results?
c. Should additional *Mycoplasma* titers be ordered as a follow-up?
d. What is the significance of the cold agglutinin titer?

3. An elderly adult patient visited the urgent care center because of a productive cough, fever, and night sweats. On examination, the patient displayed respiratory distress and bilateral lung crackling and rattling sounds. A chest x-ray revealed infiltrates in the upper lobes of both lungs. The patient was put on broad-spectrum antibiotics for suspected community-acquired pneumonia. After completing the antibiotic therapy, the patient saw a primary care provider (PCP) because the symptoms had not resolved. The patient had been diagnosed with rheumatoid arthritis (RA) 5 years ago, which was not severe enough to warrant treatment. However, 6 months before to the recent visit, the symptoms of RA worsened, and the PCP prescribed 25 mg methylprednisolone to be taken daily. The PCP ordered an interferon-γ release assay (in this case, QuantiFERON-TB Gold Plus) on the patient. The assay came back positive.

Questions

a. What disease is suggested by the patient's clinical presentation and laboratory results?
b. What factors might put the patient at increased risk for developing this disease?
c. Should additional laboratory testing be done?
d. What steps should people who've encountered the patient take?

REVIEW QUESTIONS

1. All of the following are protective mechanisms against bacteria *except:*
   a. Production of anti-microbial defense peptides
   b. Phagocytosis
   c. Activation of complement
   d. Release of lipid A from the bacterial cell

2. *Escherichia coli* plays a crucial role in vitamin K synthesis in the human intestines, demonstrating what type of relationship?
   a. Commensalistic
   b. Mutualistic
   c. Parasitic
   d. Symbiotic

3. What does the term "virulence factor" refer to in microbiology?
   a. The ability of a microorganism to cause disease
   b. The inherent capacity of an organism to always cause disease
   c. A trait that enhances the ability of a microorganism to cause disease
   d. The degree to which a microorganism can establish an infection

4. What does the term "opportunistic pathogen" refer to?
   a. A microorganism that is always harmful to the host
   b. A microorganism that only causes disease in immunocompromised individuals
   c. A microorganism that cannot cause disease
   d. A microorganism that has a high likelihood of causing disease

5. Which technique is commonly used for rapid identification of bacterial species by analyzing their protein profiles?
   a. ELISA
   b. PCR
   c. MALDI-TOF mass spectrometry
   d. SELDI-TOF mass spectrometry

6. All of the following are ways that bacteria can evade host defenses *except:*
   a. Stimulation of chemotaxis
   b. Presence of a capsule
   c. Production of toxins
   d. Lack of adhesion to phagocytic cells

7. All of the following are characteristics of streptococcal M protein *except:*
   a. It is the chief virulence factor of group A streptococci.
   b. It provokes an immune response.
   c. Antibodies to one serotype protect against other serotypes.
   d. It limits phagocytosis of the organism.

8. An ASO titer and an anti-DNaseB test are performed on a patient's serum. The ASO titer is negative, the anti-DNaseB test is positive, and both the positive and negative controls react appropriately. What can you conclude from these test results?
   a. The ASO is falsely negative.
   b. The patient likely had a recent streptococcal infection.
   c. The patient has not had a previous streptococcal infection.
   d. The patient has scarlet fever.

9. Which of the following applies to acute rheumatic fever?
   a. Symptoms begin after *S. pyogenes* infection of the throat or the skin.
   b. Antibodies to group A streptococci are believed to cross-react with heart tissue.
   c. Diagnosis is usually made by culture of the organism.
   d. All patients suffer permanent disability.

10. Which of the following is considered to be a nonsuppurative complication of streptococcal infection?
    a. Pharyngitis
    b. Pyoderma
    c. Impetigo
    d. Acute rheumatic fever

11. Which of the following is a common clinical manifestation of *Mycoplasma pneumoniae?*
    a. Mild pneumonia with lingering cough
    b. Gastric ulcers
    c. Scarlet fever
    d. Stevens-Johnson syndrome

12. *M. pneumoniae* infections are associated with the production of which antibodies?
    a. Cold agglutinins
    b. Antibodies to ATPase
    c. Antibodies to DNase
    d. Antibodies to *Proteus* bacteria

13. What is the primary target organ of *Rickettsia rickettsii* in the human body?
    a. Liver
    b. Lungs
    c. Kidneys
    d. Endothelial cells of blood vessels

14. How is *Rickettsia rickettsii* transmitted to humans?
    a. Tick bite
    b. Mosquito bite
    c. Inhalation of aerosols
    d. Skin contact with an infected person

15. Antibody testing for Rocky Mountain spotted fever may not be helpful for which reason?
    a. It is not specific.
    b. It is too complicated to perform.
    c. It is difficult to obtain a blood specimen.
    d. Testing requires two samples drawn 2 to 4 weeks apart.

16. Which of the following *best* describes the principle of the IFA test for detection of antibodies produced in Rocky Mountain spotted fever?
    a. Patient serum is applied to a microtiter plate coated with a monoclonal antibody directed against the target antigen. A detection antibody labeled with biotin and directed against the target antigen is added. After addition of a substrate, a color reaction develops, indicating the presence of the antigen.
    b. Specific antibodies in the serum sample attach to the antigens fixed to a microscope slide. In a second step, the attached antibodies are incubated with fluorescein-labeled anti-human immunoglobulin and visualized with a fluorescence microscope.

c. The serum sample is treated chemically to link the target antibodies to a fluorophore. The labeled sample is applied to a microscope slide to which the antigen has been attached. After a wash step, the slide is examined for fluorescence.
d. Patient serum is applied to a slide to which a specific antigen is bound. After a wash step, a chromogenic dye is applied that binds to the Fc region of IgG and IgM antibodies. After a second wash step, the slide is examined for fluorescence.

17. Which of the following is true regarding exotoxins and endotoxins?
a. Both endotoxins and exotoxins are highly immunogenic, allowing for the development of protective antibodies and vaccines.
b. Endotoxins have targeted activity, whereas exotoxins have systemic effects when released.
c. Endotoxins are released from the cell walls of dead bacteria, whereas exotoxins are released from live bacteria.
d. Both endotoxins and exotoxins bind to specific receptors on a bacterial cell, leading to cell lysis.

18. Characteristics of a bacterial capsule include which of the following?
a. It cannot be used for vaccine development.
b. It is composed of peptidoglycan.
c. It is an important mechanism for protecting a bacterium against ingestion by phagocytic WBCs.
d. It is what causes bacteria to stain as gram negative.

19. Which of the following best describes mycobacteria?
a. Gram-positive cocci
b. Gram-negative rods
c. Gram-positive rods
d. Acid-fast bacilli

20. Which cellular component of *Mycobacterium tuberculosis* contributes to its ability to resist phagocytosis?
a. Lipopolysaccharide (LPS)
b. Peptidoglycan layer
c. Mycolic acid layer
d. Capsule

21. Which stain is used to identify mycobacteria?
a. Gram stain
b. Ziehl-Neelsen stain
c. Giemsa stain
d. Wright stain

22. A strain of *M. tuberculosis* that is resistant to isoniazid and the three other first-line treatment drugs for tuberculosis is classified as a:
a. Drug-susceptible strain of *Mycobacterium tuberculosis* complex
b. Nontuberculosis *Mycobacterium*
c. Multi-drug resistant strain of MTB
d. Extensively drug-resistant strain of MTB

23. What is the primary advantage of the GeneXpert MTB/RIF assay in tuberculosis diagnosis?
a. Identification of *M. tuberculosis* from organisms recovered in culture
b. Detection of dead mycobacteria
c. Detection of rapidly growing mycobacteria
d. Rapid detection of *M. tuberculosis* from clinical samples

24. What do the QuantiFERON-TB Gold In-Tube test and the T-SPOT.TB test detect?
a. Antigens released by *M. tuberculosis* during a latent TB infection (LTBI)
b. Interferon (IFN)-γ released by T cells activated against TB antigens
c. Type IV hypersensitivity response to antigens found in the BCG vaccine
d. T cells responding to an active TB infection

25. A medical laboratory professional working in an acid-fast laboratory recently had a routine PPD skin test done and tested positive. An interferon-γ release assay was performed and was also positive. The technologist did not have any respiratory symptoms, and a chest x-ray showed no remarkable findings. One year ago, the technologist's PPD test was negative. Based on these results, the technologist likely:
a. Is not infected with *Mycobacterium tuberculosis*
b. Has a latent TB infection
c. Has active tuberculosis disease
d. Has multi-drug resistant TB

Chapter 20 Answer Key

Answers to Knowledge Checks

20.1 a 20.2 b 20.3 c 20.4 c 20.5 d 20.6 b

Answers to Review Questions

1. d 2. b 3. c 4. b 5. c 6. a 7. c
8. b 9. b 10. d 11. a 12. a 13. d 14. a
15. d 16. b 17. c 18. c 19. d 20. c 21. b
22. d 23. d 24. b 25. b

21 Spirochete Diseases

Rachael M. Hagerman, MA, MLS(ASCP)[CM] MB[CM]

LEARNING OUTCOMES

After finishing this chapter, you should be able to:

21.1 Describe identifying characteristics of *Treponema pallidum, Borrelia burgdorferi, Leptospira* species, and *Borrelia* species associated with relapsing fever.

21.2 Explain how syphilis, Lyme disease, leptospirosis, and relapsing fever are transmitted.

21.3 Describe the different stages of syphilis.

21.4 Discuss the principles of dark-field examination and direct fluorescent staining for *T. pallidum.*

21.5 Distinguish treponemal tests from nontreponemal (lipoidal) tests for syphilis.

21.6 Describe the principle of the following tests for syphilis: Venereal Disease Research Laboratory (VDRL), rapid plasma reagin (RPR), fluorescent treponemal antibody absorption (FTA-ABS), and *T. pallidum* particle agglutination (TP-PA).

21.7 Evaluate situations in which false-positive nontreponemal test results can occur.

21.8 Compare and contrast typical results of treponemal and nontreponemal testing during the various stages of syphilis.

21.9 Discuss the advantages and limitations of polymerase chain reaction (PCR) and enzyme immunoassay (EIA) testing for syphilis.

21.10 Explain the traditional and reverse algorithms for syphilis and discuss their advantages and limitations.

21.11 Select appropriate laboratory methods for (1) syphilis testing in specific patient scenarios, (2) cerebrospinal fluid (CSF) in neurosyphilis, and (3) congenital syphilis.

21.12 Describe early and late clinical manifestations of Lyme disease.

21.13 Discuss the role of immunoglobulin M (IgM) and immunoglobulin G (IgG) antibody responses in the diagnosis of Lyme disease.

21.14 Discuss serological methods that play a key role in the laboratory evaluation of Lyme disease and describe recommended two-tier testing algorithms.

CHAPTER OUTLINE

You can go to **fadavis.com** keyword stevens for the laboratory exercises that accompany this text.

21.15 Discuss causes of false-positive and false-negative results in serological testing for Lyme disease.

21.16 Discuss the etiology, modes of transmission, clinical presentations, and laboratory diagnosis of leptospirosis and relapsing fever.

Spirochetes are long, slender, helically coiled bacteria containing *axial filaments,* or endoflagella, which wind around the bacterial cell wall and are enclosed by an outer sheath. These gram-negative, microaerophilic bacteria exhibit a characteristic corkscrew motility. Diseases caused by these organisms have many similarities, including a localized skin infection that disseminates to several organs as the disease progresses, a latent stage, and cardiac and neurological involvement if the disease remains untreated. In this chapter, we focus on the clinical manifestations and laboratory testing for the two major spirochete diseases: syphilis and Lyme disease. Serological testing plays a key role in diagnosis of these diseases because isolation of the organisms is difficult to accomplish in the laboratory, and clinical symptoms are not always apparent. We also discuss two other clinically relevant spirochete infections that may be part of the testing repertoire of the clinical laboratory: leptospirosis and relapsing fever.

Syphilis

Syphilis is a commonly acquired spirochete disease in the United States, typically spread through sexual transmission. Although the incidence of syphilis in the United States reached an all-time low in 2000, rates have steadily increased. According to the Centers for Disease Control and Prevention (CDC) surveillance report for sexually transmitted diseases, more than 209,250 cases of syphilis were reported in the United States in 2023, representing a 61% increase over the previous 4 years. Men who have sex with men (MSM) are disproportionately affected, but disease rates among women have also increased at an alarming rate. Despite the emphasis on safe sexual practices, syphilis remains a major health problem worldwide; about 8 million new cases were reported in 2022, according to the World Health Organization (WHO). Early detection of syphilis is of major importance because treatment with antibiotics in its early stages can usually provide a cure. In this section, we discuss characteristics of the organism that causes syphilis, its clinical manifestations, and laboratory methods essential to its diagnosis.

Characteristics of *Treponema pallidum*

The causative agent of syphilis is ***Treponema pallidum,*** subspecies *pallidum,* a member of the family *Spirochaetaceae.* Organisms in this family have no natural reservoir in the environment and must multiply within a living host. Three other nonvenereal pathogens in this group are so morphologically and antigenically similar to *T. pallidum* that they require genetic sequencing to distinguish among them: (1) *T. pallidum* subspecies *pertenue,* the agent of yaws; (2) *T. pallidum* subspecies *endemicum,* the agent of bejel; and (3) *Treponema carateum,* a different species that causes pinta. Yaws is found in the tropics, pinta is found in Central and South America, and bejel is found in desert regions.

T. pallidum (which hereafter refers to the subspecies *pallidum*) varies in length from 6 to 20 µm and in width from 0.1 to 0.2 µm, with 6 to 14 coils **(Fig. 21–1).** Its outer membrane is a phospholipid bilayer that lacks lipopolysaccharide (LPS) and has very few exposed proteins. Several identified membrane proteins, called *treponemal rare outer membrane proteins (TROMPs),* have been characterized. The scarcity, phase variation, sequential variation, and posttranslational modifications of these proteins along with the use of host serum proteins as an antigen disguise appear to aid the organism in evading the host immune response.

Mode of Transmission

Pathogenic treponemes are rapidly destroyed by heat, cold, and drying, so they are almost always spread by direct contact. Sexual transmission is the primary mode of dissemination, occurring through contact of abraded skin or mucous membranes with an open lesion. About 30% to 50% of the individuals who are exposed to a sexual partner with active lesions will acquire the disease.

Congenital infections can also be transmitted during pregnancy by passage through the placenta. In utero syphilis infection is generally severe and mutilating, affecting almost every tissue of the fetus. Infants born to mothers infected with early-stage syphilis tend to have symptoms resembling secondary syphilis in adults, characterized by cutaneous lesions, nasal congestion and discharge, hepatosplenomegaly,

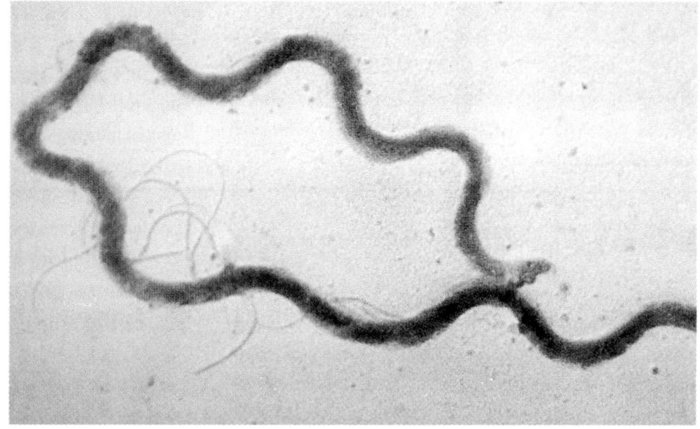

FIGURE 21–1 *Treponema pallidum.* Electron micrograph showing the coils and periplasmic flagella. *(Courtesy of CDC.)*

and central nervous system (CNS) involvement. The symptoms of early-onset syphilis generally manifest at younger than 2 years of age. Late-stage congenital syphilis occurs in infants older than 2 years when they are conceived by mothers having chronic, untreated infection. This type of manifestation corresponds to tertiary syphilis in adults, and symptoms include inflammation of the cornea, bone and tooth deformities (Hutchinson teeth), eighth-nerve deafness, and perforation of the hard palate. Manifestations of congenital syphilis range from stillbirth and neonatal death to long-term physical and physiological deformities in the surviving infants.

Other potential means of transmission include parenteral exposure through contaminated needles or blood, but this is extremely rare. For many years, the lack of transfusion-transmitted syphilis in the United States called into question the necessity of testing potential donors for presence of the disease. However, current guidelines by the American Red Cross require that people wait 12 months after treatment for syphilis before donating blood. Because syphilis can only be transmitted by means of fresh blood products, the use of stored blood components has virtually eliminated the possibility of transfusion-associated syphilis.

Knowledge Check 21-1

What structural characteristic is missing from the surface of *Treponema pallidum?*

a. TROMPs
b. LPS
c. Plasma membrane
d. Presence of coiling

Stages of the Disease

Untreated syphilis can progress through four stages: primary, secondary, latent, and tertiary.

Primary Stage

Once contact has been made with a susceptible skin site, endothelial cell thickening occurs with aggregation of lymphocytes, plasma cells, and macrophages. The initial lesion, called a **chancre,** develops between 10 and 90 days after infection, with an average of 21 days. A chancre is a firm, painless, solitary lesion characterized by raised and well-defined borders **(Fig. 21–2).** It is located where the organism entered the body and is at the location of primary sexual contact, including the penis, vagina, anus, rectum, lips, or mouth. Because they are painless, internal chancres may go undetected. The *primary stage* lasts from 3 to 6 weeks, during which time the lesion heals spontaneously.

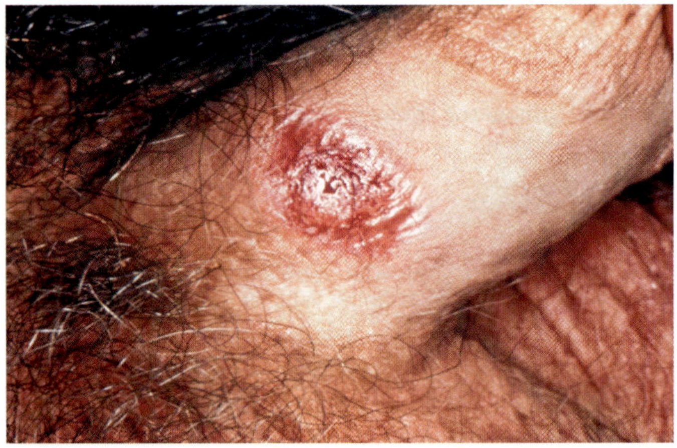

FIGURE 21–2 Primary chancre in the early stage of syphilis. *(Courtesy of the CDC/Dr. N. J. Fiumara, Public Health Image Library.)*

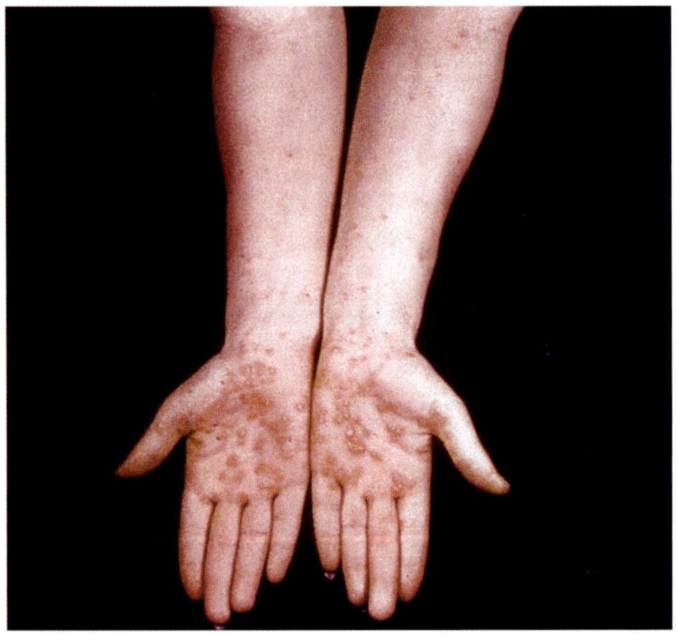

FIGURE 21–3 Skin rash characteristic of the secondary stage of syphilis. *(Courtesy of the CDC/Robert Sumpter, Public Health Image Library.)*

Secondary Stage

About 25% of patients who are untreated in the primary stage progress to the *secondary stage,* in which systemic dissemination of the organism occurs. This stage usually begins 2 to 24 weeks after the primary chancre disappears; however, in some cases, the primary lesion may still be present. Symptoms of the secondary stage include generalized lymphadenopathy (lymph node enlargement); malaise; fever; pharyngitis; and mucocutaneous manifestations, including a rash on the skin and mucous membranes that do not itch. The rash may appear on the palms of the hands and the soles of the feet; spontaneous healing occurs within a few weeks **(Fig. 21–3).** Other, less common, symptoms include condylomata lata (discolored skin lesions), alopecia (hair loss), hepatitis, and nephritis. Neurological signs, such as visual disturbances, hearing loss, tinnitus (ringing or buzzing noises in the ears), and facial weakness, appear in nearly half of patients with secondary syphilis, indicating central nervous system (CNS) involvement. Symptoms in this stage usually resolve in about 3 months but may last up to a year or recur periodically during the first few years after infection.

21-1 Clinical Correlations

The Great Imitator

Patients with syphilis can be difficult to diagnose because their clinical presentations can vary widely. Because the symptoms of syphilis can mimic those of many other diseases or conditions, the disease has often been referred to as "The Great Imitator."

Latent Stage

The *latent stage* follows the disappearance of secondary syphilis and is characterized by a lack of clinical symptoms. In the United States, it is divided into early latent (fewer than 1 year's duration) and late latent, in which the primary infection has occurred more than 1 year previously, although this is not consistent globally. In some patients, the latent stage can persist for life. While it is believed that patients are not infectious at this time, the frequency of relapses within the first year indicates that it may still be transmissible in the early latent stage. Pregnant women can pass the disease on to the fetus even if they exhibit no symptoms, regardless of the stage.

Tertiary Stage

About one-third of the people who remain untreated develop *tertiary syphilis,* which occurs most often between 10 and 30 years after the secondary stage. The disease is not transmissible in this stage but is characterized by the most severe symptoms. The three major manifestations of tertiary syphilis are gummatous syphilis, cardiovascular disease, and neurosyphilis.

Gummas are local areas of granulomatous inflammation that are most often found on bones, skin, or subcutaneous tissue. These lesions contain lymphocytes, epithelioid cells, and fibroblasts and are formed because of a type IV hypersensitivity reaction (see Chapter 14). They may heal spontaneously with scarring or remain destructive areas of chronic inflammation. They likely represent the host response to infection.

Cardiovascular complications usually involve the ascending aorta, and symptoms are caused by destruction of elastic tissue in the aortic arch. The destruction may result in aortic aneurysm, thickening of the valve leaflets causing aortic regurgitation, or narrowing of the blood vessels, producing angina pectoris.

Neurosyphilis is the complication most often associated with the tertiary stage, but it can occur any time after the primary stage and can span all stages of the disease. Immunodeficient individuals such as patients with HIV are susceptible to early neurosyphilis. During the first 2 years of infection, CNS involvement often takes the form of acute meningitis. Late manifestations of neurosyphilis in the tertiary stage include degeneration of the lower spinal cord with partial paralysis and chronic progressive dementia. These usually take more than 10 years to occur; both are the result of irreversible structural CNS damage. Fortunately, symptoms of tertiary syphilis are now very rare because of early detection and effective treatment with antibiotics such as penicillin.

Neurosyphilis, Ocular Syphilis, and Otosyphilis

Syphilis can invade the nervous system (early neurosyphilis), eyes (ocular syphilis), auditory system, and/or vestibular system (otosyphilis) during any stage of the infection and should be considered when screening patients at risk for sexually transmitted infections (STIs), not just in the tertiary stage. Early neurosyphilis manifests as meningitis, neural palsies, and stroke, often occurring during the primary and secondary stages. Ocular syphilis typically involves eye inflammation, and vision changes or loss may occur in some cases. Symptoms of otosyphilis include hearing loss, tinnitus, and dizziness. In the case of either ocular or otosyphilis, treatment should involve the appropriate medical specialists to minimize complications.

Congenital Syphilis

Congenital syphilis occurs when a pregnant woman who has early syphilis or early latent syphilis transmits treponemes to the fetus. Congenital syphilis cases in the United States increased more than threefold in recent years, with more than 3,880 cases reported in 2023. Although the disease can be transmitted at any stage of pregnancy, typically the fetus is most affected during the second or third trimester.

Often neonates have no clinical signs of disease during the first few weeks of life. Some may remain asymptomatic, but most of these infants develop later symptoms if not treated at birth. Early congenital syphilis is defined as onset of signs and symptoms before the age of 2 years. Such infants may exhibit clear or hemorrhagic rhinitis (runny nose). Skin eruptions, in the form of a maculopapular rash that is especially prominent around the mouth, palms of the hands, and soles of the feet, are also common. Other symptoms include generalized lymphadenopathy, hepatosplenomegaly, jaundice, anemia, painful limbs, and bone abnormalities. Late congenital syphilis is diagnosed after the age of 2 years, with symptoms related to bones, joints, teeth, deafness, and rash. Neurosyphilis may occur in up to 60% of infants with congenital disease.

Knowledge Check 21-2

Patients in which stage of syphilis are unable to transmit the disease to others?

a. Primary
b. Secondary
c. Latent
d. Tertiary

Nature of the Immune Response

The main body defenses against treponemal invasion are intact skin and mucous membranes. Once the skin is penetrated, *T. pallidum* replicates and spreads throughout the body. T cells and macrophages play a key role in the immune response, and $CD4^+$ and $CD8^+$ T cells are present in the primary lesions. Cytokines produced by these cells activate macrophages, and macrophage phagocytosis ultimately heals the primary chancre. The protective role of antibodies is uncertain, however, as coating the treponemes with antibodies may not bring about their destruction. *T. pallidum* can also coat itself with host proteins, delaying the recognition of the pathogen by the immune system. The rare treponemal proteins, or TROMPs, trigger complement activation, ultimately killing the organism. However, the chronic nature of the disease indicates that the organisms can evade the immune response. Treponemes may persist in the host for years if antibiotic therapy is not obtained.

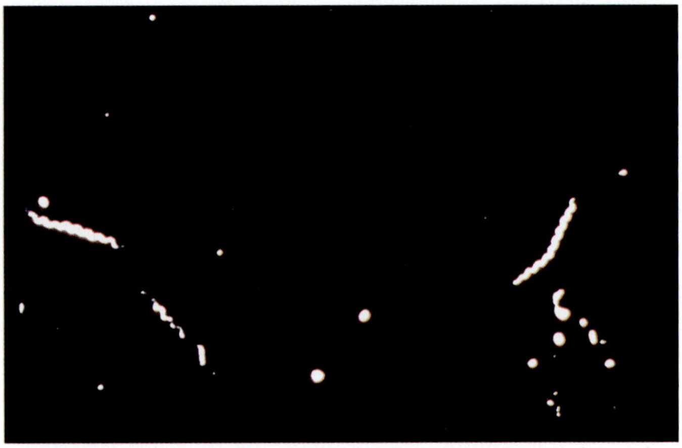

FIGURE 21–4 Using the dark-field microscopy technique, this photomicrograph revealed the presence of *Treponema pallidum* spirochetes. *(Courtesy of the CDC/Renelle Woodall, Public Health Image Library.)*

Laboratory Diagnosis

Traditional laboratory tests for syphilis can be classified into three main types: direct detection of spirochetes, nontreponemal serological tests, and treponemal serological tests. The tests vary in their ability to detect syphilis at different stages of the disease. In the text that follows, we discuss the principles and procedures of each type of testing and introduce special considerations in laboratory testing for neurosyphilis and congenital syphilis.

Direct Detection

Direct detection of spirochetes can be accomplished by dark-field microscopy or fluorescent antibody testing. The performance of either test requires the presence of active lesions and considerable expertise; thus, they are not typically performed in routine clinical laboratories.

Dark-Field Microscopy

Primary and secondary syphilis can be diagnosed by demonstrating the presence of *T. pallidum* in exudates from skin lesions. In dark-field microscopy, a dark-field condenser is used to keep all incidental light out of the field except for that captured by the organisms. It is essential to have a good specimen in the form of serous fluid from a lesion. The serous fluid is usually obtained by cleaning the lesion with sterile saline, rubbing it with clean gauze, and applying it to a microscope slide. Pathogenic treponemes are identified under a dark-field microscope by their characteristic corkscrew morphology and flexing motility **(Fig. 21–4).**

Because observation of motility is the key to identification, specimens must be examined within 20 minutes before they dry out. False-negative results can occur when there is a delay in evaluating the slides, an insufficient specimen is obtained, or the patient is pretreated with antibiotics. Thus, a negative test does not exclude a diagnosis of syphilis. An experienced microscopist should perform testing. This technique is not recommended for oral lesions, which may have morphologically identical nonpathogenic treponemes that can be confused with *T. pallidum.*

Fluorescent Antibody Testing

The use of a fluorescent-labeled antibody is a sensitive and highly specific alternative to dark-field microscopy. Testing can be performed by either a direct method, which uses a fluorescent-labeled anti–*T. pallidum* reagent, or an indirect method using antibody specific for *T. pallidum* and a second labeled anti-immunoglobulin antibody (see Chapter 11). An advantage of these methods is that live specimens are not required. A specimen can be brought to the laboratory in a capillary tube, and fixed slides can be prepared for later viewing. Treponemes can be washed off the slide even after fixing; therefore, each slide must be handled individually, and rinsing must be carefully performed. The use of monoclonal antibodies has made fluorescent antibody testing very sensitive and specific. However, results may take 1 to 2 days to obtain, and U.S. Food and Drug Administration (FDA)-approved commercial tests are no longer available in the United States.

Serological Tests

Serological testing for antibodies is key to the diagnosis of syphilis because *T. pallidum* cannot be cultured, expertise is required for direct detection, and patients may not have active lesions. Serological tests can be classified as nontreponemal or treponemal, depending on the reactivity of the antibody detected. Nontreponemal (lipoidal antigen) tests have traditionally been used to screen for syphilis because of their high sensitivity and ease of performance. However, false-positive results are common because the antigen (cardiolipin complexes) is released in the response to cell damage and is not specific for syphilis. Therefore, any positive results must be confirmed by a more specific **treponemal test,** which detects antibodies to specific *T. pallidum* surface antigens. As we discuss later, using both types of tests is also helpful in determining the disease stage.

Nontreponemal (Lipoidal Antigen) Tests

Nontreponemal tests determine the presence of an antibody that forms against cardiolipin, a phospholipid released from damaged host cells and *T. pallidum* organisms. This antibody has sometimes been referred to as **reagin** (not to be confused with the term originally used to describe immunoglobulin E [IgE]). It is found in the sera of patients with syphilis and several other diseases. An antigen complex consisting of cardiolipin, cholesterol, and phosphatidylcholine (a component of lecithin) is used in the reaction to detect the nontreponemal antibodies, which are either of the IgG or IgM class.

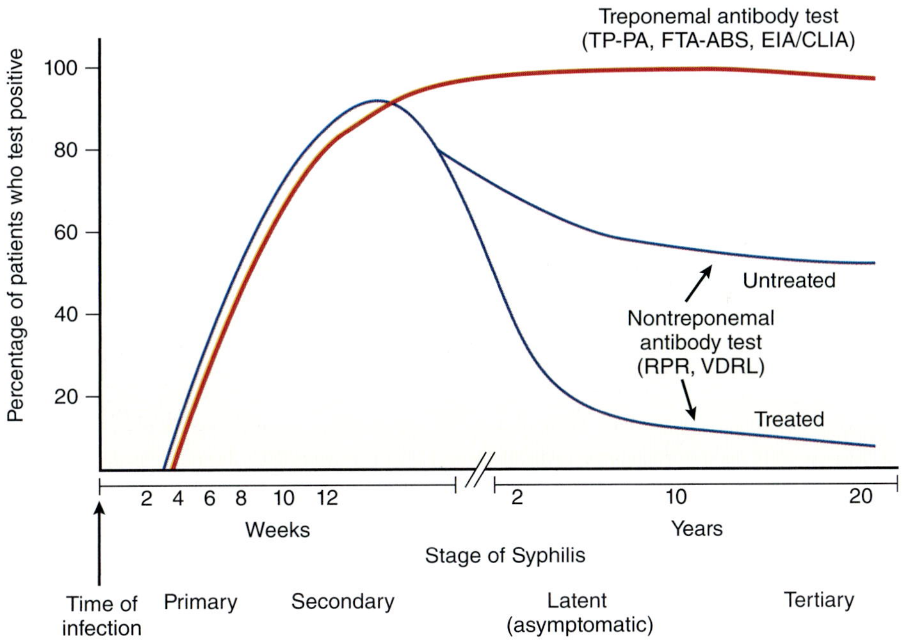

FIGURE 21–5 Typical nontreponemal and treponemal antibody patterns in syphilis. *(Adapted from Peeling RW, Ye H. Diagnostic tools for preventing and managing maternal and congenital syphilis: an overview. Bull World Health Organ. 2004;82[6]:439–446.)*

The most widely used nontreponemal tests have been the **Venereal Disease Research Laboratory (VDRL) test** and the **rapid plasma reagin (RPR) test.** These tests are based on flocculation reactions in which patient antibody complexes with the cardiolipin antigen. **Flocculation** is a specific type of precipitation that occurs over a narrow range of antigen concentrations (see Chapter 10). The antigen consists of a fleecy mass of very fine particles that clump together in a positive reaction, due to the lower antigen-antibody affinity present in the reaction.

Typical serological results for nontreponemal tests during the course of untreated and treated syphilis are shown in **Figure 21–5.** In general, nontreponemal tests become positive within 1 to 4 weeks after the appearance of the primary chancre. Titers usually peak during the secondary or early latent stages. The sensitivity for diagnosis is 62% to 78% in primary syphilis, 97% to 100% for secondary syphilis, and 82% to 100% in the early latent stage; sensitivity is not suitable for detection of tertiary syphilis. However, testing of sera from patients in the secondary stage is subject to false negatives because of the **prozone** phenomenon (antibody excess; see Chapter 10). In this case, a nonreactive pattern that is typically granular or rough in appearance is seen. If a prozone is suspected, serial twofold dilutions of the patient's serum should be made to obtain an antibody titer.

Cardiolipin antibody titers tend to decline in the later stages of the disease, even if the patient remains untreated. After several years, about 25% of untreated syphilis cases become nonreactive for reagin. This decline occurs more rapidly in people who have received treatment. A first-time infection, if in the primary or secondary stage, should show a fourfold decrease in titer by the third month following treatment and an eightfold decrease by 6 to 8 months. After successful treatment, tests typically become completely nonreactive within 1 to 2 years.

VDRL Test

The VDRL test, designed by the Venereal Disease Research Laboratories, is a qualitative and quantitative slide flocculation test for serum antibodies to cardiolipin. A modification of this method is particularly suitable for testing cerebrospinal fluid (CSF) from patients with neurosyphilis. Antigen for the tests must be prepared fresh daily in a highly regulated manner. The antigen is an alcoholic solution of 0.03% cardiolipin, 0.9% cholesterol, and 0.21% lecithin. The antigen suspension is prepared by adding the VDRL antigen with a dropper to a buffered saline solution while continuously rotating the mixture on a flat surface; attention must be paid to required rotation speed and timing. A daily calibrated Hamilton syringe is used to deliver one drop of antigen for the slide test. If the delivery is off by more than 2 drops out of 60, the syringe must be cleaned with alcohol and recalibrated.

The serum samples to be tested are heated at 56°C for 30 minutes to inactivate complement, after which 0.05 mL is pipetted into a ceramic ring of a glass slide. Three control sera—nonreactive, minimally reactive, and reactive—are pipetted into separate rings on the glass slide in the same manner. Control sera and patient samples are spread out to fill the entire ring. One drop (1/60 mL) of the VDRL antigen is then added to each ring. The slide is placed on a rotator at 180 rpm for 4 minutes, and then it is read microscopically to determine the presence of flocculation, or small clumps. The results are recorded as reactive (medium to large clumps), weakly reactive (small clumps), or nonreactive (no clumps or slight roughness). Tests must be performed at room temperature within the range of 23°C to 29°C (73°F to 85°F) because results may be affected by temperature changes: temperatures less than 23°C result in decreased reactivity, and those greater than 29°C result in increased reactivity. All sera with reactive or weakly reactive results must be tested using the quantitative slide test, in which twofold dilutions of serum ranging from 1:2

to 1:32 are initially used. The highest dilution with a reactive result is interpreted as the antibody titer. Sera yielding positive results at the 1:32 dilution are diluted further and retested.

RPR Test

The RPR test is a modified VDRL test involving macroscopic (large particle) agglutination. The cardiolipin-containing antigen suspension is bound to charcoal particles, making the test results readable by the naked eye. The suspension is stored in small glass vials, which are stable for up to 3 months after opening. The antigen is similar to the VDRL antigen, with the addition of ethylenediaminetetraacetic acid (EDTA), thimerosal, and choline chloride, which stabilize the antigen and inactivate complement so that serum does not have to be heat inactivated before use. Patient serum (approximately 0.05 mL) is placed in an 18-mm circle on a plastic-coated disposable card using a micropipette or Dispenstirs device. Cardiolipin antigen is dispensed from a small plastic dispensing bottle with a calibrated 20-gauge needle. One free-falling drop of antigen is placed onto each test area, and the card is mechanically rotated at 100 rpm for 8 minutes under humid conditions. Cards are read under a high-intensity light source; if flocculation is evident, the test is positive **(Fig. 21–6).** All reactive tests should be confirmed by retesting using doubling dilutions in a quantitative procedure, and the highest dilution with a reactive result is reported as the antibody titer.

The RPR test is more sensitive than the VDRL in primary syphilis. Automated versions of the RPR test have also been developed. These tests use digital analysis of the density and size of the flocculation complexes to determine reactivity.

Treponemal Tests

Treponemal tests detect antibody directed against the *T. pallidum* organism or against specific treponemal antigens. Typical treponemal antibody test results during various stages of syphilis are shown in Figure 21–5. Treponemal tests usually become positive before nontreponemal tests, although patients with early primary syphilis may be nonreactive. In secondary and latent syphilis, tests are usually 100% reactive. Once a patient has reactive results, they usually remain reactive for life because these tests mainly detect IgG antibodies. However, some patients may revert to a negative antibody status if they are treated very early during the course of infection or if they have advanced HIV infection. Although there are fewer false positives compared with reagin tests, reactivity is seen with other treponemal diseases, notably yaws and pinta.

Two main types of manual treponemal tests are the indirect *fluorescent treponemal antibody absorption (FTA-ABS) test* and *particle agglutination tests.* Because these tests are highly specific for syphilis, they have been used to confirm positive nontreponemal test results. More recently, automated immunoassays for treponemal antibodies have been developed. Their applications are discussed later. Qualitative point-of-care tests have also been developed that can be used by physician office laboratories and public health clinics to provide rapid results; these tests simultaneously detect antibodies to *T. pallidum* and HIV.

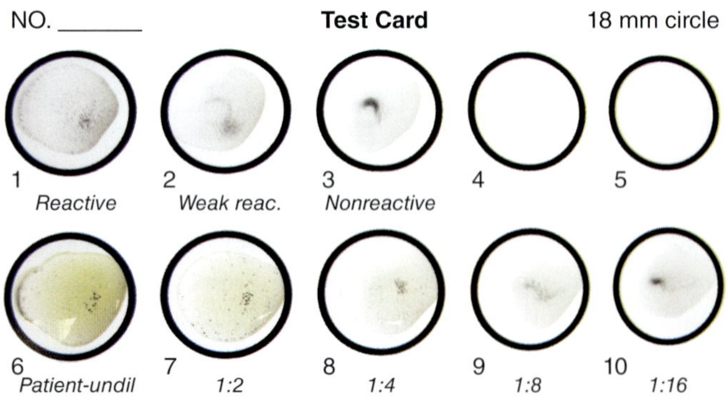

FIGURE 21–6 RPR test results. Well 1: reactive control, showing large clumps. Well 2: weakly reactive control, showing small clumps. Well 3: nonreactive control, showing slight roughness and a "tail" upon swirling. Wells 6 to 10 show results of a serially diluted sample of patient serum with a titer of 8. *(Courtesy of Linda Miller.)*

FTA-ABS Test

The **fluorescent treponemal antibody absorption (FTA-ABS) test** is one of the earliest confirmatory tests developed. In this test, a dilution of heat-inactivated patient serum is incubated with a *sorbent* consisting of an extract of nonpathogenic treponemes (Reiter strain), which removes antibodies that cross-react with treponemes other than *T. pallidum.* Diluted patient samples and controls are applied to individual wells on a test slide fixed with the *Nichols strain* of *T. pallidum.* After a 30-minute incubation at 37°C, the slides are washed and air-dried, and antibody conjugate (anti-human immunoglobulin conjugated with fluorescein) is added to each well. Slides are reincubated as before and washed to remove excess conjugate. Mounting medium is applied, and coverslips are placed on the slides, which are then examined under a fluorescence microscope.

If specific patient antibody is present, it will bind to the *T. pallidum* antigens. The antibody conjugate will, in turn, only bind where patient immunoglobulin is present and bound to the spirochetes. Slides are read under a fluorescence microscope, and the intensity of the green color is reported on a scale of 0 to 4+. No fluorescence indicates a negative test, whereas a result of 2+ or above is considered reactive. A result of 1+ means that the specimen was minimally reactive, and the test must be repeated with a second specimen drawn in 1 to 2 weeks. Experienced personnel are needed to read and interpret fluorescent test results. False-positive results, appearing as an atypical, beaded pattern of fluorescence, may occur in patients with systemic lupus erythematosus (SLE) or other autoimmune diseases. The FTA-ABS is highly sensitive and specific, but it is time consuming to perform and has been replaced in many laboratories with particle agglutination methods.

TP-PA (MHA-TP)

The **particle agglutination (PA) tests** originally used sheep red blood cells (RBCs) coated with *T. pallidum* antigen and were referred to as *MHA-TP* (microhemagglutination assay for *T. pallidum* antibody). Current PA tests for *T. pallidum,* such as the Serodia ***T. pallidum* particle agglutination (TP-PA) test,** use colored gelatin particles coated with treponemal antigens and are more sensitive in detecting primary syphilis.

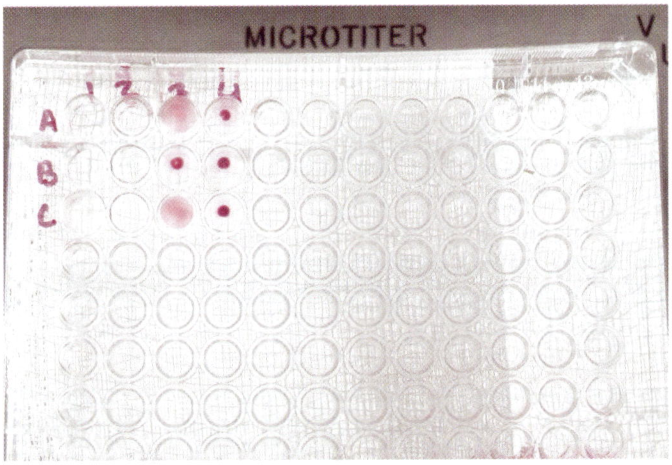

FIGURE 21–7 TP-PA test results. Row A: positive control. Row B: negative control. Row C: serum from a positive patient. *T. pallidum*–sensitized gel particles were placed in column 3 of each row, and unsensitized gel particles were pipetted into column 4 of each row. Positive wells (A3 and C3) are indicated by a diffuse mat of particles that spread over the surface of the well, whereas negative results are indicated by a compact button. *(Courtesy of Linda Miller.)*

In the Serodia TP-PA test, patient serum or plasma is diluted in microtiter plates and incubated with either *T. pallidum*–sensitized gel particles or unsensitized gel particles as a control. The presence of *T. pallidum* antibodies is indicated by agglutination of the sensitized gel particles, which bind to the antibodies to form a lattice-like structure that spreads to produce a smooth mat covering the surface of the well. If a sample is negative for the antibody, the gel particles settle to the bottom of the well and form a compact button **(Fig. 21–7).**

Knowledge Check 21-3

Which of the following is a nontreponemal test?
a. Culture
b. TP-PA
c. FTA-ABS
d. RPR

Automated Immunoassays for *T. Pallidum* Antibodies

A variety of automated immunoassays have been developed to detect antibodies to *T. pallidum*. These include enzyme immunoassays (EIAs), chemiluminescent immunoassays (CLIAs), and multiplex flow immunoassays (MFIs). EIAs have been manufactured in various formats, including one- or two-step sandwich assays, one-step competitive assays, and immune capture assays. In the sandwich assays, antibodies in the patient sample bind to recombinant *T. pallidum* antigens coated onto microtiter plate wells. An enzyme-labeled antibody or antigen conjugate and substrate are added to detect binding. In the capture immunoassay format, microtiter wells are coated with antibody to IgM or IgG and are reacted with patient serum. Antigens that are labeled with an enzyme are then added **(Fig. 21–8).** The

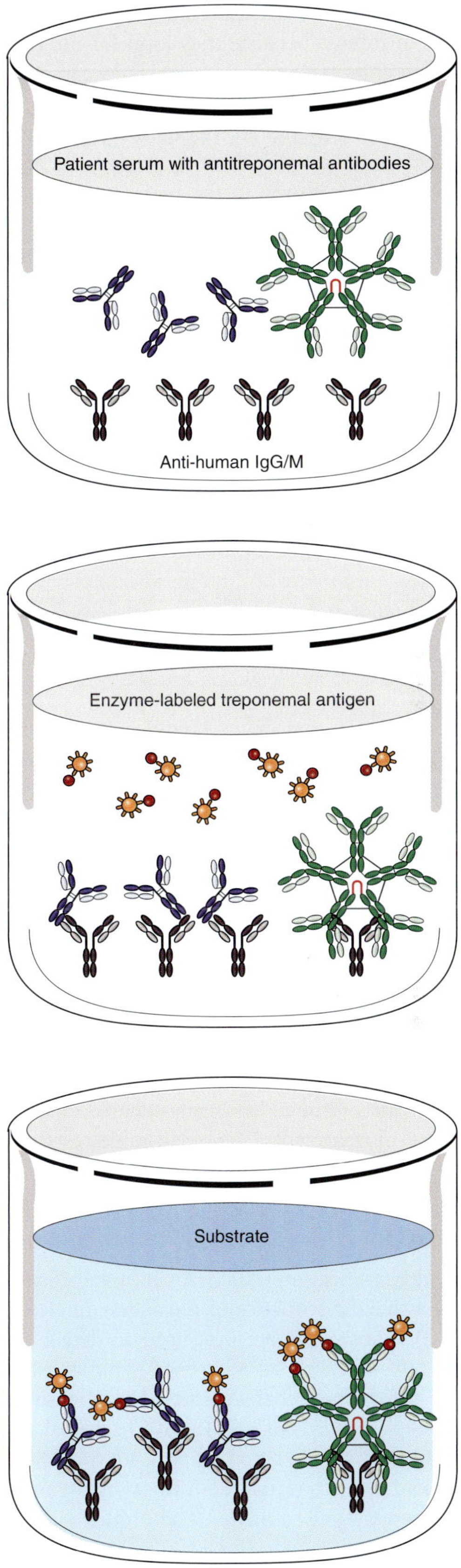

FIGURE 21–8 (A) Antibody capture enzyme-linked immunosorbent assay (ELISA) test. (B) Patient antibodies bind to anti-human IgG/IgM attached to a solid phase. (C) Only specific anti-treponemal antibody will react with enzyme-labeled antigen, producing a color change when substrate is added.

capture EIA tests are especially useful in diagnosing congenital syphilis in infants because they look for the presence of IgM, which cannot cross the placenta. They can also be used to monitor response to therapy in the early stages of syphilis because many patients are negative for IgM treponemal antibodies 6 to 12 months after treatment. In competitive EIAs, treponemal antibody in the patient sample competes with an enzyme-labeled treponemal antibody conjugate for *T. pallidum* antigens bound to microtiter plate wells. Test sensitivities of the various EIAs range from about 95% to 99%, and test specificities are 100%.

CLIAs are available as a one-step sandwich technique in which the patient sample is incubated with paramagnetic microparticles that have been coated with *T. pallidum* antigens linked to a chemiluminescent derivative. After a wash step to remove unbound material, a catalyst is added and a chemical reaction occurs, producing emissions of light if the test sample is positive. The number of relative light units (RLUs) is proportional to the amount of treponemal antibody in the sample. CLIAs have many advantages as compared with EIAs, including a higher sensitivity in the early stages of syphilis, faster performance, and more stable reagents.

MFIs involve incubation of the patient sample with microspheres coated with recombinant *T. pallidum* antigens. Microspheres that have bound immune complexes are detected after the addition of a phycoerythrin-labeled reporter antibody and are analyzed by flow cytometry. This method can simultaneously detect antibodies to multiple *T. pallidum* antigens in a small volume of sample and has a rapid turnaround time. Treponemal MFI, EIA, and CLIA yield comparable results to the FTA-ABS but have the advantage of automation.

Rapid Tests for Syphilis

Several rapid tests for syphilis have also been developed to detect treponemal antibodies, mostly in the format of immunochromatographic assays. These point-of-care tests are used mainly in resource-limited settings to enable rapid diagnosis and initiation of treatment. Combined rapid tests for syphilis and HIV have also been developed.

Molecular Testing by Nucleic Acid Amplification Tests (NAAT)

Nucleic acid amplification tests (NAATs) involve isolating and amplifying a specific sequence of *T. pallidum* nucleic acid (see Chapter 12). These tests are best used to detect the organism in exudates or swab samples from syphilis lesions. Most NAATs use polymerase chain reaction (PCR)-based methods to detect the *tp47* (*tp074*) or *polA* (*tp0105*) genes of *T. pallidum*. PCR or transcription-mediated amplification (TMA) has also been used to detect ribosomal RNA from the organism.

NAATs are extremely sensitive techniques that can detect as little as one treponeme in some clinical samples. Sensitivity is highest in patients with primary syphilis but is greatly reduced in detecting disease in secondary syphilis. Although there are no FDA-approved NAATs for syphilis at the time of this writing, use of these tests for early detection of primary syphilis looks promising for the future. NAATs may also be helpful in detecting treponemes in amniotic fluid or samples from neonates to diagnose congenital syphilis.

Clinical Applications

Nontreponemal tests are sensitive, inexpensive, and simple to perform. Thus, they have been very useful in screening for syphilis and in diagnosing patients with related symptoms or a history of sexual contact with a person who has syphilis. Because antibody titers can be determined by testing serial dilutions of the patient sample, these methods have also been useful in monitoring the progress of the disease and in determining treatment outcomes. As we noted previously, nontreponemal titers will decrease if treatment is effective; a fourfold change in titer is considered clinically significant. Their main disadvantage is that they are subject to false positives. Transient false positives may occur as a result of recent vaccinations, pregnancy, or certain infections (e.g., HIV, hepatitis, infectious mononucleosis, varicella, herpes, measles, malaria, tuberculosis). Chronic conditions causing sustained false-positive results include SLE, leprosy, IV drug use, autoimmune arthritis, advanced age, and advanced malignancy.

A reactive nontreponemal test should be confirmed by a more specific treponemal test. In pregnancy, this is especially important because nontreponemal titers from a previous syphilis infection may increase nonspecifically. Titers are considered to be nonspecifically increased if lesions are absent, the increase in titer is less than fourfold, and documentation of previous treatment is available.

Although treponemal tests are usually reactive before nontreponemal tests in primary syphilis, they suffer from a lack of sensitivity in congenital syphilis and neurosyphilis. Nontreponemal tests should be used for these purposes. Treponemal tests have been traditionally used as confirmatory tests to distinguish false-positive from true-positive nontreponemal results. They also help establish a diagnosis in late latent syphilis or late syphilis because they are more sensitive than nontreponemal tests in these stages. Treponemal tests are also used to screen blood donors for syphilis.

Testing Algorithms

The CDC published two syphilis testing algorithms: the traditional algorithm and the reverse algorithm. The CDC recommends that laboratories choose the most suitable algorithm for their situation based on their resources (cost, staff, space) and the patient population they serve.

The traditional testing algorithm for syphilis involves screening the sample with a nontreponemal test and confirming any positive results with a more specific treponemal test **(Fig. 21–9)**. This testing strategy was used in most clinical laboratories for many years.

Because of the development of sensitive, automated methods for treponemal antibodies that can be easily performed in the clinical laboratory, a change in the testing strategy for syphilis has become increasingly popular, especially among laboratories with large testing volumes. Under this "reverse sequence algorithm," the testing order is reversed from the traditional algorithm, in that patient samples are screened by

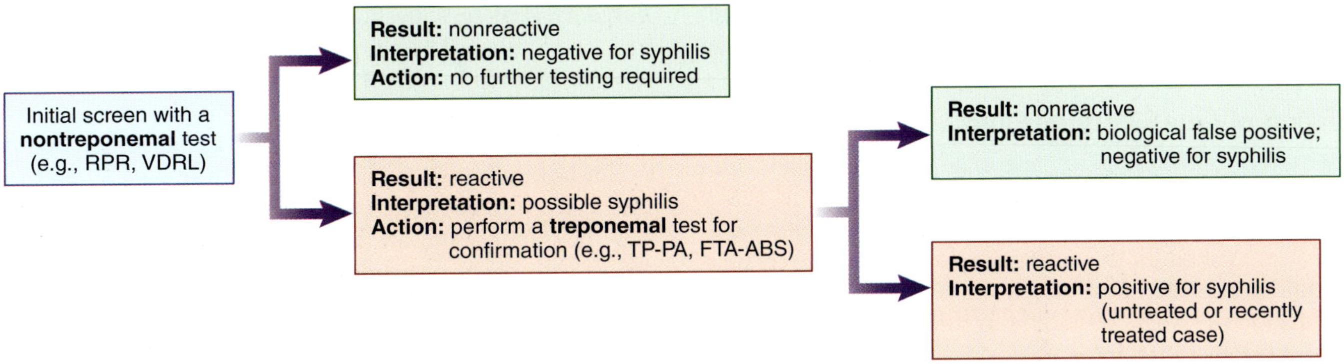

FIGURE 21–9 Traditional testing algorithm for syphilis.

an automated treponemal immunoassay, and positive results are confirmed by a nontreponemal test. The reverse algorithm has several advantages over the traditional algorithm. The first advantage is cost. Automated testing can be performed on Laboratory Information System (LIS)-interfaced high-throughput analyzers as opposed to labor-intensive manual methods, saving time and reducing errors. Also, this algorithm can potentially detect more early, late, and treated syphilis cases because of the higher sensitivity of the specific treponemal tests. In the traditional algorithm, these cases may be missed because testing stops with a negative nontreponemal test result, and the treponemal test is not performed.

In the reverse algorithm, if the initial assay is negative, no further testing is done unless early syphilis is suspected (i.e., before seroconversion). If the automated assay result is positive and the subsequent RPR is positive, the results are considered positive for syphilis. However, discrepant results can be obtained in some cases, with the initial automated test result being positive and the RPR that follows giving a negative result. This combination of results can be problematic because it could be caused by a false-positive treponemal antibody test result, a past syphilis infection, or early primary syphilis in which patients have not yet produced nontreponemal antibodies. To help distinguish between these possibilities, the CDC recommends that if laboratories use the reverse algorithm, all discrepant results should be tested reflexively using the TP-PA test as a secondary confirmatory treponemal test. If the TP-PA is positive, then late or latent syphilis or previous history of syphilis would be considered. If the TP-PA is negative, the patient would be considered negative for syphilis at the time of testing. Careful evaluation of the patient's history should be considered, and the patient may be reevaluated for syphilis at a later date **(Fig. 21–10)**.

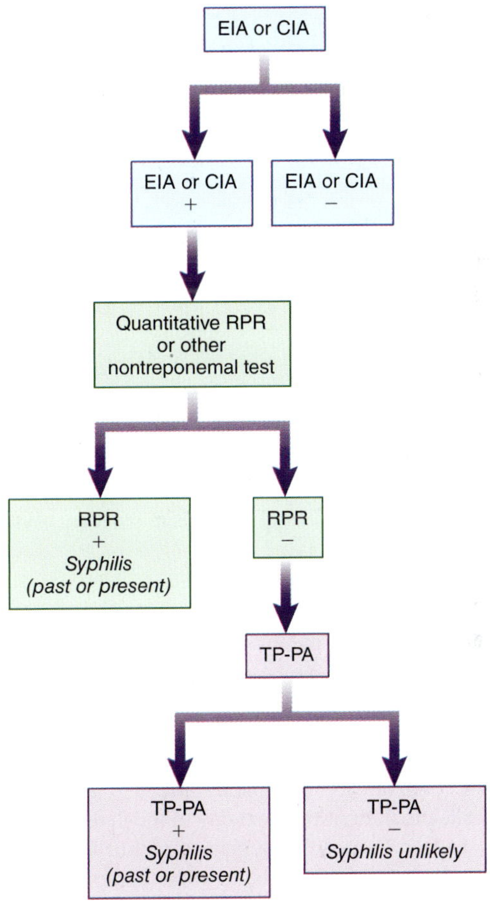

EIA = enzyme immunoassay; CIA = chemiluminescence immunoassay; TP-PA = *Treponema pallidum* particle agglutination.

FIGURE 21–10 The algorithm for reverse sequence syphilis screening involves treponemal test screening followed by nontreponemal test confirmation. The CDC recommends that discrepant results be followed by performance of the TP-PA test. *(Adapted from Centers for Disease Control and Prevention. Discordant results from reverse sequence syphilis screening: five laboratories, United States, 2006–2010. MMWR. 2011;60[5]:133–137.)*

Testing for Congenital Syphilis

Testing neonates at risk for congenital syphilis is critical, yet challenging due to the presence of maternal antibodies transferred through the placenta. Because of this, only nontreponemal tests are performed for neonatal diagnosis using newborn serum, rather than cord blood, to avoid material contamination and false-negative results due to the presence of Wharton jelly (a gelatinous connective tissue in the umbilical cord). The current recommendation is parallel testing of the mother and neonate using the same quantitative nontreponemal testing method to compare titers at birth, with follow-up testing at 3 and 6 months. Histological examination of the placenta can reveal abnormal villi and be stained with silver stain for the direct detection of spirochetes. The placenta, amniotic fluid, neonatal nasal discharge, suspicious lesions, or CSF fluid can all be tested using PCR.

Testing of Cerebrospinal Fluid

CSF is typically tested to determine whether treponemes have invaded the CNS. Such testing is usually more reliable if CNS symptoms are present. The VDRL test is the only FDA-approved method for the testing of spinal fluid to detect neurosyphilis. For VDRL CSF testing, the antigen volume used is less than in the serum test and is at a different concentration. Also, different slides are used (Boerner agglutination slides). The test is read microscopically as in the VDRL serum test. If a test is reactive, twofold dilutions are made and retested following the same protocol to determine the titer.

A positive VDRL test on CSF is diagnostic of neurosyphilis because false positives are extremely rare. However, sensitivity is low (66.7% to 85.7%); thus, many samples from patients with neurosyphilis give negative results. If a negative test is obtained, other indicators such as increased lymphocyte count and elevated total protein (45 mg/dL) are used as signs of active disease.

Treatment

Penicillin has been the treatment of choice for syphilis since its availability in the late 1940s. Infection can be easily cured by administering a single dose of intramuscular long-acting benzathine penicillin G. Doxycycline and tetracycline are other alternatives for patients who are allergic to penicillin and are not pregnant.

Critical Thinking 21-1

A patient presents to her gynecologist for an annual exam. She tells her doctor that she has had multiple sexual partners, does not regularly use protection, and has a history of several sexually transmitted infections (STI). A cervical swab was obtained for a Papanicolaou (Pap) smear, and urine and blood were collected for pregnancy and STI testing. The physician calls the patient the next day to indicate a positive pregnancy test and a positive syphilis test, but the patient is not treated with an antibiotic. In what patient scenario might a pregnant individual with a positive syphilis test not be treated?

Lyme Disease

Lyme disease was first described in the United States in 1975 when an unusually large number of cases of juvenile arthritis appeared in a geographically clustered rural area around Old Lyme, Connecticut (hence the disease name), in the summer and fall. Because of the epidemiological features of this newly described "Lyme arthritis," transmission by an arthropod vector was suggested. In 1982, the agent was isolated and identified as a new spirochete and given the name ***Borrelia burgdorferi*** after Willy Burgdorfer (first author in the original description). The clinical features of Lyme disease were soon recognized to extend beyond arthritis; it is now known to be a multisystem illness involving the skin, nervous system, heart, and joints. Lyme disease is the most common vector-borne disease in the United States; over 89,000 laboratory-confirmed cases were reported to the CDC in 2023, but thousands more are thought to have been treated for the disease based on clinical suspicion alone. According to the CDC, the number of cases in high-incidence states has remained stable but has increased in neighboring states with previously low incidence. Cases have also expanded beyond areas with high concentrations of deciduous forests into more urban areas. Increase in incidence can partially be attributed to greater awareness; however, environmental factors, such as climate change, migratory bird patterns, and increased density and distribution of reservoirs and deer populations, have expanded tick habitats.

Characteristics of *Borrelia* Species

Several species of *Borrelia* are known to be the causative agents of Lyme disease. In North America, it is exclusively *B. burgdorferi sensu stricto,* whereas in Europe, several species are known to cause Lyme disease (*Borrelia afzelii, Borrelia garinii, Borrelia sensu stricto,* and occasionally other *Borrelia* species). All share similar characteristics; for simplicity, they will be referred to as *B. burgdorferi*. The organism is a loosely coiled spirochete, 5 to 25 µm long and 0.2 to 0.5 µm in diameter. The outer membrane, which consists of glycolipid and protein, is extremely fluid and only loosely associated with the organism. Several important lipoprotein antigens, outer surface proteins (OSPs) OSP-A through OSP-F, are located in this structure and are encoded by plasmids. Surface proteins allow the spirochetes to attach to mammalian cells.

Just underneath the outer envelope are 7 to 11 *endoflagella* or *periplasmic flagella.* These run parallel to the long axis of the organism and are made up of 41-kDa subunits that elicit a strong antibody response. This immunodominant characteristic is of diagnostic importance because the host response is not only strong but also occurs very early. Unfortunately, the flagellin subunit has homology to that of other nonpathogenic and pathogenic spirochetes, notably *B. recurrentis* and *T. pallidum,* causing cross-reactivity in serological testing. Because of this, many uninfected people have low levels of antibodies to the 41-kDa protein. Although this is usually not a problem in the current diagnostic scheme of testing, it can become an issue when these people become ill with certain viruses that are known polyclonal B-cell activators (such as Epstein-Barr virus). In these cases, this normally low-level antibody increases enough to cause biological false positivity.

The organism divides by binary fission approximately every 12 hours. It can be cultured in the laboratory in a complex liquid medium (Barbour-Stoenner-Kelly) at 33°C, but it is difficult to isolate from patients. The spirochetemia (presence of spirochetes in the blood) is short-lived and is generally only found early in the illness. Cultures often must be incubated for 6 weeks or longer to detect growth and are therefore of little diagnostic utility.

Mode of Transmission

Lyme disease is maintained through a tick-rodent cycle, with the main reservoir host being the white-footed mouse *(Peromyscus leucopus)*, although in California and Oregon the spirochete is also harbored by the dusky-footed woodrat. Several types of *Ixodes* ticks serve as vectors of transmission after feeding on the rodents: *Ixodes scapularis* in the Northeast and Midwest United States **(Fig. 21–11)**, *Ixodes pacificus* in the West, *Ixodes ricinus* in Europe, and *Ixodes persulcatus* in Asia. White-tailed deer are the main host for the tick's adult stage, while humans are incidental hosts. Nymphs are responsible for most human infections; while adult ticks can transmit the disease, males do not feed and females tend to feed only on large animals, such as the white-tailed deer. Peak feeding is in the late spring, early summer, and fall, corresponding to the peak biphasic occurrence of Lyme disease. Typically, ticks must feed for more than 36 hours before the spirochete can be transmitted.

Knowledge Check 21-4

What is the vector that transmits Lyme disease?

a. Deer
b. Mouse
c. Tick
d. Woodrat

Stages of the Disease

The clinical manifestations of Lyme disease, like syphilis, occur in several stages. These have been characterized as (1) localized rash, (2) early dissemination to multiple organ systems, and (3) a late disseminated stage that often includes arthritic or neurological symptoms. These stages are not always sharply delineated; therefore, it may be easier to view Lyme disease as a progressive infectious disease that involves diverse organ systems.

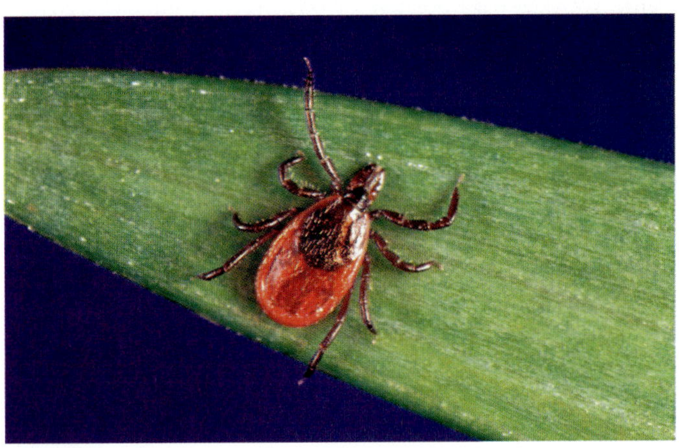

FIGURE 21–11 Adult tick *I. scapularis*, which transmits Lyme disease. *(Courtesy of the CDC/Michael L. Levin, PhD, and Jim Gathany, Public Health Image Library.)*

Localized Rash Stage

The clinical hallmark of early infection is the rash known as primary *erythema migrans* (EM, or "bull's-eye" rash), which appears between 3 and 30 days after a tick bite. EM begins as a small red papule where the bite occurred, then rapidly expands to form a large ringlike erythema and often a central area that shows partial clearing, resulting from movement of the spirochetes and the resulting inflammatory response **(Fig. 21–12).** The clinical diagnosis of early Lyme disease relies on the recognition of this characteristic rash, which should be at least 5 cm in diameter for clinical diagnosis. At this stage, the patient may be asymptomatic or have nonspecific flu-like symptoms and regional lymphadenopathy. The EM usually continues to expand for more than a week; even if untreated, it gradually fades within 3 to 4 weeks. Unfortunately, about 20% of patients do not develop the rash. At this early stage, the antibody response is minimal, and most serology results are negative.

Early Dissemination Stage

Early dissemination occurs via the bloodstream in the days to weeks after the primary EM rash. The skin, nervous system, heart, or joints may be affected. Some patients display multiple secondary skin lesions. Migratory pain often occurs in the joints, tendons, muscles, and bones, resulting in Lyme arthritis. Episodic swelling, large effusions, and inflammation occur in the large joints, predominantly the knees, and resolve with treatment. Without treatment, neurological or cardiac involvement develops in about 15% of patients within 4 to 6 weeks after the onset of infection. The most prevalent neurological sign is facial palsy, a peripheral neuritis that usually involves one side of the face. Severe headache and neck stiffness can also occur. Pain and

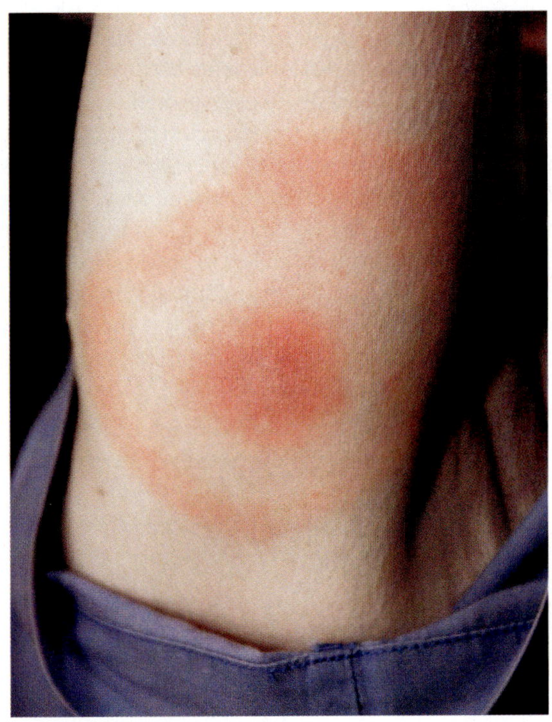

FIGURE 21–12 Erythema chronicum migrans rash, which appears after a tick bite in Lyme disease. *(Courtesy of the CDC/Jim Gathany, Public Health Image Library.)*

weakness can occur in the affected limb. Some patients develop sleep disturbances, mild chronic confusion, or difficulty with memory and intellectual functioning. Aseptic meningitis can also be seen. Lyme carditis, characterized by heart palpitations or irregular heartbeat, can also occur during the dissemination state, but its incidence appears to be declining.

Late Dissemination Stage

Late Lyme disease may develop in some untreated patients months to years after acquiring the infection. The major manifestations of late Lyme disease are arthritis, peripheral neuropathy (damage to the nerves outside of the brain and spinal cord), and encephalomyelitis (inflammation of the brain and spinal cord); the type of manifestation appears to be associated with the specific infecting *Borrelia* strain. These symptoms usually respond well to conventional antibiotic treatment, but treatment-resistant arthritis has been associated with particular *HLA–DRB* alleles. Despite resolution of objective manifestations of *Borrelia* infection after antibiotic treatment, a small percentage of patients develop chronic fatigue, concentration and short-term memory problems, and musculoskeletal pain, referred to as *posttreatment Lyme disease syndrome*. These symptoms can last longer than 6 months in some cases and may be related to the dysregulated inflammatory response triggered by the spirochetes.

Nature of the Immune Response

The immune response in Lyme disease is highly variable and complex. A well-documented humoral and cellular response is known to exist. Phagocytosis of the spirochete releases lipoproteins and intracellular pathogen-associated molecular patterns (PAMPs) that trigger the production of pro-inflammatory cytokines and chemokines, further enhancing the immune response and possibly inducing arthritic states. The organism can evade the alternative complement pathway by capturing host-derived complement-regulatory proteins, but once antibodies have been produced, the classical pathway is activated. However, the effectiveness of these responses is questionable and not necessarily protective because late Lyme disease occurs despite high levels of circulating antibody and cellular responses, demonstrating an ability to reduce the numbers of spirochetes present but not completely eliminate them. The persistently high levels of both IgM and IgG throughout infection and reduced IgG subclass switching suggest a predominantly T-independent antibody response, preventing affinity maturation and the development of memory and long-term plasma cell production. Unbalanced activation of helper T (T_H) and regulatory T (Treg) cell populations results in an imbalance of pro- and anti-inflammatory cytokines that facilitates cardiac and arthritic disease states.

Laboratory Diagnosis

The diagnosis of Lyme disease is a clinical one, with laboratory testing used as supporting evidence. Unfortunately, clinical diagnosis is often difficult. If the characteristic rash is present, this can be used as a presumptive finding, but as many as 20% of patients do not develop or do not recognize the rash. Direct isolation of the organism from skin scrapings, spinal fluid, or blood is extremely low; therefore, neither culture nor molecular techniques are used as a routine diagnostic tool.

The antibody response varies and may not be detectable until 3 to 6 weeks after the tick bite. The IgM response occurs first, followed by the IgG response, which does not peak until the third and fourth weeks of infection. Serial antibody concentrations cannot be used to determine disease progression because IgM levels remain elevated throughout the active infection, and IgG persists for life. In most cases of acute early Lyme disease (first 2 weeks), serological testing is too insensitive to be diagnostically helpful. If symptomatic patients are tested in fewer than 7 days after infection, seropositivity is only about 30%. Therefore, the decision to start treatment for early Lyme disease must be made before seroconversion (detection of specific antibodies in the blood), similar to many acute infectious diseases. However, untreated seronegative patients having symptoms for 6 to 8 weeks are unlikely to have Lyme disease, and other possible diagnoses should be pursued. Antibiotic therapy begun shortly after the appearance of EM may delay or inhibit the antibody response.

The CDC recommends a two-tiered testing algorithm to provide laboratory support for the diagnosis of Lyme disease **(Fig. 21–13)**. The *standard two-tiered testing algorithm (STTT)* has been used since 1995. Using the STTT, patients with clinical evidence of Lyme disease are screened with an enzyme immunoassay (EIA) or immunofluorescence assay (IFA) detecting IgM, IgG, and/or both. If the first serology test is negative, no further testing is performed; if it is positive or equivocal/indeterminant, an immunoblot is performed on that specimen to confirm the result. If the symptoms have been present for less than 30 days, both IgM and IgG should be analyzed in the immunoblot; if present for greater than 30 days, only IgG should be evaluated.

The STTT is highly specific but has low sensitivity in detecting early Lyme disease. These limitations have led to the development of alternative testing strategies, including a *modified two-tiered testing algorithm* (MTTT) (see Fig. 21–13). In this approach, symptomatic patients are first tested with a sensitive immunoassay that uses purified *Borrelia* peptide antigens. Samples with positive or borderline results are retested with an immunoassay that uses different *Borrelia* antigens for confirmation; the FDA must approve the combination of the paired immunoassays (most commonly, automated ELISAs). The MTTT demonstrates comparable specificity to the STTT and increased sensitivity in detecting early Lyme disease. Because the automated immunoassays are easier to perform and interpret than the immunoblot, clinical laboratories are increasingly using the MTTT.

Lyme disease testing should not be performed in the absence of supporting clinical evidence. A positive test performed under these circumstances has a low positive predictive value, even when done in an endemic area, whereas it rises to nearly 100% when clinical symptoms and history are present and consistent with Lyme disease. In the following sections, we discuss some of the laboratory procedures used in Lyme disease testing.

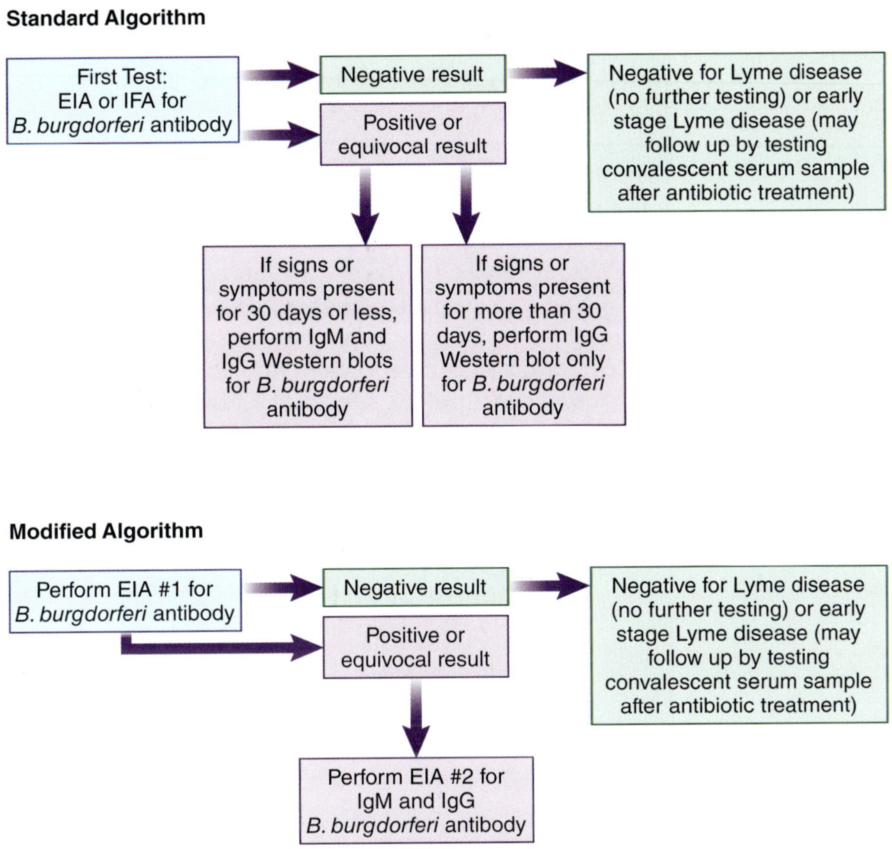

FIGURE 21–13 Two-tiered testing for Lyme disease. *(Adapted from Centers for Disease Control and Prevention [https://www.cdc.gov/lyme/media/pdfs/2024/05/Suggested-Reporting-Language-Interpretation-and-Guidance-Regarding-Lyme-Disease-Serologic-Test-Results.pdf] and Branda JA, Strle K, Nigrovic LE, Lantos PM, Lepore TJ, et al. Evaluation of modified 2-tiered serodiagnostic testing algorithms for early Lyme disease. Clin Infec Dis. 2017;64:1074–1080.)*

Immunoassays

The indirect IFA was the first type of immunoassay used to evaluate the antibody response in Lyme disease. In this method, doubling dilutions of patient serum were incubated with microscope slides coated with cultured *Borrelia* spirochetes, and antibody to the organism was detected with a fluorescent-labeled anti-human globulin. Because of the manual format and subjective interpretation of the results, the IFA has largely been replaced by automated immunoassays.

The most commonly used immunoassays for *Borrelia* antibodies have enzyme-linked immunosorbent assay (ELISA)-based formats (see Chapter 11); CLIA methods have also been developed. Automated ELISAs yield timely, objective results and are easily implemented in clinical laboratories. For these reasons, ELISAs are widely used in the initial evaluation of patients for Lyme disease and for confirmation in the MTTT algorithm, as we discussed previously. These tests can detect IgM only, IgG only, or both IgM and IgG. Newer generation ELISAs that detect antibodies against the recombinant peptides, VIsE C6 (derived from the variable major protein-like sequence in the *B. burdorferi* outer membrane) and pepC10 (derived from OSP-C) have increased sensitivity and specificity, as compared to older methods.

As we discussed earlier, immunoassays have decreased sensitivity during the early stages of Lyme disease when patients may not have mounted a sufficient antibody response, causing false-negative results. Also, false positives can occur due to antibody cross-reactivity from autoimmune diseases or other infections (e.g., syphilis, other treponemal diseases such as yaws and periodontal disease, relapsing fever, leptospirosis, infectious mononucleosis). Use of a two-tiered testing algorithm increases the accuracy of the test results.

Immunoblot

Immunoblotting, or Western blotting, has been used as a confirmatory test for samples that initially test positive or equivocal by EIA or IFA. As we mentioned previously, it has been used as the second test in the STTT scheme for Lyme disease.

The Lyme disease immunoblot is very complex. The technique involves transfer of recombinant *Borrelia* antigens to a nitrocellulose membrane, followed by incubation with patient serum and then an anti-human immunoglobulin (either anti-IgG or anti-IgM) labeled with an enzyme. Further incubation with the enzyme's substrate allows for visualization of any antibody that has bound to a particular antigen. The reactions appear as bands of specific molecular weights **(Fig. 21–14)**.

Ten proteins are used in the CDC-recommended interpretation of this test. They are designated by their molecular weights: 18, 23, 28, 30, 39, 41, 45, 58, 66, and 93 kDa. For a result to be considered positive for the presence of specific IgM antibody, two of the following bands must be present: 23 (OSP-C), 39, and 41 (flagellin) kDa. An IgG immunoblot is considered positive if any 5 of the 10 bands previously listed are positive. Because of the complexity of the Lyme immunoblots, testing and interpretation of blots should be done only

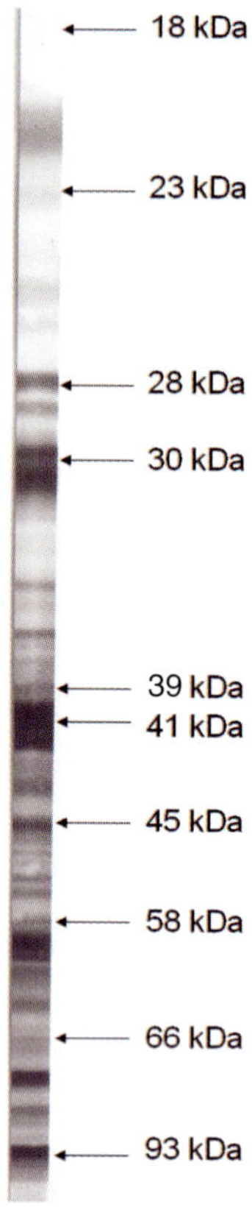

FIGURE 21–14 Immunoblot for Lyme disease.

in qualified laboratories that follow CDC-recommended evidence-based guidelines for immunoblot interpretation.

Polymerase Chain Reaction (PCR)

PCR has also been developed to detect specific *B. burgdorferi* Osp-A plasmid and flagellin genes directly from clinical samples. PCR tests are typically based on hybridization of labeled probes for the *B. burgdorferi* genes with patient DNA (see Chapter 12).

While PCR is more specific than antibody testing, it is not recommended for initial testing because of its low sensitivity, and as of this writing, there are no FDA-approved assays. False-negative results may occur because the number of organisms in body fluids from Lyme disease patients is often low, and PCR inhibitors may be present in patient samples. Thus, a negative PCR does not rule out Lyme disease.

However, the PCR may be helpful in certain scenarios, such as testing blood early in infection before development of antibody responses, testing synovial fluid for Lyme arthritis, testing skin biopsies from patients with an atypical rash, or testing for reinfection. In such situations, PCR may be useful in conjunction with antibody tests to support a Lyme disease diagnosis.

Treatment

Borrelia is sensitive to several orally administered antibiotics, including doxycycline, amoxicillin, cefuroxime, ceftriaxone, and azithromycin. Oral doxycycline is the first treatment of choice for patients with early Lyme disease who are not pregnant. IV antibiotic therapy is required for patients with neurological symptoms, cardiac involvement, or arthritis that does not respond to oral therapy. Prophylactic treatment with doxycycline may be offered to adults and children older than 8 years of age who are at high risk for contracting the infection, if the tick is identified as an *Ixodes* spp., the bite occurred in an endemic area, and the tick was attached for more than 36 hours.

A human vaccine made with the OSP-A surface antigen was approved by the FDA in 1999, but some recipients reported side effects (although association with the vaccine was not confirmed); consequently, sales of the vaccine declined, and it was discontinued in 2002. There are renewed efforts to create a new vaccine, but as of this writing, no vaccine has been approved for clinical use.

Knowledge Check 21-5

In the MTTT algorithm, the immunoblot is:

a. Not used in either stage
b. Used in the first stage
c. Used in the second stage
d. Used in both stages

Critical Thinking 21-2

A patient presents to a primary care physician with a bull's-eye rash on the left leg just above the ankle and complaints of arthritic pain in the left ankle and knee. The patient indicated they had been hiking along the Appalachian Trail in Connecticut last weekend. A skin biopsy was taken from the leg, and blood was collected. The direct exam was negative for spirochetes, and the Lyme ELISA was negative for both IgM and IgG. How do you explain these results? Should the patient be treated?

Leptospirosis

Leptospirosis is caused by bacteria of the genus ***Leptospira.*** It is more prevalent in temperate zones of the world with a warm climate. The incidence is higher in livestock and dairy farming communities. It is mainly a zoonotic infection commonly associated with occupational and recreational activities. Coming into contact with infected animals, especially rat-infested surroundings, poses increased exposure for veterinarians, dairy farmers, slaughterhouse workers, sewer cleaners, and miners. In the United States, most leptospirosis cases are associated with exposure during recreational water activities.

Characteristics

Organisms belonging to the genus *Leptospira* ("leptospires") are thin, flexible, and tightly coiled spirochetes. They are 0.1 μm wide and 6 to 20 μm long with pointed ends bent into a typical hook-like shape. Unlike *Treponema* and

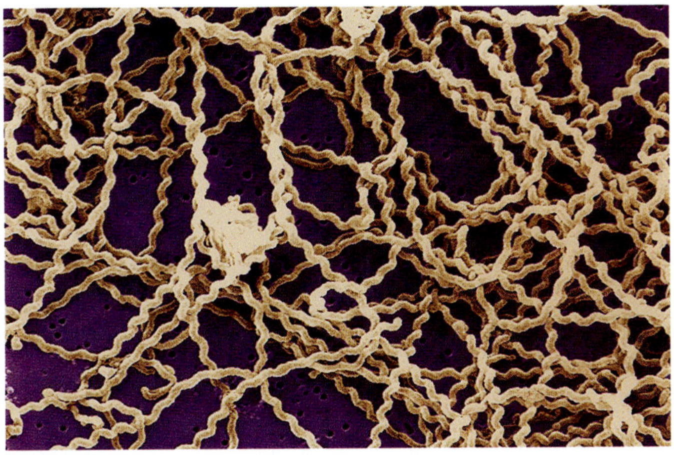

FIGURE 21–15 Scanning electron microscope (SEM) image shows many corkscrew-shaped *Leptospira* spirochetes atop a 0.1-μm polycarbonate filter. *(Courtesy of the CDC/Rob Weyant and Janice H. Carr, Public Health Image Library.)*

Borrelia organisms, the spirals of *Leptospira* are so close together that they tend to appear similar to a chain of cocci **(Fig. 21–15)**.

The genus *Leptospira* was originally divided into two main species, namely, pathogenic saprophytes, *L. interrogans*, and environmental saprophytes, *L. biflexa*. However, better distinction can be achieved by serotyping. There are more than 200 serovars of *L. interrogans* and more than 60 for *L. biflexa*. Leptospires are obligate aerobes that grow optimally at a temperature range of 28°C to 30°C. They can be grown in artificial culture media such as Fletcher semisolid medium, Ellinghausen-McCullough-Johnson-Harris (EMJH) semisolid medium, or Stuart liquid medium.

Mode of Transmission

Leptospires are naturally found inhabiting the renal tubules of infected animals such as rodents, dogs, pigs, horses, and livestock and, thus, are shed in the urine of these animals. The organisms can survive for weeks to months in urine-contaminated water and mud. Humans are exposed through mucous membranes, conjunctiva, skin abrasions, or ingestion when they come into contact with urine-contaminated water from rivers, streams, sewage, or floodwater. The risk of transmission increases by wading, swimming, or boating in floodwater or fresh water that may be contaminated with animal urine. Exposure to leptospirosis can be avoided by not wading or swimming in potentially contaminated water bodies, especially after heavy rainfall or flooding. Protective clothing such as rubber boots, gloves, and waterproof coveralls should be worn in situations involving occupational exposure.

Stages of the Disease and Treatment

The incubation period in leptospirosis varies between 2 to 30 days, but most cases manifest 5 to 14 days after exposure. The clinical presentation of the illness is generally abrupt, starting with a nonspecific febrile episode of headache, myalgia, nausea, vomiting, diarrhea, and a characteristic conjunctival suffusion (redness of the mucous membrane covering the eye). Illness may be biphasic, with the patient briefly recovering from mild illness but then developing more severe disease with renal, hepatic, pulmonary, and CNS involvement. Severe systemic disease involving renal failure and jaundice caused by hepatic failure is referred to as **Weil disease.** Patients with severe illness have a fatality rate of 5% to 15%. In pregnant women, leptospirosis can cause abnormalities, death, or abortion of the fetus.

Penicillin and doxycycline are the drugs of choice for treatment of leptospirosis. Early treatment reduces the severity and duration of the illness. Studies have shown that prophylaxis with a weekly dose of oral doxycycline is considered effective for people in high-risk environments.

Laboratory Diagnosis

Leptospires can be demonstrated in blood or serum samples in the first week of illness by dark-field, immunofluorescent, or phase contrast microscopy, but these techniques are not recommended because of their low sensitivity. Serology is the most common method to diagnose leptospirosis, followed by molecular techniques. During the first week of illness, whole blood and serum are the preferred samples, and afterward, a serum and/or urine sample should be submitted for testing. IgM screening assays are available in the form of ELISA, ImmunoDOT, and lateral flow tests. Positive screening tests should be confirmed by a **microscopic agglutination test (MAT)**, which is the gold standard for diagnosing leptospirosis. In this method, dilutions of patient serum are combined with cultured leptospires, and the degree of agglutination is observed under a dark-field microscope to determine the antibody titer. Ideally, acute and convalescent serum samples collected 7 to 14 days apart are tested by the MAT. This test is available only at regional or national reference laboratories. PCR assays are also available at the CDC and some commercial laboratories. The key advantage of PCR is quick turnaround time and prompt treatment of positive cases.

Relapsing Fever

Relapsing fever is caused by several species of *Borrelia* and is categorized into three groups based on their vector: soft tick relapsing fever (STRF), caused by *B. hermsii, B. turicatae*, and other *Borrelia* species; hard tick relapsing fever (HTRF), caused by *B. miyamotoi;* and louse-borne relapsing fever (LBRF), caused by *B. recurrentis*. While HTRF is found in the same geographical distribution as Lyme disease, STRF is found more frequently in the western mountainous states of the United States and parts of Texas; however, both are associated with outdoor activities. LBRF is not found in the United States, unless people have traveled to an endemic region in

Africa, and is associated with overcrowding and poor personal hygiene.

Characteristics

The *Borrelia* spirochetes are microaerophilic, grow optimally at temperatures between 33°C and 35°C, and share the same physiological characteristics as those of Lyme disease.

Mode of Transmission

STRF is transmitted through soft-bodied ticks of the *Ornithodoros* genus. These ticks take brief painless feedings, lasting less than an hour, typically at night. Most cases are associated with rodent-infested lodging and less commonly with spelunking (cave exploration). While these ticks are found globally, they are usually located in mountainous regions in the western United States. Prevention involves removing rodent nests and limiting tick access to bedding.

HTRF is transmitted through the same black-legged ticks that transmit Lyme disease, *I. scapularis* and *I. pacificus*. Thus, HTRF has the same geographical distribution, feeding patterns, and prevention mechanisms as Lyme disease, the only difference being that the peak incidence for HTRF occurs in August.

LBRF is spread mainly through human body louse and, rarely, head lice. Spread is associated with poor living conditions typically associated with war and social disruption; there are no animal hosts. Prevention is the same as other louse-borne illnesses and involves improving personal hygiene, not sharing bedding and clothes, and using lice-killing medications.

Stages of the Disease and Treatment

Signs and symptoms of all forms of relapsing fever include fever, headache, chills, muscle and joint aches, and nausea, although these differ in the time of onset and frequency of relapse. STRF appears 4 to 21 days after the tick bite, with the fever lasting up to 3 days, and relapse occurring several times at weekly intervals. HTRF symptoms appear 2 weeks after tick exposure, with the fever lasting from 3 to 6 days and, despite its name, no relapse. LBRF has the same pattern as STRF; however, there are fewer relapses. Tetracyclines, β-lactams, and macrolids are the preferred treatments for relapsing fever.

Laboratory Diagnosis

STRF and HTRF can be diagnosed using thick and thin Giemsa-stained blood smears, similar to malaria, as they are microscopically present and abundant during febrile episodes; however, blood collection must take place when the patient has a fever. LBRF can also be detected in stained blood smears, but only in symptomatic patients early in the infection. Because of cross-reactivity with syphilis and Lyme disease, there are no approved serological assays to diagnose relapsing fever. PCR assays are available; however, there are no standardized protocols, and they are typically only used in research facilities.

Knowledge Check 21-6

B. miyamotoi causes:
a. Leptospirosis
b. STRF
c. HTRF
d. LBRF

KEY CONCEPTS

Introduction

- Syphilis, Lyme disease, leptospirosis, and relapsing fever are caused by spirochetes.
- Spirochetes are distinguished by the presence of axial filaments that wrap around the cell wall inside a sheath and give the organisms their characteristic corkscrew motility.

Syphilis

- Syphilis is caused by the organism *Treponema pallidum,* subspecies *pallidum*. The disease is acquired by direct person-person contact, usually through sexual transmission.
- Syphilis has four main clinical stages:
    - The *primary stage* is characterized by the presence of a painless ulcer called a *chancre* at the site of initial contact.
    - An untreated patient may progress from the primary stage to the *secondary stage,* in which systemic dissemination of the organism occurs, and symptoms such as generalized lymphadenopathy, malaise, sore throat, and skin rash appear.
    - Disappearance of the secondary stage is followed by a lengthy *latent stage* in which patients are usually free of clinical symptoms.
    - About one-third of the people who remain untreated develop *tertiary syphilis*. This late-stage disease is characterized by three major clinical manifestations: granulomatous inflammation (gummas), cardiovascular disease, and neurosyphilis. Early diagnosis and treatment help to prevent later complications.
- Direct laboratory diagnosis of syphilis involves detecting the organism from a lesion by using dark-field microscopy, fluorescence microscopy, or PCR. Serological testing plays a major role in syphilis diagnosis, especially if an active lesion is not present.
- Nontreponemal serological tests (i.e., the VDRL and RPR) detect antibody to cardiolipin, also known as *reagin*. Because these tests are fairly sensitive and simple to perform, they have traditionally been used to screen for syphilis. However, they lack specificity, so specimens with positive results must be tested with a more specific treponemal antibody test for confirmation.

- Treponemal tests detect antibody against *T. pallidum*. They are more specific and sensitive in early stages of the disease. Traditional treponemal antibody tests include the FTA-ABS and particle agglutination (TP-PA).
- Treponemal antibodies remain detectable for life, whereas nontreponemal titers decline after successful treatment.
- More recent developments in syphilis testing include EIA, CLIA, and PCR. EIA and CLIA test for antibody to specific treponemal antigens, and antibody differentiation by class is possible. For large-volume testing, an automated EIA or CLIA is commonly used as a screening test, followed by confirmation with an RPR test, and possibly, a TP-PA test if there are discrepant results from the first two tests. This testing sequence is known as the *reverse screening algorithm*.

Lyme Disease

- Lyme disease is the most common vector-borne infection in the United States. The organism responsible is the spirochete *Borrelia burgdorferi*, which is transmitted by the deer tick.
- Although an expanding red rash is often the first symptom noted in Lyme disease, the disease can be characterized as a progressive syndrome that can disseminate to diverse organ systems, including the skin, nervous system, heart, and joints. Despite antibiotic treatment, a small percentage of patients continue to have fatigue; concentration and short-term memory problems; and musculoskeletal pain, which may last 6 months or longer. These symptoms may be caused by persistence of the infection.
- IgM and IgG antibodies to *B. burgdorferi* cannot usually be detected until 3 to 6 weeks after symptoms initially appear. A two-tier testing protocol is used that involves screening with an IFA or EIA and follow-up of equivocal or positive tests with immunoblotting (in the standard algorithm) or a different EIA (in the modified algorithm). All serological findings must be interpreted carefully in conjunction with clinical findings.

Leptospirosis

- Leptospirosis is a zoonosis associated with exposure to water contaminated with animal urine. It is caused by spirochetes of the genus *Leptospira* and has its highest incidence in tropical and subtropical regions of the world.
- Symptoms of severe *Leptospira* infection include fever, headache, myalgia, conjunctivitis, jaundice, and combined liver and renal failure, a condition referred to as *Weil disease*.
- The microscopic agglutination test (MAT) is the gold standard confirmatory method in the laboratory diagnosis of leptospirosis.

Relapsing Fever

- Relapsing fever (RF) is caused by several species of *Borrelia* bacteria and is classified into three groups based on the vector: soft tick relapsing fever (STRF), hard tick relapsing fever (HTRF), and louse-born relapsing fever (LBRF).
- RF symptoms include fever, headache, chills, muscle and joint aches, and nausea; the frequency of relapses varies with the type of RF. Various antibiotics are used to treat the disease.
- Diagnosis of RF involves examination of Giemsa-stained blood smears, and possibly PCR. There are no approved serological tests for RF as of this writing.

Study Guide: Comparison of Tests Used for the Diagnosis of Syphilis

TEST	ANTIGEN	ANTIBODY	COMMENTS
Direct Microscopic			
Dark-field	*T. pallidum* from patient	None	Requires active lesion with live organisms; must have good specimen, experienced laboratorian; inexpensive
Fluorescent antibody	*T. pallidum* from patient	Anti-treponemal antibody with fluorescent tag	Requires active lesion; more specific than dark-field exam; specimen does not have to contain live organisms
Nontreponemal			
VDRL	Cardiolipin	Anti-cardiolipin (reagin) in patient serum	Microscopic flocculation; may be used for screening, treatment monitoring, CSF testing; false positives are common

RPR	Cardiolipin	Anti-cardiolipin (reagin) in patient serum	Macroscopic flocculation with charcoal particles; more sensitive than VDRL in primary syphilis; used for screening, confirmation in the reverse algorithm, and treatment monitoring; false positives are common
Treponemal			
FTA-ABS	Nichols strain of *T. pallidum*	Anti-treponemal antibody in patient serum	Confirmatory; specific, sensitive; may be negative in primary stage
Serodia TP-PA (formerly, MHA-TP)	Gel particles sensitized with *T. pallidum* sonicate (formerly sensitized sheep RBCs)	Anti-treponemal antibody in patient serum	Easier to perform than FTA-ABS
EIA, CLIA, MFI	Treponemal antigen	Anti-treponemal antibody in patient serum	Sensitive, automated testing provides objective results; used to screen for syphilis in many large laboratories; EIAs have been developed as competitive, sandwich, or capture immunoassays that can detect IgM or IgG antibodies
PCR	*None. T. pallidum* DNA in patient sample is amplified	None	Highest sensitivity primary-stage syphilis; availability is limited

CLIA = chemiluminescent immunoassay; EIA = enzyme immunoassay; FTA-ABS = fluorescent treponemal antibody absorption; MFI = multiplex flow immunoassay; MHA-TP = microhemagglutination assay for antibodies to Treponema pallidum; PCR = polymerase chain reaction; RPR = rapid plasma reagin; TP-PA = T. pallidum particle agglutination; VDRL = Venereal Disease Research Laboratory.

Study Guide: Comparison of Tests for the Diagnosis of Lyme Disease

TEST	ANTIGEN	ANTIBODY	COMMENTS
IFA	Whole or processed *B. burgdorferi*	Anti-*Borrelia* antibody from patient, anti-human globulin with fluorescent tag	Initial test for Lyme disease; labor intensive to perform; false positives; subjective
ELISA	Recombinant C6 peptide (conserved region of surface lipoprotein VlsE) and pepC10 (derived from OSP-C)	IgM and/or IgG antibody to *Borrelia* antigens from patient, anti-human globulin with enzyme tag	Easy to perform; highly specific; often not sensitive in early Lyme disease; may be used as initial or confirmatory test for Lyme disease
Immunoblot (Western blot)	Antigens of *B. burgdorferi* separated by molecular weight	Detects antibodies (IgG or IgM) to individual *B. burgdorferi* antigens	Technically difficult to perform; interpreting the blot can be challenging; used as a confirmatory test for Lyme disease
PCR	None. *B. burgdorferi* DNA in patient sample is amplified	None	Available in reference laboratories

EIA = enzyme immunoassay; IFA = immunofluorescence assay; PCR = polymerase chain reaction.

CASE STUDIES

1. A patient saw a physician to complain about repeated episodes of arthritis-like pain in the knees and hip joints. The patient recalled having seen a very small tick on their arm about 6 months before the symptoms developed. However, no rash was ever seen. Laboratory tests for rheumatoid arthritis and SLE were negative. An ELISA test conducted on the patient's serum for Lyme disease was indeterminate.

Questions

a. Does the absence of a rash rule out the possibility of Lyme disease?
b. What might cause an indeterminate ELISA test?
c. What confirmatory testing would help determine the cause of the patient's condition?

2. A mother who had no prenatal care appeared at the emergency department in labor. The physician safely delivered a baby who appeared to be normal. The physician obtained a blood sample from the mother for routine screening. An RPR test performed on the mother's serum was positive. The mother had no obvious signs of syphilis and denied any past history of the disease. She indicated that she had never received any treatment for a possible syphilis infection. Cord blood from the baby also exhibited a positive RPR result.

Questions

a. Is the baby at risk for congenital syphilis?
b. What is the significance of a positive RPR on a cord blood test?
c. How should the infant be managed, based on these results?
d. What is the significance of a positive RPR in pregnancy? How should it be confirmed for syphilis?

Review Questions

1. False-positive nontreponemal tests for syphilis may occur because of which of the following?
   a. Infectious mononucleosis
   b. Systemic lupus erythematosus
   c. Pregnancy
   d. All of the above

2. In the fluorescent treponemal antibody absorption (FTA-ABS) test, what is the purpose of absorption with Reiter treponemes?
   a. It removes reactivity with lupus antibody.
   b. It prevents cross-reactivity with antibody to other *T. pallidum* subspecies.
   c. It prevents cross-reactivity with antibody to nonpathogenic treponemes.
   d. All of the above

3. Which test is recommended for testing of cerebrospinal fluid to detect neurosyphilis?
   a. RPR
   b. VDRL
   c. FTA-ABS
   d. Enzyme immunoassay

4. Which syphilis stage and description are correctly matched?
   a. Primary: painless, solitary lesion
   b. Secondary: spontaneously healing chancre on the mouth
   c. Latency: thickening of the cardiac valve
   d. Tertiary: presence of rash on the palms of the hands and soles of the feet

5. Which of the following is true of nontreponemal antibodies?
   a. They can be detected in all patients with primary syphilis.
   b. These antibodies are directed against cardiolipin.
   c. Nontreponemal tests remain positive after successful treatment.
   d. The antibodies are only found in patients with syphilis.

6. Which syphilis test detects specific treponemal antibodies?
   a. RPR
   b. VDRL
   c. FTA-ABS
   d. Dark-field exam

7. Which of the following is true of treponemal tests for syphilis?
   a. They are usually negative in the primary stage.
   b. Titers decrease with successful treatment.
   c. In large-volume testing, they are often used as screening tests.
   d. They are subject to a greater number of false positives than nontreponemal tests.

8. An RPR test done on a 19-year-old patient as part of a prenatal workup was negative but exhibited a rough appearance. What should the technologist do next?
   a. Report the result out as negative.
   b. Do a VDRL test.
   c. Send the sample for confirmatory testing.
   d. Make serial dilutions and do a titer.

9. Treponemal EIA tests for syphilis are characterized by all of the following *except:*
   a. They are adaptable to automation.
   b. They are useful in monitoring antibody titers in patients with syphilis who are undergoing therapy.
   c. Subjectivity in reading is eliminated.
   d. They can be used to distinguish between IgG and IgM antibodies.

10. Which of the following tests is the most specific during the early phase of Lyme disease?
    a. IFA
    b. EIA
    c. Immunoblotting
    d. Detection of *B. burgdorferi* DNA by PCR

11. False-positive serological tests for Lyme disease may be caused by all the following *except:*
    a. Shared antigens between *Borrelia* groups
    b. Cross-reactivity of antibodies
    c. Resemblance of flagellar antigen to that of *Treponema* organisms
    d. Testing during the early stage of the disease

12. A 24-year-old patient who had just recovered from infectious mononucleosis had evidence of a genital lesion. The RPR test was positive. What should the laboratorian do next?
    a. Report out as false positive.
    b. Do a confirmatory treponemal test.
    c. Do a VDRL.
    d. Have the patient return in 2 weeks for a repeat test.

13. A 15-year-old patient returned from a camping trip. About a week after returning, the patient discovered a small red area on the leg that had a larger red ring around it. The physician had tested for Lyme disease, but the serological test was negative. What is the best explanation for these results?
    a. The patient definitely does not have Lyme disease.
    b. The test was not performed correctly.
    c. The antibody response is often below the level of detection in early stages.
    d. Too much antibody was present, causing a false negative.

14. The reverse screening algorithm for syphilis testing:
    a. Is the CDC-preferred algorithm
    b. Is more labor intensive than the "traditional" method
    c. May give false-positive results that must be resolved by doing a TP-PA test
    d. Is more prone to transcription errors in reporting

15. Dark-field microscopy for syphilis:
    a. Uses a labeled antibody for detection
    b. Is best used in the primary or secondary stages of the disease
    c. Requires that the specimen sit at room temperature for 1 hour prior to visualization
    d. Is easy to interpret

16. Which of the following specimens provides the most reliable means of detecting leptospires during the first week of infection?
    a. Urine
    b. Liver biopsy
    c. Blood
    d. Conjunctival swab

17. Which of the following statements regarding transmission of leptospirosis is *not* true?
    a. Infection can be acquired by coming into contact with urine-contaminated soil or water.
    b. People working in rat-infested areas have a high risk of contracting the infection.
    c. High-risk activities include swimming or wading in water bodies contaminated with animal urine.
    d. Person-to-person contact is a significant means of contracting the infection.

18. The gold standard method for diagnosis of leptospirosis is:
    a. Culturing the specimen on Fletcher semisolid or Stuart liquid media
    b. Enzyme-linked immunosorbent assay (ELISA)
    c. Microscopic agglutination test (MAT)
    d. Dark-field or phase contrast microscopy

19. Cardiolipin antigen is used:
    a. In a treponemal test to detect the causative agent of relapsing fever
    b. In a nontreponemal test to detect antibodies that are not specific for syphilis
    c. To agglutinate red blood cells in the TP-PA test
    d. In a nontreponemal test to detect test the causative agent of syphilis

20. While *Treponema* sp., *Borrelia* sp., and *Leptospira* sp. are all spirochete shaped:
    a. *Leptospira* sp. are so tightly coiled they often appear as cocci.
    b. Their structural proteins, such as flagella, do not cross-react, allowing a host to develop distinct antibodies unique to each species.
    c. They all contain LPS, resulting in a pink color on a Gram stain.
    d. There is no difference in the microscopic appearance of the *Treponema* sp., *Borrelia* sp., or *Leptospira* sp. spirochetes.

21. Which organism is a cause of relapsing fever?
    a. *Borrelia miyamotoi*
    b. *Borrelia burdorferi*
    c. *Letospira interrogans*
    d. *Treponema pallidum*

Chapter 21 Answer Key

Answers to Knowledge Check

21.1 b 21.2 d 21.3 d 21.4 c 21.5 a 21.6 c

Answers to Review Questions

1. d	2. c	3. b	4. a	5. b	6. c	7. c
8. d	9. b	10. d	11. d	12. b	13. c	14. c
15. b	16. c	17. d	18. c	19. b	20. a	21. a

22 Laboratory Diagnosis of Parasitic and Fungal Infections

James L. Vossler, MS, MLS^CM(ASCP)SM^CM

LEARNING OUTCOMES

After finishing this chapter, you should be able to:

22.1 Describe the three major types of parasites.

22.2 Discuss six potential outcomes of host-parasite interactions.

22.3 Explain why a host has more difficulty overcoming parasitic diseases than those caused by bacteria or viruses.

22.4 Discuss innate and adaptive immune defenses against parasites, including the role of IgE antibody and eosinophils.

22.5 Describe six strategies used by parasites to evade host defenses.

22.6 Discuss the roles of microscopy, antigen tests, antibody tests, and molecular assays in the diagnosis of parasitic infections.

22.7 Explain the role serology plays in the diagnosis of *Toxoplasma gondii* and interpret serology results for toxoplasmosis.

22.8 Describe the four types of clinical manifestations that fungi can produce.

22.9 Describe the types of immune defenses that are important in the host response to fungal infections.

22.10 Discuss the benefits and limitations of various types of laboratory tests used in the diagnosis of fungal infections.

22.11 Recognize the clinical diseases, epidemiology, and relevant laboratory results associated with aspergillosis, candidiasis, cryptococcosis, histoplasmosis, and coccidioidomycosis.

CHAPTER OUTLINE

You can go to **fadavis.com** keyword stevens for the laboratory exercises that accompany this text.

The diagnosis of parasitic and fungal infections relies on the patient's clinical symptoms, medical history, geographic location, travel history, and laboratory results. Traditionally, laboratory identification of parasitic infections has relied mainly on microscopic examination of the clinical sample. Detection of fungal infections has been based on isolating the fungus causing the infection, direct microscopic examination of the clinical sample, and histopathology. However, technological advancements have resulted in newer methods that provide improved detection of parasitic and fungal infections; these include direct antigen detection, molecular assays, proteomics, and newer serological assays.

Despite the development of newer assays, the diagnosis of parasitic and fungal infections remains a challenge for several reasons.

- In many cases, the clinical presentations overlap or are nonspecific.
- Because of the shared antigenicity of several genera and species and the use of crude antigens in some assays, cross-reactivity may occur and the ability to distinguish a specific causative agent based on serology is sometimes not possible.
- Many fungal infections are opportunistic infections that occur in people who are immunocompromised. Those individuals may not mount a humoral antibody response, limiting the utility of serologically based assays.
- Many of the parasitic diseases occur in impoverished countries where a lack of resources and expertise has hindered the development and use of serological assays.
- For many of the agents, diagnostic serological or molecular assays are not available.

In this chapter, we provide information on the immunologic aspects of parasitic and fungal infections and discuss serological and molecular assays to detect the organisms that cause these infections.

Parasitic Immunology

Our discussion of parasitic immunology begins with the different types of parasites, the diseases they cause, and possible outcomes of parasitic infections. We then describe host immune responses against parasites and the different mechanisms these organisms can use to escape the body's defenses. Finally, we discuss different types of laboratory tests used in the diagnosis of parasitic infections, focusing on toxoplasmosis as an example.

Types of Parasites

Parasites are microorganisms that survive by living on or in other organisms, referred to as *hosts*. The three main classes of parasites that can cause human disease are protozoa, helminths, and ectoparasites.

Protozoa are a diverse group of single-celled organisms that are free-living or parasitic, the latter living and multiplying on or inside hosts. For example, giardiasis, caused by *Giardia duodenalis* (also known as *G. lamblia* and *G. intestinalis*) is a protozoal infection that can occur from ingesting water or food containing cysts of the organism. The cysts may survive up to 3 months in cold water and can be spread between people and animals. Individuals infected with the organism experience diarrhea, abdominal pain, and weight loss.

Helminths, or parasitic worms, are multicellular organisms that can live either alone or in humans. Many of the adult worms can be seen with the naked eye. They include tapeworms and roundworms. Human tapeworms include *Taenia saginata* (the beef tapeworm), *Taenia solium* (the pork tapeworm), or *Dibothriocephalus latus* (previously *Diphyllobothrium latum*—the fish tapeworm). Human roundworms include *Enterobius vermicularis* (the pinworm, the most common roundworm infection in the United States), *Ascaris lumbricoides,* and *Necator americanus* (the human hookworm).

Ectoparasites live on the outside of their hosts; the flea is an example. Ectoparasites that infect humans include *Pediculus humanus capitis* (head lice), *Pthirus pubis* (pubic lice or crabs), *Sarcoptes scabiei* (scabies), and *Cimex lectularius* (the bedbug). Other ectoparasites can transmit organisms that cause infectious diseases. In most cases, they are arthropods, with ticks being the most common. For example, *Borrelia burgdorferi,* responsible for Lyme disease, is spread by the black-legged ticks *Ixodes scapularis* (or deer tick) in the northeastern, mid-Atlantic, and north-central United States, and by the western black-legged tick *Ixodes pacificus* in the Pacific Coast states. The *Plasmodium* species responsible for malaria are transmitted by the *Anopheles* mosquito through a previous blood meal taken from an infected person.

Parasitic Diseases

Parasitic diseases are most often seen in tropical and subtropical regions of the globe, where they are on the rise mainly due to increases in the population in major cities. Climate change has also contributed to the increase in parasitic diseases. Global warmth has made areas of the world that were previously uninhabitable for parasites habitable. It has also increased the range of vectors responsible for transmitting various parasites.

For example, the World Health Organization (WHO) reported that the number of malaria cases globally has increased since 2015, with an estimated 263 million cases in 2023. Whereas malaria has been well studied, the WHO has identified 20 neglected tropical diseases (NTDs) that are mainly prevalent in tropical areas, where they affect more than 1 billion people living in impoverished communities. They are caused by a variety of pathogens including viruses, bacteria, parasites, fungi, and toxins. The diseases are "neglected" because they are almost absent from the global health agenda, which aims to identify emerging diseases and disease outbreaks that pose a risk to vulnerable populations and to strengthen health care systems globally.

Parasites cause a vast majority of the NTDs. These diseases include leishmaniasis, schistosomiasis (snail fever), African trypanosomiasis (sleeping sickness), onchocerciasis (river blindness), and lymphatic filariasis (elephantiasis). In the United States, trichomoniasis, giardiasis, cryptosporidiosis, and toxoplasmosis are the most common parasitic infections.

Although effective vaccines exist for bacterial and viral agents, the development of vaccines for parasitic diseases has remained elusive because of various roadblocks. Parasites are complex organisms, many with elaborate life cycles; over time, they have developed well-honed mechanisms for immune evasion. Also, the immune responses to parasites are not fully understood. As a result, billions of people worldwide suffer from chronic parasitic infections.

Outcomes of Parasitic Infections

When an organism encounters a host, the eventual outcome depends on a variety of factors. These include the number of organisms or size of the inoculum, the organism's multiplication rate, and the organism's virulence factors. The degree to which the organism establishes an infection or is eradicated by the host depends on the organism's ability to mobilize sufficient host defenses for removal or the organism's ability to overcome those defense mechanisms.

If the parasite can establish itself in a host, one of several possible outcomes may occur: death of the host, eradication of the parasite, or as is the case in most parasitic infections, establishment of a persistent infection. The interaction and outcomes that parasites have within their hosts have been categorized into six different levels **(Table 22–1)**.

The most severe outcome is that the host is killed. The host's death may be caused by many reasons, ranging from the parasite overwhelming the host defenses to specific features of the parasite that contribute to the death of the host. One such example is *Plasmodium falciparum*. *P. falciparum* rapidly multiplies in the host and produces an erythrocyte membrane protein-1 (PfEMP1) that binds to the endothelium in the blood vessels, resulting in the small blood vessels becoming clogged. When this occurs in the brain, the result is cerebral malaria, which can be fatal.

Death of the host is not the best strategy for a parasite. If the parasite were to totally escape the host immune system and was sufficiently virulent, the parasite would kill the host on which its survival depends. If the host dies, then so does the parasite. Any parasite's survival depends on its ability to live in a peaceful manner with its host while living and feeding off the host.

Knowledge Check 22-1

Suppose a parasite colonizes a host and there is no benefit or harm to the host. This type of interaction is called:
a. Concomitant immunity
b. Sterilizing immunity
c. Commensalism
d. Symbiosis

Immune Responses to Parasites

The immune responses to parasitic infections are more complex than those associated with bacterial and viral infections, for several reasons, as described by Chandra:

1. Many parasites are multicellular.
2. Parasites are heterogeneous with respect to their life cycles and antigenic expression.
3. Many parasitic infections are chronic in nature.
4. The mechanisms by which parasites escape immune responses are significantly different from other infectious agents.
5. Many parasites develop significant genetic and antigenic changes in a relatively short period.
6. Because of their genetic makeup and other factors, individuals differ widely in their ability to handle the complex antigens found in parasites.

Defenses to parasitic infection involve both innate and adaptive immune responses. In the following sections, we discuss the defense mechanisms the host mounts against parasitic organisms.

Table 22-1 Potential Outcomes of Host-Parasite Interactions

OUTCOME	HOST-PARASITE INTERACTION	DESCRIPTION
1	Natural resistance	No invasion of host by parasite
2	Symbiosis	Colonization of host with parasite with benefit to both
3	Commensalism	Colonization of host with parasite with no benefit or harm
4	Sterilizing immunity	Parasite invades host and causes disease; host develops immunity and is cured
5	Concomitant immunity	Parasite invades host and causes disease; host develops an immune response and has some resistance to the parasite but is not cured
6	Ineffective immunity	Parasite invades host and causes disease; host does not develop resistance to the parasite and is not cured

Adapted from Playfair JHL. Effective and ineffective immune responses to parasites: evidence from experimental models. Curr Top Microbiol Immunol. 1978;80:37–64.

Innate Defenses Against Parasites

The innate or nonspecific immune response may result in the parasite's destruction and removal, thus preventing establishment of an infection. Innate immune defenses include activation of cells that may destroy the parasite by phagocytosis, release of cytokines that enhance the immune response (e.g., tumor necrosis factor alpha [TNF-α], interleukin-1 [IL-1], type I interferons, and chemokines), and activation of the complement system (see Chapters 2, 6, and 7).

Adaptive Immune Responses Against Parasites

If innate immunity is unsuccessful in eliminating the parasite, the parasite may be eliminated through activation of the adaptive immune responses. This results in specific humoral and cell-mediated responses to the parasite (see Chapter 5). In some parasitic infections, complete immunity can be achieved through the humoral immune response. Specific antibodies can damage protozoa, neutralize parasites by blocking attachment to the host cell, prevent the spread of the parasite, promote complement lysis, enhance phagocytosis, and destroy the parasite through antibody-dependent cellular cytotoxicity (ADCC).

Many parasitic infections are characterized by eosinophilia and high levels of IgE. Scientists believe that the ability to produce IgE evolved mainly to protect the host from parasitic infections. The IgE antibody binds to mast cells and basophils in the host (see Chapter 14). When specific antigen-antibody combinations occur, mast cells degranulate and release cytokines, chemotactic factors for eosinophils, histamine, prostaglandins, and other mediators. As a result, eosinophils are attracted to the infected area and are activated to destroy some parasites by degranulation or through ADCC. This mechanism is particularly important for extracellular parasites such as helminths, which are too large to be ingested by phagocytic cells.

Cell-mediated immune responses are activated to attack parasites that reside inside of host cells, such as the protozoa that cause leishmaniasis, malaria, toxoplasmosis, and cryptosporidiosis. These responses are characterized by the production of cytokines such as interferon-γ by helper 1 T (T_H1) cells, which activates macrophages and cytotoxic T (T_C) cells to destroy the intracellular parasites. Extracellular parasites, such as schistosome helminths, can activate CD4 T cells to induce delayed-type hypersensitivity, resulting in the formation of granulomas that attempt to segregate the organism and prevent its spread (see Chapter 14).

Knowledge Check 22-2

Which type of immune response is important for defense against extracellular parasites?

a. Cytokine release by suppressor T cells
b. Destruction by T_C cells
c. Opsonization and phagocytosis
d. Antibody-dependent cellular cytotoxicity (ADCC)

Parasite Survival Strategies

Parasites have developed a variety of mechanisms to evade or downregulate the host's immune response and are often able to survive in the host. The major survival strategies are antigenic concealment, antigenic variation, antigenic shedding, antigenic mimicry, immunologic diversion, and immunologic subversion. We discuss these strategies in the paragraphs that follow and summarize them in the Study Guide at the end of this chapter.

Antigen Concealment

In **antigen concealment,** parasites hide their antigens from the host after they reach their target cells. The major way in which parasites can conceal their antigens is by remaining inside of the host's cells without their antigens being displayed. If a parasite becomes sequestered within host cells, the host cannot recognize the parasite. Thus, the parasite is hidden from the immune system and protected. Examples of parasites that have an intracellular phase in their life cycle include *Plasmodium* spp., *Trypanosoma cruzi, Leishmania,* and *Cryptosporidium parvum.*

Antigenic Variation

Antigenic variation occurs when the parasite changes or varies the antigens (epitopes) it expresses, making development of an effective immune response difficult. The process begins when the host produces antibody, mainly IgM, to a parasite antigen, thereby reducing the infection. The parasite responds by altering the expression of different genes, thus changing its antigen and making the antibody ineffective. This may occur quickly, within 5 to 6 days, and can occur repeatedly over a very long period of time. The host must produce a new antibody each time an antigen change occurs.

The three main mechanisms for antigenic variation are (1) point mutations, (2) DNA rearrangement, and (3) modification of gene transcript levels. Point mutations involve a change in a single nucleotide base, changing an amino acid and resulting in a different protein antigen (see Chapter 12). DNA rearrangement and modification of gene transcript levels are referred to as **gene switching.** Organisms may carry up to 1,000 different genes that code for surface antigens, allowing for the expression of distinct surface molecules. Organisms using this mechanism can switch from the use of one gene to another, persisting while the immune system is trying to catch up with them. Gene rearrangement occurs when a gene at a site near a promoter sequence on a chromosome is replaced with a gene from a different site near the promoter sequence, allowing for that gene to be expressed. The ability to rearrange genes and rapidly change surface molecules contributes to the virulence of *Plasmodium falciparum* (a cause of malaria).

Modification at the transcript level involves the reversible expression of two different antigen genes so that the one being expressed becomes silent, and a previously inactive gene at another locus becomes activated. As a result, a different antigen is expressed. These events occur without DNA changes at the loci themselves. Examples of parasites that use this mechanism are the trypanosomes *Trypanosoma brucei* and

Trypanosoma rhodesiense—the two causes of African sleeping sickness. These bloodborne parasites can alter their surface glycoproteins to produce an unlimited group of variable antigen types.

A factor that must be considered with respect to antigenic variation is the parasite's life cycle. Compared to bacteria and viruses, most parasites have complicated life cycles. The life cycles of many parasites involve several hosts. An example is shown in Fig. 22–1, to be discussed later. A particular host may be (1) the *definitive host* that harbors the adult or sexual stage of the parasite (e.g., humans are the definitive host for *Taenia saginata* and *Taenia solium*—the beef and pork tapeworms, respectively), (2) an *intermediate host* in which the parasite lives during the larval or asexual stage (e.g., the malarial parasites in which humans are the intermediate host and the mosquito is the definitive host), or (3) an *accidental* or *dead-end host* in which a relationship is not required for reproduction of the parasite and the parasite no longer can continue with its life cycle (e.g., the dog tapeworm *Echinococcus granulosus* for which humans are an accidental host).

Different parasite antigens may be expressed, depending on the life cycle stage in the different hosts. The parasite often undergoes complex growth cycles and differentiation in preparation for transmission to its next host. In doing so, an organism's surface antigens vary considerably while in a single host. The complicated life cycles of most parasites are the main reason that mounting an effective immune response is difficult and the development of effective vaccines is hindered. For example, the *Plasmodium* species that cause malaria in humans (*P. falciparum, P. vivax, P. malariae, P. ovale,* and *P. knowlesi*) have one of the most complex life cycles. There are four different forms in the mosquito and four different forms in humans. Each of the life cycle forms expresses different antigens, delaying the effectiveness of the immune response and development of an effective malaria vaccine. It was not until fall 2023 that the WHO recommended a vaccine for

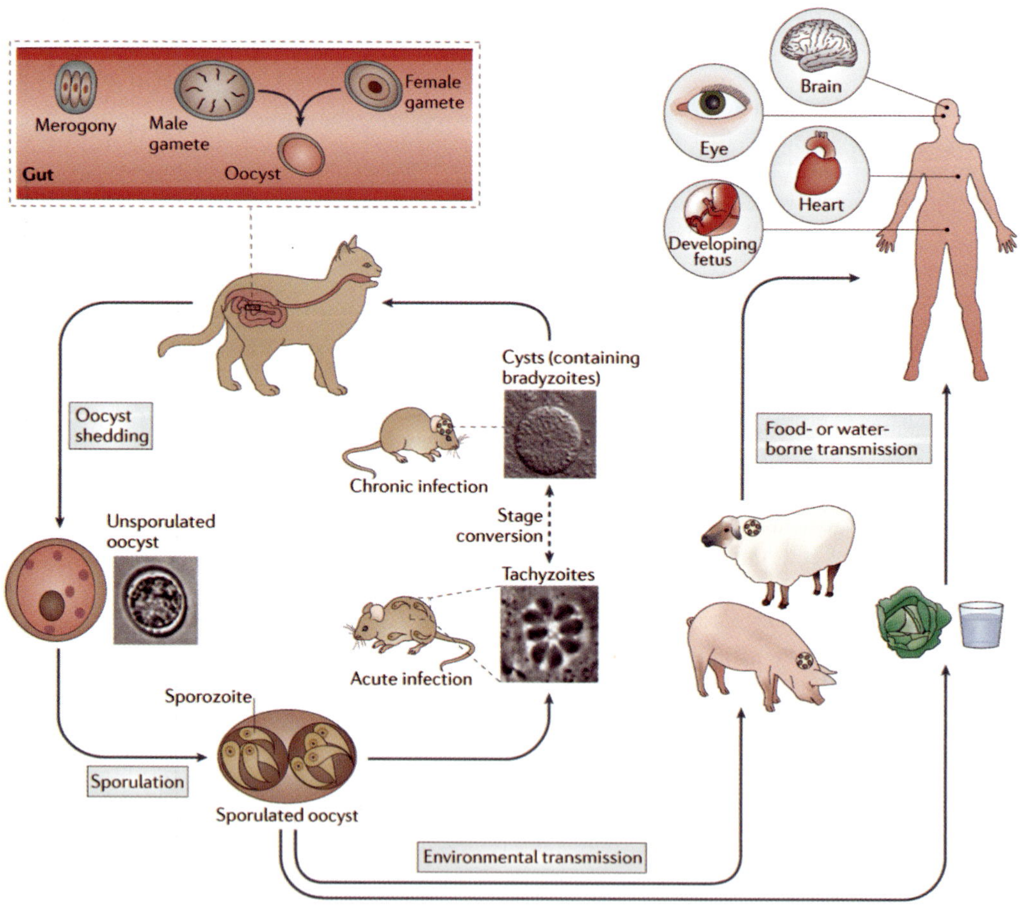

FIGURE 22–1 *Toxoplasma gondii* life cycle. Sexual replication of *T. gondii* occurs in cats, the definitive host for the parasite. *T. gondii* gametes are formed after merozoites replicate within enterocytes of the cat gut, a process known as *merogony*. The gametes fuse to form diploid oocysts, which are shed in cat feces and undergo meiosis in the environment to produce eight haploid progeny sporozoites. Asexual replication occurs in intermediate hosts such as rodents. Rapidly replicating forms called *tachyzoites* disseminate within the host during acute infection and can differentiate into slow-growing forms called *bradyzoites* inside tissue cysts. Other intermediate hosts or cats can acquire the infection by ingesting the tissue cysts, reinitiating the sexual phase of the life cycle. Oocysts can survive in the environment for a long time and develop into sporulated oocysts, which can be transmitted to intermediate hosts such as farm animals through contaminated food and water. Humans become infected by ingesting tissue cysts in undercooked meat or sporulated oocysts in contaminated water. *(Reprinted by permission from Macmillan Publishers Ltd: Nature Reviews Microbiology, 10:766–778, copyright 2012.)*

malaria prevention in children; at the time of this writing, there are no approved malaria vaccines for adults despite many years of research.

Antigenic Shedding

Some parasites exhibit **antigenic shedding,** or the casting off of antigenic material into the host environment to evade the immune system. *Entamoeba histolytica* is one example of a parasite that can shed antigens from its cell surface. Although antibody is formed against the parasite, the antibody attaches to the shed antigen rather than the parasite, allowing the parasite to escape the immune response.

Antigenic Mimicry

Antigenic mimicry occurs when the parasite expresses epitopes that are similar, if not identical, to host molecules. The similarity between host and parasitic antigens may suppress the immune response and protect the invading parasite from being recognized and eliminated by the immune system. An example is the antigenic similarity between human host antigens and those of the *Schistosoma* species. The immune response may result in host and parasite cross-reactivity, which may lead to autoimmunity, manifested by the presence of autoantibodies or T cells capable of reacting with host antigens. An autoimmune response has been linked to the cardiac and intestinal symptoms that may occur in the late stages of Chagas disease because of an infection with *Trypanosoma cruzi,* a bloodborne parasite.

Immunologic Subversion and Immunologic Diversion

Some parasites enhance their survival by modulating the host's immune system. This can be accomplished by *immunologic subversion* or *immunologic diversion.* **Immunologic subversion** is achieved by avoiding the effector mechanisms of the immune response. Effector molecules include complement and cytokines. Effector cells include plasma cells, T_H cells, and T_C cells. For example, some parasites can subvert T_C cells by producing decoy human leukocyte antigen (HLA)-like molecules. Parasites may also subvert the Fc function of antibodies by making Fc receptor homologues, or they can subvert complement by making homologues of complement control proteins (CCPs).

Immunologic diversion occurs when the parasite causes the immune system to produce proteins that redirect the attention of the immune system. For example, some parasites can cause increased production of interferon beta (IFN-β), allowing for longer parasite survival. IFN-β has been shown to decrease the ability of macrophages to kill *Leishmania* by significantly reducing the release of superoxide from these cells. Another example by which parasites can divert the immune system is seen with *P. falciparum*–infected erythrocytes (IEs), which have the potential to interact with B cells in different parts of the body, inducing them to divide and differentiate into antibody-secreting cells. The malaria parasite and some protozoa, viruses, and bacteria produce immunoglobulin-binding proteins (IBPs) that act as polyclonal B-cell activators. This results in expansion of numerous B-cell clones and in antibody production not specific for the parasite. Thus, the IBPs may act as an evasion mechanism to divert specific antibody responses.

Critical Thinking 22-1

How does a parasite's ability to adapt to transmission between hosts help it survive?

Serodiagnosis of Parasitic Diseases

Serological testing is helpful in instances where demonstration of the parasite in biological or tissue samples is not possible. Serological assays are one of two types: those that detect *antibodies* against the parasite or those detecting parasite *antigens.* The methods used in these tests include enzyme-linked immunosorbent assay (ELISA), indirect immunofluorescence (IFA), indirect hemagglutination, whole protozoan or antigen-coated particle agglutination, and lateral flow immunoassay. Previously, many of these assays used relatively crude antigens, making their sensitivity and specificity unpredictable. Advances in immunochemistry and molecular biology have allowed for the development of assays that have markedly improved sensitivity and specificity. However, assays using these newer technologies are costly and not widely available in those countries that have the highest occurrence of parasitic diseases.

Tests for Parasite Antibodies

Whereas some parasitic diseases are readily diagnosed by demonstrating the causative agent in clinical material, such as intestinal helminths, in which the worm's eggs are easily detected in fecal specimens, demonstration of other parasitic agents is difficult or not possible (e.g., toxoplasmosis). In those cases, serological assays can be very useful. **Table 22–2** indicates the usefulness of serological testing for the diagnosis of various parasitic diseases. Although serology may not be helpful in the diagnosis of some parasitic diseases, it can play a role in epidemiological investigations.

Toxoplasmosis

Toxoplasmosis, caused by the protozoan ***Toxoplasma gondii,*** is one parasite for which serodiagnosis is useful. *T. gondii* has a high prevalence around the world and can infect all species of animals and birds. An estimated 11% of the U.S. population over the age of 6 is infected with this parasite, which usually remains dormant. Reactivation may occur if the individual becomes immunosuppressed. Over 95% of toxoplasmosis cases are caused by reactivation of a latent infection.

The life cycle of *T. gondii* has three stages: the *tachyzoite,* which rapidly multiplies in the intermediate host (e.g., humans) and in nonintestinal epithelial cells of the definitive host (i.e., members of the cat family *[Felidae]*); the *bradyzoite,* which forms cysts in the host's tissues; and the *sporozoite,* which is found in oocysts **(Fig. 22–1)**. There are three routes by which *T. gondii* can be transmitted to humans: (1) Humans can become infected with *T. gondii* by eating raw or insufficiently cooked infected meat (e.g., pork, mutton, or wild game) that contains the cysts or uncooked foods that have come into contact with the infected meat. (2) Toxoplasmosis may occur when humans ingest oocysts from cat feces present

Table 22-2 Usefulness of Antibody Detection for Parasitic Diseases

SEROLOGY INDICATED	SEROLOGY MAY BE USEFUL	SEROLOGY NOT INDICATED
Amebiasis (extraintestinal) Chagas disease Clonorchiasis Cysticercosis Hydatidosis Filariasis (lymphatic; suspect cases when microfilariae cannot be identified in blood) Leishmaniasis (cutaneous and visceral) Schistosomiasis (ectopic cases; chronic cases when eggs cannot be demonstrated in feces or urine) Toxocariasis (visceral and ocular) Toxoplasmosis Trichinellosis	Amebiasis Amebic meningoencephalitis (caused by free-living amebae) Anaplasmosis/ehrlichiosis Babesiosis Malaria Paragonimiasis (eggs not detectable in sputum or feces)	Anisakiasis Ascariasis Capillariasis Cryptosporidiosis Hookworm Trichuriasis

Adapted from Maddison SE. Serodiagnosis of parasitic diseases. Clin Microbiol Rev. 1991;4(4):457–469.

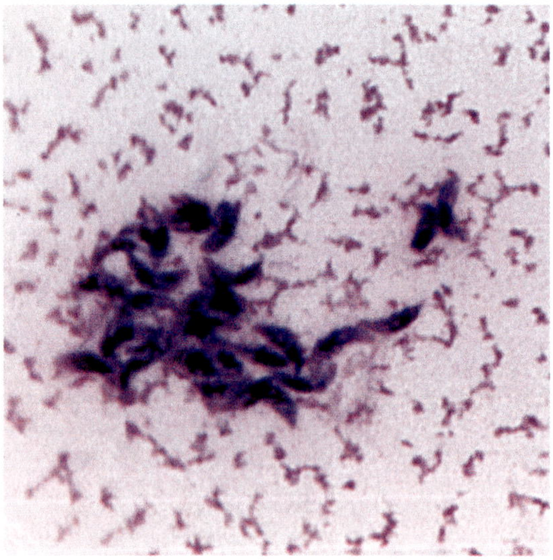

FIGURE 22–2 *Toxoplasma gondii* tachyzoites in mouse ascitic fluid stained with Giemsa stain. *(Courtesy of the CDC/Dr. L.L. Moore, Jr., Public Health Image Library.)*

in a litter box or in the soil. (3) The tachyzoites, which are observed during the primary infection, can be transmitted transplacentally to the unborn fetus **(Fig. 22–2)**. The incubation period for *T. gondii* in adults ranges from 10 to 23 days following ingestion of undercooked meat and from 5 to 20 days after ingestion of oocysts from cat feces. Following infection, the organism reproduces asexually and forms tissue cysts that remain for the life of the host.

Most initial *Toxoplasma* infections in people with a normally functioning immune system are asymptomatic or may only present with a mild lymphadenopathy. Immunity in these individuals is usually sufficient to contain the latent infection. In contrast, toxoplasmosis can cause serious symptoms in the brain and other organs in immunocompromised patients and in the developing fetus following congenital infection.

If a previously infected person becomes immunosuppressed because of human immunodeficiency virus (HIV) infection, malignancy, or immunosuppressive drugs, reactivated toxoplasmosis can occur. The tissue cysts rupture and release the active bradyzoite, which results in clinical disease. *T. gondii* infection in immunocompromised people can be severe or even fatal. In such individuals, the organism can invade the central nervous system (CNS), leading to *Toxoplasma* encephalitis.

Another concern is the organism's ability to be passed to the fetus during pregnancy. If the infection occurs before pregnancy, then the fetus is protected because of maternal antibodies. However, if a woman becomes infected just before or during pregnancy, congenital transmission of the organism can occur. Congenital toxoplasmosis may result in a miscarriage, a stillborn child, or cognitive deficits later in life. Up to one-half of pregnant women who become infected can transmit *T. gondii* across the placenta. The trimester in which the infection was acquired influences the incidence and severity of congenital toxoplasmosis. The transmission risk during the first trimester of pregnancy is 10% to 25%, whereas the transmission risk is 60% to 90% during the third trimester. *Toxoplasma* infection can result from congenital infection or infection after birth.

Laboratory Diagnosis of Toxoplasmosis

Although the diagnosis of toxoplasmosis can be made by demonstrating the parasite in stained tissue samples or cerebrospinal fluid (CSF), obtaining the appropriate specimens for these tests is difficult. Therefore, diagnosis of the infection is usually made through serological testing. Various methods have been used to detect *T. gondii* antibodies, most commonly, indirect immunofluorescence and automated immunoassays (e.g., ELISA, chemiluminescence immunoassays, multiplex bead immunoassay). A combination of IgM and IgG tests needs to be performed to determine whether an individual has been recently infected or had a previous infection with *T. gondii*. The sensitivity and specificity of different commercial kits vary, and misinterpretation of the results, particularly in determining the presence and significance of IgM antibodies, may occur. This is concerning because serological results can influence decisions regarding continuation or termination of pregnancies. IgM antibodies may persist for up to 18 months after infection with *T. gondii*. Therefore, the U.S. Food and Drug Administration (FDA) has recommended that anti-*Toxoplasma* IgM tests should be interpreted with caution and that the sole results of a single assay should not be used in determining a recent infection. The FDA and CDC have published guidelines for the interpretation of *T. gondii* serology results **(Table 22–3).**

The greatest value of testing for IgM antibodies is in determining whether a pregnant woman has had a recent infection. If no IgM antibodies are detected and only IgG is detected, a recent infection before pregnancy is unlikely. One of the problems when testing for *Toxoplasma*- IgM antibodies is that the current assays lack specificity. If only IgM antibodies are detected, additional testing should be performed. A second blood sample should be obtained from the patient 2 weeks after the first sample is collected and tested together with the first specimen. The second sample should demonstrate high levels of IgM and IgG antibodies if the first sample was collected early in the infection. If both specimens show the presence of IgM but absence of IgG, the IgM result should be considered a false positive.

When both IgM and IgG antibodies are detected and the patient is pregnant, an IgG avidity test should be performed. Determining the antibody avidity is useful in establishing whether the IgG antibodies are from a recent infection or a previous infection. As we discussed in Chapter 3, B cells evolve during the course of an immune response to produce more effective antibodies that will bind antigen with greater strength. Therefore, the presence of high-avidity IgG indicates a past infection, whereas IgG antibodies with a low avidity suggest a more recent infection. Because low-avidity antibodies may persist for a prolonged period of time, their presence does not necessarily mean that the infection was recently acquired. However, the presence of high-avidity antibodies indicates an infection for at least 3 to 5 months and does not pose a risk to the fetus.

The ELISA for IgG avidity uses a wash buffer containing urea to differentiate low-avidity from high-avidity antibodies. Antibodies with low avidity dissociate from the antigen in the presence of urea. The avidity is determined by performing the assay in duplicate using buffers with and without urea. The avidity index (AI) is determined by dividing the *T. gondii*–specific IgG signal (optical density [O.D.]) of the set washed with urea-containing buffer by the *T. gondii*–specific IgG O.D. of the set washed with non-urea buffer. AI values lower than 0.2 indicate the presence of low-avidity antibodies, values between 0.2 and 0.25 suggest intermediate avidity, and values greater than 0.25 are obtained with antibodies of high avidity.

When using serology to detect congenital toxoplasmosis, several differences exist. Because of the passive transfer

Table 22-3 General Guidelines for Interpretation of Toxoplasma gondii Serology Results

IgG RESULT	IgM RESULT	REPORT AND INTERPRETATION (EXCEPT INFANTS)
Negative	Negative	No serological evidence of infection with *Toxoplasma*.
Negative	Equivocal	Possible early acute infection or false-positive IgM result. Obtain new specimen for IgM and IgG testing. If result for the second specimen remains the same, the patient is probably not infected with *Toxoplasma*.
Negative	Positive	Possible acute infection or possible false-positive IgM result. Obtain new specimen for IgM and IgG testing. If result for the second specimen remains the same, the IgM reaction is probably a false positive.
Equivocal	Negative	Indeterminate: obtain a new specimen for testing or retest the specimen for IgG using a different assay.
Equivocal	Equivocal	Indeterminate: obtain a new specimen for IgM and IgG testing.
Equivocal	Positive	Possible acute infection with *Toxoplasma*. Obtain new specimen for IgM and IgG testing. If the result for the second specimen remains the same or if the IgG becomes positive, both specimens should be sent to a reference laboratory with experience in diagnosing *Toxoplasma* infection.
Positive	Negative	Infected with *Toxoplasma* for 6 months or longer.
Positive	Equivocal	Infected with *Toxoplasma* for probably more than 1 year or false-positive IgM reaction. Obtain a new specimen for IgM testing. If results with the second specimen remain the same, both specimens should be sent to a reference laboratory with experience in diagnosing *Toxoplasma* infection.
Positive	Positive	Possible recent infection within the past 12 months or false-positive IgM result. Send the specimen to a reference laboratory with experience in diagnosing *Toxoplasma* infection.

Adapted from Centers for Disease Control and Prevention. DPDx—Laboratory identification of parasitic diseases of public health concern: toxoplasmosis. Accessed December 6, 2024. https://www.cdc.gov/dpdx/toxoplasmosis/index.html

of IgG across the placenta, infants whose mothers are chronically infected will be born with *Toxoplasma* IgG antibodies of maternal origin. Serological diagnosis can be made 5 or 10 days after birth by demonstration of positive *Toxoplasma* IgM or IgA antibody titers, respectively, in newborn sera. Detection of anti-*Toxoplasma* IgA antibodies is more sensitive than detection of IgM antibodies. It should be noted that commercial assays currently used in the United States have not been cleared by the FDA for diagnostic testing of infants. Therefore, samples from neonates suspected of having congenital toxoplasmosis should be sent to the Toxoplasma Serology Laboratory/Sutter Health, Palo Alto, California, the site with the most experience with infant testing (see https://www.sutterhealth.org/pamf/services/lab-pathology/serology-tests; accessed July 3, 2025).

The polymerase chain reaction (PCR) for the detection of *T. gondii* nuclei acid may be helpful in diagnosing the infection in immunocompromised people who may produce low amounts of antibody. However, a negative PCR does not rule out active infection, and clinical symptoms need to be considered together with the laboratory results. PCR testing can also be done on amniotic fluid to detect a fetal infection acquired from the mother.

Knowledge Check 22-3

A patient had the following test results for *T. gondii* antibodies: IgM negative, IgG positive. What do these results indicate?

a. Acute infection with *T. gondii*
b. Past *T. gondii* infection
c. High risk for toxoplasmosis
d. Indeterminate immune status for *T. gondii*

Rapid Detection Systems to Detect Parasite Antigens

Traditionally, ELISAs have been used to detect antigens of parasites that cause human and animal infections, such as amebiasis, babesiosis, fascioliasis, cutaneous and visceral leishmaniasis, cysticercosis, echinococcosis, malaria, schistosomiasis, toxocariasis, toxoplasmosis, trichinosis, and trypanosomiasis. More recently, rapid immunochromatographic assays for detection of parasite antigens have gained widespread use in clinical laboratories.

Rapid antigen detection systems (RDTSs), also called **lateral flow assays,** are qualitative immunochromatographic methods that detect proteins or polysaccharides that are integral components of pathogens. RDTSs detect soluble antigens via their ability to bind to capture antibodies contained in a nitrocellulose strip (see Chapter 11). The clinical sample is placed on the strip and eluted by adding a few drops of buffer that contains a labeled antibody. A colored band representing the antigen-antibody complex can then be seen within minutes on the membrane. Many of the assays are stable at room temperature, easy to perform and interpret, and cost effective. One example of a widely used RDTS is shown in **Figure 22–3.**

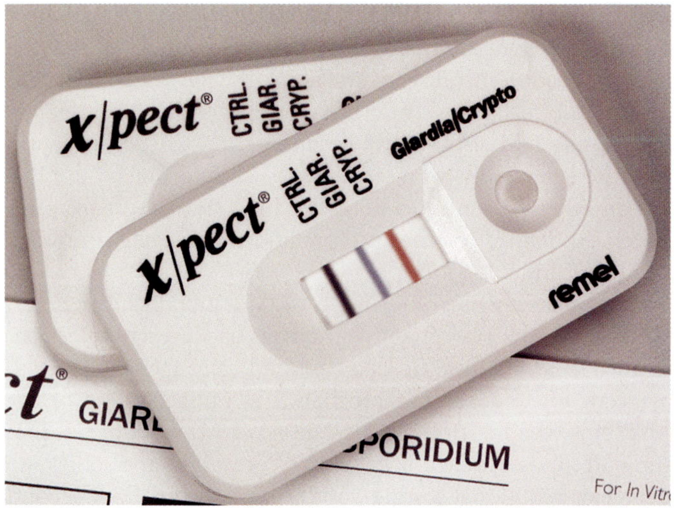

FIGURE 22–3 Remel Xpect Giardia/Cryptosporidium immunochromatographic immunoassay. The test uses sample wicking to capture *Giardia* and *Cryptosporidium* antigens on discrete test lines containing antigen-specific antibodies for each organism. *(Reprinted by permission of Thermo Fisher Scientific, Lenexa, Kansas.)*

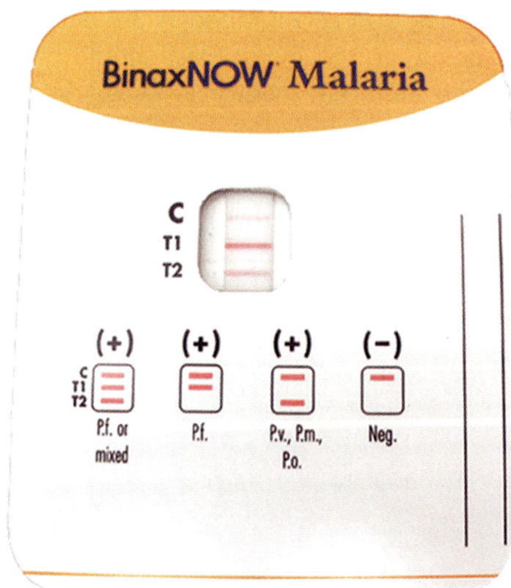

FIGURE 22–4 BinaxNOW Malaria test. The immunochromatographic assay targets the histidine-rich protein II (HRPII) antigen specific to *Plasmodium falciparum* (P.f.) and a pan-malarial antigen common to all four malaria species capable of infecting humans—*P. falciparum, P. vivax* (P.v.), *P. ovale* (P.o.), and *P. malariae* (P.m.)—circulating in human venous and capillary ethylenediaminetetraacetic acid (EDTA) whole blood. *(Reprinted by permission of BioMed Central Ltd, Malaria Journal 14;10:300, copyright 2011.)*

Because of their advantages, many RDTSs can be used in rural regions, for example, assays for the rapid diagnosis of malaria. The assays allow for differentiation between *Plasmodium vivax* and the deadlier *P. falciparum.* **Figure 22–4** shows results from the BinaxNOW Malaria test (Abbott Rapid Diagnostics), the first FDA-approved RDTS for malaria in the United States. The test detects the histidine-rich protein II (HRPII) specific to *P. falciparum* (P.f.) and a pan-malarial antigen common to all four malaria species that can infect humans—*P. falciparum, P. vivax* (P.v.), *Plasmodium ovale* (P.o.), and *Plasmodium malariae* (P.m.).

Limitations of Parasitic Serology

As with all laboratory testing, it is important to use methods that are easy to perform and cost effective. However, it is also important to consider the specificity and sensitivity of the method when choosing a procedure. Currently, there is no external proficiency testing program offered in parasitic serology except for the diagnosis of toxoplasmosis. Therefore, it is very difficult to evaluate the quality of commercial assays that are currently available. In the United States, commercial kit manufacturers must obtain FDA approval before selling their products. The FDA requires only that a new method be equivalent to a method that has already been approved. Researchers at the CDC have expressed concern that over time, the quality of new test kits may drift in a negative direction because a new kit may not be quite as good as the one used for comparison but may still receive approval.

In addition, a specific test may not detect a parasitic disease in an individual because of the inability of the assay to detect all species of the parasite causing the infection. For example, some serological tests, such as those for schistosomiasis, only detect antibodies that are species-specific. Therefore, the same sample can give either negative or positive results, depending on the species detected by the test method. Also, different types of specimens from the same patient may give conflicting results. Factors such as these can lead to an inaccurate diagnosis.

Because of the antigenic complexity of parasites, the antibody produced by a patient may not be detected because the assay uses an antigen different from the one to which antibodies have been formed. Also, the sensitivity of an assay may vary, depending on the stage and type of the patient's disease. For example, antibodies against *Plasmodium* species (malaria) rise rapidly in an acute infection but decline if the parasite becomes latent or dormant in the liver as a hypnozoite. In contrast, because of the potential for cross-reactivity of the antibodies formed in a parasitic infection, false-positive results can occur.

Although there are commercially available tests for the serological diagnosis of several parasitic agents, the number of commercial kits available in the United States is limited. In the United States, most tests are only performed by a few commercial laboratories, including Focus Technologies, Mayo Medical Laboratories, Parasitic Disease Consultants, Quest Diagnostics, and Specialty Laboratories. Most of the tests performed at these laboratories and at the CDC are produced and evaluated in-house and use reagents that are not universally standardized. Because of the differences in the reagents used in the tests, discrepant results obtained by different laboratories are commonly observed.

Molecular Methods for Diagnosis of Parasitic Disease

Although microscopic methods are how most blood and tissue parasites are detected, they have important limitations. Decreased sensitivity associated with these methods may be caused by intermittent shedding of the organism, as is seen with *Giardia lamblia,* or to low levels of the organism being present, as is observed with the bloodborne parasites such as the agents causing malaria or babesiosis. Molecular techniques are being used with increasing frequency to diagnose parasitic infections, especially in cases where unequivocal identification of the parasite cannot be made.

For example, traditional or quantitative polymerase chain reaction (qPCR) assays have been developed for some parasitic diseases, including babesiosis and malaria, and are available from commercial reference laboratories (e.g., Mayo Medical Laboratories in Rochester, Minnesota, and Focus Diagnostics in Cypress, California) and from the CDC. Many laboratories have also developed in-house assays for the identification and differentiation of parasites. Several molecular technologies, including nested multiplex PCR and loop-mediated isothermal amplification (LAMP), have the potential to detect and identify bloodborne and gastrointestinal parasites. Molecular tests are playing an increasingly important role as adjuncts to traditional diagnosis of parasitic infections and, in some cases, may even replace traditional methods as commercial companies develop molecular assays and seek FDA approval.

Fungal Immunology

Fungi are a large heterogeneous group of eukaryotic organisms that are ubiquitous in the environment. Fungi can be considered as either parasites, deriving their nutrition from living matter, or more commonly saprophytes, living off of dead and decaying matter. In the environment, fungi play an important role in maintaining the ecosystem by decomposing cellulose. Over 120,000 well-characterized fungal species exist, and new organisms are identified as advances in molecular biology allow for the detection and differentiation of fungi. Despite the number and diversity of fungi, only about 300 fungal species are potentially pathogenic to humans and animals. Fewer than 50 of these species are responsible for about 90% of all fungal infections.

When a human or animal has an infection or disease caused by a fungus, it is referred to as a **mycosis** (plural: **mycoses**). Mycoses are classified into four groups—superficial, cutaneous, subcutaneous, or systemic—based on the type and amount of tissue involvement and the host response to the pathogen. Mycotic diseases are of growing importance for several reasons: (1) Fungi are widely distributed in nature and can maintain themselves in the environment, making them difficult to eradicate. (2) Many fungi cause various clinical manifestations, ranging from invasive disease to localized infection, or allergic manifestations, as observed with *Aspergillus.* (3) Diagnosis is difficult because of the varying clinical presentations. (4) Currently, vaccines are not available. (5) There are only a limited number of antifungal agents available for treating fungal infections. (6) Most fungal infections are opportunistic in nature, and increasingly, treatment of a primary disease puts individuals at risk for opportunistic infections.

Fungi do not possess a large array of virulence factors that allow for them to be true pathogens. However, opportunistic fungal infections have risen since the advent of AIDS and increased use of immunosuppressive therapies. Fungal diseases are often the first opportunistic diseases detected in patients with AIDS. One of the most common opportunistic diseases in patients with AIDS is pneumonia caused by *Pneumocystis jirovecii* (previously *Pneumocystis carinii*). Although originally classified as a parasite, this organism has been reclassified as a fungus because it has a greater gene sequence homology with fungi than with parasites. Also, many saprophytic fungi formerly dismissed as cultural contaminants are now reported as opportunistic pathogens.

Characteristics of Fungi

Fungi are eukaryotic cells with nuclei and rigid cell walls composed primarily of chitin, glucans, mannans, and glycoproteins. Fungi can exist in two morphological states: **yeast,** which are unicellular organisms, or **mycelial fungi,** which are multicellular organisms. Yeast reproduce by budding, whereas the mycelial fungi reproduce through the production of **conidia** (i.e., spores). It should be noted that many people develop allergies to the spores and conidia produced by fungi. Although most fungi are *monomorphic* (existing in a single form), several fungi can exist as either yeast or mycelial fungi, depending on environmental conditions, and are referred to as *dimorphic* fungi.

Fungi grow more slowly than most bacteria (2 to 4 weeks versus 1 to 2 days) and have relatively simple nutritional requirements. Because most fungi are found in the environment, they prefer cooler temperatures for growth (25°C to 30°C).

Classification of Mycotic Infections (Mycoses)

Fungal infections can produce four types of clinical manifestations:

1. *Hypersensitivity.* Some people exhibit *hypersensitivity* to certain fungi. The hypersensitivity reaction generally occurs because of an allergic reaction to the spores (see Chapter 14). Hypersensitivity may occur only when a person comes in contact with the specific spores to which they are allergic, or it can occur as a chronic condition such as allergic bronchopulmonary aspergillosis (ABPA), which develops in response to the fungus *Aspergillus* (most commonly *Aspergillus fumigatus*).
2. *Mycotoxicosis.* This is a poisoning of humans and animals by food products contaminated by fungi that produce toxins from a grain substrate. Major mycotoxins include aflatoxins, deoxynivalenol, fumonisins, zearalenone, T-2 toxin, ochratoxin, and certain ergot alkaloids.
3. *Mycetismus* (mushroom poisoning). Mushrooms are classified as fungi. Mushroom poisoning can result from ingestion of toxin-producing mushrooms. Potentially deadly mushrooms include *Amanita phalloides, Amanita verna, Amanita virosa,* and certain other species that contain neurotoxins.
4. *Growth of fungi on or in the host tissue.*

Grouping fungal infections according to the body sites affected is useful, for both diagnosis and identification of the agents in the laboratory. The major groups are the following:

A. *Superficial and Cutaneous Mycoses.* These fungal infections of the skin, hair, and nails are the most common type of fungal infection. The *superficial* mycoses are restricted to the outer layers of the skin and hair and typically do not cause inflammation. These infections are cosmetic in nature and are not life threatening. *Cutaneous* mycoses involve the epidermis layer of the skin, hair, and nails. Symptoms are mainly due to the immune response causing skin inflammation, itching, and reddening. Common examples of cutaneous mycoses include *tinea corporis* (infection of body surfaces), *tinea pedis* (foot infections commonly called "athlete's foot"), *tinea cruris* (groin, inner thigh, or buttocks infections), and *tinea capitis* (scalp infections). *Tinea,* commonly referred to as "ringworm," means fungal infection of the skin, and the term after describes the body area infected. The lesions produced contain a clear area of somewhat normal skin surrounded by a circular border of inflamed skin containing red, raised, scaly areas **(Fig. 22–5).** Brittle hair and thick, broken nails can also be seen.

The organisms causing cutaneous infections live off the keratin in the epidermis and are, in most cases, noninvasive in nature. The tineas are caused by a group of closely related fungi called *dermatophytes,* which are transmitted by direct contact with an infected person or animal or by direct contact with conidia, which can germinate into fungi and cause infection. The dermatophytes causing these infections belong to one of three genera: *Trichophyton, Microsporum,* and *Epidermophyton.* Cutaneous fungal infections can also be caused by *Candida* yeast (see later section).

B. *Subcutaneous mycoses.* These infections affect the subcutaneous tissue (under the skin), where they usually form deep, ulcerated lesions. The causative agents are soil saprophytes, and acquisition of the fungal agent is generally caused by trauma to the skin, usually of the feet or legs.

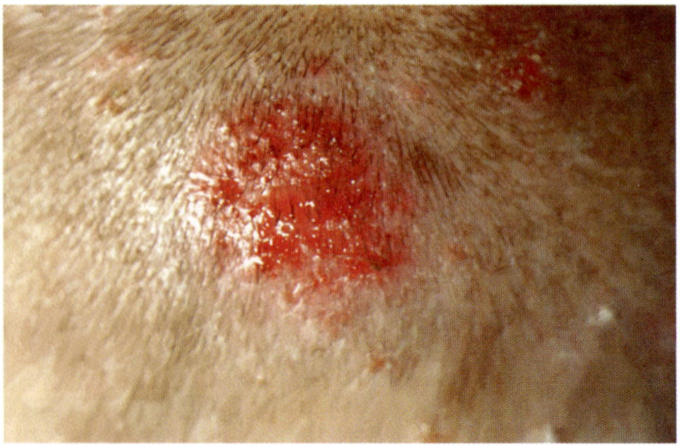

FIGURE 22–5 *Tinea capitis* (ringworm of the scalp). *(Courtesy CDC/ Dr. Lucille K. Georg.)*

C. *Systemic mycoses.* These infections involve the internal organs and spread throughout the body. They originate in the lungs and then disseminate through the blood to other locations. Although systemic mycoses are considered to be pathogenic to humans, many infected individuals are asymptomatic. Except for *Cryptococcus,* the causative agents in this group are dimorphic in nature, as they have a yeast phase at body temperature and a mold (filamentous) phase in the environment.

D. *Opportunistic mycoses.* The organisms in this group are normally not pathogenic in humans but can cause invasive infections in immunosuppressed patients, such as those who have HIV, are undergoing chemotherapy, or are receiving an organ transplant. Several agents have been long known to cause infections in immunosuppressed people, including *Candida, Aspergillus,* and the fungi causing zygomycosis (*Rhizopus* species, *Mucor* species, *Cunninghamella bertholletiae,* and *Apophysomyces elegans*).

Table 22–4 lists the most common agents associated with the various classifications. Several fungi are considered to be commensalistic in nature, including *Candida albicans* and *Malassezia furfur;* however, these organisms may cause disease or clinical symptoms in some people.

Critical Thinking 22-2

Suppose patient A has a mild urinary tract infection caused by *Candida* species. In contrast, *Candida* infection in patient B caused a severe infection of the mouth and esophagus. Explain why the clinical manifestations of *Candida* might be different in the two patients.

Immune Responses to Fungi

The most important immune defenses to fungi involve innate immunity early in the infection, especially physical barriers and phagocytosis by neutrophils, and adaptive mechanisms induced later, notably cell-mediated immunity. We discuss these and other defenses in more detail in the sections that follow.

Innate Defenses

The first line of innate defense includes the skin and mucous membranes of the respiratory, gastrointestinal, and genitourinary tracts to provide physical barriers that separate the host from the environment. Fungi possess very few factors that allow them to overcome those physical barriers; because of the nutrients and environmental conditions needed for many fungi, those mechanisms have not evolved. For example,

Table 22-4 Mycotic Infections Based on Site of Infection and Level of Tissue Involvement

CLASSIFICATION	REPRESENTATIVE AGENT	DISEASE
Superficial	*Malassezia furfur* *Exophiala werneckii* *Piedraia hortae* *Trichosporon* species	Pityriasis versicolor (skin) Tinea nigra (skin) Black piedra (hair) White piedra (hair)
Cutaneous	*Trichophyton* species *Microsporum* species *Epidermophyton floccosum*	Tinea (e.g., ringworm, athlete's foot, jock itch)
Subcutaneous	*Sporothrix schenckii* *Fonsecaea pedrosoi* *Pseudallescheria boydii*	Sporotrichosis Chromoblastomycosis Eumycotic mycetoma
Systemic	*Histoplasma capsulatum* *Coccidioides immitis* *Paracoccidioides brasiliensis* *Blastomyces dermatitidis* *Talaromyces marneffei* (previously *Penicillium marneffei*) *Cryptococcus neoformans*	Histoplasmosis (endemic in Ohio and Mississippi River valleys) Coccidioidomycosis (endemic in the southwestern United States) Paracoccidioidomycosis (endemic in Central and South America, primarily Brazil) Blastomycosis (predominantly a veterinary pathogen in Ohio and Mississippi River valleys) Talaromycosis (predominantly seen in patients with AIDS in Southeast Asia) Cryptococcosis (causes meningitis in immunosuppressed patients [e.g., AIDS])
Opportunistic	*Candida albicans* *Aspergillus* species *Rhizopus* species	Candidiasis Aspergillosis Zygomycosis
Commensalistic	*Candida albicans* *Malassezia furfur*	Urinary tract infections, vaginal yeast infections Tinea versicolor (pityriasis versicolor), dandruff, and seborrheic dermatitis

among the most common fungal infections are those caused by the dermatophytes (*Trichophyton* species, *Microsporum* species, and *Epidermophyton floccosum*). These fungi cause infections of the skin, hair, and nails because they require dead keratin for growth. Infections caused by these fungi are also sometimes known as "ringworm" or "tinea." These agents do not possess any invasive factors, and the symptoms associated with them are caused by the inflammatory response of the host.

If the fungi penetrate the physical barriers, other important innate mechanisms can attack the organism. As we discussed in Chapter 2, innate immune cells—neutrophils, macrophages, and dendritic cells (DCs)—express various pattern-recognition receptors (PRRs) that recognize specific structures on fungi called *pathogen-associated molecular patterns (PAMPs)*. After binding of these receptors to their corresponding PAMPs, neutrophils and macrophages phagocytize and kill fungal organisms, and release lysosomal enzymes and reactive oxygen species, which destroy extracellular fungi.

The PRRs include the transmembrane proteins, the **toll-like receptors (TLRs)**, and the **C-type lectin receptors (CLRs)**. Several fungal components are recognized by TLRs, including phospholipomannans and β-glucans, which are recognized by TLR2, and glucuronoxylomannans, which are recognized by CD14 and TLR4. Binding of TLRs to their corresponding PAMPs initiates cell signaling pathways that stimulate the production of type I interferons and other cytokines that promote inflammation and induce adaptive immunity.

Although TLRs play a role in the immunologic response to fungi, CLRs are central for fungal recognition and induction of innate and adaptive immune responses to fungi. Fungal cell walls consist mainly of multiple layers of carbohydrates, including mannans (cell wall polysaccharide), β-glucan, and chitins (the main component of fungal cell walls). The CLR transmembrane protein, dectin 1, recognizes β-glucans. Dectin 2 recognizes high-mannose structures common to many fungi and binds hyphal forms with higher affinity than yeast forms. People with genetic deficiencies in CLRs are highly susceptible to fungal infections.

In addition, the alternative and lectin complement pathways are activated against fungi that enter the bloodstream. The complement components released can promote opsonization to enhance phagocytosis but may not lyse fungal organisms due to their thick cell walls.

Adaptive Immune Responses

Cell-mediated immunity plays the most important role in the adaptive response to fungal infections, and patients with deficiencies in this arm of the immune system are susceptible to developing progressive fungal infections. Once the cells of the innate immune system have been activated, the cytokines and chemokines produced recruit T cells to the site of the infection and induce their activation. T_H17 cells recruit neutrophils to the site, where they can phagocytize and kill the fungi, and T_H1 cells release cytokines that can promote inflammation and activate T_C cells to kill intracellular fungi.

Although a humoral response to many fungi is stimulated, antibodies are thought to be ineffective against fungal infections. In some cases, such as aspergillosis, they may actually cause harm by inducing hypersensitivity reactions.

Laboratory Diagnosis of Fungal Infections

The incidence of invasive fungal infections has risen dramatically in the past several decades because of HIV infection and the increase in immunosuppressive therapies. The clinical diagnosis of fungal infections in many instances is difficult. The clinician must consider the patient's symptoms, history of other past or present infections, medical treatments, occupation, place of residence, and record of travel in evaluating the likely cause of a fungal infection. Laboratory methods for diagnosing fungal infections include the following:

- Isolation of the organism in the laboratory. This is the most common method to determine the cause of a fungal infection and is considered the traditional "gold standard." However, recovery is often difficult with uncommon fungi. Also, once the organism is isolated, traditional identification methods may take several weeks because of the slow growth of fungi.
- Direct examination of the clinical specimen. Potassium hydroxide (10% KOH) can be used to dissolve keratin and other cellular materials to allow for microscopic visualization of fungal elements in a specimen. India ink is used to observe encapsulated yeast such as *Cryptococcus neoformans* from CSF.
- Histopathological evidence of tissue invasion.
- Skin testing to detect a cell-mediated immune response to a fungus.
- Serological tests for fungal antigens of commonly encountered organisms. The detection of fungal antigens, including cryptococcus capsular polysaccharide, *Histoplasma* antigen, galactomannan, and β-D-glucan in body fluids, can be used for the presumptive diagnosis of some of the causative agents of a fungal infections, particularly in cases of invasive fungal infections.
- Serological tests for fungal antibodies. These are available for commonly encountered organisms, including *Candida albicans, Aspergillus* species, *Cryptococcus neoformans,* and the dimorphic fungi *Histoplasma capsulatum* and *Coccidioides immitis*. Although the humoral response to fungi is not the major defense against fungal infection, antibodies produced against the organisms may be readily detected and can be used to demonstrate current or past exposure to the agent. However, in that many fungal infections are opportunistic, serological diagnosis many times is of little value because immunosuppressed patients do not reliably produce antibodies during acute infections, and serological assays are not available for most of the opportunistic fungi. Also, in areas where a fungal agent is endemic to a geographic area, most people living in those areas will test positive for the antibodies regardless of whether or not they have an active infection.

- Molecular assays for fungal nucleic acid. Examples include peptide nucleic acid fluorescence in situ hybridization (PNA-FISH) for identification of *Candida* species in blood cultures, qPCR assays for detection of *Aspergillus* species and *P. jirovecii* from bronchial lavage fluid, and multiplex PCR coupled with a bead probe fluid array for detection of numerous species of fungi in bronchial lavage fluid or blood. Molecular methods for fungal infections continue to be developed.

Knowledge Check 22-4

Which laboratory technique is used to observe encapsulated yeast microscopically?

a. India ink preparation
b. KOH preparation
c. PNA-FISH
d. Rapid test for polysaccharide capsular antigen

Fungal Pathogens

In the following sections, we provide information on five fungal infections for which serological testing is used.

Aspergillus Species

Aspergillus is a ubiquitous fungus found worldwide in nature **(Fig. 22–6).** The genus has over 185 species and can be recovered from soil and plant material; its spores may be recovered from indoor air environments. *Aspergillus fumigatus* is the most commonly isolated species, with *Aspergillus flavus* and *Aspergillus niger* also being frequently recovered. Less commonly recovered isolates include *Aspergillus clavatus*, the *Aspergillus glaucus* group, *Aspergillus nidulans*, *Aspergillus oryzae*, *Aspergillus terreus*, and *Aspergillus versicolor.* In humans,

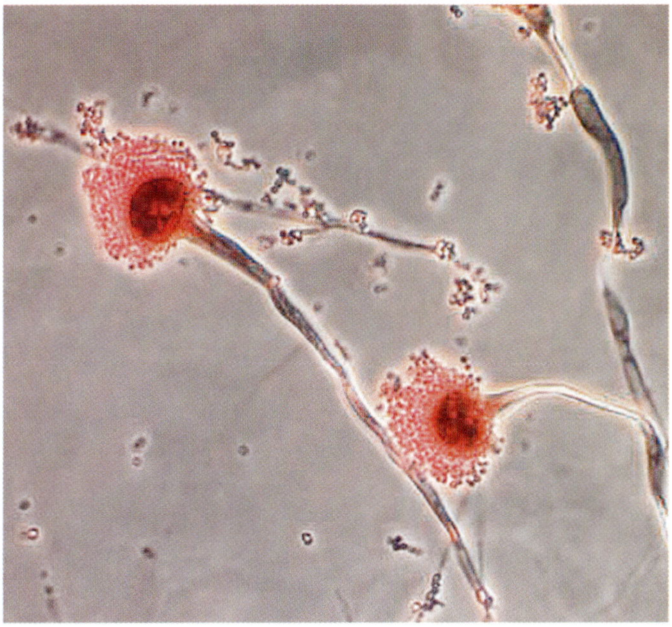

FIGURE 22–6 *Aspergillus fumigatus*, LPCB stain × 450. *(Courtesy of the CDC, Public Health Image Library.)*

Aspergillus is mainly an opportunistic pathogen causing a variety of infections. Infections in immunocompetent individuals include *Aspergillus otomycosis,* a superficial infection of the external auditory (ear) canal and auricle (otitis externa or "swimmers' ear"). *A. niger* is one of the three most common causes of otitis externa, along with two bacteria, *Staphylococcus aureus* and *Pseudomonas aeruginosa. Aspergillus* can also grow in the lung cavity, forming a solid mass of **hyphae,** which can develop into a fungus ball referred to as an *aspergilloma.* Pulmonary aspergilloma usually occurs in scarred lung tissue or in a preexisting lung cavity resulting from a previous infection, such as tuberculosis or sarcoidosis. Some fungal antigens may elicit allergic responses to *Aspergillus,* causing ABPA, which results in a long-term allergic response. ABPA is thought to be present in 1% to 2% of patients with persistent asthma and in about 7% of patients with cystic fibrosis.

Invasive forms of *Aspergillus* most frequently begin in the lung, resulting from inhalation of the conidia. The organism grows and spreads in the lung tissue. Invasive pulmonary aspergillosis (IPA) may occur in the neutropenic patient because of immunosuppression. Aspergillosis in such patients may spread from the lungs to adjacent tissues and through the blood to distant body sites.

The diagnosis of **aspergillosis** generally requires a positive tissue biopsy demonstrating the hyphae or a positive culture for *Aspergillus.* Nonculture methods may also be used to diagnose invasive aspergillosis. The detection of galactomannan in serum can be used to indicate a fungal infection and has increased the ability to diagnose invasive aspergillosis. Another assay to detect invasive fungal infections, including aspergillosis, measures β-D-glucan (BDG) in serum. BDG is a component of the cell wall of most fungi. Serological diagnosis is of limited utility because immunosuppressed patients fail to mount an antibody response, even with invasive disease. PCR, a highly sensitive method for detection of *Aspergillus* in tissue samples and bronchoalveolar lavage fluid, may be helpful in the diagnosis of invasive aspergillosis.

Candida Species

Candida spp. are yeast that may exist as commensal organisms in the human host. They are commonly found on the skin, in the gastrointestinal (GI) tract, and in the female genital tract. Of the more than 150 species of *Candida,* only a small percentage is regarded as frequently pathogenic for humans. *C. albicans* is the leading cause of human infections. Other members include *Candida guilliermondii, Candida krusei, Candida parapsilosis, Candida tropicalis, Candida pseudotropicalis, Candida lusitaniae, Candida dubliniensis,* and *Candida glabrata. Candida auris,* first seen in Japan in 2009, is an emerging yeast pathogen that is spreading at a rapid rate in U.S. health care facilities. Infections with *C. auris* are associated with a high mortality rate and are often resistant to multiple antifungal drugs.

Candida infections **(candidiasis)** rose dramatically in the United States after the introduction of antibiotics. In recent decades, *Candida* species have been the fourth most common organisms recovered from the blood of hospitalized patients in the United States. The incidence of candidemia-related hospitalizations has risen significantly in the past two decades. Invasive candidiasis is a major hospital-associated fungal disease in the United States and is associated with mortality rates of 30% to 40%. Increased use of immunosuppressive therapies, the use of advanced life-support therapies, and the incidence of HIV infection have all contributed to the increased incidence of *Candida* infections. Infections in the immunocompetent host include diaper rash, vaginitis and urinary tract infections in females, and thrush (oral candidiasis) caused by the use of broad-spectrum antibiotics. People with thrush for no obvious reason should be evaluated for AIDS. The introduction of potent antiretroviral therapy has reduced the incidence of thrush in AIDS patients. *Candida* esophagitis, pneumonia, and septicemia may be observed in the neutropenic patient because of radiation and chemotherapy or use of broad-spectrum antibiotics.

The diagnosis of *Candida* infections generally involves recovery of the causative agent. The organisms grow well in routine culture media. Direct examination of clinical material with a 10% KOH preparation may also be used to detect *Candida* species. Current recommendations include the combined detection of mannan and anti-mannan antibodies for the specific identification of *Candida* species in serum samples. These assays can be positive 6 days before blood cultures, on average. They also show a very high negative predictive value (i.e., a negative test result indicates absence of candidiasis in most patients). However, serological diagnosis of candidiasis is limited because colonization of the gastrointestinal tract or other body sites by *Candida* species can stimulate antibody production in uninfected individuals. Also, immunocompromised patients may not mount detectable antibody responses.

Over the years, various methods for serum antigens have been used to detect invasive candidiasis, including latex agglutination (LA), counterimmunoelectrophoresis, and ELISA; however, these have not proven to be useful. Molecular assays such as direct PCR of blood samples offer a sensitive means for early detection of invasive candidiasis and can differentiate between different *Candida* species.

Cryptococcus neoformans

The genus *Cryptococcus* includes 19 species of encapsulated yeasts. *C. neoformans* evolved from being a rare cause of human disease to a significant opportunistic pathogen as the population of immunocompromised patients increased. *C. neoformans* is a *saprobe* in nature, obtaining its nutrition from dead or decaying organic matter. The organism lives in certain trees and rotting wood and has frequently been isolated from soil contaminated by guano from birds (e.g., pigeons). *C. neoformans* enters the host mainly through the lungs and has a predilection for invading the CNS of the susceptible host. Although pulmonary infections are common, *Cryptococcal* meningoencephalitis (inflammation of the brain and surrounding membranes) represents the main life-threatening infection caused by *C. neoformans*. In the pre-AIDS era, cryptococcosis had an overall incidence of 0.8 cases per million persons per year. In 1992, during the peak of the AIDS epidemic, the rate in several large U.S. cities reached almost five cases per 100,000 persons per year. With the use of antiviral agents for the treatment of AIDS in developed countries, these numbers have declined.

The most important feature contributing to the organism's virulence and pathogenicity is its capsule. The capsule consists of polysaccharide containing an unbranched chain of α-1,3-linked mannose units substituted with xylosyl and β-glucuronyl groups. The capsule has many effects on the host's immune response. These include acting as a barrier to phagocytosis, preventing destruction by complement, producing antibody unresponsiveness, dysregulating cytokine secretion, interfering with antigen presentation, and enhancing HIV replication.

The two most common sites for infection with this encapsulated yeast are the lungs and CNS, with the respiratory tract being the most common portal of entry. Most cryptococcal infections are asymptomatic in people with a competent immune system, and most cases of cryptococcosis are diagnosed in individuals with compromised immune systems. Respiratory symptoms range from asymptomatic colonization of the airway to life-threatening pneumonia with evidence of an acute respiratory distress syndrome. Patients with CNS involvement generally present with subacute meningitis or meningoencephalitis. Symptoms include headache, fever, lethargy, and memory loss over several weeks. Some patients may present with an acute onset of meningitis.

The laboratory diagnosis of *Cryptococcus* infections may be done using direct microscopic examination of the clinical material, culturing for the organism, or performing serological tests. Microscopic examination of the organism can be performed by mixing the biological fluid (usually CSF) with India ink. The encapsulated yeast displaces the India ink, creating a halo around the yeast cell **(Fig. 22–7)**. Although the test is easy to perform and interpret and has high specificity, it shows poor sensitivity (50% to 80%).

Detection of cryptococcal polysaccharide antigen in serum and CSF can be performed by LA and enzyme immunoassays (EIAs). Both types of tests are more than 90% sensitive and specific. Although the LA test is a rapid and reliable serological

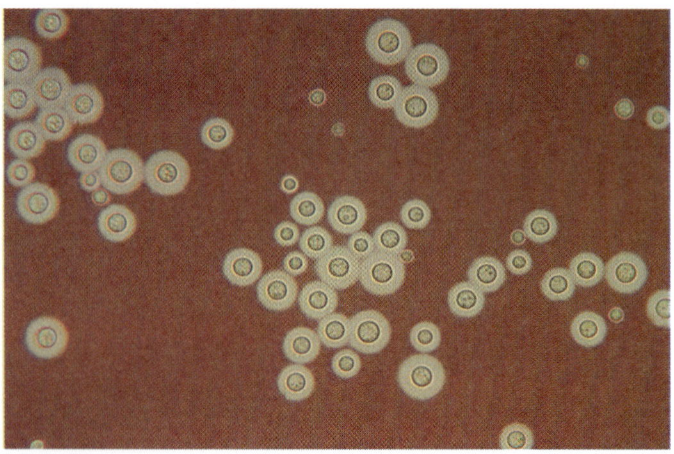

FIGURE 22–7 India ink prep showing *Cryptococcus neoformans* in CSF. The organism's large polysaccharide capsule displaces the India ink, allowing for visualization of the yeast. *(Courtesy of the CDC/ Dr. Leanor Haley, Public Health Image Library.)*

method for the diagnosis of cryptococcosis, false-positive LA test results can occur due to rheumatoid factor or other interference factors in patient samples. Pretreating the specimen with heat and pronase, or 2-mercaptoethanol, destroys these factors and reduces the incidence of false positives.

A lateral flow immunochromatographic assay (LFA) for the detection of cryptococcal antigen in CSF and serum is also available **(Fig. 22–8).** The assay can detect cryptococcal antigen in fewer than 15 minutes. The assay has a sensitivity of 100% and a specificity of 99.8% with serum samples, as well as a sensitivity of 99.3% and a specificity of 99.1% with CSF.

Measurement of cryptococcal antigen levels also has some clinical use. Serial polysaccharide antigen titers can be performed on serum or CSF. Initial high titers (1:1,024 or higher) indicate high levels of the yeast in the host and poor host immunity. Patients with high titers have a greater chance of therapeutic failure. Increasing antigen titers are usually seen with worsening of the disease, whereas declining titers are usually associated with clinical improvement. Cryptococcal antigen may be detected even months after successful therapy, so cryptococcal antigen tests should not be used to indicate cure.

Histoplasma capsulatum

H. capsulatum is a common cause of infection and is endemic in the Ohio and Mississippi River valleys. The organism is a dimorphic fungus, growing as a yeast at 35°C to 37°C and as a mycelial fungus at environmental temperatures. It is found and grows in soil under favorable conditions. The presence of bird and bat guano increases the likelihood of the organism being present in the soil. Whereas birds are not infected with the fungus, bats carry the fungus in their gastrointestinal tracts and shed it. **Histoplasmosis** (infection with *H. capsulatum*) is acquired by inhalation of mycelial fragments and microconidia. Most of the infections are self-limiting and asymptomatic. Of those who are symptomatic, pulmonary histoplasmosis, either acute or chronic, is the most frequent clinical presentation. In a primary infection, the organism disseminates to organs rich in mononuclear phagocytes. The organism can cause a potentially lethal infection in patients with preexisting conditions. The organism causes opportunistic infections in patients with weakened immune systems (e.g., people with HIV infection). Disseminated disease in the immunocompromised patient is 100% fatal if untreated. Survival rates of the acute episode exceed 80% when treated.

The definitive diagnosis of histoplasmosis is made by culture of the organism. The organism is generally recovered within 3 weeks of culture. The ability to recover the organism is affected by the number of specimens submitted for culture, the type of specimen submitted (e.g., respiratory secretions, blood, or CSF), and the severity of the infection.

Laboratory diagnosis can also be made by detecting the polysaccharide antigens of *Histoplasma* in serum or urine by ELISA. The test can also be performed on CSF or bronchoalveolar lavage fluid. Urinary antigen tests have a high specificity and sensitivity for detecting *Histoplasma* infections, even in immunosuppressed patients, such as those with AIDS.

Antibodies to the H and M glycoprotein antigens can be used to demonstrate exposure or infection with *H. capsulatum* and can be detected 3 to 6 weeks after infection in most infected people; however, immunosuppressed patients may not produce detectable antibodies. The H antibody appears after the M antibody and can be found in sera from patients during acute and/or progressive disease. The presence of both H and M antibodies indicates active infection and is conclusive for the diagnosis of histoplasmosis. The antibodies can be detected by complement-fixation assays, or more commonly by immunodiffusion. Titers between 1:8 and 1:16 are considered weakly positive and may represent past infection or may result from an immune response of healthy persons living in regions where histoplasmosis is endemic. A titer of 1:32 or greater or a fourfold increase in titer over time indicates active histoplasmosis.

Skin testing detects a cell-mediated immune response to *Histoplasma,* similar to the Mantoux tuberculin skin test, and may also determine if an individual has been exposed to the organism. The *H. capsulatum* skin test becomes positive 2 to 4 weeks after infection, when most infected people are

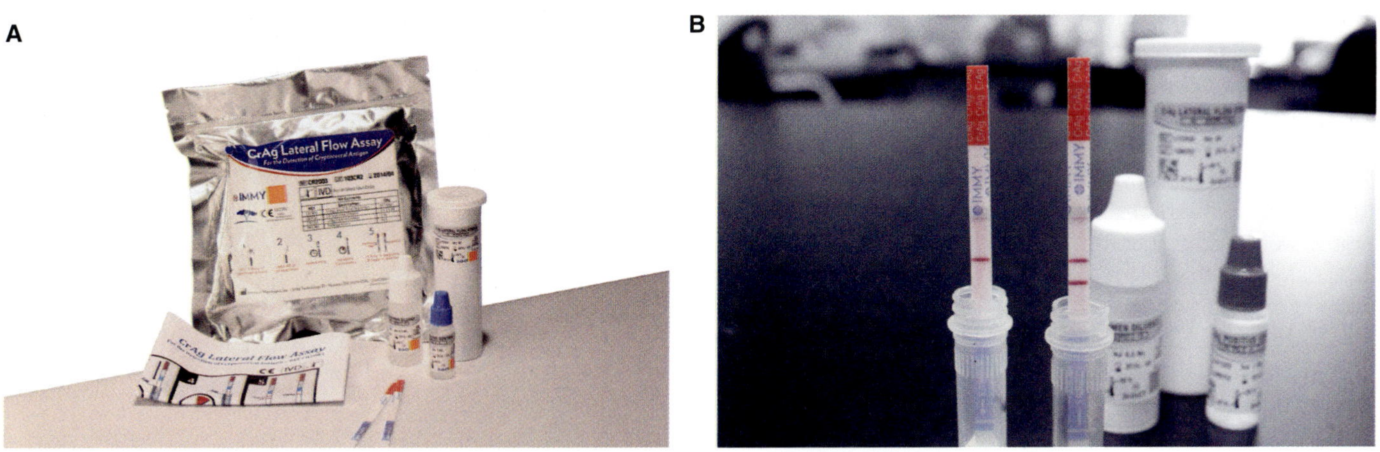

FIGURE 22–8 IMMY CrAg LFA (cryptococcal antigen lateral flow assay). (A) and (B). Kit components. The assay is a sandwich immunochromatographic dipstick assay for the qualitative and semiquantitative detection of cryptococcal antigen from CSF and serum. (B) Test results: The dipstick on the left shows one line for the control; the test sample is negative. The dipstick on the right shows two lines, indicating a valid control result and the presence of cryptococcal antigen in the test sample. *(Reprinted by permission of Immuno-Mycologics, Inc. [IMMY], Norman, Oklahoma.)*

asymptomatic. Repeat testing will usually give positive results for the rest of a person's life. Thus, in areas where the fungus is endemic, the skin test is of limited utility.

Molecular assays appear to have promise in the diagnosis of histoplasmosis; however, at the time of this writing, molecular assays for routine use are not commercially available.

Coccidioides immitis

C. immitis is a dimorphic fungus that causes **coccidioidomycosis,** also known as "valley fever." Coccidiomycosis is endemic in dry, arid regions of southwestern United States, Mexico, Central America, and South America. This is because spores from the fungus (arthroconidia) are found in the soil and dust in these areas.

In a vast majority of cases, infections result from inhaling arthroconidia that have been released into the air following a disturbance of contaminated soil and dust. A single arthroconidium can be enough to produce a naturally acquired respiratory infection. Up to two-thirds of cases caused by *C. immitis* are either inapparent or so mild as to not prompt medical evaluation. In people who become symptomatic, the clinical presentation is usually similar to a community-acquired pneumonia. About 5% to 10% of patients may develop long-term lung problems, or dissemination of the infection to other parts of the body, such as the CNS, skin, joints, and bones. Once the spores are inhaled, there is an incubation period of 1 to 3 weeks before the development of respiratory symptoms. Thus, travel history is important if the person has traveled to an endemic area.

Once coccidioidomycosis is suspected, diagnosis may be established by identifying the fungus in a clinical specimen or detecting *Coccidioides* antibodies in serum, CSF, or other body fluids. The most common way in which coccidioidomycosis is diagnosed is through serology. Although the organism can be cultured, obtaining a sputum specimen is not often possible because of the lack of sputum production in infected individuals. Also, fungal culturing is not available in outpatient settings. The use and limitations of skin testing for *Coccidioides* infection are like those for *Histoplasma.* Once positive, the skin test generally remains positive for the rest of one's life; therefore, it is of limited use for people living in endemic areas.

Complement fixation (CF), Ouchterlony immunodiffusion (ID), LA, and lateral flow immunoassay (LFA) have been the most commonly used serological methods for detecting infection (see Chapters 10 and 11 for most test principles). ID tests detect IgM antibodies to a polysaccharide from the fungal cell wall and are positive in most patients within the first 3 weeks of symptoms. The CF assay detects IgG antibodies to a chitinase antigen from the fungus. When mixed with the antigen, antibodies from patient serum form immune complexes, which bind complement. When the complement is depleted, antibody-coated red blood cells (RBCs) added to the mixture fail to lyse. CF antibodies are detected later and for longer periods than antibodies detected by ID. Therefore, CF is useful for diagnosis of both acute and chronic infection and for assessment of disease severity.

LFA and LA tests for coccidioidal antibodies are commercially available and can detect IgM or IgG antibodies. A positive LFA result is a highly sensitive indicator for *Coccidioides* infection. Although the LFA tests for IgM and IgG are more sensitive than ID, false positives have been reported. Therefore, positive EIA results, particularly positive IgM results, should be confirmed with ID or CF tests. The FDA has approved a PCR for detection of *Coccidioides* nucleic acid in lower respiratory samples, but it is not widely available at this time.

Knowledge Check 22-5

Match each fungal pathogen with its associated feature:

a. *Aspergillus* species	____ 1. Has H and M antigens
b. *Candida* species	____ 2. Cause of "valley fever"
c. *Cryptococcus neoformans*	____ 3. Hyphae can form fungus ball in the lung
d. *Histoplasma capsulatum*	____ 4. Visualized with India ink
e. *Coccidioides immitis*	____ 5. Cause of oral thrush

KEY CONCEPTS

Types of Parasites

- Parasites are microorganisms that survive by living off other organisms. The three major types of parasites are protozoa, helminths, and ectoparasites.

Parasitic Diseases

- Parasitic diseases are most often seen in tropical and subtropical regions of the globe. They are increasing in incidence because of climate change and population growth in major cities.
- Most neglected tropical diseases are caused by parasites, including leishmaniasis, schistosomiasis (snail fever), African trypanosomiasis (sleeping sickness), onchocerciasis (river blindness), and lymphatic filariasis (elephantiasis). Such diseases are almost absent from the global health agenda, which aims to identify emerging diseases and disease outbreaks and to strengthen health care systems globally.

Outcomes of Parasitic Infections

- Parasitic infections can result in eradication of the organism by the host's immune system, death of the host because of an ineffective immune response, or in most cases, establishment of persistent infection because of the host's inability to completely eliminate the organism.

Immune Responses to Parasites

- Innate defenses include activation of phagocytic cells, release of cytokines that enhance the immune response, and complement activation.
- IgE antibodies and eosinophils can destroy large extracellular parasites by ADCC, and many patients with parasitic infections have increased levels of IgE and eosinophil numbers in their blood.

- Cell-mediated immune responses, including activation of T_C cells, attack parasites that reside inside of host cells. T_H1 cells can release cytokines that induce delayed-type hypersensitivity against extracellular parasites.
- Because of their complex, multistage life cycles, immune responses to parasites are often ineffective.

Parasite Survival Strategies

- Parasites have developed six major strategies to avoid the immune system—antigenic concealment, antigenic variation, antigenic shedding, antigenic mimicry, immunologic subversion, and immunologic diversion.

Serodiagnosis of Parasitic Diseases

- Serological testing for antibodies to parasites may be helpful in cases where demonstration of the parasite in biological or tissue samples is not possible.
- Toxoplasmosis is an example of a parasitic infection for which serological testing is useful. Detection of IgG, IgM, and IgA antibodies to *T. gondii* is helpful in determining whether the infection has been acquired recently or in the past and whether an infant has acquired or is at risk of acquiring a congenital infection with the organism.
- Rapid immunochromatographic assays for detection of antigens from parasites such as *Giardia* and *Cryptosporidium* have gained widespread use in clinical laboratories.
- The use of serological assays for parasites has been limited for many reasons, including variable sensitivity and specificity, lack of proficiency testing, and low number of commercially available assays as compared to assays for other pathogens.

Molecular Methods for Diagnosis of Parasitic Diseases

- Molecular techniques such as PCR are being used with increasing frequency in the diagnosis of parasitic infections.

Characteristics of Fungi

- Fungi are eukaryotic cells with nuclei and rigid cell walls. They can exist in two morphological states: unicellular yeasts or multicellular mycelia fungi.

Classification of Mycotic Infections (Mycoses)

- Fungal infections are known as *mycoses*. They can produce hypersensitivity, mycotoxicosis (a poisoning caused by fungal toxins), mycetismus (mushroom poisoning), skin infections, or systemic infections that disseminate from the lungs or skin to other sites of the body.

Immune Responses to Fungi

- Innate defenses, including physical barriers such as the skin and attachment of phagocytic cells to pattern-recognition receptors (PRRs), are an important first line of defense against fungal infections.
- Cell-mediated immunity is the most important adaptive immune response to fungal infections.

Laboratory Diagnosis of Fungal Infections

- The diagnosis of many fungal infections relies on microscopic observation of the fungus in clinical material prepared with special techniques such as KOH treatment or India ink staining.
- Culture and growth of the fungal agent responsible for infection are considered the gold standard for diagnosis. However, recovery of some organisms may be difficult, and fungi often grow slowly.
- Detection of fungal antigens, such as cryptococcus capsular polysaccharide, *Histoplasma* antigen, galactomannan, and β-D-glucan in body fluids, can be used for presumptive diagnosis of some fungal infections, particularly in cases of invasive fungal infections.
- Serological testing for fungal antibodies can demonstrate current or past exposure to a fungus. The results should be used in conjunction with the patient's symptoms, history, and other clinical findings, as immunosuppressed individuals with an opportunistic fungal infection do not reliably produce antibodies, and people living in endemic areas will test positive for the antibodies regardless of whether or not they have an active infection.
- Molecular assays for fungal nucleic acid are available for some pathogens. Examples include PNA-FISH to identify *Candida* species in blood cultures, qPCR assays to detect *Aspergillus* species and *P. jirovecii* from bronchial lavage fluid, and multiplex PCR to detect various species of fungi in bronchial lavage fluid or blood.

Fungal Pathogens

- Important fungal infections for which laboratory tests are useful include aspergillosis, candidiasis, cryptococcosis, histoplasmosis, and coccidioidomycosis.

Study Guide: Escape Mechanisms of Parasites from Protective Host Responses

ESCAPE MECHANISM	NATURE OF RESPONSE	EXAMPLE(S)
Antigenic concealment	Intracellular survival within macrophages	*Leishmania donovani*
Antigenic variation	Random mutation Genetic recombination Gene switching Multistage parasitic life cycle	*Plasmodium species* *Plasmodium falciparum, Trypanosoma cruzi* *Trypanosoma gambiense, Trypanosoma rhodesiense* *Leishmania species*
Antigenic shedding	Shedding of surface antigens or components	*Entamoeba histolytica*
Antigenic mimicry	Incorporation of host "self" antigens into parasite surface	*Schistosoma species*
Immunologic subversion	Immunosuppression	*Schistosoma mansoni*
Immunologic diversion	Polyclonal B-cell activation	*Plasmodium species*

CASE STUDIES

1. An otherwise healthy infant developed a seizure 5 days after birth. The mother and baby returned to the hospital for evaluation. Upon examination of the infant, the physician found that the baby demonstrated chorioretinitis. Prescreening of the mother during the third trimester of pregnancy did not demonstrate the presence of antibodies against *T. gondii*. At that time, she was advised to refrain from cleaning the litter boxes of the family's two cats. Upon questioning, the mother stated that she had been cleaning the litter boxes when other family members failed to do so. The physician suspected that the child may have congenital toxoplasmosis. Serological testing of the mother and the fetus gave the following results:

	Anti–T. Gondii IgM	Anti–T. Gondii IgG
Mother	1:256	1:512
Baby	Not done	1:256

Questions

a. Evaluate the baby's status related to *T. gondii* infection.

b. What additional testing should be performed to confirm the baby's status?

2. A 60-year-old adult with a medical history of chronic obstructive pulmonary disease (COPD), diabetes mellitus, and hepatitis C was seen in the emergency department. The patient admitted to using IV drugs in the past and has been receiving inhaled steroid therapy for COPD. Nausea and severe headaches interfered with the ability to carry out normal activities. The patient also felt unbalanced and weak when standing. Head computed tomography (CT) and magnetic resonance imaging (MRI) revealed abnormalities in the cerebellum of the patient's brain. Cryptococcal meningitis was suspected. A lumbar puncture was performed, and a CSF sample was sent for laboratory testing to confirm the suspected diagnosis.

Questions

a. What clinical presentations of the patient point to a diagnosis of cryptococcosis?

b. What laboratory tests should be performed to confirm the patient's diagnosis?

REVIEW QUESTIONS

1. Compared with a host's response to a virus, overcoming a parasitic infection is more difficult for the host because of which parasite characteristics?
   a. Large size
   b. Complex antigenic structures
   c. Elaborate life cycle
   d. All of the above

2. Which of the following indicates a recent infection with *Toxoplasma gondii?*
   a. Anti-*Toxoplasma* IgM
   b. Anti-*Toxoplasma* IgE
   c. Low-avidity anti-*Toxoplasma* IgG
   d. High-avidity anti-*Toxoplasma* IgG

3. Parasites are able to evade host defenses by which of the following means?
   a. Production of antigens similar to host antigens
   b. Changing surface antigens
   c. Sequestering themselves within host cells
   d. All of the above

4. The chronic nature of parasitic infections is caused by the host's:
   a. Inability to eliminate the infective agent
   b. Type I hypersensitivity response to the infection
   c. Ability to form a granuloma around the parasite
   d. Tendency to form circulating immune complexes

5. The presence of both IgM and IgG antibody in toxoplasmosis infections suggests that the infection:
   a. Occurred more than 2 years ago
   b. Occurred more recently than 18 months ago
   c. Is chronic
   d. Has resolved

6. An increase in which of the following indicates a parasitic infection?
   a. IgA concentration
   b. IgE concentration
   c. IgG concentration
   d. IgM concentration

7. Which of the following parasites are single-celled organisms?
   a. Protozoa
   b. Helminths
   c. Ectoparasites
   d. Mycelial fungi

8. The most important adaptive defense against fungal infections is:
   a. Cellular immunity
   b. IgG antibody production
   c. IgE antibody production
   d. Complement activation

9. Clinical manifestations of fungal-related illness include:
   a. Hypersensitivity caused by fungal spores
   b. Poisoning caused by ingestion of mycotoxins
   c. Growth of fungi in or on tissue
   d. All of the above

10. Which type of assay is being increasingly adopted by clinical laboratories to detect parasitic and fungal agents because of its ease of use?
    a. ELISA
    b. Lateral flow
    c. Radial immunodiffusion
    d. Indirect immunofluorescence

11. The presence of anti-H and anti-M antibodies indicates which of the following?
    a. A previous infection with *Coccidioides immitis*
    b. A previous exposure to *Histoplasma capsulatum*
    c. An active infection with *Cryptococcus neoformans*
    d. An active infection with *Histoplasma capsulatum*

12. Antifungal antibodies may not be reliably detected in an acute infection because:
    a. Immunosuppression can reduce the humoral response to fungal agents
    b. Current assays lack specificity
    c. Antibodies are not normally formed against most fungi
    d. Antibodies tend to remain at low titer as a mycosis develops

13. False positives may be observed in latex agglutination tests for the capsular antigen of *Cryptococcus neoformans* because of:
    a. The use of serum instead of CSF
    b. Cross-reactivity with other fungal antigens
    c. The presence of rheumatoid factor in the specimen
    d. The low specificity of the assay

14. A 27-year-old patient from Ohio, diagnosed with AIDS, developed chest pains. After a short period of time, the patient also developed severe headaches with dizziness. The patient's hobby was exploring caves (a spelunker). The physician ordered a sputum culture and spinal tap, and both were positive for a yeast-like fungus. These findings are most consistent with infection by:
    a. *Candida albicans*
    b. *Coccidioides immitis*
    c. *Cryptococcus neoformans*
    d. *Histoplasma capsulatum*

15. Which serological test detects the polysaccharide capsule antigen in serum and CSF of patients with suspected infection with *Cryptococcus neoformans?*
    a. India ink test
    b. Latex agglutination (LA)
    c. Complement fixation (CF)
    d. Hemagglutination test

16. Which of the following is a nondimorphic fungus that is found in concentrated bird droppings and can readily cause meningitis in immunocompromised individuals?
    a. *Coccidioides immitis*
    b. *Candida albicans*
    c. *Cryptococcus neoformans*
    d. *Histoplasma capsulatum*

Chapter 22 Answer Key

Answers to Knowledge Checks

22.1 c 22.2 d 22.3 b 22.4 a 22.5 1-d; 2-e; 3-a; 4-c; 5-b

Answers to Review Questions

1. d 2. c 3. d 4. a 5. b 6. b 7. a
8. a 9. d 10. b 11. d 12. a 13. c 14. d
15. b 16. c

23 Serological and Molecular Detection of Viral Infections

Linda E. Miller, PhD, I, MB^CM(ASCP)SI, and Deborah Josko, PhD, MLT(ASCP)M, SM

LEARNING OUTCOMES

After finishing this chapter, you should be able to:

23.1 Describe the immune defenses that are important in protecting humans from viral infections.

23.2 Discuss mechanisms by which viruses can escape host defenses.

23.3 Correlate the presence of viral IgM and IgG antibodies with their clinical significance in detecting current infections, congenital infections, and immunity to infections.

23.4 Discuss the role of molecular tests in diagnosing and monitoring patients with viral infections.

23.5 Differentiate between the different hepatitis viruses and their modes of transmission.

23.6 Correlate the various serological markers for hepatitis with their diagnostic significance.

23.7 Explain the laboratory methods that are most commonly used to screen for, confirm, or monitor hepatitis virus infections.

23.8 Associate the following viruses with the specific diseases they cause and the laboratory tests used to diagnose them: Epstein-Barr virus (EBV), cytomegalovirus (CMV), varicella-zoster virus (VZV), rubella virus, rubeola virus, mumps virus, influenza viruses, respiratory syncytial virus (RSV), and severe acute respiratory syndrome coronavirus 2 (SARS-CoV-2).

23.9 Describe the characteristics of each of the viruses listed in Objective 23.8, their mode of transmission, and symptoms associated with disease.

23.10 Discuss the laboratory tests used to detect the viruses listed in Objective 23.8 and correlate laboratory results of these tests with their clinical significance.

CHAPTER OUTLINE

You can go to **fadavis.com** keyword stevens for the laboratory exercises that accompany this text.

23.11 Describe the laboratory methods used to test for heterophile and EBV-specific antibodies and associate results of these tests with specific diseases related to EBV infections.

23.12 Differentiate between antigenic drift and antigenic shift.

23.13 Define the acronym COVID-19.

23.14 Describe how mRNA vaccines for SARS-CoV-2 work.

Viruses are submicroscopic pathogens whose size is measured in nanometers. Their basic structure consists of a core of DNA or RNA packaged into a protein coat or capsid. In some viruses, the capsid is surrounded by an outer envelope of glycolipids and proteins derived from the host-cell membrane **(Fig. 23–1)**. It is remarkable that these tiny particles are capable of causing severe, and sometimes lethal, disease in humans, ranging from childhood infections to inflammatory diseases with a preference for a specific organ, disseminated disease (disease that has spread throughout the body) in immunocompromised patients, cancer, and congenital abnormalities.

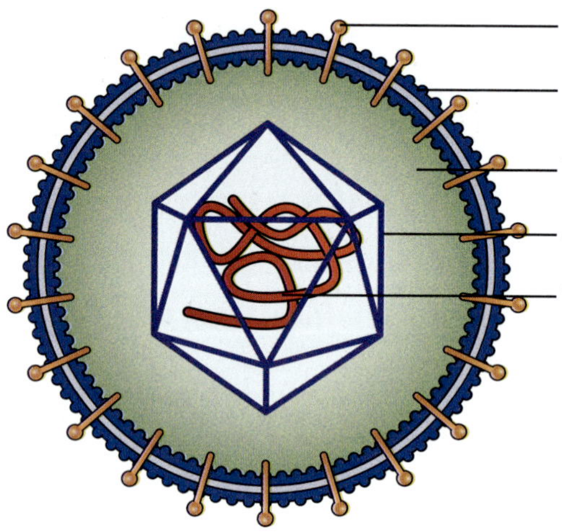

FIGURE 23–1 Basic structure of a virus.

Viruses are obligate intracellular pathogens that rely on the host cell for their replication and survival. They infect their host cells by attaching to specific receptors on the cell surface; penetrating the host cell membrane; and releasing their nucleic acid, which then directs the host cell's machinery to produce more viral nucleic acid and proteins. These components assemble to form intact viruses that are released by lysis of the cell or by budding off the cell's surface **(Fig. 23–2)**. Replication can occur quickly in cytolytic viruses that cause host cell lysis and produce acute infections, or slowly in viruses that result in chronic infections. The free virions that are generated can then infect neighboring host cells and begin new replication cycles that promote dissemination of the infection. Thus, viruses can be present in the host as both freely circulating particles and intracellular particles.

We begin this chapter by explaining the immunologic mechanisms required to attack the virus in its different states. In the remaining chapter sections, we discuss some of the most important viral infections detected by serology and molecular methods. These include the hepatitis viruses, herpes viruses, rubella, measles, mumps, influenza, RSV, and SARS-CoV-2. Laboratory tests for the human immunodeficiency virus (HIV) and human T-cell lymphotropic viruses are discussed separately in Chapter 24.

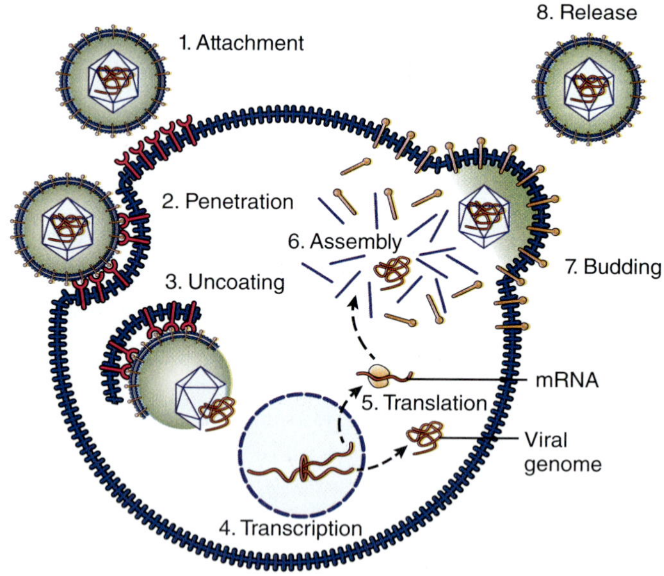

FIGURE 23–2 Basic steps of a virus life cycle. (1) Attachment of the virus to a receptor on the host cell surface. (2) Penetration, or entry of the virus into the host cell through endocytosis or other mechanisms. (3) Uncoating, or degradation of the viral capsid and subsequent release of viral nucleic acid. With some viruses, the nucleic acid integrates into the host-cell genome. (4) Transcription to produce additional viral nucleic acid. (5) Translation of viral nucleic acid to produce viral proteins. (6) Assembly of the viral components to produce intact virions. (7) Budding off the host-cell membrane or host-cell lysis results in (8) release of viral progeny. Modifications of these steps can occur with different viruses.

Immune Defenses Against Viral Infections

Successful defense against viral infections requires a coordinated effort among innate, humoral, and cell-mediated immune responses **(Fig. 23–3)**. These defenses must work together to destroy viruses in both their intracellular and extracellular states.

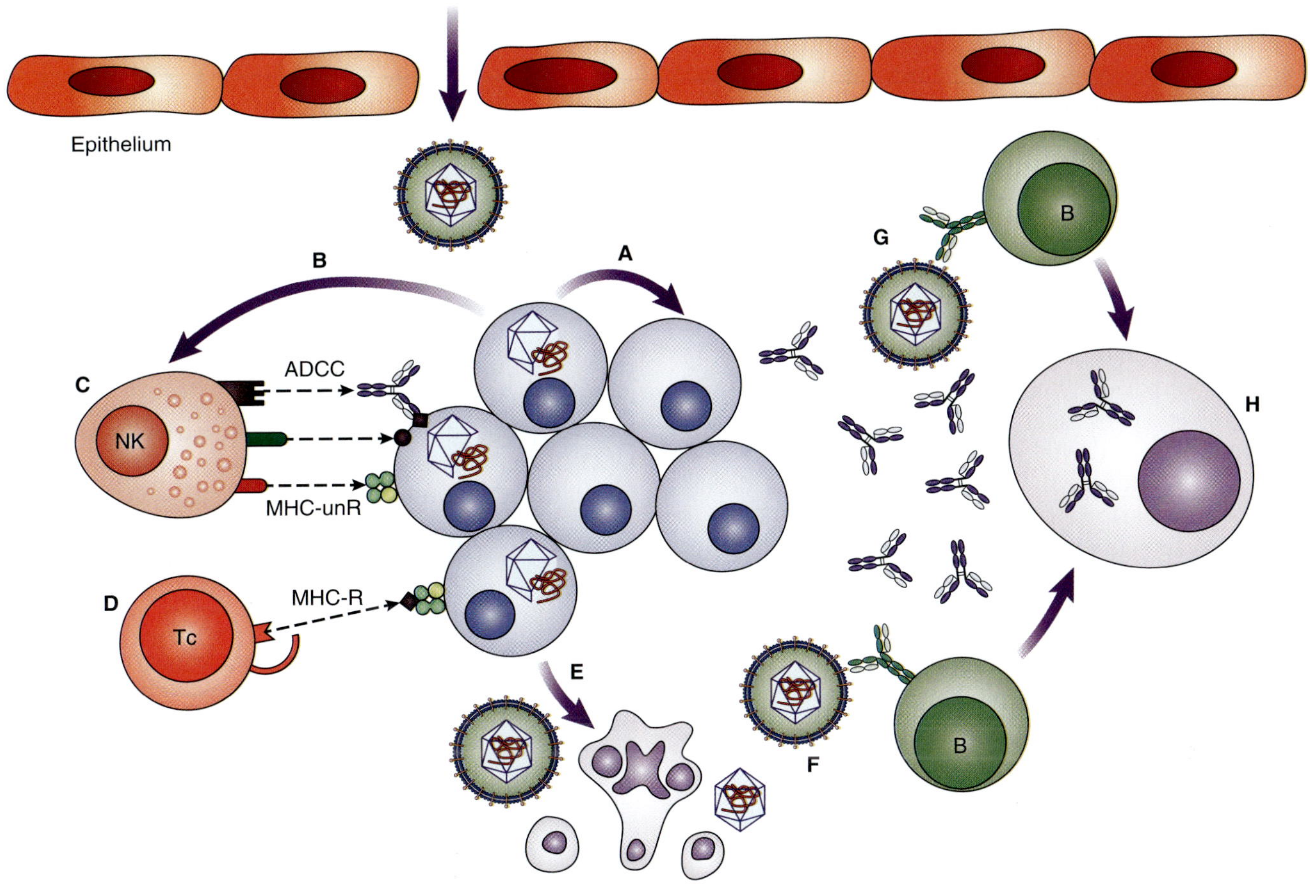

FIGURE 23–3 Immune responses to viral infection. Innate defenses provide the initial barrier to infection. Infected cells release interferons (IFNs) α and β, which (A) inhibit viral replication in surrounding cells and (B) stimulate natural killer (NK) cells. Both NK and cytotoxic T (T_C) cells destroy virus-infected host cells (C, D), resulting in the release of free virions (E). Virus-specific B cells recognize these free virions (F), as well as virions that have penetrated the epithelium (G), leading to the production of antibodies (H) that bind free virions and mediate virus neutralization, opsonization, complement activation, and antibody-dependent cellular cytotoxicity (ADCC). MHC-unR = major histocompatibility complex unrestricted; MHC-R = MHC restricted.

Innate Immunity

Innate immunity provides the first line of protection against viral pathogens. Viruses first encounter naturally occurring barriers in the body, such as the skin and mucous membranes. If they are able to invade these barriers, other innate defenses are activated when cells of the innate immune system recognize pathogen-associated molecular patterns (PAMPs) on the surface of, or within, virus-infected host cells. Two important innate defenses against viruses involve type I interferons (IFNs) and natural killer (NK) cells. Virus-infected cells are stimulated to produce IFN-α and IFN-β following recognition of viral RNA by toll-like receptors (TLRs). IFNs inhibit viral replication by inducing transcription of several genes that code for proteins with anti-viral activity—for example, a ribonuclease enzyme that degrades viral RNA. IFN-α and IFN-β also enhance the activity of NK cells, which bind to virus-infected cells and release cytotoxic proteins such as perforin and granzymes, causing the cells to die and release the viruses (see Fig. 2–7). These cell-free virions are now accessible to antibody molecules.

Antibodies

When innate defenses are insufficient in preventing viral infection, specific humoral and cell-mediated defenses are activated. Virus-specific antibodies are produced by B cells and plasma cells and can attack free virus particles in several ways. Antibodies play a key role in preventing the spread of a viral infection through neutralization. This process involves the production of antibodies that are specific for a component of the virus that binds to a receptor on the host-cell membrane. When these neutralizing antibodies bind to the virus, they prevent it from attaching to and penetrating the host cell. Secretory IgA antibodies play an especially important role in this process because they neutralize viruses in the mucosal surfaces (e.g., respiratory and digestive tracts), which often serve as entryways for the pathogens. IgM and IgG antibodies can bind to viruses in the bloodstream and inhibit dissemination of the infection. IgG antibodies also mediate phagocytosis of viruses through their opsonizing activity and facilitate destruction of viruses by antibody-dependent cellular cytotoxicity

(ADCC). Additionally, IgG and IgM antibodies activate complement, which can mediate opsonization via C3b or lyse enveloped viruses by inducing formation of the membrane attack complex. IgM antibodies may also inactivate viral particles by agglutinating them.

Cell-Mediated Immune Responses

Although antibodies can attack viruses in many different ways, they cannot reach viruses that have already penetrated host cells. Elimination of intracellular viruses requires the action of cell-mediated immunity. Type 1 helper T (T_H1) cells and cytotoxic T lymphocytes (T_C) play a key role in this mechanism of defense. T_H1 cells produce IFN-γ, which induces an anti-viral state within the virus-infected cells, and interleukin-2 (IL-2), which assists in the development of effector T_C cells. In this process, $CD8^+$ T_C cells become programmed to expand in number and attack the virus-infected cells. To recognize the virus-infected host cell, the T-cell receptor (TCR) on the T_C cell must bind to a viral antigen complexed with class I major histocompatibility complex (MHC) on the surface of the infected cell (see Chapter 5 and Fig. 23–3). CD8 is a coreceptor in this interaction. These molecular interactions stimulate the granules in the T_C cell to release a pore-forming protein called *perforin*, which produces pores in the membrane of the infected host cell, and proteases called *granzymes*, which enter the pores. These enzymes activate apoptosis in the host cell, interrupting the viral replication cycle and resulting in release of assembled infectious virions. The free virions can then be bound by antibodies. The T_C response is powerful and involves a series of cell divisions that can produce up to 50,000 times the original number of cells in a period of 1 to 3 weeks.

Viral Escape Mechanisms

Viruses can escape the host's defense mechanisms in several ways. First, viruses are rapidly dividing agents that undergo frequent genetic mutations, resulting in the production of new viral antigens that are not recognized by the initial immune response to the virus. For example, continual antigenic variation in the influenza viruses results in the emergence of novel infectious strains that require the yearly development of new vaccines to protect the population. Antigenic variation is also seen in other viruses, including rhinoviruses, which cause the common cold, and HIV, which causes AIDS.

Second, some viruses can escape the action of components of the innate immune system such as IFNs, complement proteins, or the lysosomal enzymes in phagocytic cells. For example, the hepatitis C virus (HCV) can block IFN-mediated degradation of viral RNA, and herpes simplex viruses (HSV) produce a protein that inhibits the complement pathways by binding to the complement component C3b.

Third, viruses can evade the host's defense by suppressing the adaptive immune system. Some viruses, such as the **cytomegalovirus (CMV)** and HIV, do this by reducing the expression of class I MHC molecules on the surface of virus-infected cells, making them less likely to be recognized by T_C cells. Other viruses, such as rubeola, can cause decreased expression of class II MHC molecules, resulting in reduced T_H cell activity. Some viruses can alter the function of certain cells of the immune system after directly infecting them. For example, the **Epstein-Barr virus (EBV)** causes polyclonal activation in B lymphocytes, whereas HIV suppresses the function of $CD4^+$ T_H cells. EBV can also inhibit immune responses by producing a protein that can suppress T_H1 cells because of its similarity to interleukin-10 (IL-10).

Finally, some viruses, such as CMV, **varicella-zoster virus (VZV)**, and HIV, can remain in a latent state by integrating their nucleic acid into the genome of the infected host cells. In this situation, the virus is only stimulated to replicate again if the host is exposed to other infectious agents or if the host's immune defenses decline. Latent viruses can remain silent within host cells for years because they are hidden from the immune system, although reactivation can occur later in life.

By using these evasion mechanisms, viruses have established themselves as successful human pathogens that can cause a range of mild to life-threatening diseases. Rapid, reliable laboratory detection of these pathogens is essential for early patient diagnosis and treatment. Laboratory identification also leads to prompt implementation of measures to prevent further spread of the virus to other members of the population.

Laboratory Testing for Viral Infections

As our knowledge of viruses has increased, so has the development of laboratory assays to detect viral infections. Serological and molecular tests can be easily and rapidly performed by the clinical laboratory. Therefore, they play an essential role in helping physicians establish a probable diagnosis to initiate treatment promptly. Serological tests are also important in monitoring the course of infection, detecting past infections, and assessing immune status, whereas molecular tests have enhanced our ability to detect active infection and are essential in guiding anti-viral therapy.

In general, the presence of virus-specific IgM antibodies in patient serum indicates a current or recent viral infection, whereas IgG antibodies to a virus signify either a current or past infection and, in many cases, immunity. Virus-specific IgM antibody in the newborn's serum indicates a congenital infection because IgM is actively made during fetal life. In contrast, IgG antibodies in the infant's serum are mainly maternal antibodies that have crossed the placenta. Current infections in the adult or newborn may also be detected by immunoassays for viral antigens in serum or other clinical samples or by the presence of viral nucleic acids that can be detected by molecular methods. Quantitative molecular tests are used to guide anti-viral therapy.

Knowledge Check 23-1

Which immunoglobulin plays an important role in neutralizing viruses in the mucosal surfaces by preventing viruses from attaching to and penetrating host cells?

a. IgM
b. IgG
c. IgA
d. IgE

Hepatitis Viruses

Hepatitis is a general term that means inflammation of the liver. It can be caused by several viruses and by noninfectious agents, including ionizing radiation, chemicals, and autoimmune processes. The primary hepatitis viruses affect mainly the liver and cause more than 95% of viral hepatitis. Other viruses, such as CMV, EBV, and HSV, can also produce liver inflammation, but it is secondary to other disease processes. In this section, we focus on the primary hepatitis viruses: the **hepatitis A virus (HAV)** and the **hepatitis E virus (HEV)** are transmitted primarily by the fecal-oral route, whereas the **hepatitis B virus (HBV)**, the **hepatitis D virus (HDV)**, and the **hepatitis C virus (HCV)** are transmitted mainly by the **parenteral** route (i.e., through contact with blood and other body fluids).

All hepatitis viruses may produce similar clinical manifestations. The early, or acute, stages of hepatitis are characterized by general flu-like symptoms and mild to moderate pain in the right upper quadrant of the abdomen. Progression of the disease leads to liver enlargement (hepatomegaly) and tenderness, jaundice, dark urine, and light feces.

Initial laboratory findings typically include elevations in bilirubin and in the liver enzymes, most notably alanine aminotransferase (ALT). These findings are nonspecific indicators of liver inflammation and must be followed by specific serological or molecular tests to identify the cause of hepatitis more definitively. The specific laboratory tests used to detect each type of hepatitis are listed in **Table 23–1.**

Hepatitis A (HAV)

HAV is a nonenveloped, single-stranded ribonucleic acid (RNA) virus that belongs to the *Hepatovirus* genus of the *Picornaviridae* family. Six genotypes of the virus have been identified. Genotypes I, II, and III, divided into subtypes A and B, are associated with human disease and can be detected by the same serological assays (see the text that follows). Genotype IA is the most prevalent. Hepatitis A is a common infection responsible for an estimated 1.5 million cases of hepatitis worldwide. HAV is transmitted primarily by the fecal-oral route, close person-to-person contact, or ingestion of contaminated food or water. Conditions of poor personal hygiene, poor sanitation, and overcrowding facilitate transmission. Rarely, transmission through transfusion of contaminated blood has been reported and may occur during a short period within the acute stage of infection when a high number of viral particles can be found in the source blood.

After an average incubation period of 30 days, the virus produces symptoms of acute hepatitis in most infected adults; however, most infections in children are asymptomatic. The infection does not progress to a chronic state and is usually self-limiting, with symptoms typically resolving within 2 months. Treatment is mainly supportive, involving bed-rest, nutritional support, and medication for fever, nausea, and diarrhea. Massive hepatic necrosis resulting in fulminant hepatitis (associated with rapidly progressing liver disease and failure) and death is rare and occurs mainly in those patients with underlying liver disease or advanced age.

Laboratory Testing for Hepatitis A

HAV antigens are shed in the feces of infected people during the incubation period and the early acute stage of infection, but they usually decline to low levels shortly after symptoms appear and are not a clinically useful indicator of disease. Therefore, serological tests for antibody are critical in establishing diagnosis of the infection. Hepatitis A antibodies are most commonly detected by automated enzyme immunoassays (EIAs) and chemiluminescent microparticle immunoassays. Acute hepatitis A is routinely diagnosed in symptomatic patients by demonstrating the presence of IgM antibodies to HAV **(Fig. 23–4).** IgM anti-HAV is detectable at the onset of clinical symptoms and declines to undetectable levels within 6 months in the most infected individuals. Because false-positive results can occur, the test should be reserved for symptomatic people. Tests for total HAV antibodies also detect IgM but predominantly detect IgG, which persists for life. Thus, a positive total anti-HAV test result in combination with a negative IgM anti-HAV indicates that the patient has developed immunity to the virus, either through natural infection or vaccination. Negative total anti-HAV tests can be used to identify nonimmune individuals who may have been exposed to the virus.

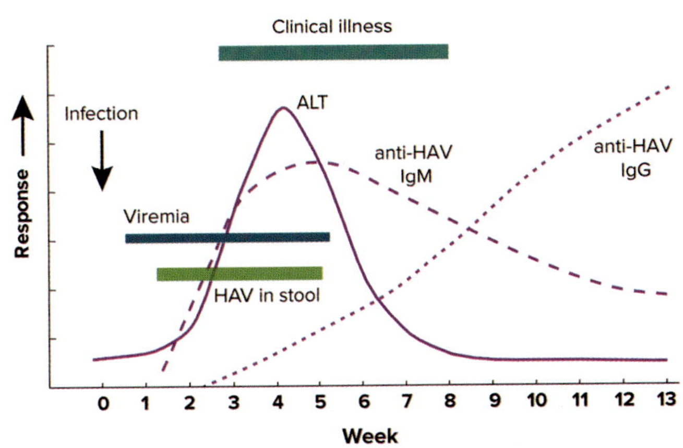

FIGURE 23–4 Hepatitis A serology. Typical patterns of IgM and IgG anti-HAV during infection and recovery. ALT = alanine aminotransferase; viremia = amount of HAV circulating in the blood. *(Figure courtesy of Centers for Disease Control and Prevention. Diagnosis and Management of Foodborne Illnesses: A Primer for Physicians and Other Health Care Professionals. MMWR 2004;53[RR-4]:17).*

Table 23–1 The Hepatitis Viruses and Their Associated Serological and Molecular Markers

HEPATITIS VIRUS	TYPE AND FAMILY	TRANSMISSION	PROGRESSION TO CHRONIC STATE	COMPLICATIONS	SEROLOGICAL AND MOLECULAR MARKERS	CLINICAL SIGNIFICANCE
Hepatitis A (HAV)	RNA *Picornaviridae*	Fecal-oral, direct contact with infectious individual Blood transfusion (rare)	No	Low risk of fulminant liver disease	• IgM anti-HAV	• Acute hepatitis A
					• Total anti-HAV	• Immunity to hepatitis A
					• HAV RNA	• Detection of HAV in clinical, food, or water samples
Hepatitis B (HBV)	DNA *Hepadnaviridae*	Parenteral, sexual, perinatal	Yes	10% to 90% of cases may develop chronic hepatitis (depending on age), with increased risk for liver cirrhosis and hepatocellular carcinoma	• HBsAg	• Active hepatitis B infection
					• HBeAg	• Active hepatitis B with high degree of infectivity
					• IgM anti-HBc	• Current or recent acute hepatitis B
					• Total anti-HBc	• Current or past hepatitis B
					• Anti-HBe	• Recovery from hepatitis B
					• Anti-HBs	• Immunity to hepatitis B
					• HBV DNA	• Acute, atypical, or occult hepatitis B; viral load may be used to monitor effectiveness of therapy

Hepatitis C (HCV)	RNA *Flaviviridae*	Parenteral, sexual, perinatal	Yes	Approximately 85% develop chronic infection, with increased risk of cirrhosis, hepatocellular carcinoma, or autoimmune manifestations	• Anti-HCV	• Current or past hepatitis C infection
					• HCV RNA	• Current hepatitis C infection; viral load may be used to monitor effectiveness of therapy; molecular tests are used to determine HCV genotype
Hepatitis D (HDV)	RNA genus *Deltavirus*	Mostly parenteral, but also sexual, perinatal; HBV infection required	Yes	Increased risk of developing fulminant hepatitis, cirrhosis, or hepatocellular carcinoma	• IgM-anti-HDV	• Acute or chronic hepatitis D
					• IgG-anti-HDV	• Recovery from hepatitis D or chronic hepatitis D
					• HDV RNA	• Active HDV infection; viral load may be used to monitor effectiveness of therapy
Hepatitis E (HEV)	RNA *Hepeviridae*	Fecal-oral Blood transfusion; vertical transmission	Yes, in immunocompromised individuals	Fulminant liver failure in pregnant women	• IgM anti-HEV	• Current hepatitis E infection
					• IgG anti-HEV	• Current or past hepatitis E infection
					• HEV RNA	• Current hepatitis E infection

Although IgM anti-HAV is the primary marker to detect acute hepatitis A, false-negative results can occur during the early phase of the infection. Molecular methods to detect HAV RNA are more sensitive in this situation. The most common format of these methods is the reverse transcriptase polymerase chain reaction (RT-PCR). Molecular methods can also be used to test samples of food or water suspected of transmitting the virus. Multiplex quantitative polymerase chain reaction (qPCR) methods that can simultaneously detect more than one type of hepatitis virus in clinical samples have also been developed.

A vaccine consisting of formalin-killed HAV was licensed in the mid-1990s to prevent hepatitis A. Currently, two inactivated single-antigen vaccines and one combination vaccine are licensed and available in the United States for hepatitis A prevention. Vaccination has resulted in a significant decrease in the number of HAV infections in the United States and other countries throughout the world. To prevent infection in unimmunized people who have been exposed to the virus, prophylactic administration of the hepatitis A vaccine or intramuscular injections of immune globulin, a sterile preparation of pooled human plasma that contains antibodies to HAV, are recommended. The vaccine is the preferred treatment for persons aged 1 to 40 years, but immune globulin can be used to prevent infection in people of any age. To be effective, these treatments must be administered within 2 weeks of exposure.

Hepatitis E (HEV)

HEV is a nonenveloped, single-stranded RNA virus that belongs to the genus *Hepevirus*, in the family *Hepeviridae*. HEV is a major cause of hepatitis worldwide. The World Health Organization (WHO) estimates that the virus causes 20 million infections, with over 3.3 million cases of acute hepatitis annually. The Centers for Disease Control and Prevention (CDC) estimate that about 70,000 deaths occur each year from HEV infections. Similar to the HAV, HEV is transmitted mainly by the fecal-oral route; however, person-to-person transmission is uncommon.

The four genotypes of the virus differ in their epidemiology and source of infection. Genotypes 1 and 2 are associated mainly with the consumption of fecally contaminated drinking water in developing regions of the world with poor sanitation, including parts of Africa, Asia, the Middle East, and Mexico. Outbreaks commonly occur in times of natural disasters such as flooding and earthquakes and can affect thousands of people. Genotypes 3 and 4 have been increasingly recognized in developed parts of the world, including Europe, North America, China, Taiwan, and Japan. HEV3 and HEV4 are zoonotic infections in which pigs are the primary host. Deer, wild boars, and other mammals are also known to harbor the virus. These infections are thought to be transmitted mainly by the consumption of infected pork and deer meat and possibly by direct contact with infected animals or fecally contaminated water. HEV has also been detected in the blood supply in several countries and can be transmitted through blood transfusions.

Although HEV infections are often silent, all genotypes can cause acute hepatitis with symptoms that are indistinguishable from other types of hepatitis. After an incubation period of 2 to 10 weeks, HEV infection in most people causes a self-limiting illness, with recovery occurring by 4 to 6 weeks. However, the infection can have severe consequences. Some patients may experience symptoms outside of the liver, including neurological syndromes, renal injury, pancreatitis, and hematologic abnormalities. Pregnant women infected with HEV1 or HEV2 have a mortality rate of 30% because of obstetric complications or development of fulminant hepatitis. The reason for this is unclear, but it may be caused by the hormonal and immunologic changes associated with pregnancy. HEV3 can result in chronic infection in immunocompromised individuals. Chronic infection can progress to liver fibrosis, cirrhosis, and liver failure, which may require liver transplantation.

Measures to prevent the infection include providing clean drinking water, improving sanitation conditions in developing countries, and in the case of HEV3, not eating undercooked meat, especially pork. A vaccine to prevent HEV1 infection has been licensed for use in China. The vaccine consists of viruslike particles that have been genetically modified to express a gene that codes for a key HEV protein. To date, no U.S. Food and Drug Administration (FDA)-cleared vaccine is available in the United States.

Laboratory Testing for Hepatitis E

Because HEV is not easily cultured, diagnosis relies on serology to detect antibodies to the virus and molecular methods to detect HEV nucleic acid. Antibodies to HEV are typically identified by sensitive EIAs that use recombinant and synthetic HEV antigens. Rapid immunochromatographic assays have also been developed. Antibody tests for HEV can detect infections with all four genotypes of the virus because there is only one viral serotype. Acute infection is indicated by the presence of IgM anti-HEV, which is detectable at clinical onset, remains elevated for about 8 weeks, and becomes undetectable in most patients by 32 weeks. HEV-specific IgG antibodies appear soon after IgM, reach peak levels about 4 weeks after symptoms develop, and persist for several years. Immunoassays for IgG anti-HEV may be performed to detect patients in the later stages of infection, determine past exposure, and identify seroprevalence of the infection in a population (i.e., the number of people who have virus-specific antibodies).

Immunocompromised persons often yield negative antibody test results; molecular testing for HEV RNA is recommended in these patients. Quantitation of HEV nucleic acid can be performed by qPCR (the gold standard for diagnosis of acute HEV infections) or a loop-mediated isothermal amplification (LAMP) assay, which is suitable for resource-limited settings because it is faster and does not require expensive equipment. These assays can be performed on blood or stool samples. HEV RNA can be detected just before clinical symptoms. It becomes undetectable in the blood about 3 weeks after symptom onset;

in the stool, it becomes undetectable at about 5 weeks. Therefore, a negative result for HEV RNA does not exclude the possibility of recent infection.

Hepatitis B

Hepatitis B is a major cause of global morbidity (disease) and mortality (death). The WHO estimates that HBV has infected 2 billion people worldwide, causing about 254 million chronic infections. In 2022, the WHO reported 1.1 million deaths because of complications from the disease (i.e., cirrhosis and hepatocellular carcinoma). The virus is highly endemic in the Far East, parts of the Middle East, sub-Saharan Africa, and the Amazon areas. In the United States, which is considered a low-prevalence area, about 2.4 million people are living with chronic HBV infections.

HBV is transmitted through the parenteral route by intimate contact with HBV-contaminated blood or other body fluids, most notably semen, vaginal secretions, and saliva. Transmission has thus been associated with sexual contact, blood transfusions, sharing of needles and syringes by IV drug users, tattooing, and occupational needlestick injury. Inapparent transmission of HBV may occur through close personal contact of broken skin or mucous membranes with the virus. Transmission of HBV may also occur via the perinatal route, from infected mother to infant, most likely during delivery.

Several measures have been introduced to prevent HBV infection, including screening of blood donors, treating plasma-derived products to inactivate HBV, implementing infection-control measures (see Chapter 8), and most importantly, immunizing with a hepatitis B vaccine. The current vaccines, consisting of recombinant hepatitis B surface antigen (HBsAg) produced from genetically engineered yeast or mammalian cells, are some of the most widely used vaccines throughout the world. Immunization has been highly successful, resulting in a significant decline in the incidence of acute hepatitis B in the United States since routine immunization was implemented in 1991. Increasingly widespread use of the vaccine will likely continue to reduce the incidence of new HBV infections worldwide. The vaccine can also be given to people thought to be exposed to the virus, along with hepatitis B immune globulin (HBIG), a preparation derived from donor plasma with high concentrations of antibodies to HBV that provides temporary protection.

Despite such preventive measures, a substantial number of HBV infections continue to occur, as we previously discussed. Infection with HBV results in an incubation period of 30 to 180 days, followed by a clinical course that varies in different age groups. Over 90% of newborns with perinatal HBV infection remain asymptomatic, whereas typical symptoms of acute hepatitis are observed in about 10% of children aged 1 to 5 years and about one-third of adolescents and adults. Symptoms may last several weeks to several months and are usually managed through bedrest and other supportive treatment. Most HBV-infected adults recover within 6 months and develop immunity to the virus, but about 1% develop fulminant liver disease. This highly fatal condition is treated with intensive life support, anti-viral drugs, and in some patients, liver transplantation.

Development of chronic HBV infection, in which the virus persists in the body for 6 months or more, occurs in the majority of infected infants, about one-third of young children, and 10% of infected adults. Chronic infection is also more likely to develop in persons who are immunosuppressed and those who have HIV. Chronic infection with the virus results in inflammation and damage to the liver and places the patient at increased risk of developing cirrhosis or hepatocellular carcinoma. Patients with chronic infection can be treated with anti-viral drugs to reduce liver inflammation and the risk of developing liver complications. Therapies consist of nucleoside analogues that inhibit the polymerase enzyme needed for viral replication and IFN-α, which enhances the immune response against the virus.

The virus responsible for hepatitis B, HBV, is a DNA virus belonging to the *Hepadnaviridae* family. Ten genotypes, designated A through J, have been identified based on nucleotide-sequence differences in their genomes. The genotypes vary in their geographic distribution, pathogenicity, and response to treatment but can be identified by the same serological assays. The intact HBV virion is a 42-nm sphere consisting of a nucleocapsid core surrounded by an outer envelope of lipoprotein. The core of the virus contains circular, partially double-stranded DNA; a DNA-dependent DNA polymerase enzyme; and the hepatitis B core antigen. A protein called the **hepatitis B surface antigen (HBsAg)** is found in the outer envelope of the virus. HBsAg is produced in excess and is found in noninfectious spherical and tubular particles that lack viral DNA and circulate freely in the blood. A nonstructural protein, the **hepatitis Be antigen (HBeAg)**, is found between the viral core and outer envelope, and released into the blood during viral replication.

These antigens, and antibodies to them, serve as serological markers for hepatitis B and have been used in the differential diagnosis of HBV infection, monitoring the course of infection in patients, assessing immunity to the virus, and screening blood products for infectivity. The levels of these markers vary with the amount of viral replication and the host's immune response. They are useful in establishing the initial diagnosis of hepatitis B and monitoring the course of infection.

Serological Markers for Hepatitis B

Serological markers for hepatitis B are listed in Table 23–1 and are described in the text that follows. Typical patterns of the markers during acute and chronic hepatitis B are shown in **Figures 23–5** and **23–6.**

HBsAg is the first marker to appear, becoming detectable 2 to 10 weeks after exposure to HBV. Its levels peak during the acute stages of infection, then gradually decline as the patient develops antibodies to the antigen and recovers. Serum HBsAg usually becomes undetectable by 4 to 6 months after the onset of symptoms in patients with acute hepatitis B. In patients with chronic HBV infection, HBsAg remains elevated for 6 months or more. Thus, HBsAg is an indicator of active

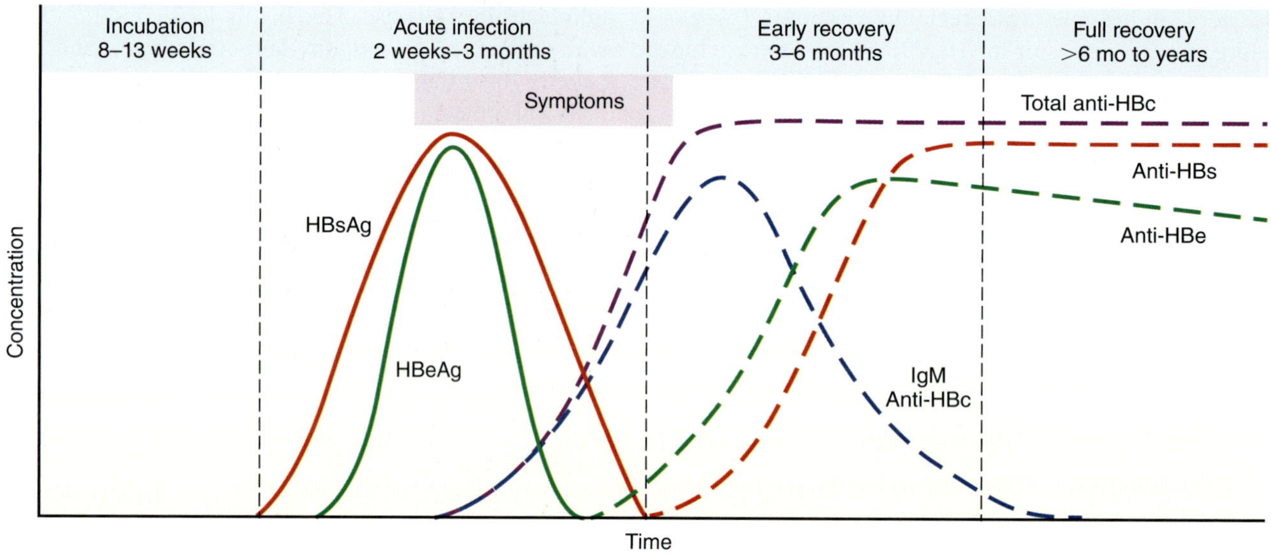

FIGURE 23–5 Typical serological markers in acute hepatitis B. Solid lines represent viral antigen concentrations, whereas dashed lines indicate antibody concentrations. Each antigen shares the same color with its associated antibody.

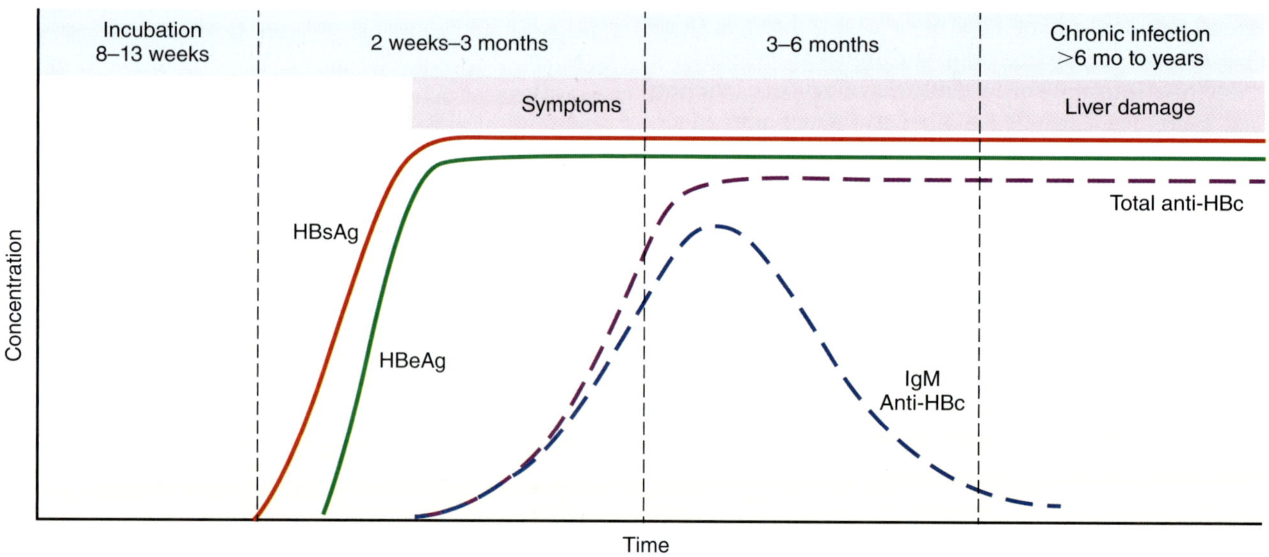

FIGURE 23–6 Typical serological markers in chronic hepatitis B.

infection and is an important marker in detecting initial infection, monitoring the course of infection and progression to chronic disease, and screening donor blood.

HBeAg appears shortly after HBsAg and disappears shortly before HBsAg in recovering patients. It may be elevated during chronic infection. This marker is present during periods of active replication of the virus and indicates a high degree of infectivity. The hepatitis B core antigen (HBc) is not detectable in serum because the viral envelope masks it.

As the host develops an immune response to the virus, antibodies appear. First to appear is IgM antibody to the core antigen, or **IgM anti-HBc.** This antibody indicates current or recent acute infection. It typically appears 1 to 2 weeks after HBsAg during acute infection and persists in high titers for 4 to 6 months and then gradually declines. IgM anti-HBc is useful in detecting infection in cases in which HBsAg is undetectable—for example, just before the appearance of antibodies to HBsAg (the "core window" period), in neonatal infections, and in cases of fulminant hepatitis. Therefore, it is used in addition to HBsAg to screen donor blood. IgG antibodies to the core antigen are produced before IgM anti-HBc disappears and then persist for the individual's lifetime. They are the predominant antibodies detected in the test for total anti-HBc and can be used to indicate a past HBV infection.

The appearance of antibodies to the HBe antigen, or **anti-HBe,** occurs shortly after the disappearance of HBeAg and indicates that the patient is recovering from HBV infection.

Antibodies to HBsAg, or **anti-HBs,** also appear during the recovery period of acute hepatitis B, a few weeks after HBsAg disappears. These antibodies persist for years and provide

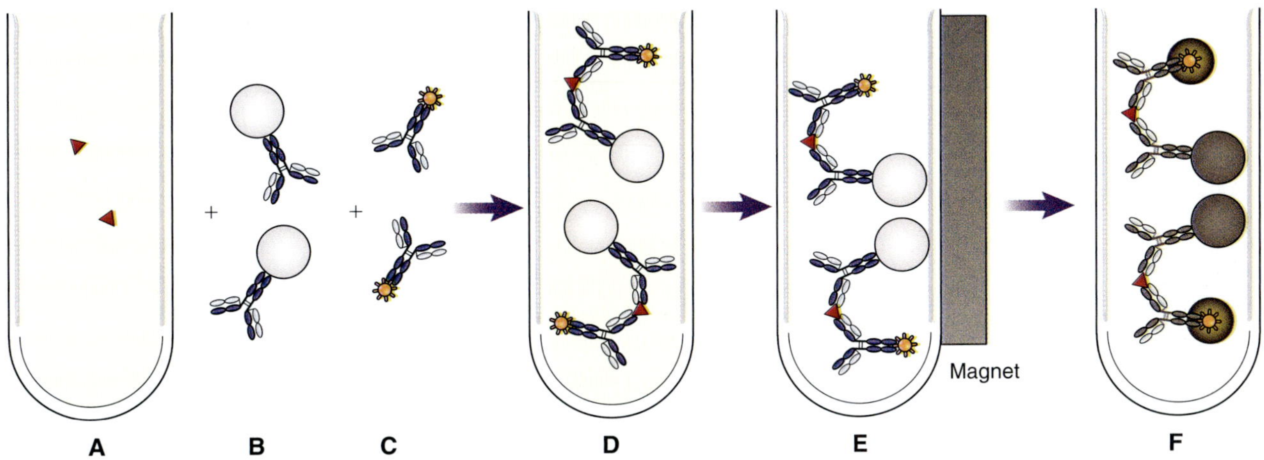

FIGURE 23–7 Detection of the HBs antigen by chemiluminescence microparticle immunoassay. (A) Patient serum or plasma containing HBsAg is mixed with (B) magnetic microparticles coated with anti-HBs and (C) acridinium-labeled anti-HBs conjugate. (D) During incubation, complexes form, with the antigen sandwiched in between the antibodies. (E) Application of a magnetic field holds the microparticles and bound reagents in the tube while unbound materials are washed away and chemiluminescent reagents are added. (F) The magnitude of light produced is measured in a luminometer and is proportional to the concentration of HBsAg in the sample.

protective immunity. Anti-HBs are also produced after immunization with the hepatitis B vaccine. Protective titers of the antibody in the serum are considered to be 10 mIU/mL or higher. Anti-HBs are not produced during chronic HBV infection, in which immunity fails to develop.

Serological markers for hepatitis B are most commonly detected by commercial immunoassays. These are available in a variety of formats, such as EIA and chemiluminescent immunoassay (CLIA). They are typically automated to ease batch testing in the clinical laboratory and have excellent sensitivity and specificity. An example of an immunoassay for detecting HBsAg is shown in **Figure 23–7.** Although these methods are highly sensitive and specific, false-positive and false-negative results can occur. Any initial positive results should be verified by repeated testing of the same specimen in duplicate, followed by confirmation with an additional assay, such as an HBsAg neutralization test or a molecular test that detects HBV DNA.

Molecular Methods for Hepatitis B

Several molecular methods have been developed to detect and quantify HBV DNA in serum or plasma and are mostly based on target amplification by qPCR or transcription-mediated amplification (TMA) (see Chapter 12). HBV DNA can be detected in the serum about 21 days before HBsAg and is a useful adjunct in detecting early acute HBV infection in certain situations, such as screening blood donors, assessing cases of occupational exposure, and evaluating patients with equivocal HBsAg test results. HBV DNA testing is also used to evaluate the effectiveness of anti-viral therapy in patients with chronic hepatitis B. Successful treatment is indicated by a 1-$\log_{10}$ reduction in HBV DNA levels by 6 months, whereas persistently elevated HBV DNA levels indicate possible drug resistance and a need to change therapy. Molecular testing is also used to diagnose atypical cases of hepatitis B originating from mutations in the HBV genome that cause HBsAg tests to be negative. Molecular methods to detect HBV genotypes and HBV mutations associated with anti-viral drug resistance can be helpful in determining optimal patient therapy.

Hepatitis D

Hepatitis D, or *delta hepatitis,* is a parenterally transmitted infection that can occur only in the presence of hepatitis B. HDV is a defective virus that requires the help of HBV for its replication and expression. The only member within the *Deltavirus* genus, HDV consists of a circular RNA genome and a single structural protein called *hepatitis delta antigen* within its core, surrounded by a viral envelope that is of HBV origin and contains the HBsAg. Currently, eight genotypes have been identified: genotype I (most common and found worldwide); genotypes I, II, and IV (Japan, Taiwan, Russia, and other eastern Asian countries); genotype III (South America); and genotypes V, VI, VII, and VIII (Africa). HDV is highly prevalent in Mediterranean Europe, the Middle East, the Amazon Basin, central Africa, and parts of Asia, and an estimated 12 to 20 million people are believed to be infected worldwide. New infections appear to be increasing in certain parts of the world.

Similar to HBV, HDV is transmitted sexually in semen or vaginal secretions; through blood by IV drug use, needlestick injuries, or transfusions; or perinatally from mother to infant. Infection with the virus can occur in one of two ways: HDV can be transmitted simultaneously as a *coinfection* with HBV, or HDV can be contracted as a *superinfection* of people who are already chronic HBV carriers. Clinically, most patients with coinfections experience an acute, self-limited hepatitis in which both viruses are cleared within a few months. Some patients may have more severe symptoms of acute hepatitis than those infected with HBV alone, but only about 2% of cases progress to a chronic state. In contrast, more than 70%

of patients with superinfections develop chronic liver disease with accelerated progression to cirrhosis and liver failure. Combinations of IFN-α and anti-viral drugs can be administered to patients with chronic or severe hepatitis D in an attempt to eradicate the virus.

Laboratory Testing for Hepatitis D

Testing for hepatitis D should be performed for all patients who are HBsAg positive and involves the detection of HDV antibodies and HDV RNA. Antibodies are detected by immunoassays using the hepatitis D antigen. The presence of IgG anti-HDV antibodies indicates exposure to the virus and can signify an acute, chronic, or past hepatitis D infection. Although IgM anti-HDV is produced during acute hepatitis D infections, its appearance may be delayed, it may persist for only a short period of time, and it may be missed. IgM antibodies to HDV can also persist during chronic infection. Serology testing for hepatitis B can be used to help distinguish HBV and HDV coinfections from HBV and HDV superinfections. In addition to being positive for HDV antibodies, patients with coinfections are positive for IgM anti-HBc, whereas patients with superinfections are positive for IgG anti-HBc.

Detection of hepatitis D has been aided tremendously by development of molecular methods to detect HDV RNA, a marker of active viral replication present in all types of active hepatitis D infections. HDV RNA testing is routinely used to confirm a positive HDV antibody screen. Molecular testing for serum HDV RNA is performed by sensitive RT-PCR assays. These assays provide quantitative results that can be used to monitor the response of patients to anti-viral therapy.

Hepatitis C

Hepatitis C is a major public health problem, with an estimated 50 million people infected worldwide and about 1 million new infections per year. It is the most common bloodborne infection in the United States, as an estimated 3.2 million people live with chronic HCV. Hepatitis C is also the most frequent cause of chronic liver infection and the leading indicator for liver transplantation in the United States.

HCV, the virus that causes hepatitis C, is responsible for most of the infections previously classified as "nonA-nonB" before the discovery of the virus in 1989. It is an enveloped, single-stranded, positive-sense RNA virus belonging to the family *Flaviviridae* and the genus *Hepacivirus*. Scientists have discovered eight different genotypes of the virus, designated 1 through 8, with more than 100 subtypes for each, indicated by lowercase letters. The genotypes differ in their geographic distribution, pathogenicity, and response to anti-viral treatment. Genotype 1, the most common, is responsible for 46% of hepatitis C infections worldwide and about 75% of HCV infections in the United States. Genotypes 1, 2, and 3 are predominant in North America, Europe, and Japan; genotypes 3 and 6 are found throughout South and Southeast Asia; genotypes 4, 5, and 7 are most common in parts of Africa; and genotype 8 is most common in India. HCV's variability and ability to undergo rapid mutations within its hosts have created difficulty in developing an effective vaccine.

Hepatitis C is transmitted mainly by exposure to contaminated blood, with IV drug use being the main source of infection. Now a rare occurrence, blood transfusion was once a major vehicle of transmission before routine screening of blood donors for HCV antibody was implemented in 1992. Organ transplantation before 1992 was also a route of transmission. Other risk factors include occupational exposures to contaminated blood, long-term hemodialysis, and unregulated body piercing or tattooing in environments such as correctional facilities where contaminated needles are likely to be used. Sexual transmission of HCV is thought to be less common but is higher in people who have had multiple sex partners or a history of sexually transmitted diseases. Perinatal transmission has been estimated to occur at a rate of about 6%.

HCV has an average incubation period of 7 weeks (range of 2 weeks to 6 months). Most infections are asymptomatic, with symptoms of acute hepatitis occurring in only about 20% of cases. Asymptomatic infection is problematic because chronic infection develops in about 70% of infected persons, and up to half of these individuals develop cirrhosis. Cirrhosis occurs slowly over a 25- to 30-year period, causing damage to the liver and posing an increased risk of developing hepatocellular carcinoma. Patients with chronic HCV infection may also develop symptoms affecting areas of the body other than the liver, including the joints, kidneys, nerves, skin, eyes, and blood vessels. Early detection would help prevent these complications, but HCV is often missed in its early stages because of the asymptomatic nature of the infection in most people.

Clearance of the infection may occur spontaneously or may require treatment with anti-viral drugs. Increased understanding of the biology of HCV has led to the development of direct-acting anti-viral drugs (DAAs) and host-targeted agents (HTAs) that inhibit specific steps of the viral replication cycle. Combination therapies using these agents are being evaluated at a rapid pace and are revolutionizing the way hepatitis C is being treated.

The laboratory plays an essential role in screening for hepatitis C, monitoring patients known to have HCV infection, and guiding therapy. The CDC recommends that screening for HCV infection be performed in all adults at least once, pregnant women, people with certain medical conditions (e.g., those who received hemodialysis, have elevated liver enzymes or HIV), people who received blood transfusions or organ transplants before testing was implemented, and infants and children born to mothers who have confirmed or probable HCV infection. The rationale behind these recommendations is that many people living with HCV infection are asymptomatic, and identifying them can lead to closer monitoring for disease progression and earlier administration of effective anti-viral treatment.

Laboratory Testing for Hepatitis C

Screening and diagnosis of hepatitis C begin with serological testing for HCV antibodies. Anti-HCV IgG is most commonly detected by sensitive EIAs or CLIAs that use recombinant and synthetic antigens developed from the conserved domains of the capsid core protein (C) and the nonstructural proteins NS3, NS4, and NS5. Alternatively, a rapid immunoblot assay can be used for point-of-care testing. Antibodies become detectable 8 to 10 weeks after HCV exposure and can remain positive for a lifetime. Thus, a reactive result can indicate the presence of a current HCV infection or a past HCV infection that has resolved. Despite the excellent specificity of these methods, false-positive results may occur because of cross-reactivity in persons with other viral infections or autoimmune disorders. Therefore, any positive results from an anti-HCV screening test should be confirmed to distinguish between the various interpretations of these results.

Current CDC guidelines recommend using a two-step sequence for diagnosis of HCV infection. When an HCV antibody test is reactive, an HCV RNA test is performed to confirm the presence of HCV. This is considered a "complete" test. However, if the HCV antibody test is reactive but the HCV RNA test is negative, this is considered an "incomplete test." Updated guidelines recommend a single-visit sample collection at the time of HCV screening to avoid incomplete testing results.

Molecular assays for HCV RNA can be classified as qualitative or quantitative. Qualitative tests distinguish between the presence or absence of HCV RNA in a clinical sample. These tests are used to confirm infection in HCV-antibody–positive patients (as previously mentioned), detect infection in antibody-negative patients who are suspected of having HCV, screen blood and organ donors for HCV, and detect perinatal infections in babies born to HCV-positive mothers. Qualitative RT-PCR and TMA methods are commercially available. These tests can detect as low as 5 IU of HCV RNA per milliliter of serum (for TMA) or 50 IU/mL HCV RNA (for RT-PCR) and become positive within 1 to 3 weeks after infection. They are generally positive at the onset of symptoms, but in some patients, they can transiently decrease to undetectable levels during the acute phase of the infection.

Quantitative tests are performed by RT-PCR or TMA. Commercial tests can detect a wide range of HCV concentrations, from about 10 IU/mL to 10 million IU/mL. They are used to monitor the amount of HCV RNA, or "viral load," carried by chronically infected patients before, during, and after anti-viral therapy. The ultimate goal of such therapy is to achieve a sustained virological response (SVR) in which the patient continuously tests negative for HCV RNA 12 or 24 weeks after therapy is completed. The initial viral load level has also been used as a prognostic tool because those with a low initial viral load are most likely to achieve an SVR.

Genotyping, to determine the exact genotype and subtype of the virus responsible for the infection, should be performed on all HCV-infected patients before anti-viral therapy. It is important to identify the patient's HCV genotype to determine the most effective treatment because HCV genotypes vary in their response to different anti-viral drugs. Due to different outcomes of treatment between the various genotypes of HCV, current strategies have focused on direct-acting anti-virals (DAAs) such as Telaprevir, Boceprevir, Grazoprevir (NS3/4A protease inhibitors), Elbasvir (an NS5A inhibitor), and Sofosbuvir (an NS5B polymerase inhibitor). Genotyping is also useful in epidemiological studies to determine the source of HCV infection in specific populations.

Genotyping is performed by RT-PCR amplification and sequencing of the target gene or RT-PCR followed by identification of the target gene with genotype-specific probes. PCR/sequencing, performed mainly by reference laboratories, is the reference method because it provides precise information about the genomic variability of the virus in patients during the course of the infection.

Knowledge Check 23-2

Which hepatitis B marker denotes a high level of infectivity?
a. HBsAg
b. HBeAg
c. HBcAg
d. HBdAg

Critical Thinking 23-1

A patient has had the following test profile for hepatitis B screening for the last 6 months:

HBsAg	Positive
HBeAg	Positive
Anti-HBcAb	Negative
Anti-HBsAb	Negative

Based on these findings, would you classify this patient as having acute or chronic HBV infection? Comment on the clinical significance of these findings.

Herpes Virus Infections

The herpes viruses are large, complex DNA viruses surrounded by a protein capsid, an amorphous tegument (structure located between the capsid and the envelope), and an outer envelope. These viruses are all capable of establishing a latent infection with lifelong persistence in the host. The *Herpesviridae* family includes eight viruses that can cause disease in humans: the herpes simplex viruses (HSV-1 and HSV-2); VZV; EBV; CMV; and the human herpes viruses HHV-6, HHV-7, and HHV-8 (associated with Kaposi sarcoma). In this section, we present the clinical manifestations and laboratory diagnosis of some of these viruses.

Epstein-Barr Virus (EBV)

The EBV is abundant in nature and causes a wide spectrum of diseases, including infectious mononucleosis (IM), lymphoproliferative disorders, and several malignancies. EBV infections most commonly result from intimate contact with salivary secretions from an infected individual. Although virus transmission can occur by other means, including blood transfusions, bone marrow and solid-organ transplants, sexual contact, and perinatal exposure, these routes appear to be much less frequent.

In developing nations and lower socioeconomic groups living under poor sanitation, EBV infections usually occur during early childhood, whereas in industrialized nations with higher hygiene standards, infections are typically delayed until adolescence or adulthood. However, by adulthood (age 40), almost 100% of people have been infected, as evidenced by the presence of EBV antibodies in their serum.

Initial infection with EBV is believed to occur in the oropharynx (the middle part of the throat), where the virus primarily infects epithelial cells and B lymphocytes. EBV binds to β1 integrins on the surface of the epithelial cells, which take up the virus by endocytosis. Inside the oropharyngeal epithelial cells, EBV enters a lytic cycle, characterized by viral replication, lysis of host cells, and release of infectious virions, until the acute infection is resolved. The virions spread to adjacent structures, including the salivary glands and tonsils. There, EBV infects B lymphocytes, which spread the virus throughout the immune system. EBV enters the B cells by binding to surface CD21, which is also the receptor for the C3d component of complement. The virus-infected B cells become polyclonally activated, proliferating and secreting several antibodies, including EBV-specific antibodies; heterophile antibodies; and autoantibodies such as cold agglutinins, rheumatoid factor, and antinuclear antibodies. In healthy people, this process is kept in check by the immune response of NK cells and specific Tc cells. However, EBV can persist in the body indefinitely in a small percentage of memory B cells, where it establishes a latent infection. In the latent state, EBV DNA exists outside of the chromosomes; in these cases, active viral replication does not occur. Periodic reactivation results in reentry of the virus into the lytic cycle, with viral shedding into the saliva and genital secretions, even in healthy, asymptomatic people.

Several antigens have been identified in EBV-infected cells that are associated with different phases of the viral infection. Antibodies to these antigens have become an important diagnostic tool. Antigens produced during the initial stages of viral replication in the lytic cycle are known as the *early antigens (EAs)*. These antigens can be further classified into two groups based on their location within the cells: EA-D, which has a *diffuse* distribution in the nucleus and cytoplasm, and EA-R, which is *restricted* to the cytoplasm only. The late antigens of EBV are those that appear during the period of the lytic cycle following viral DNA synthesis. They include the viral capsid antigens (VCAs) in the protein capsid and the membrane antigens in the viral envelope. Antigens appearing during the latent phase include the EBV nuclear antigen (EBNA) proteins, EBNA-1, EBNA-2, EBNA-3 (EBNA-3a), EBNA-4 (EBNA-3b), EBNA-5 (EBNA-LP), and EBNA-6 (EBNA-3c); and the latent membrane proteins (LMPs), LMP-1, LMP-2A, and LMP-2B **(Table 23–2)**.

The clinical manifestations of EBV vary with the host's age and immune status. Infections in infants and young children are generally asymptomatic or mild, whereas primary infections in healthy adolescents or adults commonly result in IM. More than half of patients with IM present with three classic symptoms: fever, lymphadenopathy (swollen lymph nodes), and sore throat. Symptoms usually last for 2 to 4 weeks, but fatigue, muscle aches, and need for sleep can persist for months. Treatment is mainly directed at easing symptoms. Although the associated symptoms are essential in diagnosing IM, they can also be caused by many other infectious agents, so laboratory testing plays an important role in differentiating IM from other infections.

Laboratory Testing for EBV

Characteristic laboratory findings in patients with IM include an absolute lymphocytosis (high lymphocyte count) of greater than 50% of the total leukocytes and at least 20% atypical lymphocytes **(Fig. 23–8)**. The atypical lymphocytes are predominantly activated T_C cells that are responding to the viral infection. Serological findings include the presence of a heterophile antibody and antibodies to certain EBV antigens.

By definition, **heterophile antibodies** are capable of reacting with similar antigens from two or more unrelated species. The heterophile antibodies associated with IM are IgM antibodies produced because of polyclonal B-cell activation

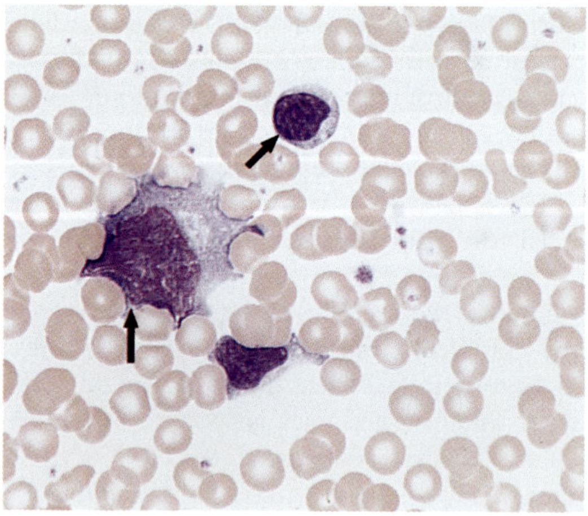

FIGURE 23–8 Atypical lymphocytes from a patient with infectious mononucleosis. Note the variation in size, nuclear:cytoplasmic ratio, and chromatin coarseness.

Table 23–2 Epstein-Barr Virus Antigens

EARLY ACUTE PHASE	LATE PHASE	LATENT PHASE
EA-R (early antigen restricted) EA-D (early antigen diffuse)	VCA (viral capsid antigen) MA (membrane antigen)	EBNA (EBV nuclear antigens): EBNA-1, EBNA-2, EBNA-3 (EBNA-3a), EBNA-4 (EBNA-3b), EBNA-5 (EBNA-LP), EBNA-6 (EBNA-3c)
		Latent membrane proteins (LMP-1, LMP-2A, LMP-2B)

and are capable of reacting with horse red blood cells (RBCs), sheep RBCs, and bovine RBCs. These antibodies are produced by 40% of patients with IM during the first week of clinical illness and by 80% to 90% of patients by the third week. They disappear in most patients by 3 months after the onset of symptoms but can be detected in some patients for 1 to 2 years. Because the heterophile antibody is present in most patients during the acute phase of illness, testing for this antibody was routinely performed to screen for IM in patients who presented with symptoms of the disease.

Rapid tests for the heterophile antibody of IM (also referred to as "Monospot") have been used for many years to test patients with disease symptoms. The original Monospot was a rapid slide agglutination method that could differentiate the heterophile antibody of IM from those produced in other conditions. In this test, serum premixed with guinea pig kidney antigen could agglutinate horse RBCs, but serum premixed with beef erythrocyte antigen could not agglutinate horse RBCs because the heterophile antibody attached to the beef RBC antigen during the first step. The antibody could then be titered by incubating serial dilutions of the patient's serum with sheep RBCs in the Paul-Bunnell test (see the Lab Exercises that accompany this text online).

These methods have been replaced by more sensitive, rapid agglutination tests or immunochromatographic assays using purified bovine RBC extract as the antigen. Although screening tests for the heterophile antibody can provide rapid results, they are not as sensitive or specific as tests for antibodies to EBV, the direct cause of IM. Negative heterophile antibody results occur in about 10% of adult patients with IM and up to 50% of children younger than 4 years old. False-positive results, although uncommon, can occur in patients with other conditions, including lymphoma, viral hepatitis, malaria, and autoimmune disease or can be caused by errors in result interpretation. Therefore, the CDC no longer recommends the Monospot test for general use; however, some clinicians may continue to order it because it is inexpensive and provides rapid results.

Testing for EBV-specific antibodies is considered the gold standard for IM diagnosis and can also be used to determine past exposure to EBV. Many different methods have been developed to detect these antibodies, including indirect immunofluorescence assays (IFAs) using EBV-infected cells, enzyme-linked immunosorbent assays (ELISA) or CLIA using recombinant or synthetic EBV proteins, and flow cytometric microbead immunoassays. All of these methods have a high level of sensitivity and specificity.

IgM antibody to the VCA is the most useful marker for acute IM because it usually appears at the onset of clinical symptoms and persists for 2 to 3 months after symptom onset. IgG anti-VCA is also present at the onset of IM but persists for life and can indicate a past infection. Antibodies to EA-D are also seen during acute IM, whereas anti-EBNA appears during convalescence. Thus, acute primary infection is typically indicated by the presence of IgM anti-VCA and anti-EA-D, as well as the absence of anti-EBNA. A summary of serological responses during acute, convalescent, and post-IM is shown in **Table 23–3.**

Some people develop chronic active EBV infection, with severe, often life-threatening IM-associated symptoms that persist or recur for more than 6 months after the acute illness. EBV can sometimes integrate its DNA into the genome of the cells it infects and transform them into cancer cells. Therefore, EBV has been associated with several malignancies, both hematologic (e.g., Burkitt lymphoma and Hodgkin disease) and nonhematologic (e.g., nasopharyngeal carcinoma and gastric carcinoma). EBV can also cause lymphoproliferative disorders in immunocompromised patients, including central nervous system (CNS) lymphomas in patients with

Table 23–3 Serological Responses of Patients With Diseases Associated With Epstein-Barr Virus

	ANTI-VCA			ANTI-EA			
Condition	IgM	IgG	IgA	EA-D	EA-R	ANTI-EBNA	HETEROPHILE ANTIBODY (IgM)
Uninfected	–	–	–	–	–	–	–
Acute IM	+	++	±	+	–	–	±
Convalescent IM	–	+	–	–	±	+	±
Past infection IM	–	+	–	–	–	+	–
Chronic active infection IM	–	+++	±	+	++	±	–
Posttransplant lymphoproliferative disease	–	++	±	+	+	±	–
Burkitt lymphoma	–	+++	–	±	++	+	–
Nasopharyngeal carcinoma	–	+++	+	++	±	+	–

EA-D = early antigen—diffuse; EA-R = early antigen—restricted; EBNA = EBV nuclear antigen; IM = infectious mononucleosis; VCA = viral capsid antigen.
Adapted from Straus SE, et al. Epstein-Barr virus infections: biology, pathogenesis, and management. Ann Intern Med. *1993;118:45, with permission.*

AIDS, X-linked lymphoproliferative disease in males with a rare genetic mutation, and posttransplant lymphoproliferative disorders (PTLD) in patients who have received hematopoietic stem cell or solid-organ transplants. These disorders result from the inability of immunosuppressed patients to control primary EBV infection, leading to massive polyclonal expansion of the EBV-infected B cells and life-threatening illness with a high rate of mortality.

EBV-associated malignancies can be diagnosed with the help of serology tests for EBV antibodies and molecular methods to detect EBV DNA in blood and tissue samples. Typical patterns of EBV antibodies seen in some of these disorders are shown in Table 23–3. Molecular tests may be more reliable than serology in immunocompromised patients, who may not demonstrate a good humoral response. qPCR is useful in monitoring viral load in transplant patients; a high or steadily increasing EBV viral load indicates the need to decrease immunosuppressive treatment and administer anti-viral therapy. Detection of EBV-encoded RNA transcripts (EBERs) by in situ hybridization is the method of choice for detecting EBV in tumor tissue.

Knowledge Check 23-3

The heterophile antibodies of IM can react with all of the following antigens *except:*

a. Guinea pig kidney antigens
b. Bovine red blood cell antigens
c. Sheep red blood cell blood antigens
d. Horse erythrocyte antigens

Critical Thinking 23-2

A teenager was seen in the emergency department with the following symptoms: cervical lymphadenopathy, sore throat, and a fever of 39°C (102.2°F). The patient also presented with hepatomegaly and splenomegaly. The physician ordered a complete blood count (CBC) with differential and a Monospot test. The CBC revealed an elevated white blood cell (WBC) count with 20% atypical lymphocytes. The Monospot was negative. How would you explain this discrepancy? What additional testing would you recommend, and what results would you expect if the patient has IM?

Cytomegalovirus (CMV)

CMV is a virus found throughout the world. Its prevalence ranges from 40% to 100%, depending on the population, and increases with age; however, crowded living conditions and poor personal hygiene facilitate spread earlier in life. Transmission of the virus can occur in various ways. CMV is spread through close, prolonged contact with infectious body secretions; intimate sexual contact; blood transfusions; solid-organ transplants; and perinatal exposure from infected mother to infant. The virus has been isolated in many body fluids, including saliva, urine, stool, vaginal and cervical secretions, semen, breast milk, and blood.

Primary, or initial, infections in healthy people are usually asymptomatic. However, some people experience a self-limiting, heterophile antibody-negative IM-like illness with fever, muscle aches, and fatigue. A small number of immunocompetent people who have other underlying disorders may develop severe CMV disease, which most commonly involves the gastrointestinal tract, CNS, and hematologic abnormalities. An immune response against CMV is stimulated, but the virus persists in a latent state in monocytes, dendritic cells, myeloid progenitor cells, and peripheral blood leukocytes. It may be reactivated at a later time in a person's life.

The clinical consequences of CMV infection are much more serious in the immunocompromised host, most notably organ-transplant recipients and patients with HIV/AIDS. CMV is the most important infectious agent associated with organ transplantation, with infections resulting from reactivation of CMV in the recipient or transmission of CMV from the donor organ. CMV infection of a previously unexposed recipient is associated with increased risk for allograft failure or graft-versus-host disease (GVHD) and poses a high risk for various complications, such as fever and leukopenia, hepatitis, pneumonia, gastrointestinal disturbances, CNS dysfunction, and retinitis. Although combination antiretroviral therapy has reduced the incidence of CMV-related illness in patients with HIV infection, CMV remains a major opportunistic pathogen in patients with low CD4 T-cell counts.

Measures can be taken to reduce the risk for CMV transmission and treat CMV infection in the immunocompromised host. Serological testing can be performed to identify CMV-positive donors so that transplantation of their organs into CMV-negative recipients can be avoided. If a CMV infection has been established in a transplant patient, immunosuppressive treatment should be reduced to the lowest dose possible. Also, a variety of anti-viral drugs are currently used to treat CMV infection and may, in some instances, be given prophylactically (i.e., before organ transplantation). Researchers are also investigating a vaccine design that involves the production of specific CMV antigens using genetic technologies. At the time of this writing, an investigational mRNA-1647 vaccine has shown promise in clinical trials. The vaccine appears to be safe, tolerable, and can induce antigen-specific immune responses across various doses.

CMV is also the most common cause of congenital infections, occurring in about 1 in every 200 newborns. Transmission of the virus may occur through the placenta, by passage of the infant through an infected birth canal, or by postnatal contact with breast milk or other maternal secretions. About one in five infants with congenital CMV infection have symptoms at birth or will develop long-term health problems. Mothers who acquire primary CMV infection during their pregnancy have a significantly higher risk of giving birth to a symptomatic or severely affected infant than do women in whom CMV was reactivated during pregnancy. Symptomatic infants present with many symptoms that reflect platelet dysfunction and CNS involvement. Ten percent of infants who are asymptomatic at birth progressively develop sensorineural hearing loss.

Laboratory Testing for CMV

Several laboratory methods have been developed to detect CMV infection; the tests recommended for use depend on the clinical situation. Assays for direct detection of the virus, such as viral culture, identification of CMV antigens, and molecular tests for CMV DNA, are necessary to detect a current CMV infection in immunocompromised patients or in neonates suspected of being congenitally infected with CMV. Serology is most beneficial in determining a past exposure to the virus, for example, in pregnant women or in patients in need of a transplant.

Isolation of the virus in culture is the traditional method of direct viral detection. In this method, human fibroblast cell lines are inoculated with CMV-infected specimens, most commonly urine, respiratory secretions, or anticoagulated whole blood. Presence of the virus is indicated by characteristic cytopathic effects (CPEs) that produce enlarged, rounded, refractile cells. Although conventional culture provides definitive results when positive, it is limited because CPEs do not appear until a few days to several weeks after inoculation, depending on the viral titer. Implementation of the rapid centrifugation-enhanced (shell vial) method has reduced the time of detection to within 24 hours after inoculation. In this assay, infected cells are grown on coverslips in shell vials and incubated with fluorescent-labeled monoclonal antibodies to CMV antigens produced early in the replication cycle. Fluorescent staining will appear in the nuclei of positive cells.

A widely used method for direct identification of CMV has been the CMV antigenemia assay, which uses immunocytochemical or immunofluorescent staining to detect the CMV lower-matrix protein pp65 in infected leukocytes from peripheral blood or cerebral spinal fluid. Following lysis of erythrocytes in the sample, the leukocytes are fixed onto a microscope slide, permeabilized, and stained with labeled monoclonal anti-pp65. Fluorescence appears in the nuclei of the infected cells, which can be counted to give quantitative results. The test can be completed in 2 to 4 hours, allowing for more rapid diagnosis and treatment of CMV infection in organ-transplant patients and people infected with HIV.

Although the antigenemia assay and shell vial culture methods are sensitive, specific, and rapid, they are labor intensive and require personnel with expertise in performing and interpreting these tests. For these reasons, they are progressively being replaced with molecular methods that detect CMV DNA or mRNA. The most widely used molecular method is qPCR because it is sensitive, simple to perform, and can provide quantitative results. PCR amplification of CMV DNA has been very useful for detecting CMV infections in HIV-infected hosts and establishing the diagnosis of CMV infection in transplant recipients. PCR also provides a more sensitive alternative to culture in diagnosing congenital CMV infections. Identification of CMV or CMV DNA in amniotic fluid after the 20th week of gestation is considered the gold standard for confirmation of fetal infection. Neonatal infection is established by detecting CMV or CMV DNA in the infant's urine during the first 10 days of life. Quantitative PCR, which detects the CMV copy number in the peripheral blood, is used to monitor the effectiveness of anti-viral treatment in immunocompromised hosts and to identify patients at risk for developing disseminated CMV disease. Increasing CMV DNA levels over time can help to distinguish an active infection from asymptomatic or latent infections.

Although serology tests for CMV have been commercially available for many years, their clinical utility is limited. The serology methods performed most commonly are semi- or fully automated EIAs that use microtiter plates or microparticle systems. Assays for CMV IgG are most useful in documenting a past CMV infection and determining if a person is at risk for future infection. For example, screening of blood and organ donors for CMV IgG is performed to identify donors who are CMV-positive so that the risk of posttransfusion/posttransplant primary CMV infection in seronegative recipients can be reduced. Screening of pregnant women for CMV IgG can determine if they have been exposed to the infection in the past or if they are susceptible to primary infection. In the latter case, the women could be educated on measures to reduce their chances of exposure while pregnant.

Although a single positive CMV IgG result indicates past exposure to the virus, conversion from a negative antibody result to a positive antibody result over time indicates a recent CMV infection. However, serial assays for CMV IgG are not routinely performed. Assays for IgM CMV antibodies have been developed but are limited in value because of the potential for false-negative results in newborns and immunocompromised patients and for false-positive results caused by other infections or the presence of rheumatoid factor. Also, IgM antibodies may not necessarily indicate primary CMV infection because they can be produced because of CMV reactivation and may persist for up to 18 months. Serological methods that distinguish CMV antibody avidity (antigen-binding strength) appear to be more useful in distinguishing a past exposure from a current primary infection. Low-avidity IgG antibodies indicate a recent infection, whereas high-avidity IgG antibodies reflect a past exposure because the avidity of the antibody increases during the course of the immune response. The presence of both IgM and low-avidity IgG antibodies can help identify pregnant women who have contracted a primary CMV infection. In cases of congenital CMV, PCR on saliva with a confirmatory test on urine is standard. This is due to the fact that CMV can be shed in breast milk, causing a false positive in saliva. Because of the limitations of serology testing, direct methods of detecting CMV infection are essential.

Knowledge Check 23-4

The standard test used to determine congenital CMV infections is:

a. EIA for IgM anti-CMV
b. IFA for IgG anti-CMV
c. PCR for CMV DNA
d. Shell vial cultures

Critical Thinking 23-3

An HIV-positive adult was exposed to cytomegalovirus by a 7-year-old child. The patient went to a physician and was tested for CMV antibodies. The doctor ordered acute and convalescent serum samples. The acute CMV antibody titer was 1:4, and the convalescent titer was 1:64. Comment on the patient's risk for developing CMV infection.

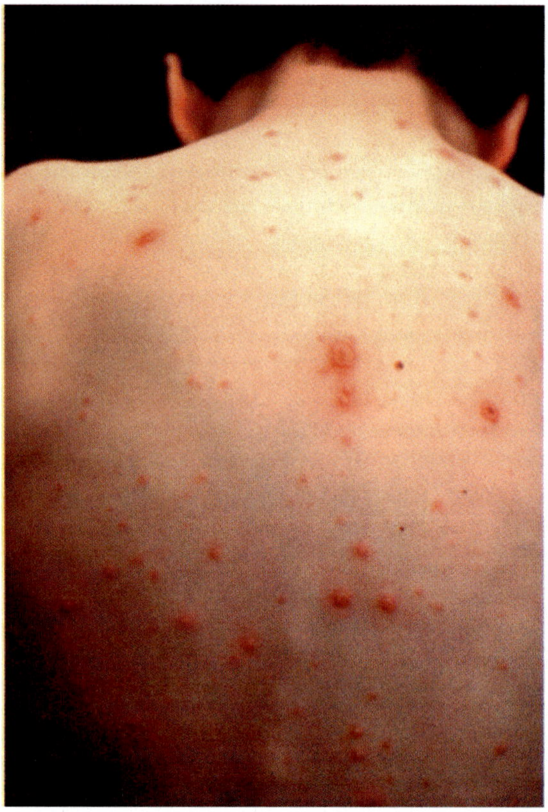

FIGURE 23–9 Vesicular lesions characteristic of chickenpox. These blister-like lesions have a pus-filled center. *(Courtesy of the Centers for Disease Control and Prevention, Public Health Image Library.)*

Varicella-Zoster Virus (VZV)

VZV is the cause of two distinct diseases: varicella *(chickenpox)* and herpes zoster *(shingles)*. It is transmitted primarily by inhalation of infected respiratory secretions or aerosols from skin lesions associated with the infection. Transplacental transmission to the fetus may also occur.

Primary infection with VZV results in varicella, a highly contagious illness characterized by a blister-like rash with intense itching and fever. Historically, most varicella cases have occurred during childhood. In a typical infection, vesicular lesions (fluid-filled blisters) first appear on the face and trunk and then spread to other areas of the body **(Fig. 23–9)**. The illness is usually mild and self-limiting in healthy children; however, in some cases, it may produce complications, the most common of which are secondary bacterial skin infections caused by scratching of the lesions. CNS involvement may occur in some cases but does not usually require hospitalization. Primary infections in adults, neonates, or pregnant women tend to be more severe, with a larger number of lesions and a greater chance of developing other complications such as pneumonia. Varicella infection in pregnant women may also cause premature labor or congenital malformations if the infection is acquired during the first trimester of pregnancy or may cause severe neonatal infection if transmission of the virus occurs around the time of delivery. Infections in immunocompromised patients are likely to result in disseminated disease, with extensive skin rash, neurological conditions (e.g., encephalitis), and other complications, including pneumonia, hepatitis, and nephritis.

During the course of primary infection, VZV is thought to travel from the skin lesions and the blood to sensory neurons, where it deposits its DNA and establishes a lifelong latent state in nerve cells in the spine, brain, and other internal organs. The host's T-cell–mediated immune response is believed to keep the virus under control during this time.

Reactivation of VZV, with active viral replication, occurs in 15% to 30% of persons with a history of varicella infection. The number of cases increases with age or the development of an immunocompromised condition, probably because of decreased cell-mediated immunity. During reactivation, the virus moves down the sensory nerve to the dermatome supplied by that nerve, resulting in eruption of a painful vesicular rash known as *herpes zoster,* or *shingles,* in the affected area. The rash may persist for weeks to months and is more severe in immunocompromised and older individuals. A significant number of patients with herpes zoster develop complications, the most common being debilitating pain in the nerves and skin that persists for weeks, months, or even years after resolution of the infection. Life-threatening complications, such as blindness, pneumonia, and internal organ involvement are more common in immunosuppressed persons.

Implementation of a vaccine consisting of a strain of live, attenuated varicella virus in the United States in 1995 has resulted in a significant decline in the incidence of chickenpox and its associated complications. In 2005, a vaccine was licensed for use in healthy children that combines the varicella vaccine with that for measles, mumps, and rubella. A recombinant (genetically engineered) zoster vaccine for shingles was licensed by the FDA in 2017. The CDC recommends that healthy adults over the age of 50 receive two doses of this vaccine 2 to 6 months apart to protect against shingles.

Laboratory Testing for VZV

Diagnosis of varicella and herpes zoster is usually based on identifying the characteristic vesicular lesions associated with the infection. Laboratory testing is most important in the diagnosis of atypical cases, such as those in which the rash is absent or delayed, and in immunocompromised patients with disseminated disease. Definitive diagnosis is based on identifying VZV or one of its products in skin lesions, vesicular fluids, or tissue. Culture of the virus and observation of characteristic CPE can be performed in several cell lines but is time consuming (4 days to 2 weeks) and may not yield productive results if clinical specimens do not contain sufficient amounts of the infectious virus. Direct immunofluorescence staining of scrapings from vesicular lesions with monoclonal antibodies directed against VZV antigens provides a rapid, more sensitive, and specific means of detecting the virus. A newer, recombinase-aided amplification-lateral flow system (RAA-LF) has also been used for the rapid detection of VZV DNA. No equipment is required, which makes this assay easier to use. Today, qPCR for VZV DNA is the laboratory method of choice for diagnosing varicella-zoster infection because it is highly accurate, sensitive, and rapid. Also, qPCR is useful in monitoring the response of immunocompromised patients to anti-viral drugs. It can be performed on a variety of samples, including vesicular fluid or scabs, skin swabs, throat swabs, cerebrospinal fluid, blood, saliva, and tissues from biopsies or autopsies.

Serology testing is of limited use in detecting current infections because accurate detection requires demonstration of a fourfold rise in antibody titer between acute and convalescent samples, a process that takes 2 to 4 weeks to perform. Testing for VZV IgM is not performed routinely for several reasons: IgM antibodies to VZV may not be detectable until the convalescent stage of illness, they cannot distinguish between primary and reactivated infection, and they may not be free of IgG antibodies when serum is processed for testing. In certain cases, IgG avidity assays may be used to differentiate between recent and past infection.

Serology is most useful in determining if immunity to VZV is present in certain people, such as health care workers, pregnant women, and patients about to undergo organ transplantation. Therefore, most serology tests detect total VZV antibody, which consists mostly of IgG. Several methods have been developed for this purpose, including ELISA, CLIA, and flow cytometric microbead immunoassays. A positive IgG result combined with a negative IgM result indicates previous vaccination or infection with VZV and protective immunity. Negative results for both IgM and IgG suggest the absence of prior VZV exposure and nonimmunity. However, a negative result does not rule out VZV infection because the serum sample may have been collected too early or the exposure may have occurred in the distant past, and antibody titers have weakened.

Knowledge Check 23-5

Which statement is true about vaccination for varicella and shingles?

a. One vaccine can prevent against both conditions.
b. There are separate vaccines for each condition.
c. There is a vaccine available for chickenpox but not for shingles.
d. There is a vaccine available for shingles but not for chickenpox.

Critical Thinking 23-4

An 18-year-old teenager who was never vaccinated and did not have chickenpox was exposed to a person who has shingles. Comment on the risk of the 18-year-old developing shingles.

Infections With Respiratory Viruses

In this section, we discuss infections with viruses that have major effects on the respiratory system—rubella, rubeola, mumps, influenza, respiratory syncytial virus, and severe acute respiratory syndrome coronavirus 2—and the serologic and molecular tests for detecting these infections.

Rubella

The **rubella virus** is a single-stranded, enveloped RNA virus of the genus *Rubivirus,* belonging to the family *Matonaviridae* (formerly *Togaviridae*). It is transmitted through respiratory droplets or transplacental infection of the fetus during pregnancy.

The virus is the cause of the typically benign, self-limited disease also known as *German measles* or *3-day measles.* Before widespread use of the rubella vaccine, this was mainly a disease of young children. However, today it occurs most often in young, unvaccinated adults. After an incubation period of 12 to 23 days, the virus replicates in the upper respiratory tract and cervical lymph nodes, then travels to the bloodstream. It produces a characteristic erythematous, maculopapular rash (flat, red areas on the skin), which appears first on the face, then spreads to the trunk and extremities, and usually resolves in 3 to 5 days **(Fig. 23–10).** Thus, rubella takes its name from the Latin term meaning "little red." In adolescents and adults, the rash is usually preceded by low-grade fever, malaise, swollen glands, and upper respiratory infection lasting 1 to 5 days. However, up to 50% of rubella infections are asymptomatic. The infection usually resolves without complications, and no specific treatment is available. A significant number of infected adult women experience joint pain and inflammation, but chronic arthritis is rare.

Rubella infection during pregnancy may have severe consequences, including miscarriage, stillbirth, or congenital rubella syndrome (CRS). The likelihood of severe consequences increases when infection occurs earlier in the

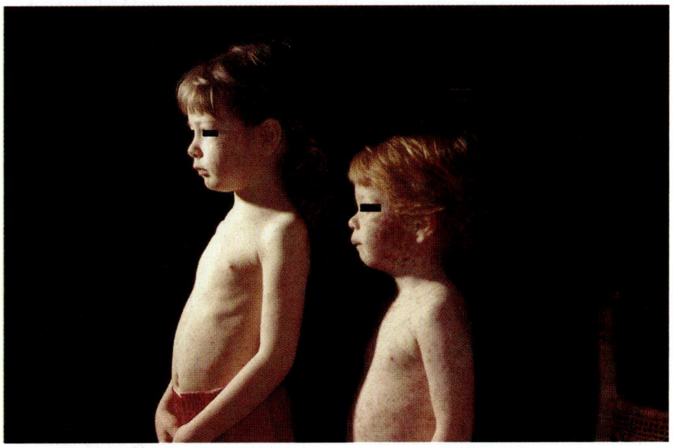

FIGURE 23–10 This image shows two young siblings, with a rash on their faces, arms, and torsos. Both had a severe case of German measles, caused by the rubella virus. *(Courtesy of the Centers for Disease Control and Prevention, Public Health Image Library.)*

pregnancy, especially during the first trimester. Infants born with CRS may present with several abnormalities, the most common of which are deafness; eye defects, including cataracts and glaucoma; cardiac abnormalities; intellectual disability; liver and spleen damage; and motor disabilities. In mild cases, symptoms may not be recognized until months to years after birth.

Scientists developed a vaccine consisting of live, attenuated rubella virus with the main goal of preventing infection of pregnant women by reducing dissemination of the virus in the population as a whole. The vaccine is part of the routine immunization schedule in infants and children and is usually given in combination with vaccines for measles and mumps (measles/mumps/rubella [MMR] vaccine) and sometimes with varicella (MMRV). Since licensure of the vaccine in 1969, the number of rubella infections and cases of CRS in the United States has dropped dramatically, with only limited outbreaks occurring, mostly among unvaccinated young immigrants to this country. However, rubella and CRS are still important health problems in parts of the world where routine immunization against the virus is not established.

Laboratory Testing for Rubella

Laboratory testing is helpful in confirming suspected cases of German measles because its symptoms may mimic those of other viral infections. It is essential in the diagnosis of CRS and in the determination of immune status in other individuals. Laboratory diagnosis of rubella infection can be accomplished by demonstrating viral RNA or detecting virus-specific antibodies. Isolation of rubella virus in conventional cell cultures is technically difficult and slow and is not performed in the routine diagnosis of rubella infection. The most widely used method for detecting rubella nucleic acid is RT-PCR (see Chapter 12). This method is a highly sensitive and specific aid in prenatal or postnatal diagnosis. Nasopharyngeal swabs are the preferred specimen types. Throat swabs and urine are also acceptable.

Serology tests are the most common means of confirming a rubella diagnosis because they are rapid, cost effective, and practical in clinical laboratory settings. The most commonly used methods for detecting rubella antibodies are ELISA, CLIA, and multiplex bead immunoassay because of their sensitivity, specificity, ease of performance, and adaptability to automation. Specific solid-phase capture ELISAs can be used to detect IgM rubella antibodies. These assays can also detect measles, mumps, rubella, and varicella antibodies simultaneously.

Primary rubella infection is indicated either by the presence of rubella-specific IgM antibodies or by a fourfold or greater rise in rubella-specific IgG antibody titers between acute and convalescent samples collected at least 10 to 14 days apart. The timing of serum collection is important because IgM antibodies to rubella do not appear in many patients until about 5 days after the onset of the rash, whereas IgG antibodies may not be detectable until 8 days after the rash. Only about 50% of patients are positive for IgM antibodies on the day that the rash appears; thus, a false-negative result can occur if the sample is obtained too early. False-positive results can also occur. Although IgM antibodies generally decline by 4 to 6 weeks, they may persist in low levels for a year or more in some cases. False-positive rubella IgM results have also been observed in people with parvovirus infections, enterovirus infections, heterophile antibodies, or rheumatoid factor. It is therefore recommended that positive IgM results, particularly in pregnant women, be confirmed by a more specific test, such as an ELISA that measures the avidity of rubella IgG antibodies, to distinguish between recent and past rubella infections. In these assays, low antibody avidity indicates a recent infection with a high risk for CRS, whereas high antibody avidity is seen in past infections, reflecting the normal change in avidity during the course of an immune response.

Laboratory diagnosis of congenital rubella infection begins with serological evaluation of the mother's antibodies and measurement of rubella-specific IgM antibodies in fetal blood, cord blood, or neonatal serum, depending on the age of the fetus or infant. To enhance the reliability of a CRS diagnosis, any positive IgM results should be confirmed by RT-PCR of rubella nucleic acid, or demonstration of persistently high titers of rubella IgG antibodies after 3 to 6 months of age.

Serology tests for rubella-specific IgG antibodies are also used to screen for immunity to rubella in populations such as pregnant women or health care workers. IgG antibodies provide immunity and persist for life. An antibody level of 10 to 15 IU/mL is considered to be protective.

Rubeola

The **rubeola virus** is a single-stranded RNA virus belonging to the genus *Morbillivirus* in the *Paramyxoviridae* family. It is a highly contagious infection that is spread by direct contact with aerosolized droplets from the respiratory secretions of infected people. After initial infection of the epithelial cells in the upper respiratory tract, rubeola virus is disseminated through the blood to multiple sites in the body, including the skin, lymph nodes, and liver.

Rubeola virus infection causes the disease commonly known as *measles*. After an incubation period of about 10 to 12 days, infected patients display symptoms of fever, cough, coryza (runny nose), and conjunctivitis (inflammation of the eyeball and eyelid membranes), which last 2 to 4 days. Early in the infection, characteristic areas known as *Koplik spots* appear on the mucous membranes of the inner cheeks or lips; these appear as gray-to-white lesions against a bright red background and persist for several days. The typical rash of measles appears about 14 days after exposure to the virus and is characterized by an erythematous, maculopapular eruption that begins on the hairline, then spreads to the face and neck and gradually moves down the body to the trunk, arms, hands, legs, and feet **(Fig. 23–11)**. The rash usually lasts 5 to 6 days.

Measles is a systemic infection that can result in complications, including diarrhea, otitis media, croup, bronchitis, pneumonia, and encephalitis. Rarely, a fatal degenerative disease of the CNS, called *subacute sclerosing panencephalitis*

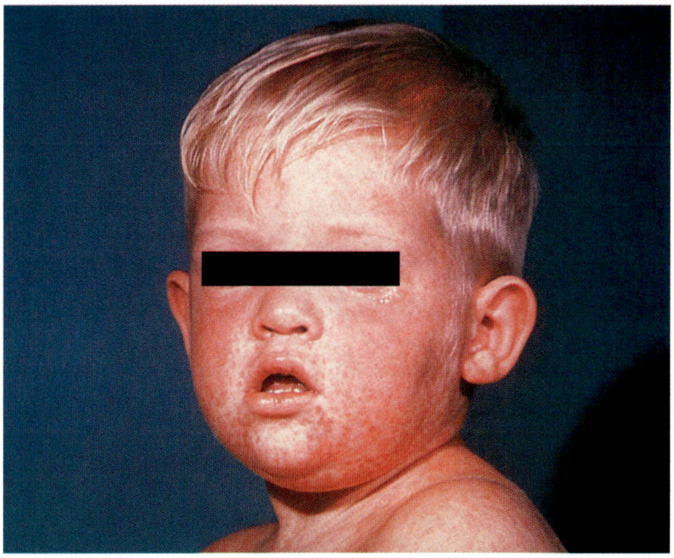

FIGURE 23–11 Characteristic rash of measles appearing on the face of a child. *(Courtesy of the Centers for Disease Control and Prevention, Public Health Image Library.)*

(SSPE), can result from persistent replication of measles virus in the brain. Measles infection during pregnancy can result in a higher risk of premature labor, spontaneous abortion, or low birth weight.

The incidence of measles has been greatly reduced in developed nations of the world since the introduction of a live, attenuated measles virus vaccine in 1968. A vaccine consisting of killed rubeola virus was originally licensed in 1963 but was ultimately ineffective because recipients developed a case of atypical measles if they were subsequently infected with the measles virus. The newer improved vaccine is used in the routine immunization schedule of infants and children, either in combination with rubella and mumps (MMR) or in combination with rubella, mumps, and varicella (MMRV). The recommended administration of the vaccine is in two doses, the first between the ages of 12 and 15 months and the second between ages 4 and 6 years. Administration of the first dose before the age of 12 months may result in vaccine failure because the presence of maternal antibodies can interfere with the infant's immune response. Although the vaccine has greatly reduced the incidence of measles, the disease continues to be a global concern, and periodic outbreaks continue to occur in the United States. Most cases in the United States and other industrialized nations are brought in by unvaccinated people from other countries and spread to persons who have refused vaccination because of religious reasons or unfounded fears of vaccine associations with disorders such as autism (see Chapter 25).

A measles diagnosis has typically been based on the patient's clinical presentation. However, the success of the U.S. immunization program in reducing the number of measles cases has decreased the ability of some physicians to recognize its clinical features. Also, atypical measles presentations can occur in people who received the earlier form of the measles vaccine, who have low antibody titers, or who are immunocompromised. Laboratory tests are therefore of value in ensuring rapid, accurate diagnosis of sporadic cases; they are also important for epidemiological surveillance and control of community outbreaks.

Laboratory Testing for Rubeola

Laboratory confirmation of rubeola infection involves detection of measles-specific antibodies in patient serum or RNA from the virus in nasopharyngeal aspirates, throat swabs, or urine. Isolation of rubeola virus in conventional cell cultures is technically difficult and slow and is not performed in the routine diagnosis of measles.

The most commonly used methods for detecting rubeola antibodies are automated ELISA, CLIA, and multiplex bead immunoassays. In patients with clinical symptoms, a diagnosis of measles is indicated by the presence of rubeola-specific IgM antibodies. IgM antibodies can be detected by 3 to 4 days after appearance of symptoms and persist for 1 to 2 months. Samples collected before 72 hours may yield false-negative results, and repeat testing is recommended in that situation. SSPE is associated with extremely high titers of rubeola antibodies.

IgG antibodies to rubeola become detectable 7 to 10 days after the onset of symptoms and persist for life. The presence of rubeola-specific IgG antibodies indicates immunity to measles because of past infection or immunization. Testing for IgG antibodies is therefore routinely performed on serum samples of individuals such as health care workers and persons with an unknown record of immunization to determine their immune status.

The CDC also recommends molecular methods to detect rubeola RNA for use in measles diagnosis and for genotyping the virus to track its source and transmission pathways. Quantitative RT-PCR is the preferred molecular technique for diagnosis as it is sensitive and capable of detecting the viral RNA within 3 days of rash appearance. The assay is most often performed on throat swabs or nasopharyngeal swabs but can also be done using urine.

Mumps

The **mumps virus,** similar to rubeola, is a single-stranded RNA virus that belongs to the *Paramyxoviridae* family (genus *Rubulavirus*). It is transmitted from person-to-person by infected respiratory droplets, saliva, and fomites, and replicates initially in the nasopharynx and regional lymph nodes. (Fomites are inanimate objects or substances that can transmit infectious organisms.) Following an average incubation period of 14 to 18 days, the virus spreads from the blood to various tissues, including the meninges of the brain, salivary glands, pancreas, testes, and ovaries, and produces inflammation at those sites. Inflammation of one or both parotid glands (a type of salivary gland), or *parotitis,* is the most common clinical manifestation of mumps **(Fig. 23–12).** The illness typically resolves in 7 to 10 days and does not require therapy other than supportive treatment to ease the symptoms, although complications in the involved tissues may occur in some patients. Mumps infection in pregnant women results in increased risk for fetal death when it occurs in the first

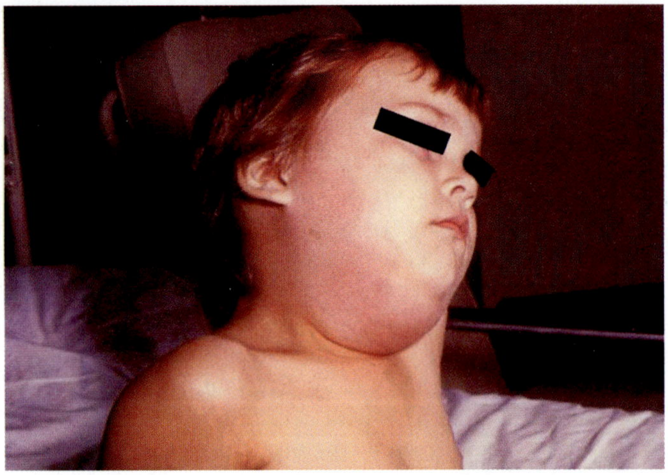

FIGURE 23–12 Parotitis characteristic of mumps. Note the swollen neck region caused by an enlargement of the child's salivary glands. *(Courtesy of the Centers for Disease Control and Prevention, Public Health Image Library.)*

trimester of pregnancy, but it is not associated with congenital abnormalities.

The number of U.S. mumps cases has declined significantly since the introduction of a live, attenuated mumps virus vaccine in 1967 and its routine use in childhood immunization schedules in 1977. The vaccine is most commonly combined with the vaccines for rubella and measles (MMR) or is used in combination with the rubella, measles, and varicella vaccines (MMRV). However, several U.S. outbreaks were reported in close-knit communities and on college campuses from 2006 to 2019. Since 2020, mumps cases significantly declined, most likely due to social distancing and safety measures put into place during the COVID-19 pandemic.

Laboratory Diagnosis of Mumps

The diagnosis of mumps is usually based on clinical symptoms, especially parotitis. The CDC recommends laboratory testing to differentiate the diagnosis from other infections that can cause parotitis. Although the mumps virus has been cultured in cell lines inoculated with a buccal (cheek cell) swab or urine sample from an infected patient, culture is time consuming and requires special facilities and experienced laboratory personnel. RT-PCR to detect viral RNA of mumps is the preferred method for confirmation of the infection because it is automated and provides faster results. The CDC recommends collection of buccal swab samples from patients with suspected mumps within a few days of symptom onset for greatest sensitivity (within 3 days is ideal). A positive result is confirmatory for mumps, but false-negative results can occur with samples that are not processed properly or collected too late. Molecular methods can also be used for genotyping the virus to track its transmission during mumps outbreaks.

The presence of IgM antibodies can support a diagnosis of acute mumps but is not confirmatory. ELISA is the most commonly used method to detect mumps antibodies. If serology is performed, the CDC recommends collection of serum samples for IgM testing 3 or more days after symptom onset to increase the likelihood of a positive result. Current or recent infection is suggested by the presence of mumps-specific IgM antibody in patient serum. Solid-phase IgM capture assays reduce the incidence of false-positive results caused by interfering factors (see Chapter 11). A negative IgM result does not rule out mumps because negative results can occur if the serum was collected too early or too late. Also, people who received any doses of the mumps vaccine tend to have lower or absent IgM antibody. Testing for IgG can be used to indicate immunity in vaccinated persons. However, IgG is not usually used in diagnosis, because acute IgG titers are often high, and a fourfold rise in IgG antibody titer between acute and convalescent-phase serum samples may not occur.

Knowledge Check 23-6

Severe consequences of congenital rubella syndrome (CRS) are most likely to occur at what stage of the pregnancy?

a. First trimester
b. Second trimester
c. Third trimester
d. Postpartum

Critical Thinking 23-5

A woman in her first trimester of pregnancy was exposed to a child with rubella. A serum sample taken 5 days after exposure showed a rubella antibody titer of 1:4, while a convalescent serum taken 2 weeks later showed a titer of 1:32. (Note: A twofold dilution was performed.)

How can these results be interpreted? What is the risk of congenital infection in the fetus?

Influenza

Influenza viruses A, B, C, and D are large, single-stranded, negative-sense RNA viruses that range from 80 to 120 nm in diameter and reside in the family *Orthomyxoviridae*. Influenza A and B are the most common and cause seasonal epidemics of the "flu" during the winter months. Influenza C is milder in comparison and does not cause human epidemics. Influenza D affects cattle and other animals and does not cause human disease.

Influenza viruses A, B, and C are classified by antigenic differences in the nucleoprotein (NP) and the matrix protein (M) of the virions. Influenza A is further divided into subtypes based on two envelope proteins, hemagglutinin (HA) and neuraminidase (NA), two matrix proteins (M1 and M2), and two nonstructural proteins (NS1 and NS2, both responsible for pathogenesis and viral replication). There are 18 different hemagglutinin subtypes and 11 different neuraminidase subtypes (H1 through H18 and N1 through N11, respectively).

The HA and NA genes of influenza A and B undergo reassortment, resulting in altered antigens and the emergence of new viral strains. The high mutation rate of the influenza viruses makes it necessary to modify vaccine formulations annually based on the most common circulating strains.

Influenza C is stable and does not undergo gene rearrangement. **Antigenic drift** occurs when genes that code for the surface proteins HA and NA gradually mutate, producing new strains of the virus with small genetic changes. These new strains are closely related and antigenically similar; therefore, antibodies most likely respond and react to the new strain, causing what is referred to as "cross-protection" between strains. Changes accumulate over time, however, leading to a decline in protection. Influenza A can also undergo **antigenic shift,** a major genetic change that occurs suddenly, yielding new HA and/or NA proteins that the body does not recognize. Antigenic shift, which occurs less frequently than antigenic drift, can result from mutations in an animal flu virus (e.g., from birds or swine) that produce a new virus capable of infecting humans for the first time.

Although influenza viruses mutate, they rarely result in a pandemic. Over the last 100 years, four pandemics have occurred due to genetic variations and mutations in viral proteins. The H1N1 influenza A pandemic of 1918 (Spanish flu) was one of the most deadly pandemics of all time, killing 50 million to 100 million people worldwide. However, influenza remains a major health concern; the CDC estimated that 41 million illnesses, 100,000 to 710,000 hospitalizations, and 4,900 to 51,000 deaths from influenza occurred annually in the United States alone between 2010 and 2023. Infections are typically seasonal, peaking during the winter months.

Influenza (flu) is a contagious respiratory infection affecting the nose, throat, and lungs. Transmission occurs from person-to-person via the spread of aerosolized respiratory droplets when an infected person sneezes or coughs. The incubation period ranges from 1 to 4 days, with a median of 2 days. The disease is usually self-limiting in most people, producing symptoms that include fever, chills, body aches, headache, congestion, and fatigue, lasting from a few days to 2 weeks. However, serious, potentially life-threatening complications (e.g., bronchitis, pneumonia) can occur in people who are immunocompromised or have certain medical conditions (e.g., asthma, chronic lung conditions, cardiovascular diseases, diabetes). Other people at risk for serious illness include those younger than 2 years old or older than 65, pregnant women, and those working or living in facilities in which there is close contact with other people (e.g., nursing homes, prisons, military barracks).

Supportive care, rest, hydration, and use of over-the-counter medications facilitate recovery in most people. In some cases, anti-viral drugs can be prescribed to alleviate symptoms and reduce the risk of progression to severe illness, and hospitalization may be required in severe infection. The best way to prevent influenza is by receiving the annual flu vaccine, which protects against influenza A and B viruses. Determining which viral strain or strains will be in circulation in the upcoming year due to antigenic drift or shift makes designing vaccines challenging. Therefore, creating a universal vaccine that can protect people against all virus strains is being researched. Other ways to prevent the flu include using an alcohol-based hand sanitizer, washing hands often with soap and water, coughing and/or sneezing into a tissue or your elbow, avoiding people who are sick with the flu, and wearing a mask.

Laboratory Testing for Influenza

Laboratory tests for influenza can detect virus in nasopharyngeal (NP), nasal, or throat swabs, NP aspirates or washes, endotracheal aspirates, or sputum, depending on the method. RT-PCR is the gold standard for identifying influenza and other respiratory viruses. Rapid molecular assays using upper respiratory samples produce results in about 15 to 30 minutes and have high sensitivity (90% to 95%) and specificity. These assays are approved by the FDA, and some are waived for point-of-care use by the Clinical Laboratory Improvement Amendments (CLIA). Rapid influenza diagnostic tests (RIDTs), based on chromatographic or fluorescent lateral flow immunoassays that detect viral antigens, can yield results in 10 to 15 minutes; however, they are not as sensitive (50% to 70%) or as accurate as rapid molecular assays. Other tests include viral cell culture (providing results in 1 to 3 days) and immunofluorescence assays for viral antigens (taking 2 to 4 hours). Serological testing for influenza antibodies is not recommended for clinical decision making but may be useful in research studies.

Respiratory Syncytial Virus (RSV)

Respiratory syncytial virus (RSV) is an enveloped, single-stranded RNA virus of the genus *Orthopneumovirus* within the Pneumoviridae family. Members of this genus include human RSV (HRSV) and human metapneumovirus. Structurally, RSV is spherical with a diameter of about 150 nm. The envelope consists of three surface transmembrane glycoproteins: G, F, and a small hydrophobic protein SH. The two major glycoproteins on the surface of the virion glycoprotein G, and glycoprotein F, are involved in the initial stages of the infection. Glycoprotein G binds to receptors on the surface of ciliated epithelial cells in the respiratory tract, and glycoprotein F then fuses with the target cell membrane, allowing the virus to enter the host cell and replicate. In the process, host cells fuse together to form syncytia, hence the name, RSV. Human RSV consists of two antigenic subtypes, RSV-A and RSV-B, which can be present simultaneously or alternate during yearly outbreaks (mostly in the fall and winter). If they cocirculate, RSV-A is usually the more predominant subtype; however, an increased prevalence of RSV-B has been reported.

RSV is transmitted by direct contact with an infected person, contact with droplets from the nose and throat of an infected person through coughing and sneezing, or touching a contaminated surface or dried respiratory secretions then transferring the virus to one's face. Once inoculated, the incubation period ranges from 2 to 8 days depending on the person's age and immune status. Individuals infected with RSV are usually contagious for 3 to 8 days and may also be contagious 1 to 2 days before when symptoms begin. It is estimated that since RSV is highly contagious, almost 100% of children will contract the virus before age 2. RSV usually causes a respiratory tract infection with mild, cold-like symptoms, including a runny nose, coughing, sneezing, wheezing, fever and decreased appetite. Hydration and over-the-counter medications can help alleviate symptoms. In most cases, anti-viral medication is not routinely recommended to combat the infection. Aerosol ribavirin and immunoglobulin injections started early in the infection may help persons with a compromised immune system. Most RSV infections are self-limiting and will resolve on their own in 1 to 2 weeks.

However, RSV infections in infants, children, and older adults can be serious and require hospitalization. Severe infections such as bronchiolitis and pneumonia can occur and are often seen in children 1 year of age or younger and in older adults. Breathing difficulties and dehydration can lead to hospitalization requiring oxygen, IV fluids, and in severe cases, intubation. People at risk include premature infants and young children with comorbidities such as congenital heart conditions, chronic lung disease, neuromuscular disorders, and compromised immune systems. Infants have much smaller airways that quickly fill up with mucus, leading to breathing problems. Adults with compromised immune systems and older adults with underlying heart disease such as congestive heart failure or lung disease, asthma, and chronic obstructive pulmonary disease (COPD) are also at great risk of developing a severe infection. According to the CDC, each year RSV leads to 2.1 million outpatient visits, over 50,000 hospitalizations, and up to 300 deaths in children younger than 5 years old, and over 60,000 hospitalizations and up to 10,000 deaths in adults 65 years and older.

Nirsevimab, a monoclonal antibody that neutralizes RSV, is available for infants and young children with compromising conditions to protect against severe RSV infection. RSV vaccination is recommended by the CDC for all adults ages 75 and older and for adults ages 60 to 74 with underlying conditions and at high risk for severe infection. Also, a vaccine is available for pregnant women at 32 to 36 weeks of pregnancy.

Laboratory Testing for RSV

The main types of laboratory tests to identify RSV are rapid antigen tests and molecular panels. Rapid tests detect RSV antigens in nasopharyngeal (NP) swab or nasopharyngeal aspirate/wash specimens from symptomatic patients. The tests are available in various formats, including lateral flow EIA point-of-care devices and automated direct fluorescent immunoassay. Antigen tests are used most commonly because they provide results in less than an hour and require only a small amount of nasal fluid. Although turnaround time is quick, the results are not as sensitive as molecular tests, especially in older children and adults who may have low viral loads.

Highly sensitive molecular tests that detect RSV nucleic acid are available in various formats, including reverse transcriptase (RT) qPCR and isothermal nucleic acid amplification assays. These tests can provide results within a few minutes to a few hours, depending on the assay. The RT qPCR assays may be part of a multiplex combination panel that also detects other respiratory viruses causing similar symptoms, such as influenza A, influenza B, and SARS-CoV-2.

Viral culture, which is costly and not widely available, and serological testing for RSV antibodies are less commonly used and performed mainly for research and surveillance.

Severe Acute Respiratory Syndrome Coronavirus 2 (SARS-CoV-2)

On December 31, 2019, the WHO learned of a cluster of viral pneumonia cases originating in Wuhan, China. The causative agent responsible for this viral outbreak was identified as a novel coronavirus called **severe acute respiratory syndrome coronavirus 2 (SARS-CoV-2).** The virus quickly spread throughout China, Europe, and the globe, becoming one of the deadliest pandemics the world has encountered. The disease caused by SARS-CoV-2 was named Coronavirus Disease 2019, commonly referred to as **COVID-19.** According to the WHO, over 760 million cases and 6.9 million deaths have been recorded worldwide since December 2019, but the actual number is thought to be higher. The disease has been responsible for over 100 million cases and over 1 million deaths in the United States alone.

Coronaviruses (CoVs) are not new viruses. Severe acute respiratory syndrome (SARS) and Middle East respiratory syndrome (MERS) coronaviruses emerged in 2002 in Guangdong Province, China, and in 2012 in Saudi Arabia, respectively. The Coronavirinae, a subfamily of the Coronaviridae, contains four genera, *Alphacoronavirus, Betacoronavirus, Gammacoronavirus,* and *Deltacoronavirus.* SARS-CoV and MERS-CoV belong to the *Betacoronavirus* lineages A and C, respectively. *Betacoronaviruses* are also called "bat-coronaviruses" since molecular studies suggest that bats may be the natural reservoir for coronaviruses, including SARS-CoV-2. Coronaviruses are termed as such because their surface projections resemble a "crown," suggestive of the "solar corona" seen on electron microscopy. CoVs contain large, linear, positive, single-stranded RNA genomes ranging from approximately 25 to 32 kb in size.

Genetic mutations have resulted in the virus's rapid evolution to create multiple variants, which the WHO have designated by Greek letters, including the original virus, alpha, followed by beta, gamma, delta, omicron, and others. As the virus mutates, new variants and their descendants continue to emerge. For example, the omicron variant has rapidly given rise to many lineages and sublineages (e.g., BA.2.86, XBB.1.9.1, EG.5, JN.1). The more recent variants are more transmissible than the original alpha virus and have caused periodic waves of infection in various parts of the world.

SARS-CoV-2 is an enveloped, single-stranded RNA virus that contains *spike (S)* glycoproteins radiating from its surface, a *nucleoprotein (N)* within the viral capsid, and the *transmembrane (M)* protein, which plays a role in viral assembly and formation of the viral envelope **(Fig. 23–13).** The S glycoprotein has two subunits: S1 and S2; S1 is an antigen that binds to the human angiotensin-converting enzyme 2 (ACE2) receptor on human cells and is responsible for membrane fusion. The ACE2 receptors provide the main portal of entry for viral invasion into host cells and are found in virtually all organs. Therefore, once the virus gains access to the host, it can infect a wide variety of cells and organs, notably the oral and nasal mucosa, nasopharynx, lungs, stomach, small intestine, colon, skin, lymph nodes, thymus, bone marrow, spleen, liver, kidney, and brain.

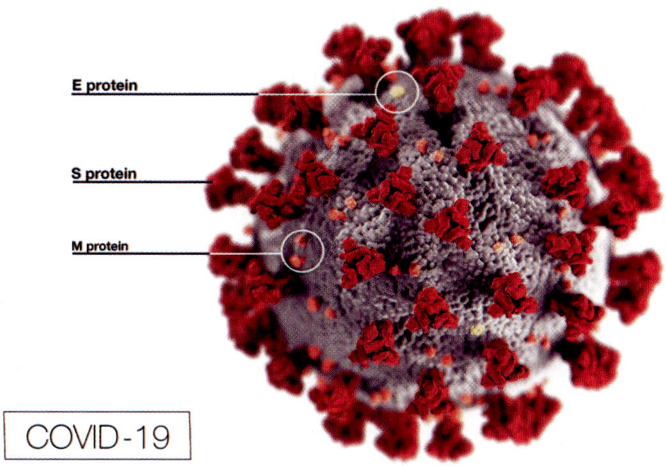

FIGURE 23–13 Structure of SARS-CoV-2, the cause of COVID-19. The E (envelope), S, and M proteins are located on the outer surface of the particle. The S proteins project out as spikes, imparting the look of a corona surrounding the virion when viewed by electron microscopy. *(Courtesy of the Centers for Disease Control and Infection/Alissa Eckert, MSMI; Dan Higgins, MAMS.)*

Transmission and Clinical Symptoms

SARS-CoV-2 is a highly communicable and infectious virus transmitted from human to human mainly by close contact and inhalation of infected respiratory droplets. It can also gain access via contact with the oral, nasal, and eye mucosa. However, contact with contaminated objects or surfaces is not thought to be a major route of transmission. The presence of SARS-CoV-2 in stool has also been reported, allowing for detection of the virus in wastewater, but transmission by the fecal-oral route does not appear to play a significant role in the spread of the infection.

Although SARS-CoV-2 can infect a wide range of cells and organs, the lungs are the primary target for infection, and disease complications can result in alveolar damage and severe respiratory distress. Signs and symptoms appear 2 to 14 days after exposure and range from asymptomatic or mild to severe depending on the person's age and immune status. Unvaccinated people, especially older individuals and those with underlying medical conditions, tend to develop more severe symptoms.

Common symptoms include fever, chills, cough, shortness of breath or difficulty breathing, fatigue, muscle or body aches, headache, new loss of taste and/or smell, sore throat, congestion, nausea or vomiting, and diarrhea. Severe symptoms include pneumonia, coughing up blood, and kidney failure. Some patients may develop "long COVID," a condition lasting weeks, months, or longer after the initial infection and characterized by extreme fatigue and respiratory, cardiac, neurological, digestive, or other symptoms. A small percentage of patients with COVID-19 developed multisystem inflammatory syndrome, a serious condition involving a massive release of cytokines and uncontrolled systemic inflammation, which can lead to acute respiratory distress, heart failure, hypotension, shock, hypercoagulation, and acute kidney injury.

Preventive Measures and Vaccines

To prevent the spread of this highly contagious, communicable disease, the CDC has issued several recommendations, including staying up to date with vaccinations (see later), wearing masks, performing hand hygiene, increasing ventilation, increasing distance between people, and socially isolating if positive for SARS-CoV-2. If an individual is exposed to a person who tested positive for SARS-CoV-2, they should follow CDC recommendations to prevent further spread of the virus and watch for development of COVID-19 symptoms such as fever, shortness of breath, and cough. At least 5 days after exposure or if the individual becomes symptomatic, they should undergo SARS-CoV-2 testing, which can be performed at home using a rapid antigen test or by undergoing testing at health care sites such as walk-in clinics, urgent care centers, pharmacies, or hospitals (see next section).

SARS-CoV-2 vaccines have had a large impact on health care. Following the onset of the pandemic, researchers worldwide were able to rapidly develop vaccines based on information about related viruses and vaccine technology. Vaccines that have been developed against SARS-CoV-2 are based on one of four designs: messenger RNA (mRNA) or DNA, protein-based, inactivated or weakened virus, and vector based (see Chapter 25 for a discussion of vaccines). The FDA has approved the use of mRNA, and more recently, protein-based vaccines, for SARS-CoV-2.

In the United States, the most used vaccines are of the mRNA format, developed by the companies Pfizer-BioNTech and Moderna, Inc. These vaccines were produced with remarkable speed, receiving approval by the FDA for Emergency Use Authorization (EUA) in December 2020. Initial administration of both vaccines involves two doses spaced 3 to 4 weeks apart. These vaccines have since been modified to protect against the original SARS-CoV-2 and/or versions of the omicron variant. Vaccine dose and timing depend on age and immune status. The vaccines are composed of synthetically produced mRNA, the genetic material used to make proteins (see Chapter 12), in this case, the spike protein of SARS-CoV-2. The mRNA is chemically modified to increase its stability and is encapsulated in lipid nanoparticles, which facilitates its entry into host cells. The mRNA enters the host cells through endocytosis and is translated into the SARS-CoV-2 spike protein, which is displayed on the host cell surface. The host's immune system recognizes the protein as foreign and begins making antibodies against it and activating T cells to fight off the infection, similar to what happens in a natural, active infection (see Chapter 4).

The neutralizing antibodies to SARS-CoV-2 induced by the vaccine are thought to prevent initial infection. Studies have shown that the mRNA vaccines generate very high antibody titers and provide excellent short-term protection, but antibody levels decrease over several months, making breakthrough infections in vaccinated individuals common. Despite this observation, the mRNA vaccines have provided long-term protection against severe disease, hospitalization, and death. Vaccine-induced $CD8^+$ T cells are thought to play a major role in preventing disease progression by destroying virally infected cells, thereby controlling replication of the virus.

Another important advancement in controlling SARS-CoV-2 infection has been the development of anti-viral medications, which are recommended for high-risk individuals who have mild to moderate symptoms associated with COVID-19. If administered within a few days of symptom onset, these medications can prevent progression to severe disease. As therapeutics and vaccine technologies continue to develop and become increasingly distributed worldwide, COVID-19 has transitioned to an endemic infection and will hopefully remain more manageable in the future.

Laboratory Testing for SARS-CoV-2

Testing is essential for an accurate COVID-19 diagnosis to differentiate it from other respiratory illnesses with similar symptoms, such as influenza. Laboratory assays to detect infection with the virus can be classified into one of three types: (1) Molecular tests to detect viral nucleic acid, (2) Viral antigen tests, and (3) Tests for antibody to the virus.

The sensitivity and specificity of these tests have improved over time. Due to the urgent need for diagnostic testing, the FDA approved many in vitro diagnostic tests for EUA; several have since received traditional FDA marketing authorization.

Specimen types used in the various molecular and antigen tests include nasopharyngeal (NP) swabs, nasopharyngeal wash/aspirates, or oropharyngeal (OP) specimens collected by a trained health care provider, a nasal mid-turbinate specimen or anterior nares specimen collected by a trained health care provider or self-collected at home, and a saliva specimen collected by the person being tested. The specimen type depends on the test kit used.

Molecular tests provide the most sensitive means of detecting a current SARS-CoV-2 infection and are highly specific. They detect viral RNA from nasal, nasopharyngeal, or oropharyngeal swabs; nasopharyngeal wash/aspirates; sputum; or saliva. The specimen type depends on the test kit used. The method of choice is quantitative RT-PCR, which targets two to three SARS-CoV-2 genes, most commonly the *N* (Nucleocapsid) genes, N1 and N2, and the RNase P (RP) gene. Most assays can produce results in 2 to 4 hours, although results usually take 1 to 3 days to be reported. Other molecular assays to detect SARS-CoV-2 nucleic acid include LAMP and TMA. Rapid molecular tests also exist but require samples to be tested individually, in contrast to the other methods, where samples can be batch-tested by automated instrumentation in highly skilled laboratories. Positive results from molecular tests indicate infection, but tests may remain positive beyond the period in which a patient is contagious (up to 90 days) because they can also detect RNA from the virus when it is no longer viable. Testing too early in the course of the infection may result in a false-negative result.

Antigen tests can also be used to identify a current infection. They detect the SARS-CoV-2 nucleocapsid or spike proteins in samples collected from nasal or nasopharyngeal swabs. Formats for antigen tests include rapid lateral flow assay, ELISA, and CLIA (see Chapter 11 for general assay principles). Rapid antigen tests are ideal for use in a variety of point-of-care settings, including physician offices, urgent care facilities, pharmacies, school health clinics, nursing homes, and drive-through testing sites. They have also become widely available as at-home over-the-counter test kits. These tests quickly identify infected individuals because they can provide results within 30 minutes. While they tend to be highly specific, they have a lower sensitivity than molecular tests and are not recommended for asymptomatic people because false-negative results can occur, especially early in the infection. Improper specimen collection or failure to accurately follow testing procedures can also lead to false-negative or false-positive results.

Serological tests detect the presence of antibodies to SARS-CoV-2 in serum, plasma, or whole blood, depending on the test kit. Test formats include ELISA, CLIA, and lateral flow assays. They detect antibodies against the nucleocapsid (N) protein, and different forms of the spike protein (S1, S1 and S2, or the receptor binding domain [RBD]). IgM, IgG, and IgA antibodies can be detected 1 to 3 weeks after infection, and IgG antibodies persist for several months in most people. The CDC does not recommend using antibody tests to diagnose a current infection because of the time it takes for antibodies to develop.

Antibodies to SARS-CoV-2 can be produced because of natural viral infection or receipt of a COVID vaccine. Therefore, in the United States and other countries where vaccines are designed to induce an immune response to the S protein, a positive test for S antibody could be the result of natural infection, vaccination, or both. In contrast, the presence of N antibody indicates a previous COVID infection, regardless of whether an individual has been vaccinated. The CDC has published tables listing different possible patterns of S- and N-antibody test results and their interpretations. Antibody levels wane over time, and a negative antibody test does not rule out a previous infection. Because immunity to the virus is not fully understood at this time, the CDC does not recommend antibody testing to assess immunity. The main applications of serological tests are to evaluate patients for donation of convalescent plasma to treat severely ill patients, to identify past COVID infections, and to evaluate immunity to the virus in populations. Antibody tests can also be used to support a diagnosis of multisystem inflammatory syndrome or other complications caused by COVID-19.

Knowledge Check 23-7

The COVID-19 vaccines most commonly used in the United States are composed of synthetically produced mRNA that codes for a SARS-CoV-2 protein. What is the target protein in these vaccines?

a. Nucleoprotein
b. Transmembrane protein
c. Spike protein
d. M protein

Critical Thinking 23-6

An adult was exposed to COVID-19 during a family wedding. The patient self-tested the next day using an at-home antigen kit. The test was negative. A few days later, the patient was symptomatic and went to a physician who ordered a PCR test. The PCR result was positive. Explain this discrepancy.

Knowledge Check 23-8

Match each virus with its major disease association:

a. Hepatitis A (HAV)	__ 1. German measles
b. Hepatitis C (HCV)	__ 2. Salivary gland inflammation
c. Epstein-Barr virus (EBV)	__ 3. COVID-19
d. Cytomegalovirus (CMV)	__ 4. Chronic liver inflammation and cirrhosis
e. Varicella-zoster virus (VZV)	__ 5. Liver inflammation transmitted by fecal-oral route
f. Rubella virus	__ 6. Most common cause of congenital infections
g. Rubeola virus	__ 7. Infectious mononucleosis
h. Mumps virus	__ 8. Shingles
i. SARS-CoV-2	__ 9. Measles
j. Influenza A	__ 10. Flu

KEY CONCEPTS

Immune Defenses Against Viral Infections

- Viruses are obligate intracellular pathogens that can produce a wide range of diseases in humans.
- Viruses can exist as either free infectious virions or intracellular particles in infected host cells. These different states require a combined effort of innate, humoral, and cell-mediated immune responses to successfully defend the host against viral infections.
- Innate defenses against viruses include the skin and mucous membranes; IFNs to inhibit viral replication; and NK cells, which release cytotoxic proteins that destroy virus-infected host cells.
- Antibodies directed against specific viral antigens can prevent the spread of viral infection by neutralizing a virus and preventing it from binding to host cells, opsonizing a virus to make it more likely to be phagocytized, activating complement-mediated mechanisms of destruction, and agglutinating viruses.
- Cell-mediated immunity is needed to eliminate intracellular viruses. Virus-specific T_C cells bind to viral antigen complexed with class I MHC on the surface of infected host cells and release cytotoxic proteins that cause the cells to undergo apoptosis.

Viral Escape Mechanisms

- Viruses have evolved in several ways to escape host defenses. These include frequent genetic mutations to produce new viral antigens; evading the action of IFNs, complement, or other components of the immune system; or suppressing the immune system. Some viruses can establish a latent state by integrating their nucleic acid into the host's genome.

Laboratory Testing for Viral Infections

- Serological tests for viral antibodies can be used to indicate exposure to a viral pathogen. In general, the presence of IgM indicates a current or recent infection or a congenital infection, if present in infant serum. The presence of IgG antibodies indicates previous exposure to a virus or immunity because of vaccination.
- Culture, antigen detection, and molecular methods for viral nucleic acid can be used to directly identify viruses in clinical samples. Molecular methods have become increasingly important in the diagnosis of viral infections and can also be used to quantitate viral load to determine the effectiveness of anti-viral therapy.

Hepatitis Viruses

- The hepatitis viruses are those whose primary effect is inflammation of the liver. Hepatitis A and E are transmitted mainly by the fecal-oral route, whereas hepatitis B, C, and D are transmitted primarily by the parenteral route. Hepatitis B, C, and D can lead to chronic infections. Vaccines have been developed to prevent hepatitis A, hepatitis B, and hepatitis E.
- Serological markers of hepatitis infections consist of virus-specific antibodies and antigens that are commonly detected by automated immunoassays.
- IgM anti-HAV antibodies indicate current or recent hepatitis A infection, whereas IgG anti-HAV antibodies are developed later in the infection and indicate immunity to hepatitis A. Likewise, IgM anti-HEV antibodies are present during current or recent hepatitis E infection, and IgG anti-HEV antibodies indicate later infection and immunity.
- Hepatitis B infection is indicated by the presence of the antigen HBsAg; HBeAg indicates high infectivity. IgM antibodies to hepatitis B core antigen are present in acute hepatitis B, whereas IgG anti-HBc is present during past or chronic hepatitis B infection. Antibodies to HBsAg (anti-HBs) indicate immunity and can be produced because of past hepatitis B infection or immunization with the hepatitis B vaccine.
- The presence of anti-HCV indicates exposure to the hepatitis C virus but cannot distinguish between a current and a past infection. Molecular tests for HCV RNA are used to confirm antibody-positive results; if positive, they indicate a current infection. Molecular tests for hepatitis C are also used to quantitate viral load to determine the effectiveness of anti-viral therapy. A third application of molecular testing is genotyping of the virus to guide decisions about therapy.
- Hepatitis D occurs as a super- or coinfection with hepatitis B and is indicated by antibodies to hepatitis D or molecular tests to detect HDV RNA. Patients with coinfections are also positive for IgM-anti-HBc, whereas patients with superinfections are positive for IgG-anti-HBc.

Herpes Virus Infections

- The Epstein-Barr virus (EBV) is the cause of infectious mononucleosis (IM), Burkitt lymphoma, Hodgkin disease, nasopharyngeal and gastric carcinomas, and lymphoproliferative disorders in immunosuppressed people.

- Most patients with IM produce heterophile antibodies, which can react with antigens from bovine, horse, or sheep RBCs. Screening for these antibodies has been done using the "Monospot" test, rapid immunochromatographic or agglutination methods that detect antibodies to bovine or horse erythrocyte antigens.
- ELISA or IFA tests for EBV-specific antibodies are recommended to confirm a diagnosis of IM. They can also be used to diagnose other EBV-associated diseases. Acute IM is indicated by the presence of IgM anti-VCA and anti-EA-D, as well as the absence of anti-EBNA.
- Molecular tests are useful in detecting EBV DNA in immunocompromised patients, who may not develop a good antibody response, and in monitoring viral load in patients with EBV-related malignancies during therapy.
- Cytomegalovirus (CMV) infection is asymptomatic in most healthy people but may cause a mononucleosis-like syndrome, disseminated infection in organ-transplant recipients and patients with HIV/AIDS, and congenital abnormalities in infants born to infected mothers.
- CMV infection is best detected by molecular assays for CMV DNA, CMV antigenemia assays for pp65 antigen, or shell vial culture. Quantitative PCR is useful in determining the CMV DNA copy number in immunocompromised hosts undergoing antiviral treatment. Serological assays for CMV antibody are most helpful in documenting a past infection in potential blood and organ donors.
- Primary infection with varicella virus causes chickenpox (varicella), whereas reactivation of the virus in nerve cells supplying the skin causes shingles (zoster). Diagnosis of current varicella virus infection is usually based on clinical findings, but detection of varicella virus DNA by qPCR may be helpful in some clinical settings. Serological methods, most commonly ELISA and CLIA, are used mainly to document immunity to varicella virus.

Infections With Respiratory Viruses

- Vaccines have greatly reduced the incidence of three childhood infections: rubella, rubeola, and mumps. Rubella infection is the cause of German measles and can result in severe congenital abnormalities if it occurs during pregnancy. Rubeola viruses cause measles, a systemic infection that can cause complications in some people. Mumps virus is the cause of mumps, whose classic feature is swelling of the parotid glands.
- Although the diagnosis of rubella, measles, and mumps is usually based on clinical findings, laboratory testing may be helpful in confirmation. Current infections may be indicated by the presence of IgM antibodies specific for the appropriate virus or by a fourfold rise in virus-specific IgG antibodies in two separate serum samples collected during the acute and convalescent phases of disease. Testing for IgG antibodies is most commonly performed to screen for immunity to these viruses. RT-PCR is useful in detecting viral RNA in patients with inconclusive serological results, in epidemiological studies, and in the detection of congenital rubella infections.
- Three viruses that cause seasonal respiratory infections are influenza A, influenza B, and RSV. Rapid antigen tests and more sensitive molecular tests are used most commonly to detect these infections. Vaccines are available to prevent infections with all three viruses. The vaccines for the influenza viruses need to be modified annually because these viruses mutate frequently by antigenic drift (and less frequently by antigenic shift).
- "Coronavirus Disease 2019," commonly referred to as COVID-19, is caused by a highly communicable and infectious virus, SARS-CoV-2. The virus is transmitted from human to human mainly by close contact and inhalation of infected respiratory droplets. The infection quickly spread throughout China, Europe, and the globe, becoming one of the world's deadliest pandemics.
- SARS-CoV-2 is an enveloped coronavirus that contains spike (S) glycoproteins on its surface, a nucleoprotein (N) within the viral capsid, and the transmembrane (M) protein, which plays a role in viral assembly and formation of the viral envelope.
- Although SARS-CoV-2 can infect a wide range of cells and organs, the lungs are the primary target for infection, and complications from the disease can result in alveolar damage and severe respiratory distress.
- CDC recommendations to prevent transmission of SARS-CoV-2 include vaccination, handwashing, masking, increasing ventilation, social distancing, and isolation of sick individuals.
- There are three types of laboratory tests for SARS-CoV-2: (1) molecular tests for viral nucleic acid to detect current infection, (2) viral antigen tests to detect current infection, or (3) tests for antibody to the virus to identify past infections and assess viral immunity in populations.
- The vaccines used most commonly in the United States are of the mRNA format, developed by the companies Pfizer-BioNTech and Moderna, Inc. The mRNA vaccines code for the spike protein of SARS-CoV-2, which is then made by cells in the recipient and induces an immune response.
- As COVID-19 therapeutics and vaccine technologies continue to develop and become increasingly distributed throughout the world, the infection has transitioned to an endemic phase.

Study Guide: Immune Defenses Against Viruses

IMMUNE DEFENSE	MECHANISM OF ACTION
Innate Defenses	First line of protection against viruses Skin and mucous membranes serve as barriers to prevent viruses from invading the body Type I IFNs inhibit viral replication NK cells bind to virus-infected host cells in a manner that is not antigen-specific and destroy the cells by releasing perforin and granzymes
Humoral Immunity	Antibodies bind to cell-free viruses and prevent them from infecting host cells by neutralizing their ability to bind to host cell receptors Antibodies also play a key role in opsonization, ADCC, and complement-mediated lysis of viruses
Cell-Mediated Immunity	T lymphocytes attack viruses in their intracellular state TH1 T helper cells produce cytokines that induce an anti-viral state and stimulate the development of Tcs Tcs bind specifically to viral antigens complexed with MHC class I on the surface of virus-infected host cells and destroy the cells by releasing perforin and granzymes

ADCC = antibody-dependent cellular cytotoxicity; Tc = cytotoxic T lymphocytes; IFN = interferon; NK = natural killer.

Study Guide: Immune Escape Mechanisms Commonly Used by Viruses

VIRAL ESCAPE MECHANISM	EXAMPLES
Acquisition of genetic mutations that result in new viral antigens	Influenza viruses, rhinoviruses, HIV
Inhibition of immunologic components	HCV blocks actions of IFNs; HSV inhibits C3b
Suppression of the immune system	CMV and HIV reduce expression of class I MHC on the surface of virus-infected cells, reducing their recognition by Tcs HIV destroys infected CD4 TH cells
Establishment of a latent state	CMV, VZV, and HIV integrate their nucleic acid into the host cell genome
Alteration of Immune System Function	EBV stimulates polyclonal B cell activation

CMV = cytomegalovirus; Tcs = cytotoxic T lymphocytes; EBV = Epstein Barr virus; HCV = hepatitis C virus; HIV = human immunodeficiency virus; HSV = herpes simplex viruses; MHC = major histocompatibility complex; VZV = varicella zoster virus.

CASE STUDIES

1. A 25-year-old adult had been experiencing flu-like symptoms, loss of appetite, nausea, and constipation for 2 weeks. The abdomen was tender, and urine was dark in color. Initial testing revealed elevations in serum alanine aminotransferase (ALT) and aspartate aminotransferase (AST) levels.

Questions

a. What laboratory tests should be used to determine if this patient has viral hepatitis?

b. If the patient tested positive for hepatitis B, which tests should be used to monitor the condition?

c. If the patient were to develop chronic hepatitis B, which markers would be present in the serum?

2. A 5-pound infant was born with microcephaly, purpuric rash, low platelet count, cardiovascular defects, and a cataract in the left eye. The infant's mother recalled experiencing flu-like symptoms and a mild skin rash early in her pregnancy. She had not sought medical attention at the time. The infant's physician ordered tests to investigate the cause of the newborn's symptoms.

Questions

a. What virus is the most likely cause of the infant's symptoms?

b. What laboratory tests would you suggest the doctor order for the mother to support your suggested diagnosis?

c. What tests should be performed on the infant's serum to support this diagnosis?

3. An adult presented to the emergency department with shortness of breath and trouble breathing, and noted a new loss of smell. The patient's vital signs revealed hypertension, rapid heart rate, oxygen saturation of 87%, and a temperature of 102.5°F.

Questions

a. Based on this information, what virus is most likely responsible for causing the patient's symptoms?

b. What laboratory tests should be ordered "STAT" to determine the patient's overall medical status?

c. What tests can be used to identify the agent causing the respiratory distress?

REVIEW QUESTIONS

1. The role of T_C cells in immune responses against viruses is to:
   a. Neutralize viral activity
   b. Promote destruction of viruses by ADCC
   c. Destroy virus-infected host cells
   d. Attack free virions

2. Viruses can escape immune defenses by:
   a. Undergoing frequent genetic mutations
   b. Suppressing the immune system
   c. Integrating their nucleic acid into the host genome
   d. All of the above

3. A patient who has developed immunity to a viral infection would be expected to have which of the following serology results?
   a. IgM^+, IgG^-
   b. IgM^-, IgG^+
   c. IgM^+, IgG^+
   d. IgM^-, IgG^-

4. A newborn suspected of having a congenital viral infection should be tested for virus-specific antibodies of which class?
   a. IgM
   b. IgG
   c. IgA
   d. IgE

5. Which of the following hepatitis viruses is transmitted by the fecal-oral route?
   a. Hepatitis B
   b. Hepatitis C
   c. Hepatitis D
   d. Hepatitis E

6. An individual with hepatomegaly, jaundice, and elevated liver enzymes has the following laboratory results: IgM anti-HAV (negative), HBsAg (positive), IgM anti-HBc (positive), and anti-HCV (negative). These findings support a diagnosis of:
   a. Hepatitis A
   b. Acute hepatitis B
   c. Chronic hepatitis B
   d. Hepatitis C

7. The serum of an individual who received all doses of the hepatitis B vaccine should contain:
   a. Anti-HBs
   b. Anti-HBe
   c. Anti-HBc
   d. Anti-HDV

8. Quantitative tests for HCV RNA are used to:
   a. Screen for hepatitis C
   b. Determine the HCV genotype
   c. Differentiate acute HCV infection from chronic HCV infection
   d. Monitor hepatitis C patients on anti-viral therapy

9. In the laboratory, heterophile antibodies can be detected by their reaction with:
   a. B lymphocytes
   b. Bovine erythrocyte antigens
   c. Guinea pig kidney antigens
   d. Epstein-Barr virus antigens

10. The presence of IgM anti-rubella antibodies in the serum from an infant born with a rash suggests:
    a. A diagnosis of measles
    b. A diagnosis of German measles
    c. Congenital infection with the rubella virus
    d. Passive transfer of maternal antibodies to the infant's serum

11. A pregnant woman is exposed to a child with a rubella infection. She had no clinical symptoms but had a rubella titer performed. Her antibody titer was 1:4. Three weeks later, the test was repeated, and her titer was 1:128. She still had no clinical symptoms. Was the laboratory finding indicative of rubella infection?
   a. No, the titer must be greater than 256 to be significant.
   b. No, the change in titer is not significant if no clinical signs are present.
   c. Yes, a greater-than-fourfold rise in titer indicates early infection.
   d. Yes, but clinical symptoms must also correlate with laboratory findings.

12. The cause of shingles is:
   a. Cytomegalovirus
   b. Rubella virus
   c. Varicella-zoster virus
   d. Epstein-Barr virus

13. The method of choice for detecting VZV infection in immunocompromised hosts is:
   a. Serology to detect virus-specific IgM antibodies
   b. Serology to detect virus-specific IgG antibodies
   c. Viral culture
   d. qPCR

14. Which of the following is true regarding laboratory testing for mumps?
   a. RT-PCR is recommended as the primary diagnostic test.
   b. Serology is necessary for confirmation of a suspected clinical case.
   c. IgM tests for mumps are highly specific.
   d. An acute infection must be confirmed by a fourfold rise in IgG titer.

15. The original strain of the COVID-19 virus was:
   a. Alpha
   b. Beta
   c. Delta
   d. Omicron

16. This virus has the ability to reduce the expression of class I MHC molecules on the surface of virus-infected cells, making them less likely to be recognized by T_C lymphocytes:
   a. CMV
   b. VZV
   c. HSV
   d. EBV

17. A classic feature of this viral infection is swelling of the parotid glands.
   a. Rubella
   b. Mumps
   c. Rubeola
   d. Varicella-zoster

18. In order to develop a hepatitis D infection, one must also be infected with:
   a. Hepatitis A
   b. Hepatitis B
   c. Hepatitis C
   d. Hepatitis E

19. The "gold standard" for detecting SARS-CoV-2 is:
   a. EIA
   b. IFA
   c. RT-PCR
   d. Chemiluminescence

20. The appearance of *Koplik spots* on the mucous membranes of the inner cheeks or lips is characteristic of this viral infection:
   a. Rubella
   b. Rubeola
   c. Epstein-Barr
   d. Coronavirus

21. The most sensitive type of laboratory tests to identify and monitor viral infections are:
   a. IgG antibody assays
   b. Rapid antigen assays
   c. Molecular assays
   d. ELISA/EIA assays

22. Which SARS-CoV-2 protein plays a role in viral assembly and formation of the viral envelope?
   a. Nucleoprotein
   b. Spike protein
   c. Transmembrane protein
   d. Vpu protein

23. Which of the following symptoms correlates with "long-term" SARS-CoV-2 effects?
   a. Shortness of breath and difficulty breathing
   b. Cardiac and neurological involvement
   c. Sore throat and digestive issues
   d. Loss of taste and fever

24. mRNA COVID vaccines give host cells instructions to make copies of which viral protein?
    a. Spike protein
    b. Transmembrane protein
    c. Nucleoprotein
    d. Vpu protein

25. Which is the most accurate and sensitive assay for detecting influenza A?
    a. Viral culture
    b. RIDTs
    c. RT-PCR
    d. Serological assays

26. Which commonly used method is the *most* sensitive when testing for RSV?
    a. Viral culture
    b. Rapid antigen detection tests
    c. Serological tests for RSV antibody
    d. RT-PCR

Chapter 23 Answer Key

Answers to Knowledge Checks

23.1 c 23.2 b 23.3 a 23.4 c 23.5 b 23.6 a
23.7 c 23.8 1-f; 2-h; 3-i; 4-b; 5-a; 6-d; 7-c; 8-e; 9-g; 10-j

Answers to Review Questions

1. c 2. d 3. b 4. a 5. d 6. b 7. a
8. d 9. b 10. c 11. c 12. c 13. d 14. a
15. a 16. a 17. b 18. b 19. c 20. b 21. c
22. c 23. b 24. a 25. c 26. d

24 Laboratory Diagnosis of Human Retroviruses

Linda E. Miller, PhD, I, MB^{CM}(ASCP)SI, and
Audrey Grimaldi, DHSc, MS, MLS(ASCP)

LEARNING OUTCOMES

After finishing this chapter, you should be able to:

24.1 Identify hallmark features of the Retroviridae family and pathologically significant virus members.

24.2 Describe the classification system used to identify HIV isolates.

24.3 Explain the conditions under which transmission of HIV can occur.

24.4 Describe the structure of the HIV, including pertinent antigens and the genes that encode them.

24.5 Outline the replication cycle of HIV, beginning with entry of the virus into host cells.

24.6 Describe the host's immune responses to HIV and the effects of HIV on the immune system.

24.7 Describe the clinical manifestations of HIV infection.

24.8 Explain the Centers for Disease Control and Prevention (CDC) classification system for HIV infection.

24.9 Discuss anti-retroviral treatments and the impact they have had on HIV infection.

24.10 Discuss the current CDC-recommended algorithm for screening for HIV infection, and its advantages and limitations as compared with the previous algorithm.

24.11 Discuss the principles and clinical uses of conventional immunoassays and rapid tests for HIV infection.

24.12 Describe the principle of the Western blot test for HIV antibody, interpretation of the results, and limitations of the test.

24.13 Discuss the benefits and limitations of point-of-care testing (POCT) and testing in a nonclinical setting for HIV.

24.14 Discuss reasons for false-positive and false-negative results in HIV antibody testing.

24.15 Explain the principle and clinical utility of flow cytometric methods for CD4 T-cell enumeration.

CHAPTER OUTLINE

You can go to **fadavis.com** keyword stevens for the laboratory exercises that accompany this text.

24.16 Discuss the role of qualitative and quantitative nucleic acid tests in the detection and diagnosis of HIV.

24.17 Describe the molecular techniques performed for HIV viral load testing and drug-resistance testing and their clinical utility.

24.18 Select appropriate methods for HIV testing of infants and children younger than 18 months of age.

24.19 Discuss the characteristics and clinical significance of HTLV 1 and 2, including transmission and effects on the host immune system.

24.20 Describe the diseases associated with HTLV-1 infection.

24.21 Describe the similarities and differences between HTLV and HIV infections.

24.22 Discuss the laboratory methods used to test for HTLV 1 and 2.

The retrovirus family Retroviridae is composed of a large diverse group of RNA viruses that primarily infect vertebrates. Retroviruses are prevalent throughout nature and found in a wide array of vertebrate hosts. This family of viruses has a highly unique replication cycle in which their genetic information, contained in the form of RNA, is reverse transcribed into DNA upon entry into the host cell. Retroviruses contain an RNA-dependent DNA polymerase called **reverse transcriptase,** that guides synthesis of their RNA into viral DNA. This newly formed viral DNA is integrated into the host chromosomal DNA, leading to the formation of a provirus, which serves as the template for progeny virions. The reverse transcription of viral RNA into DNA is the defining hallmark feature of retroviruses.

The Retroviridae family consists of seven genera and over 60 different species. Many are surprisingly benign. However, they can also be associated with a variety of diseases including malignancies, immunodeficiencies, lower motor neuron disease, and acute tissue damage. In this chapter, we discuss four clinically significant members of the Retroviridae family:

- Human immunodeficiency virus type 1 (HIV-1); *Lentivirus* genus **(Fig. 24–1)**
- Human immunodeficiency virus type 2 (HIV-2); *Lentivirus* genus
- Human T-lymphotropic virus type 1 (HTLV-1) type 1; *Deltaretrovirus* genus **(Fig. 24–1)**
- Human T-lymphotropic virus type 2 (HTLV-2), *Deltaretrovirus* genus

Human Immunodeficiency Virus (HIV)

Human immunodeficiency virus (HIV) is the etiologic agent of the **Acquired Immunodeficiency Syndrome**, or **AIDS**, a disease that has posed one of the greatest medical challenges worldwide. According to the World Health Organization (WHO), at the end of 2023, about 39.9 million people were living with HIV infection, 630,000 people died from HIV-related causes, and 1.3 million people became newly infected. Since its discovery, the virus has claimed the lives of more than 40 million people worldwide. Although most infected persons reside in developing countries, HIV infection has also created a significant problem in developed nations. For example, in the United States, there were over 1.1 million cases of diagnosed HIV infection at the end of 2023 (the most recent year for which these data were available). No cure exists for HIV infection. However, with prevention measures, diagnosis, and treatment, HIV has become a manageable chronic health condition. Of the people worldwide who know they have HIV, 76% have received retroviral therapy, and 72% have suppressed viral loads.

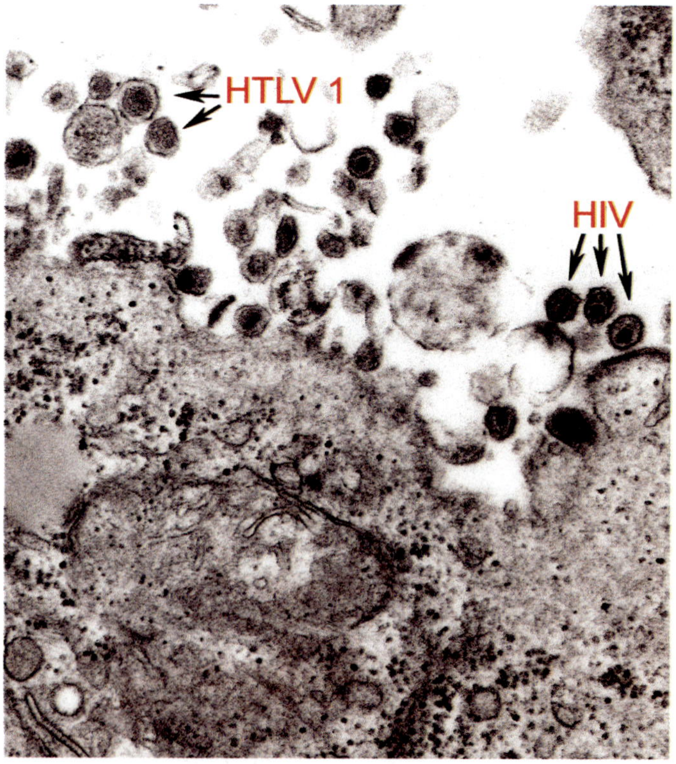

FIGURE 24–1. Transmission electron microscopic image showing HIV and HTLV-1 being produced within the same human lymphocyte from a primary culture. *(Courtesy of the Centers for Disease Control and Prevention/Cynthia Goldsmith, https://phil.cdc.gov/Details.aspx?pid=8241.)*

The virus responsible for causing AIDS, HIV-1, was identified independently by the laboratories of Drs. Luc Montagnier of France and Robert Gallo and Jay Levy of the United States in 1983 and 1984, respectively. Isolates of HIV-1 have been classified into four groups: group M (the main or major group), group O (the outlier group), and two more recently named groups, N and P. Group M viruses are responsible for most HIV-1 infections worldwide. Group M contains nine subtypes or clades, designated A, B, C, D, F, G, H, J, and K. Subtype C is the predominant subtype worldwide, whereas subtype B is the most prevalent subtype in the United States, Europe, and Australia. Groups N, O, and P occur much less frequently and are largely confined to West Africa. Many circulating recombinant forms (CRFs) exist, which are produced because of genetic recombination between two subtypes that have infected a single individual.

A related but genetically distinct virus, HIV-2, was discovered in 1986. Most HIV-2 infections have occurred in West Africa, although the virus has also been identified in patients in other parts of the world. HIV-2 is transmitted in the same manner as HIV-1 and may also cause AIDS, but it is less pathogenic and has a lower rate of transmission. Although this chapter discusses the differences between the two viruses, our focus is on HIV-1 because it is much more prevalent globally. We use the term *HIV* to refer to HIV-1, and HIV-2 is so named.

Accurate diagnosis is essential for early intervention and halting HIV spread. In this chapter, we discuss characteristics of the virus, immunologic and clinical manifestations of the disease, treatment and prevention, and laboratory techniques used to diagnose and monitor HIV infection.

HIV Transmission

Transmission of HIV occurs through one of three major routes: intimate sexual contact, contact with blood or other body fluids, or perinatally (from infected mother to fetus or infant). Most HIV cases have occurred through sexual transmission involving either vaginal or anal intercourse. Worldwide, about 85% of cases of HIV infection can be attributed to heterosexual contact, whereas in the United States, the largest number of cases has resulted from male-to-male sexual contact. The presence of other sexually transmitted diseases, such as syphilis, gonorrhea, or genital herpes, increases the likelihood of transmission by disrupting protective mucous membranes and activating immunologic cells in the genital areas.

The second route of transmission is through parenteral exposure to infected blood or body fluids, which occurs mainly through the sharing of contaminated needles by people who use IV drugs. Less frequently, transmission has occurred through blood transfusions, the use of clotting factors by hemophiliacs, occupational injuries with needlesticks or other sharp objects, or mucous-membrane contact in health care workers exposed to infectious fluids. The virus has also been acquired by transplantation of infected tissue. The incidence of infection in recipients of blood transfusions, clotting factors, and organ transplants is rare in the United States because blood and organ donors are screened for HIV.

Studies by the Centers for Disease Control and Prevention (CDC) have estimated the average risk of transmission to health care workers to be approximately 0.3% after a percutaneous exposure to HIV-infected blood and about 0.09% after a mucous-membrane exposure. Body fluids considered to be potentially infectious include blood, semen, vaginal secretions, cerebral spinal fluid, synovial fluid, pleural fluid, peritoneal fluid, pericardial fluid, amniotic fluid, saliva from dental procedures, other fluids containing visible blood, and any body fluid that cannot be differentiated from another. The transmission risk is increased in exposures involving a large quantity of blood, hollow-bore needles placed directly into an artery or vein, or deep tissue injury. The risk of infection is also increased if the source patient is in the acute or advanced stages of HIV infection, when the amount of virus circulating in the bloodstream is high.

The third route of transmission is perinatal. Transmission can occur across the placenta during pregnancy, by transfer of blood at the time of delivery, or through breastfeeding. Perinatal transmission has been markedly reduced by prenatal HIV screening, administration of anti-retroviral drugs to HIV-positive pregnant women and their newborn babies, and the use of infant formula by mothers who are infected with the virus. The WHO states that these measures have decreased the rate of perinatal transmission to less than 5%, as compared with rates of 15% to 45% in untreated mothers.

Knowledge Check 24-1

HIV transmission predominately occurs through which route?

a. Perinatal transmission
b. Parenteral exposure
c. Intimate sexual contact
d. Respiratory droplet inhalation

Characteristics of HIV

Composition of the Virus

HIV belongs to the genus *Lentivirinae* of the virus family Retroviridae. It is classified as a retrovirus because it contains ribonucleic acid (RNA) as its nucleic acid and reverse transcriptase, which transcribes the viral RNA into DNA, a necessary step in the virus's life cycle. HIV is a spherical particle, 100 to 120 nm in diameter, which contains an inner core with two copies of single-stranded RNA surrounded by a capsid (protein coat) and an outer envelope of glycoproteins embedded in a lipid bilayer. The glycoproteins are knob-like structures involved in binding the virus to host cells during the infection. **Figure 24–2** shows the structure of the HIV virion.

Structural Genes

The HIV genome includes three main structural genes—*gag*, *env*, and *pol*—and several regulatory genes. **Figure 24–3** shows the relative locations of the major HIV genes and indicates their gene products. The *gag* gene codes for p55, a precursor protein with a molecular weight of 55 kd, from which four

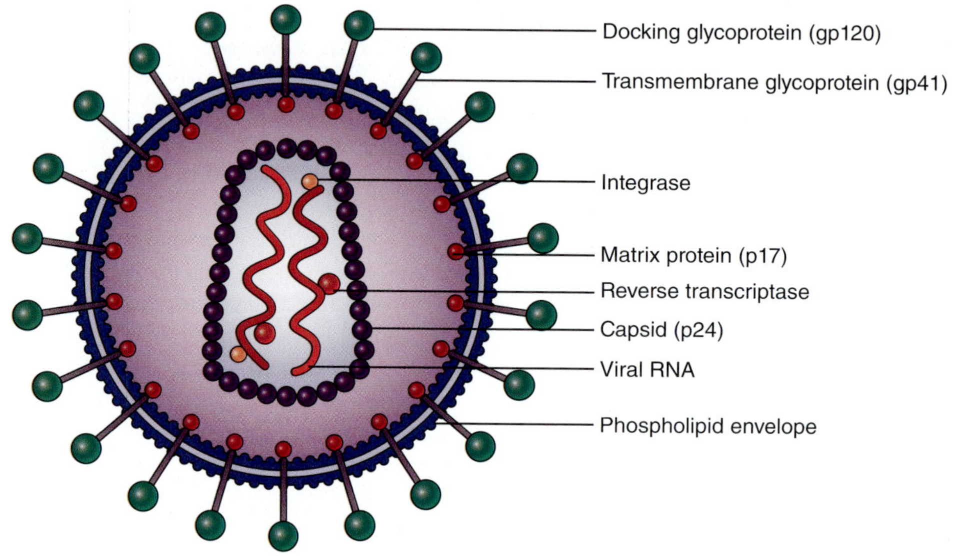

FIGURE 24–2 Structure of HIV virion, showing some of the major components. p = protein; gp = glycoprotein; the numbers refer to the molecular weights of the proteins in kilodaltons.

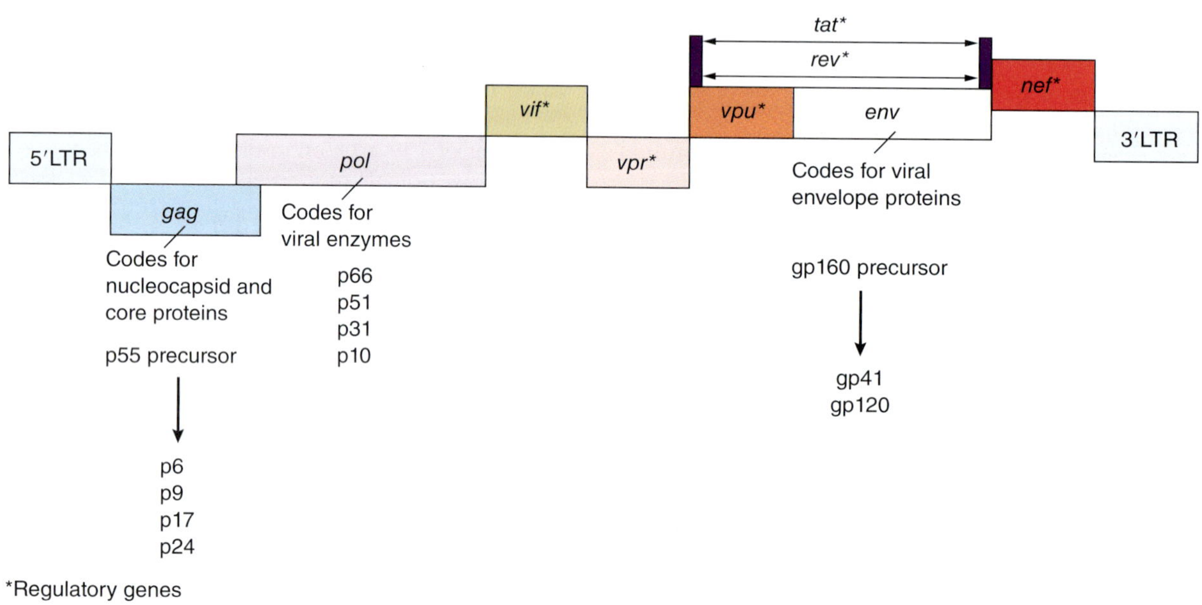

FIGURE 24–3 The HIV-1 genome. The relative locations of the major genes in the HIV-1 genome are indicated, as well as their gene products. * = regulatory genes.

core structural proteins are formed: p6, p9, p17, and p24. All four are located in the nucleocapsid of the virus. The capsid that surrounds the internal nucleic acids contains p24, p6, and p9, whereas p17 lies in a layer between the protein core and the envelope, called the *matrix,* and is actually embedded in the internal portion of the envelope.

The *env* gene codes for the glycoproteins gp160, gp120, and gp41, which are found in the viral envelope. Gp160 is a precursor protein that is cleaved to form gp120 and gp41. Gp120 forms the numerous knobs or spikes that protrude from the outer envelope, whereas gp41 is a transmembrane glycoprotein that spans the inner and outer membrane and attaches to gp120. Both gp120 and gp41 are involved in fusion and attachment of HIV to receptors on host cells.

The third structural gene, *pol,* codes for enzymes necessary for HIV replication. These include reverse transcriptase (p51); ribonuclease (Rnase H; p66), an enzyme involved in the degradation of the original HIV RNA; integrase (p31), an enzyme that mediates the integration of viral DNA into the genome of infected host cells; and a protease (p10) that cleaves precursor proteins into smaller active units used to make the mature virions. These proteins are located in the core of the virus in association with HIV RNA.

Several other genes in the HIV genome code for products that have regulatory or accessory functions. These genes include *tat* (transactivator), *rev* (regulator of expression of virion proteins), *nef* (negative effector), *vpu* (viral protein "U"), *vpr* (viral protein "R"), and *vif* (viral infectivity factor).

Although the products of these genes are not an integral part of the viral structure, they serve important functions in controlling viral replication and infectivity. The HIV gene sequence is surrounded by 5′ and 3′ long terminal repeat (LTR) regions, which also play a role in regulating expression of the genes. **Table 24–1** summarizes the major HIV-1 genes, their products, and their functions.

HIV-2 has *gag, env, pol,* and regulatory or accessory genes with similar functions to those seen in HIV-1. The homology between the genomes of the two viruses is about 50%. The *gag* and *pol* regions are most similar, whereas the *env* region differs greatly. Thus, the viruses can most easily be distinguished based on antigenic differences in their *env* proteins.

Viral Replication

In this section, we review the process by which HIV replicates **(Fig. 24–4)**.

Attachment of HIV to Host Cells. The first step in the HIV reproductive cycle occurs when the virus attaches to a susceptible host cell. This interaction is mediated through the host-cell CD4 antigen, which serves as a receptor for the virus by binding the gp120 glycoprotein on the outer envelope of HIV. Helper T (T_H) cells are the main target for HIV infection because they express high numbers of CD4 molecules on their surface and bind the virus with high affinity. Other cells, such as macrophages, monocytes, dendritic cells, Langerhans cells, and microglial brain cells, can also be infected with HIV because they have some surface CD4. HIV viruses that preferentially infect T cells are known as *T-tropic* or *X4* strains, whereas those strains that can infect both macrophages and T cells are called *M-tropic* or *R5* strains.

Coreceptor Binding and Fusion to Host-Cell Membranes. Entry of HIV into the host cells to which it has attached requires an additional binding step, involving coreceptors that promote fusion of the HIV envelope with the plasma-cell membrane. These coreceptors belong to a family of proteins known as *chemokine receptors,* whose main function is to direct white blood cells (WBCs) to sites of inflammation. The chemokine receptor CXCR4 is required for HIV to enter T lymphocytes, whereas the chemokine receptor CCR5 is required for entry into macrophages. In fact, people with a genetic mutation in the *CCR5* gene have been found to be resistant to HIV infection. Binding of the coreceptors allows for HIV entry by inducing a conformational change in the gp41 glycoprotein, which mediates fusion of the virus to the cell membrane.

Uncoating and Reverse Transcription. After fusion, the viral particle is taken into the cell, and uncoating of the particle exposes the viral genome. Action of the enzyme reverse transcriptase produces complementary DNA from the viral RNA. Double-stranded DNA is synthesized and, with the help of the HIV integrase enzyme, becomes integrated into the host cell's genome as a provirus. The provirus can remain in a latent state for a long time, during which viral replication does not occur.

Viral Gene Expression and Assembly of Intact Virions. Eventually, expression of the viral genes is induced when the infected host cell is activated by binding to an antigen or by exposure to cytokines. Viral DNA within the cell nucleus is then transcribed into genomic RNA and messenger RNA (mRNA), which are transported to the cytoplasm. Translation of mRNA occurs, with production of viral precursor proteins and assembly of viral particles. The intact virions bud out from

Table 24-1 Major HIV Genes and Their Products

GENE	PROTEIN PRODUCT	FUNCTION
gag	p17	Inner surface of envelope
	p24	Core coat for nucleic acids
	p9	Core-binding protein
	p6	Binds to genomic RNA
env	gp120	Binds to CD4 on T cell
	gp41	Transmembrane protein associated with gp120
pol	p66	Subunit of reverse transcriptase; degrades original HIV RNA
	p51	Subunit of reverse transcriptase
	p31	Integrase; mediates integration of HIV DNA into host genome
	p10	Protease that cleaves *gag* precursor
tat	p14	Activates transcription of HIV provirus
rev	p19	Transports viral mRNA to the cytoplasm of the host cell
nef	p27	Enhances HIV replication
vpu	p16	Viral assembly and budding
vpr	p15	Integration of HIV DNA into host genome
vif	p23	Infectivity factor

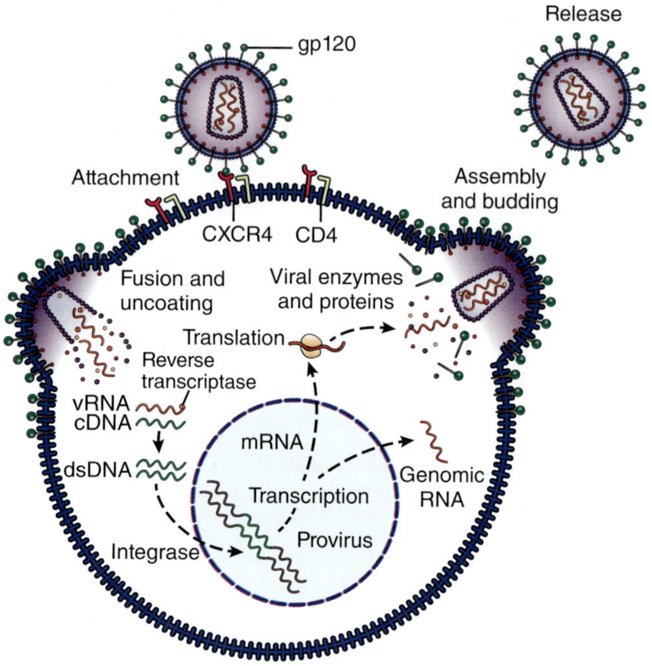

FIGURE 24–4 Replication cycle of HIV in a CD4+ T cell.

the host-cell membrane and acquire their envelope during the process. The precursor proteins are cleaved by the viral protease enzyme in the mature virus particles. These viruses can proceed to infect additional host cells. Viral replication occurs to the greatest extent in antigen-activated T_H cells.

Because viral replication occurs very rapidly and the reverse transcriptase enzyme lacks proofreading activity, genetic mutations occur at a high rate, producing distinct isolates that exhibit an extraordinary level of antigenic variation. In fact, the level of HIV diversity in a single individual can be greater than the diversity of all the influenza virus isolates throughout the world in a given year. HIV's tremendous genetic diversity hinders the host's ability to mount an effective immune response. Likewise, the high error rate of HIV reverse transcriptase and the high turnover rate of the viral population contribute to significant genetic variation of HIV-1. These properties provide opportunities for the emergence of drug-resistant strains.

Knowledge Check 24-2

Which HIV viral protein binds to CD4 on T_H cells enabling attachment between the host cell and virion?

a. gp41
b. p9
c. p24
d. gp120

Immunologic Manifestations of HIV Infection

Immune Responses to HIV

When HIV infects a healthy person, an initial burst of viral replication followed by a slowing down of virus production typically occurs as the host's immune response develops and keeps the virus in check. The initial viral replication can be detected in the laboratory by increased levels of **p24 antigen** and viral RNA in the host's bloodstream (see "Laboratory Testing for HIV Infection" section). As the virus replicates, some of the viral proteins produced within host cells form complexes with class I major histocompatibility complex (MHC) antigens and are transported to the cell surface, where they stimulate lymphocyte responses. HIV-specific CD4+ T_H cells are generated and assist humoral and cell-mediated immune responses against the virus. However, the interactions between HIV and the immune system are complex, and these responses are unable to eliminate HIV from the body.

Antibody Production. B lymphocytes are stimulated to produce antibodies to HIV, which can usually be detected in the host's serum by 6 weeks after primary infection. The first antibodies to be detected are directed against the gp41 transmembrane glycoprotein, followed by production of antibodies to the *gag* proteins such as p24, and, finally, production of antibodies to the *env, pol,* and regulatory proteins. The most immunogenic proteins are in the viral envelope and elicit the production of neutralizing antibodies. These antibodies usually appear 2 to 3 months after infection and prevent the virus from infecting neighboring cells. Antibodies to the envelope proteins have also been shown to bind to Fc receptors on natural killer (NK) cells and participate in antibody-dependent cellular cytotoxicity (ADCC)-mediated killing of HIV-infected cells. However, these antibodies may also participate in the pathogenesis of HIV infection by facilitating Fc-receptor–mediated endocytosis of opsonized virus by uninfected cells. Furthermore, dense glycosylation of the *env* proteins can mask important epitopes, and the enormous diversity of the virus poses challenges to the host in producing a protective antibody response.

Cell-Mediated Immunity. T-cell–mediated immunity is thought to play an important role in the immune response to HIV, as it does in other viral infections. CD8+ cytotoxic T (T_C) lymphocytes, also known as *cytolytic T cells* (CTLs), appear within weeks of HIV infection and are associated with a decline in the amount of HIV in the blood during acute infection. CTLs attack HIV-infected host cells by binding to HIV proteins associated with class I MHC molecules on the surface of infected cells. HIV-specific CTLs are stimulated to develop into mature, activated clones through the effects of cytokines released by activated CD4+ T_H cells, a process common to immune responses against other viruses (see Chapter 5 for details). After the CTLs bind to HIV-infected host cells, cytolytic enzymes are released from their granules and destroy the target cells. Free virions are released from the damaged cells and can be bound by antibodies. CTLs can also suppress replication and spreading of HIV by producing cytokines such as interferon (IFN)-γ, which have anti-viral activity.

Innate Defenses. Innate immune defenses may play a role in responding to HIV in the early stages of the infection. In particular, NK cells become activated during acute HIV infection and can mediate cytolysis of host cells infected with the virus. Dendritic cells recognize viral components through pattern-recognition receptors, resulting in the release of pro-inflammatory cytokines that have anti-viral effects and can activate other cells of the immune system.

Critical Thinking 24-1

Untreated HIV infection eventually leads to a progressive decline in the host's immune system. However, this immunodeficient state does not occur immediately. After initial infection, the host immune system can respond to infection and suppress viral levels. What factors contribute to this viral latency? How do humoral and cell-mediated immunity play a role in HIV viral suppression?

Effects of HIV Infection on the Immune System

Although the host's humoral and cell-mediated immune responses usually reduce the level of HIV replication, they are generally insufficient to completely eliminate the virus. This occurs because HIV has developed several mechanisms by which it can escape immune responses, notably:

- CTL and antibody responses to HIV are hindered by the virus's ability to undergo rapid genetic mutations, generating escape mutants with altered antigens toward which the host's initial immune responses are ineffective.
- HIV can downregulate the production of class I MHC molecules on the surface of the host cells it infects, protecting them from CTL recognition.
- Numerous body cells can also harbor HIV as a silent provirus for long periods, including resting $CD4^+$ T cells, dendritic cells, cells of the monocyte and macrophage lineage, and microglial cells in the brain. This proviral state protects HIV from attack by the immune system until cell activation stimulates the virus to multiply and display its viral antigens.

HIV's ability to evade the immune response results in a persistent infection that can destroy the immune system. Because the virus's prime targets are the CD4 T_H cells, these cells are most severely affected, and a decrease in this cell population is the hallmark feature of HIV infection. The gut-associated lymphoid tissue (GALT), the body's largest immune organ, is the most profoundly affected. Early in the infection, HIV causes a rapid depletion of $CCR5^+$ $CD4^+$ memory T cells in the GALT. T_H17 cells, which play an important role in the homeostasis of the epithelial cells lining the intestinal mucosa (enterocytes) and in the secretion of antimicrobial defensins, are also preferentially affected. As a result, the intestinal barrier is damaged, with leakage of microbial products such as lipopolysaccharide (LPS) into the plasma and a general state of immune activation.

HIV kills or renders CD4 T_H cells nonfunctional through various mechanisms, including loss of plasma-membrane integrity because of viral budding, destruction by HIV-specific CTL, and viral induction of apoptosis. Infected T cells turn over much more rapidly than they can be replaced, resulting in a progressive decrease in CD4 T cells during the natural course of untreated infections. In addition to reducing T-cell numbers, HIV causes abnormalities in T_H-cell function and impairs memory T_H-cell responses.

Because **CD4 T cells** play a central role in the immune system by regulating the activities of B and T lymphocytes (see Chapter 5), their destruction results in decreased effectiveness of both antibody- and cell-mediated immune responses. These effects not only apply to the immune responses directed against HIV but also to the broad range of antigens the host encounters. Dysregulated immune responses are also evident. HIV proteins actually stimulate polyclonal activation of B cells, resulting in maturational and functional defects with increased circulating immunoglobulin levels, immune complexes, and autoantibodies. However, B cells in people with HIV have a reduced ability to mount effective antibody responses after exposure to specific antigens, caused by the decrease in T-cell help.

The reduced T_H activity also affects cell-mediated immunity, resulting in a decline in CTL activity and delayed-type hypersensitivity responses to specific antigens. Altered production of cytokines and chemokines has also been seen, including increases in the levels of some cytokines during the early stages of disease, followed by declining levels of interleukin-2 (IL-2) and IFN-γ and a shift in the cytokine profile from T_H1 to T_H2 as the infection progresses toward development of AIDS. Extensive damage to the lymphoid tissues is evident late in the infection, with loss of germinal centers and follicular dendritic cells, resulting in an inability to activate T and B lymphocytes. Other immunologic abnormalities, including defective antigen presentation and oxidative burst by monocytes and macrophages and decreased NK-cell activity, have also been observed in patients with AIDS.

Clinical Symptoms of HIV Infection

HIV causes a chronic infection characterized by a progressive decline in the immune system. Although the disease manifestations vary by individual, the infection progresses through a clinical course that begins with primary, or acute, infection, followed by a period of clinical latency that eventually culminates in AIDS.

Acute (Primary) Stage

The acute, or early, stage of infection is characterized by a rapid burst of viral replication before the development of HIV-specific immune responses. The blood of infected individuals contains high levels of circulating virus, or **viremia**; therefore, HIV begins to disseminate to the lymphoid organs. There is a reduction in the peripheral blood CD4 T-cell count, but this usually returns to slightly decreased or, sometimes, normal levels. As the immune system becomes activated, an acute retroviral syndrome may develop. This syndrome, noted in 50% to 70% of patients with primary HIV infection, is characterized by flu-like or infectious-mononucleosis–like symptoms. Symptoms of the primary stage usually appear 3 to 6 weeks after the initial infection and resolve within 7 days to a few weeks. Many people, however, are asymptomatic during this stage.

Chronic Stage (Clinical Latency)

As HIV-specific immune responses develop, they begin to curtail viral replication, and patients enter a period of clinical latency. This stage is characterized by a decrease in viremia as the circulation clears the virus, and clinical symptoms are subtle or absent. However, studies have demonstrated that the virus is still present in the plasma, albeit at lower levels, and more so in the lymphoid tissues. The CD4 T-cell count remains stable for a variable period and then begins to progressively decline. A small proportion of people infected with HIV, termed *elite controllers,* have normal or mildly depressed CD4 T-cell counts and low viral loads and remain asymptomatic for many years in the absence of anti-retroviral therapy. Certain genetic factors, including HLA-B57-01 and HLA-B27-05, are thought to play a role in the ability of these individuals to mount vigorous immune responses that more effectively control replication of the virus.

AIDS

Untreated individuals will ultimately progress to AIDS, the final stage of HIV infection, characterized by profound immunosuppression with very low numbers of CD4 T cells, a resurgence of viremia, and life-threatening infections and malignancies. The rate at which people progress to the development of AIDS varies, but progression typically occurs in untreated individuals within a median time of 10 years after the initial infection. The progression rate has dramatically decreased with the use of anti-retroviral therapies (see "Treatment and Prevention" section).

The Clinical Correlations box lists the **opportunistic illnesses** considered to be indicative of AIDS. These conditions appear in immunocompromised individuals but do not usually affect people with a healthy immune system. In addition to infections and malignancies, individuals infected with HIV often demonstrate neurological symptoms resulting from the ability of the virus to infect brain cells. In early HIV infection, these symptoms may manifest as forgetfulness, poor concentration, apathy, psychomotor retardation, and withdrawal, whereas progression to late disease may result in confusion, disorientation, seizures, dementia, gait disturbances, ataxia, or paraparesis (partial lower limb paralysis).

Symptoms of AIDS in infants include failure to thrive, persistent oral candidiasis, hepatosplenomegaly, lymphadenopathy, recurrent diarrhea, or recurrent bacterial infections. Abnormal neurological findings may be present. The rate by which HIV infection progresses in children varies and may be influenced by factors such as the maturity of the immune system at the time of infection, the dose of virus to which the child was exposed, and the route of infection.

The CDC first defined AIDS as "a disease, at least moderately predictive of a defect in cell-mediated immunity, occurring in a person with no known cause for diminished resistance to that disease" (CDC, 1982). The definition has been revised several times over the years as more information has been acquired about HIV and additional laboratory tests for HIV have been developed. The CDC also published a separate case definition for HIV infection in children. The latest definition, published in 2014, contains the current guidelines at the time of this writing. It combines the case definitions for persons of all ages into a single definition that is intended to be used for surveillance of the disease. The 2014 definition bases a confirmed case of HIV infection on either laboratory criteria or clinical evidence, with laboratory results being the preferred criteria. Laboratory criteria consist of positive test results in multitest algorithms for HIV antibody or combination HIV antigen/antibody, whereas clinical evidence refers to physician documentation of HIV infection in the patient's medical record (see "Laboratory Testing for HIV Infection" section).

Clinical Correlations

Opportunistic Illnesses Indicative of AIDS (Stage 3 HIV Infection)

Bacterial infections, multiple or recurrent*
- Candidiasis of bronchi, trachea, or lungs
- Candidiasis of esophagus
- Cervical cancer, invasive†
- Coccidioidomycosis, disseminated or extrapulmonary
- Cryptococcosis, extrapulmonary
- Cryptosporidiosis, chronic intestinal (longer than 1 month's duration)
- Cytomegalovirus disease (other than liver, spleen, or nodes), onset older than 1 month of age
- Cytomegalovirus retinitis (with loss of vision)
- Encephalopathy attributed to HIV
- Herpes simplex: chronic ulcers (longer than 1 month's duration) or bronchitis, pneumonitis, or esophagitis (onset older than 1 month of age)
- Histoplasmosis, disseminated or extrapulmonary
- Isosporiasis, chronic intestinal (longer than 1 month's duration)
- Kaposi sarcoma
- Lymphoma, Burkitt (or equivalent term)
- Lymphoma, immunoblastic (or equivalent term)
- Lymphoma, primary, of brain
- *Mycobacterium avium* complex or *Mycobacterium kansasii,* disseminated or extrapulmonary
- Mycobacterium, other species or unidentified species, disseminated or extrapulmonary
- *Mycobacterium tuberculosis* of any site, pulmonary†, disseminated, or extrapulmonary
- *Pneumocystis jirovecii* (previously known as *Pneumocystis carinii*) pneumonia
- Pneumonia, recurrent†
- Progressive multifocal leukoencephalopathy
- *Salmonella* septicemia, recurrent
- Toxoplasmosis of brain, onset older than 1 month of age
- Wasting syndrome attributed to HIV

*Only among children aged younger than 6 years.

†Only among adults, adolescents, and children aged 6 years or older.

Courtesy of Centers for Disease Control and Prevention. Revised surveillance case definition for HIV infection—United States, 2014. *MMWR* 2014;63(3):1–10.

Patients who are HIV-positive are further classified into one of five stages (0, 1, 2, 3, or unknown). The stage can change for an individual patient in either direction over time. Stage 0 includes those individuals with early HIV infection who had an initial confirmed HIV-positive laboratory result followed by a negative or indeterminate HIV test result within a 6-month period. These patients can be reclassified in one of the other categories 180 days or more after initial diagnosis. Patients are classified as being in stages 1, 2, or 3 based on their peripheral blood CD4 T-cell count or percentage; if this information is missing, they are classified in the "unknown" category. The CD4 T-cell parameters used in this classification system are shown in **Table 24–2.** Stage 3 is also indicated if any of the opportunistic illnesses listed in the Clinical Correlations box are present.

Treatment and Prevention of HIV Infection

Treatment

Treatment of HIV infection involves supportive care of the associated infections and malignancies and administration of **anti-retroviral therapy (ART)** to suppress the virus's replication. Several classes of anti-retroviral drugs have been developed to treat HIV infection **(Table 24–3).** These drugs block various steps of the HIV replication cycle. Pharmacokinetic (PK) enhancers, also known as boosters, may be incorporated into the ART regimen; they do not directly target HIV but instead reduce the function of the enzyme, cytochrome P4503A4 (CYP3A4), which helps break down certain drugs. Using a PK inhibitor hinders CYP3A4's function, enabling anti-retroviral drugs to remain active in the body longer.

Table 24-2 CD4 T-Cell Parameters Used in HIV Staging

AGE ON DATE OF $CD4^+$ T-LYMPHOCYTE TEST						
	YOUNGER THAN 1 YEAR		1 TO 5 YEARS		6 YEARS OR OLDER	
STAGE	CELLS/µL	PERCENTAGE OF LYMPHOCYTES	CELLS/µL	PERCENTAGE OF LYMPHOCYTES	CELLS/µL	PERCENTAGE OF LYMPHOCYTES
1	1,500	≥34	≥1,000	≥30	≥500	≥26
2	750–1,499	26–33	500–999	22–29	200–499	14–25
3	<750	<26	<500	<22	<200	<14

The stage is based primarily on the $CD4^+$ T-lymphocyte count; the percentage is considered only if the count is missing.
Adapted from Centers for Disease Control and Prevention. Revised surveillance case definition for HIV infection—United States, 2014. MMWR *2014;63(3):1–10.*

Table 24-3 Anti-Retroviral Drugs for HIV Therapy

ANTI-RETROVIRAL DRUG CLASSIFICATION	MECHANISM OF ACTION	EXAMPLES
Nucleoside analogue reverse-transcriptase inhibitors (NRTIs)	Similar in structure to nucleosides; incorporate into HIV nucleic acid and block synthesis of viral RNA	Zidovudine, lamivudine, emtricitabine, abacavir, tenofovir
Nonnucleoside reverse transcriptase inhibitors (NNRTIs)	Bind to and inactivate reverse transcriptase	Nevirapine, doravirine, efavirenz, etravirine
Protease inhibitors (PIs)	Prevent cleavage of precursor proteins needed for assembly of HIV virions	Saquinavir, ritonavir, fosamprenavir
Integrase strand transfer inhibitors (INSTIs)	Prevent integration of HIV DNA into the host genome	Raltegravir, dolutegravir, elvitegravir
Fusion inhibitors	Block viral infection by preventing fusion of HIV with target cells	Enfuvirtide
CCR5 antagonists	Block binding of HIV to the chemokine coreceptor CCR5	Maraviroc
Postattachment inhibitors	Block binding of HIV to the CD4 surface receptor	Ibalizumab
Pharmacokinetic (PK) enhancers (or boosters)	Improve pharmacokinetic profiles of PIs and the INSTI, elvitegravir	Cobicistat

Table 24–3 summarizes the mechanisms of action of various anti-retroviral drugs. New drugs continue to be developed as advances in this area are made. Updated guidelines on the use of these drugs are available from the U.S. Department of Health and Human Services (HHS) and the WHO.

Studies have shown that treatment with multiple drugs is more effective in killing the virus and preventing viral resistance than treatment with a single drug. Therefore, potent regimens involving a combination of drugs from different anti-retroviral drug classes are the standard of treatment. The preferred initial ART regimen for a person with HIV typically includes two nucleoside analogue reverse transcriptase inhibitors (NRTIs) in combination with a third drug (an integrase strand transfer inhibitor [INSTI], nucleoside analogue reverse transcriptase inhibitor [NNRTI], or protease inhibitor [PI]), and a PK enhancer. Variations in treatment may be administered in certain situations, for example, HIV-2 infection, pediatric HIV infections, and presence of opportunistic infections.

The goal of therapy is to reduce the patient's HIV viral load to a level that is below the detectable limit of quantitative plasma viral load assays (see "Quantitative Viral Load Assays" section). This is most likely to be achieved if treatment is started early in the course of infection, and the patient can adhere to the treatment as prescribed.

ART has had a dramatic effect on the clinical course of HIV infection, as evidenced by a significant decline in the incidence of opportunistic infections, a delay in progression to AIDS, and decreased mortality in patients who have received these multidrug treatments. Before ART, the median survival time of patients with AIDS was only 26 weeks from the time of diagnosis; today, patients infected with HIV who are treated appropriately with ART can be expected to live 50 years or longer. Because of this success, ART is recommended for all people with HIV at the time of diagnosis. In addition, anti-retroviral drugs given to pregnant individuals and newborns have significantly reduced perinatal transmission of HIV, as we discussed previously. ART and avoiding breastfeeding have reduced the rate of perinatal transmission to less than 1% in developed countries of the world.

Although anti-retroviral drugs have significantly improved morbidity and mortality in people infected with HIV, they are not a cure for AIDS. This is because viral blood levels are greatly reduced in patients treated with ART, but lymphoid organs throughout their body still harbor HIV, which progressively destroys the immune system. Research is ongoing to develop additional drugs to target HIV that remains latent within infected cells.

Prevention

Several approaches for preventing initial HIV infection exist. Community-based education aimed at high-risk groups such as gay men and those who use IV drugs has provided beneficial information on reducing transmission of the virus. The CDC has published guidelines for the use of anti-retroviral drugs for pre-exposure prophylaxis (PrEP) to prevent transmission to people who are HIV-negative but at a high risk of contracting the infection, such as those who inject illicit drugs or are sexually active with partner who is infected. In addition, the CDC and the Occupational Safety and Health Administration (OSHA) have published precautions to prevent the transmission of HIV and other bloodborne pathogens in health care workers (see Chapter 8). Prophylactic therapy with anti-retroviral drugs is also offered to health care workers who may have been exposed to HIV through percutaneous or mucous-membrane contact with potentially infected blood or body fluids, in hope that early treatment will prevent infection. Because of these measures, fewer than 60 confirmed cases of occupational HIV transmission to health care workers have been recorded by the CDC.

The ultimate means of preventing HIV infection would be the development of an effective vaccine. Despite extensive research, this task has been difficult for many reasons. For example, HIV can rapidly mutate and escape immune recognition, and there is no ideal animal model in which to study vaccine effects. An effective vaccine would also need to induce mucosal immunity because HIV is usually transmitted through mucosal surfaces. It should also stimulate potent CTL and broad neutralizing antibody responses that could detect many variants of the virus. If a vaccine that can prevent HIV infection in the traditional sense cannot be developed, it is possible that a therapeutic vaccine given to already-diagnosed individuals may provide some benefits by stimulating a more effective immune response and lowering the level of viremia, thus reducing the risk of transmission to others.

Knowledge Check 24-3

Which type of anti-retroviral drug binds to and inactivates reverse transcriptase?

a. Nonnucleoside reverse transcriptase inhibitors (NNRTIs)
b. Nucleoside analogue reverse transcriptase inhibitors (NRTIs)
c. Protease inhibitors (PIs)
d. Integrase strand transfer inhibitors (INSTIs)

Laboratory Testing for HIV Infection

The laboratory plays a key role in establishing the initial diagnosis of HIV infection and in monitoring known patients for their response to ART. Also, recommendations published by the U.S. Preventative Task Force and the CDC for HIV screening, especially for those at high risk for HIV infection, have increased the number of infected individuals who are aware of their status.

Several types of laboratory tests have been used to diagnose and monitor HIV infection, including HIV antibody detection, HIV antigen detection, viral nucleic acid testing (NAT), and CD4 T-cell enumeration. In this chapter, we discuss the principles of each of these methods and their applications to HIV detection and infection monitoring. Although culturing the virus from patient samples is a definitive method of demonstrating HIV infection, it is not used in clinical settings because it is laborious, time consuming, costly, and potentially hazardous to laboratory personnel.

HIV Screening and Diagnosis

Serological tests for HIV antibody have been used in the initial diagnosis of HIV infection because most people develop antibody to the virus within 1 to 2 months after exposure. Since 1985, these tests have played a critical role in screening the donor blood supply to prevent transmission of the virus through blood transfusions or administration of blood products. Serological tests are also used in epidemiology studies to provide health officials with information about the extent of the infection in high-risk populations. These groups can then be targeted for counseling, treatment, and vaccine trials, and their medical and social concerns can be addressed.

Different serological methods have been used to test for HIV. Standard screening methods for HIV antibody have involved automated immunoassays such as the enzyme-linked immunosorbent assay (ELISA) and chemiluminescent immunoassay (CLIA) (see Chapter 11). Rapid tests can detect HIV antibody within minutes, making them an attractive alternative to standard screening methods in certain situations. Confirmatory tests are performed on samples that test positive on a screening test, to differentiate true-positive from false-positive results. The Western blot test was the standard confirmatory test for HIV for several years, but it has been replaced by newer methods for routine testing. Serological testing for p24 antigen and nucleic acid tests (NAT) for HIV RNA have been incorporated into the initial HIV testing scheme, providing for earlier and more accurate detection **(Fig. 24–5).** We discuss the principles of these methods in the text that follows, along with their use in HIV testing algorithms.

Testing Algorithms

Over the years, the CDC and the Association of Public Health Laboratories have developed algorithms that use a combination of laboratory tests performed in sequence to screen for the presence of HIV infection and resolve any discrepant results. These algorithms have been revised as improvements in laboratory testing have been made.

The CDC algorithm initially published in 2014 and updated in 2018 recommends that initial screening be performed with a combination immunoassay that detects antibodies to HIV-1 and HIV-2 as well as the HIV-1 p24 antigen. All positive specimens should then undergo additional testing with a rapid immunoassay that discriminates between HIV-1 and HIV-2 antibodies. Any samples that are reactive in the initial test and nonreactive or indeterminate in the second test should then be tested with an FDA-approved nucleic acid test (NAT) to resolve the discrepancy. Minor technical updates have occasionally been incorporated into this algorithm to provide guidance to laboratories on the use of available tests. These recommendations apply to adults and children who are older than 18 months. There are separate recommendations for children younger than 18 months, as maternal antibodies may be present that are likely to confuse the interpretation of the test results (see the section "Testing of Infants Younger than 18 months").

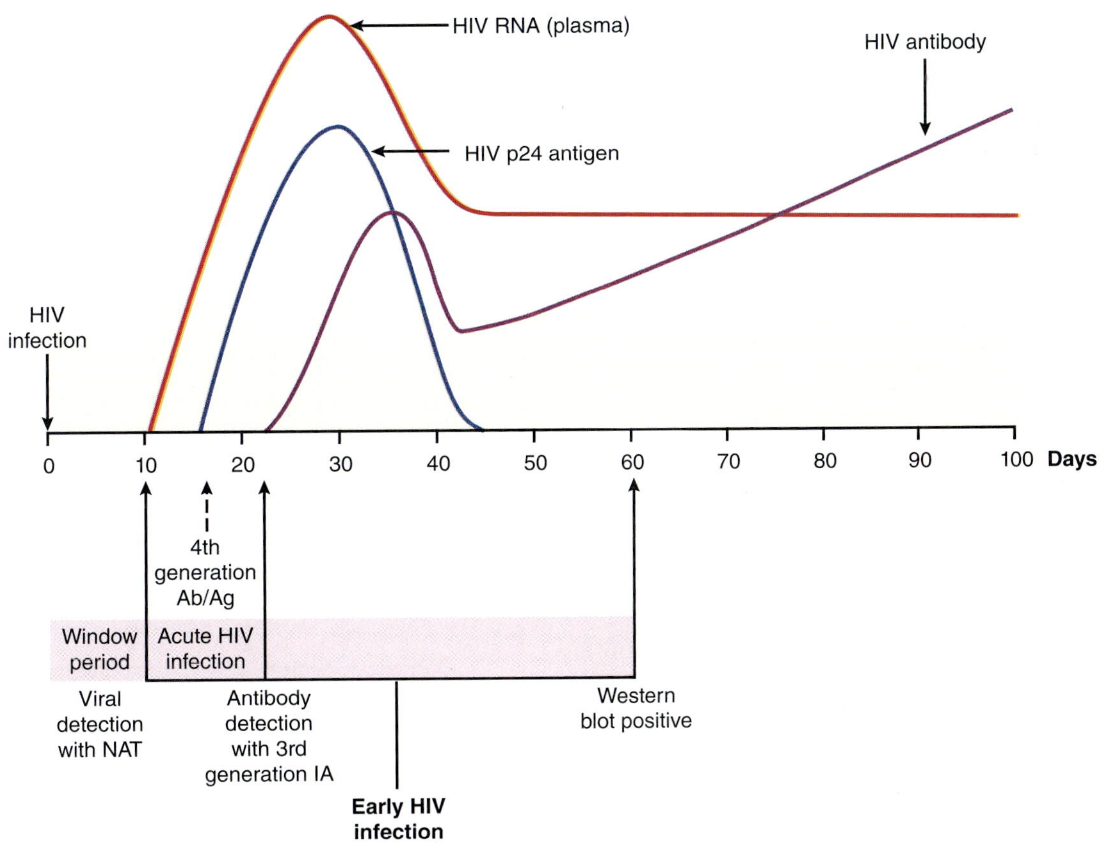

FIGURE 24–5 Appearance of HIV RNA, HIV-1 p24 antigen, and HIV antibody following HIV infection.

Figure 24–6 summarizes the main aspects of the current algorithm. This testing scheme provides significant advantages over previous algorithms. First, it allows for earlier detection of infections than prior algorithms, which initially tested for HIV antibody only, as the time between exposure and detectable results on the HIV-1/2/p24 combination assay is typically between 15 and 17 days. Second, it overcomes the limitations associated with the Western blot test, which was used previously to confirm initial positive results. The Western blot is a lengthy procedure that is typically performed only by specialized reference laboratories, and indeterminate results can occur, which can take months to resolve.

The 2014/2018 testing algorithm allows for rapid and accurate identification of HIV infection. This makes it possible to begin appropriate medical care and ART sooner in infected individuals. The 2014 testing protocol also helps to prevent additional infections by encouraging prompt initiation of counseling to reduce risky behaviors and earlier notification of sexual partners of diagnosed individuals. Incorporating an FDA-approved NAT can help resolve discrepancies between the first and second tests.

However, with any test, it is important to be aware of potential limitations. NATs have extremely high sensitivity (greater than 99%); however, any negative (nonreactive) result requires special consideration because viral replication may not be at a detectable level at the time of testing. Test results may not be reliable when the testing is performed during the *window period*, which is the time between HIV infection onset until the virus is detectable (varying from 10 to 33 days). PrEP usage may also result in low or possibly undetectable levels of HIV RNA. The CDC continues to evaluate its algorithm as additional tests become available for clinical use. Next, we discuss the principles of the major laboratory tests used in testing for HIV infection.

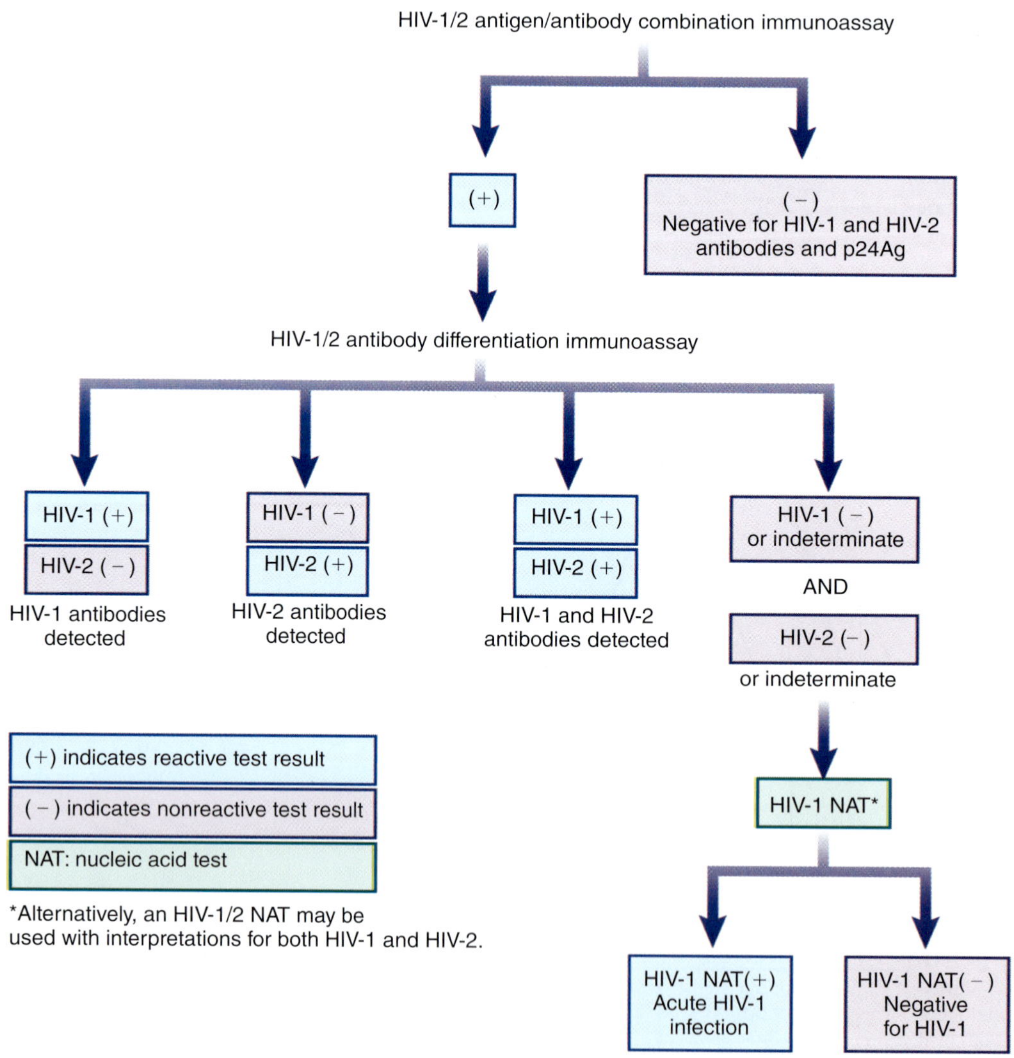

FIGURE 24–6 Laboratory HIV testing algorithm. *(Adapted from Branson BM, Owen SM, Wesolowski LG, et al. Laboratory testing for the diagnosis of HIV infection: updated recommendations. CDC Stacks. Updated 2014. Accessed December 11, 2024, http://stacks.cdc.gov/view/cdc/23447; and National Center for HIV/AIDS, Viral Hepatitis, and TB Prevention (U.S.). 2018 Quick reference guide: Recommended laboratory HIV testing algorithm for serum or plasma specimens. https://stacks.cdc.gov/view/cdc/50872. Accessed July 8, 2025.)*

Serological Test Principles

Conventional Immunoassays

Conventional immunoassays have been the cornerstone of screening procedures for HIV because they are easy to perform, can be adapted to test a large number of samples, and are highly sensitive and specific. They were first used to detect HIV antibody in the United States in 1985 in response to the need to screen donated blood. Several manufacturers have developed commercial kits to screen blood products and diagnose patients. The FDA publishes an updated list of kits approved for use in the United States. Over the years, five generations of immunoassays have been developed, resulting in improved sensitivity and specificity.

Currently, the most widely used assays are fully automated fourth-generation methods that can simultaneously detect HIV-1 antibodies, HIV-2 antibodies, and p24 antigen. Previously, separate immunoassays were used to detect the p24 antigen from the core of the HIV-1 virion as a marker of early infection. Levels of p24 in the circulation are high in the initial weeks of infection during the early burst of viral replication, providing a marker that can be detected before the appearance of HIV antibody during the acute stage of infection. The antigen becomes undetectable as antibody to p24 develops and binds the antigen in immune complexes; levels rise again during the later stages of infection when impairment of the immune system allows the virus to replicate.

Figure 24–7 illustrates the basic principle of the fourth-generation HIV-1 antibody/HIV-2 antibody/p24 antigen combination tests. These tests use a sandwich ELISA or CLIA in which patient serum is incubated with a solid phase onto which synthetic or recombinant HIV-1 antigens, HIV-2 antigens, and a monoclonal antibody to HIV-1 p24 have been attached. If antibody to HIV is in the sample, it will bind to the HIV-1 or HIV-2 antigens (or both, if both infections are present); if p24 antigen is in the sample, it will bind to the anti-p24 on the solid phase. Following a wash step to remove excess sample, a conjugate containing chemiluminescent- or enzyme-labeled anti-p24 and HIV-1/HIV-2 antigens is added. After a second incubation and wash step, the appropriate trigger solution or substrate/stop solution is added, and the relative light units released or optical absorbance is measured. Increased signal is observed if either HIV-1 or HIV-2 is present. As we

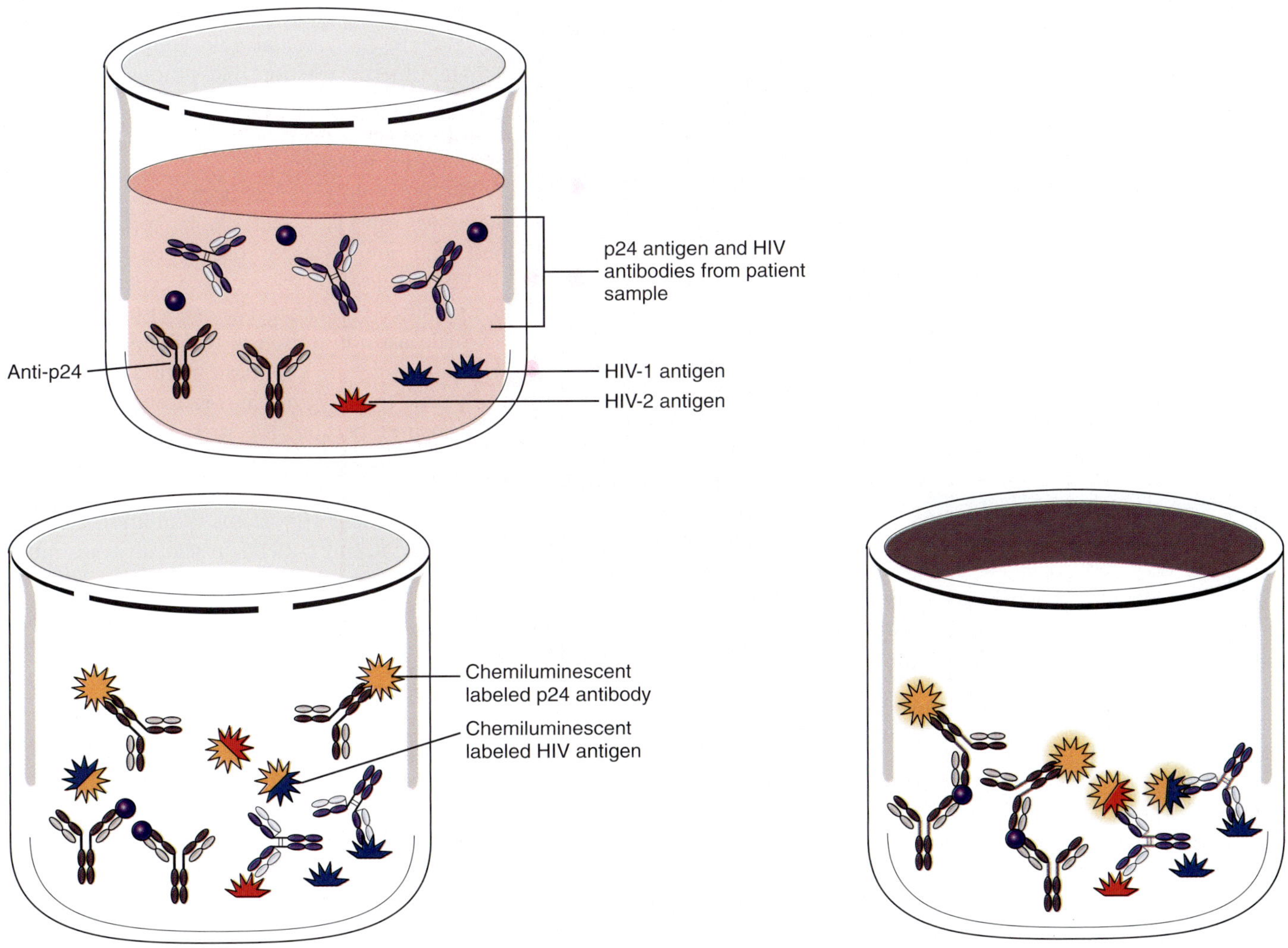

FIGURE 24–7 Principle of fourth-generation CLIA test for HIV. This test detects the HIV-1 p24 antigen as well as HIV-1 antibodies and HIV-2 antibodies.

previously mentioned, these combination assays are used in the initial step of the current CDC-recommended algorithm for HIV testing.

The FDA has also approved a fifth-generation multiplex bead immunoassay for screening for HIV infection. This assay can also detect both HIV antibodies and antigens, but in addition, it can differentiate between HIV-1 antibody, HIV-2 antibody, and p24 antigen.

Although the immunoassays used in HIV testing have a high level of sensitivity and specificity, they may sometimes give erroneous results. False-negative results for HIV antibody occur infrequently but may be caused by the collection of the test serum before the patient develops HIV antibodies (i.e., before **seroconversion**), administration of immunosuppressive therapy or replacement blood transfusion, conditions of defective antibody synthesis such as hypogammaglobulinemia, or technical errors attributed to improper handling of kit reagents. False-negative results may also occur if the patient harbors a genetically diverse, recombinant strain of HIV that is not detected by the test. The likelihood of false negatives occurring has been reduced by implementation of fourth-generation tests that can identify HIV infection several days earlier than previous tests because they detect p24 antigen in addition to HIV antibodies. This makes it possible for the infection to be diagnosed within 2 to 3 weeks after exposure. However, there are rare situations in which a patient can persistently test negative for HIV antibody despite the presence of HIV RNA.

False-positive results may also occur in these assays. These can result from several factors, including heat inactivation of the sample before testing, repeated freezing and thawing of specimens, the presence of heterophile or human–anti-mouse antibodies, passive immunoglobulin therapy, or administration of an experimental HIV vaccine to the patient. False positives can also result from specimen mix-up or mislabeling. In addition, the fourth-generation immunoassays cannot distinguish between HIV-1 and HIV-2 infection. Any positive results obtained from the initial ELISA or CLIA screen must therefore be confirmed by additional testing that can differentiate the two viruses.

Clinical Correlations

Seroconversion

By definition, seroconversion is the change of a serological test result from antibody negative to antibody positive. This occurs over time when the immune system is responding to HIV infection. Seroconversion can be detected by comparing the test results from two samples collected from the patient, the first soon after exposure to the virus and the second a few weeks later.

Rapid Tests for HIV Antibodies

Although conventional immunoassays are ideal tests for the detection of HIV antibodies in clinical laboratories that perform large-volume batch testing, they require expensive instrumentation and skilled personnel with technical expertise and may have a turnaround time of a few days. To overcome these limitations and to encourage more patients to be tested, simple, rapid methods to screen for HIV antibody have been developed. Rapid tests are easy to use and provide results within 30 minutes. They are available for use worldwide and have several applications. Rapid tests are excellent for **point-of-care testing (POCT)** such as in hospital emergency departments, clinics, and physician offices. Some tests can be used in nonclinical settings and can be purchased on the internet or in pharmacies and do not require a prescription.

The FDA has approved several commercially available rapid tests for HIV. These kits detect antibodies to HIV-1 alone or to both HIV-1 and HIV-2; they can be used on serum, plasma, whole blood samples obtained by venipuncture or fingerstick, or for some kits, oral fluid. Although each test has unique features, all are lateral flow or flow-through immunoassays that produce a colorimetric reaction in the case of a positive result. The flow-through assays require multiple steps in which the sample and reagents are added to a solid support encased in a plastic device, whereas the lateral flow assays involve a one-step procedure in which the patient sample migrates along the test strip by capillary action (see Chapter 11). With either procedure, the patient's sample is applied to a test strip or membrane containing HIV antigens. The antigen-antibody complexes bind to an enzyme-labeled conjugate or an antibody-binding (protein A) colloidal gold conjugate and are detected by a colorimetric reaction that produces a colored line or dot in the case of a positive result. Interpretation of the results is made by visual observation of the test device and does not require instrumentation.

A primary use for rapid tests has been to screen for HIV infection; these are especially suitable in certain circumstances. Rapid tests are ideal for use in resource-limited settings around the world that lack access to expensive equipment and highly trained personnel. They are also beneficial in situations in which fast notification of test results is desired. For example, rapid results are important in guiding decisions to begin prophylactic therapy with anti-retroviral drugs after occupational exposures because the therapy appears to be most effective when administered soon after exposure. Other situations in which rapid tests are advantageous include testing pregnant women whose HIV status is unknown during labor and delivery and testing patients in sexually transmitted disease clinics or emergency departments who are unlikely to return for their test results.

Although rapid tests are highly specific, false negatives and false positives can occur. Rapid tests conducted with whole blood obtained by fingerstick or oral fluid are less sensitive than those performed on plasma or serum, and a negative test result does not rule out early acute HIV infection. In addition, the specificity of rapid tests may be lower than expected when used in populations with a low prevalence for HIV. For these reasons, rapid testing should be followed by the current recommended testing algorithm whenever possible.

A rapid test that detects p24 antigen as well as HIV-1 and HIV-2 antibodies has also been approved for use in HIV screening. This POCT combo test requires whole blood, plasma, or serum and can be used to aid the diagnosis of HIV-1 and/

or HIV-2. The test can also distinguish acute HIV-1 infection from established HIV-1 infection.

In the United States, the FDA has approved one HIV test for over-the-counter, in vitro diagnostic home use. This self-test, OraQuick, is a rapid test capable of detecting HIV-1 and HIV-2 antibodies. The test requires oral fluid collected by swabbing gums, and results are obtained within 20 minutes. Nonclinical setting tests offer the advantages of convenience, privacy, and anonymity and have the potential of encouraging more widespread screening among high-risk individuals. However, false-negative results can occur because home tests are not as sensitive as conventional testing, and there is concern that some people who test positive might not seek confirmatory testing and the appropriate medical care.

As we previously discussed, a rapid immunoassay that differentiates between HIV-1 and HIV-2 has also been recommended by the CDC for confirmation of results from samples that test positive in the HIV-1 antibody/HIV-2 antibody/p24 antigen combo screen. Rapid testing has several advantages over the previously recommended Western blot test. Specifically, HIV antibodies are detected earlier, the incidence of indeterminate results is reduced, there is a shorter result-turnaround time, testing is less costly, and HIV-2 infections are detected in addition to those caused by HIV-1.

Western Blot

The **Western blot test,** or immunoblot, for HIV antibodies was introduced in 1984 and was the most common method used for confirmation of positive ELISA results from 1985 to 2014. This technique was more technically demanding than ELISA but could provide an antibody profile of the patient sample that revealed the specificities to individual HIV antigens. Patients could also be followed over time to determine if there was a change in the antibody pattern. Separate HIV-1- and HIV-2-specific Western blot tests were used to test for antibodies to each virus. The general principle of the Western blot was discussed in Chapter 11.

Because Western blot testing is highly dependent on the laboratorian's technical skill and subjective interpretation, it was generally performed only in specialized reference laboratories. For the test to be valid, a negative control run with the test should produce no bands, and the positive control should be reactive with p17, p24, p31, gp41, p51, p55, p66, and gp120/160. A negative test result for the patient sample was reported if no bands were present or if none of the bands corresponded to the molecular weights of any of the known viral proteins.

Criteria for determining a positive test result have been published by the Association of State and Territorial Public Health Laboratory Directors and CDC, the Consortium for Retrovirus Serology Standardization, the American Red Cross, and the FDA. According to these criteria, a result is considered positive if at least two of the following three bands are present: p24, gp41, and gp120/gp160 **(Fig. 24–8).**

Specimens with some of the characteristic bands but not meeting the criteria for a positive test result were considered to be *indeterminate* and were retested with a new sample obtained 4 to 6 weeks later. If the pattern converted to positive, it could be concluded that the first specimen was obtained during the early phase of seroconversion. Failure of an indeterminate test pattern to convert to positive after a few weeks strongly suggested that the pattern was caused by a false-positive test rather than HIV infection.

The Western blot was the historic gold standard for confirmation of an HIV-1 infection. However, it is no longer used for HIV diagnosis. In 2014, the CDC discontinued its recommendation for use because of its inability to detect acute infection and its potential for misclassification of HIV-2 as an HIV-1 infection. Because of its relative insensitivity, level of technical difficulty, and long turnaround time to obtain results, the CDC guidelines replaced the Western blot with a rapid HIV-1/HIV-2 antibody test as the standard method for confirming positive screening results.

Nucleic Acid Tests (NATs)

Qualitative NATs are used to determine whether a detectable level of HIV nucleic acid is present in human plasma. There are currently three FDA-approved HIV NAT tests, all of which can be used as an aid in the diagnosis of HIV. However, quantitative NAT (viral load assays) are not approved by the FDA for diagnosis unless the test has a dual claim that allows for use in both HIV-1 diagnosis and clinical management. Depending on the assay, NATs can be used to screen for infection or make an initial patient diagnosis. They can also be used to measure and monitor viral load, which assists in treatment management. They are particularly beneficial in cases where serological results are inconclusive, such as in very early infection or in the diagnosis of infants, where the presence of maternal antibodies can confuse test results.

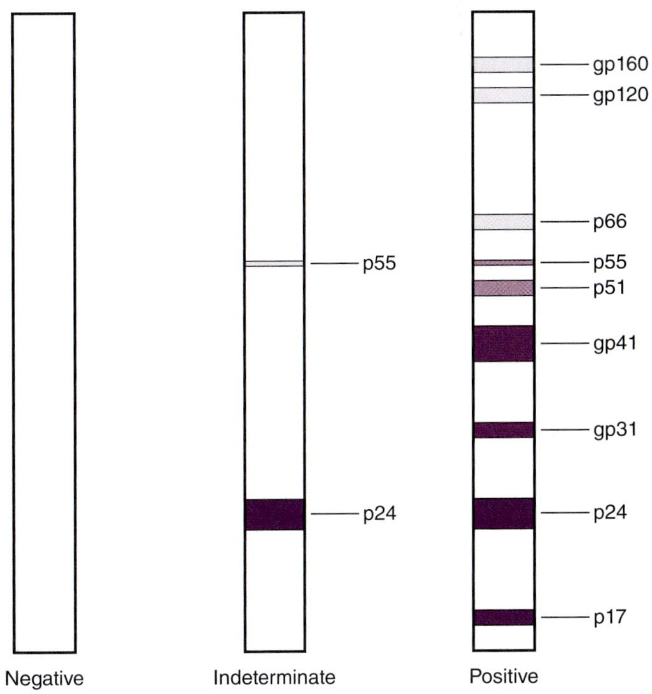

FIGURE 24–8 Western blot, showing results from a negative sample, an indeterminate sample, and a positive sample.

As we previously mentioned, NAT is an integral part of the CDC recommendations for laboratory testing for HIV. The tests are used to resolve discrepancies between a positive result in the initial antigen-antibody combo assay and the follow-up HIV-1/HIV-2 antibody differentiation assay. If the initial HIV-1 antibody/HIV-2 antibody/p24 antigen test is reactive, and the confirmatory HIV-1/HIV-2 antibody test is also reactive, the result is considered positive for HIV-1 or HIV-2, and the NAT need not be performed. However, if the HIV-1 antibody/HIV-2 antibody/p24 antigen test is reactive, but the HIV-1/HIV-2 antibody test is indeterminate or negative, then a NAT is performed. Either an HIV-1 NAT or HIV-1/-2 NAT can be performed based on the test result of the HIV-1/HIV-2 antibody differentiation test and the availability of the assay in the laboratory.

If an HIV-1 NAT is performed and reactive, the result is considered evidence for acute HIV-1 infection. In contrast, if the HIV-1 NAT is nonreactive, follow-up testing may be warranted, or a false-positive result on the initial HIV antigen-antibody combo assay may be indicated, and the result may be considered negative for HIV-1. The individual's clinical history must be considered in deciding whether follow-up is necessary.

Alternatively, some laboratories may perform an HIV-1/-2 NAT to determine the patient's status with each of the two HIV strains. Performance of a NAT may also be helpful if the HIV-1 antibody/HIV-2 antibody/p24 antigen test is nonreactive and a recent HIV exposure is suspected. It is important to take into consideration the individual's history when deciding if follow-up testing is appropriate.

HIV NATs are highly sensitive; they are able to detect HIV RNA about 10 to 12 days after infection. Methods approved by the FDA include a qualitative polymerase chain reaction (PCR)-based assay to screen donors of whole blood, blood components, or organs and a transcription-mediated amplification (TMA) assay for diagnosis (see Chapter 12).

Knowledge Check 24-4

What is an advantage of performing the HIV-1/2 antigen/antibody combination immunoassay for initial HIV infection diagnosis?

a. The assay is capable of detecting small quantities of viral nucleic acid.
b. The assay can provide an antibody profile of the patient sample that reveals the specificities to individual HIV antigens.
c. The assay allows for earlier detection of infection because the time between exposure and detectable results is shorter.
d. The assay is typically performed in reference laboratories, and result interpretation is subjective.

Disease Monitoring

Once a diagnosis of HIV infection has been established, it is essential to monitor patients over time to evaluate the effectiveness of their ART. This way, signs of disease progression can be detected early and guide decisions about further treatments. Two laboratory markers are routinely used to monitor patients with HIV infection for disease progression and guide their therapy: (1) the peripheral blood CD4 T-cell count, which is considered the best indicator of immune function in HIV-infected individuals, and (2) the HIV-1 RNA level, or "viral load," which reflects patient responses to ART. We discuss each of these laboratory markers in detail next.

CD4 T-Cell Enumeration

Destruction of the CD4 T lymphocytes is central to the immunopathogenesis of HIV infection, and a decrease in the number of CD4 T cells has long been recognized as the hallmark feature of AIDS. Therefore, enumeration of CD4 T cells in the peripheral blood has played a central role in evaluating the degree of immune suppression in HIV-infected patients. Normally, the peripheral blood CD4 T-cell count ranges from 430 to 1,800 cells/μL (on average, 1,000 cells/μL). In untreated patients, there is a progressive decline in the number of CD4 T cells during the course of infection **(Fig. 24–9).** The rate of decline varies among patients and can be rapid or gradual. As we previously discussed, the CDC classification system uses CD4 T-cell counts to place patients into various stages of HIV infection; those whose counts are below 200/μL are categorized as having stage 3 infection.

Another important clinical application of CD4 T-cell counts is to monitor the effectiveness of ART. Physicians use CD4 T-cell values to help determine whether a change in ART is needed and if prophylactic drugs for certain opportunistic infections should be administered. According to guidelines published by the HHS, a baseline CD4 T-cell measurement should be performed before the initiation of ART, then every 3 to 6 months for the first 2 years. Thereafter, annual measurements can be performed in patients whose CD4 T-cell counts have consistently remained between 300 and 500 cells/μL. More frequent testing should be performed if there is a change in the patient's clinical status. If there is a decline in the CD4 T-cell count of greater than 25%, the physician may change the ART. Patients with a CD4 T-cell count below 200/μL are placed on prophylactic therapy for *Pneumocystis jiroveci* pneumonia, and those with a count of lower than 50/μL are given prophylactic treatment for *Mycobacterium avium* complex.

The gold standard for enumerating CD4 T cells is immunophenotyping with data analysis by **flow cytometry** (see Chapter 13). In this method, fluorescent-labeled monoclonal antibodies are used to determine the CD4 T-cell percentage and absolute CD4 T-cell number in a blood sample from the patient. These values are then compared with the reference ranges (normal values) established by the testing laboratory.

The ratio of CD4 T cells to CD8 T cells may also be reported to assess the dynamics between the two T-cell populations. In HIV-infected patients, particularly those with AIDS, the large decrease in the number of $CD4^+$ T cells, along with a possible increase in $CD8^+$ cytotoxic T cells, results in an inverted ratio, or a ratio lower than 1:1.

Although flow cytometry is the accepted gold standard for enumeration of CD4 T cells, it is a costly method that requires highly skilled personnel, a stable electricity supply,

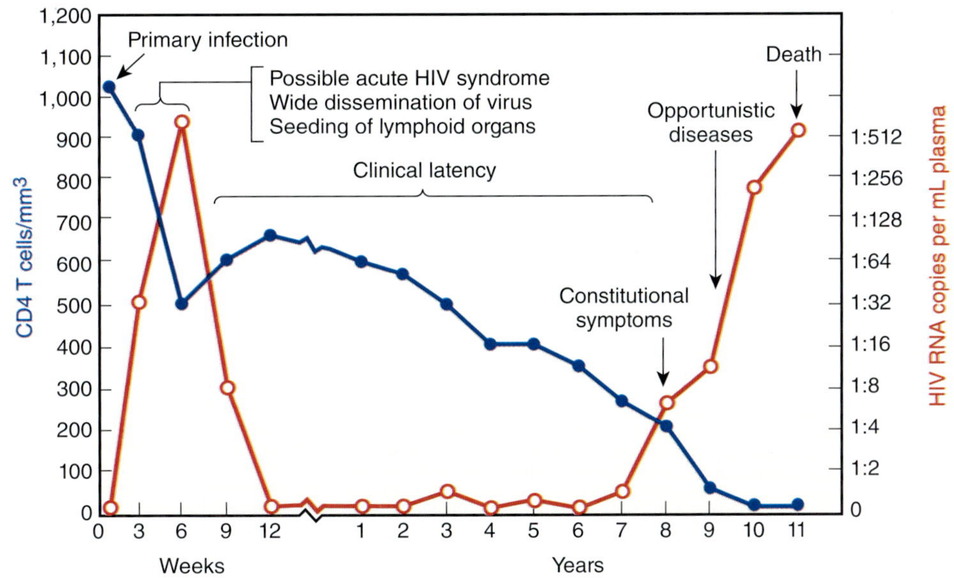

FIGURE 24–9 Typical CD4 T-cell numbers and plasma viremia during the natural course of HIV infection. *(Adapted from Pantaleo G, Graziosi C, Fauci AS. The immunopathogenesis of human immunodeficiency virus infection. N Engl J Med. 1993;328:327–335.)*

refrigeration of reagents, and regular instrument maintenance. These conditions are not available in many areas of the world. Therefore, there has been much interest in developing simpler, less expensive methods to determine CD4 T-cell measurements. This need has led to the manufacture of miniaturized flow cytometers that can be easily operated by smaller laboratories. These instruments are dedicated for CD3/CD4 measurements and use simple procedures that require a small volume of reagents.

Another major advance has been development of point-of-care devices that can be easily transported to remote regions. These devices can use blood obtained by fingerstick or venipuncture and contain stable, dried reagents that can withstand hot, humid temperatures. Disposable test cassettes are used to capture CD4$^+$ cells with labeled antibodies, and the results are analyzed by small, portable instruments that can be powered by a rechargeable battery. Lateral flow devices that do not require instrumentation have also been developed for CD4$^+$ T-cell enumeration. These methods are particularly suitable for resource-limited settings in developing countries where the incidence of HIV infection is high.

Quantitative Viral Load Assays

Quantitative **viral load tests** measure the amount of circulating HIV nucleic acid and play an essential role in helping physicians predict disease progression, monitor patient response to ART, and guide treatment decisions. The amount of HIV RNA in a patient's plasma is referred to as the "viral load" and reflects the natural history of HIV infection in that individual. HIV RNA levels become detectable about 11 days after infection and rise to very high levels shortly thereafter, during the initial burst of viral replication. Typically, over a period of a few months, the viral load drops as the individual's immune system clears viral particles from the circulation, and a stable level of plasma HIV RNA, known as the "set point," is achieved (see Fig. 24–9). In untreated people, this level can persist for a long time and then rise again later as the immune system deteriorates and the patient progresses to AIDS. In contrast, successful therapy with anti-retroviral drugs will result in a drop in the viral load to an undetectable level within a few weeks to a few months after the initiation of ART.

Information obtained from viral load tests has prognostic value. Baseline plasma viral load values obtained in patients before the start of ART are an important predictor of disease progression because higher numbers of HIV RNA copies/μL of plasma are associated with more rapid development of an AIDS-defining illness or AIDS-related death.

Viral load tests are used routinely to monitor the effectiveness of ART in HIV-infected patients and play an essential role in the clinical management of these individuals. The HHS recommends that plasma HIV RNA testing be performed before ART begins to obtain a baseline value; testing should be performed periodically thereafter to determine the effectiveness of the therapy. To obtain an accurate assessment of viral load dynamics in a single patient, it is recommended that the same assay be used for sequential viral load measurements because values may differ between different molecular tests. Patients who attain a lower number of HIV RNA copies/mL of plasma are more likely to achieve a longer treatment response. The optimal goal of therapy is to reach an undetectable level of HIV RNA, below the lower limit of detection of a currently approved viral load assay. Patients who have a persistently elevated viral load should undergo resistance testing to determine if an alternate drug regimen is needed (see "Drug Resistance and Tropism Testing" section).

Critical Thinking 24-2

A patient who was recently diagnosed as HIV-positive begins ART. Before the start of therapy, the patient has baseline HIV-1 RNA viral load testing and CD4 T-cell counts by flow cytometry performed. After ART begins, the patient's viral load and CD4 T-cell counts are monitored at 4-week intervals. The results of both tests are shown in the following table.

HIV-1 RNA VIRAL LOAD (COPIES/ML)	CD4 T-CELL COUNT (CELLS/μL)	TIME INTERVAL
125,800	380	Baseline (before ART)
11,360	440	4 weeks
1,050	450	8 weeks
794	460	12 weeks
126	462	16 weeks
<50	470	20 weeks

Why are laboratory results obtained prior to ART? What is the clinical significance of the viral load and CD4 counts at the various time intervals?

Methods

Viral load assays are based on amplification methods that increase the number of HIV RNA copies (or their derivatives) in test samples to detectable levels. Several amplification methods have been developed for this purpose, the most common being qPCR and **transcription-mediated amplification (TMA).** The basic principles of PCR and TMA are discussed briefly in the section that follows and are covered in more detail in Chapter 12.

Simpler technologies have been developed to determine HIV viral load for use in areas of the world that lack skilled laboratory personnel and the resources to purchase costly instrumentation, refrigeration, and a continuous power supply. These include point-of-care devices such as closed cartridges that can provide semiquantitative analysis with simpler instrumentation in a shorter period of time. Many of these technologies, including loop-mediated and helicase-dependent amplification, are based on isothermal reactions in which the temperature remains constant.

Polymerase Chain Reaction (PCR). Two kinds of PCR methods have been developed to detect HIV nucleic acid: the standard reverse transcriptase PCR (RT-PCR) and more recently, quantitative (real-time) PCR, also known as qPCR (see Chapter 12). A commercial RT-PCR was the first assay to be licensed by the FDA for the quantitative measurement of circulating HIV nucleic acid. Although this assay had a large impact on the management of HIV infection, it has been replaced by qPCR. Quantitative PCR is a highly sensitive, automated assay that can detect a broad range of RNA copies, from 20 to 10 million copies/mL.

In qPCR, HIV RNA is isolated from patient plasma after lysis of the virions. The RNA is treated with a thermostable DNA polymerase enzyme that has both reverse transcriptase activity and the ability to initiate DNA synthesis in the presence of the appropriate reagents. The reverse transcriptase activity of the enzyme transcribes the HIV RNA into a complementary sequence of DNA (cDNA). A portion of the cDNA is then amplified by PCR using primers that target highly conserved regions of the HIV-1 and/or HIV-2 genomes (e.g., *gag* gene). The PCR products are quantified as they are being produced by adding a fluorescent probe that binds to the amplicons during the reaction. An internal control consisting of a different nucleic acid sequence is simultaneously amplified with each sample to check for the effects of PCR inhibition and to allow for more accurate quantitation.

Transcription-Mediated Amplification (TMA). **Transcription-mediated amplification (TMA)** involves isothermal amplification of target nucleic acid. Unlike PCR, TMA is an isothermal process that does not require thermal cycling and heat-stable enzymes. Instead of using a thermocycler, a water bath or heating block is used. In TMA, RNA is amplified using reverse transcriptase and RNA polymerase. Specific primers are generated against targets of interest and include a promoter sequence for T7 RNA polymerase. The tailed primer and the target RNA are reverse transcribed (by reverse transcriptase), leading to production of a cDNA:RNA hybrid. The hybridized RNA is degraded to ssDNA, which serves as a template for reverse transcriptase to synthesize a complementary strand of DNA (along with a second primer). The newly synthesized dsDNA (which includes a binding site for RNA polymerase) is amplified with RNA polymerase to make multiple copies of RNA (see Chapter 12).

TMA produces RNA amplicons rather than DNA amplicons. RNA is more labile than DNA, reducing the chance of carryover contamination. The TMA process produces 100 to 1,000 copies per cycle, resulting in a 10-billion–fold increase within 15 to 30 minutes. TMA allows direct detection of RNA, which makes it advantageous for targeting RNA viruses, such as HIV. The high sensitivity makes it suitable for screening blood donor products. TMA is popular in clinical laboratories because the method is integrated in many commercial tests.

Drug Resistance and Tropism Testing

As we previously discussed, HIV is a rapidly replicating virus that has a high rate of mutation. Because of these properties, it is possible for drug-resistant subpopulations of the virus to emerge during the course of ART. Drug resistance has been a major reason for the failure of ART in many people. Therefore, laboratory tests have been developed to assess drug-resistance patterns; these tests have had a major impact on guiding the selection of optimal ART for individual patients.

Two types of laboratory methods can be used to test for drug resistance: *genotype resistance assays* and *phenotype resistance assays*. Genotype resistance assays are performed more frequently than phenotype resistance assays because they are less expensive, more widely available, and have a shorter turnaround time.

Genotype resistance assays detect mutations in the reverse transcriptase, protease, and integrase genes of HIV, as well as genes coding for envelope proteins that interact with entry and fusion inhibitors. These tests are available commercially and can be performed in clinical laboratory settings. In these tests, RNA is isolated from patient plasma, the desired genes are amplified by RT-PCR, and the products are analyzed for mutations associated with drug resistance by automated DNA sequencing. The nucleotide sequences of the genes of interest are identified and entered into a database, where they are compared with the corresponding sequences in wild-type HIV. The results are analyzed by commercially available software and reported qualitatively as "resistance," "possible resistance," or "no evidence of resistance" for each drug tested. Although genotyping tests have many advantages as compared with phenotypic methods, they can identify only known mutations and cannot assess the effects of combinations of individual mutations on drug resistance.

Phenotype resistance assays determine the ability of clinical isolates of HIV to grow in the presence of anti-retroviral drugs. In these assays, recombinant viruses are created by inserting the reverse transcriptase, protease, integrase, or *env* gene sequences from HIV RNA in the patient's plasma into a laboratory reference strain of HIV and transfecting the recombinant virus into mammalian cells. Varying concentrations of anti-viral drugs are incubated with the transfected cells, and the IC_{50} or IC_{90} values, or drug concentrations needed to suppress the replication of the patient's viral isolate by 50% or 90%, respectively, are calculated. These values are then compared with the IC_{50} or IC_{90} values of cells transfected with a reference strain of HIV to determine drug resistance. The major advantage of phenotypic assays is that they measure drug susceptibility directly, based on all mutations present in the patient's isolate. However, these assays are expensive and have a longer turnaround time than genotypic assays. They also involve sophisticated technologies and are only performed by a few highly specialized reference laboratories.

Both genotypic and phenotypic assays require that a viral load of at least 500 to 1,000 copies of HIV RNA/μL be present in the test sample and for the resistant virus to constitute more than 25% of the total viral population in the patient to produce detectable results. Despite these limitations, studies have shown that patients undergoing drug-resistance testing, particularly by genotyping methods, have a better chance of receiving ART regimens that are more likely to result in greater reductions in viral load. Therefore, the HHS recommends that drug-resistance testing be performed in individuals before initiating ART, in patients in whom ART has failed as evidenced by viral load values that have not been optimally reduced, and in all HIV-positive pregnant women. Genotypic testing is recommended for patients upon entry into medical care for HIV or after one to two unsuccessful treatment regimens because of its lower cost, faster turnaround time, and greater sensitivity for detecting wild-type/resistant virus mixtures. The addition of phenotypic testing is recommended when patients are thought to harbor HIV mutants with complex drug-resistance patterns.

Additional molecular tests are used to determine viral tropism and the suitability of a particular ART drug based on the HLA type of the patient. Analysis of the coreceptor tropism is used to determine whether a patient is eligible for treatment with CCR5 antagonists such as Maraviroc, which inhibits entry of HIV strains that use the CCR5 coreceptor to bind to host cells (the R5-tropic viruses). These drugs are only effective in patients who harbor these strains of HIV. Both genotypic and phenotypic tests are available for this purpose. Pharmacogenetic screening for the HLA-B*5701 allele is helpful for patients who are being considered for treatment with the nucleoside reverse transcriptase inhibitor abacavir because this allele has been associated with development of hypersensitivity to the drug. The test is typically performed by PCR amplification of the allele, followed by hybridization with sequence-specific oligonucleotide probes.

Knowledge Check 24-5

What characteristics of HIV enable the emergence of drug-resistant strains?

a. The HIV viral structure of nucleic acid surrounded by a protein coat
b. The rapid replication and high error rate of HIV reverse transcriptase
c. HIV's ability to establish viral latency
d. The binding affinity of HIV gp120 for the CD4 receptor on host cells

Testing of Infants Younger Than 18 Months

Serological tests are not reliable in detecting HIV infection in children younger than 18 months of age because of placental passage of IgG antibodies from an infected mother to the fetus. Maternal antibodies persist in the bloodstream of the infant during the first year of life (or longer in a small proportion of infants) and can confuse the interpretation of serological results from infant samples. Thus, a child born to an HIV-positive mother may test positive for HIV antibody during the first 18 months of life even though the child is not infected.

Because of the difficulties with serological testing, HIV infection in infants is best diagnosed using molecular methods. A qualitative HIV-1 RNA or an HIV-1 DNA PCR test may be used for this purpose. The latter test detects proviral DNA within the infants' peripheral blood mononuclear cells. Alternatively, quantitative HIV RNA assays using a plasma sample may be used to diagnose HIV infection in infants. Although they are less sensitive than DNA assays, RNA tests can provide a baseline viral load measurement and are more likely to detect infections with strains other than subtype B. They can also be used as a confirmatory test for infants who initially had a positive HIV DNA test.

It is recommended that nucleic acid tests for HIV be performed in infants with known perinatal exposure at the ages of 14 to 21 days, 1 to 2 months, and 4 to 6 months, and possibly at birth for infants at high risk for HIV infection. A positive test result should be confirmed by repeat testing on a second specimen because false positives can occur. Two or more negative test results (the first at older than 1 month of age and the second at older than 4 months, or two separate tests conducted after 6 months) provide evidence for the absence of HIV infection and may be confirmed by serological tests at 12 to 18 months of age. The HIV status of breastfed infants, who are continually exposed to the virus, cannot be determined accurately until breastfeeding is stopped.

The CDC and the HHS recommend that all pregnant women be tested for HIV infection so that those who are positive can be treated with ART, and their infants can be evaluated for HIV infection after birth. Prompt detection of HIV infection in newborns is important because infected infants have a better prognosis when ART is started early and can benefit from treatment with prophylactic drugs for opportunistic infections.

Critical Thinking 24-3

Suppose a woman who is HIV-positive and untreated gives birth to a child. If serology testing was performed on the infant and antibodies against HIV were detected, does this mean the infant has HIV infection? Explain your answer. What HIV tests should be performed on infants younger than 18 months of age, and when should infants with known HIV perinatal exposure be tested?

Human T-Cell Lymphotropic Viruses (HTLV)

Human T-lymphotropic viruses (HTLV) are a group of viruses recognized as oncoviruses, meaning they are capable of causing cancer, in addition to other immunosuppressive and inflammatory diseases. There are four types of HTLV; HTLV-1 and HTLV-2 are the focus of this chapter, as the other subtypes of HTLV are extremely rare. HTLV-1 is the most clinically significant. HTLV-2 is less prevalent, and a definitive correlation between the virus and disease is unclear. HTLV-3 and HTLV-4 were isolated from bushmeat hunters in Cameroon, but the numbers of infected individuals are so low their pathological role in humans is uncertain. Most people who become infected with HTLV are asymptomatic. About 95% of the patients who contract HTLV-1 will develop a chronic, asymptomatic infection. However, 5% may develop a serious and fatal outcome in the form of malignancy, inflammation, or opportunistic infection. Adult T-cell leukemia/lymphoma (ATLL) and HTLV-associated myelopathy/tropical spastic paraparesis (HAM/TSP) are significant diseases caused by HTLV-1 infection.

HTLV Transmission

HTLV-1 can be transmitted by three major routes: (1) bloodborne, mainly through transfusions containing cellular components or through IV drug abuse; (2) sexual contact, most commonly from men to women; and (3) from mother to child, mainly through breastfeeding. Prolonged breastfeeding (greater than 12 months) is associated with a high risk of mother-to-child transmission and seropositivity in more than one child of the same mother. HTLV-1 seroprevalence increases with age.

Between 5 million and 20 million people are thought to be infected with HTLV-1 worldwide. This number remains highly uncertain because systematic epidemiological investigations have not been carried out in some endemic areas. Infections in the United States and Europe have resulted mainly from immigrants from endemic areas. HTLV-1 infection is endemic in southwestern Japan, the Caribbean islands, South and Central Africa, the Middle East, Romania, parts of South America, and Papua New Guinea. The average age of patients with ATLL at time of diagnosis is about 60 years in Japan, whereas the average age of patients with ATLL in the Caribbean islands is about 45 years. The difference in age suggests that genetic and/or environmental factors may contribute to ATLL progression.

The epidemiology of HTLV-2 is different from HTVV-1. HTLV-2 infections are highest in various Native Indian populations in the Americas, a few Pygmy tribes in Central Africa, and IV drug abusers in North America and Europe. The total worldwide cases of HTLV-2 are estimated to be 6- to 12-fold lower than HTLV-1. Without sufficient and systematic epidemiological investigation, the exact numbers remain unknown.

HTLV-2 transmission has been clearly documented through transfusion of contaminated cellular blood products. Other routes are less well established, although evidence suggests with high probability that transmission is identical to that of HTLV-1. However, there may be differences in the transmission efficiency.

Characteristics of HTLV

HTLV-1 and HTLV-2 are closely related retroviruses. Both viruses have RNA as their nucleic acid and three structural genes: *gag,* which codes for viral core proteins; *pol,* which codes for viral enzymes; and *env,* which encodes proteins in the viral envelope; as well as a region called *pX,* which encodes several regulatory proteins, including Tax and Rex. Reverse transcriptase transcribes the viral RNA into DNA, which then becomes integrated into the host-cell's genome as a provirus. The provirus can remain in a latent state within infected cells for a prolonged period of time. Upon activation of the host cell, the provirus can proceed to complete its replication cycle to produce more virions. However, HTLV-1 and HTLV-2 exist predominantly in the proviral state and are spread directly to uninfected cells through a viral synapse. Additional copies of the viral nucleic acid are produced when the infected host cells replicate.

Immunologic Manifestations of HTLV

HTLV-1 preferentially infects CD4+ T lymphocytes, while HTLV-2 mainly infects CD8+ T cells. The viruses can also infect dendritic cells, monocytes, and B cells. CD8+ CTLs effectively control the proliferation of virus-infected cells in most individuals. However, inflammatory cytokines released during the immune response may contribute to the pathogenesis of HTLV-associated diseases. The risk of developing inflammatory diseases is associated with the proviral load. In addition, HTLV-1 infection of $CD4^+$ T cells can increase the production of pro-inflammatory cytokines, impair production of T_H1 cytokines necessary for cell-mediated immunity, and induce differentiation of regulatory T (Treg) cells. The differentiated Treg cells can facilitate viral persistence by suppressing the host's immune response to the virus. HTLV-1 also transforms $CD4^+$ T lymphocytes into malignant cells in a small percentage of people through mechanisms mediated by the Tax protein, resulting in increased cell proliferation and accumulation of harmful genetic mutations. Cell-mediated impairment can be significant, leading to a severe immunodeficient state.

During primary infection, antibodies develop against the core (Gag) protein (of HTLV-1). These are the first antibodies to appear and typically predominate in the first 2 months. Antibodies to Env develop later in the infection, followed by antibodies to the Tax protein. The titer of HTLV-1–specific antibodies can reach high levels during chronic infection and correlates with a high proviral load. Antibody production is useful for serology testing. However, the role of antibodies in protection of the host is unclear.

Diseases and Clinical Symptoms of HTLV

HTLV-1 is the cause of two diseases: **adult T-cell leukemia/lymphoma (ATLL)** and **HTLV-1–associated myelopathy/tropical spastic paraparesis (HAM/TSP).** ATLL can be classified into four different subtypes based on clinical manifestations: acute, T-cell non-Hodgkin lymphoma, chronic, and smoldering. Over half of patients have the acute type, an aggressive variant with a median survival of 6 months. The clinical features include skin lesions, lytic bone lesions, hypercalcemia, and pulmonary infiltrates. T-cell non-Hodgkin lymphoma, also known as the lymphomatous form of ATLL, occurs in about 20% to 25% of cases. The median survival is less than 1 year. Clinical features include lymphadenopathy, skin lesions, hypercalcemia, and hepatosplenomegaly. The chronic form accounts for about 20% of ATLL cases and has a better prognosis. The median survival is around 2 years. This type tends to be asymptomatic, and hypercalcemia is not present. The least common form is smoldering ATLL, making up about 5% of cases. Median survival is over 5 years. Clinical symptoms include skin and pulmonary lesions. However, lymphadenopathy, hepatosplenomegaly, and hypercalcemia are not present.

All four types of ATLL are characterized by a monoclonal proliferation of mature T cells that express the surface markers CD3, CD4, and CD25. The malignant cells have lobulated, "flower-shaped" nuclei that contain proviral HTLV-1 nucleic acid **(Fig. 24–10).** The lifetime risk of HTLV-1 carriers for developing ATLL is 3% to 5% and is highest in those who acquired the infection perinatally. The disease typically appears after a latent period of 20 to 30 years following initial infection. As we mentioned previously, cell-mediated

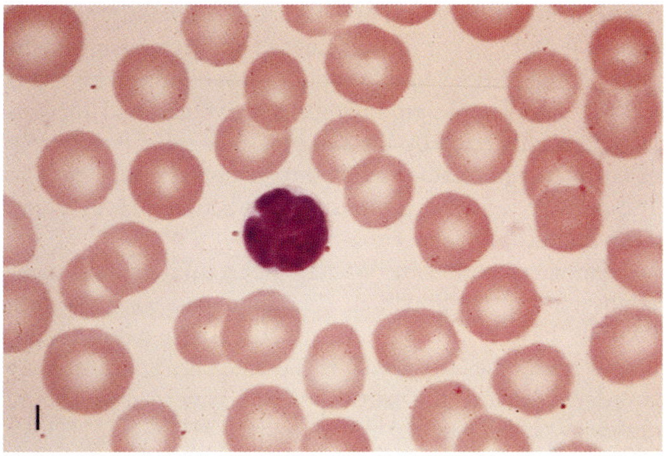

FIGURE 24–10 Flower cells typical of ATLL. Note the lobulated flower-shaped nuclei.

immunity in ATLL patients can be significantly hindered. Patients may succumb to a variety of opportunistic pathogens including various fungi, cytomegalovirus, mycobacteria, and *Pneumocystis jirovecii*.

People infected with HTLV-1 also have a 4% lifetime risk of developing a progressive neurological disorder called *HTLV-1–associated myelopathy/tropical spastic paraparesis* (HAM/TSP). The risk is highest among those who contracted the infection through sexual transmission. The disease is characterized by slowly progressive weakness and stiffness of the legs, back pain, and urinary incontinence. HTLV-1 has also been associated with various autoimmune and inflammatory disorders, including uveitis (intraocular inflammation of the eyes), infective dermatitis, myositis (inflammation of the muscles), and arthropathy (inflammation of the joints); however, a causal relationship of the virus with these conditions has not been established. It is unclear what factors influence the development and types of clinical manifestations of HTLV-1 infection, but differences in viral strains, viral load, mode of transmission, HLA haplotypes, and immune responses mounted by the host may all play a role.

The association of HTLV-2 infection with disease is unclear, and most people infected with the virus are asymptomatic. However, there is evidence that HTLV-2 may rarely be associated with a neurological disease that is similar to HAM/TSP, as well as certain hematologic and dermatologic diseases and increased incidence of infections. A close link to cancer mortality in the United States has also been identified. This evidence suggests that more research is needed to understand the pathogenicity of the virus.

Laboratory Testing for HTLV

Serological testing plays an important role in detecting HTLV-1 and HTLV-2 infections because culture of the viruses requires sophisticated techniques that cannot be performed in routine clinical laboratories. HTLV antibodies develop 30 to 90 days after exposure to the virus and persist for life. Tests for HTLV-1 and HTLV-2 antibodies are used to detect HTLV infections and to screen blood donors. The tests most commonly used for screening are ELISA or CLIA methods that incorporate recombinant antigens or synthetic peptides from both HTLV-1 and HTLV-2. Any sample producing a reactive result in the initial screen is retested by the same method and subsequently tested by a confirmatory method to reduce the incidence of false-positive results and to distinguish between HTLV-1 and HTLV-2 infection.

Commercially available Western blot assays are most commonly used for confirmation; line immunoassays (LIAs) and IFA tests have also been developed. Western blot and LIA identify antibodies to specific HTLV antigens. Specimens are considered positive if a particular band pattern representing antibodies to the gag and env proteins of HTLV-1 or HTLV-2 is obtained. According to criteria published by the WHO, for example, a sample is considered positive for HTLV-1 antibodies if visible bands are produced for one of the env proteins (either gp46 or gp62/68) *and* one of the gag proteins (p19, p24, or p53). A major problem with the Western blot and LIA methods is that indeterminate results can be obtained when a single band is observed or when multiple bands that do not meet the criteria for positivity are seen. PCR can be performed to detect HTLV-1 or HTLV-2 DNA in provirus-carrying peripheral blood mononuclear cells to clarify repeatedly indeterminate results. PCR methods can also be used to monitor the proviral load in patients with HTLV-associated diseases during therapy and to demonstrate the presence of the virus in cells from patients who are suspected of having HTLV-associated disease.

Knowledge Check 24-6

ATLL is a consequence of infection with which virus?
a. HTLV-1
b. HTLV-2
c. HTLV-3
d. HIV-1

Critical Thinking 24-4

Why should blood donors be screened for HTLV? What are the similarities and differences between HTLV and HIV infections?

KEY CONCEPTS

- The retrovirus family Retroviridae is composed of a large diverse group of RNA viruses, primarily infecting vertebrates. Some viruses in this family are human pathogens known to cause severe immunodeficiencies, inflammatory disease, and cancer. Clinically significant members include the human T-lymphotropic viruses and HIV.

Human Immunodeficiency Virus (HIV)

- Human immunodeficiency virus type 1 (HIV-1) is responsible for the majority of AIDS cases throughout the world. A related virus, HIV-2, may also cause AIDS but is generally less pathogenic.

HIV Transmission

- Transmission of HIV occurs by three major routes: (1) intimate sexual contact, (2) contact with contaminated blood or body fluids, or (3) vertical transmission from infected mother to her fetus or infant.

Characteristics of HIV

- HIV belongs to the retrovirus family, which contains RNA as the genetic material from which DNA is transcribed. HIV has three main structural genes: *gag*, which codes for the core proteins of the virus such as p24; *pol*, which codes for the enzymes reverse transcriptase, integrase, and protease; and *env*, which encodes the envelope proteins gp120 and gp41.
- The primary target cells for HIV are $CD4^+$ T lymphocytes and macrophages, which possess some surface CD4. The CD4 molecule acts as a receptor for attachment of the virus by binding to the gp120 envelope protein. After attachment, entry of the virus into the host cells is mediated by a chemokine coreceptor (CXCR4 or CCR5).

Immunologic Manifestations of HIV

- A burst of viral replication occurs after initial infection with HIV, followed by a period of latency during which viral DNA becomes integrated into the host genome as a provirus.
- Viral production slows down as the host's immune response develops and keeps the virus in check. The host produces neutralizing antibodies, which prevent the virus from infecting neighboring cells, and develops HIV-specific CTLs that lyse virus-infected target cells. Innate defenses are also activated.
- Although the immune responses of the host reduce the level of HIV replication, they are usually not sufficient to completely eliminate the virus. HIV can escape these responses by undergoing rapid genetic mutations that generate altered antigens, downregulating production of class I MHC molecules on the surface of the infected target cells, and existing in a latent proviral state.
- The hallmark feature of HIV infection is a decline in the number of CD4 T_H cells during the natural course of infection. This decline results in an immunodeficiency that affects both cell-mediated and humoral antibody responses to a variety of antigens.

Clinical Symptoms of HIV Infection

- The clinical course of untreated HIV infection begins with an acute phase in which patients may experience flu-like symptoms. This is followed by a latent, asymptomatic period that lasts an average of 10 years. The infection culminates in AIDS, which is characterized by profound immunosuppression with life-threatening opportunistic infections and malignancies.

- The 2014 CDC case definition of HIV infection is based on laboratory criteria or clinical evidence and classifies patients into one of five stages based on CD4 T-cell measurements and the presence of opportunistic illnesses.

HIV Treatment and Prevention

- Treatment with anti-retroviral therapy (ART) is recommended for all HIV-infected persons and has resulted in a significant delay in disease progression, decreased mortality, and reduction in perinatal transmission.
- Several classes of anti-retroviral drugs have been developed to block various steps of the HIV replication cycle: nucleoside analogue reverse transcriptase inhibitors, nonnucleoside reverse transcriptase inhibitors, protease inhibitors, integrase strand transfer inhibitors, fusion inhibitors, a CCR5 antagonist, and a CD4 postattachment inhibitor. These drugs are most effective when administered in combination to reduce the development of drug resistance.
- Measures to prevent HIV transmission include testing people for HIV infection, screening blood products for HIV, and education and administration of pre-exposure prophylaxis (PrEP) for high-risk individuals.

Laboratory Testing for HIV Infection

- The most current algorithm recommended by the CDC and the Association of Public Health Laboratories is to screen for HIV infection using a sequence of laboratory tests. The initial test is a fourth-generation immunoassay that simultaneously detects HIV-1 antibody, HIV-2 antibody, and p24 antigen. Positive test results must be confirmed by a rapid test that discriminates between HIV-1 antibody and HIV-2 antibody. Any samples that give discrepant results should undergo nucleic acid testing.
- Rapid screening tests for HIV antibodies are typically sensitive, lateral flow or flow-through assays that can provide results in fewer than 30 minutes. These tests are especially suitable in certain situations, including resource-limited settings, occupational exposures, labor and delivery, and clinics or emergency departments where patients are unlikely to make a return visit.
- The Western blot, which was used for many years to confirm positive HIV antibody screening test results, detects antibody specificities to individual HIV antigens. It is no longer recommended for routine diagnosis of HIV because it is labor intensive, relatively insensitive, and has a long result-turnaround time, but it may be used for confirmation in special situations.
- HIV-infected patients are routinely monitored using two laboratory measurements: CD4 T-cell enumeration and HIV viral load.
- Peripheral blood CD4 T-cell counts and percentages are an excellent indicator of immune function and are routinely measured by multicolor immunofluorescence staining followed by analysis with flow cytometry. These measurements are used to stage HIV-infected patients and to monitor patients undergoing ART. Declining numbers can indicate if there is a need to change ART or initiate prophylactic therapy for opportunistic infections.
- Qualitative nucleic acid tests can be used to screen for HIV infection or make an initial patient diagnosis. PCR and TMA are the approved methods for these purposes, respectively.
- Quantitative tests, which measure the amount of HIV nucleic acid circulating in patient plasma, are known as *viral load tests*. These tests have had an important impact on the clinical management of HIV-infected patients by allowing physicians to predict disease progression, monitor patient response to anti-retroviral therapy, and guide treatment decisions.
- Viral load tests are performed by qPCR, a quantitative real-time RT-PCR method that uses reverse transcriptase to convert HIV RNA into cDNA and then amplifies the cDNA generated; and transcription-mediated amplification (TMA), an isothermal method that produces copies of HIV RNA.
- Drug-resistance testing can be performed by genotypic assays that use molecular methods or by phenotypic assays in which HIV replication in clinical isolates is assessed in the presence of varying concentrations of anti-retroviral drugs.
- Diagnosis of HIV in neonates is more complex than testing in adults. The presence of maternally acquired antibody in newborns makes tests for HIV antibody unreliable until a child is older than 18 months.
- Nucleic acid testing is recommended for the diagnosis of HIV infection in infants younger than 18 months. Testing can be performed with a qualitative PCR that detects HIV proviral DNA in the infant's peripheral blood mononuclear cells or a qualitative test for HIV RNA in the infant's plasma. Careful monitoring of HIV-infected mothers and early testing of infants at risk are recommended to facilitate prompt medical intervention.

Human T-Cell Lymphotropic Viruses (HTLV)

- The human T-cell lymphotropic viruses, HTLV-1 and HTLV-2, are retroviruses that infect $CD4^+$ T lymphocytes. HTLV-1 is the cause of adult T-cell leukemia and lymphoma (ATLL), HTLV-1–associated myelopathy/tropical spastic paraparesis (HAM/TSP), and other inflammatory disorders.

- HTLV-2 may be associated with a HAM/TSP-like neurological disease as well as hematologic and skin disorders, but the disease associations of this virus are unclear.
- ELISA and CLIA tests are used routinely to screen blood donors for antibodies to HTLV-1 and HTLV-2 and to detect exposure to HTLV in other individuals. Positive results are confirmed by Western blot or line immunoassays. PCR for proviral DNA can be used to clarify indeterminate results and monitor viral load in patients undergoing therapy.

CASE STUDIES

1. A young adult recently discovered that their partner tested HIV-positive. The individual was concerned that they may have also contracted the infection because they had experienced flu-like symptoms 1 month ago. The person decided to visit their physician for a medical evaluation.

Questions

a. What initial laboratory test should be performed on the patient to determine if they have been exposed to HIV?

b. If the patient tests positive in the initial evaluation, what follow-up testing should be performed to confirm the results?

c. If the patient's test results are confirmed to be positive, what tests should be done to monitor the patient over time?

2. A pregnant woman had used IV drugs in the past and recently discovered that she was HIV-positive. She was concerned that her baby would also contract HIV infection and discussed this with her physician.

Questions

a. How is HIV infection transmitted from mother to infant, and what measures should be taken to reduce the risk of HIV infection to the infant?

b. Should testing for HIV antibody be performed to determine if the infant is HIV-positive after birth? Explain your answer.

c. What type of laboratory testing would be best to evaluate the infant for HIV infection after birth?

3. A 65-year-old adult from southwestern Japan with a travel history to Central Africa presented with fatigue, skin rash, hepatosplenomegaly, and enlarged lymph nodes in the neck, armpit and groin. Laboratory tests revealed hypercalcemia. The HIV-1/2 antigen/antibody combination immunoassay was negative. Serology testing revealed that the patient was positive for HTLV-1 antibodies. Flow cytometry showed T cells expressing CD3, CD4, and CD25, loss of CD7, and negative for CD8. Microscopic analysis showed abnormal lymphocytes with lobulated, "flower-shaped" nuclei. Serology and flow cytometry results ruled out Sézary syndrome or other mature T-cell lymphomas and confirmed HTLV-1 as the etiologic agent.

Questions

a. Based on the laboratory results, what disease does the patient have?

b. Based on the patient's clinical features, what subtype of the disease do they have?

c. What is the median survival for this patient? How does that compare to other disease subtypes?

d. What is the worldwide distribution of HTLV-1 and HTLV-2 infection? Where is HTLV-1 endemic? How does the patient's travel history contribute to the likelihood of infection?

REVIEW QUESTIONS

1. All of the following describe HIV *except:*
   a. It possesses an outer envelope.
   b. It contains an inner core with p24 antigen.
   c. It contains DNA as its nucleic acid.
   d. It is a member of the retrovirus family.

2. HIV virions bind to host T cells through which receptors?
   a. CD4 and CD8
   b. CD4 and the IL-2 receptor
   c. CD4 and CCR5
   d. CD8 and CCR2

3. Suppose an HIV-1/2 antigen/antibody combination immunoassay to screen for HIV infection was positive, but the HIV-1/HIV-2 antibody differentiation test was nonreactive or indeterminate for HIV-1 and HIV-2. Which of the following tests should be performed?
   a. p24 antibody
   b. Western blot
   c. CD4 T-cell measurement
   d. NAT for HIV-1 or NAT HIV-1/-2

4. The most common means of HIV transmission worldwide is through:
   a. Blood transfusions
   b. Intimate sexual contact
   c. Sharing of needles in IV drug use
   d. Transplacental passage of the virus

5. An anti-retroviral drug that blocks the synthesis of HIV RNA because of its similarity to a nucleoside is a:
   a. Nucleoside analogue reverse transcriptase inhibitor
   b. Nonnucleoside reverse transcriptase inhibitor
   c. Protease inhibitor
   d. Fusion inhibitor

6. False-negative test results in a laboratory test for HIV antibody may occur because of:
   a. Heat inactivation of the serum before testing
   b. Collection of the test sample before seroconversion
   c. Interference by autoantibodies
   d. Recent exposure to certain vaccines

7. Which of the following combinations of bands would represent a positive Western blot for HIV antibody?
   a. p24 and p55
   b. p24 and p31
   c. gp41 and gp120
   d. p31 and p55

8. The fourth-generation combination immunoassays for HIV detect:
   a. HIV-1 and HIV-2 antigens
   b. HIV-1 and HIV-2 antibodies
   c. p24 antigen
   d. HIV-1 antibodies, HIV-2 antibodies, and p24 antigen

9. The characteristic laboratory finding in HIV infection is decreased:
   a. Numbers of CD4 T cells
   b. Numbers of CD8 T cells
   c. Numbers of CD20 B cells
   d. Immunoglobulins

10. Which of the following tests is currently recommended by the CDC to confirm a positive screening test result for HIV infection?
    a. Rapid test for HIV-1 and HIV-2 antibodies
    b. Western blot
    c. Molecular testing for HIV RNA
    d. HIV viral culture

11. Which of the following tests would give the *least* reliable results in a 2-month-old infant?
    a. CD4 T-cell count
    b. ELISA for HIV antibody
    c. PCR for HIV proviral DNA
    d. p24 antigen

12. Which of the following measurements is/are routinely used to monitor patients with HIV infection who are undergoing anti-retroviral therapy?
    a. HIV antibody titer
    b. p24 antigen levels
    c. CD4 T-cell and CD8 T-cell counts
    d. CD4 T-cell count and HIV RNA copy number

13. A positive result on a screening test for HTLV-1 antibody should be:
    a. Considered highly specific for HTLV-1 infection
    b. Followed by screening test for HIV
    c. Confirmed by Western blot
    d. Validated by viral culture

14. Which disease is associated with HTLV-1 infection?
    a. AIDS
    b. Adult T-cell leukemia/lymphoma (ATLL)
    c. Diabetes
    d. Wasting syndrome

15. Which subtype of ATLL is most common and has a median survival of about 6 months?
    a. Acute type
    b. T-cell non-Hodgkin lymphoma
    c. Chronic
    d. Smoldering

16. What are the four groups into which HIV-1 has been classified?
    a. M, O, N, P
    b. A, B, C, D
    c. HIV-1A, HIV-1E, HIV-1Y, HIV-1D
    d. A, AB, ABO, O

17. How is the acute phase of HIV infection characterized?
    a. Rapid burst of viral replication before the development of HIV-specific immune responses
    b. Insidious and slow replication of HIV after the development of HIV-specific immune responses
    c. Decreased viremia with subtle or absent symptoms
    d. Profound immunosuppression with very low numbers of CD4 T cells, and a resurgence of viremia

18. According to the CDC classification system for HIV infection, which best describes stage 0?
    a. Confirmed HIV-positive adults with a CD4 T-cell counts between 200 and 499 cells/μL
    b. Confirmed HIV-positive adults with a CD4 T-cell count less than 200 cells/μL
    c. Early HIV infection with an initial confirmed HIV-positive laboratory test result followed by a positive test within a 3-month period
    d. Early HIV infection with an initial confirmed HIV-positive laboratory test result followed by a negative or indeterminate test within a 6-month period

19. Which of the following is a benefit of HIV point-of-care testing?
    a. Convenience
    b. Privacy
    c. Rapid results
    d. All of the above

20. Isothermal amplification of nucleic acid in which RNA amplicons are the final product describes:
    a. Quantitative PCR (qPCR)
    b. Transcription-mediated amplification (TMA)
    c. Western blot
    d. Lateral flow immunoassay

21. True or False: Both HTLV and HIV use reverse transcriptase to transcribe viral RNA into DNA, which then becomes integrated into the host-cell's genome as a provirus.
    a. True
    b. False

Chapter 24 Answer Key

Answers to Knowledge Check

24.1 c 24.2 d 24.3 a 24.4 c 24.5 b 24.6 a

Answers to Review Questions

1. c	2. c	3. d	4. b	5. a	6. b
7. c	8. d	9. a	10. a	11. b	12. d
13. c	14. b	15. a	16. a	17. a	18. d
19. d	20. b	21. a			

25 Immunization and Vaccines

Linda E. Miller, PhD, I, MB^{CM}(ASCP)SI

LEARNING OUTCOMES

After finishing this chapter, you should be able to:

25.1 Explain the underlying principles of active immunity, passive immunity, and adoptive immunity and provide examples of each.

25.2 Discuss the historical evolution of vaccines, from the early contributions of Edward Jenner through modern approaches to producing vaccines.

25.3 Define *vaccine, toxoid, attenuation, adjuvant, recombinant protein vaccine,* and *community (herd) immunity.*

25.4 Describe the composition of the following types of vaccines: live attenuated, inactivated, toxoid, polysaccharide, purified protein, recombinant, mRNA, and viral vector. Contrast their advantages and limitations and provide examples of each type of vaccine.

25.5 Discuss host factors, pathogen factors, and vaccine/adjuvant characteristics that influence the immune response to vaccines and determine the ways in which vaccines are administered.

25.6 List two broad categories of adjuvants, recognize examples of each, and explain the mechanisms by which they enhance the immune response to vaccines.

25.7 Contrast the benefits and adverse effects associated with vaccines.

25.8 Differentiate between IV immunoglobulin therapy and antigen-specific globulins and their clinical applications.

25.9 Differentiate between mouse monoclonal antibodies, chimeric antibodies, humanized antibodies, and fully human antibodies in terms of their structure and nomenclature.

25.10 Discuss some of the clinical applications of monoclonal antibody therapy.

25.11 Explain the benefits and limitations of passive immunization.

25.12 Discuss clinical applications of adoptive immunotherapy.

25.13 Describe the structure of chimeric antigen receptors and the clinical utility of CAR-T cells.

CHAPTER OUTLINE

You can go to **fadavis.com** keyword stevens for the laboratory exercises that accompany this text.

As we discussed in Chapter 1, **immunity** can be defined as the condition of being resistant to disease, most notably to infections. The process by which this state of protection is acquired is called **immunization.** Three types of immunity can be acquired through immunization: active, passive, and adoptive.

Active immunity results from immunization with a specific antigen by natural exposure to infection or administration of a vaccine. Adaptive, or antigen-specific, immune responses to bacteria, viruses, fungi, and parasites can all result in active immunity. For example, production of antibodies to a specific strain of group A streptococci bacteria following a streptococcal sore throat protects a person from future infection with that strain of bacteria. Active immunity is also stimulated through the administration of vaccines (see sections that follow). For example, after receiving all doses of the measles vaccine, most people develop immunity to the measles virus. In active immunity, the individual's own immune system is stimulated to mount an adaptive immune response to an antigen. The advantage of active immunization over other types of immunization is that it results in long-term memory to an antigen, providing potentially lifelong protection against the harmful effects of a pathogen.

Passive immunity results from the transfer of antibodies from immunized hosts to a nonimmune individual. This state of immunity can occur naturally, from transfer of a mother's antibodies to her fetus or infant, or artificially, through passive immunization of an individual with commercial antibody preparations. The latter application, **passive immunotherapy,** can be used to prevent or treat disease. An example of passive immunotherapy is the use of pooled human antibodies to protect a person who has an immunodeficiency disease. The main advantage of passive immunization is that it provides immediate protection to an individual who has not developed immunity to a particular antigen.

Adoptive immunity results from the transfer of cells of the immune system, usually lymphocytes, from an immunized host to a nonimmune individual. **Adoptive immunotherapy** involves the administration of immune cells to treat patients with conditions such as immunodeficiency diseases or cancer. This type of therapy can be beneficial if the cells transferred can successfully establish themselves in the recipient. An example of adoptive immunotherapy is transplantation of hematopoietic stem cells (HSCs) to restore immune function in patients with leukemia who have been treated with high doses of irradiation and chemotherapy.

The primary difference between the immunity gained by active, passive, and adoptive immunization is that in active immunity, an individual's own immune system is responding to an antigen. In passive and adoptive immunity, immunity is provided to an individual through the transfer of antibodies or cells from another source to provide immediate protection.

In this chapter, we discuss the mechanisms by which active, passive, and adoptive immunity occur in the context of their advantages and limitations. We describe clinical examples under each category so you can develop a better understanding of how knowledge of basic immunology principles can be translated into therapies that benefit humankind. We place a special focus on the topic of vaccines because their use has significantly improved the health of populations worldwide.

Knowledge Check 25-1

Active immunity differs from passive immunity in that the former involves:

a. Artificial induction of the immune response
b. Stimulation of a person's immune system by an antigen
c. Transfer of premade antibodies to a person
d. Transfer of immune cells to a person

Vaccines

A **vaccine** is an antigenic preparation that stimulates an immune response against a pathogen or disease. Vaccines containing pathogen-derived antigens are routinely given to healthy people to prevent infectious diseases from developing or producing severe medical consequences. These vaccines are a form of **immunoprophylaxis,** or the prevention of disease through immunization. Vaccines have had a tremendous impact on public health by significantly reducing the incidence of illness and death from many diseases that had devastating effects on civilization. Vaccines for cancer have been developed as **immunotherapy** for patients who already have the disease (see Chapter 17). In this section, we discuss the historical evolution of vaccines, the different forms of vaccines, how they are routinely administered, factors that affect their effectiveness, and vaccine strategies for the future.

Historical Evolution of Vaccines

As we discussed in Chapter 1, the science of immunology was born out of early observations of immunity and studies involving vaccination. The goal of these studies was to eliminate death and suffering caused by infectious diseases. Advances in science and technology during the 20th century and beyond have led to the creation of safer, more effective vaccines and remarkable success toward that goal.

Smallpox and the First Vaccine

One of the most feared diseases in ancient times was smallpox, a highly fatal illness characterized by a high fever and pustular rash. Those who survived the disease were usually left with disfiguring scars or blindness. It was noted in Greece as early as 430 BC that people who survived this infection became immune to the deadly disease. These observations led to *variolation,* the subcutaneous injection of fresh material from a skin lesion of a person recovering from smallpox into the arm or leg of a nonimmune person. Recall from Chapter 1 that in an older form of the procedure practiced in ancient China, the material was dried into a powder and inhaled by the nonimmune person. Variolation usually resulted in milder disease and recovery and was performed for centuries in Africa, India, and China. In the 18th century, the practice was introduced to Europe, where over 400,000 people died each year from smallpox, so the procedure quickly became popular. However, variolation was not without risks; 1% to 2% of the recipients developed smallpox and died, and others contracted infectious diseases such as syphilis or tuberculosis (TB) from the injected material.

These observations led to the search for a safer procedure. Farmers observed that milkmaids who had a similar but milder disease called *cowpox* were protected from contracting the deadlier smallpox. The farmers, therefore, used cellular material from the cowpox lesions of milkmaids to variolate others and observed the same protective effects without the danger of contracting smallpox **(Fig. 25–1).** The English physician Edward Jenner brought fame to this procedure when, in 1796, he injected fluid from the cowpox lesions of a milkmaid into an 8-year-old boy. When Jenner later inoculated the boy with smallpox, he did not develop the disease, showing that the method was a success. Jenner called this procedure "vaccination" after the Latin word *vacca,* meaning "cow." The protective effects induced by the vaccination were caused by **cross-reactivity** (i.e., antigenic similarity) between the viruses that caused cowpox and smallpox. This early vaccine for smallpox led to the development of the modern smallpox vaccine, which is still derived from the *vaccinia* virus that causes cowpox **(Fig. 25–2).** The vaccine was so successful that smallpox has been eradicated from the world, and the vaccine is no longer routinely administered.

The 1800s: Pasteur's Contributions to Vaccine Development

Despite the early development of the smallpox vaccine, many years passed before scientists understood that microbes were the underlying cause of infectious diseases and that components of these pathogens could be used to produce protective vaccines. Thus, it was not until 80 years after Jenner's procedure that the next vaccine was developed by the French scientist, Louis Pasteur, against chicken cholera. Pasteur subsequently developed vaccines against anthrax and rabies, which were based on the principle of attenuation. **Attenuation** involves the use of bacteria or viruses that have been weakened by exposure to conditions that modify their growth (see "Live, Attenuated Vaccines"). These weakened microorganisms do not cause disease in healthy individuals but are able to stimulate the immune response because they contain many of the same antigens as their pathogenic counterpart.

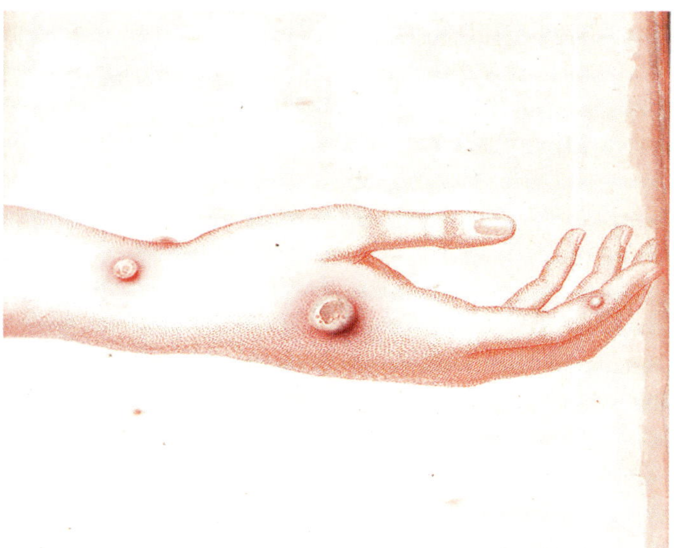

FIGURE 25–1 Color etching of a hand and wrist with cowpox lesions, from Edward Jenner's "Inquiry Into the Causes and Effects of the *Variolae Vaccinae.*" The etching shows several stages of cowpox, from early blistering to its later dimpled rupture. *(Courtesy of the National Library of Medicine, National Institutes of Health & Human Services. Bethesda, MD.)*

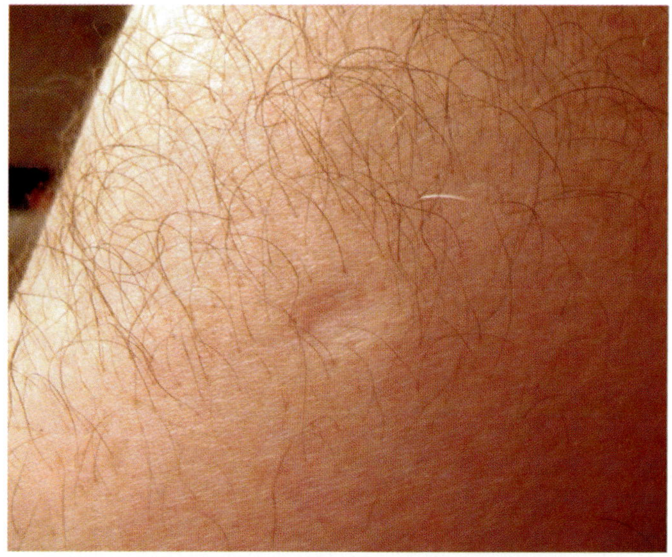

FIGURE 25–2 Evidence of smallpox vaccination. People who have received the smallpox vaccine develop a blister, which dries up and forms a scab within the first 2 weeks. They can be identified by the scar that forms at the site of injection once the scab falls off. *(Courtesy of Linda Miller.)*

The rabies vaccine, for which Pasteur is most famous, was developed in 1885. Recognizing that rabies affected the central nervous system (CNS), Pasteur prepared an attenuated vaccine by repeatedly infecting rabbits with material contaminated with rabies, recovering the rabbits' spinal cords, and exposing them to dry air to make a vaccine. After testing the vaccine on dogs, he administered his vaccine preparation to a 9-year-old boy who had been severely bitten by a rabid dog. The boy received a series of subcutaneous injections over a period of 10 days and never developed rabies **(Fig. 25–3).** Pasteur received worldwide honors for this treatment and was the first person to use the word *vaccination* in reference to all immunization procedures.

Pasteur believed that only live, attenuated organisms could be used for effective immunization, and these remain the basis for many vaccines used today. However, in the late 1800s, scientists Salmon and Smith showed that a killed suspension of *Vibrio cholerae* could provide pigeons with protection against cholera. A few years later, vaccines against human cholera, typhoid fever, and plague were developed using whole killed organisms.

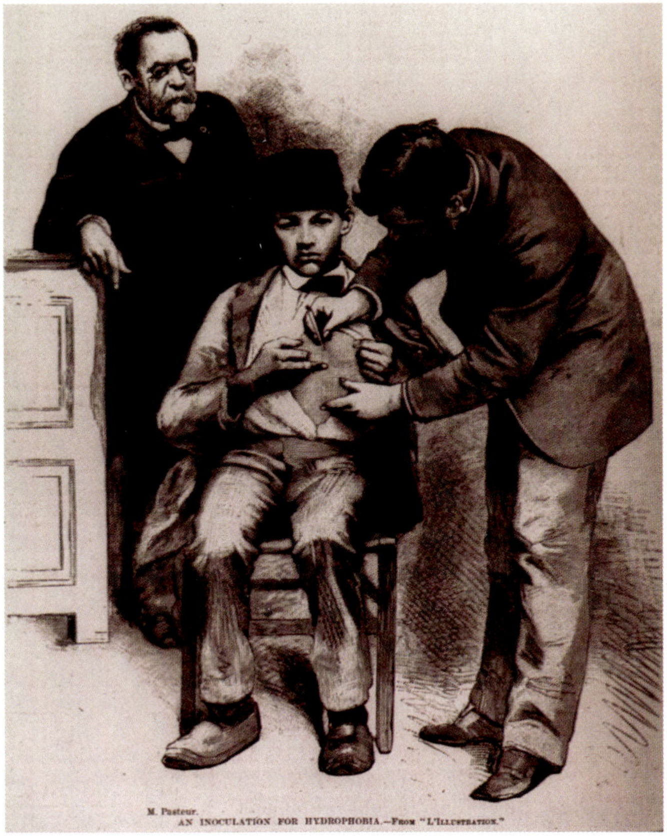

FIGURE 25–3 Louis Pasteur observes as a young boy receives an inoculation for hydrophobia (a symptom of rabies). *(Courtesy of the National Library of Medicine, National Institutes of Health and Human Services. Bethesda, MD.)*

Twentieth-Century Vaccines

The 20th century witnessed a tremendous expansion in vaccine development because of advances in scientific research and laboratory techniques. New methods of attenuating microorganisms, growing viruses in culture, inactivating bacterial toxins, and genetic engineering enabled the production of many vaccines. Following are some of the major developments during this period:

- Development of live, attenuated vaccines against tuberculosis (TB), typhoid fever, yellow fever, and influenza A (1920s to 1940s).
- Production of chemically inactivated bacterial toxins called **toxoids**, allowing for development of vaccines against diphtheria and tetanus (1920s).
- Development of attenuated viral vaccines, including those against polio, measles, mumps, rubella, and varicella (1950 to 1980).
- Use of purified bacterial polysaccharides in vaccines to prevent meningococcal meningitis, pneumococcal pneumonia, and *Haemophilus influenzae* type b (Hib) (1970s and 1980s). In the late 1980s, these vaccines were made more effective by linking the polysaccharides to a protein, forming *glycoconjugates* that can be recognized by T cells.
- Production of the first **recombinant** (i.e., genetically engineered) **protein vaccine** in 1986 against hepatitis B. The vaccine consists of purified hepatitis B surface antigen (HBsAg) made by genetically modified yeast cells that have incorporated the gene for HBsAg.

Beyond the 20th Century

The beginning of the 21st century has seen continued use and refinements in vaccine technologies:

- The first decade of the 21st century witnessed the licensure of live, attenuated vaccines for influenza, rotavirus, and herpes zoster, and multivalent, glycoconjugate vaccines for pneumococcus and meningococcus.
- Vaccines composed of genetically recombinant antigens from the human papillomavirus (HPV; the cause of cervical cancer, other genital cancers, and anal cancer) and the herpes zoster virus (the cause of shingles) were also introduced.
- In 2020, during the COVID-19 (coronavirus disease 2019) pandemic, vaccines consisting of mRNA from SARS-CoV-2 (severe acute respiratory syndrome coronavirus 2) were developed to prevent severe disease and death.

According to the World Health Organization (WHO), vaccines are available worldwide to prevent more than 25 infectious diseases. However, many diseases still present a challenge to the medical profession because they cannot be prevented by immunization. Research is ongoing to develop new vaccines that target these diseases by applying advanced genetic technologies. Later in this chapter, we discuss some of these challenges and strategies for future vaccine development.

Knowledge Check 25-2

Live, weakened microorganisms used in vaccines are:
a. Attenuated
b. Inactivated
c. Toxoids
d. Recombinant

Types of Vaccines

Vaccines routinely used for infectious diseases consist of (1) live, attenuated (nonpathogenic) microorganisms; (2) inactivated (killed) microorganisms; (3) antigenic components of microorganisms (i.e., subunit vaccines); or (4) mRNA that codes for a protein antigen of a pathogen. Refer to **Figure 25–4** and the text that follows for a presentation of the main features of each vaccine type. We also introduce newer strategies for future vaccine development in this section.

Vaccine preparations also contain preservatives, such as thimerosal, to prevent bacterial and fungal contamination, and stabilizers to maintain the activity of the ingredients. Some vaccines contain *adjuvants* to enhance the immune response (see discussion later).

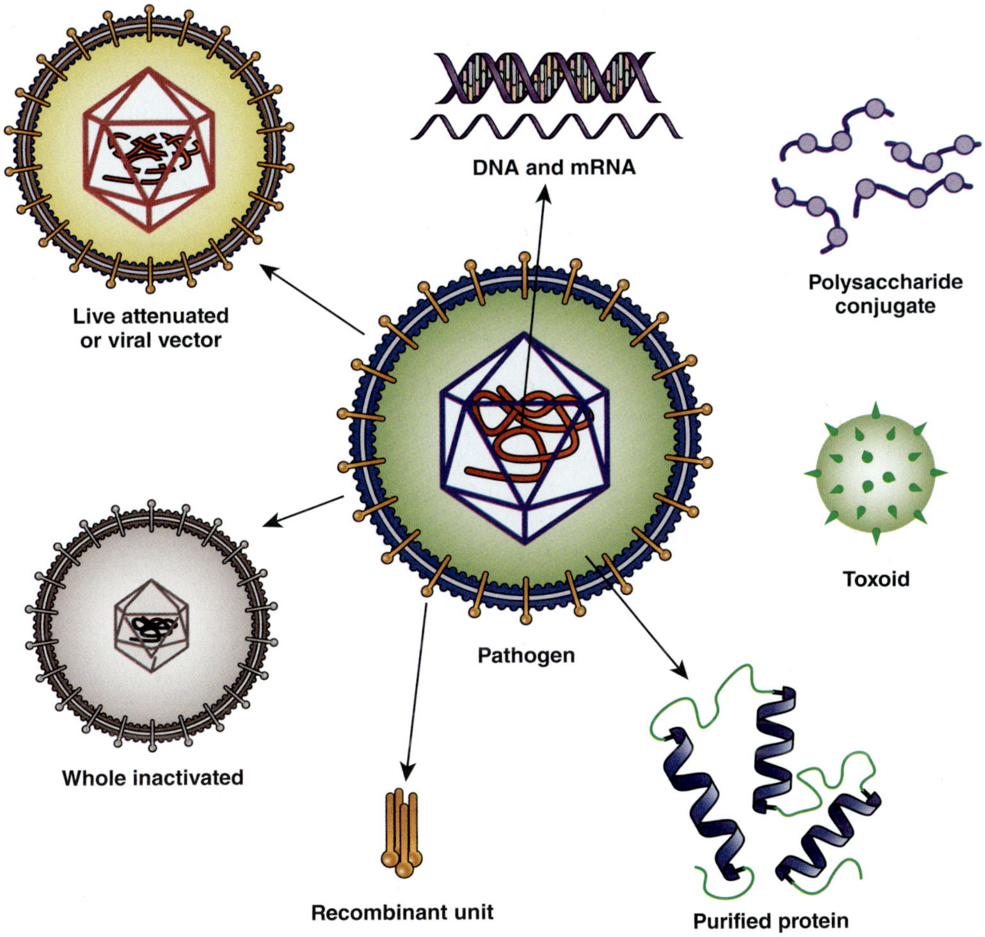

FIGURE 25–4 Major types of vaccines: attenuated, inactivated, toxoid, recombinant, DNA, mRNA, purified protein, polysaccharide conjugate, and viral vector.

Live, Attenuated Vaccines

Live, attenuated vaccines consist of viruses or bacteria that have been modified so that they lose their pathogenic properties but can still stimulate a good immune response. To prepare these vaccines, the microorganism is cultured under conditions that are different from those in the host and are unfavorable to its growth (e.g., growing bacteria in different media, growing the organism at a different temperature or in the presence of a chemical, or repeatedly passaging viruses in cell lines, a technique in which some of the cells are periodically transferred to a flask containing fresh nutrient medium). These conditions select for forms of the organism that have been genetically modified to make them weaker. Molecular techniques can also be used to create mutant forms of the organism that lack a particular gene and have lost their virulence.

Attenuated vaccines are more easily prepared against viruses than bacteria, as the latter have a more complex structure. Examples of attenuated vaccines in routine use for preventing viral infections are those for the following:

- Polio, a serious disease that causes aseptic meningitis and paralysis. In the early 1960s, Albert Sabin developed an oral polio vaccine containing three serotypes of live, attenuated poliovirus cultured in monkey kidney cells. Each **serotype** is a form of the virus that can be distinguished by specific antigens that can be identified by serological typing. Sabin's vaccine was the main poliovirus vaccine used in the United States from 1963 to 1997, before a potent inactivated polio vaccine was licensed. Although the oral polio vaccine is no longer available in the United States because of its potential for adverse effects (see "Benefits and Adverse Effects of Vaccines"), an oral vaccine is still used in some lower-income countries of the world because it is easier to administer than the inactivated vaccine, which requires injections.
- Measles, mumps, rubella, and varicella (MMR or MMRV; see Chapter 23 for disease descriptions).
- Influenza ("flu"; see Chapter 23). This form of the influenza vaccine is administered intranasally. The main antigens targeted by the vaccine are two surface glycoproteins of the influenza virus called *hemagglutinin* (H) and *neuraminidase* (N). A new attenuated influenza vaccine must be prepared each year because of the high mutation rate of the influenza viruses, which results in the synthesis of modified antigens to which people have not developed immunity. The vaccine consists of a trivalent or quadrivalent suspension containing commonly circulating antigenic strains of influenza A (H3N2) and influenza A (H1N1), plus one or two influenza B virus strains grown in embryonated hen eggs.
- Rotavirus, an intestinal virus that can cause severe diarrhea and dehydration.

Examples of live, attenuated vaccines for bacterial infections include the following:

- *Bacille Calmette-Guérin (BCG)*, a vaccine for TB developed by Albert Calmette and Camille Guérin at the Pasteur Institute in 1927 (see Chapter 20). The preparation contains an attenuated strain of *Mycobacterium bovis* grown on culture media containing increasing concentrations of bile.
- A vaccine against typhoid fever, an intestinal infection caused by *Salmonella* bacteria. The vaccine consists of a mutated strain of *Salmonella typhi* packaged into capsules that are ingested orally.

Advantages and Limitations

The main advantage of live, attenuated vaccines is that the organisms can replicate at a low level in the host and, therefore, induce strong immunity by stimulating cell-mediated immune responses in addition to humoral responses. This is especially important for viral infections because cytotoxic T cells are required to attack viruses during the intracellular phase of the viral life cycle. Because of the broad immunity induced by live, attenuated vaccines, they generally induce an effective immune response after just a single dose.

Despite these advantages, live, attenuated vaccines also have some major limitations. It is important *not* to administer vaccines containing live organisms to immunocompromised individuals. Although the organisms are attenuated, they may cause severe, disseminated, and potentially fatal infections in patients with immunodeficiency diseases or patients receiving immunosuppressive treatments. Live vaccines may also not be recommended for use in pregnant women. On rare occasions, mutations may occur in the vaccine organism, causing it to lose its attenuation and revert to the pathogenic form. This unfortunately occurred during use of the live, attenuated (Sabin) vaccine for polio, which led to the vaccine's replacement with an inactivated polio vaccine in industrialized countries. The use of genomic techniques to design live, attenuated strains that lack the genes required for pathogenicity will hopefully prevent such an occurrence in the future.

Another limitation of live, attenuated vaccines is potential interference with replication of the organism from maternal antibodies in infants, necessitating a delay in the dosing schedule (see "Factors Affecting Vaccine Effectiveness"). Finally, careful handling and storage of attenuated vaccines is very important because exposure to heat and light may destroy the live organisms, causing the vaccines to become ineffective. This requirement can pose a major problem in developing countries of the world, where refrigeration may not be readily available.

Inactivated Vaccines

Inactivated vaccines consist of intact viruses or bacteria that are killed by heat or chemical treatment so they are not pathogenic but retain their antigenic properties. Chemicals such as formaldehyde or β-propiolactone are used more often than heat treatment because they are less likely to alter the structure of the surface epitopes. Following are examples of commonly used inactivated vaccines:

- The intramuscular vaccine for polio, developed in the early 1950s by Jonas Salk. The vaccine consists of the three disease-related serotypes of poliovirus killed by chemical treatment. This form of the polio vaccine is used routinely today in developed countries of the world because of its effectiveness and safety.
- The inactivated influenza vaccines, which contain one influenza A (H3N2) virus strain, one influenza A (H1N1) virus strain, and one or two influenza B virus strains killed by chemical treatment. Many versions of these influenza vaccines are available; some use viruses grown in embryonated hen eggs, while others use virus grown in cultured mammalian cells. The vaccines are administered by intramuscular injection.
- The hepatitis A vaccine, which consists of purified hepatitis A virus (HAV) cultured in human fibroblasts and chemically inactivated. Although this vaccine was initially only given to people at high risk for contracting hepatitis A, it has been incorporated into routine childhood immunization programs to reduce the incidence of this common infection.

A major advantage of inactivated vaccines is that they can be safely given to immunocompromised people because the organisms have been killed and cannot replicate in the body. However, this property makes it necessary to provide a larger amount of antigen to stimulate an effective immune response. Two or more booster doses administered over time are often required to produce protective immunity. The repeated doses induce a memory response, with a shorter lag time before antibody production, and higher, more persistent antibody titers (see Chapter 3). Because the inactivated organisms do not infect host cells, these vaccines mainly induce a humoral immune response, with little or no cell-mediated immunity.

Subunit Vaccines

Subunit vaccines consist of one or more purified components of a pathogen that can stimulate an immune response. In general, this type of vaccine has a high safety profile because whole organisms are not used; however, booster doses and adjuvants (see later section) are required to produce a strong, protective immune response. The forms of subunit vaccines routinely used are toxoids, capsular polysaccharides, purified proteins, and recombinant protein antigens.

Toxoid Vaccines

The pathology of some bacterial diseases, such as diphtheria and tetanus, is caused by a single exotoxin. **Toxoids** are bacterial exotoxins that have been chemically inactivated so that they cannot cause harm to the host but retain their ability to stimulate an immune response. Toxoids are used in vaccines to induce the production of antibodies that can bind to exotoxins and neutralize their effects. Toxoid vaccines are routinely used to protect against the following:

- Diphtheria, a contagious, life-threatening infection of the upper respiratory tract. The vaccine consists of a formaldehyde-inactivated toxin from the causative organism, *Corynebacterium diphtheriae*.

- Tetanus, a serious infection that affects the nervous system. The vaccine consists of a formaldehyde-inactivated toxin from the causative organism, *Clostridium tetani.*
- Pertussis ("whooping cough"). Inactivated toxin from the bacterium *Bordetella pertussis* is part of the acellular pertussis vaccine (see "Purified Protein Vaccines").

The vaccines for diphtheria, tetanus, and pertussis are available singly or in combinations known as *DTaP, TdaP, DT,* or *Td,* depending on the amounts of diphtheria, tetanus, and acellular pertussis components.

Polysaccharide Vaccines

Some bacteria have a hydrophilic polysaccharide capsule that covers their outer membrane and allows them to resist phagocytosis and other immune defenses (see Chapter 20). Vaccines against encapsulated bacteria contain purified capsular polysaccharides that stimulate antibody production to facilitate clearance of the organisms through opsonization or complement-mediated lysis. Because the structure of these capsular antigens varies with different bacterial serotypes, these vaccines contain multiple polysaccharide types to ensure an immune response that provides broad protection. Examples of polysaccharide vaccines in routine use are those against the following:

- *Streptococcuvs pneumoniae,* the cause of pneumococcal pneumonia. Different forms of the vaccine are available for children and adults; they each contain polysaccharides from multiple *S. pneumoniae* serotypes.
- *Hemophilus influenzae* type b (Hib), which was a major cause of pneumonia and meningitis in infants and young children before the vaccine was implemented. The vaccine is composed of the polyribosylribitol phosphate component of the Hib capsule conjugated to a protein carrier.
- *Neisseria meningitidis,* an important cause of bacterial meningitis, especially in young people living in close quarters such as dormitory buildings. A vaccine consisting of five purified bacterial capsular polysaccharides (A, B, C, Y, W-135) from *N. meningitidis* is available for persons 10 to 25 years old.

A problem with polysaccharide antigens is that they do not induce a good immune response, especially in infants and older adults, two populations that are at high risk for severe consequences of encapsulated bacterial infections. This is because polysaccharides are T-independent antigens that stimulate IgM production with no immunoglobulin class-switching or long-term memory response (see Chapter 5). This problem has been overcome by using *glycoconjugates,* polysaccharide antigens linked to a carrier protein such as tetanus toxoid. The conjugates induce a more effective immune response by activating helper T (T_H) cells, resulting in immunoglobulin class-switching, production of polysaccharide-specific IgG antibodies, and generation of memory cells.

Purified Protein Vaccines

This type of vaccine uses proteins derived from a pathogen. One such vaccine protects against pertussis, a serious respiratory disease also known as "whooping cough" because of the characteristic whooping sound patients make while trying to breathe during violent coughing fits. The vaccine is made from purified proteins of *Bordetella pertussis* and has fewer side effects than the previous vaccine made from whole bacterial cells. It is combined with the vaccines for diphtheria and tetanus (see "Toxoid Vaccines"). Purified protein vaccines stimulate good antibody responses but do not induce cytotoxic T-cell responses.

Recombinant Protein Vaccines

Several protein vaccines are made using recombinant DNA technology. In these methods, the gene coding for a specific protein antigen from a pathogenic microorganism is isolated and incorporated into the genome of nonpathogenic yeast or mammalian cells. The genetically modified cells are cultured in large quantities and produce the desired antigen, which is then purified by conventional biochemical methods **(Fig. 25–5).** In this way, vaccines can be produced in a cost-effective manner that does not require the culture of pathogenic organisms and produces fewer side effects in recipients. Examples of recombinant protein vaccines are those for the following:

- Hepatitis B. The vaccines contain recombinant hepatitis B surface antigen (HBsAg; see Chapter 23).
- Human papillomavirus (HPV), a cause of cervical cancer, other genital cancers, anal cancer, and oropharyngeal cancer. These vaccines contain recombinant L1 major capsid proteins from nine HPV virus types (including types 16 and 18) that are highly associated with anal-genital cancers.
- Varicella-zoster virus (VZV), the cause of shingles. The vaccine contains recombinant VZV envelope glycoprotein E antigen.
- Influenza. This form of the influenza vaccine contains recombinant haemagglutinin (HA) proteins of three to four commonly circulating strains of influenza A and influenza B viruses.
- Respiratory syncytial virus (RSV). The vaccine contains recombinant RSV surface protein F.

Messenger RNA (mRNA) Vaccines

Messenger RNA (mRNA) vaccines work by instructing the host's cells to make the vaccine antigen. As we discussed in Chapter 12, mRNA carries the genetic code in DNA from the nucleus to the cytoplasm, where it is translated into the amino acid sequence of a protein. To make an mRNA vaccine, the DNA sequence for the desired protein antigen is identified and cloned in bacterial plasmids to produce millions of copies. The corresponding mRNA sequence is transcribed from the DNA in the laboratory, purified to remove contaminants, and processed to improve stability. It is then packaged into lipid nanoparticles to prevent its degradation and facilitate its uptake by host cells. After the vaccine is injected intramuscularly, the mRNA is engulfed by the host's antigen-presenting cells (APCs), where it is translated into the designated protein by ribosomes in the cytoplasm. The protein is complexed with a major histocompatibility complex (MHC) molecule and transported to the cell surface, where it is presented to T cells and stimulates an immune response.

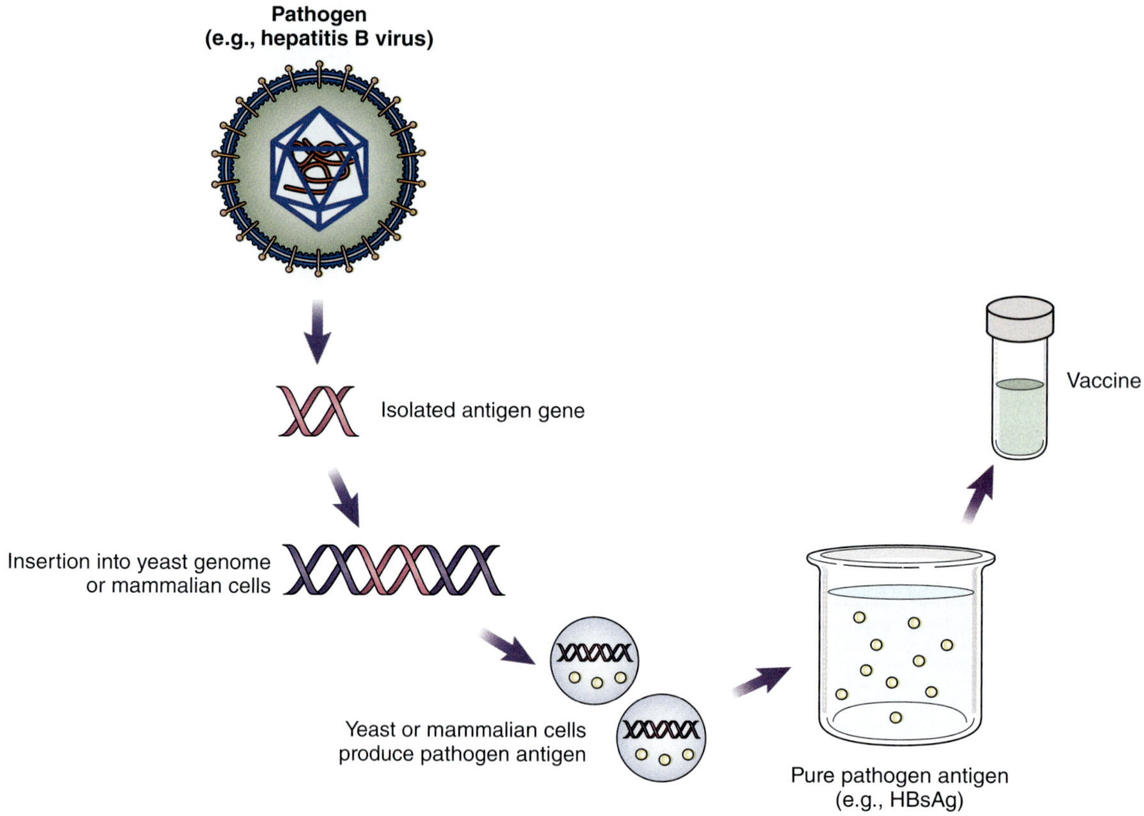

FIGURE 25–5 Production of a recombinant vaccine. The gene that codes for a pathogen-derived antigen is identified and cloned in yeast or mammalian cells, which produce large amounts of the pathogen antigen when they multiply in culture. The antigen is retrieved and purified to make the vaccine.

At the end of 2020, mRNA vaccines were approved by the U.S. Food and Drug Administration (FDA) for emergency use for severe acute respiratory syndrome coronavirus 2 (SARS-CoV-2), the cause of the pandemic disease COVID-19. The vaccine, which contains mRNA coding for the outer spike protein of the virus, has had a tremendous impact on reducing the incidence of severe disease and death caused by the virus **(Fig. 25–6).** Studies are under way to evaluate the use of mRNA vaccines in preventing other infectious diseases and in treating cancer.

The mRNA-based vaccines have several advantages: they can be manufactured rapidly and inexpensively, they do not contain infectious material, and they generate strong immune responses. Also, the mRNA is degraded quickly and cannot integrate into the host genome. However, they require cold storage and can produce inflammatory reactions in some individuals.

Viral Vector Vaccines

Viral vector vaccines use a genetically modified nonpathogenic virus, such as an adenovirus, to deliver the genetic code for a vaccine antigen to host cells. The vector enters host cells and inserts the genetic material, which instructs the cells to produce the vaccine antigen. A strong immune response is induced, but vaccine design is complex, the vaccines cannot be given to immunocompromised people, and the vaccines have reduced effectiveness in people who have been previously exposed to the viral vector and developed an immune response against it. Viral vector vaccines for SARS-CoV-2 have not been approved in the United States but have been used in other countries. Viral vector vaccines have also been designed to prevent other infectious diseases, such as dengue and Ebola.

Knowledge Check 25-3

Match each disease with the type of vaccine used to prevent it:

a. Measles	____ 1. Conjugated polysaccharide
b. Tetanus	____ 2. Inactivated
c. *Haemophilus influenzae* type b	____ 3. mRNA
d. Polio	____ 4. Toxoid
e. COVID-19	____ 5. Attenuated
f. Hepatitis B	____ 6. Recombinant

Factors Affecting Vaccine Effectiveness

Vaccine effectiveness is determined by the ability to protect people against infection, symptomatic illness, hospitalization, and death. The main factors that influence vaccine efficacy are related to the host, the pathogen, and the vaccine. Immunization experts consider these factors when deciding how a vaccine should be administered to achieve an optimal immune response.

Host Factors

The main host factors that experts consider in determining how a vaccine is administered include a person's age,

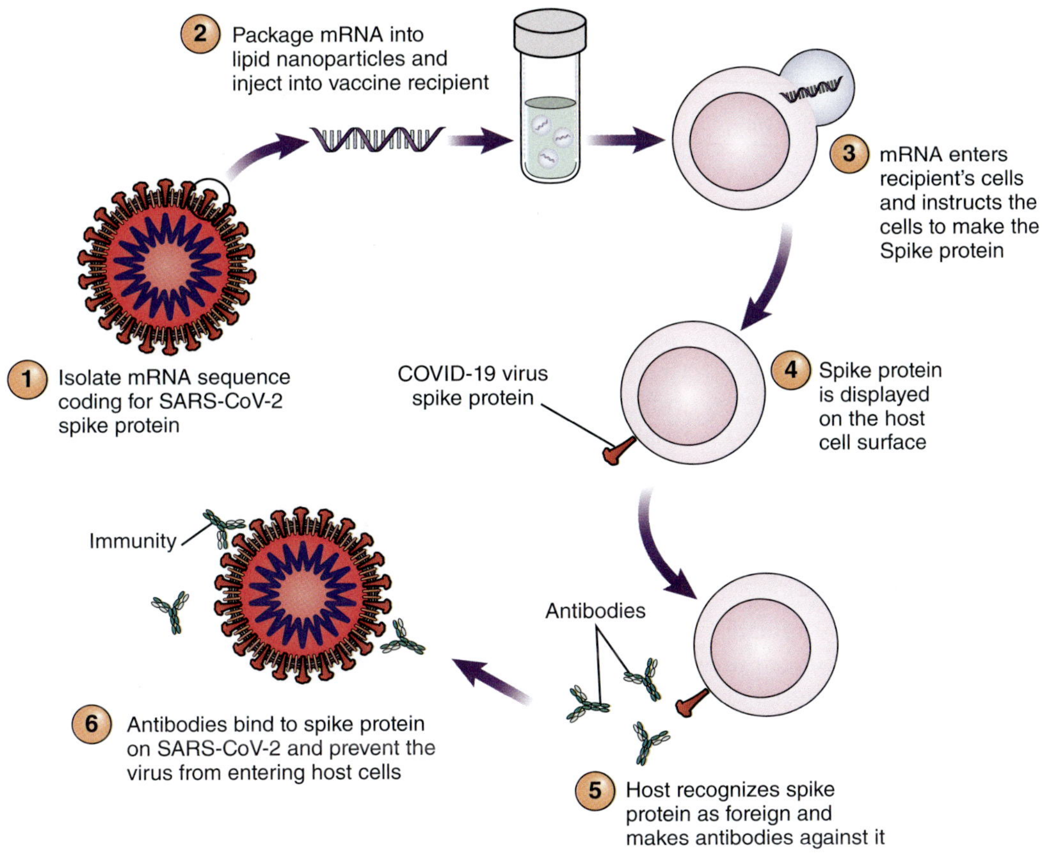

FIGURE 25–6 Principle of mRNA vaccine for COVID-19. The mRNA contains the genetic code for the SARS-CoV-2 virus spike protein. It instructs the host's APCs to make the spike protein, which is then displayed on the cell surface and induces a strong immune response.

presence of certain medical conditions, previous exposure to the antigen, and other factors that could interfere with antibody production. Other characteristics that can influence an individual's immune response to a vaccine are their genetic makeup, sex, nutritional status, gut microbiota, and obesity.

Age is an important factor in determining how a vaccine should be provided to people in a population. Older adults and infants typically show reduced immune responses to vaccines and may require stronger vaccine doses or repeated administration of a vaccine to achieve optimal immunity.

Thus, age-related recommendations for routine vaccine administration are based on the risk of contracting a disease and the recipient's ability to respond to the vaccine. In the United States, vaccination schedules recommended by the Centers for Disease Control and Prevention's (CDC) Advisory Committee on Immunization Practices (ACIP) are categorized according to age. The schedules are revised annually by the ACIP in consultation with the American Academy of Pediatrics (AAP) and the American Academy of Family Physicians (AAFP). See https://www.cdc.gov/vaccines for up-to-date schedules and additional information about vaccines. As of this writing, some age-related recommendations are:

- Begin immunization against hepatitis B soon after birth because the hepatitis B virus may have been transferred through the placenta.
- Begin vaccines for diphtheria, pertussis, tetanus, rotavirus, *H. influenzae* type b, polio, and streptococcal pneumonia at 2 months of age, followed by booster shots periodically through the first 18 months of life to achieve optimal immunity, because the infant's immune system is immature. Additional doses of some of these vaccines are recommended during childhood, adolescence, and/or adulthood to maintain high antibody titers.
- Give the live, attenuated vaccine for measles, mumps, and rubella at 12 to 15 months of age because maternal antibodies that have passed through the placenta limit replication of the attenuated viruses and interfere with the infant's immune response.
- Give vaccines for meningococcal meningitis and HPV at 11 to 12 years of age because the risk for contracting these infections is greater during adolescence.
- Give other vaccines, such as those for varicella zoster (the cause of shingles) and pneumococcal pneumonia, later in adulthood because the natural decline of immune function in older individuals makes them more susceptible to developing these infections.

The recommendations may be revised in special situations. For example, additional vaccine doses may be recommended for people who are immunocompromised or have chronic diseases that make them less capable of mounting an effective immune response. Also, people who are immunocompromised should not receive live, attenuated vaccines (see "Benefits and Adverse Effects of Vaccines" section). A few vaccines, such as those for typhoid fever or yellow fever, are recommended only for people traveling to areas of the world where there is a high incidence of these diseases.

Pathogen Factors

Some viruses, notably influenza A virus, influenza B virus, and SARS-CoV-2, have high mutation rates. Therefore, vaccine formulations for these pathogens must be modified annually based on the most common circulating strains.

Nature of the Vaccine and Adjuvants

The vaccine type is another important factor influencing the quality of the immune response. In general, the most immunogenic vaccines consist of live, attenuated organisms that can replicate in the host, and the least immunogenic vaccines consist of purified components (subunits) derived from the pathogen. Vaccine antigens with a low level of immunogenicity require an adjuvant (see discussion that follows).

Adjuvants

An **adjuvant** is a substance that is administered together with a vaccine antigen to produce a stronger immune response. Adjuvants are used in vaccines to increase antibody titers and, for some vaccines, to also stimulate cell-mediated immunity. Effective adjuvants can reduce the dose of antigen needed in a vaccine, decrease the number of inoculations required, and increase the speed and duration of the immune response.

Diverse molecules can function as vaccine adjuvants, including emulsions, mineral salts, microbial products, small molecules, microparticles, and liposomes. Adjuvants can be broadly classified as *immunostimulants* (also known as *immunopotentiators*) or *antigen delivery systems.*

Immunostimulants bind to pattern-recognition receptors on APCs, such as the toll-like receptors (TLRs) to activate the cell-signaling pathways of the innate defense system (see Chapter 2). This leads to maturation and activation of the APCs, enhancing their ability to release cytokines and present antigens to T cells in humoral or cell-mediated immune responses.

Antigen delivery systems function as carrier molecules for antigens and enhance their uptake by APCs. Depending on the type, these adjuvants can (1) slowly release the antigen, prolonging its availability to the immune system; (2) recruit more immune cells to the injection site; and/or (3) protect the antigens from enzymatic degradation. Examples of adjuvants that function as antigen delivery systems are aluminum salts, oil-in-water emulsions (liquid dispersions of oil droplets stabilized with surfactants), and microparticles.

Table 25–1 presents examples of adjuvants, their description, and vaccines into which they are incorporated. Some vaccines contain more than one adjuvant.

Knowledge Check 25-4

One mechanism by which adjuvants boost the immune response to vaccines is by:

a. Inhibiting innate cells
b. Quickly releasing antigen to immune cells
c. Recruiting immune cells to the injection site
d. Breaking down the antigen into pieces that can be recognized by lymphocytes

Table 25-1 Examples of Adjuvants

ADJUVANT	DESCRIPTION	VACCINE EXAMPLES
Aluminum salts	Most commonly used adjuvant; contains one or more of the following: amorphous aluminum hydroxyphosphate sulfate (AAHS), aluminum hydroxide, aluminum phosphate, potassium aluminum sulfate ("alum")	Diphtheria, tetanus and pertussis (acellular); *Haemophilus influenzae* type b conjugate; hepatitis A inactivated; hepatitis B recombinant; human papillomavirus recombinant; meningococcal group B recombinant; pneumococcal polysaccharide conjugate; poliovirus inactivated
AS01B	An oil-in-water emulsion containing monophosphoryl lipid A (MPL) and QS-21, a natural compound derived from the Chilean soapbark tree	Herpes zoster recombinant
CpG 1018	A cytosine-phosphate-guanine (CpG) oligodeoxynucleotide that acts as an immunostimulant by binding to TLR9	Hepatitis B recombinant
Freund's complete/incomplete adjuvants	Oil-in-water emulsions with/without killed mycobacteria	Used only in animal studies because of undesirable side effects in humans
Matrix-M	Saponins from the soapbark tree (*Quillaja saponaria* Molina) combined with cholesterol and phospholipid in nanoparticles	COVID-19 recombinant
MF59	An oil-in-water emulsion containing squalane, a naturally occurring plant oil	Influenza recombinant

Challenges and Future Directions in Vaccine Development

Although vaccines have been highly successful in preventing many infections, effective vaccines do not exist for other diseases that cause major illnesses and death in the world. These diseases are caused by viruses, bacteria, and parasites that have complex mechanisms of pathogenesis. They may display antigen variability through genetic mutations or multistage life cycles or have developed other methods to escape attack by the immune system.

For example, the immune system's ability to eliminate HIV is hampered by the virus's capacity to infect and kill $CD4^+$ T cells, integrate into the host genome, and rapidly mutate (see Chapter 24). BCG, the vaccine for TB, is not optimally effective because mycobacteria can establish a carrier state and become reactivated during periods of immune suppression (see Chapter 20). *Plasmodium falciparum*, the cause of malaria, has posed a challenge for vaccine development through its ability to alter its surface antigens in the different stages of its complex life cycle. After many years of research, two vaccines with partial effectiveness have been approved for malaria, but studies aim to develop vaccines that provide better protection. Other infections that have posed a global challenge for effective vaccine development include hepatitis C, Epstein-Barr virus (EBV), cytomegalovirus (CMV), herpes simplex, rhinovirus, and leishmaniasis.

Scientists are studying new vaccine designs and developing new adjuvants in attempts to conquer such diseases. Researchers are using molecular techniques to identify antigens that can be formulated with potent adjuvants to produce vaccines that will stimulate a long-lasting, broad humoral response and effective T-cell responses. Several future vaccines will likely be based on mRNA technology or live, recombinant nonpathogenic viral vectors that carry genes from a pathogen. Global vaccine success will also depend on developing better ways to transport and store vaccines in areas of the world that do not have refrigeration and methods of vaccine administration that do not use conventional needles and syringes (e.g., by nasal spray or patches with very tiny needles). Hopefully, these approaches will help accelerate the development of new, effective vaccines against major global diseases in the next generation.

Benefits and Adverse Effects of Vaccines

Although there may be some adverse effects associated with vaccines, these are usually mild and greatly outweighed by their benefits.

Benefits

Vaccines are recognized as one of the greatest medical achievements. Because of routine immunization, smallpox and two of the three poliovirus serotypes been have been eradicated worldwide. Infectious diseases that were once leading causes of illness and death, such as diphtheria and measles, have a greatly reduced incidence today, especially in developed nations. The estimated numbers of cases of selected vaccine-preventable diseases in the United States before and after implementation of their corresponding vaccines are shown in **Table 25–2.** Worldwide, it is estimated that childhood vaccines prevent about 4 million deaths each year.

Immunization benefits the individuals receiving the vaccine and also reduces the risk of nearby unvaccinated persons contracting the infectious disease. When a sufficient

Table 25-2 Estimated Number of Cases of Selected Vaccine-Preventable Diseases in the United States Annually

DISEASE	ANNUAL NUMBER OF CASES IN PREVACCINE ERA	REPORTED ANNUAL CASES POSTVACCINE[a]
Diphtheria	>21,000	0
Haemophilus influenza b	20,000	3,042
Hepatitis A	>117,000	5,726
Hepatitis B (acute)	>66,000	2,044
Measles	>530,200	48
Mumps	>162,300	189
Pertussis	>200,700	2,166
Polio	>16,300	0
Rubella	>47,700	7
Smallpox	>29,000	0
Tetanus	580	28
Varicella	>4,000,000	3,496

[a]*Data from 2021. (Table adapted from CDC nationally notifiable diseases and conditions, United States, annual tables. Accessed October 7, 2024. https://wonder.cdc.gov/nndss/static/2021/annual/2021-table1.html; and Roush SW, Murphy TV. Historical comparisons of morbidity and mortality for vaccine-preventable diseases in the United States.* JAMA. *2007; 298:2155–2163.)*

proportion of people in a population have been immunized, unvaccinated individuals, such as newborns and patients who are immunocompromised, receive some protection because there is little chance for the disease to spread in the community. This concept of extending protection to others in the population is known as **community immunity** or **herd immunity** and is of great importance to public health (**Fig. 25–7**).

Adverse Effects

Vaccines can produce undesirable effects in previously healthy people, but fortunately, most of these are not severe. These can be local, systemic, or allergic. A local inflammatory response of pain, redness, and swelling at the injection site is frequently reported because the innate immune system is stimulated by the vaccine antigen or adjuvant. Systemic reactions such as mild fever, chills, irritability, fatigue, headache, and muscle/joint aches are also common after injection, but these generally resolve within 72 hours.

Allergic reactions are less common and may occur in response to vaccine additives such as preservatives, stabilizers, or antibiotics. These can be in the form of type I (IgE-mediated) or type IV (delayed/contact dermatitis) hypersensitivity (see Chapter 14). Anaphylactic reactions are rare, occurring in about one case per 1 million vaccine doses. A skin reaction from local immune complex formation (type III hypersensitivity) has been reported in some people after receiving a tetanus booster shot due to residual antibodies from previous tetanus immunization.

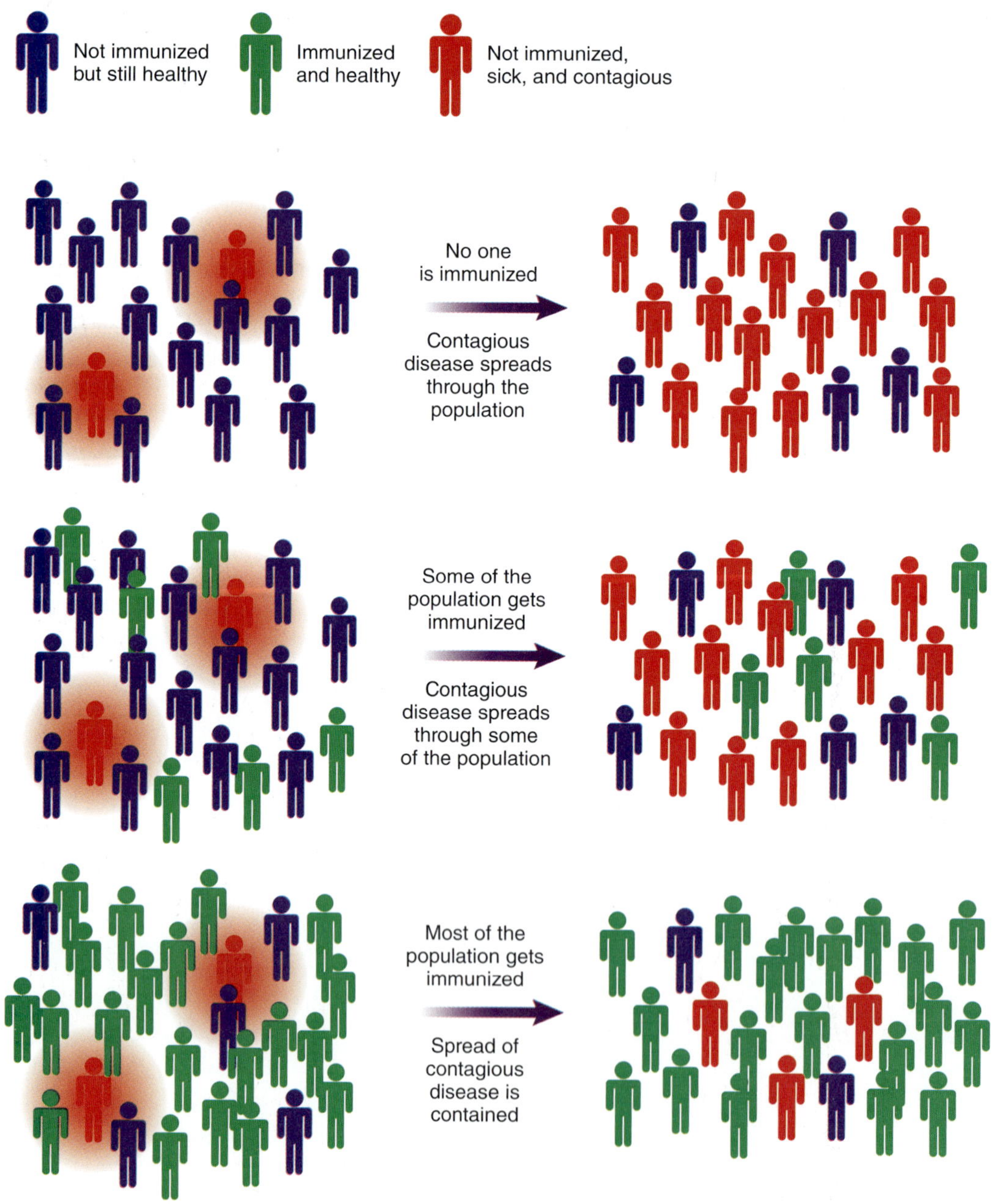
Not immunized but still healthy
Immunized and healthy
Not immunized, sick, and contagious
No one is immunized
Contagious disease spreads through the population
Some of the population gets immunized
Contagious disease spreads through some of the population
Most of the population gets immunized
Spread of contagious disease is contained

FIGURE 25–7 Community immunity ("herd immunity"). *(Adapted from the National Institute of Allergy and Infectious Diseases. Accessed October 7, 2024. https://www.nih.gov/about-nih/what-we-do/science-health-public-trust/perspectives/building-trust-vaccines.)*

People with inherited primary immunodeficiency diseases or acquired deficiencies secondary to other conditions (e.g., HIV infection, hematologic malignancies, treatment with immunosuppressive drugs or radiation) require special consideration (see Chapter 19). Administering live vaccines is contraindicated in severely immunocompromised people because the attenuated organisms have the potential to replicate uncontrollably and cause severe, disseminated disease. For example, when the smallpox vaccine was in routine use, it caused a highly fatal condition in infants with severe combined immunodeficiency disease (SCID), involving progressive spread of necrotic lesions from the site of vaccine injection to adjacent areas of the skin, bone, and internal organs. The CDC publishes specific recommendations for vaccination of persons with altered immunocompetence.

Other adverse effects associated with vaccines are rare and are published by the CDC in vaccine-specific information sheets. Concerns about vaccine safety have been fueled by a flawed research study of a link between the MMR vaccine and autism by Andrew Wakefield and colleagues in 1998 and the spread of misinformation about vaccines through social media. Fears such as these and religious or personal objections against immunization have caused some people to delay or refuse vaccination for themselves or their children. This concept, referred to as **vaccine hesitancy,** has been defined by the WHO as the "delay in acceptance or refusal of vaccination despite availability of vaccination services" (WHO, 2025). Anti-vaccine public sentiments can result in lower-than-optimal vaccine coverage, leaving many people in the population unprotected against serious diseases. This situation, coupled with importation of diseases by unvaccinated people immigrating into a country, can lead to outbreaks of diseases that would normally be preventable, such as measles and pertussis. High vaccine coverage is essential to preventing such outbreaks and maintaining a healthy population.

Critical Thinking 25-1

Explain why influenza infections are common in the United States despite the wide availability of influenza vaccines.

Passive Immunization

Passive immunity results from the transfer of preformed antibodies to an unimmunized host. Antibodies can be transferred naturally to a fetus or infant in two ways:

1. A pregnant woman's IgG antibodies pass through the placenta to her unborn fetus.
2. Maternal immunoglobulin A (IgA) antibodies in breast milk and colostrum are ingested by the infant during the nursing process (see Chapter 3 and **Fig. 25–8**).

These antibodies protect the newborn against pathogens to which the mother has developed immunity after natural infection or vaccination. IgG antibodies protect the infant during its first few months of life, a time when the baby's own immune system is immature and has not yet encountered many antigens. IgA antibodies provide mucosal immunity, an important mechanism for attacking pathogens at their portals of entry into the body. Antibodies can also be passively transferred to a host as a means of immunoprophylaxis or immunotherapy.

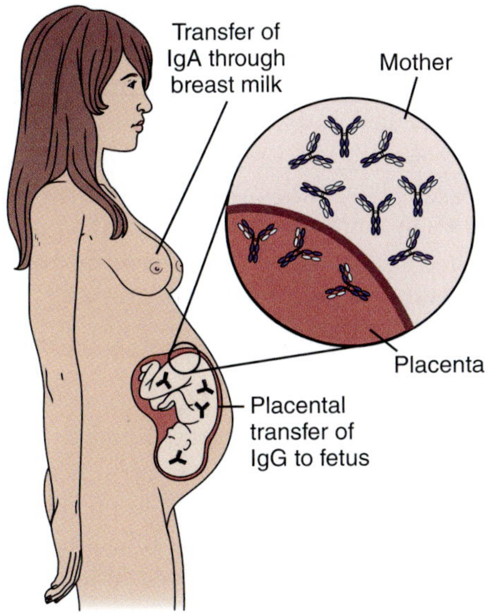

FIGURE 25–8 Passive immunity is transferred from a mother to her fetus or infant through the placenta (IgG) or breast milk (IgA).

Passive Immunotherapy

In passive immunotherapy, patients are treated with antibody preparations to manage or prevent disease. Human immunoglobulin preparations can provide passive immunity to patients who are antibody deficient and to people who have been exposed to a pathogen but have not developed immunity through vaccination or natural infection. Passive immunotherapy can also be used for cancer, autoimmune diseases, and other chronic inflammatory disorders. Three types of antibody preparations can be administered in passive immunotherapy: IV immunoglobulin (IVIG), antigen-specific globulins (hyperimmune globulin and Rh immune globulin), and monoclonal antibodies.

IV Immunoglobulin Therapy (IVIG)

IVIG, which has also been referred to as *standard human immune serum globulin* or *gamma globulin,* is a sterile preparation of concentrated antibodies made from pooled plasma of 1,000 to 100,000 healthy donors who test negative for bloodborne diseases. The plasma is enriched for immunoglobulins by precipitation in cold ethanol, then purified by chromatography, and treated to inactivate or remove viruses to further ensure safety of the preparation.

IVIG consists mostly of IgG; IgM and IgA are present in insignificant quantities because of their lower serum concentrations and rapid half-lives (see Chapter 3). The preparation contains antibodies specific for many antigens to provide general humoral protection against a variety of pathogens.

Therefore, IVIG is routinely administered intravenously (into a vein) or subcutaneously (under the skin) as a prophylactic treatment to restore IgG levels and prevent infections in immunodeficient patients who are unable to produce sufficient amounts of antibodies (see Chapter 19).

Interestingly, IVIG can also be used to suppress inflammation in several autoimmune and chronic inflammatory disorders, including immune-mediated thrombocytopenia (ITP), Kawasaki disease, multifocal motor neuropathy, and chronic inflammatory demyelinating polyneuropathy. IVIG appears to modulate inflammation in several ways, which vary in different diseases. The mechanisms of IVIG include binding to and neutralizing circulating autoantibodies; binding to and blocking activated complement proteins such as C3a and C5a; saturating Fc receptors on phagocytic cells to prevent engulfment of immune complexes; inducing anti-inflammatory cytokine release; suppressing B-cell proliferation; and enhancing regulatory T-cell populations.

Antigen-Specific Globulins

Hyperimmune globulins and Rh immune globulin are antigen-specific immunoglobulins used in passive immunotherapy. **Hyperimmune globulins** are prepared from pooled serum of human donors who have developed immunity against a particular pathogen after a recent infection or vaccination. These preparations contain a high concentration of antibody against a pathogen or its product and provide immediate protection to people who have potentially been exposed to the pathogen but have not been immunized. The preparation's potency is ensured by determining the antibody titer through laboratory testing. Hyperimmune globulins have been developed for various infectious diseases, including hepatitis A, hepatitis B (hepatitis B immune globulin; HBIG), varicella zoster, rabies, tetanus, and RSV.

Specific immune globulins for some antigens have also been prepared from animal sera, usually horse serum. Examples include tetanus, diphtheria, and botulism anti-toxins, and antisera against snake venoms. **Anti-toxins** are antibodies that specifically bind to epitopes on bacterial toxins and protect against their harmful effects by neutralizing their activity.

Rh immune globulin (RhIg), as we discussed in Chapter 14, is specific for the Rh-D antigen on red blood cells (RBCs). It is given to Rh-negative women during pregnancy to prevent hemolytic disease of the newborn. RhIg is believed to inhibit the production of anti-Rh antibodies by the mother toward paternally derived Rh-D antigens on the fetus' RBCs.

Monoclonal Antibodies

Monoclonal antibodies, as we discussed in Chapter 3, are derived from a single clone of B cells; therefore, they have exquisite specificity for a particular epitope of an antigen. Because of their high specificity, they are ideal agents of passive immunotherapy and have revolutionized medicine. Monoclonal antibodies are used to treat a wide variety of conditions, including hematologic malignancies, solid tumors, autoimmune disorders, cardiovascular disease, transplant rejection, and allergic asthma. We presented some of the clinical applications of monoclonal antibody therapy in Chapters 14, 15, and 17.

As we discussed in Chapter 3, monoclonal antibodies were originally developed using mouse B cells to produce hybridomas that secreted antibody to the desired antigen. When these monoclonal antibodies were used as therapeutic agents in humans, immune responses were likely to occur to the foreign epitopes on the mouse immunoglobulins, resulting in the production of *human anti-mouse antibodies (HAMAs)*. HAMAs significantly limited the usefulness of the monoclonal antibody therapy because they caused type I (anaphylactic) or type III (immune complex) hypersensitivity reactions.

Mouse monoclonal antibodies produced by traditional hybridoma technology are denoted by the suffix, "-**o***mab*." Over the years, recombinant DNA technology has enabled scientists to produce monoclonal antibodies that have an increasingly larger human component, making them less likely to trigger an adverse immune reaction **(Fig. 25–9):**

- *Chimeric antibodies* (denoted by the suffix, "-**xi***mab*"; e.g., rituximab): These antibodies consist of a mouse-derived immunoglobulin variable region combined with a human-derived constant region.
- *Humanized antibodies* (denoted by the suffix, "-**zu***mab*"): These antibodies contain human sequences except for the antigen-binding complementarity-determining regions, which are mouse derived.
- *Human monoclonal antibodies* (denoted by the suffix "-**u***mab*"): These antibodies are made entirely of human sequences and are becoming more widely available. They can be produced by different molecular techniques,

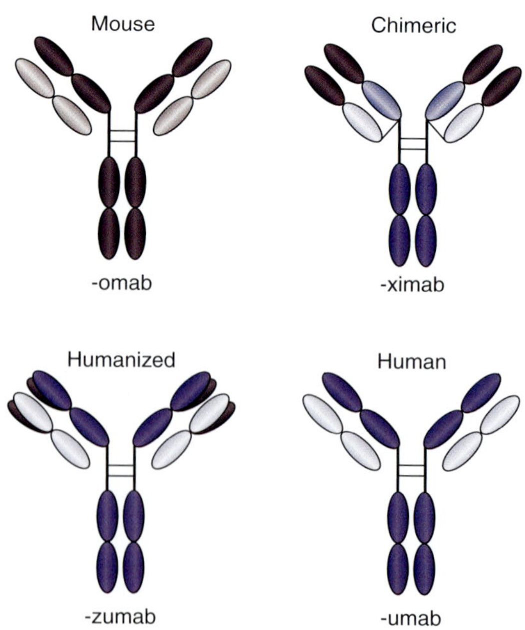

FIGURE 25–9 The four types of monoclonal antibodies. The black regions represent protein sequences derived from mouse genes, and the blue regions represent protein sequences coded for by human genes.

including phage display (a technique in which genes coding for a specific antibody molecule are cloned in bacteriophages—viruses that infect bacteria); transgenic mouse technologies in which the immunoglobulin genes of interest are incorporated into genetically modified mice; creation of hybridoma lines that secrete fully human antibodies; and the cloning of immunoglobulin genes from single isolated B cells.

Other modifications of monoclonal antibodies have also been developed for use in certain conditions. These include using Fab fragments to enhance antibody effectiveness or penetration into the tissues, producing antibody conjugates to direct drugs or toxins to tumor cells, and fusing two immunoglobulin chains with different antigen specificities to bring two cell types close together (e.g., cytotoxic T cells and tumor cells; see Chapter 17).

A list of monoclonal antibody therapies approved by the FDA and the European Medicines Agency (EMA) or undergoing review is available online from The Antibody Society. Examples of monoclonal antibodies used in passive immunotherapy are listed in **Table 25–3**.

Knowledge Check 25-5

Monoclonal antibodies are ideal agents of passive immunotherapy because they:

a. Induce a memory response
b. Do not cause adverse reactions
c. Are directed against a single epitope
d. Are easy to manufacture

Advantages and Limitations of Passive Immunization

The main advantage of passive immunization is that it provides immediate immunity to the host. The antibodies are already present in the serum being transferred; thus, there is no delay in waiting for the recipient's own immune system to be activated by antigen (see Chapter 3). Immediate protection from passive immunotherapy is especially beneficial in preventing disease in persons whose immune systems are deficient or immature and in unimmunized individuals who have been exposed to a harmful antigen.

Table 25-3 Examples of FDA-Approved Monoclonal Antibodies Used for Immunotherapy

NAME[a]	TYPE	SPECIFICITY	KEY DISEASE INDICATION(S)
Adalimumab (Humira)	Human	TNF-α	Reduces inflammation in rheumatoid arthritis, juvenile idiopathic arthritis, psoriatic arthritis, ankylosing spondylitis, Crohn disease, ulcerative colitis, plaque psoriasis, hidradenitis suppurativa
Alemtuzumab (Campath, Lemtrada)	Humanized	CD52	Destroys malignant cells in chronic lymphocytic leukemia and multiple sclerosis
Basiliximab (Simulect)	Chimeric	CD25 (IL-2 receptor)	Prevents kidney transplant rejection
Bevacizumab (Avastin)	Humanized	Vascular endothelial growth factor (VEGF)	Inhibits blood vessel formation in colorectal cancer, non–small-cell lung carcinoma, renal cell carcinomas, glioblastoma
Daratumumab (Darzalex)	Human	CD38	Destroys malignant cells in multiple myeloma
Ipilimumab (Yervoy)	Human	CTLA-4	Blocks inhibition of T-cell activation in melanoma by binding to CTLA-4
Omalizumab (Xolair)	Humanized	IgE	Binds to IgE to reduce allergic symptoms in asthma, nasal polyps, chronic hives, food allergies
Pembrolizumab (Keytruda)	Humanized	PD-1	Blocks PD-1 receptor on T cells, allowing T-cell activation in melanoma, non–small-cell lung cancer, Hodgkin lymphoma, Merkel cell carcinoma, and other cancers
Rituximab (Rituxan)	Chimeric	CD20	Binds to and destroys B cells in non-Hodgkin lymphoma, chronic lymphocytic leukemia, rheumatoid arthritis, granulomatosis with polyangiitis, microscopic polyangiitis
Trastuzumab (Herceptin)	Humanized	HER2	Targets malignant cells that overexpress HER2 (e.g., certain types of breast cancer, gastric adenocarcinoma, gastroesophageal junction adenocarcinoma)

[a]Brand names are in parentheses. CD = cluster of differentiation; CTLA-4 = cytotoxic T-lymphocyte–associated protein 4; HER2 = human epidermal growth factor receptor 2; IgE = immunoglobulin E; PD-1 = programmed cell death protein 1; TNF = tumor necrosis factor.

Situations in which passive immunization is helpful include the following:

- During natural transfer of antibodies from a mother to her fetus or infant through the placenta or breast milk; the child is provided with immediate protection to a variety of pathogens until their own immune system can mature.
- Preventing infections in antibody-deficient patients with IVIG therapy.
- Preventing severe disease from RSV by injection of the RSV monoclonal antibody (nirsevimab) in infants younger than 8 months born to unvaccinated mothers during the RSV season, and for children between 8 and 19 months old who are at high risk for severe RSV disease.
- Preventing tetanus in an unvaccinated person who had contact with soil that was potentially contaminated with tetanus-causing bacteria.
- Preventing hepatitis B in a health care worker who had an accidental needlestick involving blood from a patient whose infection status is positive or unknown.
- Preventing death in people who have been bitten by a poisonous snake or an animal with rabies.

However, passive immunity is only temporary. The duration of the immunity is limited by the biological half-life of the immunoglobulins (21 to 28 days for IgG). Memory lymphocytes are not generated, so an individual will not be protected if exposure to the same antigen occurs at a later time in life. Another limitation of passive immunization is that hypersensitivity reactions, although rare with human immunoglobulin preparations, can occur frequently after therapy with animal serum.

Critical Thinking 25-2

Explain why patients with antibody immunodeficiencies require repeated, periodic treatments with Ig therapy to be adequately protected.

Adoptive Immunotherapy

Passive immunization provides humoral immunity to a recipient; in contrast, adoptive immunotherapy involves transferring *cells* of the immune system to increase the cell-mediated immune response. The transferred cells can be derived from a donor individual or from the recipients themselves (i.e., autologous). They may be naturally derived or genetically engineered to target a particular antigen.

Clinical Applications of Adoptive Immunotherapy

Adoptive immunotherapy can provide generalized immunity or antigen-specific immunity. A common general application of adoptive immunotherapy involves transplantation of bone marrow or peripheral blood hematopoietic stem cells (HSCs) to provide immune cell populations to patients with certain immunodeficiency diseases (see Chapter 19). Autologous or allogeneic HSCs can also restore the immune system in patients with certain malignancies who have been treated with chemotherapy and a high dose of total body irradiation (e.g., multiple myeloma, non-Hodgkin lymphoma, acute leukemias).

Clinical applications of antigen-specific adoptive immunotherapy have mainly focused on treatment of patients with cancer. This type of immunotherapy is based on studies in animals, and later in humans, which demonstrated that lymphocytes activated by IL-2 in vitro can mount cytolytic immune responses against tumor cells when they are adoptively transferred to individuals with cancer.

As we discussed in Chapter 17, adoptive immunotherapy for cancer involves transferring one of two types of cells:

- **Tumor-infiltrating lymphocytes (TILs):** These are lymphocytes isolated from a tumor mass in the body. The TILs are activated in vitro by incubation with dendritic cells from the patient, expanded in culture with IL-2, and infused into the patient's bloodstream (see Fig. 17–14). TIL therapy has induced good clinical responses in patients with malignant melanoma who have not responded to other treatments and is being studied for its effectiveness for other solid tumors.
- **CAR T cells** (chimeric antigen receptor T cells): CAR T cells are genetically modified peripheral blood T cells that express high-affinity T-cell receptors (TCRs) for specific tumor antigens. Unlike naturally occurring TCRs, the TCRs of CAR T cells can bind to a tumor antigen in the absence of an MHC molecule. Thus, they are not MHC restricted and can be used to treat many patients with a particular type of tumor rather than being limited to patients with a specific human leukocyte antigen (HLA) type.

While the structure of CAR–T-cell receptors can vary, they generally have four components **(Fig. 25–10):**

- An *antigen-binding domain,* consisting of antigen-specific single-chain variable fragments of a monoclonal antibody molecule linked together (i.e., linked variable heavy [V_H] and variable light [V_L] fragments)
- A *spacer domain,* which provides flexibility to the antigen-binding domain, allowing it to interact effectively with the antigen
- A *transmembrane domain,* which anchors the receptor to the T-cell membrane and allows interactions to occur between the extracellular and intracellular parts of the receptor
- An *intracellular signaling domain,* consisting of the CD3ζ chain and costimulatory molecules such as CD28 and CD137, which transmit signals inside the cell to promote T-cell activation

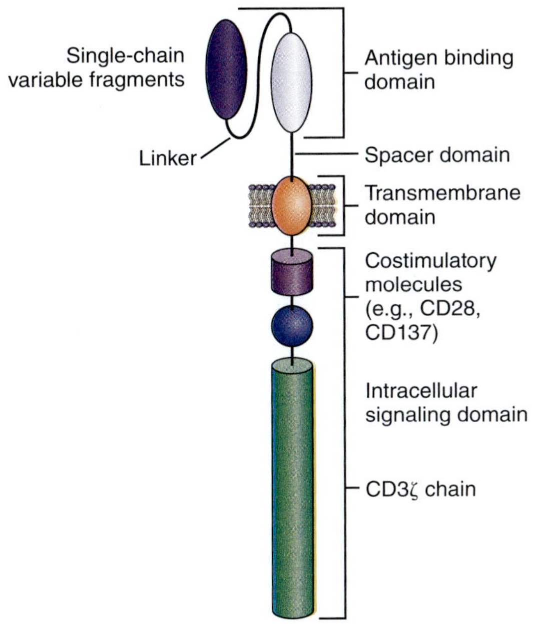

FIGURE 25–10 Structure of a CAR–T-cell receptor. Key components of the receptor include linked single-chain variable fragments from a monoclonal antibody that will bind to a tumor antigen, a spacer region to allow flexible movement of the molecule, a transmembrane domain, and an intracellular signaling domain.

At the time of this writing, CAR–T-cell therapies that target the CD19 or CD38 antigens have been FDA approved for patients with certain B-cell malignancies and advanced multiple myeloma, respectively, for whom other treatments have not been effective. Studies are under way to determine if CAR–T-cell therapy can be used for other blood cancers and solid tumors. Research is also being conducted to determine if other forms of genetically modified T cells or natural killer (NK) cells can be used.

While adoptive immunotherapy can provide long-lasting protection if the transferred cells become established in the recipient, it can be associated with significant side effects. For example, the recipient's own immune cells must be depleted prior to the therapy to ensure its success. Transplantation of allogeneic HSCs can cause graft-vs-host disease if the donor and recipient are not HLA matched (see Chapter 16). Also, adoptive immunotherapy is expensive and highly personalized. Efforts are under way to provide funding and improve techniques to reduce the cost of this treatment so that it can be expanded to larger numbers of patients, including those with other conditions.

Knowledge Check 25-6

A main advantage of CAR T cells is that they are not:

a. Antigen specific
b. MHC restricted
c. Associated with significant side effects
d. Expensive

KEY CONCEPTS

Introduction

- Immunity is the condition of resistance to a disease. Immunization is the process by which immunity is acquired. The three types of immunization are active, passive, and adoptive.
- Active immunization involves stimulating an individual's own immune system to mount an adaptive immune response to an antigen. This can occur after a natural infection or receiving a vaccine.
- Passive immunization involves the transfer of antibodies from an immune host to a nonimmune individual. Passive immunity can result from transfer of maternal antibodies to a fetus or infant or from administration of commercial antibody preparations to treat patients with certain diseases.
- Adoptive immunity is achieved by transferring cells of the immune system to a nonimmune individual.
- Active immunity takes time to develop but provides long-lasting protection to the individual because it generates immunologic memory. Passive immunity provides immediate protection but is short lived because antibody titers decline at a rate determined by the biological half-life of the immunoglobulins. Adoptive immunity provides long-lasting protection if the cells become established in the recipient.

Vaccines

- A vaccine is an antigen preparation that stimulates an immune response.
- Vaccines containing a pathogen-derived antigen suspension are administered to healthy people to prevent infectious diseases and are thus a form of immunoprophylaxis.
- Vaccines for cancer are used as immunotherapy for patients who already have the disease.

Historical Evolution of Vaccines

- In 1796, Dr. Edward Jenner was the first to publicize the procedure of vaccination by using material from cowpox skin lesions to immunize against the deadly disease smallpox.
- In the 1800s, Louis Pasteur used attenuated, or weakened, microorganisms to produce vaccines against chicken cholera, anthrax, and rabies.
- In the 20th century, vaccine development grew exponentially because of new methods to attenuate microorganisms, produce toxoids, and grow viruses in cell culture. The first recombinant vaccine, produced by genetic engineering, was developed in the latter part of the 20th century.
- Vaccine developments continue in the 21st century. Notably, mRNA vaccines were developed to prevent severe disease and death from SARS-CoV-2 during the COVID-19 pandemic.

Types of Vaccines

- Vaccines to prevent infectious diseases may be composed of live, attenuated (weakened, nonpathogenic) microorganisms; inactivated (killed) microorganisms; antigenic subunits such as toxoids, polysaccharides conjugated to a protein, purified or recombinant antigens; mRNA that codes for a pathogen antigen; or nonpathogenic viral vectors that carry the genes for a pathogen antigen to host cells.
- Toxoids are bacterial toxins that have been inactivated so that they are no longer pathogenic but are still immunogenic.
- Live, attenuated vaccines induce a strong immune response because the organisms can replicate in the recipient and stimulate both humoral and cell-mediated immunity. However, they cannot be given to immunocompromised people, in whom they can produce severe disease.
- Inactivated and subunit vaccines can be given to immunocompromised people because they do not contain live organisms. They mainly stimulate humoral immunity and generally require booster doses and adjuvants to generate a protective immune response.
- mRNA vaccines can be manufactured rapidly, do not contain infectious material, and generate strong immune responses, but they may produce inflammatory reactions in some people.
- Viral vector vaccines induce a strong immune response, but they have a complex design, cannot be given to immunocompromised people, and may have reduced effectiveness in people previously exposed to the virus.

Factors Affecting Vaccine Effectiveness

- The vaccine's ability to protect people against illness, hospitalization, and death is influenced by the recipient's age, immune status and other factors, the pathogen's characteristics, and the type of vaccine. To obtain an optimal immune response, vaccines must be administered according to recommended schedules.
- Adjuvants are substances that are often included in vaccines to increase the immune response to the target antigens. Some adjuvants are immunostimulants that bind to innate receptors on APCs, increasing their ability to release cytokines and present antigens to T cells. Others are antigen delivery systems (e.g., aluminum salts and oil-in-water emulsions) or carrier molecules that enhance antigen uptake by APCs by prolonging antigen release, recruiting immune cells, and protecting antigens from degradation.

Challenges and Future Directions in Vaccine Development

- Vaccine development for many pathogens has been challenging due to factors such as complex pathogen life cycles, frequent genetic mutations and antigen variability, and other mechanisms of escaping the immune response.
- Global success of vaccination will depend on creating new vaccine designs, discovering new adjuvants, using needleless ways to give vaccines, and developing improved ways to store and transport vaccines to areas of the world that do not have refrigeration.

Benefits and Adverse Effects of Vaccines

- Vaccines are one of the greatest medical achievements, preventing millions of severe illnesses and deaths worldwide.
- Vaccines protect both the individuals who have received the vaccines and their close unvaccinated contacts, a concept known as "community immunity" or "herd immunity."
- Vaccines can cause side effects such as local inflammation at the injection site, mild systemic reactions, and rarely, hypersensitivity reactions. Live vaccines should not be administered to patients with immunodeficiency disorders because they can replicate uncontrollably and cause disseminated disease.
- Vaccine hesitancy is the delay or refusal to accept available vaccines due to fears about vaccine safety, personal or religious beliefs, and misinformation about vaccines. This has led to outbreaks of preventable diseases. High vaccine coverage is needed to provide optimal protection to a population.

Passive Immunization

- Passive immunity can result from natural transfer of maternal IgG antibodies through the placenta to the fetus or by transfer of IgA antibodies to an infant through breast milk.
- Immunity can also be transferred passively during immunotherapy using commercial antibody preparations.

Passive Immunotherapy

- Patients with humoral immunodeficiencies are routinely treated with IV immunoglobulin (IVIG) therapy, prepared from pooled serum of many donors and containing numerous antibodies, to provide protection against a variety of pathogens.
- IVIG can also suppress inflammation in patients with autoimmune and chronic inflammatory disorders by neutralizing autoantibodies, blocking complement, preventing phagocytosis of immune complexes, inducing anti-inflammatory cytokines, suppressing B-cell proliferation, or enhancing regulatory T cells.

- Hyperimmune globulins contain antigen-specific antibodies from pooled serum preparations. They can provide immediate protection against a particular pathogen or venom in nonimmune individuals who have had recent contact with a pathogen or who have been bitten by a poisonous snake.
- Anti-toxins are antibodies directed against toxins from pathogenic bacteria. They can be isolated from the serum of laboratory animals that have been injected with such a toxin and used to prevent diseases such as tetanus, diphtheria, and botulism by passive immunization.
- Rh immune globulin is a type of passive immunotherapy that contains antibody to the RBC antigen, Rh-D. It is given to Rh-negative pregnant women to prevent hemolytic disease of the newborn in infants who possess a paternally derived Rh-D antigen.
- Monoclonal antibodies have specificity for a particular antigenic epitope. They are used as therapeutic agents for cancers, autoimmune diseases, and various other conditions.
- Monoclonal antibodies were originally 100% mouse derived because they were produced by hybridoma technology. Advances in genetic technologies have allowed scientists to make hybrid antibodies that consist partially of mouse protein and partially of human protein. These antibodies can be characterized as chimeric ("-ximab"), humanized ("-zumab"), or fully human ("-umab"), depending on the amount of the human component. Administration of these antibodies reduces the chance that the recipients will produce human anti-mouse antibodies (HAMAs) and develop hypersensitivity reactions.

Advantages and Limitations of Passive Immunization

- Passive immunization provides immediate humoral immunity to the recipient because the antibodies are preformed.
- However, passive immunity is temporary, being limited by the IgG half-life of 21 to 28 days. Memory responses are not formed. Hypersensitivity reactions can develop in some people, usually as a result of therapy with animal serum.

Adoptive Immunotherapy

- Adoptive immunotherapy involves transferring cells of the immune system to provide immunity.

Clinical Applications of Adoptive Immunotherapy

- Examples of adoptive immunotherapy include administration of HSCs to patients with immunodeficiency diseases or hematologic malignancies treated with high doses of chemotherapy and irradiation; treatment of patients with melanoma with autologous IL-2 activated TILs; and CAR–T-cell therapy for selected B-cell malignancies and advanced multiple myeloma.
- CAR T cells are genetically modified peripheral blood T cells with high-affinity TCRs that are not MHC restricted. The receptors consist of an antigen-binding domain, a spacer domain, a transmembrane domain, and an intracellular signaling domain.
- Adoptive immunotherapy can provide long-lasting protection if the cells become established in the recipient, but it is a costly, highly personalized therapy that may have significant side effects.

Study Guide: Major Features of Active Immunity, Passive Immunity, and Adoptive Immunity

	MECHANISM	EXAMPLES	ADVANTAGES	LIMITATIONS
Active Immunity	Activation of humoral and cell-mediated responses by an individual's own immune system after exposure to an antigen	Natural infection with a pathogen Immunization with a vaccine	Long-term immunologic memory to the antigen is generated	Delay in initiation of the immune response
Passive Immunity	Transfer of antibodies from immunized individual(s) to a nonimmune individual	Passage of IgG through the placenta, from a pregnant woman to the fetus Passage of IgA through breast milk, from mother to infant Intravenous immunoglobulin therapy Hyperimmune globulins Antitoxins Rh-immune globulin Monoclonal antibodies	Provides immediate protection to the recipient	Immunity is temporary, declining with the half-life of the antibodies Immunologic memory is not generated Hypersensitivity can develop, especially when sera of animal origin are used

Adoptive Immunity	Transfer of cells of the immune system to nonimmune individuals	Hematopoietic stem cell (HSC) transplantation Adoptive immunotherapy with activated TILs or CAR-T cells to cancer patients	Can provide long-lasting protection if cells are established in the recipient Can transfer cell- mediated immunity	Patient's own immune cells must be depleted to increase chance of successful HSC therapy Allogeneic cells may cause graft vs host disease Therapy is highly personalized, expensive, and associated with significant side effects

Study Guide: Characteristics of Different Vaccine Types

VACCINE TYPE	COMPOSITION	EXAMPLES	ADVANTAGES	LIMITATIONS
Attenuated	Live pathogens that have been weakened by growth under modified culture conditions	BCG (Bacillus Calmette Guérin) Typhoid fever Oral polio (Sabin) Measles (rubeola) Mumps German measles (rubella) Chickenpox (varicella) Influenza (nasal mist) Rotavirus	Induces both humoral and cell-mediated immunity Effective in inducing immunity after a single dose	Cannot be administered to immunocompromised individuals Rare potential to mutate to a pathogenic form Maternal antibodies can interfere with infant's immune response to the vaccine Requires careful handling and storage
Inactivated	Killed microorganisms	Intramuscular polio (Salk) Influenza (intramuscular) Hepatitis A	Can safely be given to immunocompromised individuals	Stimulates humoral immunity but little or no cell-mediated immunity May require two or more booster doses to produce protective immunity
Subunit	One or more purified components of a pathogen	Toxoids Purified proteins Polysaccharides Recombinant antigens	Induces an immune response to the pathogenic component(s) of a microorganism Safer than administering an intact organism	Requires two or more booster doses to produce protective immunity Requires an adjuvant to increase immunogenicity Must contain multiple antigens if a broad immune response is desired
a. **Toxoids**	Bacterial toxins that have been chemically inactivated so that they are not pathogenic	Diphtheria Tetanus	See information for subunit vaccines in this table	Requires two or more booster doses to produce protective immunity Requires an adjuvant to increase immunogenicity
b. **Purified Components**	Biochemically purified components of a microorganism	Pertussis (whooping cough)	See information for subunit vaccines in this table Produces fewer side effects than whole bacteria	See information for subunit vaccines in this table

c. Polysaccharides	Biochemically purified polysaccharide from bacterial capsule	Streptococcal pneumonia *Haemophilus influenzae* type b Neisserial meningitis	See information for subunit vaccines in this table	See information for subunit vaccines in this table Requires conjugation to a carrier protein to induce IgG production and long-term immunity
d. Recombinant Antigen	Protein produced by genetically modified nonpathogenic bacteria, yeast, or mammalian cells	Hepatitis B Human papilloma virus Influenza Varicella zoster (shingles) Respiratory syncytial virus (RSV)	Highly purified protein that is safer than administration of intact organism	See information for subunit vaccines in this table Cannot be used to produce antigens other than proteins
Messenger RNA (mRNA)	mRNA encoding a pathogen antigen, packaged in nanoparticles	SARS-Co-V2 (COVID-19)	Does not contain infectious material Generates strong immune responses Can be manufactured rapidly	May produce inflammatory reactions in some people
Viral vector	Genetically modified nonpathogenic virus (e.g. adenovirus) that carries the genetic code for a vaccine antigen to host cells	SARS-Co-V2 Dengue Ebola	Induces a strong immune response	Vaccine design is complex Cannot be given to immunocompromised people May have reduced effectiveness in people previously exposed to the viral vector Not approved in the U.S.

CASE STUDIES

1. A 2-year-old child has made numerous visits to a doctor because of recurring respiratory and ear infections. An immunologic workup revealed that the child had a low number of B cells and decreased immunoglobulin concentrations. Based on these results, the child was diagnosed with an antibody immunodeficiency disease.

Questions

a. What childhood vaccines could safely be administered to this child? What is the composition of these vaccines?

b. What childhood vaccines should not be administered to this child? Why?

c. How can children such as the one in this case be protected against the diseases for which they are unable to receive vaccination?

2. Suppose an unvaccinated staff member of a health care facility was accidentally exposed to hepatitis B from a needlestick injury in which the source patient tested positive for the virus.

Questions

a. What type of passive immunization could be administered, and what is the main benefit of this treatment?

b. If the staff member received this treatment and did not develop hepatitis B, would they be immune to this virus 10 years from now? Why or why not?

REVIEW QUESTIONS

1. Suppose a person develops antibodies in response to a streptococcal pharyngitis infection. This is an example of:
   a. Active immunity
   b. Passive immunity
   c. Adoptive immunity
   d. Immunoprophylaxis
2. Which of the following illustrates passive immunity?
   a. Development of high antibody titers in a healthy person after receipt of the hepatitis B vaccine
   b. Recovery of a patient from a hepatitis A infection
   c. Passage of IgG antibodies through the placenta of a pregnant woman to her fetus
   d. Transfer of tumor-infiltrating lymphocytes to a cancer patient
3. Which of the following is *not* a characteristic of passive immunity?
   a. Transfer of antibodies
   b. Occurs naturally or because of therapy
   c. Provision of immediate protection
   d. Development of long-term memory
4. What was one of the major contributions of Louis Pasteur to vaccine development?
   a. Development of the smallpox vaccine
   b. Use of attenuated microorganisms in vaccines
   c. Inactivation of bacterial toxins for vaccines
   d. Discovery of recombinant vaccine antigens
5. The antigenic component of the hepatitis B vaccine consists of a:
   a. Live, attenuated virus
   b. Inactivated virus
   c. Cryptic antigen
   d. Recombinant antigen
6. Which of the following describes the properties of a toxoid?
   a. Both pathogenic and immunogenic
   b. Pathogenic but not immunogenic
   c. Not pathogenic but immunogenic
   d. Neither pathogenic nor immunogenic
7. Suppose a vaccine was available in two forms: attenuated and inactivated. What is an advantage of the attenuated form?
   a. It can be used in immunocompromised patients.
   b. It induces both humoral and cell-mediated immunity.
   c. There is no interference of the immune response in infants by maternal antibodies.
   d. It does not require special handling and storage to maintain its effectiveness.
8. What factor(s) influence the effectiveness of a person's immune response to a vaccine?
   a. Age of the recipient
   b. The individual's immune status
   c. The nature of the vaccine
   d. All of the above
9. Chimeric antigen receptors in CAR T cells are composed of:
   a. α and β chains of the TCR in complex with CD3
   b. α and β chains of the TCR in complex with class I MHC
   c. Single-chain variable fragments of a monoclonal antibody complexed with class I MHC
   d. Single-chain variable fragments of a monoclonal antibody complexed with CD3 and costimulatory molecules
10. When one person becomes immunized by receiving a series of vaccine injections according to schedule, the resulting protection extends to that person's nearby contacts. This concept is known as:
    a. Immunologic memory
    b. Neighborhood immunity
    c. Herd immunity
    d. Contagious immunity
11. Which preparation would you recommend to treat a patient with an antibody deficiency?
    a. Monoclonal antibody
    b. IV immunoglobulin
    c. Hyperimmune globulin
    d. Animal serum antitoxin
12. Immunoglobulins consisting of a mouse-derived variable region combined with a human-derived constant region are known as:
    a. Monoclonal antibodies
    b. Chimeric antibodies
    c. Humanized antibodies
    d. Fully human antibodies
13. HAMAs are:
    a. Mouse-derived antibodies that have been used for therapy
    b. Monoclonal antibodies with therapeutic benefits
    c. Human antibodies that are produced against mouse proteins
    d. Anti-toxins that can provide immediate immunity

14. What is a major characteristic of adoptive immunotherapy?
    a. It involves the transfer of cells to deliver immunity.
    b. It involves the transfer of cytokines to deliver immunity.
    c. It can only occur in the presence of autologous cells.
    d. Its purpose is to increase the humoral immune response.

15. Infusion of TILs into a cancer patient is an example of:
    a. Active immunity
    b. Adoptive immunity
    c. Passive immunity
    d. Natural immunity

16. Aluminum salts are used in vaccines to:
    a. Activate cell-signaling pathways of innate immunity
    b. Preserve vaccine stability
    c. Increase antigen uptake by APCs
    d. Decrease vaccine side effects

17. Monoclonal antibodies can be used to treat:
    a. Cancer
    b. Autoimmune disorders
    c. Allergic asthma
    d. All of the above

Chapter 25 Answer Key

Answers to Knowledge Checks

25.1 b 25.2 a 25.3 1-c, 2-d, 3-e, 4-b, 5-a, 6-f
25.4 c 25.5 c 25.6 b

Answers to Review Questions

1. a 2. c 3. d 4. b 5. d 6. c 7. b
8. d 9. d 10. c 11. b 12. b 13. c 14. a
15. b 16. c 17. d

Glossary

Accreditation: The process by which an external agency evaluates an institution or program to ensure that it meets an established set of professional standards.

Accuracy: The ability of a test to obtain the expected result (i.e., the true value of an analyte).

Acid-fast bacilli: A term used to describe mycobacteria, based on their ability to resist decolorization with acid alcohol during Gram-staining, because of their cell wall composition.

Acquired immunodeficiency syndrome (AIDS): A disease caused by HIV that affects the immune system.

Activation unit: The combination of complement components C1, C4b, and C2b that form the enzyme C3 convertase, whose substrate is C3.

Active immunity: Immunity resulting from natural exposure to an infectious agent or administration of a vaccine.

Acute phase reactants: Normal plasma proteins that rapidly increase or decrease in concentration by at least 25% during an inflammatory response.

Acute rejection (AR): A type of rejection that occurs days to weeks after transplantation as a result of cellular mechanisms and antibody formation.

Acute rheumatic fever: A disease that develops in some patients as a sequel to a group A streptococcal infection, characterized by the presence of antibodies that cross-react with heart tissue.

Adaptive immunity: The form of immunity mediated by T and B lymphocytes; it is characterized by specificity for an antigen and the ability to remember a prior exposure to the antigen, resulting in an increased response to the antigen upon repeated exposure.

Adaptive type 1 regulatory T (Tr1) cells: CD4$^+$ T cells induced from antigen-activated naive T cells under the influence of interleukin-10. These cells exert suppressive activities.

Adjuvant: A substance administered with an antigen to enhance the immune response.

Adoptive immunity: Immunity resulting from the transfer of cells of the immune system (usually lymphocytes) from an immunized host to a nonimmune individual.

Adoptive immunotherapy: Administration of immune cells to treat patients with conditions such as immunodeficiency diseases or cancer.

Adult T-cell leukemia/lymphoma (ATLL): A T-cell malignancy caused by human T-lymphotropic virus type 1 (HTLV-1).

Affinity: The initial force of attraction that exists between a Fab site on an antibody and one epitope or a determinant site on the corresponding antigen.

Affinity maturation: Process during the immune response whereby somatic mutations in B cells result in immunoglobulin receptors that can bind the antigen more strongly.

Agammaglobulinemias: Immunodeficiency diseases in which antibody levels in the blood are significantly decreased.

Agglutination: The process by which particulate antigens such as cells aggregate to form large complexes when a specific antibody is present.

Agglutination inhibition: An agglutination reaction based on competition between antigen-coated particles and soluble patient antigens for a limited number of antibody-combining sites. Lack of agglutination is a positive test result.

Agglutinin: An antibody that causes clumping or agglutination of the cells that triggered its formation.

Allele: An alternate form of a gene that codes for a slightly different form of the same protein product.

Allelic exclusion: The expression of an allele on only one chromosome of a chromosome pair.

Allergen: An antigen that triggers a type I hypersensitivity response (i.e., an allergy).

Allergy immunotherapy (AIT): Therapy involving administration of increasing doses of an allergen with the goal of inducing immune tolerance to the allergen.

Alloantigen: An antigen that is found in another member of the host's species and that is capable of eliciting an immune response in the host.

Allograft: Tissue or cells transferred from an individual into another individual of the same species with a different genetic composition.

Allotype: A minor variation in amino acid sequence in a particular class of immunoglobulin molecules that is inherited in a Mendelian fashion.

Alpha-fetoprotein (AFP): A serum tumor marker that is commonly elevated in patients with primary hepatocellular carcinoma and nonseminomatous testicular cancer.

Alpha1-antitrypsin (AAT): An acute phase protein that inhibits proteases released from white blood cells and regulates the expression of pro-inflammatory cytokines.

Alternative pathway: A pathway of complement activation that does not involve antigen-antibody complexes. This pathway is triggered by constituents of microorganisms.

Amplification: Copying of nucleic acids to increase the amount available for detection.

Analyte: The substance being measured in an immunoassay.

Analytic sensitivity: The lowest measurable amount of an analyte.

Analytic specificity: An assay's ability to generate a negative result when the analyte is not present.

Anamnestic response: The memory, or secondary, immune response.

Anaphylatoxin: A small peptide formed during complement activation (C3a and C5a) that causes increased vascular permeability, contraction of smooth muscle, and release of histamine from basophils and mast cells.

Anaphylaxis: An acute, life-threatening type I hypersensitivity response to an allergen that simultaneously involves multiple organs.

Anergy: A state of immune unresponsiveness to a specific antigen.

Annotation: The process of searching databases of variants and phenotypic associations to identify significant and reportable alterations.

Antagonism: Effect that occurs when the action of one cytokine counteracts the activity of another cytokine.

Antibodies: Antigen-specific glycoproteins produced by B lymphocytes and plasma cells in response to a foreign substance. Antibodies are also known as *immunoglobulins*.

Antibody-dependent cellular cytotoxicity (ADCC): The process of destroying antibody-coated target cells by natural killer cells, monocytes, macrophages, and neutrophils, all of which have receptors for the Fc portion of an antibody.

Antibody-drug conjugates: Antibody that is attached to a toxin or radioisotope to help specifically destroy cancer cells.

Anti-centromere antibodies: Autoantibodies that bind to proteins in the centromere (the middle region of a chromosome where the sister chromatids are joined); associated with limited cutaneous systemic sclerosis (i.e., CREST syndrome).

Anti-cyclic citrullinated peptide antibody (anti-CCP or ACPA): Autoantibodies to proteins that contain an atypical amino acid called *citrulline* (a modified arginine), produced by granulocytes and monocytes. This antibody is highly specific for rheumatoid arthritis.

Anti-DNase B: An antibody directed against DNase B, an enzyme secreted by group A streptococci that can degrade DNA; testing for the antibody is performed to aid in the diagnosis of poststreptococcal sequelae.

Antigen: A molecule that is capable of binding specifically to an antibody or lymphocyte receptor during an immune response.

Antigen concealment: Means by which parasites hide their antigens from the host by remaining inside of the host's cells without their antigens being displayed.

Antigen-dependent phase: The final phase of B-cell development, which occurs when a B cell is stimulated by an antigen and undergoes transformation to a blast stage, resulting in the formation of memory cells and antibody-secreting plasma cells.

Antigen-independent phase: The first phase of B-cell development in the bone marrow, which results in mature B cells that have not yet been exposed to antigen.

Antigen presentation: The process by which degraded peptides within cells are transported to the plasma membrane with major histocompatibility class (MHC) molecules so that T cells can then recognize them.

Antigenic drift: The process by which viruses undergo gradual genetic mutations, producing different but similar surface proteins.

Antigenic mimicry: A mechanism by which parasites express epitopes that are similar or identical to host molecules, thus protecting the parasite from being recognized and eliminated by the immune system.

Antigenic shedding: A mechanism by which parasites can evade the immune system by shedding surface antigens that bind to the host's antibodies and cells.

Antigenic shift: A major change in a virus's genetic makeup that occurs suddenly, producing new viral strains with proteins that the immune system does not recognize.

Antigenic variation: A change in parasite antigens due to genetic modifications that allows them to escape the immune response.

Anti-glomerular basement membrane (anti-GBM) disease: An autoimmune disease characterized by production of antibodies to the basement membranes in the kidneys and lungs; formerly known as *Goodpasture syndrome*.

Anti-HBe: Antibody to a protein located between the outer envelope and core of the hepatitis B virus.

Anti-HBs: Antibody to the hepatitis B surface antigen that is located in the outer envelope of the virus.

Anti-histone antibodies: Autoantibodies to histones, which are nucleoproteins found in chromatin. Elevated levels are associated with drug-induced lupus.

Anti-neutrophil cytoplasmic antibody (ANCA): Autoantibodies produced against proteins in the neutrophil granules; these antibodies are strongly associated with vascular inflammatory syndromes.

Anti-nuclear antibodies (ANAs): Autoantibodies produced to different components of the nucleus in systemic lupus erythematosus, other systemic autoimmune rheumatic diseases, and other conditions. Examples include antibodies to DNA, histones, extractable nuclear antigens, and centromere proteins.

Anti-phospholipid antibodies: A heterogeneous group of autoantibodies that bind to phospholipids or phospholipid-protein complexes.

Anti-retroviral therapy (ART): Therapeutic drugs that suppress the replication of a retrovirus such as HIV.

Anti-RNP antibody: Autoantibodies directed against ribonucleoprotein (RNP), which consists of several nonhistone proteins complexed to a small nuclear RNA called *U1-nRNP*. These antibodies are found in some patients with systemic autoimmune rheumatic diseases.

Anti-toxin: Antibody used in passive immunization for the purpose of neutralizing a bacterial toxin.

Apoptosis: A noninflammatory process of cell death characterized by cell shrinkage, nuclear chromatin condensation, and formation of small structures that are phagocytized by macrophages.

Arthus reaction: A type III hypersensitivity skin reaction that occurs when an individual has a large amount of circulating antibody and is exposed to the antigen intradermally, resulting in localized deposition of immune complexes.

ASO titer: A test for the diagnosis of poststreptococcal sequelae, based on the combination of the group A streptococcal enzyme, streptolysin O, with anti-streptolysin O in patient serum.

Aspergillosis: An opportunistic fungal infection predominantly caused by *Aspergillus fumigatus*.

Ataxia-telangiectasia (AT): An autosomal recessive syndrome characterized by a combined defect of cellular and humoral immunity, nervous system abnormalities with poor muscle control, and capillary swelling.

Atopy: An inherited tendency to develop allergic reactions to naturally occurring substances by producing specific IgE antibodies.

Attenuation: A process of producing nonpathogenic bacteria or viruses for use in vaccines. These organisms have been weakened by treatment with a chemical, exposure to elevated or cold temperatures, or repeated passage in cell culture.

Atypical hemolytic uremic syndrome (aHUS): A rare genetic disorder associated with defects in complement regulation that cause microvascular thrombosis, hemolytic anemia, low platelet count, and acute renal failure.

Autoantibodies: Antibodies produced against antigens found in an individual's own cells, tissues, or organs.

Autoantigens: Antigens that belong to the host and do not elicit an immune response under normal circumstances (i.e., self-antigens).

Autocrine: Effect produced by a cell that stimulates the same cell.

Autograft: Tissues removed from one location of an individual's body and reintroduced in another location in the same individual.

Autoimmune diseases: Disorders in which damage to body organs results from the presence of autoantibodies or autoreactive T cells.

Autoimmune hemolytic anemia: An autoimmune disorder in which patients produce antibodies that destroy their own red blood cells.

Autoimmune hepatitis (AIH): Autoimmune disease in which patients produce antibodies that damage the liver; formerly known as *chronic active hepatitis*.

Autoimmune liver disease: An autoimmune disease that mainly affects the liver, including autoimmune hepatitis (AIH), primary biliary cholangitis (PBC), and primary sclerosing cholangitis (PSC).

Autoimmune regulator (AIRE): A transcription factor that induces expression of peripheral tissue antigens in the thymus to aid in the negative selection of T cells directed against self-antigens.

Autoimmune thyroid diseases (AITDs): Autoimmune diseases that affect the function of the thyroid gland, caused by the formation of antibodies or sensitized T cells; include Hashimoto disease and Graves disease.

Autoinflammatory disorders: Immunodeficiencies caused by inappropriate activation of innate immunity, resulting in recurrent fevers and systemic inflammation.

Automatic sampling: Automatic pipetting of a sample that is programmed into an instrument for testing of that sample.

Autoverification: The process by which a laboratory analyzer performs an automated comparison of patient results with predetermined, preapproved criteria programmed into the instrument.

Avidity: The strength with which a multivalent antibody binds a multivalent antigen; a measure of the overall stability of an antigen-antibody complex.

B-cell receptor (BCR): An immunoglobulin on the surface of a B cell that binds to a specific antigen during the immune response.

B lymphocyte: Cell derived from the bone marrow, which plays a key role in the humoral immune response; it develops into a plasma cell that produces a specific antibody.

Bacille Calmette-Guérin (BCG) vaccine: A vaccine consisting of attenuated strains of *Mycobacterium bovis*, used to prevent infection with *M. tuberculosis* in some parts of the world.

Basophil: A type of white blood cell (WBC) found in peripheral blood, containing granules that release substances that are involved in allergic reactions.

Batch analyzer: An instrument that permits analysis of several different samples at the same time and provides access to the samples for the formation of subsequent reaction mixtures.

Bence Jones proteins: Monoclonal immunoglobulin light chains found in the urine of some patients with multiple myeloma, Waldenström macroglobulinemia or amyloidosis.

Benign: Tissue that is not malignant.

Bi-specific T-cell engagers (BiTEs): Monoclonal antibodies that have two antigen binding sites, one for a tumor antigen and the other for a T-cell marker such as CD3; they are used in immunotherapy to facilitate T-cell killing of the tumor cells of interest.

Bioassays: Assays that measure the biologic activities of proteins such as cytokines.

Biohazard: A biological substance that poses a threat to human health, for example, contaminated blood or body fluids.

Biohazardous material: Patient specimens that may contain potentially harmful infectious agents or items that have come into contact with them.

Bioinformatics: Field of study that combines biology, computer science, statistics, mathematics, and other information sciences to develop and use methods to analyze large sets of biological data.

Biotin: A vitamin of the B-complex family that has an affinity for streptavidin; the complex is used for labeling in some types of immunoassays.

Bloodborne pathogens (BBPs): Pathogens such as HIV and the hepatitis B virus that can be transmitted by contact with contaminated blood or blood products.

Bone marrow: The tissue in the central cavities of most bones, which functions in the generation of hematopoietic cells and B-cell maturation.

***Borrelia burgdorferi*:** A spirochete bacterium that causes Lyme disease.

Bruton tyrosine kinase (Btk) deficiency: An X-linked recessive immunodeficiency disease that results in a lack of mature B lymphocytes and decreased immunoglobulins.

Bystander lysis: A phenomenon that occurs in complement activation when C3b becomes deposited on host cells, making them a target for destruction by phagocytic cells.

C-reactive protein (CRP): An acute phase protein that increases rapidly following infection or trauma to the body. It acts as an opsonin to enhance phagocytosis and activates complement after binding to phosphocholine or another component of pathogens.

C-type lectin receptors (CLRs): Pattern recognition receptors on white blood cells (WBCs) that bind to mannan and β-glucans in fungal cell walls.

C1 inhibitor (C1-INH): A glycoprotein that acts to dissociate C1r and C1s from C1q, thus inhibiting the first active enzyme formed in the classical complement cascade.

C3 glomerulopathy (C3G): Diseases involving complement dysregulation causing inflammation of the renal glomeruli.

C3 nephritic factors (C3NeFs): Autoantibodies that cause uncontrolled complement activation by stabilizing C3 convertase.

C4-binding protein (C4BP): A protein in the complement system that serves as a cofactor for factor I in the inactivation of C4b.

Calculated panel reactive antibody (cPRA): Proportion of potential transplant donors in a hypothetical donor pool possessing one or more HLA antigens to which the recipient has antibodies; a calculation that determines the likelihood that a donor and recipient will be incompatible based on HLA frequencies in a large donor population.

Cancer: A disease characterized by the presence of a malignant tumor.

Cancer antigen 125 (CA 125): A glycosylated protein that is used clinically as a marker for ovarian cancer.

Cancer vaccines: Vaccines that have been developed for the purpose of preventing or treating cancer by stimulating the body's immune defenses.

Candidiasis: An opportunistic fungal infection caused by *Candida albicans* and other *Candida* species.

Capture (sandwich) immunoassays: Immunoassays that detect an antigen by its ability to bind to an antibody attached to a solid phase as well as a detector antibody that contains a label, such as an enzyme.

CAR T cells: Genetically modified T cells possessing a chimeric antigen receptor that binds without major histocompatibility complex restriction to an antigen that can serve as a target for adoptive immunotherapy.

Carcinoembryonic antigen (CEA): An oncofetal protein that may be elevated in patients with colorectal and other cancers.

Carcinogenesis: The process by which a cell is transformed into a malignant tumor.

Carcinomas: Malignant tumors derived from the skin or epithelial linings of internal organs or glands.

Cathelicidins: A group of anti-microbial peptides with broad-spectrum anti-microbial activity.

CD4 T cell: Type of lymphocyte that provides help to B cells to initiate antibody production (helper T cell) or that inhibits the immune response (regulatory T cell).

CD40L deficiency: An X-linked recessive deficiency in the CD40 ligand (i.e., CD154) molecule on T cells needed for B-cell activation in the T-dependent antibody response, resulting in increased IgM and decreased levels of the other immunoglobulin classes.

Celiac disease: An autoimmune disease affecting the small intestine and other organs.

Cell cycle: The sequence of events that occurs between cell divisions and consists of the following phases: G1 (Gap 1), S (DNA synthesis), G2 (Gap 2), and M (Mitosis).

Cell-mediated immunity: A type of adaptive immunity in which T cells produce cytokines that help to regulate innate and adaptive immune responses.

Central tolerance: Destruction of potentially self-reactive T and B cells as they mature in the thymus or bone marrow, respectively.

Ceruloplasmin: An acute phase reactant that acts as the principal copper-transporting protein in human plasma.

Chain of infection: A continuous link between six elements—an infectious agent, a reservoir, a portal of exit, a means of transmission, a portal of entry, and a susceptible host.

Chain termination sequencing: A modification of the DNA replication process, which uses modified nucleotide bases called *dideoxynucleotide triphosphates* (ddNTPs), also known as *Sanger sequencing*. When these are incorporated into the growing DNA chain, synthesis stops.

Chancre: A firm, painless, solitary lesion that develops at the site of initial contact in syphilis.

Chemical Hygiene Plan: A plan that identifies appropriate work practices, standard operating procedures, and safety considerations in regard to the use of chemicals in the laboratory.

Chemiluminescence: The production of light energy by a chemical reaction.

Chemiluminescent immunoassay: A technique that uses a chemiluminescent label attached to either an antigen or antibody. Light is emitted because of a chemical reaction and indicates that antigen-antibody combination has taken place.

Chemiluminescent microparticle immunoassay (CMIA): A heterogeneous immunoassay that uses a chemiluminescent tag and antibody-coated microparticles as a reagent.

Chemokines: A large family of homologous cytokines that promote migration of white blood cells through chemotaxis.

Chemotaxin: A protein or other substance that acts as a chemical messenger to produce chemotaxis.

Chemotaxis: The directed migration of cells along the concentration gradient of a chemical attractant.

Chromosome: Structure in the nucleus that carries genetic information, consisting of DNA complexed with nuclear proteins.

Chronic granulomatous disease (CGD): An immunodeficiency inherited in either an X-linked or autosomal recessive fashion that results in the inability of neutrophils to produce the reactive forms of oxygen needed for normal bacterial killing.

Chronic mucocutaneous candidiasis (CMC): Immunodeficiency involving a selective defect in the immune response to *Candida* organisms.

Chronic rejection: Rejection of a graft that usually occurs after the first year of transplantation and results from progressive fibrosis of blood vessels in the grafted tissue.

Class I MHC (HLA) molecules: Proteins coded for by genes at three loci (HLA—A, B, C in humans) in the major histocompatibility complex. They are expressed on all nucleated cells and are important to consider in the transplantation of tissues.

Class II MHC (HLA) molecules: Proteins coded for by the HLA-DR, HLA-DP, and HLA-DQ loci of the major histocompatibility complex in humans. They are found on antigen-presenting cells—monocytes, macrophages, dendritic cells, B lymphocytes, and thymic epithelial cells—and are important to consider in the transplantation of tissues.

Class switching: The production of immunoglobulins other than IgM by daughter cells of antigen-exposed B lymphocytes.

Classical pathway: A series of steps involved in the activation of complement that begins with antigen-antibody binding.

Clinical and Laboratory Standards Institute (CLSI): An organization that develops clinical laboratory testing standards based on input from industry, government, and health care professionals.

Clinical Laboratory Improvement Amendments (CLIA): Federal regulatory standards that apply to all clinical laboratory testing in the United States.

Clonal deletion: The process of eliminating clones of lymphocytes that would be capable of an autoimmune response.

Clonal expansion: Proliferation of lymphocytes during an immune response to create a population of identical cells, all capable of responding to the same antigen.

Clonal selection: Stimulation of B or T lymphocytes with specificity for a particular antigen to proliferate to produce a clone of identical cells to enhance the immune response.

Clonal selection hypothesis: A theory postulated to explain the specificity of antibody formation, based on the premise that each B lymphocyte is genetically programmed to produce a specific type of antibody and is selected to proliferate by contact with an antigen.

Cloned enzyme donor immunoassay (CEDIA): A homogeneous competitive immunoassay that uses a β-galactosidase enzyme that has been genetically engineered in two parts: acceptor and donor.

Cluster of differentiation (CD) markers: Antigenic markers on leukocytes that are identified by groups of monoclonal antibodies expressing common or overlapping reactivity.

Clustered regularly interspaced short palindromic repeats (CRISPRs): Repeated DNA sequences in microbial DNA that are interrupted by spacer sequences matching regions extracted from invading plasmids or viruses; used in the laboratory for DNA analysis and genome editing.

Coagglutination: A type of reverse passive agglutination in which bacteria (e.g., *Staphylococcus aureus*) serve as the inert particle to which antibodies are attached.

Coccidioidomycosis: A fungal disease caused by *Coccidioides immitis* that is endemic to the southwestern United States and may be characterized by primary pulmonary infection.

Codon: A three-base nucleotide sequence in mRNA that codes for one of the 20 amino acids or a stop signal.

Coefficient of variation (CV): The average distance of each data point in a normal distribution from the mean. It is expressed as a percentage of the mean.

Cold agglutinins: Autoantibodies that react with antigens on the surface of red blood cells at temperatures below 37°C, typically formed in response to certain infections (e.g., *Mycoplasma pneumoniae*) and B-cell or plasma cell lymphoproliferative disorders.

Colony-stimulating factors (CSFs): Cytokines that promote hematopoiesis; they are needed for the expansion and differentiation of leukocytes and erythrocytes in the bone marrow.

Commensalistic: A relationship between two species of organisms in which there is no benefit or harm to either organism.

Commission on Laboratory Accreditation (COLA): An accreditation agency that helps laboratories meet CLIA and other federal regulations.

Common variable immunodeficiency (CVI): A heterogeneous group of immunodeficiency disorders that usually appear in patients between the ages of 20 and 30 years. It is characterized by a deficiency of one or more classes of immunoglobulins.

Community immunity: Concept of extending protection to unvaccinated individuals by reducing spread of an infection when a significant proportion of individuals in the population have been immunized; also known as *herd immunity.*

Companion diagnostics: Tests that provide information needed to identify patients who would most likely benefit from a particular therapy.

Comparative genomic hybridization (CGH): A microarray assay that detects gains or losses of chromosomal material throughout the genome.

Competitive immunoassay: An immunoassay in which unlabeled antigen and labeled antigen compete for a limited number of binding sites on reagent antibody.

Complement: A series of proteins that are normally present in serum and whose overall functions are mediation of inflammation and destruction of foreign cells.

Complement-dependent cytotoxicity (CDC) test: Serological test for HLA typing based on lymphocyte death resulting from attachment of HLA-specific antibody and complement activation.

Complement receptor type 1 (CR1): A cell-bound regulator of complement activation. It assists in degrading C3b and C4b and mediates transport of C3b-coated immune complexes to the liver and spleen.

Complementarity-determining regions (CDRs): Hypervariable amino acid sequences in the chains of an antibody molecule or T-cell receptor that form the antigen binding site.

Complementary: The relationship between the bases in two nucleotide strands; cytosine and guanine can only pair with each other, and adenine can only pair with thymine (in DNA) or uracil (in RNA).

Complementary or copy DNA (cDNA): A DNA sequence made from ribonucleic acid (RNA) using the enzyme reverse transcriptase and nucleotide base-pairing rules.

Conformational epitope: Key antigenic site that results from the folding of one peptide chain or multiple chains, bringing certain amino acids from different segments of a linear sequence or sequences into close proximity with each other so that they can be recognized together.

Congenital syphilis: The transfer of syphilis from an infected mother to her fetus during pregnancy.

Conidia: Asexual reproductive structures produced by fungi at the tip of hyphae; also known as *spores.*

Constant region: The carboxy-terminal segment of an antibody molecule that consists of a polypeptide sequence found in all molecules of the same (sub)class. The region is responsible for the biological functions that play a role in immune defense against an antigen.

Contact dermatitis: A delayed hypersensitivity reaction caused by T-cell sensitization to low molecular weight compounds that come in contact with the skin, such as nickel and poison ivy.

Control mean: The average of all data points.

Coombs reagent: An anti-human immunoglobulin reagent used to enhance the detection of immunoglobulin G (IgG) antibodies in blood bank testing.

Coronaviruses: A family of RNA viruses with surface projections that resemble a crown seen with electron microscopy; they cause respiratory tract infections that may be severe in some people.

Cortex: The outermost layer of the thymus (which contains immature T cells) or the lymph nodes (in which follicles containing B cells are found).

COVID-19: Coronavirus disease 2019, caused by SARS-CoV-2.

CREST syndrome: A subset of scleroderma named after its five major features: calcinosis, Raynaud phenomenon, esophageal dysmotility, sclerodactyly, and telangiectasia; also known as *limited cutaneous systemic sclerosis.*

Crossmatch: Incubation of donor lymphocytes with recipient serum to determine the presence of antibodies that could mediate rejection of a potential transplant.

Cross-reactivity: A phenomenon that occurs when an antibody reacts with an antigen that is structurally similar to the original antigen that induced production of the antibody.

Cryoglobulins: Immunoglobulins of the IgM or IgG class that precipitate at cold temperatures, causing occlusion of blood vessels in the extremities if a patient is exposed to the cold.

Cryptococcosis: A fungal disease caused by *Cryptococcus neoformans* and characterized as a pulmonary infection that may spread to the central nervous system and the brain.

Cyst: Inactive form of a parasite that can transmit infection.

Cytogenetics: The branch of genetics devoted to the study of chromosomes.

Cytokine cascade: A series of steps whereby the secretion of a cytokine by a cell activates target cells to produce additional cytokines.

Cytokine network: An interconnected system of cytokine-cell interactions that influences an immune response.

Cytokine profile: A group of cytokines characteristically made by a particular cell population or detected in a cytokine assay.

Cytokine release syndrome (CRS): A severe, often fatal condition resulting from dysregulation of cytokine synthesis and massive overproduction of cytokines; also known as a *cytokine storm or hypercytokinemia.*

Cytokine storm: A severe, often fatal condition resulting from dysregulation of cytokine synthesis and massive overproduction of cytokines; also known as a *cytokine release syndrome or hypercytokinemia.*

Cytokines: Small proteins that act as chemical messengers that affect the function or activity of other cells, especially cells of the immune system.

Cytomegalovirus (CMV): A virus in the herpes family that may cause a mononucleosis-like syndrome in healthy people, a life-threatening illness in immunocompromised patients, or congenital infections.

Cytotoxic T (Tc) cells: T cells that bear the CD8 marker and function to kill virus-infected cells and tumor cells by triggering apoptosis.

Damage-associated molecular patterns (DAMPs): Substances released by stressed, injured, or transformed cells that are recognized by pattern recognition receptors (PRRs) on host cells. Examples include heat-shock proteins, altered membrane phospholipids, and DNA.

Decay-accelerating factor (DAF): A glycoprotein found on peripheral red blood cells (RBCs), endothelial cells, fibroblasts, and epithelial cell surfaces that is capable of dissociating the C3 convertases formed by all three pathways of complement.

Defensins: A class of small proteins produced by cells of the innate immune system and epithelial cells of the skin and mucous membranes which have broad-spectrum anti-microbial activity against bacteria and other pathogens.

Delayed hypersensitivity: Type IV or T-cell–mediated hypersensitivity; so named because its manifestations are not seen until 24 to 48 hours after exposure to the inducing antigen.

Delta check: A quality assurance procedure that compares a patient's test results with their previous results.

Dendritic cells: Tissue cells covered with long membranous extensions resembling nerve cell dendrites; these cells capture antigens by phagocytosis or endocytosis and, upon activation, present them to T cells in the adaptive immune response.

Deoxyribonucleic acid (DNA): The nucleic acid whose sugar is deoxyribose. It is the primary genetic material of all cellular organisms and DNA viruses.

Dermatomyositis (DM): A systemic autoimmune rheumatic disease that involves the skin and muscles.

Diagnostic sensitivity: The proportion of people who have a specific disease or condition and who have a positive test result.

Diagnostic specificity: The proportion of people who do not have a disease or condition and who have a negative test result.

Diapedesis: The process by which cells move from the circulating blood to the tissues by squeezing through the wall of a blood vessel.

DiGeorge syndrome: A congenital defect of the third and fourth pharyngeal pouches of the embryo, affecting development of the heart, parathyroid glands, facial features, and thymus, resulting in a T-cell deficiency; also known as *22q11.2 deletion syndrome, velocardiofacial syndrome, Shprintzen syndrome,* and *conotruncal anomaly face syndrome.*

Digital PCR (dPCR): A type of polymerase chain reaction that provides absolute quantification of the number of DNA molecules in a sample.

Diluent: One of two entities needed for making up a solution. It is the medium into which the solute is added.

Dilution factor: A numerical value representing the extent to which a solution has been diluted. It is often expressed as a fraction or ratio.

Direct agglutination: A clumping of cells that occurs when antibodies react with antigens that are naturally found on the surface of the cells.

Direct allorecognition: Pathway in which a transplant recipient's T cells recognize intact HLA molecules on the donor's cells.

Direct antiglobulin test (DAT): A technique to determine in vivo attachment of antibody or complement to red blood cells, using anti-human globulin to cause a visible agglutination reaction.

Direct immunofluorescence assay: A technique to identify a specific antigen using an antibody that has a fluorescent tag attached.

Domains: Globular regions in the three-dimensional structure of an antibody molecule, each consisting of approximately 110 amino acids.

Double-negative (DN) thymocyte: Stage in the development of T cells when neither CD4 nor CD8 is expressed.

Double-positive (DP) thymocyte: Stage in the development of T cells when both CD4 and CD8 antigens are expressed.

Double-stranded DNA (dsDNA) antibodies: Autoantibodies produced against double-stranded DNA that are diagnostic for systemic lupus erythematosus (SLE).

Dual-parameter dot plot: A histogram that depicts cells based on two different characteristics, one of which is plotted on the *x*-axis and the other on the *y*-axis.

Ectoparasites: Multicelled parasitic organisms that live on the skin of the host.

Effector cells: Mature, functional T lymphocytes or B lymphocytes that carry out the functions of immune responses.

Electrochemiluminescence immunoassay (ECLIA): A modified chemiluminescence immunoassay in which an antibody reagent is labeled with ruthenium, which is oxidized at the surface of an electrode and releases light when it is returned to its reduced state.

Electronic quality control: A method that monitors the accuracy and functionality of a test system through electronic signals or internal checks within a laboratory instrument itself, rather than using liquid control samples.

Electrophoresis: The separation of molecules in an electrical field based on differences in charge and size.

ELISA: See *Enzyme-linked immunosorbent assay.*

ELISpot: A bioassay that detects the frequency of cultured cells that secrete a particular cytokine.

Endocrine: Internal secretion of substances, such as hormones or cytokines, directly into the bloodstream that causes systemic effects.

Endotoxin: A component of the cell walls of gram-negative bacteria, which consists of the portion of lipopolysaccharide (LPS) called *lipid A.* Endotoxin is a potent stimulator of cytokine release that can lead to septic shock.

Endpoint method: A technique in which antigen is allowed to react with antibody until the point of equivalence is reached (e.g., radial immunodiffusion).

Enzyme: A protein that acts as a catalyst for a specific biochemical reaction; commonly used as a label in immunoassays.

Enzyme immunoassay (EIA): An assay that uses an enzyme label to detect an antigen-antibody reaction; the enzyme acts on a substrate to produce a colored product, light, or fluorescence.

Enzyme-linked immunosorbent assay (ELISA): An immunoassay that uses an enzyme label on one of the reactants.

Enzyme-multiplied immunoassay technique (EMIT): A homogeneous immunoassay based on the principle of change in enzymatic activity as a specific antigen-antibody interaction occurs in solution.

Eosinophils: White blood cells (WBCs) that contain reddish-orange granules on Wright-stained blood smears and are involved in allergic reactions, defense against large parasites, and release of cytokines that regulate immune responses.

Epigenetic: Modifications in gene expression that are not caused by changes in the nucleotide sequence of DNA.

Epitope: A key portion of an immunogen against which the immune response is directed; also known as an *antigenic determinant.*

Epitope spreading: An expansion of an immune response to unrelated antigens, which may be involved in the development of autoimmunity.

Epstein-Barr virus (EBV): A DNA virus of the herpesvirus family that causes infectious mononucleosis, Burkitt lymphoma, Hodgkin disease, nasopharyngeal and gastric carcinomas, and lymphoproliferative disorders in immunosuppressed people.

Erythropoietin (EPO): A colony-stimulating factor that increases red blood cell (RBC) production in the bone marrow.

Examination variable: A factor that can affect test results during performance of a test, including reagents and test procedure, instrument calibration and maintenance, personnel requirements, technical competence, and interpretation of QC data; formerly known as an *analytical variable.*

Exons: The protein coding sequences in DNA or RNA.

Exotoxin: Potent protein released from living bacteria (mostly gram-positive) that causes harm to the host by binding to a specific cellular receptor.

Extensively drug-resistant tuberculosis (XDR-TB): Tuberculosis caused by bacterial strains of *M. tuberculosis* that are resistant to isoniazid and other first-line treatment drugs.

External controls: Known standardized samples tested along with patient samples to verify the accuracy and precision of a test.

External quality assessment (EQA): The testing of unknown samples received from an outside agency.

Extractable nuclear antigens (ENAs): Small nuclear proteins associated with uridine-rich RNA that can stimulate the production of autoantibodies; examples are Sm and RNP.

Extrinsic parameters: In flow cytometry, properties of a cell such as a surface protein that require addition of a fluorescent-labeled antibody for their detection.

Fab fragments: Fragment of an immunoglobulin molecule obtained by papain cleavage that consists of a light chain and one-half of a heavy chain held together by disulfide bonding; it contains the antigen binding site.

F(ab′)2 fragment: Fragment of an immunoglobulin molecule obtained by pepsin cleavage that contains two antigen binding sites; it consists of two Fab regions held together by disulfide bonds in the hinge area.

Factor H: A control protein in the complement system that acts as a cofactor with factor I to break down C3b formed during complement activation.

Factor I: A serine protease that cleaves C3b and C4b formed during complement activation; a cofactor is required for these reactions.

False negative: A laboratory result that occurs when a person has a specified condition, but the test for that condition is negative.

False positive: A laboratory result that occurs when a person does not have a specified condition, but the test for the condition is positive.

Fc fragment: Fragment of an immunoglobulin molecule obtained by papain cleavage that consists of the carboxy-terminal halves of two heavy chains held together by disulfide bonds. This fragment spontaneously crystallizes at 4°C.

Ferritin: An acute phase reactant whose main function is the storage of intracellular iron.

Fibrinogen: An acute phase reactant that is converted to fibrin in the coagulation cascade and forms clots in the bloodstream.

Flocculation: A type of precipitation reaction in which immune complex formation happens over a narrow range of antigen concentrations, resulting in fine particulate precipitants.

Flow cytometry: An automated system in which single cells in a fluid are analyzed in terms of their intrinsic light-scattering characteristics and evaluated for their extrinsic properties after the addition of fluorescent-labeled antibodies or probes.

Fluorescence in situ hybridization (FISH): A technique used to identify a specific region of DNA in a chromosome through binding of fluorescent-tagged complementary DNA probes.

Fluorescent anti-nuclear antibody (FANA) testing: Testing to identify the presence of antibody to nuclear antigens, using a human epithelial cell line fixed to a microscope slide and a fluorescent-labeled anti-human immunoglobulin.

Fluorescent treponemal antibody absorption (FTA-ABS) test: A confirmatory test for syphilis, which detects antibodies to *Treponema pallidum* by using anti-human immunoglobulin with a fluorescent label.

Fluorochrome: See *fluorophores.*

Fluorophores: Compounds that absorb energy from an incident light source and convert that energy into light of a longer wavelength and lower energy as the excited electrons return to the ground state.

Follicular helper T (TFH) cell: A subpopulation of helper T cells that remains in the lymph nodes, where they interact with B cells to assist in antibody production.

Fomites: Inanimate objects that can become contaminated with an infectious agent (e.g., from contact with a human specimen) and transmit the agent to a new host.

Forward scatter (FSC): In flow cytometry, light scatter measured in a forward direction at a slight angle from the axis of the laser beam, which indicates the size of a cell.

Fungi: Organisms made up of eukaryotic cells with rigid walls composed of chitin, mannan, and sometimes cellulose.

Gate: In flow cytometry, a defined boundary placed around a population of interest to analyze various parameters (extrinsic and intrinsic) of the cells contained within the selected region.

Gel electrophoresis: Method of separating either proteins or DNA based on their size and electrical charge. Samples are placed in wells in the gel and exposed to an electrical current.

Gene expression microarrays: Microarrays that use RNA from a test sample (e.g., tumor tissue) to analyze the expression of multiple genes and compare the results to a reference sample (e.g., normal tissue).

Gene switching: A mechanism used by parasites to evade the host's immune system by rearranging DNA and modifying gene transcript levels to vary synthesis of surface antigens.

Genes: Specific sequences of nucleotides in chromosomes that carry information for a protein or a noncoding RNA molecule.

Genetic code: A set of three nucleotides that code for one amino acid.

Genome: The entire set of genes in an organism.

Genomics: The study of all the genes in an organism.

Genotype resistance assays: Tests that detect mutations in viral genes that can render viruses resistant to anti-viral drugs.

Germinal center: The interior of a secondary follicle in lymphoid organs, where B-cell proliferation and transformation into plasma cells and memory cells takes place.

Globally Harmonized System (GHS): An international system that standardizes the classification of hazardous chemicals and the symbols used for these hazards on labels and in safety data sheets.

Goodpasture syndrome: An autoimmune disease characterized by the presence of an autoantibody to collagen in the glomerular (kidney) or alveolar (lung) basement membranes; also known as *anti-glomerular basement membrane disease.*

Graduated pipette: A pipette that has markings at regular increments all along its length to allow for varying amounts of liquid to be measured.

Graft-vs-host disease (GVHD): A condition that results when immunocompetent cells in a hematopoietic cell transplant mount an immune response against the tissues of a genetically dissimilar recipient.

Granulocyte colony-stimulating factor (G-CSF): A cytokine produced by fibroblasts and epithelial cells that enhances the production of neutrophils.

Granulocyte-macrophage colony-stimulating factor (GM-CSF): A cytokine produced by T cells and other cell lines that stimulates increased production of granulocytes and macrophages.

Granulocytes: White blood cells that contain numerous granules in their cytoplasm; neutrophils, eosinophils, basophils, and mast cells are the cell types in this category.

Granulomas: Organized clusters of inflammatory cells formed in some type IV hypersensitivity reactions.

Granulomatosis with polyangiitis (PGA): An autoimmune disease involving inflammation of the small- to medium-sized blood vessels and the production of anti-neutrophil cytoplasmic antibody (ANCA); formerly known as *Wegener granulomatosus.*

Graves disease: An autoimmune disease characterized by hyperthyroidism caused by the presence of antibody to thyroid-stimulating hormone receptors. Binding of antibody to the receptors results in excessive release of thyroid hormones.

Group A streptococcus (GAS): Gram-positive, catalase-negative cocci often found in pairs or chains that are responsible for several diseases, ranging from pharyngitis to necrotizing fasciitis; i.e., *Streptococcus pyogenes.*

Gummas: Localized areas of granulomatous inflammation on bones, skin, and subcutaneous tissue seen in tertiary syphilis.

Hairy cell leukemia: Chronic leukemia characterized by the formation of large mononuclear cells with irregular cytoplasmic projections found in bone marrow.

Haplotype: A set of genes that are located close together on a chromosome and are usually inherited as a single unit.

Hapten: A simple chemical group that can bind to an antibody once it is formed but that cannot stimulate antibody formation unless bound to a larger carrier molecule.

Haptoglobin: An acute phase reactant that binds irreversibly to free hemoglobin released by intravascular hemolysis.

Hashimoto thyroiditis: An autoimmune disease that results in hypothyroidism caused by the presence of cytotoxic T cells and autoantibodies to anti-thyroglobulin and thyroid peroxidase, which progressively destroy the thyroid gland.

Heavy (H) chains: The larger chains in an immunoglobulin molecule. Each immunoglobulin monomer consists of two heavy chains paired with two light chains.

Heavy chain diseases: B-cell lymphomas characterized by the production of monoclonal immunoglobulin heavy chains that are not attached to light chains.

Helminths: Parasitic worms, such as flatworms, tapeworms, or roundworms.

Helper T (TH) cells: Lymphocytes that express the CD4 antigen and secrete cytokines that provide help to B cells in antibody production and activate other cells in cell-mediated immune responses. They are classified into several subpopulations based on the types of cytokines they secrete.

Helper Type 1 (TH1) cells: A subset of helper T cells that secretes IFN-γ and IL-2 and is mainly responsible for cell-mediated immune responses against intracellular pathogens.

Helper Type 2 (TH2) cells: A subset of helper T cells that secretes IL-4, IL-5, and IL-13 and whose main function is to activate B cells, mast cells, and eosinophils in immune responses against extracellular parasites.

Helper Type 17 (TH17) cells: A subset of helper T cells that plays an important role in defense against bacterial and fungal infections and secretes IL-17 to recruit neutrophils to the site of infection. TH17 cells also enhance inflammation in pathological autoimmune responses.

Hemagglutination: An antigen-antibody reaction that results in the clumping of red blood cells.

Hemagglutination inhibition: A test for detecting antibodies to certain viruses, based on lack of RBC agglutination that results from antibody neutralizing the virus.

Hematopoiesis: Process by which blood cells are produced from multipotent hematopoietic stem cells in the bone marrow.

Hematopoietic growth factors: Cytokines that stimulate proliferation, differentiation, and maturation of the blood cell lineages from bone marrow progenitor cells.

Hemolytic disease of the fetus and newborn (HDFN): A cytotoxic reaction that destroys an infant's red blood cells (RBCs) because of placental transfer of maternal antibodies to Rh or other RBC antigens.

Hemolytic titration (CH50) assay: An assay that determines complement-activating ability by measuring the amount of patient serum required to lyse 50% of a standardized concentration of antibody-sensitized sheep erythrocytes.

Hepatitis: Inflammation of the liver that can be caused by several viruses as well as noninfectious factors, such as radiation, exposure to chemicals, or autoimmune diseases.

Hepatitis A virus (HAV): An RNA virus that can cause hepatitis; transmitted by the fecal-oral route, close person-to-person contact, or ingestion of contaminated food or water.

Hepatitis B surface antigen (HBsAg): An antigen on the surface envelope of the hepatitis B virus, the first marker to appear in hepatitis B infection.

Hepatitis B virus (HBV): A DNA virus that can cause hepatitis; it is transmitted by intimate contact with contaminated blood or other body fluids, sexual contact, or perinatally.

Hepatitis Be antigen (HBeAg): Protein located between the outer envelope and core of the hepatitis B virus.

Hepatitis C virus (HCV): An RNA virus that can cause hepatitis; it is transmitted sexually or through contaminated blood or needles.

Hepatitis D virus (HDV): An RNA virus that can cause hepatitis; it requires the presence of hepatitis B virus (HBV) for its replication and expression.

Hepatitis E virus (HEV): An RNA virus that can cause hepatitis; it is transmitted by the fecal-oral route or ingestion of contaminated food or water.

Herd immunity: Concept of extending protection to unvaccinated individuals by reducing spread of an infection when a significant proportion of individuals in the population have been immunized; also known as *community immunity.*

Hereditary angioedema (HAE): A disease characterized by swelling of the extremities, the skin, the gastrointestinal tract, and other mucosal surfaces because of a deficiency in the complement inhibitor C1NH.

Heteroantigen: An antigen of a species different from that of the host, such as other animals, plants, or microorganisms.

Heterogeneous immunoassay: An immunoassay that requires physical separation of bound and free components; this can be achieved by different methods, including centrifugation, binding to solid-phase material, or magnetic separation.

Heterophile antibody: Antibody that is capable of reacting with similar antigens from two or more unrelated species; commonly found in patients with infectious mononucleosis.

Heterophile antigen: An antigen that is either identical or closely related to an antigen in unrelated plants or animals so that antibody to one will cross-react with antibody to the other.

High-dose hook effect: Limitation of immunoassays caused by excess antigen in the patient sample (e.g., a tumor antigen), causing falsely decreased detection, and leading to an analyte concentration reading that appears to be low or normal (i.e., a postzone effect).

Hinge region: The flexible portion of the heavy chain of an immunoglobulin molecule located between the first and second constant regions. This allows the molecule to bend so that the two antigen binding sites can operate independently.

Histamine: A vasoactive amine released from mast cells and basophils during an allergic reaction.

Histoplasmosis: An infection caused by the fungus *Histoplasma capsulatum*.

HLA antibody screen: Test for HLA antibodies in transplant recipients that could potentially react with the donor graft.

HLA genotype: The HLA allele composition in an individual.

HLA matching: The pairing up of a transplant donor and recipient based on similarity of HLA antigens or alleles.

HLA phenotype: The HLA antigen composition of an individual.

HLA typing: Laboratory testing used to identify the HLA antigens or genes in a transplant candidate or donor.

Hodgkin lymphoma (HL): A malignant disease that typically begins in one lymph node and is characterized by the presence of Reed-Sternberg cells, giant multinucleated cells that are usually transformed B lymphocytes.

Homogeneous immunoassay: An immunoassay in which the antigen-antibody reaction occurs in solution, and separation of free and bound components is not needed.

HTLV-associated myelopathy/tropical spastic paraparesis (HAM/TSP): A progressive neurological disorder caused by HTLV-1.

Human chorionic gonadotropin (hCG): A hormone that is synthesized by trophoblasts and used as a marker for tumors of the ovaries, testes, and trophoblast cells; it is also used to detect pregnancy.

Human epidermal growth factor receptor 2 (HER2): A transmembrane receptor that binds human epidermal growth factor; it is overexpressed in some breast cancers and other cancer types.

Human immune serum globulin (HISG): A sterile preparation of concentrated antibodies made from pooled serum of thousands of donors; used as a prophylactic treatment in patients with antibody deficiencies.

Human immunodeficiency virus (HIV): A retrovirus that is the etiologic agent of AIDS.

Human leukocyte antigen (HLA): Protein coded for by the human major histocompatibility class (MHC) genes that has essential roles in the immune response and the rejection of foreign transplants.

Human T-cell lymphotropic virus type 1 (HTLV-1): An RNA retrovirus that causes adult T-cell leukemia/lymphoma and HTLV-associated myelopathy/tropical spastic paraparesis.

Human T-cell lymphotropic virus type 2 (HTLV-2): An RNA retrovirus thought to be associated with neurological disease, certain hematologic and dermatologic diseases, and an increased incidence of infections.

Humoral immunity: A type of adaptive immunity resulting from substances circulating in body fluids (i.e., antibodies).

Hybridization: Complementary binding of two single-stranded nucleic acid segments, as in binding of a probe with a known nucleic acid sequence to an unknown piece of DNA.

Hybridoma: A cell line resulting from the fusion of a myeloma cell and a B cell. The line is maintained in tissue culture and produces a monoclonal antibody, which is specific for a single antigen epitope.

Hydrodynamically focused: The use of two streams of fluid in flow cytometry to align cells or particles so that they pass single file through the intersection of the laser light source.

Hyper IgE syndromes: Immunodeficiencies characterized by elevated serum IgE, increased eosinophils, eczema, and frequent skin abscesses and lung infections.

Hyperacute rejection: Rejection of tissue that occurs within minutes or hours following transplantation because of pre-existing antibodies to ABO and HLA antigens in the graft recipient.

Hypercytokinemia: An often fatal condition involving dysregulation and massive production of cytokines, producing hyperstimulation of the immune response; also known as *cytokine release syndrome* or *cytokine storm*.

Hyperimmune globulins: Preparations of pooled serum of human donors who have a high antibody titer against a pathogen or its product, for use in passive immunization to provide immediate protection to unimmunized people.

Hypersensitivity: An exaggerated immune response to a typically harmless antigen that results in tissue injury, disease, or death.

Hyphae: Filamentous tubular branching structures characteristic of some fungi.

Hypogammaglobulinemia: Low levels of immunoglobulins in the blood.

Idiotypes: The variable portions of each light and heavy immunoglobulin chain that are unique to a particular immunoglobulin molecule. This region forms the antigen binding site.

IgM anti-HBc: Antibody that is the first to appear in hepatitis B infection. It is of the IgM class and is directed against the core antigen of the virus particle.

Immature B cell: A phase in the growth of B cells characterized by the appearance of IgM antibody monomers on the cell surface.

Immediate hypersensitivity: Reaction to an allergen that occurs within minutes to a few hours after exposure to the inducing antigen.

Immune adherence: The ability of phagocytic cells to bind complement-coated particles.

Immune checkpoint inhibitors: Monoclonal antibodies that enhance patients' T-cell responses to tumors by blocking inhibitory pathways that inactivate T cells; examples include antibodies to CTLA-4, PD-1, and PD-L1.

Immune thrombocytopenic purpura (ITP): A disorder in which antibodies develop against platelets; previously known as *idiopathic thrombocytopenic purpura*.

Immunity: The condition of being resistant to infection.

Immunization: The process by which immunity is acquired.

Immunoassays: Assays that use immune reactions to detect and measure proteins such as antibodies or cytokines.

Immunoblotting: A technique used to identify antibodies to complex antigens. It involves electrophoresis of the antigen mixture followed by transfer of the pattern to a durable test membrane for reaction with patient serum (i.e., a Western blot).

Immunochromatography: A rapid technique in which the analyte is applied at one end of a membrane and migrates toward the distal end, where it combines with an antibody to produce results that can be visualized in minutes.

Immunodeficiencies: Inherited or acquired disorders in which a part of the body's immune system is missing or dysfunctional.

Immunoediting: A process by which genetic and other changes in tumor cells allow them to develop resistance to immune defenses.

Immunofixation electrophoresis (IFE): A semiquantitative gel precipitation technique in which proteins are first separated by electrophoresis, then incubated with antibodies to individual proteins that are added directly to the gel surface; used commonly to identify monoclonal immunoglobulins.

Immunofluorescence assay (IFA): Test used to identify cellular antigens or antibodies to those antigens using an antibody labeled with a fluorescent tag.

Immunogen: A substance that is capable of inducing an adaptive immune response.

Immunogenicity: The ability of an immunogen to stimulate an immune response.

Immunoglobulin (Ig): Glycoprotein in the serum portion of the blood that is a major component of humoral immunity (i.e., an antibody).

Immunohistochemistry (IHC): A type of in situ hybridization in which labeled antibodies bind to clinically significant protein targets (e.g., tumor markers) expressed in tissue.

Immunologic diversion: A mechanism by which parasites enhance their survival in the host by inducing the production of proteins that divert the attention of the immune system.

Immunologic memory: Ability of the adaptive immune system to respond more rapidly and effectively after re-exposure to the same antigen.

Immunologic subversion: A mechanism by which parasites can avoid the effector mechanisms of the immune response by producing proteins that act as homologues of various components of the immune system.

Immunologic tolerance: A state of immune unresponsiveness directed against a specific antigen.

Immunology: The study of the immune system and its reactions to foreign substances.

Immunometric assay: An immunoassay in which antibody to the target antigen is bound to the solid phase; also known as a *capture* or *sandwich* immunoassay.

Immunophenotype: The combined presence or absence of specific antigens on a cell.

Immunophenotyping: Identifying cells according to their surface antigen expression.

Immunoprophylaxis: The use of immunization to prevent disease.

Immunosubtraction (immunotyping): A procedure that uses capillary electrophoresis to identify monoclonal immunoglobulin components.

Immunosuppressive agents: Drugs or antibodies used to suppress an immune response (e.g. an antigraft immune response to transplanted tissue).

Immunosurveillance: The mechanisms by which the immune system patrols the body for the presence of cancerous or precancerous cells and eliminates them before they become clinically evident.

Immunotherapy: Treatment that uses the ability of the immune system to destroy tumor cells.

Immunotoxins: Antibodies conjugated to toxins to help destroy cancer cells; also called *antibody-drug conjugates.*

Immunoturbidimetry: A technique for determining the concentration of particles in a solution based on the change in absorbance, caused by a reduction in light intensity that occurs when an incident beam is passed through a solution in which antigen-antibody complexes are forming.

Impetigo: A skin infection characterized by vesicular lesions on the extremities that become pustular and crusted, caused by bacteria such as group A streptococci.

In situ hybridization (ISH): Molecular assays that detect targets "in place" as they appear in tissues, cells, and subcellular structures.

Inborn errors of immunity: A diverse group of inherited conditions caused by abnormalities in single genes that affect immune function; also known as *primary immunodeficiency diseases.*

Indigenous microbiota: See *microbiota.*

Indirect allorecognition: Pathway by which the immune system recognizes foreign HLA antigens on a donor graft; it involves the uptake, processing, and presentation of foreign HLA proteins by the recipient's antigen-presenting cells (APCs) to the recipient's T cells to produce antibodies and cell-mediated responses against the graft.

Indirect antiglobulin test (IAT): A laboratory method that detects in vitro binding of antibody to red blood cells (RBCs); it is used in typing patient RBCs for specific blood group antigens and in crossmatching blood to prevent a transfusion reaction.

Indirect ELISA: A noncompetitive enzyme immunoassay that detects an antibody in the test sample that binds to a solid-phase antigen and an enzyme-labeled antibody reagent.

Indirect immunofluorescence (IIF) assay: A technique to identify an antibody or antigen in a test sample by using two reagent antibodies: one that is specific for the antigen (i.e., the primary antibody) and a second that is labeled with a fluorescent tag and is specific for the primary antibody (e.g., an anti-human immunoglobulin).

Individualized quality control plan (IQCP): An alternative CLIA QC option that provides equivalent quality testing to meet the CLIA regulations for moderate and high complexity tests and provider-performed microscopy procedures.

Infection control: Procedures used to control and monitor infections occurring within health care facilities.

Infectivity: An organism's ability to establish an infection; the proportion of individuals exposed to a pathogen through horizontal transmission (i.e., person-to-person contact) who will become infected.

Inflammasomes: Protein complexes that contain enzymes that cleave precursors of the pro-inflammatory cytokines, interleukins IL-1β and IL-18, to generate their active forms and induce death of host cells infected with intracellular pathogens; inappropriate activation may contribute to some autoinflammatory disorders.

Inflammation: Cellular and humoral mechanisms involved in the overall reaction of vascularized tissue to injury or invasion by an infectious agent.

Inflammatory myopathies (IMs): A group of systemic autoimmune diseases characterized by chronic inflammation of the skeletal muscles and progressive muscle weakness.

Influenza: A contagious respiratory infection ("the flu") caused by influenza viruses.

Innate lymphoid cells (ILCs): Family of cells that contribute to innate immunity and tissue remodeling; ILCs are morphologically and functionally similar to T cells but do not possess antigen-specific receptors.

Innate (natural) immunity: The ability to resist infection by mechanisms existing in the body prior to contact with antigen (e.g., anatomical barriers, phagocytic cells, cytokines). Innate responses are not antigen specific and do not result in immunologic memory.

Integrins: Molecules on certain leukocytes that cause adhesion to vascular endothelial cells.

Interferon gamma release assays (IGRAs): In vitro methods that detect latent tuberculosis infection by measuring the production of IFN-γ by patient T cells that have been stimulated with *Mycobacterium tuberculosis*–specific antigens.

Interferons (IFNs): Cytokines produced by T cells and other cells that inhibit viral replication or act as immune regulators.

Interleukins (IL-): A diverse group of cytokines produced by leukocytes and other cells that regulate adaptive immune responses and the inflammatory process.

Internal controls: Internal monitoring systems built into the test system to monitor the sufficient addition of a patient sample or reagent.

Intrinsic parameters: Light-scattering properties in flow cytometry that are a part of a cell, such as size and granularity.

Introns: The noncoding sequences found between the exons in DNA or RNA.

Invariant chain (Ii): A protein that associates with human leukocyte antigen (HLA) class II antigens shortly after they are synthesized to prevent interaction of their binding sites with any endogenous peptides in the endoplasmic reticulum.

Isoelectric focusing (IEF): A laboratory technique in which proteins are separated based on differences in their isoelectric point (pI), or the pH at which a molecule is electrically neutral.

Isograft (syngeneic graft): Graft that involves the transfer of tissue between two genetically identical members of the same species.

Isohemagglutinins: Naturally occurring antibodies that agglutinate red blood cells (RBCs) of other individuals of the same species; in humans, they are directed against the A or B antigens on RBCs.

Isothermal: An amplification process using a reaction that proceeds at a single temperature.

Isotype switching: A genetically driven process by which B cells change their antibody production from IgM to another immunoglobulin class.

Isotypes: Unique amino acid sequences that are common to all immunoglobulin molecules of a particular class or subclass in a given species.

J (Joining) chain: A glycoprotein with a molecular weight of 15,000 that links immunoglobulin monomers together. J chains are found only in immunoglobulin M (IgM) and secretory IgA molecules.

Job syndrome: An inherited immunodeficiency disease characterized by high levels of circulating IgE, decreased T helper cells, defective neutrophil chemotaxis, recurrent infections, and distinct facial features.

Kappa (κ) chain: One of two types of immunoglobulin light chains; they are present in about two-thirds of all immunoglobulin molecules.

Karyotype analysis: A test used to examine the chromosomes in a cell sample for numerical or structural abnormalities.

Lambda (λ) chain: One of two types of immunoglobulin light chains; they are present in about one-third of all immunoglobulin molecules.

Laminar flow: In flow cytometry, the concept by which cells or particles move parallel to the sheath fluid and do not mix with it.

Lancefield group: A means of classifying streptococci based on differences in their cell wall carbohydrate.

Latent tuberculosis infection (LTBI): Asymptomatic infection with *Mycobacterium tuberculosis* that may convert to active tuberculosis in some people at a later time.

Lateral flow assays (LFAs): Immunochromatographic assays for rapid antigen detection.

Lattice: A stable complex that results from the combination of antibody molecules with multivalent antigens and produces a visible reaction.

Law of mass action: A law used to mathematically describe the equilibrium relationship between the reactants and the products of a reaction. It can be applied to antigen-antibody relationships.

Lean system: A system used in the laboratory that focuses on the elimination of waste using the 6S rules to allow a facility to do more with less and at the same time increase customer and employee satisfaction.

Lectin pathway: A pathway for complement activation initiated by binding of mannose-binding lectin to mannose or related sugars on bacteria, yeast, viruses, and some parasites.

***Leptospira* species:** Spirochete bacteria that cause leptospirosis.

Leptospirosis: Infection caused by tightly coiled spirochete bacteria called *leptospires*.

Leukemias: Malignancies that originate from hematopoietic cells in the bone marrow and migrate to the peripheral blood.

Leukocytes: White blood cells (WBCs).

Leukotrienes (LT): A class of secondary mediators released from mast cells and basophils during type I hypersensitivity reactions.

Light (L) chains: The smaller peptide chains in an immunoglobulin molecule; they are bound to the larger chains by disulfide bonds. The two types of light chains are called *kappa* and *lambda*.

Linear epitope: A sequence of amino acids on a single polypeptide chain that acts as a key antigenic site.

Loop-mediated amplification (LAMP): An isothermal DNA amplification technique in which specially designed primers self-hybridize to form loops, which then serve as primer binding sites for further amplification.

Lyme disease: A disease caused by infection with spirochete bacteria from the *Borrelia* genus.

Lymph nodes: Secondary lymphoid organs located throughout the body whose purpose is to filter lymphatic fluid from the tissues and act as a site for processing foreign antigens.

Lymphocyte: The key type of white blood cell involved in the adaptive immune response; the three major types of lymphocytes are T cells, B cells, and NK cells.

Lymphoid: Relating to lymphocytes or the tissues from which they are produced.

Lymphomas: Cancers of the lymphoid cells that usually arise in the lymph nodes and other lymphoid tissues and proliferate to form solid tumors.

Macrophage colony-stimulating factor (M-CSF): A cytokine that induces growth of hematopoietic cells destined to become monocytes and macrophages.

Macrophages: White blood cells in the tissues that engulf and kill microbes and present antigens to T cells.

Major histocompatibility complex (MHC): The genes that control expression of a large group of proteins originally identified on leukocytes but now known to be found on all nucleated cells in the body. These proteins play an important role in antigen recognition and stimulate graft rejection.

MALDI-TOF: Matrix-associated laser desorption ionization time-of-flight mass spectrometry, a technique used to analyze proteins to identify a substance or microorganism in a sample.

Malignant: A descriptive term for cancerous tumors that can invade nearby organs and circulate to other parts of the body.

MALT (mucosal-associated lymphoid tissues): Lymphoid tissue found in the gastrointestinal, respiratory, and urogenital tracts.

Mannose-binding lectin (MBL): A protein in the blood that binds to mannose on bacteria and other pathogens to initiate the lectin pathway of complement activation.

Mast cells: Tissue cells that resemble basophils and play a role in allergic reactions.

Medulla: Inner layer of the thymus (containing mature T cells) or the lymph nodes.

Membrane attack complex (MAC): The combination of complement components C5b, C6, C7, C8, and C9 that becomes inserted into the target-cell membrane, causing lysis.

Membrane cofactor protein (MCP): A protein found on all epithelial and endothelial cells that helps to control complement-mediated lysis by acting as a cofactor for factor I–mediated cleavage of C3b.

Membrane inhibitor of reactive lysis (MIRL): A complement regulator that blocks formation of the membrane attack complex by preventing C9 from inserting into the cell membrane.

Memory cells: Long-lived progeny of an antigen-activated B or T cell that are able to respond to antigen more quickly than the parent cell.

Messenger RNA (mRNA): A complementary copy of DNA that carries the genetic information for the amino acid sequence of a protein.

Metastasis: The ability of cells to break away from the original tumor mass and spread through the blood to nearby or distant sites in the body.

MHC restriction: The positive selection of thymocytes that will only interact with the major histocompatibility complex (MHC) antigens found on host cells.

MIA: see *Multiplex immunoassay.*

Microarray: A technology that enables simultaneous analysis of thousands of genes in a sample by hybridization with a panel of molecular probes that are complementary to portions of specific genes or chromosome regions; the probes are spotted onto separate locations on a small glass slide or nylon membrane.

Microbiome: The collection of microorganisms that live on or in the body, including bacteria, viruses, yeast, and fungi.

Microbiota: Symbiotic microorganisms that reside on and colonize specific body sites, also known as *normal flora.*

Micropipette: Mechanical pipette that delivers volumes in the microliter (µL) range; used when very small volumes are needed.

Microsatellite instability: A change in the number of microsatellites (short repeated DNA sequences) caused by replication errors resulting from mutations in DNA mismatch repair genes; associated with certain types of cancer.

Microscopic agglutination test (MAT): A technique that is the gold standard for diagnosing leptospirosis.

Minor histocompatibility antigens (mHAs): Non-HLA proteins that can induce a weak graft rejection response when introduced into an individual possessing a different polymorphic variant.

Mitogen: A substance that stimulates mitosis in all T cells or all B cells, regardless of antigen specificity.

Mixed connective tissue disease (MCTD): An autoimmune disorder characterized by overlapping features of limited cutaneous systemic sclerosis (SSc), systemic lupus erythematosus (SLE), polymyositis, and rheumatoid arthritis.

Mixed lymphocyte reaction (MLR): An in vitro assay that measures the proliferation of responder T cells to non-self antigens in a potential transplant donor.

Molecular mimicry: The similarity between an infectious agent and a self-antigen that causes antibody formed in response to the former to cross-react with the latter.

Monoclonal: Derived from a single clone of identical cells.

Monoclonal antibody: An antibody derived from a single antibody-producing cell that has been cloned or duplicated; it is directed against a specific epitope on an antigen.

Monoclonal gammopathies: Disorders in which a clone of plasma cells causes overproduction of a single immunoglobulin component called a *paraprotein;* also known as plasma cell dyscrasias.

Monoclonal gammopathy of undetermined significance (MGUS): A premalignant plasma cell disorder characterized by the presence of monoclonal immunoglobulin in the serum, a plasma cell count of less than 10% in the bone marrow, and absence of clinical features. Some cases may eventually progress to multiple myeloma.

Monocytes: The largest white blood cells in peripheral blood; they migrate to the tissues to become macrophages.

Multi-drug resistant TB (MDR-TB): Tuberculosis caused by *M. tuberculosis* that is resistant to the first-line treatment drugs, isoniazid and rifampin.

Multiple myeloma: A malignancy of mature plasma cells that results in a monoclonal increase in an immunoglobulin component, most commonly IgG.

Multiple sclerosis (MS): An autoimmune disease in which the myelin sheath of axons becomes progressively destroyed by activated T cells and antibodies to myelin proteins.

Multiplex immunoassay (MIA): An automated immunoassay that uses a mixture of polystyrene beads conjugated with different antigens or antibodies as the solid phase and a fluorescent-tagged antibody to simultaneously detect multiple antibodies or antigens in a sample by flow cytometry; also known as *fluorescent microbead immunoassay.*

Mumps virus: A single-stranded RNA virus that causes mumps, a disease characterized by swelling of the parotid glands.

Mutation: A change in the nucleotide sequence in DNA.

Mutualistic: A relationship between a human host and microbial species in which both organisms benefit.

Myasthenia gravis (MG): An autoimmune disease characterized by progressive muscle weakness caused by formation of antibody to acetylcholine receptors in skeletal muscle or to other proteins in the neuromuscular junction.

Mycelial fungi: Multicellular fungi that are made up of intertwined hyphae and reproduce through the production of spores.

***Mycobacterium tuberculosis* complex (MTB complex):** A group of 11 different species within the genus *Mycobacterium,* including *M. tuberculosis.*

Mycoplasma pneumoniae: A small gram-negative bacterium that lacks a cell wall and is the cause of upper respiratory tract infections and an atypical pneumonia.

Mycosis (mycoses): Infection(s) or disease(s) caused by fungi.

Myeloid cells: Neutrophils, eosinophils, basophils, monocytes, and most dendritic cells.

Natural killer (NK) cells: A type of lymphocyte functioning in innate defenses by destroying altered host cells such as tumor cells and virus-infected cells.

Negative predictive value: The percentage of all negatives in a serological test that are true negatives; the probability that a person with a negative screening test does not have the disease being tested for.

Negative selection: The process by which T cells that can respond to self-antigen are destroyed in the thymus.

Neoantigens: Tumor-specific antigens created as a result of mutations in proto-oncogenes, tumor suppressor genes, or unrelated genes; also known as *mutation-derived tumor antigens.*

Neoplasm: An abnormal cell mass; a tumor.

Nephelometry: A technique for determining the concentration of particles in a solution (i.e., free antigen, free antibody, and antigen-antibody complexes) by measuring the light scattered at a particular angle from the incident beam as it passes through the solution.

Neutrophil: A white blood cell with a multilobed nucleus and a large number of neutral staining granules on a blood smear treated with Wright stain. Its main functions are phagocytosis and destruction of foreign particles during innate inflammatory responses.

Neutrophil extracellular traps (NETs): Structures extruded from activated neutrophils into the extracellular environment, where they trap and kill bacteria, fungi, and parasitic cells.

Next-generation sequencing (NGS): A technique that is able to sequence large numbers of DNA templates simultaneously (massively parallel sequencing), yielding hundreds of thousands of short nucleotide sequences in a single run.

Noncompetitive immunoassay: An immunoassay in which the analyte in the patient sample does not compete with a labeled analyte for its respective antibody or antigen. The amount of label measured is directly proportional to the amount of antigen or antibody in the test sample.

Non-Hodgkin or lymphocytic lymphomas (NHL): A wide range of cancers of the lymphoid tissue, of which B-cell lymphomas represent the majority.

Nontreponemal tests: Serological tests for syphilis that detect antibody to cardiolipin instead of specific anti-treponemal antibody.

Nontuberculosis mycobacteria (NTM): *Mycobacterium* species that does not belong to the *Mycobacterium tuberculosis* complex group.

Nucleic acid: A sequence of nucleotides that carries the genetic information for a protein; DNA or RNA.

Nucleolus: A prominent structure within the nucleus where transcription and processing of ribosomal RNA and assembly of the ribosomes take place.

Nucleoside: A unit of DNA or RNA composed of a deoxyribose or ribose sugar and a nitrogen base.

Nucleosome antibodies: Autoantibodies against DNA-histone complexes (also known as nucleosomes or deoxyribonucleoprotein [DNP]).

Nucleotide: A unit of DNA or RNA composed of a phosphorylated deoxyribose or ribose sugar and a nitrogen base.

Occupational Safety and Health Administration (OSHA): A federal agency that monitors and enforces safety regulations for workers.

Oncofetal antigens: Antigens that are expressed in the developing fetus and in rapidly dividing tissue, such as that associated with tumors, but that are absent in normal adult tissue.

Oncogene: Gene that encodes a protein capable of inducing cellular transformation.

Oncology: The medical field that specializes in cancer diagnosis and treatment.

Opportunistic illnesses: Infections or malignancies that mostly occur in individuals who are immunocompromised.

Opsonins: Serum proteins that attach to a foreign substance and enhance phagocytosis (from the Greek word meaning "to prepare for eating"); e.g., IgG, C3b.

Opsonization: Coating of a foreign antigen with antibody or complement to enhance phagocytosis.

Ouchterlony double diffusion: A qualitative gel precipitation technique in which both antigen and antibody diffuse out from wells cut in a gel. The pattern obtained indicates whether the antigens are identical, nonidentical, or partially identical in terms of their reactivity with an antibody.

Oxidative burst: An increase in oxygen consumption in phagocytic cells, which generate oxygen radicals that kill engulfed microorganisms.

p24 antigen: A structural core antigen that is part of HIV.

Paracortex: The region between the follicles and the medulla in the lymph nodes where T cells are mainly found.

Paracrine: Secretions such as cytokines that only affect target cells in close proximity.

Paraprotein (M protein): A single immunoglobulin component produced by a malignant clone of plasma cells in immunoproliferative diseases.

Parasites: Microorganisms that survive by living on or in another organism.

Parasitic: Relationship in which an organism causes harm to its host.

Paratope: An antigen binding site on an antibody molecule.

Parenteral: Mode of transmission other than through the intestinal tract, most notably bloodborne transmission.

Paroxysmal nocturnal hemoglobinuria (PNH): A disease characterized by complement-mediated hemolysis of erythrocytes resulting from a deficiency of the glycophospholipid anchor that attaches decay-accelerating factor to red blood cells.

Particle agglutination (PA) tests: Agglutination tests that use antigen-coated gel particles or red blood cells to detect antibody to *Treponema pallidum.*

Particle-based multi-analyte technology (PMAT): An automated immunoassay that uses paramagnetic microparticles coupled to different antigens and fluorescence to simultaneously detect multiple antibodies.

Passive agglutination: A reaction in which particles coated with antigens not normally found on their surfaces clump together because of their combination with antibody.

Passive immunity: A type of immunity that results from the transfer of antibodies from immunized hosts to a nonimmune individual.

Passive immunodiffusion: A precipitation reaction in a gel in which antigen-antibody combination occurs by means of diffusion in a gel medium in the absence of an electrical current.

Passive immunotherapy: Passive immunization of an individual with commercial preparations of antibodies formed by other hosts to prevent or treat a disease.

Pathogen-associated molecular patterns (PAMPs): Structural patterns of carbohydrates, nucleic acids, or bacterial peptides on microorganisms that are recognized by pathogen recognition receptors (PRRs) on the cells of the innate immune system.

Pathogenicity: The inherent capacity of an organism to cause disease.

Pattern recognition receptors (PRRs): Receptors on cells of the innate immune system that bind to pathogen-associated molecular patterns on pathogenic microorganisms.

Periarteriolar lymphoid sheath (PALS): White pulp of splenic tissue, which is made up of lymphocytes, macrophages, plasma cells, and granulocytes. It surrounds the central arterioles.

Peripheral tolerance: Destruction or suppression of lymphocytes that could respond to self-antigens in the secondary lymphoid organs.

Personal protective equipment (PPE): Items such as gowns, masks, gloves, and face shields used to protect the body from infectious agents.

Phagocytosis: Engulfment of cells or particulate matter by neutrophils, macrophages, or other cells; from the Greek word *phagein,* meaning "cell eating."

Phagolysosome: The structure formed by the fusion of cytoplasmic granules and a phagosome during the process of phagocytosis.

Phagosome: A vacuole formed within a phagocytic cell as pseudopodia surround a particle during the process of phagocytosis.

Phenocopies of primary immunodeficiencies: Defects in the immune system that result from somatic mutations or autoantibodies directed against cytokines, resulting in clinical manifestations that resemble those of inherited immunodeficiencies.

Phenotype resistance assays: Tests that determine the ability of clinical isolates of a virus (e.g., HIV) to grow in the presence of anti-viral drugs.

Pipeline: The combination of nucleic acid base calling, quality assessment, data extraction, trimming, assembly, alignment, variant calling, and matching, performed by software programs.

Plasma cell: Fully differentiated B cell that actively secretes antibody.

Plasma cell dyscrasias: Immunoproliferative diseases characterized by overproduction of a single immunoglobulin component by a clone of plasma cells; also known as *monoclonal gammopathies.*

Plasmids: Self-replicating extrachromosomal genetic elements located in the cytoplasm of a bacterium, with a limited number of genes that can be transferred between bacteria.

Pleiotropy: A property by which a single gene or protein (e.g., a cytokine) has multiple effects. For example, a cytokine may affect the activities of more than one kind of cell and have more than one kind of effect on the same cell.

Point-of-care testing (POCT): Testing performed at or near the site of patient care.

Polyclonal: Derived from many clones of cells. Polyclonal antibodies are derived from many clones of B cells or plasma cells and are therefore diverse in terms of their antigen specificity.

Polymerase chain reaction (PCR): A technique of amplifying tiny quantities of nucleic acid using a heat-stable polymerase enzyme and a primer pair that is specific for the DNA sequence desired.

Polymorphism: One of two or more different forms of a specific DNA or protein sequence shared by at least 2% of individuals in a population (e.g., HLA genes).

Polymyositis (PM): A systemic rheumatic autoimmune disorder that involves inflammation of the skeletal muscles.

Positive predictive value: The percentage of all positives in a serological test that are true positives; the probability that a person with a positive screening test has the disease being tested for.

Positive selection: The process of selecting immature T lymphocytes for survival in the thymus based on their ability to interact with self-MHC class I or class II molecules.

Postexamination variable: A process that affects the reporting of results and correct interpretation of data; formerly called *postanalytical variable.*

Postexposure prophylaxis (PEP): Course of preventive treatment provided after exposure to potentially infectious organisms.

Poststreptococcal glomerulonephritis (PSGN): A condition that damages the glomeruli of the kidneys, caused by an immune response to a recent streptococcal infection in some patients.

Postzone: Lack of a visible reaction in an antigen-antibody combination, caused by extreme excess of antigen.

PPD test: A skin test that detects exposure to *Mycobacterium tuberculosis* using a purified protein derivative from cultures of the organism.

Pre-B cell: The stage of development of a B cell where the heavy chain part of the antibody molecule is present.

Precipitation: The combination of soluble antigen with soluble antibody to produce visible insoluble complexes.

Precipitins: Antibodies that participate in a precipitation reaction.

Precision: The ability to consistently reproduce the same result upon duplicate or repeated testing of the same sample.

Preexamination variable: A factor that can affect test results that occurs before the actual testing of the specimen and includes test requests, patient preparation, timing, specimen collection, handling, and storage; formerly known as a *preanalytical* variable.

Preventive maintenance (PM): Regular, scheduled maintenance performed proactively to ensure optimal test performance by keeping laboratory instruments in excellent condition.

Primary antibody response: The initial response to a foreign antigen, characterized by a long lag phase, a slow rise in antibody production, and mostly IgM.

Primary biliary cholangitis (PBC): An autoimmune disease that involves progressive destruction of the intrahepatic bile ducts; formerly known as *primary biliary cirrhosis.*

Primary follicles: In lymphoid tissue, clusters of B cells that have not yet been stimulated by antigen.

Primary immunodeficiency diseases (PIDs): Inherited diseases in which part of the immune system is absent or dysfunctional.

Primary lymphoid organs: The organs in which lymphocytes mature: these are the bone marrow and the thymus.

Primers: Short DNA sequences used to hybridize specifically to a particular target DNA to help initiate replication of the DNA.

Pro-B cell: A stage in B-cell development in which rearrangement of the genes that code for the heavy chain region of an antibody molecule occurs.

Probe: A labeled single-stranded nucleic acid with a known sequence that is used to identify the presence of a complementary DNA or RNA sequence in an unknown sample.

Procalcitonin: An acute phase protein made by C-cells in the thyroid gland, which functions to lower calcium levels in the blood; precursor of the hormone, calcitonin.

Proficiency testing: The laboratory testing of unknown samples received from an outside agency.

Pro-inflammatory: Ability to promote inflammation (e.g., pro-inflammatory cytokines).

Properdin: A protein that stabilizes the C3 convertase generated in the alternative complement pathway.

Prostate-specific antigen (PSA): A glycoprotein produced specifically by epithelial cells in the prostate gland; used as a marker for prostate cancer.

Proteome: The total complement or set of proteins expressed by an organism or cell.

Proteomics: The field of study that involves identification and quantification of the array of proteins present in a sample.

Proto-oncogenes: Normal genes that stimulate cell proliferation and growth; mutations can convert these genes into cancer-promoting oncogenes.

Protozoa: A diverse group of single-celled organisms that can be free-living or live and multiply inside of human hosts.

Provider-performed microscopy procedures (PPMPs): Microscopy tests performed by a physician, midlevel practitioner, or dentist.

Prozone: Lack of a visible reaction in antigen-antibody combination caused by the presence of an extreme excess of antibody. This may produce a false-negative test result.

Pyrosequencing: A DNA sequencing method that relies on the generation of light when nucleotides are added to a growing strand of DNA.

Quality assessment (QA): The overall process of guaranteeing quality patient care. It involves the continual monitoring of the entire test process from test ordering and specimen collection through reporting and interpreting results.

Quality control (QC): The materials, procedures, and techniques that monitor the accuracy, precision, and reliability of a laboratory test.

Quality control plan (QCP): A plan that establishes control procedures to reduce the possibility of reporting an inaccurate patient test result.

Quality indicators: Measurements developed by each laboratory to determine if the quality system essentials are being met.

Quality management (QM): The overall process of guaranteeing quality patient care.

Quality management system (QMS): All the laboratory's policies, processes, procedures, and resources needed to achieve quality testing.

Quality system essentials (QSEs): Methods to meet the requirements of regulatory, accreditation, and standard-setting organizations.

Quantitative PCR (qPCR): A molecular test involving accumulation of a polymerase chain reaction (PCR) product in real time during amplification of a nucleic acid sequence.

Radial immunodiffusion (RID): A precipitation technique in which antibody is uniformly distributed in the support gel, and antigen is applied to a well cut into the gel. As the antigen diffuses out from the well, antigen-antibody combination occurs until the zone of equivalence is reached, producing a precipitin ring around the well.

Radioimmunoassay (RIA): A technique used to measure small concentrations of an analyte, using a radioactive label on one of the immunologic reactants.

Random-access analyzer: An analyzer that can analyze many test samples and perform several different tests for any one sample.

Rapid antigen detection system (RDTS): See *lateral flow assays.*

Rapid immunoassays: Membrane-based tests based on immunochromatography and commonly used for point-of-care testing.

Rapid plasma reagin (RPR) test: A rapid slide test for syphilis that detects antibody to cardiolipin through macroscopic agglutination.

Rate nephelometry: A technique that measures the rate of light scattering after the reagent antibody is added to a sample containing patient antigen. The rate change is directly related to antigen concentration if the concentration of antibody is kept constant.

Reactivation tuberculosis: Development of active tuberculosis disease after a long period of latent TB infection.

Reactive nitrogen species (RNS): Group of molecules formed in activated phagocytic cells when nitric oxide interacts with reactive oxygen species, causing cell injury and death.

Reactive oxygen species (ROS): Unstable, highly reactive molecules that contain oxygen (e.g., superoxide anion, hydrogen peroxide). They are generated in activated phagocytic cells during the oxidative burst and are toxic to phagocytized microbes.

Reagin: An antibody formed during the course of syphilis that is directed against cardiolipin released from damaged host tissues and not against *Treponema pallidum*.

Recognition unit: The C1qrs complement complex. The complex must bind to at least two Fc regions on antibody molecule(s) to initiate the classical complement cascade.

Recombinant protein vaccine: A vaccine produced by cloning the gene coding for the vaccine antigen into the genome of bacteria, yeast, or cultured cells.

Redundancy: A phenomenon that occurs when different cytokines have the same effect.

Reference interval: The range of values found in healthy individuals who do not have the condition detected by the assay.

Regulatory T (Treg) cells: A type of T cell that suppresses the actions of B cells and other T cells; Tregs play an important role in suppressing the immune response to self-antigens and other undesirable immune responses.

Relapsing fever: A group of diseases caused by several species of *Borrelia,* characterized by recurring episodes of fever, headache, chills, muscle and joint aches, and nausea.

Reliability: The ability to maintain both precision and accuracy in laboratory testing.

Reportable range: The range of values that generate a positive result for the specimens assayed by the test procedure.

Respiratory syncytial virus (RSV): An RNA virus that causes respiratory infections which may become severe in infants and elderly adults.

Restriction endonucleases: Enzymes that cleave DNA at specific recognition sites that are typically four to six base pairs long.

Restriction fragment length polymorphisms (RFLPs): Variations in nucleotides within DNA that change where restriction enzymes cleave the DNA. This results in different-size pieces of DNA and an altered electrophoretic pattern.

Retroviridae: A large, diverse family of RNA viruses that use reverse transcriptase in their replication cycle inside of host cells.

Reverse passive agglutination: A reaction in which carrier particles coated with antibody clump together because of a combination with antigen.

Reverse transcriptase: An enzyme produced by certain RNA viruses to convert viral RNA into complementary DNA.

Rheumatoid arthritis (RA): An autoimmune disease that affects the synovial membrane of multiple joints. It is characterized by the presence of the autoantibodies *anti-CCP* and *rheumatoid factor.*

Rheumatoid factor (RF): An antibody, most commonly of the IgM class, that is directed against the Fc portion of IgG; produced by patients with rheumatoid arthritis and other conditions.

Ribonucleic acid (RNA): The nucleic acid containing the sugar ribose. It is the primary genetic material of RNA viruses and plays a role in transcribing genetic information in cells.

Ribosomal RNA (rRNA): A type of RNA that serves as an important structural and functional component of the ribosomes.

Rickettsiae: Small gram-negative fastidious bacteria that are obligate intracellular parasites and are responsible for diseases such as Rocky Mountain spotted fever and typhus.

Rocky Mountain spotted fever (RMSF): A disease caused by infection with *Rickettsia rickettsii.*

Root cause analysis (RCA): A problem-solving protocol used to identify the causes of adverse events in a health care setting.

Rubella virus: An RNA virus that causes German measles and congenital infection.

Rubeola virus: A single-stranded RNA virus that causes measles.

sC5b-9: See *soluble membrane attack complex (sMAC).*

S protein: A control protein in the complement cascade that interferes with binding of the C5b67 complex to a cell membrane, thus preventing cell lysis.

Safety Data Sheet (SDS): A document that contains information on physical and chemical characteristics of a substance, fire and explosion potential, reactivity, health hazards, primary routes of entry, exposure limits and carcinogenic potential, precautions for safe handling, spill cleanup, and emergency first aid information.

Sandwich immunoassay: An immunoassay in which the target antigen is bound both to a capture antibody on the solid phase and a labeled detector antibody; also known as a *capture* or *immunometric* immunoassay.

Sarcomas: Cancers derived from bone or soft tissues such as fat, muscles, tendons, cartilage, nerves, and blood vessels.

Scarlet fever: An illness with a characteristic rash and fever that is caused by the erythrogenic toxins released from group A streptococcal bacteria.

Secondary antibody response: A second or memory response to an antigen, characterized by a shortened lag period, a more rapid rise in antibody, and higher serum antibody levels that persist for a longer period of time.

Secondary follicles: In lymphoid tissue, clusters of B cells that are proliferating in response to a specific antigen.

Secondary immunodeficiencies: Immunodeficiencies that are acquired as a result of other conditions, such as certain infections, malignancies, autoimmune disorders, and immunosuppressive therapies.

Secondary lymphoid organs: Organs that include the spleen, lymph nodes, appendix, tonsils, and other mucosal-associated lymphoid tissue where contact with foreign antigens takes place.

Secretory component (SC): A protein that is synthesized by epithelial cells and added to IgA molecules to facilitate their transport to mucosal surfaces.

Selectins: Adhesion molecules on the surface of the vascular endothelial cells that bind to integrins on leukocytes in the blood to mediate initial interaction with the cells during processes such as inflammation.

Self-tolerance: The ability of the immune system to accept self-antigens and not initiate a response against them.

Sensitization: (1) The combination of antibody with a single antigenic determinant on the surface of a cell without agglutination. (2) Induction of an immune response.

Serial dilution: A series of dilutions that decrease the concentration of an antibody in regular amounts by using the same dilution factor for each step.

Seroconversion: Change of a serological test result from antibody negative to antibody positive from samples obtained during the course of an immune response.

Serological pipette: A graduated or measuring pipette that has marks all along its length all the way down to the tip.

Serology: The study of the fluid components in the blood, especially antibodies.

Serotype: A group of related bacteria or viruses that share specific antigens that can be identified by serological testing.

Serum: The liquid portion of the blood minus the clotting factors.

Serum amyloid A (SAA): A family of acute phase proteins that activate macrophages and transport cholesterol from the plasma to the site of infection, where it is used in tissue repair.

Serum sickness: A type III hypersensitivity reaction that results from the production of antibodies to animal serum used in passive immunization.

Severe acute respiratory syndrome coronavirus 2 (SARS-CoV-2): An RNA virus that causes COVID-19.

Severe combined immunodeficiency (SCID): A group of inherited, life-threatening diseases caused by a lack of mature T cells, causing defects in cell-mediated and antibody responses that result in overwhelming infections and death in infancy if not treated successfully.

Shift: An abrupt change in the mean that may be caused by a malfunction of an instrument, a loss of calibration, or a new lot number of reagents.

Side scatter (SSc): Light scattered at 90° from the light source in a flow cytometer that indicates the complexity of a cell, determined by characteristics such as granularity.

Single nucleotide polymorphisms (SNPs): Variants of a particular DNA sequence involving a single base pair; these variations are shared by at least 1% of a population and result in the generation of different alleles.

Single nucleotide variants (SNV): Variants of a particular DNA sequence involving a single base pair.

Single-parameter histogram: Plot of a chosen parameter or measurement on the *x*-axis against the number of events on the *y*-axis.

Single-positive (SP) stage: A stage in T-cell development characterized by the presence of surface CD4 or CD8 but not both markers.

Single-step, competitive, immunochromatographic method: A rapid immunoassay in which antigen in a patient sample is added to a membrane containing detection antibody adsorbed onto colloidal gold or colored latex particles.

Six Sigma: A method used by health care organizations to reduce variables and decrease errors.

Sjögren syndrome: A systemic rheumatic autoimmune disease characterized by the presence of dry eyes and a dry mouth.

Skin-associated lymphoid tissue (SALT): Lymphoid tissue in the epidermal layer of the skin.

Sm antigen: An extractable nuclear antigen; autoantibodies to Sm are specific for systemic lupus erythematosus.

Soluble membrane attack complex (sMAC): Soluble form of the complement membrane attack complex that can be measured in the blood; also known as *sC5b-9*.

Solute: The substance being diluted (e.g., serum) during preparation of a dilution.

Spirochetes: Long, slender, helically coiled bacteria containing flagella that wind around the bacterial cell wall and exhibit a characteristic corkscrew motility.

Spleen: The largest secondary lymphoid organ in the body, located in the upper left quadrant of the abdomen. Its function is to remove aged cells and foreign antigens from the blood.

SS-A/Ro: An extractable nuclear antigen consisting of small, uridine-rich RNA complexed to cellular protein; found in a significant percentage of patients with Sjögren syndrome.

SS-B/La: An extractable nuclear antigen consisting of small, uridine-rich RNA complexed to cellular protein; found in a significant percentage of patients with Sjögren syndrome.

Standard deviation (SD): A measurement statistic that describes the average distance of each data point in a normal distribution from the mean.

Standard of care: The attention, caution, and prudence that a reasonable person in the same circumstances would exercise in performing laboratory testing.

Standard Precautions (SPs): Guidelines describing personnel protection that should be used for the care of all patients, including hand hygiene, gloves, mask, eye protection, face shield, gown, respiratory hygiene, patient-care equipment, environmental control, linens, handling needles, and taking care to prevent injuries.

Streptavidin (SAv): A bacterial protein that has a strong affinity for biotin; the complex is used for labeling in some types of immunoassays.

Streptococcus pyogenes: Group A streptococci; gram-positive cocci that have several clinical manifestations, including pharyngitis, impetigo, scarlet fever, acute rheumatic fever, and poststreptococcal glomerulonephritis.

Streptolysin O: A protein capable of lysing red blood cells and white blood cells, produced by some groups of streptococci.

Superantigens: Microbial proteins that can act as potent T-cell mitogens because they bind to both class II MHC molecules and T-cell receptors, regardless of antigen specificity.

Surrogate light chain: Two short polypeptide chains noncovalently associated with each other that appear before actual light chains are formed by a developing B cell.

Symbiotic: A relationship in which two species live together, often maintaining a long-term, but not necessarily a beneficial, interaction (e.g., a bacterium and a human).

Synergy: Effect of cytokines that complement and enhance each other's effects.

Syngeneic graft: The transfer of tissue or organs between genetically identical individuals such as identical twins; also called an *isograft*.

Syphilis: A sexually transmitted disease caused by the spirochete bacterium *Treponema pallidum*.

Systemic lupus erythematosus (SLE): A chronic inflammatory autoimmune disease characterized by the presence of anti-nuclear antibodies. Symptoms often include swelling of the joints, an erythematous rash, and deposition of immune complexes in the kidneys.

Systemic sclerosis (SSc): A systemic autoimmune rheumatic disease characterized by excessive fibrosis and vascular abnormalities that affect the skin, joints, and internal organs; also known as *scleroderma*.

Targeted therapies: Small molecule inhibitors and monoclonal antibodies that specifically target molecules needed for growth and survival of cancer cells.

T-cell receptor (TCR): Receptor on the surface of T lymphocytes that recognizes complexes of an antigen bound to a self-MHC molecule; composed of two polypeptide chains, usually an α chain and a β chain.

T-cell receptor excision circles (TRECs): Small circles of DNA removed during normal TCR gene rearrangements that occur during T-cell development; the number of TRECs indicates the number of T cells in blood samples taken from newborns to screen for T cell deficiencies.

T-dependent antigen: An antigen that requires T-cell help in order for B cells to respond.

T-independent antigens: Antigens that are able to elicit antibody formation in the absence of helper T cells.

T lymphocytes: Cells that mature in the thymus. They play important roles in cell-mediated immunity and produce cytokines that assist humoral immune responses.

Terminal complement complex (TCC): The membrane attack complex formed in the final steps of the complement pathways, consisting of C5b6789.

Tertiary syphilis: The last stage of syphilis that appears months to years after secondary infection. It is characterized by granulomatous inflammation, cardiovascular disease, and central nervous system involvement.

Tetrapeptide: The basic four-chain unit common to all immunoglobulin molecules, consisting of two large heavy chains and two smaller light chains.

The Joint Commission (TJC): An independent body that certifies and accredits health care organizations in the United States.

Thrombotic microangiopathies (TMAs): A group of disorders characterized by RBC destruction, decreased platelets, and organ damage caused by formation of tiny blood clots in the capillaries and small arteries; includes thrombotic thrombocytopenic purpura and atypical hemolytic uremic syndrome (aHUS), which is complement mediated.

Thymocytes: Immature lymphocytes in the thymus that undergo differentiation to become mature T cells.

Thymus: A small, flat, bilobed organ in the chest cavity of humans, which serves as the site for differentiation of T cells.

Thyroglobulin (Tg): A large iodinated glycoprotein from which the active thyroid hormone triiodothyronine (T3) and its precursor, thyroxine (T4), are synthesized.

Thyroid peroxidase (TPO): An enzyme that oxidizes iodine ions to form the iodine atoms that are incorporated into thyroglobulin to facilitate the synthesis of the thyroid hormones T3 and T4.

Thyroid-stimulating hormone (TSH): A hormone produced by the pituitary gland that binds to specific receptors on the thyroid gland, causing thyroglobulin to be broken down into secretable T3 and T4; also known as *thyrotropin*.

Thyroid-stimulating hormone receptor antibodies (TRAbs): Antibodies that are directed against the receptor for thyroid-stimulating hormone (TSH). Some of these antibodies are associated with Graves disease and result in overstimulation of the thyroid gland, while others prevent TSH from binding to its receptor and cause decreased thyroid function.

Thyroid-stimulating immunoglobulins (TSIs): Autoantibodies directed against the thyroid-stimulating hormone (TSH) receptor, which are responsible for the hyperthyroidism seen in Graves disease.

Thyrotoxicosis: A condition caused by overproduction of thyroid hormones, as seen in Graves disease.

Thyrotropin-releasing hormone (TRH): A hormone secreted by the hypothalamus that acts on the pituitary gland to induce the release of thyroid-stimulating hormone (TSH).

Tissue transglutaminase (tTG): An intestinal enzyme that converts the glutamine residues in gliadin to glutamic acid; autoantibodies to tTG are commonly produced in patients with celiac disease.

Titer: A number that represents the relative concentration of an antibody. It is the reciprocal of the highest dilution in which a positive antigen-antibody reaction occurs.

Toll-like receptors (TLRs): A class of pathogen recognition receptors on human leukocytes and other cell types that recognize microorganisms and aid in their destruction in the innate immune response.

Toxoid: A chemically inactivated bacterial toxin used in some vaccines.

Toxoplasma gondii: The protozoal organism that causes toxoplasmosis, an infection that can have severe consequences in immunocompromised people and congenitally infected infants.

TP-PA test: See *Treponema pallidum particle agglutination (TP-PA) test.*

Transcription: The process of generating a complementary mRNA strand from DNA during protein synthesis.

Transcription-mediated amplification (TMA): A nucleic acid amplification technique in which a complementary DNA copy is made of the original RNA and used to produce millions of RNA copies.

Transfer RNA (tRNA): A type of RNA that carries the amino acids specified by mRNA to the ribosomes during protein synthesis.

Transforming growth factor-β (TGF-β): A cytokine that induces antiproliferative activity in various cell types and downregulates the inflammatory response.

Transient hypogammaglobulinemia of infancy (THI): A condition characterized by prolonged low immunoglobulin levels in infants that usually normalizes spontaneously by 2 to 6 years of age. It is believed to be caused by delayed maturation of one or more components of the immune system.

Translation: The process by mRNA is converted into amino acid sequences during protein synthesis.

Transporters associated with antigen processing (TAP1 and TAP2): Proteins that are responsible for the adenosine triphosphate (ATP)-dependent transport of newly synthesized short peptides from the cytoplasm to the lumen of the endoplasmic reticulum for binding to class I HLA antigens.

Trend: A gradual change in the mean in one direction that may be caused by a gradual deterioration of reagents, controls, or instrument performance.

Treponema pallidum: A spirochete that is the causative agent of syphilis.

***Treponema pallidum* particle agglutination (TP-PA) test:** A particle agglutination test that detects antibodies to *Treponema pallidum* to aid in the diagnosis of syphilis.

Treponemal tests: Serological tests for syphilis that detect antibodies directed against *Treponema pallidum*.

True negative: A laboratory result that occurs when a person does not have a specified condition, and the test for that condition is negative.

True positive: A laboratory result that occurs when a person has a specified condition, and the test for the condition is positive.

Tumor: An abnormal cell mass that can be either benign or malignant.

Tumor-associated antigens (TAAs): Antigens that are present on some types of normal cells but are overexpressed or abnormally expressed by cancer cells.

Tumor-infiltrating lymphocytes (TILs): Lymphocytes within a tumor mass that are able to react with antigens on tumor cells to help destroy them.

Tumor markers: Biological substances found in increased amounts in the blood, body fluids, or tissues of patients with a specific type of cancer.

Tumor microenvironment: The immune cells, fibroblasts, molecules, and blood vessels that surround the cancer cells in a tumor.

Tumor necrosis factor (TNF): Family of cytokines that regulate diverse immunologic functions, including inflammation, expression of adhesion molecules on vascular endothelial cells, cell proliferation, cell survival, tissue degeneration or regeneration, and apoptosis.

Tumor-specific antigens (TSAs): Antigens that are unique to tumor cells.

Tumor suppressor genes: Genes that control the entry of cells into the cell cycle and prevent cells from completing the cycle if they contain damaged DNA or other abnormalities. Mutations in these genes can cause unregulated cell proliferation and contribute to tumor growth.

Turnaround time (TAT): The amount of time required between the point at which a test is ordered by a health care provider and the results are reported to the health care provider.

Type 1 diabetes mellitus (T1D): A chronic autoimmune disease characterized by insufficient insulin production, caused by progressive destruction of the beta cells of the pancreas.

Type I hypersensitivity: An allergic reaction in which antigen-specific IgE antibody binds to mast cells and basophils, triggering degranulation and the release of chemical mediators; also known as *anaphylactic hypersensitivity*.

Type II hypersensitivity: An immune reaction in which IgG or IgM antibodies are produced to cell surface receptors, causing damage, dysfunction, or overstimulation of the function of the cells; also known as *antibody-mediated cytotoxic hypersensitivity.*

Type III hypersensitivity: An immune reaction in which IgG or IgM antibodies react with soluble antigens to form small complexes that deposit in the tissues and activate complement to induce inflammation; also known as *complex-mediated hypersensitivity.*

Type IV hypersensitivity: A cell-mediated response involving the release of cytokines that induce inflammation and tissue damage 24 to 72 hours after contact with an antigen; also known as *delayed hypersensitivity.*

Typhus: Diseases characterized by fever, rash, and a cough caused by *Rickettsiae* bacteria.

Vaccine: Most often, an antigen preparation derived from a pathogen that is administered to healthy individuals to produce immunity to an infectious disease. Cancer vaccines use tumor antigens to stimulate an immune response in some people known to have cancer.

Vaccine hesitancy: Delay in, or refusal of, vaccination despite available vaccination services.

Variable region: The amino-terminal region of an immunoglobulin that has a unique amino acid sequence and is responsible for the antigen specificity of an antibody.

Variables: Factors, which, if changed or altered, can affect test results.

Variant: A change in the nucleotide sequence of DNA.

Varicella-zoster virus (VZV): A herpes virus that causes chickenpox and zoster (i.e., shingles).

Venereal Disease Research Laboratory (VDRL) test: A flocculation test for the cardiolipin antibody produced in syphilis patients; an example of a nontreponemal test.

Viral load tests: Quantitative tests for nucleic acid from viruses such as HIV. These tests are used to predict disease progression and to monitor the effects of anti-viral therapy.

Viremia: The presence of a virus circulating in the blood.

Virulence: A quantitative trait of an organism that refers to the extent of pathology it can cause when it infects a host.

Virulence factors: Characteristics of a microorganism that can increase its pathogenicity by contributing to its ability to establish itself in the host, invade or damage host tissue, or evade the host immune response.

Volumetric pipette: A pipette that is marked and calibrated to deliver only one volume of a specified liquid.

Waldenström macroglobulinemia: An immunoproliferative disease caused by a malignancy of lymphocytes that results in production of an IgM paraprotein.

Wegener granulomatosis (WG): See *granulomatosis with polyangiitis (PGA).*

Weil disease: Severe systemic leptospirosis involving renal and hepatic failure.

Western blot: A technique that involves separation of antigens in a complex mixture (e.g., antigens from a pathogen) by electrophoresis, followed by transfer or blotting of the antigen pattern to a supporting membrane for reaction with test serum. It has been used as a confirmatory test for some infections (e.g., HIV, Lyme disease); also known as an *immunoblot.*

Wiskott-Aldrich syndrome (WAS): A rare X-linked recessive syndrome characterized by immunodeficiency, eczema, and thrombocytopenia.

X-linked agammaglobulinemia: See *Bruton tyrosine kinase (Btk) deficiency.*

Xenograft: The transfer of tissue from an individual of one species to an individual of another species, such as animal tissue transplanted to a human.

Yeast: A unicellular form of certain fungi that reproduces asexually by budding, in which the parent cell divides into two unequal parts.

Zone of equivalence: The point in an antigen-antibody reaction at which the number of multivalent sites of antigen and antibody are approximately equal, resulting in an optimal antigen-antibody reaction (e.g., precipitation).

Selected References*

**A complete list of references is available in the online resources at FADavis.com*

Chapter 1: Introduction to Immunity and the Immune System

Abbas AK, Lichtman AH, Pillai S. *Cellular and Molecular Immunology.* 10th ed. Elsevier; 2022:11–40.

Bioexplorer. History of immunology. Accessed January 27, 2025. http://www.bioexplorer.net/history_of_biology/immunology/

Harmening DM, Woslager CJ, Del Toro CL. Morphology and maturation of human blood cells. In: Harmening DM, Hutson LM. *Clinical Hematology and Fundamentals of Hemostasis.* 6th ed. F.A. Davis; 2024:1-42.

HCDM. Molecule information. Accessed January 27, 2025. https://hcdm.org/index.php/molecule-information

Mirza KM. Hematopoiesis. In: Keohane E, Otto CN, Walenga JM, eds. *Rodak's Hematology: Clinical Principles and Applications.* 6th ed. Elsevier/Saunders; 2020:43–61.

Chapter 2: Innate Immunity

Abbas AK, Lichtman AH, Pillai S. *Cellular and Molecular Immunology.* 10th ed. Elsevier; 2022:61–101.

ARUP Consult. Inflammatory Markers. Accessed January 27, 2025. https://arupconsult.com/content/inflammatory-markers

Güleç UG, Turgut YB, Turgut M. Acute phase proteins. In: N. Rezaei, ed. *Encyclopedia of Infection and Immunity.* Vol. 4. Elsevier; 2022:206–214.

Mantovani A, Garlanda C. Humoral innate immunity and acute-phase proteins. *N Eng J Med.* 2023;388(5):439–452.

Sameer AS, Nissar S. Toll-like receptors (TLRs): structure, functions, signaling, and role of their polymorphisms in colorectal cancer susceptibility. *BioMed Res Int.* 2021;2021:1157023. https://doi.org/10.1155/2021/1157023

Chapter 3: Antibody Structure and Function

Abbas AK, Lichtman AH, Pillai S. *Cellular and Molecular Immunology.* 10th ed. Elsevier Health Sciences (US); 2022:102–121.

Bayer V. An overview of monoclonal antibodies. *Semin Oncol Nurs.* 2019;35(5):150927. https://doi.org/10.1016/j.soncn.2019.08.006

Burnet FM. A modification of Jerne's theory of antibody production using the concept of clonal selection. *Aust J Sci.* 1957;20:67–69.

Owen JA, Punt J, Stranford SA, Jones PP, Owen JA. *Kuby Immunology.* 8th ed. WH Freeman and Company; 2019:75–83, 205–235, 760–762.

Schroeder HW, Cavacini L. Structure and function of immunoglobulins. *J Allergy Clin Immunol.* 2010;125(2S2):S41–S52.

Chapter 4: Nature of Antigens and the Major Histocompatibility Complex

Abbas AK, Lichtman AH, Pillai S. *Cellular and Molecular Immunology.* 10th ed. Elsevier; 2022:123–150.

Fiorillo MT, Paladini F, Tedeschi V, Sorrentino R. HLA class I or class II and disease association: catch the difference if you can. *Front Immunol.* 2017 Nov 7;8:1475. https://doi.org/10.3389/fimmu.2017.01475

Koch J, Tampe R. The macromolecular peptide-loading complex in MHC class I-dependent antigen presentation. *Cell Mol Life Sci.* 2006;63:653–662.

Murphy KP, Weaver C, Berg L. *Janeway's Immunobiology.* 10th ed. W. W. Norton & Company; 2022:217–258.

Owen JA, Punt J, Stranford SA, Jones PP. *Kuby Immunology.* 8th ed. WH Freeman and Co.; 2019:249–288.

Chapter 5: Adaptive Immunity

Abbas AK, Lichtman AH, Pillai S. *Cellular and Molecular Immunology.* 10th ed. Elsevier; 2022:187–286.

Meng X, Yang B, Suen WC. Prospects for modulating the CD40/CD40L pathway in the therapy of the hyper-IgM syndrome. *Innate Immun.* 2018;24(1):4–10.

Murphy K, Weaver C, Berg LJ. *Janeway's Immunobiology.* 10th ed. W. W. Norton & Company; 2022:141–216, 347–452.

Parham P. *The Immune System.* 5th ed. W. W. Norton & Company; 2022:163–210.

Smith JA, Yuen BTK, Purtha W, et al. Aire mediates tolerance to insulin through thymic trimming of high-affinity T cell clones. *Proc Natl Acad Sci U S A.* 2024 May 14;121(20):e2320268121.

Chapter 6: Cytokines

Abbas AK, Lichtman AH, Pillai S. *Cellular and Molecular Immunology.* 10th ed. Elsevier; 2022:88–100, 235–247, 549–553.

Berraondo P, Sanmamed MF, Ochoa MC, et al. Cytokines in clinical cancer immunotherapy. *Br J Cancer.* 2019;120:6–15.

Cusabio Technology LLC. Cytokines. Accessed January 27, 2025. https://www.cusabio.com/cytokines/Cytokine-Family.html

Hughes CE, Nibbs RJB. A guide to chemokines and their receptors. *FEBS J.* 2018;285(16):2944–2971. https://doi.org/10.1111/febs.14466

Liu C, Chu D, Kalantar-Zadeh K, George J, Young HA, Liu G. Cytokines: from clinical significance to quantification. *Adv Sci.* 2021;8(15):e2004433. https://doi.org/10.1002/advs.202004433

Chapter 7: The Complement System

Antonucci L, Thurman JM, Vivarelli M. Complement inhibitors in pediatric kidney diseases: new therapeutic opportunities. *Pediatr Nephrol.* 2024;39(5):1387–1404.

Barnum S, Schein T. *The Complement Facts Book.* Elsevier; 2018.

Brodszki N, Frazer-Abel A, Grumach AS, et al. European Society for Immunodeficiencies (ESID) and European Reference Network on Rare Primary Immunodeficiency, Autoinflammatory and Autoimmune Diseases (ERN RITA) complement guideline: deficiencies, diagnosis, and management. *J Clin Immunol.* 2020;40:576–591.

Freeley S, Kemper C, Le Friec G. The "ins and outs" of complement-driven immune responses. *Immunol Rev.* 2016;274(1):16–32.

Holers VM. Complement and its receptors: new insights into human disease. *Annu Rev Immunol.* 2014;32:433–459.

Chapter 8: Safety and Quality Management

Centers for Disease Control and Prevention. Updated U.S. public health service guidelines for the management of occupational exposures to HBV, HCV, and HIV and recommendations for postexposure prophylaxis. Updated May 23, 2018. Accessed January 28, 2025. https://stacks.cdc.gov/view/cdc/20711

Centers for Medicare and Medicaid Services, Department of Health and Human Services. Clinical Laboratory Improvement Amendments, proficiency testing and PT referral booklet. September 2017. Accessed January 28, 2025. https://www.cms.gov/Regulations-and-Guidance/Legislation/CLIA/Downloads/CLIAbrochure8.pdf

Occupational Safety and Health Administration. Bloodborne Pathogens standard 1910.1030. Accessed July 17, 2025. https://www.osha.gov/laws-regs/regulations/standardnumber/1910/1910.1030/

Strasinger SK, DiLorenzo MS. *The Phlebotomy Textbook.* 4th ed. F.A. Davis; 2019:43–69, 443–461.

Strasinger SK, DiLorenzo MS. *Urinalysis and Body Fluids.* 7th ed. F.A. Davis; 2021:49–70.

Chapter 9: Principles of Serological Testing

Ashwood ER, Bruns DE. Clinical evaluation of methods. In: Burtis CA, Bruns DE, eds. *Tietz Fundamentals of Clinical Chemistry and Molecular Diagnostics.* 7th ed. Elsevier Saunders; 2015:32–39.

Dugan K, Warning E. Basic principles and practices of clinical chemistry. In: Bishop ML, Fody EP, Van Siclen C, et al., eds. *Clinical Chemistry: Principles, Techniques, and Correlations.* 9th ed. Jones & Bartlett Learning; 2023:2–37.

Estridge BH, Reynolds AP. *Basic Clinical Laboratory Techniques.* 5th ed. Thomson Delmar Learning; 2008:85–96.

Krishnan KU, Adisesh M, Navaneethakrishnan L, Manjunathan R. Calibration of micropipettes through gravimetric solution and its beneficial impact on research. *Biotechnol Ind J.* 2019;15(4):195.

Lo SF. Principles of basic techniques and laboratory safety. In: Burtis CA, Bruns DE, eds. *Tietz Fundamentals of Clinical Chemistry and Molecular Diagnostics.* 7th ed. Elsevier Saunders; 2015:107–128.

Chapter 10: Precipitation and Agglutination Reactions

Csako G. Immunofixation electrophoresis for identification of proteins and specific antibodies. *Methods Mol Biol.* 2012;869:147–171.

Fahey JL, McKelvey EM. Quantitative determination of serum immunoglobulins in antibody-agar plates. *J Immunol.* 1965;94:84.

Mancini G, Carbonara AO, Heremans JF. Immunochemical quantitation of antigens by single radial immunodiffusion. *Immunochem.* 1965;2:235.

Pincus MR, Lifshitz MS, Bock JA. Analysis: principles of instrumentation. In: McPherson RA, Pincus MR, eds. *Henry's Clinical Diagnosis and Management by Laboratory Methods.* 23rd ed. Elsevier Saunders; 2017:33–59.

Van Oss CJ, Precipitation and agglutination. *J Immunoassay.* 2000;21(2–3):143–164.

Chapter 11: Labeled Immunoassays

Cinquanta L, Fontana DE, Bizzaro N. Chemiluminescent immunoassay technology: what does it change in autoantibody detection? *Auto Immun Highlights.* 2017;8(1):9.

Engvall E, Perlmann P. Enzyme-linked immunosorbent assay, ELISA. 3. Quantitation of specific antibodies by enzyme-labeled anti-immunoglobulin in antigen-coated tubes. *J Immunol.* 1972;109(1):129–135.

Li J, Wagar EA, Meng QH. Comprehensive assessment of biotin interference in immunoassays. *Clin Chim Acta.* 2018;487:293–298.

Thermofisher Scientific. Overview of Western blotting. Accessed April 16, 2024. https://www.thermofisher.com/us/en/home/life-science/protein-biology/protein-biology-learning-center/protein-biology-resource-library/pierce-protein-methods/overview-western-blotting.html#detection

Werfen. Systems Aptiva. PMAT method. Accessed June 7, 2024. https://www.werfen.com/na/en/autoantibody-testing/aptiva

Chapter 12: Molecular Diagnostic Techniques

Hu T, Chitnis N, Monos D, Dinh A. Next-generation sequencing technologies: an overview. *Hum Immunol.* 2021;82(11):801–811.

Jiang F, Doudna JA. CRISPR-Cas9 structures and mechanisms. *Annu Rev Biophys.* 2017;46:505–529.

Navarro E, Serrano-Heras G, Castaño MJ, Solera J. Real-time PCR detection chemistry. *Clin Chim Acta.* 2015;439:231–250.

Tagliaferro SS, Zejnelagic A, Farrugia R, Wettinger SB. Comparison of DNA extraction methods for samples from old blood collections. *Biotechniques.* 2021;70(5):243–250.

Zhu H, Zhang H, Xu Y, Laššáková S, Korabečná M, Neužil P. PCR past, present and future. *Biotechniques.* 2020;69(4):317–325.

Chapter 13: Flow Cytometry and Laboratory Automation

Appold K. Checklist for buying a chemistry analyzer. *Clin Lab Prod.* 2013(Nov);12–15.

BD Biosciences. Fluorochrome/laser reference poster. Accessed July 17, 2025. https://www.bdbiosciences.com/content/dam/bdb/marketing-documents/Multicolor_Fluorochrome_Specs.pdf

Herold NC, Mitra P. Immunophenotyping. In: *StatPearls.* StatPearls Publishing. Updated May 1, 2023. Accessed January 29, 2025. https://www.ncbi.nlm.nih.gov/books/NBK558927/

Moon TC, Legrys VA. Teaching method validation in the clinical laboratory science curriculum. *Clin Lab Sci.* 2008;21(1):19–24.

Pincus MR, Lifshitz MS, Bock JL. Analysis: principles of instrumentation. In: McPherson RA, Pincus MR, eds. *Henry's Clinical Diagnosis and Management by Laboratory Methods.* 23rd ed. Elsevier Saunders; 2017:33–59.

Chapter 14: Hypersensitivity

Abbas AK, Lichtman AH, Pillai S. *Cellular and Molecular Immunology.* 10th ed. Elsevier; 2022:436–478.

Ansotegui IJ, Melioli G, Canonica GW, et al. IgE allergy diagnostics and other relevant tests in allergy, a World Allergy Organization position paper. *World Allergy Organ J.* 2020;13:100080. http://doi.org/10.1016/j.waojou.2019.100080

Belknap R, Daley CL. Interferon gamma release assays. *Clin Lab Med.* 2014;34:337–349.

Harmening DM, Rhees JR, Green R. Hemolytic anemias. In: Harmening DM, Hutson LM, eds. *Clinical Hematology and Fundamentals of Hemostasis.* 6th ed. F.A. Davis; 2024: 283–311.

Usman N, Annamaraju P. Type III hypersensitivity reaction. In: *StatPearls.* StatPearls Publishing. Updated May 22, 2023. Accessed January 29, 2025. https://www.ncbi.nlm.nih.gov/books/NBK559122/

Chapter 15: Autoimmune Diseases

Ameer MA, Chaudhry H, Mushtaq J, et.al. An overview of systemic lupus erythematosus (SLE) pathogenesis, classification, and management. *Cureus.* 2022 Oct 15;14(10):e30330. https://doi.org/10.7759/cureus.30330

Bonroy C, Vercammen M, Fierz W, et al. Detection of antinuclear antibodies: recommendations from EFLM, EASI and ICAP. *Clin Chem Lab Med.* 2023;61(7):1167–1198. https://doi.org/10.1515/cclm-2023-0209

Bossuyt X, Cohen Tervaert J-W, Arimura Y. Revised 2017 international consensus on testing of ANCAs in granulomatosis with polyangiitis and microscopic polyangiitis. *Nature Rev Rheum.* 2017;13:684–692.

Damoiseaux J, Andrade LEC, Carballo OG, et al. Clinical relevance of HEp-2 indirect immunofluorescent patterns: the International Consensus on ANA Patterns (ICAP) perspective. *Ann Rheum Dis.* 2019;78:879–889.

Pisetsky DS. Pathogenesis of autoimmune disease. *Nat Rev Nephrol.* 2023;19:509–524. https://doi.org/10.1038/s41581-023-00720-1

Chapter 16: Transplantation Immunology

Gebel HM, Bray RA, Nickerson P. Pre-transplant assessment of donor-reactive, HLA-specific antibodies in renal transplantation: contraindication vs. risk. *Am J Transplant.* 2003;3:1488–1500.

Goker H, Haznedaroglu IC, Chao NJ. Acute graft-vs-host disease: pathobiology and management. *Exp Hematol.* 2001;29:259–277.

Health Resources and Services Administration. Donation and transplantation statistics. Accessed June 7, 2025. https://bloodstemcell.hrsa.gov/data/donation-and-transplantation-statistics

Singh N, Samant H, Hawby A, Samaniego M. Biomarkers of rejection in kidney transplantation. *Curr Opin Organ Transplant.* 2018;23:1–8.

Siu JHY, Surendrakumar V, Richards JA, Pettigrew GJ. T cell allorecognition pathways in solid organ transplantation. *Front Immunol.* 2018;9:2548.

Chapter 17: Tumor Immunology

American Cancer Society. Biomarker tests and cancer treatment. Accessed January 30, 2025. https://www.cancer.org/cancer/diagnosis-staging/tests/biomarker-tests.html

Hanahan D. Hallmarks of cancer: new dimensions. *Cancer Discov.* 2022;12(1):31–46. https://doi.org/10.1158/2159-8290.CD-21-1059

National Cancer Institute. What is cancer? Accessed January 29, 2025. https://www.cancer.gov/about-cancer/understanding/what-is-cancer

Quraish RU, Hirahata T, Quraish AU, Ul Quraish S. An overview: genetic tumor markers for early detection and current gene therapy strategies. *Cancer Inform.* 2023;22:11769351221150772. https://doi.org/10.1177/11769351221150772

Waldmann AD, Fritz JM, Lenardo MJ. A guide to cancer immunotherapy: from T cell basic science to clinical practice. *Nat Rev Immunol.* 2020;20(11):651–668. https://doi.org/10.1038/s41577-020-0306-5

Chapter 18: Immunoproliferative Diseases

Alaggio R, Amador C, Anagnostopoulos I, et al. The 5th edition of the World Health Organization classification of haematolymphoid tumours: lymphoid neoplasms. *Leukemia.* 2022;36(7):1720–1748.

Craig FE, Foon KA. Flow cytometric immunophenotyping for hematologic neoplasms. *Blood.* 2008;111(8):3941–3967.

Ekpa QL, Akahara PC, Anderson AM, et al. A review of acute lymphocytic leukemia (ALL) in the pediatric population: evaluating current trends and changes in guidelines in the past decade. *Cureus.* 2023;15(12):e49930.

Falini B, Marino G, Lazzi S. A comparison of the International Consensus and 5th World Health Organization classifications of mature B-cell neoplasms. *Leukemia.* 2023;37:18–34.

Munir F, Hardit V, Sheikh IN, et al. Classical Hodgkin lymphoma: from past to future—a comprehensive review of pathophysiology and therapeutic advances. *Int J Mol Sci.* 2023;24(12):10095.

Chapter 19: Immunodeficiency Diseases and Inborn Errors of Immunity

Aiuti A, Roncarolo MG, Naldini L. Gene therapy for ADA-SCID, the first marketing approval of an ex vivo gene therapy in Europe: paving the road for the next generation of advanced therapy medicinal products. *EMBO Mol Med.* 2017;9(6):737–740.

Bousfiha A, Moundir A, Tangye SG, et al. The 2022 update of IUIS phenotypical classification for human inborn errors of immunity. *J Clin Immunol.* 2022;42(7):1508–1520. https://doi.org/10.1007/s10875-022-01352-z

Immune Deficiency Foundation. Types of PI. Accessed January 29, 2025. https://primaryimmune.org/understanding-primary-immunodeficiency/types-of-pi

Knight V, Heimall JR, Chong H, et al. A toolkit and framework for optimal laboratory evaluation of individuals with suspected primary immunodeficiency. *J Allergy Clin Immunol Pract.* 2021;9(9):3293–3307.e6. https://doi.org/10.1016/j.jaip.2021.05.004

Wang JJF, Dhir A, Hildebrand KJ et al. Inborn errors of immunity in adulthood. *Allergy Asthma Clin Immunol.* 2024;20:6. https://doi.org/10.1186/s13223-023-00862-8

Chapter 20: Laboratory Detection of Bacterial Infections

Bae W, Park KU, Song EY, et al. Comparison of the sensitivity of QuantiFERON-TB Gold In-Tube and T-SPOT.TB according to patient age. *PLOS ONE.* 2016;11(6):e0156917.

Centers for Disease Control and Prevention. Clinical and laboratory diagnosis for Rocky Mountain spotted fever. Accessed January 30, 2025. https://www.cdc.gov/rocky-mountain-spotted-fever/hcp/diagnosis-testing/

Litwin CM, Litwin SE, Hill HR. Diagnostic methods for group A streptococcal infections. In: Detrick B, Schmitz JL, Hamilton RG, eds. *Manual of Molecular and Clinical Laboratory Immunology.* 8th ed. ASM Press; 2016:394–403.

Tille PM. *Bailey and Scott's Diagnostic Microbiology.* 15th ed. Mosby Elsevier; 2022:77–163.

Waites KB, Bébéar C. Mycoplasma and ureoplasma. In: Carroll KC, Pfaller MA, eds. *Manual of Clinical Microbiology.* 12th ed. ASM Press; 2023:1219–2035.

Chapter 21: Spirochete Diseases

Ghanem KG, Ram S, Rice PA. The modern epidemic of syphilis. *N Engl J Med.* 2020;382(9):845–854. https://doi.org/10.1056/nejmra1901593

John TM, Taege AJ. Appropriate laboratory testing in Lyme disease. *Cleve Clin J Med.* 2019;86(11):751–759. https://doi.org/10.3949/ccjm.86a.19029

Kullberg BJ, Vrijmoeth HD, van de Schoor F, Hovius JW. Lyme borreliosis: diagnosis and management. *BMJ.* 2020;369:m1041. https://doi.org/10.1136/bmj.m104

Papp JR, Park IU, Fakile Y, et al. CDC laboratory recommendations for syphilis testing, United States, 2024. *MMWR Recomm Rep.* 2024 Feb 8;73(RR-1):1–32. https://doi.org/10.15585/mmwr.rr7301a1

Rajapakse S. Leptospirosis: clinical aspects. *Clin Med.* 2022;22(1):14–17. https://doi.org/10.7861/clinmed.2021-0784

Chapter 22: Laboratory Diagnosis of Parasitic and Fungal Infections

Centers for Disease Control and Prevention. DPDx—laboratory identification of parasites of public health concern. Accessed January 30, 2025. https://www.cdc.gov/dpdx/diagnosticprocedures/index.html

Centers for Disease Control and Prevention. Toxoplasmosis: laboratory diagnosis. Accessed January 30, 2025. https://www.cdc.gov/dpdx/toxoplasmosis/index.html

Chandra RK. Immune responses in parasitic diseases. Part B: mechanisms. *Rev Infect Dis.* 1982;4(4):756–762.

Fida M, Wengenack NL, Theel ES. General approaches for direct and indirect detection and identification of fungi. In: Carroll KC, Pfaller MA, eds. *Manual of Clinical Microbiology.* 13th ed. ASM Press; 2023:2–12.

Parija SC. Superficial, cutaneous and subcutaneous mycoses. In: Parija SC, ed. *Textbook of Microbiology and Immunology.* Springer, Singapore; 2023:957–971. https://doi.org/10.1007/978-981-19-3315-8_66

Chapter 23: Serological and Molecular Detection of Viral Infections

Abbas AK, Lichtman AH, Pillai S. Immunity to microbes. In: *Cellular and Molecular Immunology.* 10th ed. Elsevier Saunders; 2022:363–387.

Centers for Disease Control and Prevention. *Epidemiology and Prevention of Vaccine-Preventable Diseases.* 14th ed. 2021. Accessed January 29, 2025. https://www.cdc.gov/pinkbook/hcp/table-of-contents/index.html

Centers for Disease Control and Prevention. COVID-19. Accessed January 30, 2025. https://www.cdc.gov/covid/site.html#hcp

Dienstag JL. Acute viral hepatitis. In: Loscalzo J, Fauci A, Kasper D, Hauser S, Longo D, Jameson J, eds. *Harrison's Principles of Internal Medicine.* 21st ed. McGraw-Hill education; 2022. Accessed January 30, 2025. https://accessmedicine.mhmedical.com/content.aspx?bookid=3095&sectionid=264532564

Lupo J, Truffot A, Andreani J, et al. Virological markers in Epstein-Barr virus-associated diseases. *Viruses.* 2023;15(3):656. https://doi.org/10.3390/v15030656

Chapter 24: Laboratory Diagnosis of Human Retroviruses

Association of Public Health Laboratories. Suggested reporting language for the HIV laboratory diagnostic testing algorithm 2018. Accessed January 30, 2025. https://www.aphl.org/aboutAPHL/publications/Documents/ID-2019Jan-HIV-Lab-Test-Suggested-Reporting-Language.pdf

Bangham C, Matsuoka M. Human T-cell leukemia virus types 1 and 2. In: Howley PM, Knipe DM, Whelan S, et al., eds. *Fields Virology Volume 3: RNA Viruses.* 8th ed. Wolters Kluwer; 2023:1064–1126.

Centers for Disease Control and Prevention. HIV. Accessed January 30, 2025. https://www.cdc.gov/hiv/index.html

Fauci AS, Folkers GK, Lane H. Human immunodeficiency virus disease: AIDS and related disorders. In: Loscalzo J, Fauci A, Kasper D, Hauser S, Longo D, Jameson J. eds. *Harrison's Principles of Internal Medicine.* 21st ed. McGraw-Hill education; 2022.

U.S. Department of Health and Human Services. Guidelines for the use of antiretroviral agents in adults and adolescents with HIV. Accessed January 30, 2025. https://clinicalinfo.hiv.gov/en/guidelines/hiv-clinical-guidelines-adult-and-adolescent-arv/whats-new

Chapter 25: Immunization and Vaccines

Ahmad U, Khan Z, Ualiyeva D, et al. Chimeric antigen receptor T cell structure, its manufacturing, and related toxicities: a comprehensive review. *Adv Cancer Biol Metastasis.* 2022;4:2667–3940. https://doi.org/10.1016/j.adcanc.2022.100035

Centers for Disease Control and Prevention. Vaccines and immunizations. Accessed January 30, 2025. https://www.cdc.gov/vaccines/index.html

Chaudhary N, Weissman D, Whitehead KA. mRNA vaccines for infectious diseases: principles, delivery and clinical translation. *Nat Rev Drug Discov.* 2021;20:817–838. https://doi.org/10.1038/s41573-021-00283-5

College of Physicians of Philadelphia. Vaccine timeline. Accessed January 30, 2025. https://historyofvaccines.org/history/vaccine-timeline/timeline

Novaretti MC, Dinardo CL. Immunoglobulin: production, mechanisms of action and formulations. *Rev Bras Hematol Hemoter.* 2011;33(5):377-82. https://doi.org/10.5581/1516-8484.20110102

World Health Organization. Vaccine hesitancy: a growing challenge for immunization programmes. Accessed July 9, 2025. https://www.who.int/news/item/18-08-2015-vaccine-hesitancy-a-growing-challenge-for-immunization-programmes

Answer Key

Chapter 1: Introduction to Immunity and the Immune System

Answers to Critical Thinking

1–1 Such a virus is HIV (see Chapter **24**). CD4 is a key surface marker on helper T cells, which produce many cytokines that are necessary for adaptive immune responses. As a result, the patient would be deficient in both cell-mediated and humoral antibody responses.

1–2 Bruton tyrosine kinase (Btk) deficiency is an X-linked genetic disorder characterized by the inability to produce mature B lymphocytes. Mature B cells normally populate the follicles of the lymph nodes and are transformed into germinal centers after contact with antigen. As a result of the deficiency, patients are unable to produce antibodies; thus, the humoral arm of adaptive immunity is affected.

Answers to the Case Studies

1. a. Because the swelling has occurred within 3 days, it is most likely caused by an innate immune response. The adaptive immune response takes longer to develop because it depends on lymphocytes recognizing and responding to a specific antigen. Swelling, redness, and pus are caused by an innate inflammatory response to bacteria and accumulation of dying neutrophils and debris in the tissue.

1. b. There may be neutrophils, macrophages, and dendritic cells present.

2. a. The adaptive immune system is characterized by specificity and memory. The response is more rapid and effective each time an individual is exposed to the same antigen. Thus, with a serious disease such as tetanus, getting a booster shot of a similar but harmless substance will stimulate the immune system each time a booster is given. Restimulating the adaptive immune response provides greater protection than the innate immune system on its own, which could possibly be overwhelmed by pathogens such as the bacteria that cause tetanus.

2. b. The most important cells in a response to a vaccine are the cells involved in adaptive immunity, namely, T cells and B cells. Memory T cells will help B cells to divide and develop into plasma cells in a very short time if the individual is re-exposed to the bacteria that cause tetanus in the future.

Chapter 2: Innate Immunity

Answers to Critical Thinking

2–1 Neutrophils are an essential component of the innate immune response to bacteria, as they are a major type of white blood cell involved in phagocytosis. The defect in the patient's neutrophilic granules could affect their ability to fuse with phagosomes to form phagolysosomes and/or their ability to subsequently destroy engulfed bacteria if their contents lacked functional proteolytic enzymes. As a result, the patient would be expected to experience severe, recurrent bacterial infections. Such a deficiency, Chédiak-Higashi syndrome, is discussed in Chapter **19**.

2–2 While some increase in C-reactive protein (CRP) after surgery is expected, the very high CRP concentration along with the patient's clinical presentation indicate that a postsurgical complication, such as a bacterial infection, has occurred. The erythrocyte sedimentation rate and procalcitonin levels would also be expected to increase, and the neutrophil count would likely be elevated. Bacterial culture and susceptibility testing would provide definitive proof of infection and would indicate the type of antibiotic therapy that should be administered.

Answers to Case Studies

1. a. Edema (swelling) is one of the five cardinal signs of inflammation. The other signs are heat, redness, pain, and loss of function.

1. b. During inflammation, white blood cells (WBCs) are attracted to the inflammatory site, and cytokines are released that increase production of WBCs from precursors in the bone marrow. The largest increase would be expected for the neutrophils.

1. c. C-reactive protein and prolactin are acute phase reactants that rise rapidly during an inflammatory response. The results of the laboratory tests that measure these proteins can be available within 30 minutes, providing doctors with information that would prompt them to begin treatment with antibiotics. If they had waited for the culture results before they initiated treatment, the patient's outcome may have been much worse.

2. a. Although the patient's cholesterol levels were within normal limits for both HDL and total cholesterol, some studies have found an association between elevated C-reactive protein (CRP) and a higher risk of a future heart attack. Higher fibrinogen levels are also associated with an increased risk for a future cardiovascular event, although increased fibrinogen is not as great a risk factor as increased CRP. A rise in both of these acute phase reactants indicates an underlying inflammatory process. Such a process is associated with atherosclerosis, a condition that damages coronary blood vessels. The spouse should encourage the patient to follow a healthy diet and to lose weight through exercise.

Chapter 3: Antibody Structure and Function

Answers to Critical Thinking

3–1 Selective IgA deficiency is a common immunodeficiency disorder. Because IgA protects the mucosal surfaces by binding to pathogens and preventing them from penetrating farther into the body, these patients may have an increased incidence of respiratory and gastrointestinal infections.

3–2 Antigen-specific IgM along with low levels of IgG in a symptomatic patient supports the presence of an active infection with the virus. These results would be present if the patient were mounting a primary antibody response to the virus.

Answers to Case Studies

1. a. The presence of IgM only is an indicator of an early acute infection. IgM is the first antibody to appear, followed by IgG. In a reactivated case of infectious mononucleosis, a small amount of IgM might be present, but IgG would also be present. Thus, the patient is encountering the virus for the first time.

1. b. In a secondary response, the memory cells triggered by the first exposure to the virus would cause IgG to be produced in a much shorter time in the primary response. The secondary response is also characterized by a greater increase in IgG compared with the amount of IgM.

2. a. The increase in IgE is an indicator that the cold symptoms may actually be caused by an allergy. This is especially evident in the springtime when pollen levels are high. The child should be tested for allergies to specific antigens to determine the cause of the symptoms. Treatment with anti-histamine drugs and avoidance of the allergen will help to relieve the symptoms.

2. b. Chronic respiratory infections may be caused by a decrease or lack of IgA, but this is not the case here. Normal levels of IgG, IgM, and IgA indicate that this child is not immunocompromised.

Chapter 4: Nature of Antigens and the Major Histocompatibility Complex

Answers to Critical Thinking

4–1 Denaturation causes a change in tertiary structure of a protein, altering the positions of amino acids on the exterior surface of the protein and changing its shape. This is most likely to alter the epitopes recognized by B-cell receptors. Since denaturation does not change the amino acid sequence (primary structure) of the protein, it will not alter the peptide antigens presented on major histocompatibility complex molecules for recognition by T-cell receptors. Denaturation is used to inactivate toxins (like tetanus toxin) or pathogens (such as influenza virus), rendering them safe for use in vaccines. In these cases, the degree of denaturation is minor and causes only slight changes in structure, so that important B-cell epitopes are preserved.

4–2 Toll-like receptor **4** is the target innate receptor of AS**04**. By adding AS**04** to vaccines, a stronger immune response is mounted than by the vaccine antigens alone. In a sense, AS**04** *tricks* the immune system into acting as if a bacterial infection is under way, and the result is stronger immune protection against the corresponding bacteria.

4–3 The major histocompatibility complex (MHC) peptide-binding cleft is a tertiary protein structure. The amino acids in the groove that bind to the peptide antigen do not follow each other in a linear sequence but are separated by intervening amino acids that form helix, strand, and loop segments. These parts interact with each other to make up the overall three-dimensional structure of the MHC molecule. In doing so, they bring some of the amino acids that are distant from each other together in the position of the peptide-binding groove.

Answers to Case Studies

1. a. Because every child inherits one haplotype (set of genes) from the mother and one from the father, 50% of the human leukocyte antigens would match the mother, and 50% would match the father. It would not be more than that unless the mother and father have at least one antigen in common.

1. b. According to the genetics law of independent assortment, there would be a 1:4 chance that the sister would be an exact match, a 1:2 chance that a sister would share half of the same alleles, and a 1:4 chance that a sister would share no alleles, having received the opposite haplotype from each parent.

1. c. It is possible that a cadaver kidney may actually be a better match, if neither sister is an exact match. The most important alleles to match are HLA-A, HLA-B, and HLA-DR. If a cadaver match has more than one allele in common with the recipient at each of these loci, then it would be a closer match.

2. a. Of all the different antigens that have been purified by the other scientists working on the project, proteins generally make the best immunogens. This is because of all the biomolecules listed, only protein antigens can be processed and presented to T cells. B cells can respond to essentially all of the listed biomolecules—but an effective antibody response requires cooperation between T cells and B cells.

2. b. Antigen alone is often insufficient to stimulate an immune response. For this reason, the zombie plague vaccine should be formulated with an adjuvant. Incorporating an adjuvant into the inoculum will stimulate an innate immune response and may also keep the antigen concentrated at the site of vaccination. Both of these adjuvant properties will help strengthen the response against the zombie pathogen antigen.

Chapter 5: Adaptive Immunity

Answers to Critical Thinking

5–1 Only a few lymphocytes possess receptors that recognize and respond to any given infection. It takes time for these lymphocytes to proliferate to combat the infection.

5–2 T1D–associated insulin gene mutations interfere with the ability of AIRE to initiate expression of insulin antigens in thymic cells. This prevents negative selection of insulin-reactive T cells, allowing them to mature and exit the thymus. Ultimately, these cells target the insulin-producing pancreatic β cells, leading to their destruction.

Answers to Case Studies

1. a. The normal CD19⁺ cell count indicates that there is not a lack of B cells. The low CD4⁺ T-cell count indicates that there is a decrease in helper T (TH) cells.

1. b. Helper T (TH) cells are necessary for an antibody response to T-dependent antigens. The decreased CD4⁺ count means that B cells are not activated by TH cells, and class switching to IgG does not occur. Memory B cells are not produced either. Thus, the decrease in TH cells severely limits antibody production, resulting in increased bacterial infections.

2. a. CD8⁺ T cells are responsible for destroying cancer cells and intracellular pathogens like viruses. In contrast, antibodies can only exert their effects on extracellular antigens. Thus, if an individual's cytotoxic T cells were not functioning properly, they would be more susceptible to certain kinds of infections and to cancer.

Chapter 6: Cytokines

Answers to Critical Thinking

6–1 These symptoms are the result of a cytokine storm caused by dysregulation of cytokine synthesis, leading to overproduction of pro-inflammatory cytokines. IL-1β, TNF-α, and IL-6 should be included in the test panel, as these are highly associated with an inflammatory state. Studies have shown that elevations in IL-6 are the most profound, and that IL-6 levels are the best indicator of disease severity and risk of death.

6–2 Sample handling is extremely important in cytokine immunoassays. It is likely that the laboratorian's results were much lower than the comparison laboratory's results for the same samples because IL-2 was degraded during prolonged storage of the samples in the refrigerator or freeze-thawing of the samples prior to testing by the laboratorian.

Answers to Case Study

1. a. G-CSF.

1. b. IFN-γ and IL-2.

1. c. IL-4, IL-5, and IL-13.

Chapter 7: The Complement System

Answers to Critical Thinking

7–1 Measuring C1q and C2 levels could be helpful. Deficiencies in either of these classical pathway components, while rare, can also lead to lupus-like symptoms.

7–2 There are two possible reasons. The first, and more likely reason if the patient was showing symptoms of aHUS, is that the disease was causing complement activation. If there was poorly controlled complement activity causing damage to the kidneys, complement would be consumed, and there would not be sufficient complement to give a normal CH50. The overactivation of complement due to the disease would be expected to lead to increased C5 cleavage and sC5b-9. The second reason, consistent with the patient not demonstrating any symptoms, would be how the samples were handled prior to testing. If the serum sample (for the CH50) and EDTA plasma sample (for sC5b-9) were not frozen, this could lead to ex vivo complement activation, which would produce the same laboratory results.

Answers to Case Studies

1. a. Levels of C3 and C4 are normal, indicating that a deficiency of one or more of the membrane attack components are involved. Although a lack of C1q or C2 cannot absolutely be ruled out, the fact that the alternative pathway is also affected is an additional indicator that the components common to both pathways, C5 through C9, are the ones involved. Because defense against encapsulated bacteria such as meningococci is reduced if there is a decrease in C5 through C9, the patient's symptoms are in agreement with this conclusion.

1. b. Measuring the individual components C5 through C9 should be performed to confirm the actual deficiency. C8 deficiency, in particular, is associated with susceptibility to Neisserian infections that can cause meningitis.

2. a. Although the abdominal pain and vomiting could be caused by several infectious agents, the normal white blood cell count decreases the likelihood of a bacterial infection. The accompanying swelling of the hands and legs may be an indicator of a possible inflammatory problem associated with continuous activation of the complement system. Because this has been a recurring problem, the likelihood of an immune problem is increased. Because the total serum protein is within the normal range, it is unlikely that the deficiency is from lack of antibody production. A decrease of one complement component would not be apparent on a total protein determination.

2. b. Reduced levels of both C4 and C2 could be caused by inheritance of defective genes for both components. However, the possibility of that is extremely rare. A more plausible explanation is that the deficiency of both C2 and C4 is caused by overconsumption rather than a lack of production. The normal level of C1q indicates it is likely not an acquired complement deficiency.

2. c. A lack of C1-INH would result in increased C1q and overconsumption of C4 and C2. As this is the most common deficiency of the complement system, this represents a likely explanation for the patient's symptoms, which are characteristic of C1-INH deficiency. This can be verified by testing for C1-INH.

Chapter 8: Safety and Quality Management

Answers to Critical Thinking

8–1 The laboratorian may have developed a latex allergy. Other more serious conditions can occur, such as a delayed hypersensitivity reaction appearing 24 to 48 hours after exposure, or an immediate hypersensitivity reaction characterized by facial flushing and breathing difficulties. The situation can be resolved by immediately sanitizing the hands after removing the gloves and replacing latex gloves with nitrile or vinyl gloves.

8–2 Yes. The absorbent material to separate the specimens and absorb the contents of the primary container in case of leakage or breakage is missing. The primary container must be enclosed in a secondary container with sufficient absorbent material. Specimens for public transport are required to have triple packaging: a primary container, a secondary leakproof container with sufficient absorbent material, and an outer container of rigid material.

8–3 Trends in quality control results are a systemic error that may be caused by a gradual deterioration of the reagents, control deterioration, or deterioration of the instrument. The laboratorian should check the outdates on the reagents and controls, open and test new controls and reagents, and check the preventive maintenance records for the instrument.

Answers to Case Studies

1. a. Gloves should never be removed when working with patient specimens. When they are, hands should be washed right away using the correct procedure. Any contamination of the laboratory bench should be treated with sodium hypochlorite, and the paper towels should be disposed of in the regulated medical waste container. Because the supervisor's lab coat was disposable and became contaminated, it should be discarded in the regulated medical waste container and replaced with a new coat. Pipetting should have been done behind a Plexiglass shield because this would have prevented the spill onto the lab coat.

1. b. Reservoir. The hands and contaminated fomites (laboratory coat and laboratory bench) that contain blood are ideal reservoirs for infectious agents.

1. c. To break the chain, disinfect the work area with a 1:10 sodium hypochlorite solution and sanitize hands to kill the infectious agent and eliminate the reservoir.

2. a. Take corrective action.

b. Take corrective action.

c. Accept.

d. Take corrective action.

3. a. Incident (variance) report.

b. The Joint Commission

4. 2, 1, 2, 3, 2, 2

Chapter 9: Principles of Serological Testing

Answers to Critical Thinking

9–1 Dilution of tube 3 = Dilution of tube 1 × $(1/df)^2$ = ½ × ½ × ½ = 1:8 [df = dilution fold]

9–2 Diagnostic specificity = 167/(167 + 33) = 83.5%

Answers to Case Studies

1. a. The serological pipette must be emptied completely to obtain the correct volume because it is marked to contain (TC) rather than to deliver (TD). Therefore, the last drop should have been blown out of the pipette using a bulb or an automatic pipette filler, or the measurement should have been from point to point, as in filling the pipette up to the 0.8-mL mark and then letting it drain to the 0.9-mL mark.

1. b. The 1.9 mL of diluent was not correct. To make a 1:40 dilution with 0.1 mL of serum, the calculations are as follows:

$$1/40 = 0.1/x$$

$$x = 4.0 \text{ mL (This represents the total volume.)}$$

4.0 – 0.1 = 3.9 mL of diluent to make a 1:40 dilution.

2. a. 80

b. 5

c. 95

d. 20

e. 80/(80 + 20) = 80/100 = 0.8 × 100% = 80%

f. 95/(95 + 5) = 95/100 = 0.95 × 100% = 95%

g. 80/(80 + 5) = 80/85 = 0.94 × 100% = 94%

h. 95/(95 + 20) = 95/115 = 0.83 × 100% = 83%

i. This is a measure of the positive predictive value, which in this case is 94%. Therefore, there is a 94% chance that the patient's positive test result is truly positive.

Chapter 10: Precipitation and Agglutination Reactions

Answers to Critical Thinking

10–1 The negative result could be caused by the prozone phenomenon. The patient could be producing a very high amount of antibody (prozone), resulting in a prozone effect. In this situation, the measles antigen reagent used in the assay is in much lower concentration than the patient's antibody, resulting in a lack of cross-linking and a false-negative test result. To compensate for the prozone effect, a serial dilution of the patient sample can be performed to reach the zone of equivalence to allow for the detection of the measles antibody. Alternatively, the patient may have been tested too early in the course of the infection, before antibody can be detected. To see if this is the case, another serum sample from the patient could be collected a few days later and tested for IgM.

10–2 Since C-reactive protein (CRP) circulates in the bloodstream and does not naturally occur on a cell surface, a direct agglutination assay cannot be used. Because CRP is an antigen, not an antibody, an indirect agglutination assay cannot be used because this type of assay uses particles coated with antigens to detect antibodies in the patient sample. Reverse passive agglutination would be the most appropriate type of agglutination assay to detect CRP. Reverse passive agglutination assays use inert particles coated with antibodies to detect antigens. To detect CRP, inert particles coated with CRP antibodies are mixed with the patient sample and form immune complexes with CRP. The test can be performed by manual assays, or more commonly, by automated particle-enhanced immunoassays.

Answers to Case Studies

1. a. *Shigella sonnei*.

1. b. Direct agglutination, as the antigen is naturally occurring on *Shigella* bacteria.

2. a. The *Treponema pallidum* particle agglutination assay test is a particle agglutination test used to detect antibodies to *T. pallidum*, the bacterium that causes syphilis. In this test, dilutions of patient serum are incubated with gel particles that have been sensitized with *T. pallidum* antigen, and the wells are examined for agglutination. A smooth mat of particles covering the well indicates that a lattice has been formed and thus represents a positive result.

2. b. If the 1:40 result was negative and the 1:80 result was positive, this is an example of a prozone phenomenon, in which there is an excess of antibody molecules in the 1:40 dilution that inhibited lattice formation, but equivalence was reached when the antibody was diluted 1:80.

2. c. The positive result indicates that the patient has been exposed to *T. pallidum* but cannot differentiate between a current infection and a past exposure. This would have to be determined by performing additional laboratory tests and taking a thorough medical history.

Chapter 11: Labeled Immunoassays

Answers to Critical Thinking

11–1 In the indirect assay design, rubella antigen would be attached to a solid phase, such as wells of a microtiter plate. When patient serum is incubated with the solid phase, if rubella antibody is present, it will bind to the antigen. Excess serum proteins are removed by washing, then an enzyme-labeled anti-human immunoglobulin reagent would be added and would bind to the patient antibody. After another wash step, the appropriate substrate would be added and would react with the enzyme to create a colored product.

11–2 This is an example of cross-reactivity. *Borrelia miyamotoi* and *Borrelia burgdorferi* are both spirochete bacteria that cause tick-borne illnesses. *B. miyamotoi* possesses antigens that are similar to the C6 antigen (a synthetic peptide derived from a protein in the outer membrane of *B. burgdorferi*), which is commonly used in EIA tests for *B. burgdorferi* antibodies. Because EIAs are used as the initial test for *B. burgdorferi* antibodies and can produce false-positive results such as the one presented here, an additional method is required to confirm the results (see Chapter 21).

Answers to Case Study

1. a. This is an example of a high-dose hook effect (also called *antigen excess* or *postzone effect*). It occurs commonly in immunoassay measurements of tumor markers. The tumor marker concentration generally reflects the tumor burden: large tumors tend to generate very high concentrations of the test marker in the blood. This causes the value to fall outside of the reportable range of the test method, leading to loss of the linear relationship between the detected signal and the analyte concentration.

1. b. Dilute the patient sample. In this case, the technologist prepared a 1:10 dilution of the sample, based on the patient's first reported value (1,250 U/mL) and the test assay reportable range. This is illustrated by the two test results performed on instrument B at the patient's 3-month follow-up. The initial test result from instrument B before dilution was 110 U/mL. After making a 1:10 dilution, the instrument result is 95 U/mL. Accounting for the dilution factor, the final reported result is 950 U/mL, indicating that the original undiluted sample result of 110 U/mL performed on instrument B was falsely low because of antigen excess. If the diluted test result had instead been 5 U/mL for a final value of 50 U/mL, this could reflect successful treatment of the patient.

1. c. Immunoassay manufacturers often develop capture and detection antibodies using slightly different epitopes so that the reagent antibodies detect different parts of the test marker molecule. The lack of standardization across different manufacturer methods means that test results may not be equivalent in the same person simply because the methods are different. For this reason, it is essential to have reference interval (normal range) cutoffs determined for each method. In this case, the cutoff value for instrument A is 38 U/mL, whereas it is 55 U/mL for instrument B. Ideally, the same instrument/method should be used to measure the patient's tumor marker concentration for serial (repeat) testing to ensure the results are correctly interpreted.

1. d. If the original laboratory (test method) could not be used for follow-up, the manufacturer-specific cutoff value should be used to interpret the test result.

Chapter 12: Molecular Diagnostic Techniques

Answers to Critical Thinking

12–1 Fixation preserves tissue morphology for immunohistochemistry and pathological analysis, but fixatives used for this purpose can damage nucleic acids. For this reason, it is important to assess nucleic acid integrity to ensure accurate test results free of false negatives or other artifacts. The longer product is more likely to be damaged or degraded than the short product. Based on the reverse relationship between Ct and quantity, the short product is likely to have a lower Ct value than the long product. A difference of 50 would indicate a lower DNA integrity and a lower quantity of the long product caused by degradation. The DNA in this case would not be of acceptable quantity for use. If the long product Ct is close to the short product Ct (e.g., a difference of three cycles), the DNA is likely to be of good quality and can be used for subsequent molecular testing.

12–2 The likely reason for the run failure was inadequate DNA input due to the use of spectrophotometry, rather than fluorometry, to quantify input DNA. Spectrophotometry measurement is based on single nucleotides, which can overestimate the DNA concentration, especially if the DNA is degraded, as is likely here. Fluorometry measures intact DNA bound by the fluorescent dyes. The enzymatic DNA fragmentation used in this protocol is more sensitive to DNA input compared to mechanical fragmentation. Success depends on accurate quantification of intact DNA.

Fluorometric quantification of the barcoded products before sequencing should have revealed the inadequacy. Low library concentration can lead to insufficient cluster density for dye imaging on the flow cell. The quality and quantification of the library should be performed using methods recommended by the instrument manufacturer.

12–3 Failed or compromised amplification will result in loss of detection of an allele (allelic dropout). If one allele of a heterozygous locus has insufficient amplification, the locus would appear to be homozygous (having only one allele for the trait). Depending on the sequencing test, a missed allele could influence interpretation of inherited disease risk, therapeutic strategy, or transplant management.

Answers to Case Studies

1. a. The most common fixative, 10% buffered formalin, causes intermolecular and intramolecular cross-linking (covalent attachment) of proteins that produce changes in protein structure and solubility. These effects influence the degree of epitope recognition by test antibodies. Protein cross-linking is partially reversible by antigen-retrieval methods. Heating, acid treatment, and proteolytic agents break protein cross-links and expose antigenic sites. There is some variation in the quality of antigen preservation with various agents. The preservation of antigenicity is an important consideration when choosing a fixative.

1. b. Tissue that expresses PD-L1, such as tonsil, would be a positive control for recognition of the epitope by the primary antibody. There should be no staining reaction in most lymphocytes, nor in superficial epithelial cells, providing an internal negative control. Cultured cells from cell lines expressing PD-L1 are provided with reagent sets and should also be included with each run as a standard for the reagents provided. Tumor tissue that gives no staining but contains tumor-associated macrophages/immune cells that may express PD-L1 could also provide an internal positive control. An adjacent section cut from the test tissue run without addition of the primary antibody is a negative control for reagent quality and specificity.

Ideally, the control tissues are processed with the test tissue. Control tissues processed differently from the test tissue validate reagent performance but do not verify the tissue preparation. If staining of positive control tissue is not satisfactory, or if unwanted staining occurs in negative controls, all results with the patient specimen should be considered invalid.

2. a. Choice ii. The amplification control should always be positive to demonstrate that the polymerase chain reaction is working and to avoid false negatives. Since the amplification control did not work, the current results are not interpretable. A reagent blank (no template) control is included to detect contamination. The previous results do not necessarily predict that the current test results should be positive.

2. b. Choice i. Since the amplification control is positive, the polymerase chain reaction is working, and the result is a true negative. The reagent blank (no template) control, not the amplification control, is used to detect contamination. The previous results may be reviewed for interpretation of the result but do not predict a positive result in the current sample.

2. c. No. The analytical sensitivity of the test is 50 copies/mL, meaning that there may be fewer than 50 copies/mL present that will not be detected by the test method. Since the patient was previously determined to be HIV positive, a residual low level of viral copies could still be present after treatment. The results should be reported as "less than 50 copies/mL" to indicate the capacity of the test to detect low-level presence of HIV.

Chapter 13: Flow Cytometry and Laboratory Automation

Answers to Critical Thinking

13–1 The experimental panel needs to include antigens that differentiate B-cell lineage (see Chapter 5). These could include CD10, CD19, CD20, CD22, κ chains, and λ chains. The panel should also include antigens that differentiate B-cell maturity. CD34 is commonly used to detect progenitor cells, and CD10 is used to identify immature B cells. CD45 should always be included in experiments to aid in gating cell populations. Fluorochromes should be chosen for each antigen with its cell surface density in mind. High-density antigens should be paired with dim fluorochromes and low-density antigens with bright fluorochromes. An example of a panel could be as follows: CD45 PerCP, CD19 APC, CD34 FITC, CD10 PE.

13–2 Lymphocyte subset analysis starts by gating around only the lymphocytes. Fluorescent-labeled antibodies are added to the sample to differentiate the lymphocyte populations—B cells, T cells, and natural killer cells. Using absolute counts, patient values can be compared to normal reference ranges to determine if there is a decrease in any specific lymphocyte populations. Immunodeficiency disorders affect certain populations of lymphocytes; for example, a decrease in B cells may point physicians to Bruton tyrosine kinase deficiency, while a decline in T cells may indicate HIV infection.

13–3 (a) The analyzer's operational type is a continuous random access; therefore, several tests can be performed on any one sample. In this scenario, serum is an acceptable specimen for both assays. Therefore, one sample can be used for both *Toxoplasma gondii* IgM and rubella virus IgG analysis. (b) Recall from Chapter 11 that enzyme immunoassays using a noncompetitive indirect method will produce a signal intensity that is directly proportional to the amount of analyte present. In this scenario, if the validation specimen has high levels of antibody, the medical laboratory professional should expect to see raw data results with a strong signal (larger colorimetric reading). If the validation specimen has low levels of antibody, the raw data results should show a weaker signal (smaller colorimetric reading).

Answers to Case Studies

1. a. The result may represent an error of specificity given that the newer instrument is getting positive results on specimens that were negative by the older method. However, the newer instrument could be more sensitive than the older one, so these could actually be positive samples.

1. b. To resolve this discrepancy, known positive and negative controls should be run. The positive controls need to include those at the lower limit of detection, as well as more highly positive samples. This would help to determine if the new instrument is actually more sensitive rather than lacking in specificity.

2. a. The pattern in panel A indicates that the majority of lymphocytes are B cells because they are $CD19^+$. The population most affected appears to be $CD3^+$, or T cells. Panel C indicates that the $CD3^+CD4^+$ cell count is very low.

2. b. Helper T cells are necessary to provide help to B cells so they can respond by making antibodies. Thus, the child is unable to make enough IgG in response to potential pathogens they might encounter in the environment.

2. c. This child should be tested for HIV, a virus that destroys $CD4^+$ T cells.

Chapter 14: Hypersensitivity

Answers to Critical Thinking

14–1 A total IgE concentration of 100 KU/L or less is considered to be normal in adults. However, more information is needed to determine the clinical significance of the patient's IgE level, as values vary widely among patients and may not correlate with the presence of allergy. Clinical symptoms of the patient must be considered before making a diagnosis. In addition, skin prick tests and allergen-specific IgE tests are recommended instead of total IgE testing for routine evaluation of patients with suspected allergies because they provide more specific information.

14–2 If no agglutination is obtained in the DAT and IAT tests, commercially prepared antibody-coated RBCs (check cells) must be added to the reaction. If the AHG in the tube is working properly, it will bind to the antibody and agglutinate the check cells.

14–3 The patient's exposure to *M. tuberculosis* cannot be determined from the test results because the mitogen tube minus the background signal (NIL) was not greater than or equal to 0.50 IU/mL. The result would be reported as "Indeterminate." The low result in the mitogen tube was likely caused by failure of the patient's cells to respond to the T-cell mitogen because of immunosuppression. Improper collection of the patient's sample into the test tubes could also be the cause of a low response in the mitogen tube.

Answers to Case Studies

1. a. An increase in eosinophils is typically found in allergic individuals. Interleukins released by stimulated TH1 cells are involved in the recruitment of eosinophils from the bone marrow. Although there are other causes of eosinophilia, such as a parasitic infection, an increased number most often indicates an allergic reaction.

1. b. A skin prick test can be performed to determine which allergens the patient is sensitized to. The patient would know their results immediately because a positive test would be indicated by formation of wheal-and-flare reactions within 20 minutes at the site(s) of injection. If the patient is unable to discontinue any anti-histamines they might be taking, or if an unblemished area of skin in their forearm or back could not be found, a solid-phase immunoassay for allergen-specific IgE could be performed.

1. c. A solid-phase immunoassay for total IgE could be performed to monitor the patient's response to allergen immunotherapy. If the therapy is successful, the IgE concentration in the patient's serum should decrease to a level within the reference age for patients of the same age.

2. a. A positive DAT indicates that the red blood cells (RBCs) are coated with either antibody or complement components. These components could damage some of the patient's RBCs by type II hypersensitivity, causing the symptoms.

2. b. The most likely cause of the positive DAT is the presence of an antibody of the IgM class. It might be an anti-I, triggered by *Mycoplasma pneumoniae*. This is a cold-reacting antibody.

2. c. A DAT that is only positive with anti-C3d indicates that only complement products are present on the RBCs. This is a further indication that the antibody is an IgM antibody because it does not remain on the cells at 37°C but does trigger complement activation, which can cause the cell destruction.

Chapter 15: Autoimmune Diseases

Answers to Critical Thinking

15–1 The patient's doctor likely suspects systemic lupus erythematosus (SLE). Antibodies to double-stranded DNA are highly specific for SLE and can produce a homogeneous pattern. To strengthen the diagnosis, the doctor should order a laboratory test for anti-ds DNA antibodies. These antibodies can be tested for by a solid-phase immunoassay or an indirect immunofluorescence assay using *Crithidia luciliae* as the substrate. Antibody titers can be determined by testing dilutions of the patient serum and can be used along with other tests such as serum complement levels to monitor disease activity over time.

15–2 The patient's symptoms and laboratory results point to Graves disease, an autoimmune disorder affecting the thyroid gland. To confirm the diagnosis, tests for antibodies to the TSH receptor (TRAbs), thyroglobulin (Tg), and thyroid peroxidase (TPO) should be performed. TRAbs are specific for Graves disease and cause hyperthyroidism by binding to TSH receptors and stimulating the thyroid gland to produce excess

T4. Many patients with Graves disease also make Tg and TPO antibodies, but these are not disease specific.

Answers to Case Studies

1. a. A positive RF and ANA, as seen in this case, along with the patient's symptoms, suggest an autoimmune rheumatic disease.

1. b. The decreased RBC count may be caused by an autoantibody directed against RBCs, often associated with lupus.

1. c. Two diseases that should be considered in the differential diagnosis are rheumatoid arthritis (RA) and systemic lupus erythematosus (SLE). Testing for anti-CCP should also be performed, as this antibody is highly specific for RA; the result was negative in this case. An IIF for ANAs should be done, and dilutions of the patient's serum should be used to determine the antibody titer. The serum should also be tested for antibodies to specific nuclear antigens by ELISA or multiplex bead immunoassay. In this case, these tests were positive for anti-dsDNA and anti-Sm antibodies, indicating a diagnosis of SLE.

2. a. The patient's symptoms, enlarged thyroid gland, high TSH, and low FT4 levels are indicators of Hashimoto thyroiditis.

2. b. Tests for autoantibodies to thyroglobulin (Tg) and thyroid peroxidase (TPO) should be performed. Most patients with Hashimoto disease have TPO antibodies, and many have Tg antibodies.

2. c. Graves disease is also an autoimmune illness that affects the thyroid, but it is characterized by hyperthyroidism, with symptoms of nervousness, insomnia, restlessness, and weight loss. Patients with Graves disease have decreased or undetectable TSH and high FT4. Many Graves disease patients have TPO and Tg antibodies, but the presence of TSH receptor antibodies (TRAbs) is diagnostic for the disease.

Chapter 16: Transplantation Immunology

Answers to Critical Thinking

16–1 The paired HLA results indicate that a host-vs-graft reaction is more likely. The donor shares the A*23:01 allele with the patient (who is homozygous A*23:01); thus, the donor's cells should not mount an immune reaction since there is no mismatch that is recognized. In contrast, the recipient will recognize the donor A*03:01 as foreign and thus may elicit a host-vs-graft immune response.

16–2 One would expect a positive crossmatch to both donor T and B cells. HLA class I antigens are expressed on all nucleated cells; therefore, the patient antibody should bind to both T cells and B cells.

Answers to Case Studies

1. a. The most compatible donor for this patient would be friend 2. Sibling 1 has the B35 antigen for which the patient possesses HLA antibody. Sibling 2 also has the B35 antigen and is also ABO incompatible. Friend 1 is ABO incompatible. Friend 2 is ABO identical and does not express the HLA-B35 antigen and is thus the most appropriate donor.

2. a. Maybe; one cannot be sure that an unrelated donor has the same alleles at each locus, even if they have the same low-resolution type.

2. b. The physician requested high-resolution HLA to determine if the donor and recipient had the same alleles at each locus. Serological typing (phenotyping) provides low-resolution results, as indicated. The best outcome for a transplant occurs if the recipient and donor are HLA matched at the allele level. High-resolution typing of the donor was performed and indicated presence of the alleles HLA-A*02:05 and HLA-B*44:03. Thus, the donor and recipient were actually mismatched for two alleles. Based on this finding, this donor was declined, and an additional search was conducted.

Chapter 17: Tumor Immunology

Answers to Critical Thinking

17–1 A small percentage of ovarian tumors do not produce CA 125. However, a more likely explanation for the result is that ovarian cancer is often diagnosed in its late stages, when the tumor mass is large and producing a high amount of CA 125. A large excess of CA 125 could produce a high-dose hook effect in an immunoassay, resulting in a falsely decreased CA 125 level. If this were the case, repeating the test with diluted patient serum would produce an accurate result in the linear range of the assay.

17–2 The immune checkpoint therapy was initially successful in allowing T-cell anti-tumor responses to occur by blocking binding of the PD-L1 molecule on the tumor cells to PD-1 on the patient's T cells. However, some cancer cells remained after the therapy. Malignant cells are able to rapidly divide, increasing the chance for DNA replication errors and genetic mutations. Some of these mutations could have resulted in decreased expression of PD-L1 on the tumor cell surface, allowing those tumor cells to become resistant to the therapy and grow in the presence of the drug.

Answers to Case Studies

1. a. If no further CA 15-3 is being produced by tumor tissue, levels will decrease to within the reference range. Because CA 15-3 levels did not decrease to this level, residual tumor is suspected.

1. b. HER2 overexpression on the patient's tumor indicates that monoclonal anti-HER2 therapy may be successful.

1. c. Because the tumor lacks estrogen and progesterone receptors, hormone-suppressing therapy is unlikely to improve prognosis.

2. a. The source of PSA is the prostate gland.

2. b. Although the patient's PSA increased to above the reference interval, there was only a slight increase from the prior year's value. Also, the ratio of free PSA/total PSA did not indicate a high likelihood of finding prostate cancer, and the digital rectal exam did not detect any obvious sign of malignancy. Because PSA increases with age and prostate enlargement, benign prostatic hypertrophy is likely, and further PSA testing after a waiting period may be warranted in lieu of a prostate biopsy. The decision as to whether to have a biopsy should be made by the patient after a discussion with the doctor.

Chapter 18: Immunoproliferative Diseases

Answers to Critical Thinking

18–1 Differences between normal and malignant white blood cells based on observation of morphology alone can be subjective. Flow cytometry has added much detail to the traditional microscope-based laboratory evaluation of hematologic malignancies. Detection of cell surface markers provides insight into the lineage and maturation stage of the malignant cell type, which can be used to make a more accurate diagnosis. Molecular and cytogenetic analyses detect genetic mutations and chromosomal abnormalities in the cells, providing doctors with a more precise diagnosis and information about the patient's prognosis, which they can use to select the most effective therapy for the patient. Both the World Health Organization and the International Consensus Classification incorporate these methods into their classification schemes.

18–2 Lymphocyte maturation and activation are affected by proteins involved in somatic recombination and cell signaling, and receptors and ligands that promote cell proliferation and survival (e.g., the IL-2 receptor). Immunodeficiency diseases such as severe combined immunodeficiency (discussed in Chapter 19) are characterized by genetic defects that prevent lymphocyte survival and proliferation. Understanding these diseases can give insights into mechanisms that can be specifically targeted by drugs to inhibit proliferation or survival of leukemic clones.

18–3 Disruption of the bone marrow space in hematologic malignancies destroys the environment that supports production of normal white blood cells, thus weakening immunity. Treatment of leukemias and lymphomas involves a growing number of targeted molecular therapies intended to inhibit growth or survival of malignant cells. Not unlike standard chemotherapy, these treatments impact normal hematopoietic cells as well as the tumor. In leukemias and lymphomas in particular, the cells most affected are the normal cells of the immune system. Disruption of the immune system by therapeutic regimens, overall suppression of the immune system by the tumor, and insufficient production of immune cells, all increase the risk to patients for developing potentially life-threatening infections.

Answers to Case Studies

1. a. The high IgG level indicates that a monoclonal gammopathy is probably present, most likely, multiple myeloma. The patient's back pain, age, and presence of anemia are also consistent with a diagnosis of multiple myeloma.

1. b. The diagnosis could be confirmed by performing a bone marrow biopsy because having more than 10% plasma cells in the bone marrow is one of the diagnostic criteria for multiple myeloma. Radiographs could reveal the presence of lytic bone lesions responsible for the patient's back pain. Also, serum protein electrophoresis (SPE) could be used to detect a monoclonal band, and immunofixation electrophoresis (IFE) would be used to identify the suspected monoclonal IgG in the patient's serum and possibly detect Bence Jones proteins in the urine. Free light chain assays can be used to determine the concentration of monoclonal light chains in the serum and the κ/λ ratio. A serum monoclonal protein concentration of greater than 3 g/dL and a urinary monoclonal protein greater than 200 mg/day indicate the presence of multiple myeloma.

2. a. Although hairy cell leukemia (HCL) cells are not generally seen in the bone marrow, the hematologic bone marrow studies describe malignant cells characteristic of HCL. Splenomegaly is often seen in patients with HCL.

2. b. The patient's abnormal cells were positive for CD20, CD25, and CD103. CD103 is a sensitive and specific marker for HCL. Although not tested for in this patient, CD123 is also a specific marker for HCL.

Chapter 19: Immunodeficiency Diseases and Inborn Errors of Immunity

Answers to Critical Thinking

19–1 Previously made maternal IgG antibodies cross the placenta during pregnancy and provide protection against bacterial infections during the infant's first few months of life. After birth, maternal IgG decreases according to its half-life (~23 days), so that by about 6 months of age, the remaining levels are no longer protective. While the infant is making some IgG at this age, its humoral immune system is not fully developed.

19–2 Patient medical and family history, which were not provided in the scenario, would be important in determining the cause of the patient's condition. The patient may have a secondary immunodeficiency resulting from environmental factors, such as a condition that suppresses the immune system (e.g., diabetes) or previous treatment with antibiotics or immunosuppressive therapy. Less common explanations for the negative test result are that the patient has a hereditary form of chronic mucocutaneous candidiasis that was not detected by the gene panel used, or a phenocopy of an inborn error of immunity caused by production of autoantibodies to IL-17 or IL-22.

Answers to Case Studies

1. a. The patient's recurrent bacterial infections, low lymphocyte count, and absence of a gamma band on SPE indicate an immunodeficiency disease, most likely Bruton tyrosine kinase deficiency. This condition results from inheritance of an X-linked recessive gene and affects males almost exclusively.

1. b. Measurement of serum IgA, IgM, and IgG levels should be performed to determine if all classes of antibody are absent. Enumeration of B and T lymphocytes should be determined by flow cytometry. In Btk deficiency, B-cell development is affected, and $CD19^+$ lymphocytes are decreased, but T-cell numbers are normal.

1. c. The patient should be treated with Ig replacement therapy and antibiotics.

2. a. Region 4 best represents the IFE pattern that would be seen for this patient.

2. b. Note the lighter IgG and light chain bands in region 4 as compared to the normal control (specimen 1). Also, only faint IgA or IgM bands are visible. Specimen 2 contains a monoclonal IgG κ protein. Specimen 3 is a concentrated 24-hour urine specimen that contains albumin. The patient's IFE results correlate with the clinical history, SPE result, and reduced Ig levels, indicating an antibody deficiency.

Chapter 20: Laboratory Detection of Bacterial Infections

Answers to Critical Thinking

20–1 The patient may have had a previous skin infection caused by group A streptococcus; such patients usually produce antibodies to DNase B but not to streptolysin O, in contrast to patients who initially had streptococcal pharyngitis. Also, about 15% of patients with acute rheumatic fever do not develop ASO antibodies; some of these patients may be positive for anti-DNase B.

20–2 The patient likely has a drug-resistant strain of *Mycobacterium tuberculosis* contracted during their recent travel to a country where such strains are more prevalent. Because the patient did not respond to the first-line drugs (isoniazid, rifampin, pyrazinamide, and ethambutol), second-line drugs should be administered. However, these drugs are more expensive, have an increased likelihood of side effects, and require prolonged treatment as compared to treatment for nonresistant strains of MTB.

20–3 There are limitations on laboratory tests for detection of acid-fast bacilli (AFB). The sensitivity of AFB stains ranges from 45% to 75%, so a negative smear does not rule out the presence of AFB in the specimen. Also, mycobacteria are slow-growing organisms; depending on the number of bacilli in the sample, growth in culture may not be observed for a month or more. In cases where there is clinical suspicion of active tuberculosis, but negative AFB smears and culture, highly sensitive molecular testing should be performed to detect *Mycobacterium tuberculosis* genes.

Answers to Case Studies

1. a. Poststreptococcal glomerulonephritis (PSGN).

1. b. *Streptococcus pyogenes* (group A streptococci).

1. c. Streptococcal antigen-antibody complexes may deposit in the glomeruli of the kidneys, or antibody formed against the organisms may cross-react with antigens in the glomeruli. These immune responses stimulate an inflammatory response that causes damage to the glomeruli, leading to renal impairment and function. The rapid GAS test was negative because the patient did not present with pharyngitis and the organism is no longer present in the throat.

1. d. A urinalysis is helpful because microscopic hematuria is typically present in children with acute PSGN. The proteinuria rarely exceeds 3+ by dipstick; however, massive proteinuria and a nephrotic picture may be observed in a small percentage of patients.

1. e. The ASO titer was negative, as may be seen in patients with PSGN. The anti-DNAse B titer was above the reference range, indicating a positive result and confirming the diagnosis of PSGN.

2. a. *Mycoplasma pneumoniae.*

2. b. The patient has only been ill for several days and has not had time to mount a serological response to the causative agent. IgG levels suggest that the patient had a previous exposure to the organism, and the level may represent residual immunoglobulin G (IgG) from an earlier exposure.

2. c. Definitive diagnosis of *M. pneumoniae* requires documented seroconversion by paired specimens obtained 2 to 4 weeks apart, measuring both IgM and IgG antibodies to the organism. A fourfold rise in IgG levels is considered diagnostic.

2. d. Cold agglutinin titers used for the diagnosis of *M. pneumoniae* infections are not very specific or very sensitive. Testing for cold agglutinins is no longer recommended for the detection of *M. pneumoniae* infections because the development of cold agglutinins occurs in other conditions, including some viral infections and collagen vascular diseases. Although not specific for *M. pneumoniae* infection, a high cold agglutinin titer in a patient with community-acquired pneumonia symptoms (greater than 1:64) is likely to be caused by *M. pneumoniae.*

3. a. The patient's clinical symptoms, along with suggesting bacterial pneumonia, are consistent with tuberculosis. The clinical presentation along with the patient's age suggest reactivation tuberculosis due to a latent TB infection (LTBI). The QuantiFERON-TB Gold test measures the release of interferon-γ if a patient has latent or active tuberculosis caused by *M. tuberculosis.*

3. b. Methylprednisolone, an immunosuppressive corticosteroid drug used to treat RA, would put the patient at increased risk for developing LTBI, as they would not be able to mount an effective immune response against *M. tuberculosis*. In LTBI, healthy hosts mount a strong immune response that contains but does not eliminate the infection. The likelihood of developing reactivation TB from a LTBI is estimated to be between 5% and 10%. Risk factors for developing active disease include HIV/AIDS, transplantation with immunosuppressant therapy, chronic renal failure and hemodialysis, and use of corticosteroids. Immigrants from countries with a high TB prevalence are also at a higher risk of developing reactivation TB.

3. c. Given the patient's clinical presentation and laboratory finding, sputum cultures for AFB should be ordered. Current protocol is the collection of three samples collected 12 hours apart. An AFB stain should also be done on the specimen. The AFB stain is used rather than a Gram stain because the mycolic acid in the cell wall of mycobacteria resists decolorization with acid alcohol. Some laboratories perform a PCR assay directly from the processed specimen that can detect *M. tuberculosis* as well as drug resistance testing.

3. d. The patient's contacts should be identified, including health care personnel and people who were in the waiting rooms at the urgent care center and the PCP's office. Those individuals should have either a TB skin test or an interferon-γ release assay performed. Current guidelines for contacts with an initially negative IGRA recommend repeating the IGRA at 6 to 10 weeks after TB exposure and repeating the TB skin test after 8 to 10 weeks.

Chapter 21: Spirochete Diseases

Answers to Critical Thinking

21–1 The patient likely had a history of treated syphilis infection. If the laboratory ran a reverse algorithm for syphilis, the treponemal test would have been performed first, which would have been positive from her prior history, and the follow-up RPR would have been negative if there was no active infection. The RPR should be repeated in 3 months to verify that she indeed does not have a new active infection.

21–2 It is common to not isolate any spirochetes from serum or tissues, as the organism number is very low and the spirochetes are motile; therefore, direct detection is not recommended for diagnosis. Likewise, the patient has likely not seroconverted yet, as it takes at least 3 weeks for antibody to be detected; if the ELISA were repeated in another 3 to 4 weeks, it would likely be positive for both IgM and IgG. The patient should be treated with an antibiotic immediately, however, as they are presenting with erythema migrans and have spent time in an endemic region.

Answers to Case Studies

1. a. Almost 25% of individuals with Lyme disease do not exhibit the characteristic rash; therefore, its absence does not rule out the possibility of the disease.

1. b. There are several conditions that can cause false-positive results in ELISA testing, including syphilis, other treponemal diseases, infectious mononucleosis, and autoimmune diseases such as rheumatoid arthritis. Thus, low levels of antibody might indicate one of these other diseases. However, false-negative results in Lyme disease are also possible because of a low level of antibody production, especially early in the disease. Therefore, an indeterminate test neither rules out nor confirms the presence of Lyme disease.

1. c. If there is a history of tick bite and patient symptoms are consistent with Lyme disease, then a confirmatory Western blot or another EIA should be performed. The Western blot is fairly specific for Lyme disease. If 5 of 10 protein bands specific for *Borrelia burgdorferi* IgG antibodies are positive, this confirms the presence of Lyme disease.

2. a. Although it is possible that the mother's positive RPR test could be a false positive, it is also likely that the mother is in the latent stage of syphilis, with no obvious signs of the disease. Although syphilis is not sexually transmitted during this stage, it can be transmitted from a mother to her unborn child. Many infants do not show clinical signs of the disease at birth; however, if infected and untreated, a large percentage of babies develop later symptoms, including neurological deficits such as blindness and mental retardation.

2. b. A positive RPR on cord blood could be from transplacental passage of the mother's IgG antibodies. A titer should be performed on the cord blood and a serum sample obtained from the infant in several weeks. If infection is present in the infant, the titer will remain the same or increase. An IgM capture assay could also be performed. The presence of specific anti-treponemal IgM would indicate that the infant had been exposed to *Treponema pallidum* because IgM antibodies do not cross the placenta.

2. c. Because there is a good chance that the infant is at risk for congenital syphilis, immediate treatment with penicillin can prevent neurological and other consequences.

2. d. A positive RPR test indicates the presence of antibodies against host-cell cardiolipin complexes. As these antibodies are not specific to syphilis and can be produced during pregnancy and certain other conditions, syphilis diagnosis should be confirmed by doing a treponemal-specific test such as the TP-PA or FTA-ABS.

Chapter 22: Laboratory Diagnosis of Parasitic and Fungal Infections

Answers to Critical Thinking

22–1 Many parasites have complex life cycles that require multiple host species to survive and reproduce. For example, *Plasmodium* species causing malaria in humans require the mosquito as the definitive host (in which sexual reproduction occurs) and humans as the intermediate host (in which asexual reproduction occurs). Antigenic variation allows such parasites to express different epitopes in each life cycle stage in each host, making an effective immune response difficult.

22–2 *Candida albicans* is a commensal organism that is normally nonpathogenic. Patient A is likely a person with a normal, functional immune system, whereas patient B is likely immunocompromised, allowing the organism to spread as an opportunistic infection and cause more severe symptoms.

Answers to Case Studies

1. a. It cannot be determined by the test results available whether the baby has congenital toxoplasmosis. The IgG antibodies in the newborn may reflect maternal antibodies that crossed the placenta. The presence of IgG antibodies in the newborn may reflect either past or recent infection in the mother. IgM antibodies may persist for up to 18 months after infection with *Toxoplasma gondii*. Thus, the greatest value of testing for IgM antibodies is in determining whether a pregnant woman has had a recent infection. If no IgM antibodies are detected and only IgG is detected, this excludes a recent infection before pregnancy. The presence of IgG and IgM in the mother may indicate a recent infection.

1. b. Tests for IgA and IgM antibodies are commonly used for the diagnosis of infection in the newborn. If IgG, IgM, and IgA are detected, a diagnosis of congenital toxoplasmosis is established. If IgG antibodies are detected but serological test results for IgM and IgA antibodies are negative, follow-up serological testing in suspected cases is indicated. Maternally transferred antibodies usually decrease and disappear within 6 to 12 months. Established infection in the mother can also be indicated by the presence of high avidity IgG antibodies.

2. a. Most patients with symptomatic cryptococcosis have an underlying immunocompromised condition. Such conditions include AIDS, prolonged treatment with corticosteroids, organ transplantation, advanced malignancy, diabetes, and sarcoidosis. The clinical symptoms and outcome of cryptococcal meningitis vary, in part because of the related underlying medical conditions and the immune status of the host. The most common symptoms are headache, altered mental status, personality changes, confusion, lethargy, and coma. Nausea and vomiting are also common and are caused by increased intracranial pressure. Onset of the disease is often subacute and worsens over several weeks. The patient in this case was immunosuppressed because of long-term steroid use and presented with severe headaches, gait instability, and weakness upon standing.

2. b. The simplest diagnostic test is an India ink test on the patient's CSF. Because of the large polysaccharide capsule produced by the organism, the India ink is displaced, allowing for visualization of the yeast. The serological tests for cryptococcal antigen in serum and CSF are highly sensitive and specific for the diagnosis of invasive disease. Immunochromatographic assays may also be used to detect the capsular antigen in serum and CSF.

Chapter 23: Serological and Molecular Detection of Viral Infections

Answers to Critical Thinking

23–1 This patient has been positive for HBsAg and HBeAg and has not developed antibodies to these antigens during the last 6 months. The patient is therefore in a chronic carrier state. Carrier states lead to a risk of liver cirrhosis and hepatic carcinoma due to liver destruction and damage caused by the virus.

23–2 The findings suggest a diagnosis of infectious mononucleosis because of the patient's clinical symptoms and increase in atypical lymphocytes. However, false-negative Monospot results can occur in some patients. The suspected diagnosis of infectious mononucleosis (IM) should be confirmed by testing for EBV-specific antibodies. In acute IM, the expected results would be positive for IgM and IgG anti-VCA and anti-EA-D; anti-EBNA would be negative.

23–3 The patient has HIV and is immunocompromised. The acute and convalescent serum samples showed more than a fourfold rise in titer; therefore, the patient is at risk of developing a primary cytomegalovirus infection.

23–4 Shingles is caused by reactivation of the varicella-zoster virus within a host who previously had chickenpox. If the teenager acquired the virus, it would manifest as chickenpox (i.e., a primary infection), not shingles (reactivation of a previous infection).

23–5 Since there was at least a fourfold rise in titer between the acute and convalescent samples and the mother is not immune to rubella, the risk is high for congenital infection in the fetus, especially since she is in her first trimester of pregnancy.

23–6 At-home COVID-19 antigen tests are less sensitive than PCR and are therefore less likely to detect the SARS-CoV-2 virus. This is especially true early in an infection or in people who do not have COVID-19 symptoms.

Answers to Case Studies

1. a. The patient's clinical symptoms and increased liver function enzymes indicate inflammation of the liver. To determine whether the inflammation is the result of viral hepatitis and to identify the cause, the following tests should be ordered: (1) IgM anti-HAV to screen for hepatitis A, (2) HBsAg to screen for hepatitis B, (3) IgM anti-HBc to screen for hepatitis B in the core window period when HBsAg is absent, and (4) anti-HCV to screen for hepatitis C.

1. b. To monitor hepatitis B infection, testing for HBsAg and HBeAg should be performed periodically to determine how long the infection is persisting and the relative infectivity of the patient. Tests for anti-HBe and anti-HBs are performed to indicate whether the infection has resolved and whether immunity has been established, respectively.

1. c. In chronic hepatitis B, HBsAg persists in the serum for more than 6 months. Total anti-HBc is also present; HBeAg may or may not be present, depending on the degree of disease progression. Anti-HBe and anti-HBs are usually not present but may have a delayed appearance in people who eventually recover.

2. a. Many viruses can produce congenital abnormalities in an infant born to a mother infected during pregnancy. These include cytomegalovirus, rubella virus, and varicella-zoster virus. The infant's symptoms and mother's history suggest infection with rubella virus.

2. b. Ideally, the mother would have been tested at the time of illness during her pregnancy for rubella antibodies. Demonstration of rubella-specific IgM antibody, seroconversion from negative to positive for rubella antibody, or a fourfold rise in antibody titer would have indicated an active rubella infection. However, because this was not done, the mother could be tested for rubella-specific IgG antibody, which would indicate if rubella exposure occurred. Tests that measure the avidity of the IgG antibody can be performed to distinguish between a recent infection (low avidity) and a past infection (high avidity).

2. c. The infant's serum should be tested for rubella-specific IgM antibody, preferably with an IgM antibody capture enzyme immunoassay. IgM antibodies, which cannot pass through the placenta, would have been produced by the fetus as a result of active rubella infection. IgG antibodies, in contrast, are derived mainly from the mother's serum as a result of passive transfer through the placenta. Viral culture or reverse transcriptase polymerase chain reaction should be used to confirm positive IgM results.

3. a. Several different viruses and bacteria can cause respiratory distress. The fact that the patient experienced a new loss of smell most likely points to an infection with SARS-CoV-2. This virus causes fever, shortness of breath, difficulty breathing, and decreased oxygen saturation levels in addition to high blood pressure and a rapid heart rate.

3. b. Several laboratory tests should be ordered "STAT" to assess the entire clinical picture. An arterial blood gas test should be performed to measure the pH and oxygen and carbon dioxide levels in the blood; a complete blood count (CBC) and differential can provide information about whether the infection is bacterial or viral in nature. An increase in lymphocytes is most often seen in viral infections, in contrast to an increase in neutrophils, which indicates a bacterial infection. A comprehensive metabolic panel (CMP) gives electrolyte information and kidney and liver function parameters.

3. c. PCR can be performed to differentiate between SARS-CoV-2, influenza, and respiratory syncytial virus, all of which can cause respiratory distress. A nasopharyngeal swab sample should be collected and sent for PCR; this test is highly sensitive and can provide results in 2 to 4 hours. Rapid antigen tests can also be done, which will provide a result in 15 to 30 minutes but are not as sensitive as molecular assays.

Chapter 24: Laboratory Diagnosis of Human Retroviruses

Answers to Critical Thinking

24–1 Antibodies and cell-mediated immune responses can initially keep viral replication in check. Antibodies can attach only to virions circulating freely outside of host cells, whereas cytotoxic T lymphocytes (CTLs) can attack host cells harboring viruses internally. $CD8^+$ CTLs appear within weeks after HIV infection and can attack HIV-infected host cells. Meanwhile, B lymphocytes are stimulated to produce antibodies against HIV. Antibodies are first developed against gp41 within 6 weeks after exposure, followed by antibodies to gag proteins (such as p24). The highly immunogenic viral envelope proteins elicit the production of neutralizing antibodies, which appear 2 to 3 months after infection. These neutralizing antibodies prevent the virus from infecting neighboring cells.

24–2 After patients are initially diagnosed with HIV, a baseline viral load and CD4 T-lymphocyte count are obtained. Baseline values direct specific treatment with anti-retroviral therapy (ART). ART consists of a combination of various anti-retroviral drugs. Certain factors, including baseline values, guide clinical decisions about the specific drugs that should be administered to the patient. Equally important, the baseline values serve as prognostic indicators and alert clinicians to the potential effectiveness of an ART regimen. They also alert clinicians to the potential emergence of drug-resistant HIV genotypes. Genotype and phenotypic testing can be performed to determine if the ART regimen needs to be modified.

The decrease in viral load and increase in CD4 counts at the time intervals listed indicate that the ART regimen is working effectively for this patient. Typically, if ART is successful, there is a significant viral load reduction (typically within 2 to 4 weeks). Once the viral load has been reduced to undetectable levels, the testing interval frequency will decrease. With effective ART, viral loads may drop to undetectable levels within 16 to 24 weeks.

According to U.S. Department of Health and Human Services guidelines, a baseline CD4 T-cell measurement should be performed before the initiation of ART, then every 3 to 6 months for the first 2 years. Thereafter, annual measurements can be performed in patients whose CD4 T-cell counts have consistently remained between 300 and 500 cells/μL. Typically, the CD4 T-cell count may increase as much as 50 to 100 cells/uL within the first 4 weeks of ART (and up to 3 months of treatment), followed by a more gradual but steady increase thereafter. The rate of change can vary in different patients.

24–3 It cannot be determined if HIV infection is present in the infant because serological testing is not a reliable method for detecting HIV infection in children younger than 18 months old. Most subclasses of IgG are capable of crossing the placenta because they can bind to receptors for the Fc region of IgG molecules on placental tissue. This enables receptor-mediated endocytosis and transportation to fetal blood. Maternal antibodies persist in the infant's bloodstream for about a year and sometimes even longer. Thus, molecular methods are more accurate than serology testing for testing infant serum. An HIV-1 DNA test or a qualitative HIV-1 RNA test may be performed. It is recommended that nucleic acid testing for HIV be performed on infants with known perinatal exposure at the ages of 14 to 21 days, 1 to 2 months, and 4 to 6 months, and possibly at birth (for those at high risk for HIV infection).

24–4 Although HIV-1 is much more prevalent than HTLV-1 infection, HTLV-1 is still a threat to public health, with millions of infections occurring worldwide. Both retroviruses are capable of infecting CD4 T cells and eventually leading to immunodeficiencies. Both viruses establish viral latency, and people may not be aware they are infected. If left untreated, patients can develop serious complications. Without treatment, most people with HIV will develop AIDS. Alternatively, HTLV-1 infection can lead to ATLL or HAM/TSP. Most people living with HTLV-1 will develop chronic and asymptomatic infection, while 5% will progress to develop a severe and fatal outcome in the form of malignancy, inflammation, or opportunistic infection.

Answers to Case Studies

1. a. The physician should order a fourth-generation ELISA, which simultaneously detects antibodies to HIV-1, antibodies to HIV-2, and p24 antigen. Alternately, the physician could perform a rapid EIA for HIV antibody to obtain a fast result and order a fourth-generation ELISA to verify the result.

1. b. If the fourth-generation ELISA was positive, a rapid test for HIV-1 and HIV-2 antibodies should be performed to confirm the results and distinguish between infection by the two viruses.

1. c. If it is determined that the patient truly has HIV infection, the CD4 T-cell counts should be monitored periodically to assess the effects of the virus on the immune system. In addition, the patient should be placed on anti-retroviral therapy, and the effectiveness of the therapy should be evaluated by periodically performing viral load assays to monitor the amount of HIV RNA in the plasma.

2. a. HIV infection is transmitted from mother to infant by three routes: (1) passage through the placenta during pregnancy, (2) exposure to maternal blood during the delivery process, or (3) through breast milk. To reduce the risk of transmission, anti-retroviral therapy should be administered to the mother during her pregnancy and to the infant after birth. Also, the mother should be advised not to breastfeed her baby.

2. b. Testing the infant's serum for HIV antibody would yield confusing results. This is because the IgG HIV antibodies in the mother's serum would pass through the placenta during the pregnancy and be detectable in the infant's serum. The result would be a false positive if the infant was not HIV-infected.

2. c. Because of the problems associated with antibody testing, molecular methods are preferred to make a diagnosis of HIV infection in infants younger than 18 months of age. The preferred molecular test is a PCR that detects the presence of proviral HIV DNA in the infant's peripheral blood mononuclear cells. Alternately, a quantitative HIV RNA test could be performed on the infant's plasma.

3. a. Based on the HTLV-1 serology, flow cytometry, and microscopy results and the patient's symptoms, the most likely diagnosis is ATLL from HTLV-1 infection.

3. b. The hypercalcemia, skin lesions, hepatosplenomegaly, and lymphadenopathy indicate T-cell non-Hodgkin lymphoma, which accounts for about 20% to 25% of all ATLL cases.

3. c. The median survival for this subtype is less than 1 year. It is an aggressive form of ATLL, along with the acute subtype, which has a median survival rate of less than 6 months. The chronic subtype accounts for about 20% of all cases with a median survival of about 2 years. Hypercalcemia is not present in the chronic form, and patients tend to be asymptomatic. The last subtype, referred to as the smoldering form, accounts for only 5% of cases and has a median survival rate of over 5 years.

3. d. About 5 to 20 million people are thought to be infected with HTLV-1 and HTLV-2 worldwide. HTLV-1 infection is endemic in southwestern Japan, the Caribbean islands, South and Central Africa, the Middle East, Romania, parts of South America, and Papua New Guinea. The patient lives in an HTLV-1 endemic region. The travel history along with the presenting symptoms are significant for the suspicion of HTLV-1 infection.

Chapter 25: Immunization and Vaccines

Answers to Critical Thinking

25–1 Although influenza vaccines are widely available in the United States, in some years, the vaccine antigens may not be sufficiently matched to the influenza viruses circulating at the time, as the viruses have a high mutation rate. Also, some people may not have an optimal immune response to the vaccine because of their age or presence of medical conditions that affect the immune system. To prevent influenza infections, a high percentage of individuals need to be vaccinated to protect themselves and the people around them; vaccine hesitancy will reduce the level of protection in a population.

25–2 In IVIG therapy, patients are treated with a standard preparation of pooled immunoglobulins to prevent infections. Because this is a form of passive immunotherapy, the protection provided is temporary because memory cells are not produced, and the Ig levels in the preparation decline according to their half-life (28 days or less). Thus, repeated treatments are needed to restore Igs to protective levels.

Answers to Case Studies

1. a. The child could safely receive vaccines that do not contain a live component. These include the vaccines for hepatitis B and RSV (recombinant antigens); diphtheria and tetanus (toxoids); pertussis, *Haemophilus* influenza b, and pneumococcus (subunit vaccines); and polio, hepatitis A, and influenza (vaccine formulations containing inactivated virus).

1. b. The child could not receive any live, attenuated vaccines because the organisms in these vaccines, although weakened, could not be controlled by the child's immune system and could cause serious, disseminated infections. Such vaccines include those against the viral diseases: measles, mumps, rubella, varicella, and rotavirus and the nasal mist form of the influenza vaccine.

1. c. The child could be protected against these infections by receiving regular injections of IVIG, a preparation of pooled serum from other individuals, which contains numerous premade antibodies. Family members and close friends of the child should make sure they are up to date on their own immunizations. By preventing development of these diseases in themselves, they are ensuring that they cannot pass the pathogen along to the child. This concept, whereby protection against infectious diseases is extended to others in a population, is known as "community immunity" or "herd immunity."

2. a. Hepatitis B-specific hyperimmune globulin, consisting of a high concentration of antibody to the hepatitis B virus, should be used to prevent the infection in the staff member. Because this preparation is derived from people who have previously been exposed to hepatitis B, the antibodies are premade and provide immediate protection when they are administered soon after exposure to the pathogen.

2. b. Although the hyperimmune globulin provides immediate protection, it is only temporary because the antibody titers decline over time, according to the half-life of the immunoglobulin molecules. The half-life for IgG, which constitutes most of the preparation, is 21 to 28 days. To achieve long-term immunity without actually acquiring the infection, the staff member would need to be immunized with the hepatitis B vaccine. The vaccine, consisting of recombinant hepatitis B surface antigen, would stimulate an immune response and generate memory lymphocytes that could quickly be reactivated in case of a later exposure.

Index

References followed by the letter "f" are for figures, "t" are for tables, and "b" are for boxes.